Allergic Diseases of Infancy, Childhood and Adolescence

Edited by

C. WARREN BIERMAN, M.D.

Clinical Professor of Pediatrics, University of Washington School of Medicine;
Chief, Division of Allergy, Children's Orthopedic Hospital and
Medical Center, Seattle, Washington

and

DAVID S. PEARLMAN, M.D.

Clinical Professor of Pediatrics, University of Colorado Medical School;
Senior Staff Physician, Department of Pediatrics, National
Jewish Hospital and Research Center/National Asthma Center,
Denver, Colorado

1980

W. B. SAUNDERS COMPANY

Philadelphia / London / Toronto

W. B. Saunders Company: West Washington Square
Philadelphia, PA   19105

1 St. Anne's Road
Eastbourne, East Sussex BN21 3UN, England

1 Goldthorne Avenue
Toronto, Ontario M8Z 5T9, Canada

Library of Congress Cataloging in Publication Data

Main entry under title:

Allergic diseases of infancy, childhood, and adolescence.

1. Pediatric allergy.   I. Bierman, Charles Warren, 1924–
   II. Pearlman, David S. [DNLM: 1. Hypersensitivity — In
   infancy and childhood. WD300 A4313]

RJ386.A43   618.9′29′7   79–3915

ISBN 0–7216–1726–3

Allergic Diseases of Infancy, Childhood and Adolescence   ISBN 0-7216-1726-3

Last digit is the print number: 9   8   7   6   5   4   3   2   1

To my parents, Margery and Linn C. Bierman, my wife, Joan, and my daughters, Margot, Karen, Charlotte, and Barbara.

C. Warren Bierman

To my late father, Benjamin Norman Pearlman, and to my mother, Sylvia, my wife, Doris, and my children, Michael and Melanie.

David S. Pearlman

CONTRIBUTORS

JOHN A. ANDERSON, M.D.
Director, Allergy and Clinical Immunology Training Program, Henry Ford Hospital; Clinical Assistant Professor of Pediatrics and Communicable Diseases, University of Michigan; Head, Division of Allergy and Clinical Immunology, Department of Medicine, Henry Ford Hospital, Detroit, Michigan.
Drug Allergies

CHARLES S. AUGUST, M.D.
Associate Professor of Pediatrics, University of Pennsylvania School of Medicine; Acting Director, Division of Allergy and Clinical Immunology, Children's Hospital, Philadelphia, Pennsylvania.
Diseases of Erythrocytes, Leukocytes, and Platelets

JOSEPH A. BELLANTI, M.D.
Professor of Pediatrics and Microbiology, Georgetown University School of Medicine, Washington, D.C.
Immunogenetics

WILLIAM E. BERGER, M.D.
Attending Staff Physician, Bridgeport Hospital and St. Vincent's Medical Center, Bridgeport, Connecticut.
Chemical Mediators of Inflammation

BERNARD A. BERMAN, M.D.
Assistant Clinical Professor of Pediatrics, Tufts University School of Medicine; Director of Pediatric Allergy, St. Elizabeth Hospital; Consultant in Allergy, Carney Hospital, Boston Floating Hospital, and Kennedy Memorial Hospital, Boston, Massachusetts.
Injection Therapy

C. WARREN BIERMAN, M.D.
Clinical Professor of Pediatrics, University of Washington School of Medicine; Chief, Division of Allergy, Children's Orthopedic Hospital and Medical Center, Seattle, Washington.
Injection Therapy
Diseases of the Nose
Asthma

CHARLES D. BLUESTONE, M.D.
Professor of Otolaryngology, University of Pittsburgh School of Medicine; Director, Department of Otolaryngology, Children's Hospital of Pittsburgh, Pittsburgh, Pennsylvania.
The Ear in Upper Respiratory Tract Disease

JEROME M. BUCKLEY, M.D.
Clinical Associate Professor of Pediatrics, University of Colorado Medical Center; Senior Staff Physician, Department of Pediatrics, National Jewish Hospital and Research Center/National Asthma Center, Denver, Colorado.
Pulmonary Function Testing
Controlling the Environment

REBECCA H. BUCKLEY, M.D.
Professor of Pediatrics and Immunology, Duke University School of Medicine; Chief, Division of Allergy, Immunology and Pulmonary Diseases, Department of Pediatrics, Duke Medical Center, Durham, North Carolina.
IgE Antibody

H. PETER CHASE, M.D.
Associate Professor of Pediatrics, University of Colorado School of Medicine; Attending Physician, University of Colorado Medical Center, Denver Children's Hospital, and Denver City and County Hospital, Denver, Colorado.
Nutritional Considerations

VICTOR CHERNICK, M.D., F.A.A.P., F.R.C.P. (Can.)
Professor, Department of Pediatrics,

University of Manitoba; Head, Section of Respirology, Children's Hospital, Winnipeg, Canada.
Lower Respiratory Tract Disease

DENNIS L. CHRISTIE, M.D.
Clinical Assistant Professor, Section of Pediatric Gastroenterology, Mason Clinic, University of Washington School of Medicine; Head, Gastroenterology Clinic, Children's Orthopedic Hospital and Medical Center, Seattle, Washington.
Gastrointestinal Tract Diseases

JAMES M. CORRY, M.D.
Instructor in Clinical Pediatrics, Washington University School of Medicine; Associate, Children's Consultation Services, Inc., St. Louis, Missouri.
Disorders of Complement and Phagocyte Function

LLOYD V. CRAWFORD, M.D.
Clinical Professor of Pediatrics; Chief— Allergy Section, The University of Tennessee Center for the Health Sciences; Attending Physician, LeBonheur Children's Medical Center, Memphis, Tennessee.
Allergy Diets

ROBERT J. DOCKHORN, M.D.
Clinical Professor of Pediatrics and Medicine, University of Missouri Medical School; Adjunct Clinical Professor of Pediatrics, University of Kansas School of Medicine; Director of Allergy and Immunology Teaching and Chief of Allergy and Immunology, Children's Mercy Hospital, Kansas City, Missouri.
Genitourinary Problems

JAMES A. DONALDSON, M.D.
Professor of Otolaryngology, University of Washington; Attending staff member, University Hospital and Children's Orthopedic Hospital and Medical Center, Seattle, Washington.
Diseases of the Ear
Diseases of the Nose

JACQUELINE DUPONT, Ph.D.
Professor of Food and Nutrition, Iowa State University, Ames, Iowa. Visiting Professor, University of Colorado School of Medicine, Denver, Colorado.
Nutritional Considerations

JAMES G. EASTON, M.D.
Director, Allergy-Immunology Training Program, Kaiser Foundation Hospital;

Clinical Professor of Pediatrics, University of California, Los Angeles, California.
Anaphylaxis
Insect Allergy

PEYTON A. EGGLESTON, M.D.
Associate Professor of Pediatrics, University of Virginia School of Medicine; Attending Pediatrician, University of Virginia Hospital, Charlottesville, Virginia.
Obstructive Diseases of the Larynx and Trachea
Exercise-Induced Asthma

ABRAHAM H. EISEN, M.D., F.R.C.P. (Can.)
Assistant Clinical Professor of Pediatrics, University of Texas Medical School; Attending Physician, Hermann Hospital and Texas Children's Hospital, Houston, Texas.
Eosinophils
Eosinophilia

ELLIOT F. ELLIS, M.D.
Professor and Chairman, Department of Pediatrics, State University of New York at Buffalo; Pediatrician-in-Chief, Children's Hospital of Buffalo, Buffalo, New York.
Acute Bronchopulmonary Infections

HELEN M. EMERY, M.D.
Senior Fellow, Division of Arthritis and Immunology, Department of Pediatrics, University of Washington School of Medicine, Seattle, Washington.
Rheumatic Diseases

HOWARD FADEN, M.D.
Assistant Professor of Pediatrics, State University of New York at Buffalo; Associate Attending Physician, Children's Hospital of Buffalo, Buffalo, New York.
Acute Bronchopulmonary Infections

S. LANCE FORSTOT, M.D., F.A.C.S.
Assistant Professor of Ophthalmology, University of Colorado School of Medicine; Ophthalmologist, University Hospital, Denver General Hospital, and Veterans Administration Hospital, Denver, Colorado.
Diseases of the Eye

OSCAR L. FRICK, M.D., Ph.D.
Professor of Pediatrics and Director, Allergy-Immunology Research Laboratory, University of California-San Francisco; Attending Pediatrician, University of

California-San Francisco Medical Center, San Francisco, California.
Controversial Concepts and Techniques

GILBERT A. FRIDAY, M.D.
Clinical Associate Professor of Pediatrics, University of Pittsburgh School of Medicine; Attending Physician, Children's Hospital of Pittsburgh, Mercy Hospital, St. Clair Memorial Hospital, and St. Francis General Hospital, Pittsburgh, Pennsylvania.
Headache

VINCENT A. FULGINITI, M.D.
Professor and Head, Department of Pediatrics, University of Arizona; Director, Clinical Pediatrics, University Hospital; Consultant, Tucson Medical Center, Tucson, Arizona.
Immunization

CLIFTON T. FURUKAWA, M.D.
Clinical Assistant Professor, Departments of Pediatrics and Medicine, University of Washington School of Medicine; Attending Physician, University of Washington Affiliated Hospitals, Seattle, Washington.
Host Defense Mechanisms
Psychologic Aspects of Allergic Disease

STANLEY P. GALANT, M.D.
Associate Professor of Pediatrics, University of Utah College of Medicine, University of Utah Medical Center, Salt Lake City, Utah.
Food Allergens

ERWIN W. GELFAND, M.D., F.R.C.P. (Can.)
Professor of Pediatrics, University of Toronto; Senior Scientist, Hospital for Sick Children, Toronto, Ontario, Canada.
Organization of the Immune System

JEFFREY M. GREENE, M.D.
Instructor in Pediatrics and Acting Director, Immunology Clinic, University of Pennsylvania School of Medicine, Philadelphia, Pennsylvania.
Diseases of Erythrocytes, Leukocytes, and Platelets

KENNETH M. GRUNDFAST, M.D.
Assistant Professor of Otolaryngology, University of Pittsburgh School of Medicine; Staff Otolaryngologist, Children's Hospital of Pittsburgh, Pittsburgh, Pennsylvania.
Upper Respiratory Tract Disease

DOUGLAS C. HEINER, M.D., Ph.D.
Professor of Pediatrics, UCLA School of Medicine; Chief, Division of Immunology and Allergy, Harbor General Hospital Campus, Torrance, California.
Non-IgE Antibody in Disease

LESLIE HENDELES, Pharm.D.
Associate Professor, College of Pharmacy; Clinical Pharmacist, Pediatric Allergy Clinic, University of Iowa, Iowa City, Iowa.
Pharmacologic Management

BETTINA C. HILMAN, M.D.
Professor of Pediatrics and Chief of Allergy-Pulmonary Section, Department of Pediatrics, Louisiana State University School of Medicine, Louisiana State University Hospital Full-time faculty; Academic staff member, Schumpert Medical Center, Shreveport, Louisiana.
Surgery in Allergic Patients

J. ROGER HOLLISTER, M.D.
Assistant Professor of Pediatrics, University of Colorado Medical Center; Senior Staff Physician, National Jewish Hospital and Research Center, Denver, Colorado.
Tests to Diagnose Collagen-Vascular Disease

WILLIAM ALLEN HOWARD, M.D.
Clinical Professor of Pediatrics, George Washington University School of Medicine; Senior Advisory Staff in Pediatrics and Allergy and Immunology, Children's Hospital National Medical Center, Washington, D.C.
Medical Evaluation

ALVIN H. JACOBS, M.D.
Emeritus Professor of Dermatology and Pediatrics, Stanford University School of Medicine; Consultant in Dermatology, Children's Hospital of Stanford, Palo Alto, California.
Atopic Dermatitis

RICHARD B. JOHNSTON, Jr., M.D.
Chairman, Department of Pediatrics, National Jewish Hospital and Research Center/National Asthma Center; Professor of Pediatrics, University of Colorado School of Medicine, Denver, Colorado.
Disorders of Complement and Phagocyte Function

DOUGLAS E. JOHNSTONE, M.D.
Co-Director, Pediatric Allergy Clinic and Training Program and Clinical Professor of Pediatrics, Strong Memorial Hospital, University of Rochester School of Medicine and Dentistry; Consultant in Pediatric Allergy, Genesee Hospital and Northside General Hospital, Rochester, New York.
Prevention of Allergic Disease

GUINTER KAHN, M.D.
Director, Pediatric Dermatology Seminars, Parkway General Hospital, Miami, Florida.
Diagnosis and Treatment of Skin Disorders

ILDY M. KATONA, M.D.
Research Fellow, Georgetown University School of Medicine, Washington, D.C.
Immunogenitics

ROGER M. KATZ, M.D.
Associate Clinical Professor of Pediatrics, UCLA School of Medicine; Co-Director of Allergy-Immunology, UCLA Department of Pediatrics and UCLA Center for Health Sciences, Los Angeles, California.
Chronic Cough

EDWIN L. KENDIG, Jr., M.D., Sc.D. (Hon.)
Professor of Pediatrics, Medical College of Virginia, Health Sciences Division, Virginia Commonwealth University; Director, Child Chest Clinic, Medical College of Virginia Hospitals; Director, Department of Pediatrics, St. Mary's Hospital, Richmond, Virginia.
Obstructive Diseases of the Larynx and Trachea

MICHEL KLEIN, M.D.
Assistant Professor of Pathology and Director, Immunology Laboratory, Toronto Western Hospital, Toronto, Ontario, Canada.
Organization of the Immune System

WILLIAM T. KNIKER, M.D.
Professor of Pediatrics and Microbiology, University of Texas Health Science Center at San Antonio; Head, Division of Immunology and Allergy, Bexar County Hospital, Robert B. Green Medical Center, and Santa Rosa Medical Center, San Antonio, Texas.
Disorders of Antibody and Cell-Mediated Immunity

MANUEL LOPEZ, M.D.
Clinical Assistant Professor of Medicine, Tulane University Medical School, New Orleans, Louisiana. Member of Active Staff, Sacred Heart Hospital, Pensacola, Florida.
Nonimmune Environmental Factors in Allergic Disease

MICKEY J. MANDEL, M.D.
Clinical Assistant Professor of Pediatrics and Medicine, University of Colorado Medical School; Attending Dermatologist, General Rose Hospital, Children's Hospital, and Mercy Hospital, Denver, Colorado.
Skin Disorders

HERBERT C. MANSMANN, Jr., M.D.
Professor of Pediatrics; Associate Professor of Medicine; Director, Division of Allergy and Clinical Immunology, Thomas Jefferson Medical College, Philadelphia, Pennsylvania.
Allergy Tests

F. STANFORD MASSIE, M.D.
Associate Clinical Professor of Pediatrics, Medical College of Virginia, Health Sciences Division, Virginia Commonwealth University; Attending Physician, Pediatrics and Allergy, Medical College of Virginia Hospitals and St. Mary's Hospital of Richmond, Richmond, Virginia.
Hypersensitivity Pneumonitis and Pulmonary Reactions to Drugs

KENNETH P. MATHEWS, M.D.
Professor of Internal Medicine, University of Michigan Medical School; Consultant in Allergy, Wayne County General Hospital and Ann Arbor Veterans Administration Hospital, Ann Arbor, Michigan.
Inhalant Allergens

RAWLE M. MCINTOSH, M.D.
Professor of Pediatrics and Medicine, University of Colorado Medical Center; Staff Physician, National Jewish Hospital and Research Center/National Asthma Center, Denver, Colorado. (Deceased)
Renal Diseases

D. LEE MILLER, M.D.
Clinical Assistant Professor of Pediatrics, University of Pittsburgh School of Medicine; Attending Physician, Children's Hospital of Pittsburgh, Mercy

Hospital, St. Clair Memorial Hospital, and St. Francis Hospital, Pittsburgh, Pennsylvania.
Headache

MICHAEL E. MILLER, M.D.
Professor of Pediatric Immunology, UCLA School of Medicine; Chief, Division of Immunology and Hematology/Oncology, Harbor-UCLA Medical Center, Torrance, California.
Developmental Immunity

HELEN G. MORRIS, M.D.
Associate Professor of Medicine, University of Colorado Medical School; Endocrinologist, National Jewish Hospital and Research Center/National Asthma Center, Denver, Colorado.
Endocrine Aspects of Allergy

HAROLD S. NELSON, M.D.
Associate Clinical Professor of Medicine, University of Colorado School of Medicine; Chief, Allergy-Immunology Service, Fitzsimons Army Medical Center, Denver, Colorado.
Pregnancy and Allergic Disease

JERRY L. NORTHERN, Ph.D.
Professor, Department of Otolaryngology, University of Colorado Health Sciences Center; Head, Audiology Division, University Hospital, Denver, Colorado.
Diagnostic Tests in Ear Disease

HANS D. OCHS, M.D.
Associate Professor, Department of Pediatrics, University of Washington School of Medicine; Attending Physician, University Hospital, Children's Orthopedic Hospital and Medical Center, Seattle, Washington.
Host Defense Mechanisms

MICHAEL J. PAINTER, M.D.
Associate Professor of Neurology and Pediatrics, University of Pittsburgh School of Medicine; Attending Physician, Children's Hospital of Pittsburgh and Magee Women's Hospital, Pittsburgh, Pennsylvania.
Headache

JOHN WILLIAM PAISLEY, M.D.
Assistant Professor of Pediatrics, University of Colorado School of Medicine; Consultant, Pediatric Infectious Disease, University of Colorado Medical Center; Director of Inpatient Services, Department of Pediatrics, Denver General Hospital, Denver, Colorado.
Infection and Allergy

FRANK PARKER, M.D.
Professor and Chairman, Department of Dermatology, University of Oregon Health Sciences Center; Attending Physician, Portland Veterans Administration Hospital, Portland, Oregon.
Contact Dermatitis

DAVID S. PEARLMAN, M.D.
Clinical Professor of Pediatrics, University of Colorado Medical School; Senior Staff Physician, National Jewish Hospital and Research Center/National Asthma Center, Denver, Colorado.
Controlling the Environment
Asthma

WILLIAM E. PIERSON, M.D.
Clinical Professor of Pediatrics, University of Washington School of Medicine; Co-Director, Allergy Division, Children's Orthopedic Hospital and Medical Center, Seattle, Washington.
Diseases of the Ear
Diseases of the Nose

DANA P. RABIDEAU, M.D.
Assistant Attending Physician/Assistant Professor of Medicine, Rush Medical College, Rush-Presbyterian-St. Luke's Medical Center, Chicago, Illinois.
Renal Diseases

GARY S. RACHELEFSKY, M.D.
Associate Clinical Professor, UCLA School of Medicine; Co-Director, Pediatric Allergy Clinic, UCLA School of Medicine, Los Angeles, California. Director, Allergy Clinic, Santa Monica Hospital, Santa Monica, California.
Atopic Dermatitis
Diseases of the Paranasal Sinuses

THOMAS A. ROESLER, M.D.
Clinical Instructor of Psychiatry, University of Washington School of Medicine; Attending Physician, Children's Orthopedic Hospital, Seattle, Washington.
Psychologic Aspects of Allergic Disease

JOHN E. SALVAGGIO, M.D.
Henderson Professor of Medicine, Tulane Medical Center; Visiting Physician, Charity Hospital; Consulting Physician, Veterans Administration Hospital; Staff Physician, Tulane University Hospital, New Orleans, Louisiana.
Nonimmune Environmental Factors in Allergic Disease

JANE G. SCHALLER, M.D.
Professor of Pediatrics, University of Washington School of Medicine, Seattle, Washington.
Rheumatic Diseases

ROBERT H. SCHWARTZ, M.D.
Professor of Pediatrics, University of Rochester, School of Medicine and Dentistry; Pediatrician, Strong Memorial Hospital, Rochester, New York.
Nonallergic Chronic Pulmonary Disease

JOHN C. SELNER, M.D.
Associate Clinical Professor of Pediatrics, University of Colorado Medical School, Denver, Colorado.
Endocrine Aspects of Allergy

GAIL G. SHAPIRO, M.D.
Clinical Associate Professor of Pediatrics, University of Washington School of Medicine; Attending Physician, University of Washington Hospital and Children's Orthopedic Hospital and Medical Center, Seattle, Washington.
Urticaria and Angioedema
Diseases of the Paranasal Sinuses

SHELDON C. SIEGEL, M.D.
Clinical Professor of Pediatrics, UCLA School of Medicine; Co-Director of the Pediatric Immunology-Allergy Training Program, UCLA School of Medicine, Los Angeles, California.
Chronic Upper Respiratory Tract Infections and Otitis Media

F. ESTELLE R. SIMONS, M.D., F.R.C.P. (Can.), F.A.A.P.
Assistant Professor, Department of Pediatrics, University of Manitoba; Head, Section of Allergy and Clinical Immunology, Children's Hospital, Winnipeg, Canada.
Lower Respiratory Tract Disease

RAYMOND G. SLAVIN, M.D.
Professor of Internal Medicine, St. Louis University School of Medicine; Attending Physician, St. Louis University, Cardinal Glennon Hospital, John Cochran V.A. Hospital, and St. Louis City Hospital, St. Louis, Missouri.
Epidemiologic Aspects of Atopic Disease

R. MICHAEL SLY, M.D.
Professor of Child Health and Development, George Washington University School of Medicine and Health Sciences; Director of Allergy and Immunology, Children's Hospital National Medical Center, Washington, D.C.
Allergy and School Problems

LAURIE JOAN SMITH, M.D.
Assistant Chief of Allergy and Immunology Service, Walter Reed Army Medical Center; Assistant Professor, Uniformed Services University of the Health Sciences; Clinical Consultant, National Institute of Health, Washington, D.C.
Epidemiologic Aspects of Atopic Disease

WILLIAM R. SOLOMON, M.D.
Professor of Internal Medicine, University of Michigan Medical School; Attending Physician, University Hospital; Consultant in Allergy, Wayne County General Hospital, Ann Arbor Veterans Administration Hospital, and University of Michigan Student Health Service, Ann Arbor, Michigan.
Pollen and Fungus Allergens

J. F. SOOTHILL, M.D.
Professor of Child Health; Chief, Division of Immunology, Institute of Child Health, University of London, London, England.
Prevention of Allergic Disease

JOSEPH F. SOUHRADA, M.D., Ph.D.
Associate Professor of Medicine, University of Colorado Medical Center; Staff member, National Jewish Hospital and Research Center/National Asthma Center, Denver, Colorado.
Pulmonary Function Testing

E. RICHARD STIEHM, M.D.
Professor of Pediatrics, University of California School of Medicine; Attending Pediatrician, UCLA Center for the Health Sciences, Los Angeles, California.
Therapy of Immunodeficiency

ROBERT C. STRUNK, M.D.
Assistant Professor of Pediatrics, University of Colorado Medical School; Senior Staff Physician, National Jewish Hospital and Research Center/National Asthma Center, Denver, Colorado.
Chemical Mediators of Inflammation

ANDOR SZENTIVANYI, M.D.
Chairman, Department of Pharmacology and Therapeutics; Professor of Pharmacology and Therapeutics, University of South Florida College of Medicine, Tampa, Florida.
Constitutional Basis of Atopic Disease

PAUL P. VanARSDEL, Jr., M.D.
Professor of Medicine and Head, Section of Allergy, University of Washington School of Medicine; Attending Physician, University Hospital, Seattle Veterans Administration Hospital, and Seattle Public Health Hospital; Consultant, Children's Orthopedic Hospital and Medical Center, Seattle, Washington.
Fever

VICTOR C. VAUGHAN, III, M.D.
Professor of Pediatrics, Temple University School of Medicine; Attending Physician, St. Christopher's Hospital for Sick Children; Senior Fellow in Medical Evaluation, National Board of Medical Examiners, Philadelphia, Pennsylvania.
Introduction

ALAN A. WANDERER, M.D.
Volunteer Staff Member, National Jewish Hospital and Research Center/National Asthma Center; Clinical Assistant Professor, University of Colorado Medical Center; Chief of Allergy and Immunology, Mercy Hospital; Allergy Consultant, Kaiser-Permanente Medical Plan, Denver, Colorado.
Physical Allergy

MILES WEINBERGER, M.D.
Associate Professor of Pediatrics and Pharmacology; Chairman, Pediatric Allergy and Pulmonary Division, University of Iowa Hospital and Clinics, Iowa City, Iowa.
Pharmacologic Management

WILLIAM LEE WESTON, M.D.
Associate Professor of Dermatology and Pediatrics, Chairman, Department of Dermatology, University of Colorado Health Science Center, Denver, Colorado.
Skin Disorders

JOSEPH F. WILLIAMS, Ph.D.
Associate Professor of Pharmacology and Therapeutics, University of South Florida College of Medicine, Tampa, Florida.
Constitutional Basis of Atopic Disease

PREFACE

Allergy is one of the most common causes of acute and chronic childhood disease. It is the leading cause of school absenteeism for chronic conditions of the respiratory tract and is responsible for a wide range of problems for the child and family. It may cause physical disability, may interfere with the normal psychosocial development of the child and often creates severe social and economic difficulties for the family as well. Unfortunately, allergy is a misunderstood and mysterious area of medicine for many physicians. On the one hand, it commonly is invoked as the basis for numerous types of symptoms for which no other explanation is apparent. On the other hand, allergic disease often is not recognized and, even when recognized, is managed inappropriately. This book was conceived and developed for physicians who provide primary patient care and addresses itself to diagnosis and treatment of those disorders, symptoms, complexes, and signs in the pediatric age range in which the question of "allergy" may arise.

The terminology of allergy suffers from divergent and often vague usage, in itself obstructing recognition and treatment of allergic disease. The term "allergy" was coined in 1906 by von Pirquet following his recognition with Bela Schick that antibodies could cause as well as ameliorate disease. The term, taken from the Greek *allos* ("change in the original state") referred to the concept that encounter with a foreign substance induced an alteration in specific responsiveness, so that subsequent contact with that substance was heightened (hypersensitivity) or decreased (hyposensitivity or immunity). Eventually, an association was recognized between immune factors and various clinical syndromes, leading to the idea that these disorders had an immune basis; in this context "allergy" came to refer only to the hypersensitive (adverse) manifestations of the immune response, and the terms "allergic disease" and "allergic disorder" came into use. Current understanding of the pathogenesis of many of these disorders, however, differs from earlier concepts on which the terms were based, and the terms "allergy" or "allergic" often are more confusing than helpful.

Accordingly, we have adopted the following definitions for "allergy" in this book:

An *allergic reaction* is the adverse consequence of a specific immune event, that is, of the interaction between antigen and antibody or sensitized lymphocytes.

An *allergic disorder (disease)* is a complex of symptoms and signs in which immune events are thought frequently to play a major role. It should be recognized that in some individuals with an allergic disease, immune events may not be of major importance or may not participate in the disease at all and, further, that even when "allergy" is an important factor in the disease, it may not be the underlying basis of the disease (see Chapter 14 and chapters that deal with individual disorders).

Atopy (from the Greek, *atopos,* or "strangeness"), another term that requires definition, was first used by Coca and Cooke over 50 years ago with reference to a group of diseases (seasonal rhinitis, perennial rhinitis, asthma) that shared certain clinical features, suggesting a common basis for these disorders. Sulzberger later argued for the inclusion of infantile eczema ("atopic dermatitis") as well. The occurrence of a specific skin-sensitizing substance ("atopic reagin"), now considered to be principally IgE antibody, was recognized in a high proportion of individuals with atopic disorders and was believed to contribute to the pathogenesis of the disorder in such individuals. Though frequently associated, there is considerable evidence that atopic disease can be independent of IgE antibody.

We have chosen, therefore, to consider *atopy* in terms of a constellation of complexes of symptoms and signs that exhibit certain features in common: a familial (and presumably hereditary) basis, an end-organ hypersensitivity to a variety of chemical mediators of inflammation, and precipitation or aggravation of the complex by various mechanisms, only one of which may involve IgE antibody. Thus, involvement of IgE antibody is not a required characteristic of an atopic disorder. Conversely, the capacity to produce IgE antibody, known to be present in many individuals without any other feature of atopy, does not in itself warrant the designation "atopic." Thus, atopic disorders are considered to represent a subgroup of allergic disorders, which include perennial and seasonal allergic rhinitis, asthma, and atopic dermatitis.

This book is for the practicing physician, and its orientation, therefore, is practical. Some sections may appear at first glance to be academic considerations of physiology, biochemistry, and immunology, but they provide background information necessary for a rational approach to diagnosis and treatment of allergic disease. Also included is consideration of various nonallergic conditions that exhibit features sometimes confused with "allergy" and a consideration of disorders in which a *deficiency* in immune mechanisms may result in disease. In addition, an attempt has been made to reference individual chapters broadly, including review articles and in some cases additional general references on the subject matter covered. We hope that the information and the manner in which it is provided not only will foster more intelligent diagnosis and therapy of allergy but, in so doing, also will encourage the physician to deal more effectively with allergic diseases of infancy, childhood, and adolescence.

C. WARREN BIERMAN, M.D.
DAVID S. PEARLMAN, M.D.

INTRODUCTION

Victor C. Vaughan, III, M.D.

The recorded history of allergic disorders is almost as old as the recorded history of man. Asthma was known to the ancients, as well as the concept that one man's food may be another's poison. The modern perspective with regard to allergy began to be formed early in the 19th century, when Bostock (1819) gave the first modern description of hay fever; a few years later Blackley proved hay fever to be a pollenosis and reported the first confirmatory diagnostic tests, including (in 1873) the first skin test. The recognition that asthma and hay fever and certain other clinical syndromes were related to an altered reactivity of the body, often excited by environmental particles, foods, or other conditions, led to a long and exciting period during which the practice of the clinical allergist was dominated by the quest for the identity of those inciting factors.

Immunology is much younger conceptually than allergy. It had its birth in the late 19th century in studies of bacterial infection and resistance, in studies of resistance to snake venom, in the development of antisera against diphtheria and other scourges, and in the description of anaphylaxis. The link between allergy and immunology was forged early in the 20th century by a host of investigators too numerous to list but whose names include Arthus, Calmette, Cooke, Noon, Richet, Schick, Schloss, Theobald Smith, von Behring, and von Pirquet. Richet described *anaphylaxis* (1902) and became the father of modern experimental immunology; von Pirquet invented the word *allergy* (1906) to describe *altered reactivity*; Leonard Noon first (1911) injected an extract of allergen to treat hay fever by *desensitization* (hyposensitization). The next half century was dominated by a clinical orientation among allergists, based on the concepts developed in these early years. The fundamental notion of allergy was that altered reactivity was based upon prior exposure and that its management was to identify and avoid the inciting factors or to desensitize against those inciting factors when they cannot be avoided altogether and when an effective extract could be prepared.

The romance between allergy and immunology began almost a century ago, and the marriage at its diamond jubilee seems secure, but recent studies have both put the relationship on a more solid conceptual and experimental basis and revealed areas in which appeals to immunology for understanding of allergic problems have failed to find adequate responses. New techniques and new rigors in the scientific study of allergic diseases are changing our perceptions of their natures and are calling upon us to modify or abandon time-honored notions with respect to allergic and related immunologic problems.

The development of sophisticated immunologic tests and their correlation with traditional clinical observation and allergic testing have indicated that

xv

some patients with clinical allergy by traditional definitions have no substantial evidence of an immunologic disorder nor any clear-cut sign that traditional measures are likely to be helpful. For such patients, traditional management is to be regarded as unacceptably costly, intrusive, and futile. For them, management with drug therapy may be the only effective present recourse; the same will be true for many other patients who have more traditional forms of allergy. The advances in pharmacologic therapy in the past quarter century have aided in this differentiation and management.

Hyposensitization began to be used in 1911 in the treatment of hay fever. The process was long known as "desensitization" and still may be for some allergists, though it is clear that when wheal and flare reactivity is part of the response to a skin test, this reactivity may not much abate as symptoms are controlled by the injection of extracts. Recent rigorous experimental studies have sharply revised our notions of the effectiveness of this time-honored procedure. The anecdotal evidence of nearly two generations of clinical allergists has supported the procedure with enthusiasm, but studies using modern criteria for statistical reliability and validity were not done until nearly 40 years after desensitization was first introduced. These studies and others that have followed have validated the procedure statistically but have also raised problems as to how the procedure should be properly used in the particular patient. For example, the results of an early study might be interpreted as suggesting that *all* the statistically significantly beneficial effects of desensitization in a study group might have represented major impact on the symptoms of a relatively small subgroup of those who were treated. We are left to wonder how to identify reliably those patients who will and those who will not benefit from or need this form of treatment.

It is clear that attitudes towards allergic diseases are in a state of rather rapid change. Our attitudes towards skin testing and immunization therapy (desensitization or hyposensitization) are more conservative than a decade ago, and with the refined chemical techniques that allow us to accurately measure the levels of drugs (and especially of theophylline) in the blood, we have entered a new era in management of asthma. Cromolyn and corticosteroids also have roles to play in this new development. All of these developments are discussed in detail in the pages that follow, and the contributors to this volume will indicate our present conceptualization of the relationship between the basic sciences and the clinical conundrum known as allergy and will show us where we are sometimes served best by immunology, sometimes best by pharmacology, and sometimes best by an empiric common sense rooted in decades of clinical practice.

Nothing in the foregoing comments should be construed as suggesting that the allergist or any other physician should abandon in any major respect the traditional plan of study of allergic children, which is to attempt through complete and creative history-taking to identify events or substances precipitating symptoms of allergic disorders. Skin tests have a place in the study of certain children. Some constraint on exposure to inciting agents is appropriate, and prophylactic constraints often may also be useful. But any of these processes may become cost-ineffective when pushed to the point where the frustration of physician, child, or parents outweighs relief of tolerable symptoms or to the point where guilt and depression are generated by the failure of intense efforts to abate symptoms that nothing can control. Even though for many years skillful conventional allergic management has brought comfort or relief to millions, we must be ready to test and retest our notions as to what best fits the individual patient and must be ready as soon as possible to identify those patients for whom non-immunologic therapy is the only kind required or likely to be helpful.

When value systems are in rapid evolution, it is helpful to have substantial reviews such as this volume to bring us to the advancing edge of a changing field and show us where we are, what is going on, and what likely lies ahead. We may guess that what lies ahead for allergic children and their families is continued progress in clinical immunology, clinical physiology, clinical pharmacology, and clinical psychology of child development. This continuing progress will tell us with ever more confidence what allergic children need and how to provide it for them.

CONTENTS

DISEASES OF HOST DEFENSE

IMMUNOPHARMACOLOGY OF ALLERGIC DISEASE

ETIOLOGY AND PATHOGENETIC CONSIDERATIONS IN ALLERGIC DISEASE

GENERAL MANAGEMENT OF ALLERGIC DISEASE

DISORDERS THAT MAY INVOLVE IMMUNE MECHANISMS

Erwin W. Gelfand, M.D.
Michel Klein, M.D.

1

Functional Organization of the Immune System

Components of the Lymphoreticular System*

Erwin W. Gelfand, M.D.

ORGANIZATION

Long before the specific functions of lymphocytes were identified, an important role in inflammatory and immune reactions was recognized based on their abundance in a number of chronic inflammatory conditions or tumor-bearing tissues. Although most familiar as a circulating white cell, lymphocytes constitute the major cell type in the thymus, spleen, lymph node, and Peyer's patches of the gastrointestinal tract. These organs serve as principal sites of proliferation and development of cells involved in immune responses.

Thymus. The thymus plays a strategic role in the development and maintenance of immunologic integrity. It arises from the ventral portions of the third and fourth pharyngeal pouches; between the seventh and tenth week of gestation, it descends from the neck into the upper and anterior compartments of the mediastinum. The organ is largest at birth in relation to total body size. With increasing age, thymic tissue de-

creases in amount and becomes infiltrated with fatty tissue.

The thymus is highly organized, consisting of numerous lobules and a well demarcated outer cortex and an inner medulla. The cortex contains densely packed cells, indistinguishable from small lymphocytes. The medulla contains small thymocytes, but these are more dispersed than in the cortex. Prominent in the medulla are the reticulo-epithelial cells that form Hassall's corpuscles (Fig. 1–1). Immunologically competent lymphocytes and the lymphoid histology and corticomedullary demarcation characteristic of the mature thymus are achieved by 10 to 12 weeks of fetal life. The number of Hassall's corpuscles increases during fetal life.

Spleen. The spleen develops during the fifth week of intrauterine life. It is organized so that lymphocyte-rich areas are located primarily in close proximity to small arterioles. This so-called "white pulp" is a cylindrical structure surrounding the central arteriole and constitutes a periarteriolar lymphocyte sheath (PALS) (Fig. 1–2). This sheath is populated chiefly by thymus-derived (T cell) lymphocytes; the follicle and germinal center adjacent to the PALS

*Supported by the Medical Research Council of Canada [Grant MT–4875]

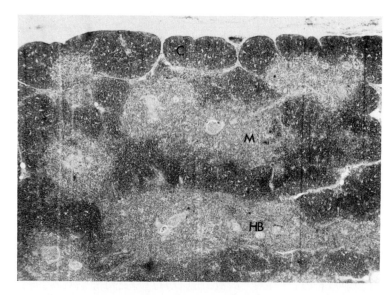

FIGURE 1–1. Photomicrograph of the thymus. C = cortex; M = medulla; HB = Hassall's bodies.

represent the B cell area of the spleen. Following antigenic stimulation, blast-like cells appear throughout the white pulp. In contrast to lymph nodes, in which immune stimulation comes mainly from locally-derived lymph-borne antigens, antigenic stimulation of the spleen is blood-borne.

Lymph Nodes. Lymph nodes are situated along the path of collecting lymphatics, with efferent lymphatics from the nodes joining to enter the venous circulation. In the newborn period, lymph nodes are small and require antigenic stimulation, e.g., by microorganisms, before they take on their characteristic appearance. Morphologically the node can be divided into cortical, paracortical, and medullary areas (Fig. 1–3). The cortex contains aggregates of lymphoid cells called follicles, in the middle of which there is the germinal center. The follicles constitute the B cell area of the node and are absent, for example, in congenital X-linked agammaglobulinemia. The paracortical zone contains postcapillary venules, through which the blood supply to the node passes; lymphocytes infiltrating this area are primarily T cells. The medulla or medullary cord zone contains numerous plasma cells. Following antigenic stimulation, there is generalized nodal hypertrophy with large lymphocytes and blast-like cells accumulating in the cortex, enlargement of the primary follicles, formation of secondary follicles, and an increase in numbers of plasma cells.

Gastrointestinal Tract. The mammalian gastrointestinal system, including the liver, is a major contributor to the immune ca-

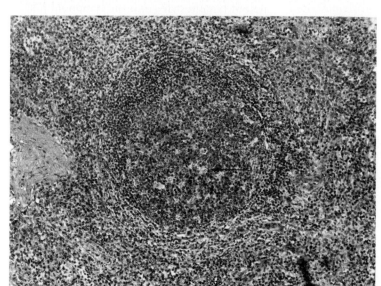

FIGURE 1–2. Photomicrograph of the spleen, illustrating the periarteriolar lymphocyte sheath. The arrow indicates the central arteriole.

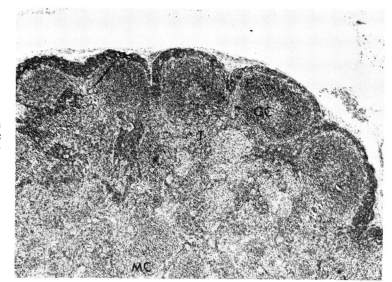

FIGURE 1–3. Photomicrograph of a lymph node. F = follicle; GC = germinal center; T = paracortex; MC = medullary cords.

pacity of the individual. The lymphoid components of the mature gastrointestinal tract consist of intraepithelial lymphocytes, Peyer's patches, and plasma cells.

Peyer's patches are groups of subepithelial lymphoid follicles located in the mucosa of the small intestine (Fig. 1–4). They are recognizable by the twenty-fourth week of gestation and increase in size and number during the first two decades of life. It has been shown in animals that these accumulations of lymphoid cells are initially populated by T cells; later B lymphocytes increase in number, eventually constituting about 30 percent of the lymphocyte population. The function of the Peyer's patches is not known, but it appears unlikely that they represent the mammalian equivalent of the avian bursa of Fabricius (a gut-associated organ in birds that appears largely responsible for generating B lymphocytes).

Plasma cells are distributed homogeneously throughout the lamina propria of the small gut. Their appearance coincides with colonization of the gut by microorganisms. Plasma cells containing all five classes of immunoglobulin have been demonstrated; but IgA-containing cells predominate, reflecting the role of IgA as the major immunoglobulin class in the secretory immune system.

Bone Marrow. The bone marrow is the principal source of lymphoid precursor cells in postnatal life. The pluripotent hemopoietic precursor cells (stem cells) within the marrow cavity have the capacity to differentiate into erythrocytes, granulocytes, megakaryocytes, monocytes, and T or B lymphocytes. The lymphocytes consti-

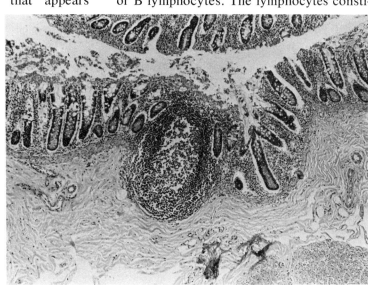

FIGURE 1–4. Photomicrograph of the small intestine, illustrating the Peyer's patch.

tute 10 to 20 percent of all nucleated cells in bone marrow. Although few mature T cells reside in the marrow, mature B lymphocytes and fully-differentiated immunoglobulin-secreting plasma cells are abundant in the mature individual. Plasma cells are less apparent in neonates and infants.

CELLS INVOLVED IN THE IMMUNE RESPONSE

Lymphoid Cells

The basis of the immune response resides in the ability of subpopulations of lymphoid cells to recognize and react in a specific manner to the wide variety of antigens normally encountered. These responses have been separated into reactions directly mediated by cells *(cell-mediated immunity)* and responses mediated by antibody *(humoral immunity)*. The effects of thymectomy and bursectomy in animals, as well as clinical observations, suggest that one subpopulation of lymphocytes, thymus-dependent or *T lymphocytes,* are responsible for cell-mediated immune reactions, whereas thymus-independent (bursa-dependent; bone-marrow derived) or *B lymphocytes* are the precursors of plasma cells that are responsible for the secretion of antibody. This two-component concept of the immune system is supported by differences in pathways of differentiation, organization of lymphoid tissues, morphology, antigenic markers, as well as function.

Differentiation of the lymphoid precursor cells proceeds in two discrete stages. In the first stage, pluripotent hematopoietic stem cells, which originate in the yolk sac during the first trimester of fetal life and subsequently are found in fetal liver and then fetal bone marrow, differentiate into cells committed to a particular pathway. Depending on the microenvironment, these committed progenitor cells can differentiate into red blood cells, granulocytes, megakaryocytes, monocytes, or lymphocytes. In the second stage, cells committed to the development of the lymphoid system mature along one of the two recognized pathways.

T LYMPHOCYTES

Differentiation. Differentiation of the T lymphocyte system is dependent upon and regulated by the thymus (Gelfand et al., 1978). Lymphoid precursors enter this epithelial organ, where, under the specific inductive influences of this microenvironment, they undergo rapid proliferation. The thymus acts on T cell differentiation in at least two ways:

(1) It promotes the transformation of pre-thymic precursor cells into functional post-thymic cells. Factors controlling lymphoid cell differentiation and expansion within the thymus are not well understood, but both cell-cell contact with the epithelial cells and thymic humoral factor(s) may be required (Miller, 1961). During this phase of differentiation, the cells acquire new surface membrane markers and increasing functional capacity.

(2) Following migration of post-thymic cells to the peripheral lymphoid tissues, thymic humoral factors may continue to modulate and further expand these cells populations (Stutman and Good, 1973). In the peripheral blood, T lymphocytes constitute the major population of circulating lymphocytes; in peripheral lymphoid tissues, they occupy the paracortical region of the lymph nodes, the periarteriolar lymphocyte sheath of the spleen, and the interfollicular tissue spaces of Peyer's patches along the gastrointestinal tract.

The presence of thymic humoral factors was suggested originally by Miller and colleagues, who demonstrated immune reconstitution of thymectomized animals by implantation of thymic tissue in cell-impermeable diffusion chambers (Osoba and Miller, 1963). More recent work has shown that thymic extracts, e.g., prepared from calf thymus, can induce the appearance of specific T cell markers on subpopulations of murine lymphocytes (Komuro and Boyse, 1973; Scheid et al., 1973). We have shown that the source of a similar human factor is derived from the thymic epithelial cells and not the thymocytes themselves (Pyke and Gelfand, 1974). Incubation of T cell precursors from human bone marrow or fetal liver with supernatant fluid from long-term cultures of human thymic epithelium results in the appearance of both E-rosetting cells, a marker of human T cells *(vida infra),* and functional differentiation (Gelfand et al., 1978). We proposed that the initial stages of T cell differentiation in man require cell-cell contact with the thymic epithelial stroma, whereas at later stages, thymic humoral factors alone may be sufficient to promote maturation. A wide variety of thymic humoral factors or thymus-replacing factors have been extracted or isolated in various species. These include thymosin, thymopoietin, and thymic epithelial cell conditioned medium. These substances appear to share certain properties, but they have been isolated in relatively impure states. Their mechanisms of action remain, at best, poorly understood.

Functional Properties of T Cells. Although the immune system can be considered as a two-component system, one involving humoral immunity (antibody) and another based on more direct participation of immunocompetent cells (cell-mediated immunity), it must be emphasized that this separation is somewhat artificial. That is, in most immune responses, there is a striking interdependence of humoral and cell-mediated immunity.

Immunocompetent T lymphocytes are involved in cell-mediated immunity either as the effector cells in a particular response or as the initiators or regulators of the reactions. Thus, T lymphocytes play a major role in tumor immunity, transplant rejection, and immunity to facultative intracellular organisms. T lymphocytes are responsible for the initiation of delayed hypersensitivity skin test reactions and are involved in contact sensitivity. Absence of T lymphocytes or of functionally competent T cells is associated with recurrent and severe infections from viruses, fungi, or unusual pathogens such as *Pneumocystis carinii;* failure to thrive; and susceptibility to graft-versus-host disease. T lymphocytes actually consist of a number of distinct subsets, all presumably thymic-dependent in origin. As maturation proceeds, these subsets express different defined functions, cell surface markers, and surface antigens. Distinct T cell subsets have been identified in mice, and, recently, several T cell subsets have been delineated in humans: for example, *helper T cells,* which trigger, or *suppressor T cells,* which interfere with or suppress, antibody responses.

Identification of T Cells

The ability to identify and recognize T cells or B cells in peripheral blood or lymphoid tissues has contributed immensely to our understanding of disorders of the immune system. Although most of these assays give no specific information regarding the functional capacity of these cells, they do provide the means for the nosologic classification of lymphoid cells and for identifying disorders in which responsible cells are present but nonfunctional, versus diseases in which entire cell populations may be absent. Table 1–1 lists these assays, which also are described below.

SURFACE RECEPTORS

1. *E-rosette assay.* Human T lymphocytes are capable of spontaneously binding sheep red blood cells to form "rosettes" (Fig. 1–5) (International Union Report, 1975). This capacity appears to be due to the presence of a surface glycoprotein receptor that is found on virtually all thymocytes and mature peripheral blood T cells. Approximately 60 to 80 percent of peripheral blood lymphocytes possess a receptor for sheep erythrocytes. A modification of this technique may be applied to outline T cell areas in lymphoid tissues (Silviera et al., 1972). There are a number of modifications in the way the assay is performed, some of which may be used to define T cell subpopulations. We have used the drug theophylline to identify two functionally distinct T cell subpopulations: a subset that loses the ability to bind sheep red cells in the presence of theophylline and a population that continues to bind sheep red cells in the presence of the drug (Limatibul et al., 1978).

TABLE 1–1 IDENTIFICATION OF PERIPHERAL BLOOD T CELLS

Marker	Assay	Population of T cells
RECEPTORS		
SRBC	E rosette	Virtually all
C3	EAC rosette	<5%
Fc–IgM	EA–IgM rosette	65–80%
Fc–IgG	EA–IgG rosette	~ 20%
HISTOCHEMISTRY		
Esterase	α (or β) naphthyl esterase	~ 70–80% show 1–2 dots in cytoplasm

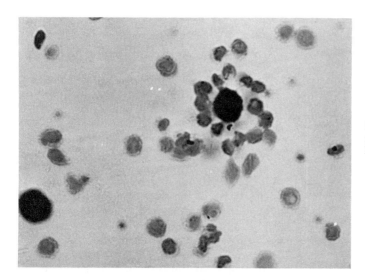

FIGURE 1–5. Identification of an E-rosetting T cell and a non-rosetting lymphocyte.

2. *Fc receptors*. Most peripheral blood T lymphocytes also have been shown to carry a receptor for either the Fc portion of IgM (Tμ cells) or for the Fc portion of IgG (Tγ cells) (Moretta et al., 1975). Sixty-five to 80 percent of peripheral blood T cells that bind sheep erythrocytes have a receptor for IgM. As will be discussed below, these different populations are characterized also by their abilities to subserve distinctive immune functions (Moretta et al., 1977; Shore et al., 1978).

3. *C3 receptor*. A very small population of T cells — perhaps immature, precursor T cells — appear to carry a receptor for the third component of complement (Shore et al., 1979). These cells are found in proportionately greater numbers in thoracic duct lymph. In contrast to B lymphocytes, which have a receptor for both C3b and C3d, the receptor on T lymphocytes is restricted to C3d.

T Cell Antigens

Antisera, specific for a surface antigenic marker for T cells, can be produced by immunization of animals with human T cells (generally thymocytes) and absorption of the antisera with non–T cells. Such antisera can be used to identify T cells either by using immunofluorescent analysis or complement-dependent cytotoxicity (Touraine et al., 1974).

Histochemistry

Nonspecific esterase staining of peripheral blood cells distinguishes two cell types. Characteristically, monocytes can be identified by the fact that their entire cytoplasm

stains. The majority of T cells, on the other hand, can be identified by the presence of one or two discretely stained dots in the periphery of the cytoplasm (Fig. 1–6) (Ranki et al., 1976).

Tests of T Cell Function

There are many tests of considerable value in assessing the functional capacity of T lymphocytes and their ability to mediate cell-mediated immune reactions. Tests of most importance are listed in Table 1–2 and summarized below.

In Vivo

1. *Lymphocyte count*. Systematic evaluation of the T cell system involves examination of the peripheral blood smear. Normally, peripheral blood contains greater than

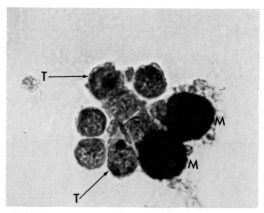

FIGURE 1–6. α-Naphthyl esterase staining of peripheral blood mononuclear cells. M = darkly staining monocytes; T = single dots in cytoplasm of T lymphocytes.

TABLE 1–2 TESTS OF T CELL FUNCTION

In vivo
  Peripheral blood lymphocyte count and morphology
  Delayed hypersensitivity skin test responses
  Allogeneic skin graft rejection

In vitro
  Lymphocyte proliferation in response to lectins, antigens, or allogeneic cells
  Lymphokine production
  Helper/suppressor cell activity

2000 lymphocytes/mm^3; a minimum of 10 percent of these are small lymphocytes.

2. *Delayed hypersensitivity skin tests.* Although there have been major advances in our attempts to assess cell-mediated immunity *in vitro*, the simple intradermal skin test remains a useful tool for measuring cell-mediated immune functions. Positive delayed reactions (erythema and induration) to various microbial extracts imply normal thymus-dependent immunity. Inability to react to a battery of normally encountered antigens is termed "anergy." Delayed hypersensitivity skin testing is of relatively little value during the first years of life, when lack of adequate exposure to antigens available for testing may account for nonreactivity.

3. *Graft rejection.* Rejection of a third party or allogeneic skin graft within 14 to 28 days is indicative of a functionally intact T cell system.

In Vitro

1. *Lymphocyte proliferation.* Following interaction with plant lectins or specific antigens, resting lymphocytes undergo blast transformation and mitosis. The addition of radiolabeled thymidine to the cultures and later extraction of newly synthesized radiolabeled DNA permits evaluation of the degree of stimulation. The plant lectins, phytohemagglutinin, concanavalin A, or pokeweed, are nonspecific mitogens and activate a large proportion of lymphocytes, whereas specific antigens (e.g., PPD, tetanus toxoid) stimulate only a small proportion of cells. Allogeneic cells also activate lymphocytes in the mixed lymphocyte culture (MLC). The MLC is a special example of antigen stimulaton since responding cells do not need prior sensitization (Plate and McKenzie, 1973). Lymphocyte proliferative responses predominantly, if not exclusive-

ly, reflect the response of T lymphocytes (Boldt et al., 1975).

2. *Lymphokine production.* Following activation by specific antigen or nonspecific mitogens, T lymphocytes release or secrete a number of biologically active factors, collectively called "lymphokines." These include migration inhibition factor (MIF) and interferon (David, 1971). Lymphokines are important mediators of cell-mediated immunity and serve to amplify the host's immune response. In general, lymphokines are not produced in response to antigens that fail to elicit a delayed skin test reaction.

3. *Helper/suppressor cell activity.* As will be discussed below, *in vitro* and *in vivo* assays of immunoglobulin synthesis are T cell dependent. The presence of helper T cells or suppressor T cells can be evaluated in these assays (Moretta, 1977a; Dosch et al., 1978).

B LYMPHOCYTES

Differentiation. As differentiation of the T cell system is taking place within the thymus, differentiation of B lymphoid precursor cells, destined to become mature antibody-secreting plasma cells, is occurring in other sites. Concepts of B lymphocyte differentiation (Fig. 1–7) are based primarily on studies carried out in birds and rodents (Kincade and Cooper, 1971). The developmental pathway of stem cells to the B lymphocyte stage has been best studied in the chicken, in which the maturation of B cells begins with the migration of progenitor cells to a specific microenvironment within the bursa of Fabricius, an outpouching of the hindgut. This population rapidly expands, and as the cells mature, they leave the bursa (Cooper et al., 1971); immunoglobulin-bearing B lymphocytes enter the circulation and occupy the lymphoid follicles and medullary cords of lymph node tissue and the red pulp and germinal centers of the spleen. The series of steps leading to clonal diversity in this sequence of events is unclear; but by whatever mechanism, following contact with antigen, B lymphocytes proliferate and differentiate into antibody-secreting cells (Cooper and Lawton, 1974).

Despite considerable effort, the existence of a bursal analogue in mammals has not been demonstrated. Attempts to identify the gut-associated lymphoid tissue as a pos-

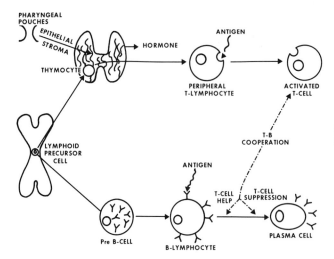

FIGURE 1–7. Differentiation of the lymphoid system.

sible site have been unrewarding, and suspicions now are directed at either the bone marrow, fetal liver, or spleen as the potential site.

Functional Properties of B Cells. B lymphocytes and their progeny, plasma cells, mediate humoral immunity by producing various kinds of proteins with antibody activity. The interdependence of the B cell and T cell systems is emphasized by a requirement for immunocompetent T cells in the maturation of B lymphocytes to the plasma cell stage.

Identification of B Cells, B Cell Precursors, and Their Progeny (Table 1–3)

SURFACE RECEPTORS (FIG. 1–8)

1. *Surface immunoglobulin.* The detection of immunoglobulin on lymphocyte membranes has served as a valuable marker of B lymphocytes in man; B lymphocytes are defined as cells that bear surface immunoglobulin (Pernis et al., 1970; Fro-

land et al., 1971). With conventional techniques, plasma cells generally do not behave as if they possess surface immunoglobulin (sIg). Pre–B cells also lack sIg but can be identified by the presence of cytoplasmic immunoglobulin (Pearl et al., 1978).

sIg–bearing B lymphocytes can be identified through a variety of techniques. The most commonly used method is direct immunofluorescence with fluorochrome-labeled anti-immunoglobulin antisera and counting these cells in a fluorescence microscope (International Union Report, 1975). Most investigators agree that IgM and IgD are the predominant immunoglobulin classes on human peripheral blood B lymphocytes, coexisting on the same cell, and represent 5 to 10 percent of the total number of peripheral blood lymphocytes (Pernis, 1977). Other methods of identifying B lymphocytes are more complex; many involve radiolabeling techniques.

2. *C3 receptor.* B lymphocytes carry a receptor for the activated third component

TABLE 1–3 IDENTIFICATION OF PERIPHERAL BLOOD B LYMPHOCYTES

Marker	Assay	Population of B Cells
RECEPTORS		
sIg	Direct immunofluorescence	5–15% of peripheral blood lymphocytes: sIgM and sIgD predominate
C3	EAC rosette	Most B lymphocytes
Fc-IgG	EA–IgG rosette Aggregated IgG	Most B lymphocytes
Mouse RBC	MRBC rosette	Most B lymphocytes
EB virus	Direct immunofluorescence	Most B lymphocytes
B CELL ANTIGENS		
Ia	Indirect immunofluorescence using heterologous or alloantisera	Most B lymphocytes

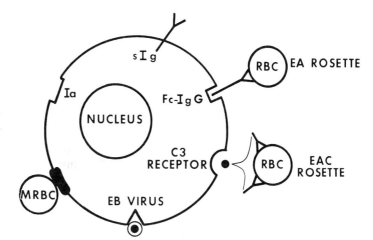

FIGURE 1–8. Schematic representation of surface receptors on human B lymphocytes.

of complement and can be identified by a rosetting technique similar to the E-rosetting technique used to identify T cells (Bianco et al., 1970). To avoid confusion with E(T cell)-rosettes, ox red cells coated with IgM antibody in the presence of complement (EAC) generally are used in this assay (International Union Report, 1975).

3. *Fc receptor.* A receptor for the Fc portion of IgG also can be detected on B cells, using fluorochrome-labeled aggregated IgG (Dickler and Kunkel, 1972) or a rosette technique using ox red cells coated with IgG antibody (EA) (International Union Report, 1975).

On the basis of what has been said earlier, it is obvious that the presence of many of these receptors are of doubtful value as selective B cell assays (also see Table 1–4). Monocytes carry C3 and Fc receptors (see below) and, as mentioned, T cell subpopulations may have Fc receptors for IgG or IgM. Some of the confusion may be eliminated by using double marker assays in attempting to identify the lineage of a particular cell (Shore et al., 1979).

4. *Mouse red blood cells.* Human B lymphocytes also can be identified by their ability to bind mouse RBC (Gupta and Grieco, 1975).

5. *Epstein-Barr (EB) virus.* Human B lymphocytes carry a receptor for EB virus; it is the presence of this receptor that enables B lymphocytes to be immortalized in long-term culture (Jondal and Klein, 1973).

B CELL ANTIGENS. Human B lymphocytes (and monocytes) carry the gene products for a group of HLA-linked, serologically defined, surface alloantigens, which can be detected using sera obtained from multiparous or multi-transfused individuals (Möller, 1976). These antigens, known as Ia antigens, are thought to play a vital role in the genetic control of the immune response (see Chapter 3). Specific anti-Ia antisera are important reagents for identifying and characterizing B cells and their progeny.

Tests of B Cell Function. B cells and their progeny, plasma cells, are responsible for the functions of humoral immunity, through the production of plasma proteins (immunoglobulins) that have antibody activity. Antibody activity refers to the specific combination with the substance (antigen) that elicited their formation. The immunoglobulins represent an extremely heterogeneous group of proteins. The quantitation, structure, physicochemical, and biologic properties of these proteins will be considered at a later point in this chapter. Their function, namely antibody activity,

TABLE 1–4 COMPARISON OF MARKERS ON HUMAN PERIPHERAL BLOOD MONONUCLEAR CELLS

	Monocytes	T cells	B cells
sIg	−	−	+
EA–IgG	+	+	+
EA–IgM	−	+	−*
Aggregated IgG	+	−	+
EB virus	−	−	+
E rosette	−	+	−
EAC	+	±†	+
Nonspecific esterase‡	+	+	−
Mouse RBC	−	−	+

*Some B lymphocytes may demonstrate IgM receptors.

†Only 1 to 2 percent T cells.

‡Monocytes – diffuse cytoplasmic staining; T cells – discrete cytoplasmic dots.

TABLE 1–5   TESTS OF B CELL FUNCTION

In vivo
  Presence of immunoglobulins of all five classes
  Schick test, isohemagglutinins
  Antibody response following immunization
  Presence of plasma cells

In vitro
  Plaque-forming cell assays

can be assessed *in vivo* or *in vitro*. Major tests for B cell function are listed in Table 1–5 and summarized below.

In Vivo. Normally, antibodies arise in response to foreign antigenic substances introduced into the body. So-called "natural antibodies," for example, anti-A or anti-B isohemagglutinins, arise in a similar manner, emerging as a result of immunization with cross-reacting antigens. Major sources of such cross-reacting substances include microorganisms (coliforms) that colonize the gastrointestinal tract, and foods of plant origin.

Active immunization with any antigen elicits a detectable antibody response in most normal individuals. The most convenient antigens to use, since most individuals have received prior immunization, include tetanus, polio, and diphtheria. Diphtheria antibody can be determined easily using the Schick test. The presence of antibodies can be estimated prior to and following a booster injection to evaluate immunologic memory.

In Vitro. Several assays are currently available for determining the capacity of an individual's lymphocytes to synthesize specific antibodies following *in vitro* incubation of the cells with antigen. These assays take the form of a plaque assay wherein specific antigen is coupled to indicator red cells. In the presence of cells that secrete antibody and following the addition of complement, the red cells lyse, leaving a hemolytic plaque with the antibody-secreting cell in the center (Dosch and Gelfand, 1979).

Non–Lymphoid Cells

Mononuclear Phagocytes. The mononuclear phagocytes include the circulating peripheral blood monocytes and tissue macrophages. Monocytes are derived from precursor cells in the bone marrow, whereas tissue macrophages are derived

from blood monocytes and the local proliferation of macrophages. Although primarily phagocytic in function, these cells can bind antigen and antigen-antibody complexes through their surface receptors for the Fc portion of IgG and C3 (International Union Report, 1975). There is a growing awareness of the role of these cells, particularly through antigen processing, in a number of immune responses, including T cell proliferation and antibody synthesis (Möller, 1978a).

Polymorphonuclear Leukocytes. Granulocytes are capable of migrating toward stimuli such as bacterial products, tissue proteases, and complement components (see Chapter 5). These cells bind and ingest appropriately opsonized materials following attachment of these materials to the cell surface via receptors for IgG or C3. Eosinophils also are phagocytic and can ingest antigen-antibody complexes. They play an important role in allergic phenomena and in host defense against parasitic infestation (see Chapter 12). Circulating basophils and tissue mast cells contain a number of biologically active components, including histamine and heparin. As targets for IgE, these cells also play an important role in allergic phenomena (see Chapter 11).

CELL COOPERATION

The requirement for cell cooperation between thymus-derived T cells, B cells, and macrophages was established by showing that no cell population alone could mount an immune response, whereas the presence of all three cell populations enabled the response to develop. Although B cells are the precursors of antibody-secreting cells, they require T cells to direct their terminal differentiation to the secretory or plasma cell stage. These cellular interactions are complex and a number of mechanisms have been postulated to explain the interrelationships (Feldmann, 1973).

A large body of evidence supports the hypothesis that both T cells and B cells possess specific receptors for antigen and cooperate, for example, in the elaboration of an antibody response. For B cells, sIg appears to serve as the specific receptor for antigen. Specific T cell receptors have not been well defined, and the nature of T cell interaction with macrophages remains enigmatic (Möller, 1978 a). Heterogeneity within the T cell population has been demonstrated, with at least two major subsets delineated. Helper T cells promote the differentiation of B cells into antibody secreting cells, whereas suppressor T cells impede or interfere with this process (Benacerraf, 1978). In humans, helper cells appear to be theophylline-resistant and bear receptors for the Fc portion of IgM: suppressor cells are theophylline-sensitive and bind IgG (Shore et al., 1979). Helper cell effects also may be mediated by humoral products released from activated helper T cells.

Thymus Dependency of Antigens

In the murine system, antigens vary in their degree of dependence on T cell interactions for elicitation of antibodies. Thus, certain antigens have been designated as *thymus-independent* and include polysaccharide antigens. Other antigens such as erythrocytes and soluble proteins are *thymus-dependent*. Production of certain classes of immunoglobulins also exhibit various degrees of T cell dependency: IgM antibodies may be least influenced by the absence of a thymus; the synthesis of IgG and IgE are more dependent on the presence of T cells (Katz and Benacerraf, 1972).

In humans, the distinction between thymus-dependent or thymus-independent antigens is less obvious, and there is little evidence *in vivo* or *in vitro* for the ability of B cells alone to mount an antibody response. The degree of T cell involvement in B cell responses to different antigens therefore is likely to vary only on a relative basis.

Genetic Control of the Immune Response

The immune response is under precise genetic control. This control can be expressed at all levels, including antigen recognition, antigen processing, or the cooperative interactions occurring between T cells, B cells, and macrophages. The roles of immune response genes, linked to the major histocompatibility locus, have been described best in highly inbred mice and guinea pigs (Möller, 1978 b). Similar control, linked to the HLA system in man, also has been postulated, particularly in view of the association of certain disease states with specific HLA haplotypes (Dausset and Svejgaard, 1977).

In the animal models, histocompatibility-linked immune response (Ir) genes control responses to thymic-dependent antigens; in mice the relationships between the H-2 complex and Ir genes are well defined. These are further discussed in Chapter 3. No such linkage for thymus-independent antigens has been identified. Histocompatibility-linked Ir genes are expressed on all cell types involved in the immune response and are concerned primarily with interactions between these cell types. The nature of these interactions remains unclear, but it appears that cell-cell contact is not mandatory since soluble products, for example, from activated T cells, can replace T cells in some reactions. Despite the present lack of clarity of the mode of action of the products of the major histocompatibility complex, it is likely that their function is expressed through participating T cell subsets (helper cells and suppressor or regulator cells) and that the response in a given individual is determined by the balance between these individual influences.

Regulation of IgE Production

The cellular and molecular control mechanisms involved in IgE antibody production are complex and only beginning to be unraveled (Tada, 1975) (also see Chapter 9). The basic constituents of the immune components involved in IgE production include the IgE B lymphocyte precursors of antibody-secreting cells, macrophages, and T lymphocytes. These cells as discussed above form a regulatory network of feedback loops, with the T lymphocytes playing a central role in this control. There are both helper and suppressor T cells capable of mutually interacting with one another as well as with the IgE B cells. Among these immune components, there is evidence that the major histocompatibility gene products contribute in a significant way to the development of allergic responses.

In one scheme of IgE production (Fig. 1–9), it is postulated that macrophages process antigen and, via interaction (through Ir gene products) with helper T cells, lead to activation of the helper T cells, which in turn facilitate the differentiation of IgE B cells to mature antibody-secreting plasma cells (Katz, 1978). These

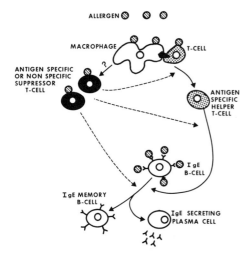

FIGURE 1–9. Schematic representation of the cellular regulation of IgE production.

interactions may involve direct cell-cell contact or soluble T cell factors. Antigen-specific or non–antigen-specific suppressor T cells can interfere with these events, conceivably at several levels: the activation of helper T cells, interactions with the B lymphocytes, or in the actual process of differentiation of the B lymphocytes to the plasma cell stage. Various investigators have demonstrated a significant negative

regulatory role of suppressor T cells in the production of IgE antibodies in rodents. Thus, low doses of irradiation or cyclophosphamide, which reduce suppressor T cell effects, administered to several strains of mice prior to primary immunization result in substantial and selective enhancement of IgE antibody production (Chiorazzi et al., 1977). These manipulations can reconstitute the IgE response in genetically-determined low responder mice. In turn, a decrease in amounts of IgE produced can be accomplished by the passive transfer of T cells.

This may suggest that a low IgE responder phenotype does not reflect a genetic inability of certain strains to respond, but rather reflects their genetic capability to actively suppress IgE production. The expression of the allergic phenotype, therefore, may result from the diminished capacity of such individuals to effectively suppress IgE production. Effective immunotherapy for such individuals may be through the induction of antigen-specific suppressor cells. The selective induction of such specific suppressor cells has been accomplished using urea-denatured antigens in appropriate concentrations (Takatsu and Ishizak, 1976a and b).

References

Benacerraf, B.: Suppressor T cells and suppressor factor. Hosp. Practice 13:65, 1978.

Bianco, C., Patrick, R., and Nussenzweig, V.: A population of lymphocytes bearing a membrane receptor for antigen-antibody-complement complexes. J. Exp. Med. 132:702, 1970.

Boldt, D. H., MacDermott, R. P., and Jorolan, E. P.: Interaction of plant lectins with purified human lymphocyte populations: Binding characteristics and kinetics of proliferation. J. Immunol. 114:1532, 1975.

Chiorazzi, N., Fox, D. A., and Katz, D. H.: Hapten-specific IgE antibody responses in mice. Conversion of IgE "nonresponder" strains to IgE "responders" by elimination of suppressor T-cell activity. J. Immunol. 118:54, 1977.

Cooper, M. D., Kincade, P. W., and Lawton, A. R.: Thymus and bursal function in immunologic development: A new theoretical model of plasma cell differentiation. In Kagan, B. M., and Stiehm, E. R. (eds.): Immunologic Incompetence. Chicago, Year Book Medical Publishers, 1971, p. 81.

Cooper, M. D., and Lawton, A. R.: The development of the immune system. Sci. Am. 231:58, 1974.

Dausset, J., and Svejgaard, A. (eds.): HLA and Disease. Copenhagen, Munksgard, 1977.

David, J. R.: Mediators produced by sensitized lymphocytes. Fed. Proc. 30:1730, 1971.

Dickler, H., and Kunkel, H. C.: Interaction of aggregated gammaglobulin with B-lymphocytes. J. Exp. Med. 136:191, 1972.

Dosch, H. M., and Gelfand, E. W.: Antigen-induced regulation of the PFC response in man. In Fauci, A. S., and Ballieux, R. E. (eds.): In vitro Induction and Measurements of Antibody Synthesis in Man. New York, Academic Press, 1979, pp. 121–139.

Feldmann, M.: Cellular components of the immune system and their cooperation (T and B cells). Transplant Proc. 5:43, 1973.

Froland, S., Natvig, J. L., and Berdaz, P.: Surface bound immunoglobulin as a marker of B-lymphocytes in man. Nature 234:251, 1971.

Gelfand, E. W., Dosch, H. M., and Shore, A.: The role of the thymus and thymus microenvironment in T-cell differentiation. In Golde, D. W., Cline, M. J., Metcalf, D., and Fox, C. F. (eds.): Hematopoietic Cell Differentiation. New York, Academic Press, 1978, pp. 277–293.

Gupta, S., and Grieco, M. H.: Rosette formation with mouse erythrocytes: Probable marker for human B lymphocytes. Int. Arch. Allergy Appl. Immunol. 49:734, 1975.

International Union of Immunological Societies Report — July 1974. Identification, enumeration and isolation of B and T lymphocytes from human peripheral blood. Clin. Immunol. and Immunopath. 3:584, 1975.

Jondal, J., and Klein, G.: Surface markers on human B and T lymphocytes. II. Presence of Epstein-Barr virus receptors on B lymphocytes. J. Exp. Med. 138:1365, 1973.

Katz, D. H., and Benacerraf, B.: The regulatory influence of activated T-cells on B cell responses to antigen. Adv. Immunol., 15:1, 1972.

Katz, D. H.: Control of IgE antibody production by suppressor substances. J. Allergy Clin. Immunol. 62:44, 1978.

Kincade, P. W., and Cooper, M. D.: Development and distribution of immunoglobulin-containing cells in the chicken: An immunofluorescent analysis using purified antibodies to μ,γ and light chains. J. Immunol. 106:371, 1971.

Komuro, K., and Boyse, E. A.: Induction of T-lymphocytes from precursor cells in vitro by a product of the thymus. J. Exp. Med. 138:479, 1973.

Limatibul, S., Shore, A. H., Dosch, H-M., and Gelfand, E. W.: Theophylline modulation of E-rosette formation: An indicator of T-cell maturation. Clin. Exp. Immunol. 33:503, 1978.

Miller, J. F. A. P.: Immunological function of the thymus. Lancet 2:748, 1961.

Möller, G. (ed.): Biochemistry and biology of Ia antigens. Transplant Rev., Volume 30. Copenhagen, Munksgard, 1976.

Möller, G. (ed.): Role of macrophages in the immune response. Immunological Reviews, Volume 40, Munksgard, Copenhagen, 1978a.

Möller, G. (ed.): Ir genes and T-lymphocytes. Immunological Reviews, Volume 38, Munksgard, Copenhagen, 1978b.

Moretta, L., Ferrarini, M., Durante, M. L., and Mingari, M. C.: Expression of a receptor for IgM by human T-cells in vitro. Eur. J. Immunol. 5:565, 1975.

Moretta, L., Webb, S. R., Grossi, C. E., Lydyard, P. M., and Cooper, M. D.: Functional analysis of two human T-cell subpopulations: Help and suppression of B-cell responses by T-cells bearing receptors of IgM or IgG. J. Exp. Med. 146:184, 1977.

Osoba, D., and Miller, J. F. A. P.: Evidence for a humoral thymus factor responsible for the maturation of immunological faculty. Nature 199:653, 1963.

Pearl, E. R., Vogler, L. B., Okos, A. J., Crist, W. M., Lawton, A. R., and Cooper, M. D.: B-lymphocyte precursors in human bone marrow: An analysis of normal individuals and patients with antibody deficiency states. J. Immunol. 120:1169, 1978.

Pernis, B., Forni, L., and Amante, L.: Immunoglobulin spots on the surface of rabbit lymphocytes. J. Exp. Med. 132:1001, 1970.

Pernis, B.: Lymphocyte membrane IgD. Immunol. Rev. 37:210, 1977.

Plate, J. M. D., and McKenzie, I. F. C.: B-cell stimulation of allogeneic T-cell proliferation in mixed lymphocyte cultures. Nature 245:247, 1973.

Pyke, K. W., and Gelfand, E. W.: Morphological and functional maturation of human thymic epithelium in culture. Nature 251:421, 1974.

Ranki, A., Totterman, T. H., and Hayry, P.: Identification of resting human T & B lymphocytes by acid a-naphthyl acetate esterase staining combined with rosette formation with Staphylococcus aureus strain Cowan I. Scand. J. Immunol. 5:1129, 1976.

Scheid, M. P., Hoffmann, J. K., Komuro, K., Hammerling, U., Abbott, J., Boyse, E. A., Cohen, G. H., Hooper, J. A., Schulof, R. S., and Goldstein, A. Z.: Differentiation of T-cells induced by preparations from thymus and by non-thymic agents. The determined state of the precursor cell. J. Exp. Med. 183:1027, 1973.

Shore, A., Dosch, H-M., and Gelfand, E. W.: Expression and modulation of C3 receptors during early T-cell ontogeny. Cellular Immunology 45:157, 1979.

Shore, A., Dosch, H-M., and Gelfand, E. W.: Induction and separation of antigen-dependent T-helper and T-suppressor cells in man. Nature 274:586, 1978.

Silviera, N. P. A., Mendes, N. F., and Tolnai, M. E. A.: Tissue localization of two populations of human lymphocytes distinguished by membrane receptors. J. Immunol. 108:1456, 1972.

Stutman, O., and Good, R. A.: Thymus hormones. Contemporary Topics in Immunobiology. 2:299, 1973.

Tada, T.: Regulation of reaginic antibody formation in animals. Prog. Allergy 19:122, 1975.

Takatsu, K., and Ishizaka, K.: Reaginic antibody formation in the mouse. Depression of ongoing IgE antibody formation by suppressor T-cells. J. Immunol. 117:1211, 1976a.

Takatsu, K., and Ishizaka, K.: Reaginic antibody formation in the mouse. Induction of suppressor T-cells for IgE and IgG antibody responses. J. Immunol. 116:1257, 1976b.

Touraine, J. L., Incefy, G. S., Touraine, F., Rho, Y. M., and Good, R. A.: Differentiation of human bone marrow cells into T lymphocytes by in vitro incubation with thymic extracts. Clin. Exp. Immunol. 17:151, 1974.

Immunoglobulins*

Michel Klein, M.D.

Antibody activity is found in a system of multichain proteins, called immunoglobulins (Ig), which are synthesized specifically in response to antigenic exposure. Although antigenically and electrophoretically heterogeneous, they are found mainly in the β and γ-globulin fractions of the serum. Immunoglobulins are multifunctional: they combine with antigen through their antibody sites in a "lock and key" fashion and, through a separate distinct region of the macromolecule, mediate various effector functions such as complement activation, attachment to cells, control of catabolic rates, and transfer across specialized membranes.

Antibody activity evolved with the emergence of vertebrates, which developed a sophisticated adaptive immune system in response to antigenic challenge. The complexity of this humoral immune system increased with the appearance of the mammals, which acquired the ability to synthesize various kinds (classes) of immunoglobulins. The emergence of these new immunoglobulin isotypes corresponded to a specialization in their biologic functions, performed in combination with various types of cells involved in the immune response and with the complement system. In this context, immunoglobulins appear to act as molecular transducers, capable of transferring specific information from a polyantigenic environment to the body's defense mechanisms.

Most of the knowledge on the antigenic nature, chemical structure, and functional properties of antibody molecules comes from studies on monoclonal immunoglobulins and Bence Jones proteins, isolated from sera or urine of patients with lymphoproliferative diseases. Monoclonal proteins are produced

*Supported by the Medical Research Council of Canada (Grant MT–4259).

TABLE 1-6 PHYSICOCHEMICAL PROPERTIES OF HUMAN IMMUNOGLOBULINS

Ig	Heavy chain	S(a)	M.W.(b)	M.W. (H chain)	Number of domains (c)	CHO(d) (%)	S(e)	J(f)	Allotypic markers	Half-life (days)	Distribution (% IV(g))
IgG1	γ_1	7S	145,000	50,000	4	2–3	–	–	G1m	21	45
IgG2	γ_2	7S	145,000	50,000	4	2–3	–	–	G2m	20	45
IgG3	γ_3	7S	170,000	60,000	4	2–3	–	–	G3m	7	45
IgG4	γ_4	7S	145,000	50,000	4	2–3	–	–		21	45
IgM	μ	19S	970,000	65,000	5	12	–	+		10	80
IgA1	α_1	7S	160,000	56,000	4	7–11	–	–		6	42
IgA2	α_2	7S	160,000	52,000	4	7–11	–	–	A2m	6	42
sIgA*	α_1, α_2	11S	385,000	52–56,000	4	7–11	+	+		–	–
IgD	δ	7S	180,000	69,000	4	9–14	–	–		3	75
IgE	ϵ	8S	190,000	72,000	5	12	–	–		2	50

Notes:
(a) Sedimentation coefficient (Svedberg units)
(b) Molecular weight of the native immunoglobulin (daltons)
(c) Number of domains of the corresponding heavy chain
(d) Carbohydrate content
(e) Secretory piece
(f) J piece
(g) Intravascular distribution
* Secretory IgA

TABLE 1-7 MAJOR EFFECTOR FUNCTIONS OF HUMAN IMMUNOGLOBULINS*

Biologic Property	IgG1	IgG2	IgG3	IgG4	IgM	IgA1	IgA2	IgD	IgE
Mean serum concentration (mg/ml)	9	3	1	0.5	1.5	3.0	0.5	0.03	0.00005
Complement activation									
Classic pathway	++	+	++	–	++++	–	–	–	–
Alternative pathway	(+)	(+)	(+)	(+)	–	(+)	(+)	–	(+)
Binding to macrophages	++	±	++	+	(+)	–	–	–	(+)
Binding to B lymphocytes	++	–	++	–	(+)	+	?	–	+
Binding to T lymphocytes (T-subsets)	+	ND	ND	ND	++	+	?	–	–
Binding to neutrophils	+	–	++	(-)	–	+	+	–	–
Binding to mast cells	–	–	–	+	–	–	–	–	++++
Placental transfer	++	±	++	+	–	–	–	–	+
Selective appearance at mucosal surfaces	–	–	–	–	+	+++	+++	ND	+

*Results indicated in parentheses need to be confirmed.

by a single clone of malignant plasmacytes and are synthesized and secreted in large quantities. They are structurally homogeneous and are chemically and functionally identical to their normal counterparts.

CLASSES OF IMMUNOGLOBULINS

Normal "polyclonal" immunoglobulins are antigenically heterogeneous. By raising heterologous monospecific antisera against various monoclonal human immunoglobulins, it has been possible to identify five distinct classes by simple precipitin reactions in agar. These classes are characterized by their unique antigenic specificity (isotype) and are designated: IgG, IgA, IgM, IgD, and IgE. Each of these five classes is found normally in different concentrations and distribution in body tissues. Each has distinct physicochemical features and has evolved to play specific biologic roles. Some of these properties are listed in Tables 1–6 and 1–7.

IgG is the major class of immunoglobulin in normal serum. Antibody of this class is the predominant type produced in response to a secondary antigenic challenge, although it is produced on primary challenge as well. It is present in significant concentrations in both the vascular and extravascular spaces. IgG has a molecular weight of 150,000, corresponding to a sedimentation coefficient of 7S. IgG antibodies are extremely heterogeneous in charge and have electrophoretic mobilities ranging from the α_2 to the slow γ regions.

Although IgA is the second most abundant immunoglobulin in serum, it is the main antibody of the external secretory system. It is present selectively at mucosal surfaces and is found in significant amounts in saliva, tears, and colostrum, as well as in tracheobronchial, gastrointestinal, and genitourinary secretions.

IgM is a 19S macromolecule with a molecular weight of 900,000; it is a euglobulin with β electrophoretic mobility. Because of its large size, its distribution is virtually restricted to the intravascular space. IgM antibodies are synthesized largely during a primary immune response, and antibodies of this class generally are the first detectable in a primary response.

IgD exists in serum in low concentration. Its physiologic role is unclear. A major role of the molecule may be to act as a B cell antigen receptor that modulates the humoral response.

IgE is present in trace amounts in normal serum and can be detected only by radioimmunoassay. It is part of an extraordinary biologic amplification system. Through its propensity to induce mediator activation and release, and despite its low serum concentration, this antibody (also referred to as reaginic or skin-sensitizing antibody) is responsible for severe allergic reactions (see Chapter 9).

Subclasses of Immunoglobulins. By antigenic analysis, minor isotypic differences have been detected within a given class of immunoglobulin. These antigenic differences define subclasses within immunoglobulin classes. Thus, four IgG subclasses (IgG1, IgG2, IgG3, and IgG4) have been characterized, and two IgA subclasses (IgA1 and IgA2) have been identified. To date, only one isotype each has been described for IgM, IgD, and IgE immunoglobulins. The existence of additional isotypes in these last categories has been suggested but not established.

As will be discussed below, the subclass antigenic specificity reflects subtle differences in the heavy chain primary structure and correlates with the functional specialization of the molecule. For example, IgG4 molecules do not fix the first component of complement, whereas the other three IgG subclasses do; the half-life of IgG3 is significantly shorter than that of the other three subclasses; the concentration of IgA2 is selectively increased in external secretions (see Tables 1–6 and 1–7).

MOLECULAR STRUCTURE OF IMMUNOGLOBULINS

Chain Structure of Monomeric Immunoglobulins

The basic structure of monomeric immunoglobulins is a four-chain unit, consisting of two identical heavy (H) chains and two identical light (L) chains. These polypeptide chains are held together by noncovalent forces and covalent disulfide bridges. A schematic diagram of a fully assembled immunoglobulin, corresponding to the structural formula $(HL)_2$, is shown in Figure 1–10. All L chains have the same molecular weight (22,500), whereas the molecular weight of H chains varies from 53,000 to 70,000, depending on the isotype.

As previously mentioned, H chain isotypic determinants define both the class and the

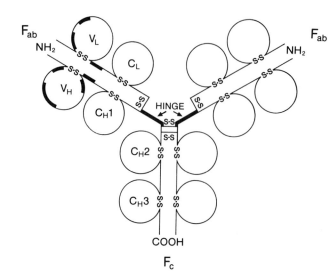

FIGURE 1–10. Multichain structure of human IgG, showing both inter- and intra-chains disulfide bridges, homology regions, and complementarity-determining (antigen-binding) regions, located on the variable portions of the H (V_H) and the L (V_l) chains (thick lines). The hinge region is denoted by the heavy solid bars.

subclass of the parent molecule. The H chain of each class is designated by a small Greek letter corresponding to the Roman letter. Thus, IgG molecules have two γ chains; IgA — two α chains; IgM — ten μ chains; IgD — two δ chains; and, IgE — two ϵ chains. H chains belonging to the same class are more than 90 percent homologous in amino acid sequence, whereas the degree of sequence homology between H chains of different classes is less than 50 percent. Antigenic differences between H chains of different subclasses reflects the existence of a limited number of amino acid substitutions and variations in the position and the number of interchain disulfide bridges. For example, IgG1 and IgG4 heavy chains are linked by two disulfide bonds, whereas IgG2 and IgG3 have four and eleven inter-heavy chain disulfide bridges, respectively. One allotypic form of the IgA2 subclass A2m(1) has an unusual structural feature: it lacks disulfide bridges between the H and L chains, whereas the antithetical allotype IgA2 subclass A2m(2) resembles IgA1 molecules.

Antigenic analyses of L chains isolated from monoclonal immunoglobulins and of Bence Jones proteins (which are free immunoglobulin L chains found in the urine of patients with myeloma) led to the characterization of two L chain isotypes; kappa (κ) and lambda (λ). While only one kappa isotype has been described to date, five lambda chain isotypes have been identified. Each of the major λ isotypic determinants, "Oz" and "Kern," arises from a single amino acid interchange in the constant region of lambda chains.

Each heavy chain isotype is capable of combining with each light chain isotype to form a fully assembled monomer of immunoglobulin of a given class. Hybrid molecules with one κ and one λ chain are never found.

Polymeric Immunoglobulins

Certain classes of immunoglobulins exist primarily as oligomers of the basic monomeric subunit $(HL)_2$. IgM is a pentamer $(H_2L_2)_5$, formed by covalent association of five subunits of 180,000 molecular weight each (Fig. 1–11). A small percentage of serum IgA exists in the form of dimers and trimers, whereas the majority of secretory

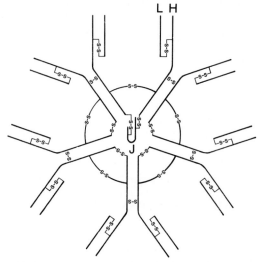

FIGURE 1–11. Schematic diagram of human IgM pentamer, showing inter-subunits, disulfide bridges, and the possible location of the J-piece.

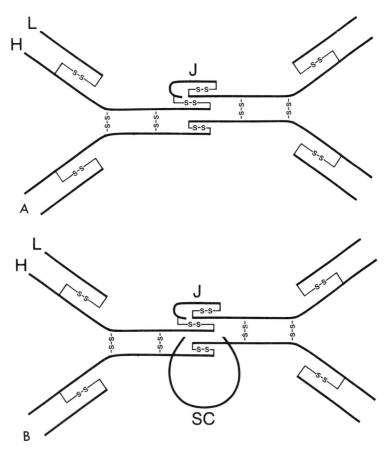

FIGURE 1–12. *A,* Schematic diagram of human serum IgA dimer. The model utilizes the clasp configuration proposed by Koshland (1975, Advan. Immunol. 22:232). *B,* Secretory IgA dimer. The location of the secretory component (SC) is hypothetical.

IgA molecules are dimeric (Fig. 1–12*A* and *B*). Polymerization of monomeric IgM and IgA subunits occurs through the formation of inter-subunit disulfide bridges between their penultimate half-cystines. In addition, all these oligomeric molecules possess an extra polypeptide chain of 15,000 daltons, called joining or J-chain. There is one mole of J per mole of oligomer. Although the mode of linkage of the J-chain to an oligomeric protein is not clear, it seems that one molecule of J-chain binds two monomers in a given oligomer. As a result of their polyvalency, oligomeric immunoglobulins have a greater avidity (affinity) than do monomeric immunoglobulins for antigens with repetitive determinants. This is a major reason why IgM antibodies agglutinate red cells and bacteria more efficiently than do IgG antibodies.

Proteolytic Cleavage of Immunoglobulins

By treating rabbit 7S antibody molecules with purified papain, R. R. Porter obtained three fragments of similar size (50,000 daltons each). Two of them were shown to be antigenically and structurally identical, and consisted of an intact light chain and the N-terminal half of the H chain (Fd fragment). Since these fragments were capable of combining specifically with one molecule of the immunizing antigen, they were called Fab fragments (fragment antigen binding). Fab fragments are monovalent antibody fragments that do not precipitate the corresponding antigen. In contrast, the third fragment was shown to be a covalent dimer of the two C-terminal halves of the heavy chains and had no antigen binding activity. Since this fragment was able to crystallize, it was called Fc (crystallizable fragment). Similar fragments have been obtained with human IgG molecules (see Fig. 1–10).

Another proteolytic enzyme, pepsin, gives different cleavage products; the major 5S fragment, which has two combining sites and consists of two Fab-like fragments linked by the interheavy chain disulfide bridges, is called $F(ab')_2$. This divalent fragment can still precipitate the antigen.

The stretch of amino acids joining the Fab arm to the Fc region contains the cysteinyl residues involved in the covalent linkage of the two heavy chains. This region, which is rich in proline, is referred to as the hinge

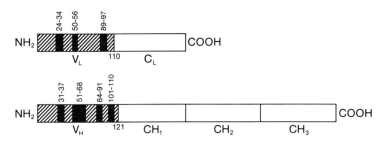

FIGURE 1–13. Schematic representation of hypervariable regions (solid area), framework regions (hatched area), and constant regions (white area) of light (above) and heavy (below) polypeptide chains. Approximate residue positions corresponding to the three complementarity-determining regions of the light chain and the four hypervariable regions of the heavy chain are numbered from the N-terminus.

region. The hinge region allows a certain degree of flexibility of the two Fab arms relative to the Fc portion, so that the overall shape of the molecule can vary from a T-shaped to a Y-shaped configuration (see Fig. 1–10).

Primary Sequence: Constant, Variable, and Hypervariable Regions

Comparison of amino-acid sequences available for human H and L chains has revealed that each type of chain can be divided into two regions; one constant (or C) region and one variable (or V) region, as illustrated in Figure 1–13.

The C-region sequence of a given isotype determines its antigenic specificity (class and subclass). Thus, all γ_1 chain constant regions or similarly all κ light chain constant regions are identical, except for minor allotypic variations that will be discussed later.

In contrast the N-terminal sequence has been found to vary from one chain to another when several chains are compared. Each chain, belonging to a given isotype, therefore, has a unique variable region. There are three sets of variable regions, designated V_H, V_κ, and V_λ, which are associated with H chains, kappa chains, and lambda chains, respectively. Further analysis of the primary structure of each family of V regions showed that these variable regions contain stretches of sequence exhibiting a high degree of variability within a much less variable framework. As indicated in Figure 1–13, L chain V regions (V_L) have three hypervariable regions, while V_H regions possess four hypervariable regions. The characterization of relatively constant framework regions within V_H and V_L regions led to the definition of V-region subgroups. V regions belonging to the same subgroup are 70 to 90 percent homologous in amino-acid sequence, whereas homology between different subgroups is only between 50 and 70 percent. Four V_H subgroups (V_{HI}, V_{HII}, V_{HIII} and V_{HIV}) have been identified.

The last is exclusively associated with μ heavy chains. Four V_κ and five V_λ subgroups have been described.

As a result of intracellular assembly of H and L chains, V_H and V_L regions are brought together to form a cavity which constitutes the antigen binding site. Random association of large number of H and L chains with different V regions therefore is an important factor in the generation of antibody diversity. The normal population of immunoglobulins consists of a wide variety of antibody molecules that share the same pool of constant regions but are unique within their antigen binding sites. In contrast, immunoglobulins belonging to different classes may carry an identical combining site, for instance, IgM and IgG molecules produced by plasma cells originating from the same clone.

Polypeptide Domains and the Tertiary Structure of Immunoglobulins

Each immunoglobulin polypeptide chain can be divided into two (L chain) or four (H chain) more or less equivalent areas containing approximately 110 amino acid residues each. Each of these areas or "domains" has a great deal of similarity (homology) in amino acid sequence with each other, and appears to have originated from a common ancestral polypeptide. The homology in primary structure has implications with regard to the structural conformation of the polypeptide. In particular, there is an invariable periodicity of cysteine residues involved in the formation of an intrachain disulfide bridge which causes a loop in each homology region (see Figure 1–10), and in so doing preserves the tertiary (globular) structure of the various domains. Thus, each immunoglobulin appears to be formed as a linear series of compact domains, folded in a characteristic manner, and linked by loose stretches of amino acids. The characteristic folding of these domains into similar compact globules appears to be of great importance both structurally and functionally, for it has been shown to be highly preserved throughout evolution.

GENETIC MARKERS: ALLOTYPES

Allotypes are genetically-controlled antigenic markers on immunoglobulin polypeptide chains. Each allotype represents a set of allelic antigens encoded in one genetic locus and inherited as dominant autosomal characters in a Mendelian fashion. All allotypic markers in man are located in the constant regions of the molecule. They are found on κ chains and on γ and α heavy chains and are designated Km, Gm, and Am, respectively. In contrast, allotypic specificities have been found associated with the V regions of all classes of immunoglobulins in the rabbit. Although in most instances allotypic markers are still defined serologically, in some cases the allotypic expression correlates with particular amino acid substitutions in the primary sequence of the polypeptide chain. For example, the Km (I) specificity is characterized by a valine at position I53 and a leucine at position I9I, whereas the expression of Km (3) allotype requires an alanine and a valine at these two positions, respectively. Allotypes have been found to be restricted to a certain H chain subclass and therefore the addition of the subclass number to the notation has been recommended. To date, four groups of heavy chain associated allotypes (G1m, G2m, G3m, and A2m) have been described and correspond to antigenic markers located on $\gamma_1, \gamma_2, \gamma_3$, and α_2 heavy chain constant regions, respectively. Certain allotypes can be localized precisely within one domain of the heavy chain. For instance, G1m(a+) and G1m(a−) are allotypic markers on the CH_3 domain of γ_1 chains, whereas G1m (z) and G1m (f) are located on the CH_1 domain of the same chain.

A diploid cell has two genes at one locus. In an individual homozygous for one allotypic locus, all immunoglobulins which belong to the subclass expressing the allotype will share the same allogypic specificity. On the other hand, if an individual is heterozygous for antithetical (i.e., mutually exclusive) allotypes, such as G1m (z) and G1m (f), for example, both markers will be expressed, but on two different populations of IgG1 molecules.

Structural genes for κ, λ, and H chains are distributed in three unlinked gene clusters, called translocons. Within each cluster, V and C structural genes exist at separate loci. Each immunocompetent cell produces only one allotype, but not both, in a heterozygous individual. This phenomenon is called allelic exclusion. The mechanism by which one of the two alleles is inactivated is not understood.

FUNCTIONAL DIFFERENTIATION OF IMMUNOGLOBULINS

The C regions of H chains of human immunoglobulin classes and subclasses differ in number of domains, structure of the hinge region, carbohydrate content, and ability to form polymers. The structural evolution of human H chain isotypes has resulted in a corresponding functional differentiation. Nevertheless, the preservation of common functions among different classes of immunoglobulins probably implies the conservation of common structures. It has been hypothesized that each domain originated by duplication of a primordial gene and evolved independently in order to perform discrete biologic functions. Table 1–8 summarizes the relationships between IgG domain structure and their respective functions. As previously discussed, the antigen binding site results from the pairing of V_H and V_L domains, whereas the effector functions of the molecule are mediated by sites in the Fc region.

Nature of the Antigen Binding Site

The antibody combining site results from the noncovalent assembly of H and L chain variable regions. An Fv fragment, consisting of the two paired V regions, has been shown to have the same binding affinity as the combining site in the parent protein. Also, it has been demonstrated that amino acids involved in the formation of the antigen binding site are present in the hypervariable regions of both chains of the antibody molecule. The complementarity-determining regions (or hypervariable regions) of the molecule are brought together upon folding to form a cleft, which constitutes the combining site. Antigen binding involves various different hypervariable regions, located both on the H chain and on the L chain of the antibody molecule. The number of residues and hypervariable regions contributing to the

TABLE 1–8 STRUCTURE–FUNCTION RELATIONSHIPS IN IgG DOMAINS

Domain	Function
$V_H + V_L$	Antigen binding site Noncovalent stabilization of H-L interaction
$CH_1 + C_L$	Covalent H-L assembly Noncovalent stabilization of H-L interaction
Hinge Region	Covalent H-H assembly Flexibility of the Ig molecule
CH_2	Interaction with Clq Control of catabolic rate
CH_3	Noncovalent H-H assembly Cytophilic site for monocytes and macrophages (phagocytosis)
$CH_2 + CH_3$	Cooperative binding site for: Neutrophils (phagocytosis) Placental syncytiotrophoblasts (passive transfer) K cells (ADCC) Staphylococcal Protein A*

*The property of certain IgG subclasses (IgG_1, IgG_2, IgG_4) to bind Protein A from *Staphylococcus aureus* has been used to purify IgG_3 subclass proteins or to remove residual IgG from $F(ab')_2$ preparations.

binding site varies from one immunoglobulin to another.

The specificity of binding of an antigen results from a close interaction between the antigenic determinant and the complementary amino-acid side chains which form the antibody active site. This stereochemical interaction involves noncovalent forces such as hydrophobic bonds, electrostatic interactions, hydrogen bonding, and van der Waals forces. The binding affinity of the antibody molecule for its antigen will depend on the nature and the number of these noncovalent interactions. High affinities will correspond to a marked decrease in the overall free energy of the antigen-antibody system. Studies with monoclonal antibodies have shown that a combining site with a known specificity could also recognize structurally-related antigens, although with a lower affinity. As listed in Table 1–9, antibodies raised against 2,4-dinitrophenyl-L-lysine can discriminate between the two optical isomers of the hapten and bind cross-reacting DNP analogs, but with 10 to 100 times less affinity than the homologous ligand. Cross-reactivity also has

been observed between unrelated antigenic determinants. A limited number of homogeneous antibodies can bind DNP and menadione, both with a significant affinity. This observation suggests that two different subsites may exist in the antibody active site. Nevertheless, the degree of multispecificity of an antigen binding site is still uncertain, and more work is needed to assess its physiologic significance.

Each antibody molecule has a unique combining site formed by the folding of the complementarity-determining regions that are exposed at the surface of the Fab fragment. Therefore, each combining site has an individual antigenic specificity, called the *idiotype*. Idiotypes must be clearly distinguished from allotypes — which are genetic markers common to many immunoglobulins with different combining activities. Antibod-

TABLE 1–9 SPECIFICITY OF THE ANTIGEN BINDING SITE

Ligand	Relative Affinity
2,4-dinitrophenyl-L-lysine O_2N—〈benzene, NO_2〉—NH—$(CH_2)_4$—C〈COO^-, NH_3^+〉	1.0
2,4-dinitrophenyl-D-lysine O_2N—〈benzene, NO_2〉—NH—$(CH_2)_4$—C〈COO^-, NH_3^+〉	0.5
2,4-dinitrophenol O_2N—〈benzene, NO_2〉—OH	0.01
2,4-dinitroaniline O_2N—〈benzene, NO_2〉—NH_2	0.1
p-mononitroaniline O_2N—〈benzene〉—NH_2	0.0003

Note: Antibodies were raised against 2,4-dinitrophenyl-L-lysine. As judged by their relative affinities, they can discriminate between optical isomers of DNP-lysine. Note the contribution of lysine groups and of nitro and amino groups.

ies can be raised against idiotypic determinants and these antibodies have been used to demonstrate that idiotypes correlate with the antibody specificity of the combining site. Thus anti-idiotypic antisera raised against a monoclonal antibody with a known specificity (e.g., anti-phosphorylcholine) would not react with normal immunoglobulins, but would cross-react with homogeneous antibodies exhibiting the same antibody specificity.

Anti-idiotypes also have proven useful in elucidating the nature of the T cell antigen receptor, which bears V_H determinants, and to establish the monoclonality of human lymphoproliferative disorders by demonstrating that surface Ig on all malignant lymphocytes in a given patient express the same idiotype.

The L chain dimer of the Bence Jones protein is similar in structure to a Fab fragment. Certain Bence Jones L chain dimers have been shown to bind hapten-like molecules with a weak affinity. It has been speculated, therefore, that L chain dimers may carry a primitive antigen binding site.

Light chains can be cleaved into their V and C regions by limited proteolysis. Using this approach, it has been possible to demonstrate that the sensitivity of Bence Jones proteins to heat denaturation is a property of their V region. Similarly, it has been shown that the V region also is responsible for the cryoprecipitation of certain Bence Jones proteins at low temperature and for the formation of amyloid fibrils in primary amyloidosis.

Effector Functions of Immunoglobulins

Biologic functions of immunoglobulins, such as complement activation, transport across specialized membranes, interaction with cell-surface receptors, and a protecting role at the mucosal surface, are associated with specific sites on the Fc portion of immunoglobulins.

Complement Fixation and Activation. Activation of complement by IgG or IgM antibodies in antigen-antibody complexes begins with binding of C1q (see Chapter 5). Monomeric IgG1 and IgG3 bind C1q with a low affinity, whereas IgG2 is less active and IgG4 does not interact at all with this first component of complement. The inability of IgG4 to fix C1q probably is due to an interaction of the Fab arm hindering the ac-

cessibility to the C1q binding site (which actually is present on a nearby area on the Fc portion of the molecule). A minimum of two IgG antibody molecules is necessary to activate the C1 macromolecular complex. Because of its polyvalency, pentameric IgM binds C1q with a greater intrinsic affinity than does IgG. The affinity for C1 is increased markedly when IgG or IgM antibodies are complexed to an antigen or are nonspecifically aggregated. C1q binding has been shown to be an exclusive property of the $C\gamma2$ domain of IgG1 H chains, whereas the C1q binding site on IgM molecules has been located on the $C\mu4$ domain.

Although it is accepted that IgA antibodies do not activate complement by the classic pathway (see Chapter 5), aggregated monoclonal IgA in large concentration and their Fc fragments in fact may be capable of interacting with C1q. IgD and IgE myeloma, however, does not appear to activate the classic complement pathway.

The activation of the alternative complement pathway (Chapter 5) by antigen-antibody complexes is controversial: data supporting an activation by aggregated human IgG, IgA, and IgE are contradictory. Nevertheless, deposition of IgA, C3, and properdin in tissue of patients with anaphylactoid purpura, IgA nephropathy, and bullous pemphigoid suggest a possible activation of the alternative pathway by specific IgA antibodies.

Interaction with Cellular Receptors. A wide variety of cells can interact with the Fc portion of several classes and subclasses of human immunoglobulins through specialized Fc receptors on the cell surface.

INTERACTION WITH MONOCYTES, MACROPHAGES, AND NEUTROPHILS. Monomeric human IgG1 and IgG3 antibodies bind to monocyte and macrophage membrane receptors with a relatively high affinity through specific sites on their Fc fragments. In contrast, IgG2 and IgG4 have been reported to have much lower affinity or be devoid of binding ability. Immune complexes containing IgG antibodies have a much greater avidity for the cell surface receptor than does the noncomplexed (unaggregated) antibody. The binding of immune complexes to monocyte and macrophage Fc receptors triggers phagocytosis and therefore plays a major role in the clearance of invading antigens. Similarly, binding studies of monomeric human IgG to neutrophils showed that only IgG1 and IgG3 proteins have a significant binding affinity for neutrophil Fc receptors, whereas aggregated IgG proteins of all four subclasses, as well as antigen-antibody complexes, interact with neutrophils and thus promote phagocytosis and the release of lysozomal enzymes.

The Cγ3 domain of IgG1 possesses a primary binding site for monocytes and macrophages, whereas the integrity of the quaternary structure of the Fc region is necessary for the binding of IgG to neutrophil Fc receptors. Thus, there are differences in cellular Fc receptors among various cell types.

The binding of monomeric IgM subunits and IgE molecules to macrophages and the interaction of aggregated myeloma IgA proteins with neutrophils also have been reported. The physiologic role of these interactions is not known.

INTERACTION WITH B AND T LYMPHOCYTES. B lymphocytes bear an Fc receptor capable of recognizing monomeric IgG1 and IgG3 with a weak affinity but have little or no affinity for IgG2 and IgG4. When complexed with antigen, the avidity of IgG for B cells is markedly increased. Because of this, human red cells sensitized with anti-Rh antibodies or aggregated IgG have been used extensively as B cell surface markers. Certain malignant clones of B cells also possess an Fc receptor for IgM molecules, and a lymphoblastoid cell line has been shown to bear IgE-Fc-receptors. Although a role in feedback regulation has been proposed for the IgG-Fc-receptor interaction at the B cell level, the physiologic function of the various B lymphocyte immunoglobulin receptors remains unclear.

The majority of normal peripheral T cells (80 percent) express a surface receptor for a site on the Fc fragment of IgM. These Fc μ(+) T cells have been shown to be helper T cells. (The affinity of this receptor towards the Fc (5μ) fragment is high [$K_A \simeq 10^9$ M^{-1}].) A different and much smaller subset of T suppressor lymphocytes (6 to 10 percent) bears a receptor specific for the Fc portion of IgG molecules.

IgA receptors have been described on both B and T lymphocytes; but the biologic significance of the presence of these receptors on lymphocytes has not been determined.

INTERACTION WITH K CELLS. A subpopulation of non–B non–T mononuclear cells (K cells) is responsible for antibody-dependent cell-mediated cytolysis (ADCC). K cells have been shown to kill target cells coated with human IgG1, IgG3, and possibly IgG2 antibodies.

INTERACTION WITH MAST CELLS AND BASOPHILS. IgE molecules bind with high affinity to mast cell and basophil Fc receptors ($K_A \simeq 10^9$ M^{-1}). One consequence of this high-affinity interaction is that IgE antibodies are quasi-irreversibly attached to the cell membrane. Antigen (allergen)-bridging of two membrane-bound molecules of IgE antibodies results in the release of vasoactive amines, in particular histamine, which are responsible for the clinical manifestations of immediate-type allergic reactions (see Chapters 9 and 11). Homocytotropic IgG also can interact with IgE receptors, although with a much lower affinity.

INTERACTION WITH PLACENTAL SYNCITIOTROPHOBLASTS. Humoral protection of the newborn against infections during the first month of life is provided by maternal IgG antibodies transferred to the fetus *in utero*. The transmission of IgG across the placental barrier requires as an initial step the binding of immunoglobulins to the syncitiotrophoblast membrane through receptors for specific sites on the Fc fragment of the immunoglobulin molecule. The relative affinity of membrane receptors for IgG subclasses has been found to be: IgG1 = IgG3 > IgG4 >> IgG2. Thus, little maternal IgG2 antibody reaches the newborn. The binding site on the Fc portion of the IgG molecules is a cooperative site apparently formed jointly by the Cγ_2 and the Cγ_3 regions. Other classes of immunoglobulins do not interact with syncitiotrophoblasts and are not transported across the placental barrier (see Chapter 2).

Selective Secretion at Mucosal Membranes — The Secretory Immune System. Whereas IgG is the major immunoglobulin class in the serum, IgA is the predominant antibody found in secretions. The proportion of IgA2 molecules in secretions is significantly increased (50 percent) as compared to its relative concentration in serum (20 percent of total IgA). The characteristic structural feature of secretory IgA (sIgA) is a covalent dimer (or a trimer in a much lower proportion), containing one mole of J piece and one mole of specific polypeptide chain, called secretory component (SC) (see Figure 1–12 B).

The protective role of IgA antibodies at mucosal surfaces is not fully understood. Because sIgA is a polyvalent antibody, it binds efficiently to bacteria, neutralizes viruses,

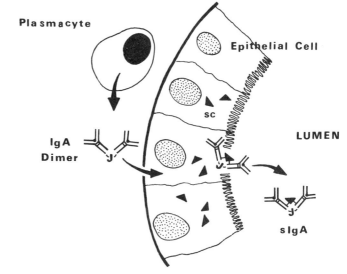

FIGURE 1–14. Schematic drawing depicting the synthesis of secretory IgA (sIgA). Dimeric IgA secreted by plasma cells passes through the epithelial cells, where it becomes associated with the secretory piece and is subsequently released in the lumen.

and thus prevents their adsorption to mucosal cellular surfaces. That specific IgA antibodies contribute to local immunity is demonstrated by such observations as the fact that immunity to cholera correlates with the titer of coproantibodies but not with serum antibody levels. The role played by secretory component is unclear. There is evidence that secretory component, which is synthetized in epithelial cells lining the mucosal surface, is involved in the vectorial transport of polymeric IgA secreted by mucosal plasmocytes, from the mucosae to the lumen (Fig. 1–14). Secretory component also may protect the sIgA molecule from proteolytic attack since sIgA is extremely resistant to enzymatic cleavages *in vitro*. In addition, recent experiments suggest that secretory component may be a surface receptor for IgA on the membrane of hepatocytes and epithelial cells.

Mucosal synthesis of IgM and IgE antibodies also occurs. Pentameric IgM antibodies raised by local immunization contain one mole of secretory component and exhibit strong antibacterial activity. IgE antibodies synthesized locally in gastrointestinal and respiratory secretions also may play a protective role at mucosal surfaces, in addition to their potential role in adverse (allergic) reactions (see Chapter 9).

BIOSYNTHESIS OF IMMUNOGLOBULINS

L chain and H chain isotypes are encoded in separate genes. Immunoglobulin domains of H and L chains are further separate portions of each gene. The genome concerned with immunoglobulin biosynthesis consists of multiple tandem sets of redundant "V" genes and tandem sets of corresponding "C" genes (one for each isotype). V-C integration occurs by an unknown mechanism; the integrated DNA then gives rise to cytoplasmic RNA which codes for an H or L polypeptide chain. Translation into polypeptide chains occurs on membrane-bound polyribosomes and is regulated by direct feedback by the intracellular immunoglobulin pool. The newly synthesized H and L chains move into the cisternae of the rough endoplasmic reticulum and are vectorially released into the cisternal space. The pathway of covalent assembly depends upon the H chain isotype.

Glycosylation of immunoglobulin H chains occurs in a sequential fashion at specific subcellular sites as the molecule is synthesized, assembled, transported through the cytoplasm, and secreted. Addition of the branch and terminal sugars (galactose, fucose, and sialic acid) seems to be required for transport and secretion of IgM molecules but is not necessary for IgG secretion. It has been suggested that IgG remains enclosed within membrane vesicles throughout its intracytoplasmic transport; these vesicles are assumed to fuse with the cytoplasmic membrane with subsequent release of immunoglobulin by reverse pinocytosis.

Polymerization of IgM and IgA 7S subunits occurs at a late stage of their intracellular transport, almost concomitantly with secretion. The J piece, which is not associated with intracellular monomers, may initiate their polymerization by a disulfide-interchange mechanism prior to secretion.

A given plasma cell synthesizes only a single type of L chain and a single type of H chain. Therefore, all antibody molecules produced within one plasmacyte are identical. Expansion of a clone of plasmacytes leads to the production of large quantities of an electrophoretically homogeneous immunoglobulin. In myelomas, this can be observed as a monoclonal spike on electrophoresis of serum.

The production of a fully-assembled IgG molecule depends on the availability of H and L chains. In normal plasmacytes, there is a slight excess of free L chains over H chains. This excess of L chains is secreted in the serum and excreted in the urine as a normal polyclonal L chain proteinuria. This unbalanced synthesis explains the massive urinary excretion of monoclonal Bence Jones proteins frequently seen in patients with myeloma.

Defective immunoglobulin biosynthesis may occur in neoplastic plasmacytes. A defect in secretion results in an intracellular accumulation of the monoclonal protein seen in nonsecreting myeloma. Some myeloma variants lose the ability to produce both H and L chains (nonproducing myeloma) or fail to synthesize H chains only ("L-chain disease"). Another group of synthetic aberrations includes the synthesis of defective H chains which cannot combine with L chains ("heavy-chain disease") or are depleted of one Fc domain, and that of isolated L chain domains (V_L or C_L).

METABOLISM OF IMMUNOGLOBULIN

The catabolic mechanisms by which immunoglobulins are removed from the circulation are poorly understood. IgG is one of the longest-lived serum proteins; its half-life is approximately 21 days, except that of the IgG3 subclass which is markedly shorter (see Table 1–6). Although IgG and IgA have similar synthetic rates, the serum concentration of IgA is four-fold lower than that of IgG because of its rapid clearance. IgM has a synthetic rate only one-fifth that of IgG and a fractional catabolic rate two-fold faster. The very low IgD level in human serum results from a slow synthesis and an extremely rapid clearance. Thus, IgD is one of the shortest-lived serum proteins.

Two general mechanisms are responsible for the clearance of immunoglobulins. The first involves filtration-reabsorption processes at the kidney level. For example, free monomeric light chains are readily filtered through the glomeruli because of their small molecular weight and are excreted in the urine. It is only when these light chains are synthesized in very large quantities or form unusual tetramers, or when a patient has a renal insufficiency, that free circulating light chains can be detected in the serum. The second includes the binding of normal Ig to Fc receptors and the uptake of chemically, enzymatically, and physically modified Ig by receptor-mediated clearance mechanisms. *In vivo* or *in vitro* modifications of Ig increase their fractional catabolic rates and are responsible for what is referred to as immunoglobulin "aging." Catabolism of Fc fragments is similar to that of the parent IgG. Control of the catabolic rate of IgG1 molecules has been shown to be a property of the CH_2 domain, which bears carbohydrate moieties. Clearance of Fab or $F(ab')_2$ fragments are 50- to 100-fold faster than that of intact IgG. Modification of the Fc portion of IgG, which enables intravenous administration for therapy, also usually results in shortening its half-life in serum (see Chapter 7).

TESTS FOR MEASUREMENT OF IMMUNOGLOBULINS

Electrophoresis. Because of the heterogeneity in electric charge of serum proteins, it is possible to separate serum into several protein components that differ in electrophoretic mobility. Most immunoglobulins migrate as gamma globulins, some as beta globulins. Paper or, more recently, other stabilizing media (such as cellulose acetate) have been used for such separation. Following migration in an electrical field, the proteins "band" in characteristic positions and can be identified and quantified following staining, using optical techniques that measure density of protein stain. Electrophoretic techniques are only grossly quantitative, allowing identification of large increases or decreases mainly in IgG, and to a lesser extent IgM and IgA. Monoclonal gammopathies (myeloma, Waldenström's macroglobulinemia) generally are detectable by this method.

Immunodiffusion. The major method of quantitation of serum immunoglobulins is through immunoprecipitation in a semisolid medium. In the most commonly used technique, specific antiserum to a given immunoglobulin (e.g., anti-IgG) is impregnated in agar gel; serum containing immunoglobulin is placed in a hole cut in the impregnated gel, and allowed to diffuse into the gel. The area or diameter of the precipitin ring (containing immunoglobulin and anti-immunoglobulin) that forms is measured, and can be related through appropriate standards to the concentration of that specific immunoglobulin in serum. This test is utilized for measurement of IgG, IgA, and IgM concentrations in serum; a modification of this test also is capable of measuring IgD, which ordinarily is present in extremely low concentration in serum. IgE is present in concentration too low to be detected by standard immunoprecipitation techniques, and is assayed instead by radioimmunoassay (described in Chapter 9). Normal serum concentrations of the major immunoglobulins are found in Chapter 2.

Immunoelectrophoresis. Separation of serum components on the basis of electric charge can be enhanced by first electrophoresing serum in an agar medium, then reacting the electrophoretically separated serum components against an antihuman serum by immunodiffusion. The result of this process is separation of serum into over two dozen distinct and identifiable protein components. The technique is only semiquantitative, and can identify the presence or absence of IgM, IgA, and IgG, as well as indicate gross increases or decreases in the concentration of these immunoglobulins. It also is useful in identifying paraproteins (e.g., monoclonal IgG, IgA, or IgM gammopathy). Accurate quantitation of immunoglobulins, however, requires immunodiffusion techniques of the type described previously.

Other Techniques. Variations in immunodiffusion and immunoelectrophoretic techniques enable determination of low concentrations of immunoglobulins in body fluids. Nephelometry, a technique of measuring turbidity or cloudiness of serum, can be used to determine immunoglobulin concentration after specific anti-immunoglobulin antiserum has been added. An advantage of this technique is its susceptibility to automation. Radioimmunoassays have been used mainly in the measurement of materials present in concentrations too low to lend them-

TABLE 1–10 SENSITIVITY OF QUANTITATIVE TESTS MEASURING ANTIBODY NITROGEN OF HIGH–AVIDITY ANTIBODY

Test	mg Ab N/ml or Test
Precipitin reactions	3–20
Immunoelectrophoresis	3–20
Double diffusion in agar gel	0.2–1.0
Complement fixation	0.01–0.1
Radial immunodiffusion	0.008–0.025
Bacterial agglutination	0.01
Hemolysis	0.001–0.03
Passive hemagglutination	0.005
Passive cutaneous anaphylaxis	0.003
Antitoxin neutralization	0.003
Antigen-combining globulin technique (Farr)	0.0001–0.001
Radioimmunoassay	0.0001–0.001
Enzyme-linked assays	0.0001–0.001
Virus neutralization	0.00001–0.0001
Bactericidal test	0.00001–0.0001

From Bellanti, J. A.: Immunology II. Philadelphia, W. B. Saunders Co., 1978, p. 214.

selves to visible precipitation (e.g., measurement of hormones and measurement of IgE). Ultracentrifugation, chromatography, and other techniques are available for characterizing and separating immunoglobulins, but are largely investigative tools.

Measurement of Specific Antibody. Identification and qualification of antibody depends, first, on the ability of antibody to combine specifically with its corresponding antigen and, second, on a method of detecting this interaction. Most tests of antibody function depend upon some observable phenomenon (e.g., precipitation) that is a consequence of antigen-antibody interaction, but does not measure the primary event (antigen-antibody binding) itself. Description of the numerous kinds of tests available for measurement of antibody function is beyond the scope of this chapter. It is important to note, however, that the kind of test useful for antibody measurement is dependent upon numerous factors, including antibody as well as antigen concentration, the physicochemical properties of the antigen, physicochemical and biologic properties of the antibodies to be assayed, and the "sensitivity" of the assay system. Table 1–10 is a partial list of tests used to measure antibody and their relative limits of sensitivity for antibody detection.

General References

Bellanti, J. A. (ed.): *Immunology II*. Philadelphia, W. B. Saunders Co., 1978.

Dorrington, K. J., and Painter, R. H.: Biological activities of the constant region of immunoglobulin G. *Progress in Immunology III*. Amsterdam, North-Holland Publishing Company. 1977, p. 298.

Immunoglobulin E. *Immunological Reviews, 41*. Copenhagen, Munksgaard, 1978.

Lamm, M. E.: Cellular aspects of Immunoglobulin A. Adv. Immunol. *22*:223, 1976.

Nisonoff, A., Hopper, J. E., and Spring, S. B. (eds.): *The Antibody Molecule*. New York, Academic Press, 1975.

Porter, R. R.: The hydrolysis of rabbit γ-globulin and antibodies with crystalline papain. Biochem. J., *73*:119, 1959.

Putnam, F. W. (ed.): *The Plasma Proteins, Structure, Function and Genetic Control*. New York, Academic Press, 1976.

Underdown, B., and Dorrington, K. J.: Immunoglobulins, structure and function. *In* Movat, M. Z. (ed.): *Inflammation, Immunity and Hypersensitivity. Cellular and Molecular Mechanisms*. New York, Harper and Row Publisher, 1979, p. 163.

Weigert, M., Gatmaitman, L., Loh, E., Schilling, J., and Hood, L.: Rearrangement of genetic information may produce immunoglobulin diversity. Nature *276*:785, 1978.

Michael E. Miller, M.D. 2

Developmental Immunity

The growing understanding in recent years of the functional status of neonatal host defense mechanisms has led to a re-thinking of previous concepts of neonatal responsiveness to foreign substances. Contrary to earlier beliefs, it is now clear that the normal neonate is not "immunologically null" but has a variety of "specific" and "nonspecific" mechanisms available for combating foreign microorganisms.

THE NEONATAL T CELL SYSTEM

Several techniques have been utilized to measure numbers of T cells present at or around the time of birth (Miller, 1979). T cells have been identified in human thymuses ranging from 11 to 26 weeks gestational age, but improved methods will be necessary in order to determine when T cells originate during fetal development. Cord blood contains a lower *percentage* of T cells than blood of older children or adults, as measured by the sheep cell roseting technique (see Chapter 1). The total *number* of T cells in cord blood generally is greater than in adult blood, however, due to the normal absolute lymphocytosis of the newborn period. Recent studies suggest that the neonate has a relatively greater level of suppressor T cell activity than that found in older children or adults. If true, this has major clinical implications. For example, immunization with pneumococcal or other recently developed vaccines may be relatively ineffective during the early

months of life. Why the newborn should have a relative excess of suppressor activity, and at what age this activity becomes normal, are yet to be understood.

The presence of normal numbers of T cells does not necessarily imply normal function. Though techniques for measuring specific T cell functions are limited, studies of neonatal T cells indicate that, in general, functional ontogeny correlates with the quantitative data, both developing early in fetal life. A summary of current data on chronology of T cell functions is provided in Table 2–1. Information about lympho-

TABLE 2–1 T CELL FUNCTIONS IN THE HUMAN FETUS

Function	Fetal Age First Reported
Antigen recognition	12 weeks
Antigen binding	10 to 30 weeks
Cell-mediated lympholysis	7 months (not studied earlier)
Antibody-dependent cyto-toxicity (may not be T cell function)	Cord blood (not studied earlier)
Graft-versus-host reactivity	13 weeks
Mitogenic stimulation	12 to 22 weeks
Antigenic stimulation	Newborns (not studied earlier)
Lymphotoxin production	Cord blood (not studied earlier)
Interferon production	Indeterminate

Modified from Miller, M. E.: *Host Defenses in the Human Neonate.* New York, Grune & Stratton, Inc., 1978.

kine production by neonatal T cells is of particular interest. Production of at least three lymphokines may be diminished in neonatal T cells — lymphotoxin, immune interferon, and macrophage inhibitory factor (MIF).

THE NEONATAL B CELL SYSTEM

Ontogeny. As with the T cell system, better methods have improved our ability to study the development of the B cell system. In the case of B cells, major advances have come through the development of highly specific antisera to individual immunoglobulin classes (Lawton et al., 1972). Since B cells express class-specific immunoglobulins upon their surfaces, individual B cell classes can be detected through the use of panels of fluorescent-labeled antisera. Two major observations have derived from such studies: *First,* in most studies, IgM-bearing B cells are the first type detected in the human fetus; detection has been as early as 9.5 to 10 weeks gestation. B cells emerge in a sequence of IgM, followed by IgG and IgA. IgD follows IgM; its relationship to the emergence of IgG and IgA B cells varies. These studies negate the hypothesis that IgD was the first immunoglobulin to appear during fetal life and that it was a necessary antecedent to the appearance of IgM. This stage of B cell development appears to be an antigen-independent process and occurs as part of normal embryogenesis. *Second,* B cell development appears to involve at least two distinct stages (Raff et al., 1976; Gathings et al., 1976). In the first stage, lymphoid cells termed "pre-B cells" contain intracellular (cytoplasmic) immunoglobulins but lack detectable surface immunoglobulins. In the second stage, mature B cells can be identified by the presence of surface immunoglobulins. Gathings and co-workers found IgM-containing pre-B cells in fetal liver cells from a 7.5-week-old human fetus, but were unable to detect surface positive immunoglobulin cells of any type. Both pre-B and mature B cells were identified in fetuses ranging from 9.5 to 12.5 weeks gestational age.

The recognition of these stages of B cell development is of more than academic interest, for it suggests that a sequence of developmental defects may result in impaired B cell function in children afflicted with hypogammaglobulinemia due to blocks at different stages of development. These may include absence of B cells, failure of B cells to express immunoglobulins, and failure of B cells to secrete immunoglobulin. (see Chapter 6). The second stage of B cell differentiation involves expansion of the now developed class-specific clones of B cells. Unlike the initial phase, this is an antigen-dependent process, thereby differing markedly from one fetus to the next according to the antigenic experience of the fetus. Similarly, the degree of general lymphoid tissue development varies significantly, depending upon the amount of antigenic stimulation occurring during fetal life and after birth. Animals raised in germ-free environments, for example, show delayed development of lymphoid organs in comparison with those raised in normal environments (Thorbecke, 1959).

Several sources may provide antigenic stimulation of the fetus. The fetus may be sensitized by *placental transfer of antigens to which the mother has been exposed.* For example, anti-salmonella antibody has been identified in 75-day-old (approximately midgestation) lamb fetuses (Sterzl and Silverstein, 1967). This antibody was high molecular weight, probably IgM and therefore of fetal origin, presumably reflecting sensitization of the fetal lamb by salmonella antigens absorbed from the maternal gut. In genetically inbred rats, Gill and co-workers (1977) studied the maternal-fetal immunologic interaction by immunizing the mothers with an aggregated synthetic polypeptide prior to mating. Some of the newborns showed an antibody response to the antigen, thereby suggesting that placental transfer had occurred. In another part of their study, lymphocyte reactivity to a panel of five antigens was studied in 48 human maternal-fetal pairs. On occasion, cord blood lymphocytes of fetal origin were found to react to antigens that, for unknown reasons, failed to elicit a response from corresponding maternal lymphocytes, suggesting that the fetal cells were sensitized by the transplacental passage of antigen. A number of investigators have elicited skin test reactions in newborns against common allergens and tuberculoprotein, presumably transferred to the fetus across the placental barrier. Such studies are extremely complex and difficult to interpret, and direct evidence of transfer of antigen from mother to fetus must, therefore, await confirmation. The implication of stimulation of the fetal lymphoid system by transplacental transfer of antigen is most important, however, since it may provide a means of manipulating the fetal immune response and, perhaps, influencing the immune response in later life.

The *amniotic fluid* constitutes a second potential source of fetal antigen exposure. In experimental studies, Richardson and Connor (1972) injected brucella antigen into the amniotic fluid of fetal lambs in late gestation. Offspring demonstrated both primary and secondary immune responses to brucella antigen. When twin fetuses in separate amniotic fluid sacs were present, only the fetus sensitized by amniotic fluid injection (and subsequent ingestion of antigen) developed antibody. Little is known of the significance of this route of antigen exposure in human fetuses.

Intrauterine infection from organisms such as rubella virus, cytomegalovirus, *Treponema pallidum* and *Toxoplasmosa gondii* also leads to increased production of IgM antibody by the fetus (Alford, 1971). In addition, an infection acquired at or shortly after birth stimulates IgM synthesis. The postnatal IgM level must be significantly greater than that expected physiologically to be considered a significant indicator of intrauterine infection, however, since IgM levels rise rapidly after birth (probably as a result of bacterial colonization of the gastrointestinal tract).

FETAL IMMUNOGLOBULIN PRODUCTION

Antibody Responses. Studies on the antibody response in fetal lambs produced a major contribution in this area (Sterzl and Silverstein, 1967). Indwelling catheters were placed in the cervical vessels of fetal lambs, thereby permitting injection of antigens into the fetal circulation and periodic withdrawal of blood samples for antibody measurements without further surgical intervention. A variety of antigens were administered, including bacteriophage ϕX 174, ferritin, egg albumin, and salmonella. These studies revealed that the fetal lamb was able to produce antibodies against most of the antigens long before birth, and that there was a stepwise maturation or "hierarchy" of antigen responsiveness. In

other words, the fetal lambs developed the ability to respond to each of the antigens at different stages of gestation. Thus, antibodies to phage appeared by day 35 to 41 of gestation, antibodies to ferritin were first observed at day 66, and antibody to egg albumin at day 125. Anti-salmonella antibody had not appeared in fetuses by term (150 days). More recent studies have demonstrated a similar stepwise maturation in the opossum and the rat.

The interpretation of this hierarchy of antigen responsiveness has major implicatons in the understanding of mechanisms of the fetal immune response. The initial explanation — that the stepwise development of antibody responses to various antigens reflected the development of separate clones of antibody-producing cells—has little evidence to support it. An alternative hypothesis for which there are supportive data relates to stepwise maturation of antigen-processing cells, such as macrophages. Various antigens, for example, may not stimulate antibody production until development of mechanisms for their degradation by macrophages and subsequent presentation to the antibody-producing B cells. Antibody responses in newborn sheep, mice, and rats are increased by the addition of adult macrophages, but not by adult lymphocytes (Blaese et al., 1970; Argyris, 1968).

Immunoglobulins. The human fetus produces little *IgG*. Serum levels remain below 100 mg/dl until approximately 17 weeks of gestation, at which time a gradual and steady increase occurs. By term, the fetal IgG level usually exceeds the maternal level by 5 to 10 percent. *IgA* has been detected in 30-week-old human fetuses. Only limited synthesis occurs, so serum levels seldom are in excess of 5 mg/dl. Little, if any, IgA is transferred across the placenta. Most newborns beyond 30 weeks of gestation have low but detectable *IgM* measurable in cord serum. Buckley and co-workers (1969) reviewed the results of seven studies of cord blood IgM levels and found that mean levels varied from 5.8 to 15.8 mg/dl; the two standard deviation limit levels varied from 1 to 10 mg/dl (lower limit) to 12.9 to 27.4 mg/dl (upper limit). In premature infants, IgM levels usually are slightly lower than in term infants, but not in a predictable fashion. The proportion of infants with no detectable cord IgM increases with decreasing gestational age. There is no known clinical significance to the absence of cord IgM. In contrast, as discussed before, an elevated cord IgM indicates intrauterine antigenic stimulation, often the result of intrauterine infection. *IgD* also does not cross the placenta and usually is not detectable in cord blood. When present, IgD levels are 5 to 30 percent of the normal adult level of 3 mg/dl. Maternal IgD levels tend to increase in pregnancy. *IgE* does not cross the placenta (Bazaral et al., 1971). The development and clinical significance of the IgE system is discussed in Chapter 9.

THE ANTIBODY RESPONSE OF THE NEONATE

A number of circulating factors may inhibit or suppress the neonatal antibody response. Transplacentally acquired maternal antibody inhibits active antibody formation in the newborn period. For example, infants with passively acquired diphtheria antitoxin or poliomyelitis antibodies have decidedly diminished responses when given diphtheria toxoid or inactivated poliomyelitis vaccine. Inhibition can be overcome for certain potent antigens at least (e.g., tetanus) by employing larger antigen doses, more frequent immunizations, or by using adjuvants. Other humoral factors may exert an immunosuppressive effect upon neonatal antibody production. Bilirubin, for instance, can suppress antibody responses to pertussis, diphtheria, tetanus, and *E. coli* until 1 year of age (Nejedla, 1970).

The studies by Smith and Eitzman (1964) of antibody responses to *Salmonella* flagellar (H) antigens and somatic (O) antigens illustrate the antibody response of the human newborn. Passively acquired maternal antibody influenced immune responsiveness: only those children without detectable maternal antibody or with titers (less than 1:20) exhibited antibody responses. Most premature and term neonates with passively acquired *Salmonella* agglutinins were able to produce antibodies to flagellar (H) antigens when immunized with *Salmonella* vaccine, but older infants (greater than 13 days) were more responsive than newborn infants. The response was not related to maturity, since over half of the prematures (less than 2500 gm birth weight) produced flagellar agglutinins in titers of at least 1:10 by day 7 following immunization, and more than 80 percent had responded by day 14. In many instances, the titers of flagellar agglutinins were comparable to those found in adults. Dancis and coworkers (1953), utilizing diphtheria toxoid, found that a small proportion of full-term and premature neonates immunized with toxoid during the first week of life developed diphtheria antitoxin within one month. All premature infants responded when immunized with diphtheria toxoid at their estimated birth dates. The antigenic stimulus supplied by the bacterial flora acquired at birth seems to play a major role in the development of the antibody response.

Smith and Eitzman (1964) also found premature or full-term neonates rarely developed agglutinins to the somatic O antigen, in contrast to H agglutinins, whereas immunized older children and adults developed O agglutinins by day 14. The capacity to produce agglutinins to O antigens developed between 3 to 9 months of age. Even though the assay technique used in measuring O agglutinins is less sensitive than that used for measuring H agglutinins, it is evident that a significant difference exists in the ability of neonates to respond to those two antigens. Whether immunologic or nonimmunologic (processing) maturational factors are responsible for the different reactions to these antigens is not clear, however.

The antibody response to H antigen also followed a sequential development similar to that seen in the adult. The first antibody activity to appear in the neonates was found in the macroglobulin fraction, probably IgM, followed by the appearance of activity in the IgG fraction. Although the heterogeneity of response was similar to that seen in the adult, the newborns differed in the timing of the appearance of activity in the IgG fraction. IgM was present exclusively in the neonates for prolonged periods, up to 20 to 30 days following immunization, whereas adults showed IgG-antibody activity at 5 to 15 days. The prolonged transition from IgM to IgG antibody in neonates has been found to last until 1 to 6 months of age.

PASSIVE IMMUNITY IN THE NEWBORN

The fetus receives IgG antibodies passively via the placenta, and the breast-fed infant in addition receives secretory antibodies (which are not absorbed) via the oral route. Passively acquired maternal IgG antibodies confer the neonate with protection against certain disorders such as measles, rubella, meningococcal infections, streptococcal disease, and *H. influenzae* infection; some protection against certain other infections (such as vaccinia, varicella, pertussis, tetanus, diphtheria) also may result. However, since protective IgG antibodies to these agents do not persist in high titer, only recently infected or immunized mothers provide such protection to their infants. Certain maternal antibodies to antigens of gram-negative organisms such as *E. coli* and salmonellae reside chiefly within the IgM class and do not cross the placenta; consequently, the infant does not receive all of the mother's antibodies to these organisms. Gitlin and co-workers (1973) postulated that this deficiency of IgM may be responsible, at least in part, for the unusual susceptibility of newborns to infection with gram-negative organisms. However, IgG antibodies to somatic antigens of gram-negative organisms do cross the placenta and can provide protection for most infants.

It should be recognized that *lack* of placental transfer of certain maternal IgM antibodies is advantageous to the neonate. For example, the presence of maternal IgM isoagglutinins (natural anti-A and anti-B) in the infant would result in ABO hemolytic disease in every ABO incompatible maternal-newborn pair.

Role of Human Milk in Host Defense

Human milk has long been postulated to play an important role in the enhancement of neonatal host defenses. In 1621, in his "Anatomy of Melancholy," Burton observed, "From a child's nativity, the first ill accident that can likely befall him in this kind, is a bad nurse. . . ." In 1908, Leiner, in describing 43 infants with diffuse seborrheic dermatitis, diarrhea, recurrent infection, and failure to thrive, noted that 41 of the infants were breast fed. He found that clinical improvement resulted upon changing the afflicted infant to bottle feeding or, occasionally, to a wet nurse. Leiner postulated that the milk of the natural mother contained some toxic substance(s) resulting in the clinical abnormalities. Although current findings suggest a different explanation (Miller and Nilsson, 1970; Nilsson, Miller, and Wyman, 1974), the concept is deeply rooted that human milk may have beneficial and, under certain circumstances, adverse consequences to neonatal host defense.

Breast-fed infants have fewer infections of the gastrointestinal tract than infants fed a variety of artificial formulas. Winberg and Wessner (1971) also observed an increased incidence of septicemia in infants whose intake of breast milk decreased before the symptomatic period, suggesting that septicemia was not simply the result of poor suckling by the children. While breast feeding may protect the infant, the mechanisms by which protection occurs have not been characterized.

Antibodies. Although passage of intact milk antibodies through the entire gastrointestinal tract has been demonstrated occasionally, the role of breast milk antibodies in neonatal host defense is not clear. Breast-fed infants appear more resistant than bottle-fed infants to infection with attenuated poliomyelitis virus during the first 10 days of life; nevertheless, antibody responses following polio immunization are equivalent in breast-fed and bottle-fed infants. Classes and levels of antibodies against specific organisms differ in serum and breast milk. The colostral antibody system acts as an active component of the immune system, and appears to be part of a unique gut-breast immune system with important functions separate from the circulating immune system.

Other Non-cellular Factors in Breast Milk. The intestinal environment of breast-fed infants inhibits the proliferation of enteropathogenic bacteria and favors the emergence of bifidobacteria. Breast-fed infants tend to produce large amounts of acetic and lactic acid in their guts, which results in relatively low stool pH levels. This may, in turn, inhibit the growth of *Shigella* organisms and *E. coli* (Miller, 1979b). Various other proteins present in human milk such as lactoferrin, lysozyme, and an antistaphylococcal substance may aid in the response of breast-fed infants to infection.

Cellular Components of Milk. Viable cells present in colostrum and milk may be important in protecting the infant. Human milk contains an average of 1 to 2 $\times$ 10^6 leukocytes per ml of exosecretion, of which approximately 85 percent are monocytes or

TABLE 2-2 LEVELS OF IMMUNOGLOBULINS IN SERA OF NORMAL SUBJECTS, BY AGE

Age	IgG		IgM		IgA		Total Immune Globulin	
	mg/dl	Percent of Adult Level	mg/dl	Percent of Adult Level	mg/dl	Percent of Adult Level	mg/dl	Percent of Adult Level
Newborn	1031 ± 200*	89 ± 17	11 ± 5	11 ± 5	2 ± 3	1 ± 2	1044 ± 201	67 ± 13
1 to 3 mo	430 ± 119	37 ± 10	30 ± 11	30 ± 11	21 ± 13	11 ± 7	481 ± 127	31 ± 9
4 to 6 mo	427 ± 186	37 ± 16	43 ± 17	43 ± 17	28 ± 18	14 ± 9	498 ± 204	32 ± 13
7 to 12 mo	661 ± 219	58 ± 19	54 ± 23	55 ± 23	37 ± 18	19 ± 9	752 ± 242	48 ± 15
13 to 24 mo	762 ± 209	66 ± 18	58 ± 23	59 ± 23	50 ± 24	25 ± 12	870 ± 258	56 ± 16
25 to 36 mo	892 ± 183	77 ± 16	61 ± 19	62 ± 19	71 ± 37	36 ± 19	1024 ± 205	65 ± 14
3 to 5 yr	929 ± 228	80 ± 20	56 ± 18	57 ± 18	93 ± 27	47 ± 14	1078 ± 245	69 ± 17
6 to 8 yr	923 ± 256	80 ± 22	65 ± 25	66 ± 25	124 ± 45	62 ± 23	1112 ± 293	71 ± 20
9 to 11 yr	1124 ± 235	97 ± 20	79 ± 33	80 ± 33	131 ± 60	66 ± 30	1134 ± 254	85 ± 17
12 to 16 yr	946 ± 124	82 ± 11	59 ± 20	60 ± 20	148 ± 63	74 ± 32	1153 ± 169	74 ± 12
Adults	1158 ± 305	100 ± 26	99 ± 27	100 ± 27	200 ± 61	100 ± 31	1457 ± 353	100 ± 24

*One standard deviation.

From Stiehm, E. R., and Fudenberg, H. H.: Serum levels of immune globulins in health and disease. Pediatrics 37:715, 1966. Values shown were derived from measurements made in 296 normal children and 30 adults. Levels were determined by the radial diffusion plate method using specific rabbit antisera to human immunoglobulins.

macrophages and 11 percent are small lymphocytes consisting of T and B cells in equiproportions (Diaz-Jouanen and Williams, 1974; Beer, 1975). Although hyporesponsive to a variety of nonspecific mitogens, milk lymphocytes respond to certain antigens, notably K1 antigen of *E. coli,* even though peripheral blood lymphocytes from the same mother are totally unresponsive. This may explain the lower incidence of K1 *E. coli* meningitis in breast-fed infants. Mohr (1973) tested the cutaneous reactivity to tuberculin of infants who were breast fed, either by tuberculin-negative or tuberculin-positive mothers. A greater proportion of breast-fed offspring of tuberculin-positive mothers reacted with positive skin tests.

Macrophages in human milk also may play an important role in host defense. Necrotizing enterocolitis is a disease seen primarily in premature, low birth-weight infants, but uncommonly in breast-fed infants. Barlow and co-workers (1974) have developed a model in the newborn rat subjected to daily hypoxia that resembles human necrotizing enterocolitis. Such animals routinely die if formula fed but not if breast fed. Macrophages present in rat milk are the critical protective factors.

Frozen breast milk from "milk banks" unfortunately does not contain viable macrophages, and immunoglobulins are destroyed as well if the milk has been autoclaved. Frozen breast milk thus does little to enhance the host defenses of the infant.

SKIN REACTIVITY AND INFLAMMATORY RESPONSE

Since many assays of inflammatory-immune function depend upon some form of skin response, it must be recognized that an abnormal cutaneous response can be due to abnormal skin reactivity as well as to defective inflammatory or immune function. Gaisford (1955) found that infants immunized with BCG developed a positive Mantoux test in 14 to 21 days, as in the adult, but that the intensity of the reaction was diminished by comparison. Also infants under 1 year of age were found to develop less contact sensitivity to a Rhus allergen, pentadecylcatechol, than adults.

Uhr, Dancis, and Neumann (1960) studied the development of delayed type (contact) hypersensitivity in premature and term neonates exposed to 2,4-dinitrochlorobenzene (DNCB). Reactions developed in all of the control subjects, and in two of five term neonates and three of ten prematures studied. The reactions in the neonates were less intense than those in the older infants, but the histology of the lesions was qualitatively similar to that seen in contact-type hypersensitivity in the adult. Responses to sensitization did not correlate with the weight of the premature or the full-term neonates. The authors concluded that newborns have the capacity to develop cell-mediated immunity at or shortly after birth but that the response is uneven, partly due to a diminished ability to maintain an inflammatory response at this age.

Many neonatal animals exhibit poor inflammatory responses to dermal infections and have a reduced capacity to localize such infections. They also demonstrate delayed migration of neutrophils and mononuclear cells. The skin of human newborns responds poorly to irritation and fails to localize inflammation when compared with the skin of older children (Eitzman and Smith, 1959). Studies of cutaneous inflammation in human neonates by the Rebuck-Crowley "skin window" method also have demonstrated a relatively delayed and less intense shift from the predominantly polymorphonuclear to the mononuclear phase than in adults (Eitzman and Smith, 1959; Bullock et al., 1969). Skin homografts applied to human infants at birth are rejected, although more slowly than in adults (Fowler, Schubert, and West, 1960).

Sterzl and Hrubesova (1959) demonstrated passive transfer of tuberculin skin test reactivity from skin test–negative piglets to adult pigs by sensitizing neonatal leukocytes. Salvin, Gregg, and Smith (1962) immunized guinea pigs during the first two weeks of life with diphtheria toxoid. Although the neonatal guinea pigs failed to show cutaneous reactivity to toxoid, their leukocytes were able to passively transfer cutaneous reactivity to toxoid to adult guinea pigs.

In most studies of humans, newborns fail to accept sensitized cells or manifest a delayed allergic skin test reaction after receiving sensitized cells. Fireman, Kumate, and Gitlin (1970) studied PPD reactivity in infants between one and two days of age born of mothers with positive tuberculin tests. No reactivity to PPD by skin test or in lymphocyte culture was found in any infant. Passive transfer of PPD reactivity with leukocytes or leukocyte transfer factor from PPD-positive mothers was studied in neonates of both PPD-positive and PPD-negative mothers. Infants who received either intact leukocytes or transfer factor from PPD-positive donors showed increased activity to PPD in *in vitro* lymphocyte cultures, as assessed by blast transformation or incorporation of ³H-thymidine into nucleoprotein. By contrast, these infants showed no *in vivo* response to PPD skin testing. When leukocytes from three infants who had failed to develop a delayed skin test after passive sensitization were injected into PPD-negative adult recipients, two of three of the latter became PPD-positive. The investigators then administered BCG to the passively sensitized infants as well as to a group of normal non-sensitized infants. *In vivo* skin and *in vitro* leukocyte responses to PPD were not different in the two groups. The development of the *in vitro* leukocyte response to PPD preceded the development of *in vivo* skin reactivity by one to three weeks. These studies demonstrate that the neonatal lymphocyte is capable of responding immunologically to antigen, despite the absence of a skin test response.

In addition to the decreased cutaneous responsiveness of newborn skin, defects have been observed in the phagocyte and complement system of neonates (Miller, 1979*a* and *b*). While the degree to which these individual deficiencies contribute to the overall diminished skin response is unclear, it is highly probable that some (or all) of them play a role. These areas are covered in detail elsewhere in this text, and only information relevant to the newborn period is summarized here.

Phagocytic Functions. In the presence of adequate concentrations of adult serum, *phagocytosis* by isolated neonatal leukocytes is normal. In low concentrations of serum, however, neonatal polymorphonuclear leukocytes (PMN's) are less effective phagocytes than adult PMN's. In general, PMN's from premature infants are less effective phagocytes than those from term infants. This deficiency in phagocytic activity of neonatal PMN's may be clinically significant.

Most investigators have found normal *bactericidal* activity in neonatal PMN's, though further studies should be done when more sensitive methods are available. Recent studies revealed no difference between bactericidal activities of human monocytes from infants and adults toward *S. aureus* or *E. coli*. *Chemotactic activity* of neonatal PMN's has been found deficient towards chemotactically active materials generated from normal pooled serum by incubation with either *S. aureus*, *E. coli* or antigen-antibody complexes. Several studies of neonatal monocyte chemotaxis have indicated a relative deficiency of neonatal monocyte chemotaxis, whereas normal responses were found in one study. Neonatal PMN's also exhibit markedly decreased *membrane deformability* over control PMN's, i.e., neonatal PMN's are much more rigid cells. This may relate to deficient neonatal PMN leukocyte chemotaxis.

Complement. C1q, C2, C3, C4, C5, C3PA, and total hemolytic levels in newborns all have been reported to be low compared to adult levels. It is emphasized that measurement of complement components by immunochemical or hemolytic methods may fail to reveal gross defects of biologic activity.

Ontogeny of complement has been studied by three basic approaches: (1) synthesis of complement components by isolated fetal tissues *in vitro,* (2) demonstration of maternal-fetal discordance of genetic type when genetic polymorphisms exist, and (3) identification in fetal serum of a component that the mother is genetically deficient in. Such studies indicate that most complement components are synthesized early in fetal life, at or slightly preceding the time of onset of immunoglobulin synthesis. In several species, including man, there is little or no placental transfer of maternal complement to the fetal circulation.

Opsonic deficiencies in sera from premature and term infants have been demonstrated by a number of workers. The nature of the opsonic defect(s) in neonatal sera remains unclear and may be due to more than a single factor. Potential factors that may be involved include IgM, IgG, C3, C5, and C3PA. Generation of *chemotactic factors* from fresh, whole serum of full-term neonates by various methods is markedly deficient compared with similarly treated normal adult sera.

References

Alford, C. A., Jr.: Immunoglobulin determinations in the diagnosis of fetal infection. Pediatr. Clin. North Am. *18*:99, 1971.

Argyris, B. F.: Role of macrophages in immunological maturation. J. Exp. Med. *128*:459, 1968.

Barlow, B., Santulli, T. V., Heird, W. C., Pitt, J., Blanc, W. A., and Schullinger, J. N.: An experimental study of acute neonatal enterocolitis — the importance of breast milk. J. Pediatr. Surg. *9*:587, 1974.

Bazaral, M., Orgel, H. A., and Hamburger, R. N.: IgE levels in normal infants and mothers and an inheritance hypothesis. J. Immunol. *107*:794, 1971.

Beer, A. E.: Immunologic benefits and hazards of milk in the maternal-perinatal relationship: Natural transplantation of leukocytes during suckling in necrotizing enterocolitis in the newborn infant. *In* Moore, T. D. (ed.): Report of the Sixty-eighth Ross Conference on Pediatric Research. Columbus, Ross Laboratories, 1975, pp. 48–53.

Blaese, R. M., Henrichon, M., and Waldmann, T. A.: Ontogeny of the immune response: The afferent limb (abstract). Fed. Proc. *29*:699, 1970.

Buckley, R. H., Younger, J. B., and Brumley, G. W.: Evaluation of serum immunoglobulin concentrations in the perinatal period by use of a standardized method of measurement. J. Pediatr. *75*:1143, 1969.

Bullock, J. D., Robertson, A. F., Bodenbender, M. T., Kontras, S. B., and Miller, C. E.: Inflammatory response in the neonate re-examined. Pediatrics *44*:58, 1969.

Dancis, J., Osborn, J. J., and Kunz, H. W.: Studies of immunology of the newborn infant. IV. Antibody formation in the premature infant. Pediatrics *12*:151, 1953.

Diaz-Jouanen, E. P., and Williams, R. C.: T and B lymphocytes in human colostrum. Clin. Immunol. Immunopathol. *3*:248, 1974.

Eitzman, D. V., and Smith, R. T.: The non-specific inflammatory cycle in the neonatal infant. Am. J. Dis. Child. *97*:326, 1959.

Fireman, P., Kumate, J., and Gitlin, D.: Development of delayed hypersensitivity in neonates (abstract). Excerpta Med. (Amst.), Sect. VII. International Congress of Allergology, No. 211, 1970.

Fowler, R., Jr., Shubert, W. K., and West, C. D.: Acquired partial tolerance to homologous skin grafts in the human infant at birth. Ann. N.Y. Acad. Sci. *87*:403, 1960.

Gaisford, W.: Protection of infants against tuberculosis. Br. Med. J. *2*:1164, 1955.

Gathings, W. E., Cooper, M. D., Lawton, A. R., and Alford, C. A., Jr.: B cell ontogeny in humans. Fed. Proc. *35*:393, 1976.

Gill, T. J. III, Rabin, B. S., Kunz, H. W., Davis, B. K., and Taylor, F. H.: *In* Dayton, D. H., and Cooper, M. D. (eds.): *The Development of Host Defenses.* New York, Raven Press, 1977, p. 287.

Gitlin, D., Rosen, F. S., and Michael, J. G.: Transient 19S gamma-deficiency in the newborn infant and its significance. Pediatrics *31*:197, 1963.

Lawton, A. R., Self, K. S., Royal, S. A., and Cooper, M. D.: Ontogeny of B-lymphocytes in the human fetus. Clin. Immunol. Immunopathol. *1*:104, 1972.

Leiner, C.: Erythrodermia desquamation (universal dermatitis of children at the breast). Br. J. Child. Dis. *5*:244, 1908.

Miller, M. E.: The immunodeficiencies of immaturity. *In* Stiehm, E. R., and Fulginiti, V. A. (eds.): *Immunologic Disorders in Infants and Children,* 2nd Ed. Philadelphia, W. B. Saunders Co. 1979*a*.

Miller, M. E.: Innate immunity. *In* Stiehm, E. R., and Fulginiti, V. A. (eds.): *Immunologic Disorders in Infants and Children,* 2nd Ed. Philadelphia, W. B. Saunders Co., 1979*b*.

Miller, M. E., and Nilsson, V. R.: A familial deficiency of the phagocytosis enhancing activity of serum related to a dysfunction of the fifth component of complement (C5). New Engl. J. Med. *282*:354, 1970.

Mohr, J. A.: The possible induction and/or acquisition of cellular hypersensitivity associated with ingestion of colostrum. J. Pediatr. *82*:1062, 1973.

Nejedla, A.: The development of immunological factors in infants with hyperbilirubinemia. Pediatrics *45*:102, 1970.

Nilsson, U. R., Miller, M. E., and Wyman, S.: A functional abnormality of the fifth component of complement (C5) from human serum of individuals with a familial opsonic defect. J. Immunol. *112*:1164, 1974.

Raff, M. C., Megson, M., Owen, J. J. T., and Cooper, M. D.: Early production of intracellular IgM by B-lymphocyte precursors in mouse. Nature *259*:224, 1976.

Richardson, M., and Conner, G. H.: Prenatal immunization by the oral route: Stimulation of *Brucella* antibody in fetal lambs. Infect. Immunol. *5*:454, 1972.

Salvin, S. B., Gregg, M. B., and Smith, R. F.: Hypersensitivity in newborn guinea pigs. J. Exp. Med. *115*:707, 1962.

Smith, R. T., and Eitzman, D. V.: The development of the immune response — Characterization of the response of the human infant and adult to immunization with Salmonella vaccines. Pediatrics *33*:163, 1964.

Sterzl, J., and Hrubesova, M.: Attempts to transfer tuberculin hypersensitivity to young rabbits. Folia Microbiol. (Praha) *4*:60, 1959.

Sterzl, J., and Silverstein, A. M.: Developmental aspects of immunity. Adv. Immunol. *6*:337, 1967.

Thorbecke, G. J.: Some histological and functional aspects of lymphoid tissue in germfree animals. I. Morphological studies. Ann. N.Y. Acad. Sci. *78*:237, 1959.

Uhr, J. W., Dancis, J., and Neumann, C. G.: Delayed-type hypersensitivity in premature neonatal humans. Nature (London) *187*:1130, 1960.

Winberg, J., and Wessner, G.: Does breast milk protect against septicemia in the newborn? Lancet *1*:1091, 1971.

GENERAL

Miller, M. E.: *Host Defenses in the Human Neonate.* New York, Grune and Stratton, Inc., 1978.

3

Ildy M. Katona, M.D.
Joseph A. Bellanti, M.D.

Immunogenetics

Immunogenetics is the study of those processes involved in the immune response that may have a genetic basis. In recent years the existence of immune response genes that control specific immune responsiveness to a variety of antigens has become apparent. Several genes also have been identified that appear to influence interactions among the myriad of cells and cell products that constitute the immune system. Other genes have been determined to control the transmission of antigenic specificities from generation to generation. In light of these recent developments, a contemporary definition of immunogenetics includes the study of all factors that control immune responsiveness to foreign material, as well as the transmission of antigenic specificity from generation to generation.

CLINICAL IMPORTANCE OF IMMUNOGENETICS

A knowledge of genetic influences on specific immune responses or on antigenic specificities may, at first, seem far removed from the application of immunology to clinical medicine. An understanding of these phenomena, however, is assuming increased clinical importance because the genetic variability from individual to individual appears to form the basis for determining susceptibility to infection and the predisposition to many of the allergic (atopic) and other hypersensitivity diseases, the autoimmune diseases, and possibly even malignant diseases.

Knowledge of genetics also provides immediate tools for the physician in the diagnosis, treatment, and prevention of disease. The usefulness of information on the pedigree, or family history, is not to be underestimated in the diagnostic approach to common problems seen in clinical practice, as well as to the less common defects of the immune system.

A knowledge of genetic factors controlling the antigenic specificities of the ABO, Rh and HLA systems is of clinical importance. In addition to forming the basis for understanding of hemolytic disease of the newborn, transfusion reactions, and factors involved in transplantation of tissues and organs, a recent association between histocompatibility type and rheumatoid, malignant, immune, atopic and other diseases in man has been uncovered that presents new and exciting diagnostic possibilities. In atopic disease specifically, there is evidence for an association between (ragweed) hayfever, IgE antibody to ragweed, and markers for immune response genes closely linked to the histocompatibility system.

PRINCIPLES OF IMMUNOGENETICS

The immune system consists of a highly complex network of cellular and soluble factors, the activities of which are extensively interdependent and interrelated. At least several of the interactions between these factors are under genetic control.

The Major Histocompatibility Complex

The major histocompatibility complex (MHC) in mammals is a single genetic region that determines the histocompatibility antigens that are present on the surface of most body cells other than erythrocytes. Histocompatibility antigens are unique for each individual, except in identical twins. This uniqueness of "self" is accompanied by an exquisite host sensing mechanism that triggers the genetically controlled immune response to "foreignness."

The numerous histocompatibility antigens differ in their ability to elicit an immune response in a grafted recipient. In man, one set of antigens, which were first detected on the surface of white blood cells, provides by far the strongest barrier to successful transplantation. These antigens are called HLA (human leukocyte) antigens. The "A" of HLA refers to the first system of this kind recognized in the human. Human cells contain 46 chromosomes, as 23 pairs: one set maternal in origin, the other paternal. Subunits of chromosomes, genes, contain DNA and code for synthesis of a particular protein. The position or gene location on the chromosome is called the "gene locus." Different genes that occur at the same locus are called "alleles."

Four loci identified in a single region on chromosome six form the major histocompatibility complex in man. These loci are designated HLA-A, HLA-B, HLA-C, and HLA-D. Products of three of these regions (HLA-A, HLA-B, HLA-C) on the cell surface are detected by serologic reagents and are therefore referred to as *serologically defined* (SD). The fourth, HLA-D, can be detected by mixed lymphocyte culture only and is referred to as a *lymphocyte-defined* (LD) antigen (Fig. 3–1). The gene alleles possible for each of these four loci are numerous, and the number recognized is increasing constantly. Presently 19 alleles are recognized for the A locus, 26 for the B locus, and 6 for the incompletely characterized C locus. So complex is this system that there are 65,052 different genotypes possible.

MHC of Mice (H-2)

The H-2 region, located on the seventeenth chromosome in the mouse, is homologous to the HLA system of man. Our knowledge of the H-2 region of the mouse is much greater than our knowledge of the HLA system, facilitated by study of genetically homogeneous mice produced by intensive inbreeding (brother to sister mating). The four histocompatibility loci of H-2 are K, D, I, and Ss-Slp (see Fig. 3–2).

The K and D Regions. These regions are homologous to the HLA-B and HLA-A in man; they code for antigens that can be detected on the cell surface by antisera and are

MHC Man (HLA)

Nomenclature of HLA

NEW	OLD	ORIGINAL
HLA-A	SD1	1st locus
HLA-B	SD2	2nd locus
HLA-C	SD3	3rd locus
HLA-D	LD1	—

FIGURE 3–1. Schematic representation of the human major histocompatibility complex (MHC), illustrating chromosomal loci (HLA) and their gene products and the lymphocyte detectable (LD) and serologically detectable (SD) antigens. (From Bellanti, J. A.: *Immunology II.* Philadelphia, W. B. Saunders Co., 1978, p. 90.)

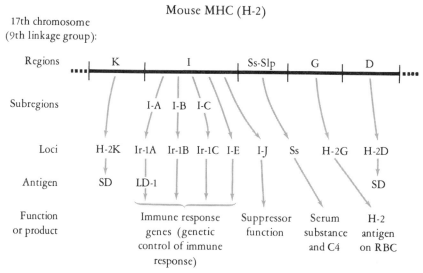

FIGURE 3–2. Schematic representation of the mouse MHC (H-2), depicting regions, subregions, loci, antigens, and their gene functions and products. (From Bellanti, J. A.: *Immunology II*. Philadelphia, W. B. Saunders Co., 1978, p. 83.)

known as serologically defined (SD) antigens. These antigens have been characterized as beta$_2$ microglobulin. During graft rejection, these antigens are recognized by cytotoxic T-lymphocytes. When cells are treated with viruses or chemical haptens, they seem specifically to alter SD antigens. Altered SD antigens then are recognized as foreign and are attacked by cytotoxic T-lymphocytes. It is hypothesized that the modified SD regions present a new antigenic determinant to the T-lymphocyte and hence are recognized as an altered or "nonself" (see Fig. 3–3). A second hypothesis, called the "dual recognition" hypothesis, postulates that cytotoxic T-lymphocytes require dual recognition signals via reception for the specific antigen and the SD antigen.

I Region. The I region in the mouse controls many major immune phenomena. The antigens on the cell surface coded by genes from this region (Ir genes) are called Ia (I region associated) antigens. Ia antigens are lymphocyte defined and differ from SD antigens in tissue distribution and function. Whereas products of the K and D regions are located on all cells, except erythrocytes, Ia antigens are located only on lymphocytes, macrophages, and on Langerhans cells in the skin. In man Ia antigens seem to be encoded by genes within or near the HLA-D region.

Ia antigens control immune responses to specific antigens, recognition of antigen presented by the macrophages, helper and suppressor function of T-lymphocytes, interac-

tion between T and B cells, and antibody production by B-lymphocytes.

Genetic Control of Complement. The Ss-Slp region of the major histocompatibility complex in the mouse controls the synthesis of the fourth component of complement (C4). This region specifically controls the synthesis of two serum proteins, Ss (serologically detected serum protein) and Slp (the sex-limited protein), which in turn influence C4 synthesis.

INHERITANCE OF HISTOCOMPATIBILITY ANTIGENS

Ir genes are transmitted in an autosomal dominant pattern. The transmission of the histocompatibility complex follows the Mendelian principles of genetics. Figure 3–4 shows a pedigree in which X and X' are representative of the MHC complex present on the pair of mother's chromosomes and Y and Y' represent the MHC complex present on the father's chromosomes. It can be seen how the genotypes of the grandparents are transmitted to the parents and the grandchildren.

HISTOCOMPATIBILITY AND DISEASE

The first disease recognized to be associated with HLA was Hodgkin's disease (1967). Since that time numerous associations be-

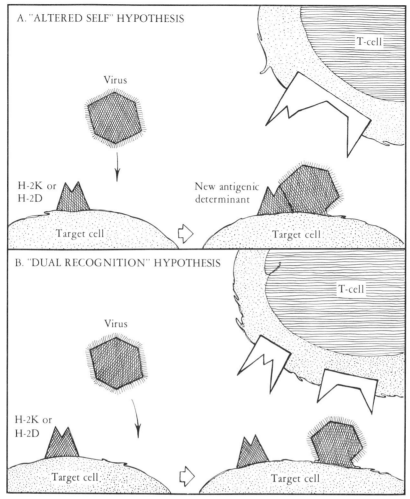

FIGURE 3–3. Schematic representation of two hypotheses of genetic restrictions concerned with recognition of virus-infected target cells by cytotoxic lymphocytes. (From Bellanti, J. A.: *Immunology II*. Philadelphia, W. B. Saunders Co., 1978, p. 84.)

tween HLA and specific diseases have been identified (Table 3–1). Interestingly, investigation of HLA patterns and various disease states has resulted in associating diseases that previously were only vaguely clinically connected and has established subcategories in other diseases. A characteristic common to virtually all diseases associated to date

FIGURE 3–4. Family pedigree, showing inheritance of histocompatibility antigens. (From Bellanti, J. A.: *Immunology II*. Philadelphia, W. B. Saunders Co., 1978, p. 94.)

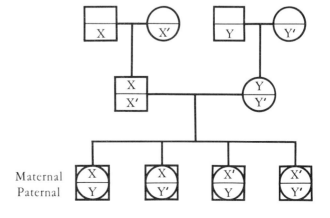

TABLE 3–1   HLA ANTIGENS AND DISEASE ASSOCIATIONS

HLA ANTIGENS	DISEASES	HLA FREQUENCY		RELATIVE RISK FACTORS
		Patients (Positive Reaction, Per Cent)	Controls (Positive Reaction, Per Cent)	
Group 1: Certain Associations				
HLA-B27	Ankylosing spondylitis	81–96	4–8	121
	Reiter syndrome	60–96	4–14	40
	Acute anterior uveitis	55	4	24
	Juvenile rheumatoid arthritis	42	6	11.5
	Psoriatic arthritis	63	8	4.7
	Yersinia arthritis	91	14	*
HLA-B8	Gluten-sensitive enteropathy and celiac disease	77–88	20–30	11* 8†
	Grave disease	*	*	11.5
	Myasthenia gravis	38–65	18–31	4.5
	Dermatitis herpetiformis	58–84	17–33	4.3
	Chronic active hepatitis	68	18	3.6
HLA-Bw15	Insulin-dependent	36	10	31
HLA-B8	diabetes mellitus	*	*	16
HLA-A3	Multiple sclerosis	32–40	18–27	24
HLA-B7		35–39	25–26	12
HLA-B18		*	*	12
HLA-B13	Psoriasis vulgaris	11–27	2–5	5
HLA-Bw17		19–36	4–16	4.8
Group 2: Probable Associations				
HLA-B8 and HLA-Bw15	Systemic lupus erythematosus			
HLA-B13	Pemphigus			
HLA-A3	Idiopathic autoimmune hemolytic anemia			
HLA-A3 and HLA-B7	Poliomyelitis			
HLA-B5	Behçet disease			
Group 3: Possible Associations				
HLA-A2 and HLA-B12	Acute lymphoblastic leukemia			
HLA-A2	Chronic glomerulonephritis			
HLA-A2, decreased	Periodontitis			
HLA-Bw35	Infectious mononucleosis			
HLA-B14	Leprosy			
HLA-A10	Hodgkin disease (patients > 45 years of age)			

*In adults.
†In children.
From Ritzmann, S. E.: HLA patterns. J.A.M.A., *236*:2305, 1976.

with certain HLA types is the implication of autoimmune mechanisms in the pathogenesis of the disease.

Diseases Associated with HLA-B27. A group of clinical entities, characterized by arthritis of the sacroiliac joint, extremities, and spine and the absence of rheumatoid factor, have been found to have a distinct association with B27 antigen. All of these diseases can be familial. The most striking histocompatibility association occurs in ankylosing spondylitis, in which more than 90 percent of the affected individuals have HLA-B27. For individuals with B27, the relative risk of disease is about 200 times that of B27-negative individuals. However, using the highest risk estimates, less than 20 percent of B27-positive individuals develop clinical disease. This raises the question of what other factors are important in susceptibility to the disease.

Diseases Associated with HLA-B8. A number of diseases, characterized in general by chronic inflammation, aberrant immune responses, and a familial occurrence, have been associated with B8 antigen. These include gluten-sensitive enteropathy, dermatitis herpetiformis, chronic active hepatitis, myasthenia gravis, diabetes mellitus, and several chronic endocrinopathies. B8 has been found in 45 percent of patients with childhood diabetes and adult insulin-dependent diabetes. An increased incidence of B15 antigen has also been found in these patients. By contrast, there have been no demonstrable HLA associations with insulin-*independent* diabetes.

In general, there appears to be an association of HLA-B8 with a general expression of allergy (D. Marsh, unpublished observations). There are also associations between specific IgE responses to highly purified antigens with either A locus or B locus specificities, e.g., Ra5 with DW2 and B7, Ra3 with A2 and rye grass 1 with B8 (DW3) specificities. In addition to these specific associations the overall expression of allergy appears to be controlled by an IgE regulating gene where low IgE is dominant.

Theories of HLA Relationship to Disease. There are three possible explanations of how HLA is related to disease. *First,* the HLA genes themselves may alter the cell's configuration, making it more vulnerable to specific disease. *Second,* the HLA genes may not be responsible for disease susceptibility per se, but susceptibility may be closely linked to a gene controlling some other trait, such as immune responsiveness. From an immunologic standpoint, this hypothesis is the most attractive since Ia genes closely linked to histocompatibility complex have been related to viral oncogenesis in the mouse. *Third,* certain HLA types may have enabled the host to survive various epidemics in the past, though now the immune advantages of their HLA systems have become disadvantages in regards to development of autoimmune diseases. The unequal distribution of the HLA types in the population would be compatible with this postulation. The greater frequency of individuals with certain HLA types might reflect their greater survival rate during smallpox, cholera, or bubonic plaque epidemics, but these genes do not protect from the autoimmune diseases.

Further understanding of HLA and Ir genes can lead to both better clinical diagnostic methods and an increased knowledge of fundamental disease processes.

References

Bach, F. H., and Van Rood, J. I.: The major histocompatibility complex. N. Engl. J. Med., *295*:806, 872, 927 (three part series), 1976.

Bellanti, J. A.: *Immunology II.* Philadelphia, W. B. Saunders Co., 1978, pp. 78–94.

Katz, D. H., and Benacerraf, B.: *The Role of Products of the Histocompatibility Gene Complex in the Immune Response.* New York, Academic Press, 1976.

Marsh, D. G., and Bias, W. B.: The genetics of atopic allergy. *In* Samter, M. (ed.): *Immunologic Diseases.* 3rd ed. Boston, Little, Brown and Company, 1978, pp. 819–831.

Ritzmann, S. E.: HLA patterns and disease associations. J.A.M.A. *236*:2305, 1976.

Schaller, J. G., and Omenn, G. S.: The histocompatibility system and human disease. J. Pediatr. *88*:913, 1976.

Shreffler, D. C., and David, C. S.: The H-2 major histocompatibility complex and the I immune response region: Genetic variation, formation and organization. Adv. Immunol. *20*:125, 1976.

4

Vincent A. Fulginiti, M.D.

Immunization

At one time a child routinely experienced and hopefully survived the "normal" infectious diseases of early life, and in doing so, gained immunity to the separate infectious agents. This chapter deals with the use of immunizations to induce immunity and thus to avoid the mortality and morbidity of natural disease.

ACTIVE IMMUNITY

Most immunizing procedures attempt to mimic nature by evoking an active immune response that resembles the response following infection by the natural disease. To be effective, a vaccine must more than simply induce an immune response; it must evoke the *quality* and *quantity* of the immune response sufficient for effective resistance to the virulent agent. Attenuated measles virus vaccine meets this criterion and protects most persons against measles. By contrast, parainfluenza virus vaccines developed to date have failed to evoke a protective active immunity despite induction of some immune responses. For lasting immunity, B and/or T cell "memory" must be induced. Pertussis vaccine fails to do this, thus periodic "booster" immunizations are necessary to maintain protection.

PASSIVE IMMUNITY

In nature, an infant derives protection against some infectious diseases through transfer of maternal IgG antibody across the placenta. This type of protection is passive, affording only temporary relief from infection; once maternal antibody is metabolized, the infant reverts to a more susceptible state.

Based upon this natural model, medical practice has sought to duplicate such passive immunity. Initially, sera from animals treated with specific infectious agents were infused into susceptible individuals who were exposed to the infectious agent or in whom disease was established. Only limited success was achieved with this method, owing to restricted specificity of antisera; limited content of immune reactants involved in immunity; limited effectiveness, especially when administered late in incubation or after disease appearance; and hypersensitivity reactions to the foreign animal proteins.

As technology and knowledge in immunology soared after World War II, human gamma globulins were prepared that were known to contain a variety of antibodies. Polio, measles, and hepatitis were among the diseases modified or prevented by the administration of pooled gamma globulin of adult origin. Using increasingly sophisticated techniques, manufacturers provided gamma globulins selected for a specific level of a specific antibody or from adult volunteers deliberately "boosted" by specific vaccines. Gamma globulins with high antibody content against tetanus toxin, measles, pertussis, mumps, and other agents came into general use.

All such globulins have certain characteristics in common:

They are a concentrated solution of electrophoretically similar globulins, usually prepared by cold alcohol fractionation (Cohn's method). The standard concentration is 16.5 grams per dl.

They contain a high concentration of IgG, with little IgA and IgM (less than 1 gm per dl).

They contain a variety of antibodies, based upon the immune experience of the adults from whom the pool was obtained. Despite a specific label, antibodies other than that named are included, although not necessarily titered.

They must be given by intramuscular injection. Deliberate or inadvertent intravascular administration may be associated with anaphylactic or anaphylactoid reactions.

Dimers and other complexes of IgG form during storage, increasing likelihood of reactions in recipients.

The pooling of all genetic types of IgG can evoke an immune response in the recipient against those genetic types different from his own.

Generic practical considerations in the use of any gamma globulin preparation include:

The dose of gamma globulin is not uniform; it varies for each clinical preparation and for the specific clinical circumstances of its use. These variables must be known for effective use of the antibody contained in the preparation.

Intradermal testing with gamma globulin is not advised. It is unnecessary and may, in fact, be misleading because intradermal inoculation may result in a wheal and flare reaction which does *not* indicate sensitivity to intramuscular administration.

Whenever an active immunizing antigen and gamma globulin containing the corresponding antibody are administered simultaneously, the effect of the antigen may be decreased by neutralization of antigen in the host. It may be wise in some situations to administer additional doses of the antigen to ensure adequate antigenic stimulation.

OTHER PASSIVE ANTIBODY

Animal Sera. Traditionally animal sera, usually equine but occasionally from other species, has been utilized as a source of antibody for humans. Particular preparations differ, not only in their antibody content, but (presumably) also in their specific equine or other animal antigens.

Development of sensitivity to animal serum is a major limiting factor in the use of antibody from animal serum. This is of particular importance in using horse serum. The possibility of hypersensitivity must be considered each time the use of animal serum is contemplated, and appropriate medications to treat anaphylactic reactions must be available for instant use. Serum sickness develops later in a high proportion of recipients of horse serum.

Table 4–1 lists the steps in testing for sensitivity to horse serum or other animal serum.

Human Plasma or Serum. On rare occasions, serum or plasma may be collected from a single human for specific transfer to another human. Such serum or plasma is selected on the basis of known or predicted specific antibody content. Examples include postvaccination plasma in the treatment of complications of smallpox vaccination and post-zoster plasma in the prevention of varicella in the immunodepressed individual. A major problem with such biologic material is the possible transmission of hepatitis viruses.

PRACTICAL CONSIDERATIONS IN IMMUNIZATION

Increasing numbers of vaccines, antiserums, and gamma globulin preparations are becoming available. They differ in composition, form, stability, route of administration, and how they should be used. It is essential that the practitioner carefully read the informational brochure provided by the manufacturer before administering the preparation to a patient.

There is no "typical" vaccine, but the following types of components are common. The extent of this list points out the complexities of some vaccines and the difficulty in attributing an unusual reaction to a specific component.

The Principal Antigen. This may be whole bacteria, bacterial products (e.g.,

TABLE 4–1 ADMINISTRATION OF HORSE SERUM OR SERUM FROM OTHER ANIMAL SOURCES

I. Obtain history of:
  A. Allergy in general
  B. Receipt of horse serum in past
  C. Allergic reaction to horse serum or to horse dander (allergy to horse dander does not *necessarily* indicate allergy to horse serum).
II. Perform skin tests.* A tourniquet and emergency medication must be available for immediate use if necessary. See Chapter 52 for treatment of anaphylaxis.
  A. Administer scratch test, using undiluted serum first.
  B. If negative, proceed to intradermal testing, using 0.05 ml of 1:100 saline dilution of serum.
  C. Reduce dose to 0.05 ml of 1:1000 in allergic individuals; if negative, proceed to 1:100 dilution.
  D. Appearance of a wheal in 10 to 30 minutes that is larger in size than wheal of the saline control indicates hypersensitivity.
III. Procedure for administering serum
  A. History and skin tests negative:
    Give appropriate intramuscular dose
    or
    Give 0.5 ml serum intravenously slowly in 10 ml fluid; with no reaction in 30 minutes, give remainder of dose as 1:20 dilution.
  B. History *or* skin test positive:
    Give 1.0 ml of 1:10 dilution subcutaneously; with no reaction, give intramuscularly or intravenously as above.
  C. History *and* skin test positive (*use horse serum only if* **imperative**):
    1. Establish an intravenous line and keep open with normal saline.
    2. Give 0.05 ml of 1:20 dilution subcutaneously.
    3. With no reaction, increase subcutaneous dose every 15 minutes as follows:

       0.1 ml of 1:10 dilution
       0.3 ml of 1:10 dilution
       0.1 ml of undiluted
       0.2 ml of undiluted
       0.5 ml of undiluted
       remainder of dose

    4. If there is a local reaction at any stage, reduce dose by one half, and proceed again. With any systemic manifestations, treat appropriately, reduce serum dose to one-tenth of the provoking dose, and increase by threefold increments.

*Conjunctival tests are unreliable due to irritant effect; it is recommended that they not be used.

toxins or hemolysins), whole viruses, or substructures of viruses.

Host-Derived Antigen. These are proteins or other constituents of host tissue that are carried along with or intimately associated with the virus particles.

Altered Antigens. Distorted proteins and other substances may become incorporated into vaccines as a result of the complex changes associated with the effects of virus infection on the cells in which the virus is grown.

Preservatives and Stabilizers. A variety of chemical compounds are employed to prevent bacterial growth or to maintain the desired antigen in a stable form. Typical are thimerosal (Merthiolate) and glycerine.

Antibiotics. Trace amounts may be present in viral vaccines that have been prepared in media containing antibiotics. Various antibiotics are employed, and the "same" vaccine prepared by different manufacturers may vary in the specific antibiotics used.

Menstruum. All vaccines are solutions or suspensions. The fluid phase may consist simply of saline, or it may be as complex as the tissue culture media employed in virus growth.

Unwanted or Unknown Constituents. Despite elaborate precautions in preparing vaccines, viruses or other antigens may be included that are not wanted; they may not even be detectable.

Adjuvants. A variety of substances may be used to enhance the antigenic effect of the principal antigen. Materials such as alum, aluminum phosphate, and aluminum hydroxide are in use; others (e.g., mineral oil, peanut oil) show potential. The purpose of these materials is to retain the antigen at the depot site and to release it slowly, thus enhancing the immune response by allowing prolonged contact.

Adjuvant, or depot type, vaccines are preferred because they provide more prolonged immunity and greater antigenic stimulation with fewer systemic reactions than are observed with rapidly absorbed fluid antigens.

Antigens vary in their ability to produce the desired immune response. In some, this ability is weak and, in others, strong. In addition, the host response may be poor or absent for any given antigen. For this reason, some children who receive a usually adequate dose of an effective antigen at the proper time will simply not respond and may contract the disease if exposed naturally. For example, measles vaccine regularly fails to induce protection in 3 to 5 percent of children over 15 months of age. If these children are exposed subsequently to the natural disease, they may develop measles. This should not condemn any particular antigen, since it does protect the vast majority of recipient children.

Factors important in achieving the desired immune response include the dose of vaccine, the route of administration, the scheduling, the clinical condition of the patient, and the temporal association of administration of a single vaccine with other biologicals.

The appropriate dose and route of administration for any vaccine are determined during the development process. The dose, for instance, should produce an immune response in all, or almost all, recipients, yet should not be harmful, uneconomical, or impossible to administer. The physician should follow the manufacturer's recommendations on the package insert.

The scheduling of immunizations is crucial and is discussed in the sections on specific immunizations. Circumstances may warrant administration of a given vaccine coincident with or shortly after exposure to the corresponding disease, as with rabies or live measles virus vaccine, in which the incubation period of the disease is longer than the incubation period of the corresponding vaccine. Some vaccines require booster doses because the immunizing agent fails to invoke long-term immunity. The precise timing of these additional doses is determined by both theory and experience.

Immunization plays an important role in preventive health care and should be adapted to the needs and health of the patient. For instance, in a patient suffering from or recovering from viral illness, a live virus vaccine may be ineffective because of the presence of another virus, or because interferon induced by another virus can inhibit effective immunization. Further, the side effects or primary effect of the vaccine can complicate or intensify an already present or impending illness.

Pre-existent CNS disease poses a specific therapeutic dilemma. The patient with any one of a variety of diseases that affect the central nervous system may have severe CNS reactions, specific or nonspecific, to vaccines. The therapeutic dilemma arises because these patients are also susceptible to the systemic and CNS effects of the natural infectious diseases. Thus it is at once hazardous to immunize and necessary to do so. Decisions concerning these risks must be made individually. In general, patients with a static CNS lesion may be immunized, whereas patients with active CNS disease should not be.

Vaccines are frequently combined to facilitate immunization. Early experimental results suggested that there were limits to the responsiveness of an individual to multiple antigens; that specific combinations of agents, particularly viruses, appeared to inhibit the efficacy of one or more of the constituents of the combination; and that additive adverse effects occurred. However, in practice certain vaccine combinations have been used successfully. For example, DPT and oral polio vaccine, a combination of six separate antigens, are given together with no discernible decrease in immune response or increase in adverse consequences. Also, measles, mumps, and rubella viruses are administered in various combinations, including all three together, without ill consequences or diminished effect.

Sequential administration of vaccines has the potential for interference. Thus care must be taken to space vaccines appropriately. Most live viral vaccines have the potential for stimulating interferon production, which may decrease immunity to subsequent viral antigens. Only specific studies can establish the optimal spacing of diverse inactivated and live antigens.

Vaccines for immunization are designed to deliver as specific an antigen as possible without introducing extraneous organisms. Environmental bacteria, especially those that have colonized the recipient's skin, and hepatitis virus are the greatest risks. To prevent introduction of such agents, precautions are taken in the manufacture, transport, storage, and administration of biologicals. For the most part, the physician can assume that the product is sterile when he receives it. His responsibility is to ensure proper storage and sterile administration of the vaccine. Most physicians prefer individually packaged disposable sterile syringes and needles. Aseptic technique must be used in treating the surface of the vaccine vial and the skin of the recipient. For specific recommendations, consult the American Academy of Pediatrics Report of the Committee on Infectious Diseases (1977).

Another practical consideration is the

procedure used to minimize the risks associated with the adjuvant or depot type vaccines. As mentioned before, these products contain substances (alum, aluminum hydroxide, aluminum phosphate) to "hold" the antigens in place and release them slowly for maximal effect. All such products must be placed deep in a large muscle mass, since leakage into subcutaneous or dermal tissues may result in irritation and necrosis (so-called sterile abscess or cyst). Most experts recommend the Z method of injection (by drawing the skin over the injection site laterally, the tract of administration springs aside when the skin is released at the end of injection). A small amount of air in the syringe, enough to eject all of the product into the tissue, can prevent deposit of adjuvant along the injection tract.

The preferred site of intramuscular injections is the anterolateral thigh (vastus lateralis muscle), in order to avoid sciatic nerve damage that may occur in intragluteal injections, or the deltoid or triceps muscle mass (in older children and adults). Aspiration is essential before injection to avoid intravenous administration.

Possible Reactions to Vaccines. There are relative contraindications to administering some vaccines. Certain disease states, especially immunodeficiency involving B or T cell defects, are associated with high risk of infection by attentuated live viruses. Thus, patients with congenital immunodeficiency states or acquired deficiencies, such as lymphatic and other malignancies or collagen vascular diseases, and patients receiving immunosuppressive drugs such as steroids, antimetabolites, and cell poisons are especially vulnerable to such infections.

Allergic diseases pose special problems in immunization. Since many vaccines are prepared in tissues that contain materials to which patients may react allergically, the physician must be aware of the potential allergic risk of each vaccine. This information is available in the vaccine's package insert. Not only should the physician obtain a detailed history of the potential for hypersensitivity to any of the components of the vaccine, he must also have equipment on hand to treat allergic reactions if they occur (see Chapter 52).

In doubtful cases, a skin test may be useful to rule out allergy to the vaccine or its components. Material for a skin test may be prepared by diluting the vaccine 1:100

with normal saline. If a scratch test is negative, an intradermal test should be performed, injecting 0.02 ml of diluted vaccine intracutaneously and observing for a wheal and flare reaction in 15 minutes. With a negative test, it is appropriate to proceed with the immunization. If the skin test is equivocal, an additional test should be performed with a 1:10 solution. On some occasions, it may be wisest to forego the vaccine because of a history of definite sensitivity. For example, if the only vaccine product available is known to contain penicillin, and an individual has a history of a serious penicillin reaction, the physician may prefer to avoid immunization with that product altogether. If there is no alternative vaccine, the patient should be apprised of the risks of immunization as well as the consequences of not being immunized. If there is a compelling reason for immunization, it should be performed in the hospital, using fractional dosages with an intravenous infusion running and emergency equipment on hand.

Local reactions often are not due to hypersensitivity; in fact, they are usually due to irritation. In pediatric practice it is common to reduce the dose of a vaccine to avoid such irritant reaction. Any individual dose may be reduced by 50 percent or more, but, of course, the total number of doses of vaccine must be increased so that the total recommended amount of antigen is given.

VACCINES, SERA, AND GAMMA GLOBULINS IN COMMON USE

Diphtheria

Rationale for Active Immunization. Diphtheria is caused by infection with *Corynebacterium diphtheriae.* Multiplication of the organism is less important in disease than is the local elaboration and systemic distribution of a powerful exotoxin. Toxin production is associated with strains of the organisms infected with a specific bacteriophage.

Immunity to diphtheria is related to the presence of adequate quantities of antitoxin. Immunization is predicated on inducing continued levels of circulating antitoxin and on providing a large supply of cells capable of synthesizing additional antitoxin rapidly.

Immunizing Antigen. Immunization is provided by a chemically altered toxin, diphtheria toxoid. This product is produced at two levels of potency, singly and in combination with other antigens, i.e., tetanus (DT—diphtheria-tetanus, adult) and pertussis (DPT). Primary immunization of children younger than 6 years is accomplished with preparations containing 7 to 25 Lf units of toxoid. This concentration is too toxic for older children and adults; a preparation containing not more than 2 Lf of toxoid is used instead. The usual preparations are adsorbed to an aluminum-type adjuvant to provide maximal stimulation of antibody function. Though fluid toxoid is available, indications for its use are limited (see below). Since toxoid is alum-adsorbed, it must be given deep into a substantial muscle mass.

Some individuals either naturally infected or immunized with toxoid are exquisitely sensitive to subsequent doses of diphtheria toxoid. To detect such sensitivity in adults, the toxoid sensitivity test (Zeller-Moloney) should be employed. Fluid diphtheria toxoid is injected intracutaneously (0.1 ml of 1:50 or 1:100 dilution in saline), and the site is observed at 24 hours. A positive test indicates hypersensitivity, is presumptive of immunity, and contraindicates administration of toxoid in any amount. A reaction of

TABLE 4–2 RECOMMENDED SCHEDULE OF IMMUNIZATIONS TO BE INCORPORATED INTO WELL CHILD CARE

Age	Vaccines
2 months	DTP,[1] TOPV[2]
4 months	DTP, TOPV
6 months	DTP, (TOPV)[3]
12 months	PPD[4]
15 months	MMR[5]
18 months	DTP, TOPV
4–7 years	DTP, TOPV
14–16 years	Td[6]
Every 10 years	Td

[1]DTP = Diphtheria and tetanus toxoids combined with pertussis vaccine.
[2]TOPV = Trivalent (types I, II & III) and attenuated, live poliovirus vaccine.
[3]The third dose of vaccine can be administered in those states which have records of importation of polio.
[4]Intermediate strength tubercular test advised for routine screening.
[5]Measles, mumps and rubella live, attenuated viruses in combination.
[6]Td = "Adult" type containing *less* diphtheria toxoid than TD or pediatric type. Do not use latter in individuals older than 7 years.

TABLE 4–3 RECOMMENDED SCHEDULE OF IMMUNIZATIONS FOR INFANTS AND CHILDREN LESS THAN 7 YEARS OF AGE NOT IMMUNIZED IN INFANCY

Time	Vaccine
First visit	DTP,[1] TOPV,[2] PPD[4]
1 month later	MMR[5]
2 months later	DTP, TOPV
4 months later	DTP, TOPV
10–16 months later or preschool	DTP, TOPV
14–16 years old	Td[6]
Every 10 years	Td[6]

Notes: refer to Table 4–2.

erythema (and, on occasion, induration) may persist. A negative test (no reaction at the test site) indicates no hypersensitivity, no immunity, and the necessity for diphtheria immunization.

Immunity. Immunization with diphtheria toxoid does not provide 100 percent protection among recipients. The best experimental data suggest five to ten times less chance of diphtheria in the immunized person than in the unimmunized. Also, severe cases are fewer and deaths rarely occur in fully immunized individuals. In the past, the Schick test has been used to determine immunity or susceptibility, but it is rarely used today.

Immunity to diphtheria persists longer than previously thought. Booster doses were recommended every 4 to 6 years; it is now suggested that a 10-year interval between doses is adequate. Schedules for immunization are listed in Tables 4–2, 4–3 and 4–4.

Special Circumstances. If Td (tetanus-diphtheria, adult type) is not available, hy-

TABLE 4–4 RECOMMENDED SCHEDULE FOR CHILDREN AND ADULTS OLDER THAN 7 YEARS NOT PREVIOUSLY IMMUNIZED

Time	Vaccine
First visit	Td, TOPV,[1] PPD
1 month later	MMR[2]
2 months later	Td, TOPV
8–14 months later	Td, TOPV
Age 14–16 years and/or every 10 years	Td

[1]TOPV should not be used in individuals older than 18 years (see text).
[2]May be modified by definite history of specific disease(s).

persensitivity to toxoid is determined by the Zeller-Moloney test. If the test is positive, immunity is assumed and toxoid is not administered. If results are negative, susceptibility is assumed and either diphtheria toxoid or pediatric DT is administered.

For children with CNS lesions or with a history of CNS reactions to previous DPT, DT is administered in fractional doses, 0.05 to 0.1 ml, extending the series to five or more doses.

If a patient survives diphtheria, *no immunity is conferred. Therefore, a primary series of immunization should be administered*. If a fully immunized person is exposed to diphtheria, 0.5 ml of toxoid is administered as DT or Td, depending on age.

Adverse Effects of Immunization. Sensitivity or toxic reactions to diphtheria toxoid are rare in infants and children. However, increasing age and exposure to toxoid can result in a hypersensitive state. Severe local reactions can occur with further doses of full-strength (7 to 25 Lf) toxoid. Adult Td containing 2 Lf of toxoid or less should be used in individuals without a history of reaction. With history of reaction to diphtheria toxoid–containing products, the Zeller-Moloney test should be performed or no further toxoid given.

Systemic reactions, including anaphylaxis, have been reported rarely.

Passive Immunization. Diphtheria antitoxin is prepared in horses. It is used both in prophylaxis and therapy of diphtheria and is available in vials of 1,000, 10,000, 20,000 and 40,000 units.

Prophylaxis. 10,000 units are administered to unimmunized, exposed, susceptible persons who cannot be kept under surveillance. It is preferable to avoid administration of antitoxin. Instead, daily examination, throat cultures for *C. diphtheriae* with penicillin administered to those with positive cultures, and toxoid administration should be employed.

Therapy. The use of antitoxin is empiric. It should be administered as soon as diphtheria is diagnosed clinically, even before positive cultures are obtained. Suggested doses are as follows: pharyngeal or laryngeal diphtheria (48 hours), 20,000 to 40,000 units; nasopharyngeal, 40,000 to 60,000 units; extensive diseases ($>$ 72 hours), 80,000 to 120,000 units; brawny neck edema, 80,000 to 120,000 units; and cutaneous lesions, no antitoxin. These doses are strictly empiric and may be modi-

fied based on site and size of membrane involved, severity of toxic symptoms, and duration of illness.

Cervical adenitis frequently reflects toxin absorption: softness of the nodes and diffuse node involvement indicate moderate to severe toxicity. Antitoxin should be administered intravenously as early as possible following sensitivity testing. Since diphtheria antitoxin is horse serum, the reader is referred to Table 4–1 on testings for horse serum sensitivity. *Remember that antimicrobial therapy is not a substitute for antitoxin*. Rather, the two should be used together.

Tetanus

Rationale for Active Immunization. Tetanus is caused by the neurotoxicity of a potent exotoxin elaborated by *Clostridium tetani*, which produces infection upon entry into a wound.

Sixty to 300 cases of tetanus have occurred annually throughout the United States in the past 15 years; the mortality rate has been 40 to 70 percent. Immunization is aimed at developing antitoxic immunity in the same way as immunity to diphtheria is developed. Immunization against tetanus provides personal protection; it does not provide any community protection.

Immunizing Antigen. Tetanospasmin, the *C. tetani* toxin, is chemically modified to form a potent antigen with minimal toxicity for immunization. Tetanus toxoid is used alone or in combination with diphtheria toxoid (DT, Td) and pertussis vaccine (DPT). It is one of the most effective antigens used in immunization, virtually assuring total protection for a person who receives a complete primary series.

Immunity. Disease protection is due to antitoxin entirely. In an adequately immunized individual, as little as 0.01 IU/ml of antitoxin is protective. Primary immunization is so effective that protective levels have been observed as long as 35 years after primary immunization. In persons whose antitoxin levels fall below the protective level, a booster dose results in a prompt recall antibody response. Boosters are recommended every ten years to ensure protective levels of antitoxin in the circulation.

Special Circumstances. In patients who

survive tetanus, *full primary immunization, utilizing a schedule appropriate for age, should be administered, since the natural disease does not confer immunity.*

Adverse Effects of Immunization. Although tetanus toxoid evokes a potent antibody response, it is an extremely safe biological, associated with few local or systemic reactions if used according to recommended schedules. *A severe local necrotizing Arthus-type reaction can occur in the individual who receives too many doses at too frequent intervals.* Abundant antibody present in the serum combines with recently injected antigen to produce toxoid-antitoxin complexes that destroy vascular channels and initiate a brisk inflammatory response.

Passive Immunization. Tetanus antitoxin is now administered as specific immune human globulin. Horse serum is no longer necessary. The tetanus immune globulin (TIG) is supplied in vials containing 250 units and is identical in all respects to all human gamma globulin except in its measured tetanus antitoxin content.

Prophylaxis. In treating tetanus-prone injuries (defined as severe trauma, deep penetrating wounds, or any trauma [including surgical] that is associated with potential *C. tetani* contamination) several factors determine the use and dose of TIG. If the wound has not been treated for 24 hours and is infected, TIG should be administered to both the immunized and the unimmunized. Also, in any tetanus-prone injury, TIG administration is recommended regardless of immune status. In the previously immunized, TIG is administered in conjunction with a booster dose of toxoid, given with separate syringes in different sites to avoid neutralization. In the unimmunized, tetanus toxoid primary immunization is begun and arrangements are made for completion. The dose of TIG is 4 units per kg of body weight intramuscularly, to a maximum of 250 units. Higher doses may be used for persons with highly contaminated or extensive wounds.

Therapy. The exact dose of TIG is not known. At least 140 units per kg of body weight intramuscularly is recommended. More may be given if the disease is severe.

Pertussis

Rationale for Active Immunization. Between 1700 and 9700 cases of pertussis have been reported yearly in the past decade. Most experts agree that the reported incidence falls far short of the actual incidence.

Pertussis occurs throughout the United States. It is a disease primarily of infancy, although adolescents and young adults do experience the disease. Complications and death — mainly due to CNS lesions, pneumonia and other pulmonary diseases, and electrolyte disturbances — are usually confined to early infancy. Because this disease is prevalent early in life, immunization programs have been designed to provide protection as early as immunologically feasible, beginning in the first months of life.

Pertussis immunization has been curtailed beyond age 7 because the adverse reactions to pertussis vaccine in late childhood and adult life are believed to be worse than the disease. Also, the disease was thought to be confined to infancy and childhood, thereby arguing against later pertussis immunization. In recent years, however, localized epidemics of pertussis have been reported among adult contacts (family and health workers) of infants with pertussis. Some individuals feel that physicians, nurses, and others likely to encounter pertussis should receive booster doses (0.25 ml) of pertussis vaccine.

Immunizing Antigen. Pertussis vaccines are among the least well defined of immunizing biologicals. Pertussis vaccine consists of killed pertussis organisms and fragments of organisms. The precise antigen or antigens responsible for protection are not known. Attempts have been made to "purify" pertussis vaccines, but the vagaries of potency continue to mandate the use of whole-bacteria products.

Pertussis vaccine can be administered alone or in combination with diphtheria and tetanus toxoids. It is prepared as both a "plain" preparation and one adsorbed to alum. The adjuvant (alum) vaccine contains 4 protective units per 0.5 ml dose, whereas the plain vaccine contains slightly more antigen. There is little practical use for plain pertussis vaccine; it offers no advantages immunologically and does not improve safety.

Immunity. Although several antigens have been characterized in *Bordetella pertussis* and several antibodies have been identified in humans after exposure to these antigens, the precise mechanism of immunity to pertussis is not known and the role of other immune mechanisms, e.g., cell-mediated immunity, has not been explored.

Virtually complete immunity follows an attack of the natural disease; rarely do second cases of bacteriologically proved disease occur in the same individual. Protection following vaccine is relatively short-lived; booster doses are required to maintain immunity. Schedules for immunization are given in Tables 4-2, 4-3, and 4-4.

Complicating assessment of immunity is the occurrence of the pertussis syndrome caused by agents other than *B. pertussis*. Parapertussis has been estimated to account for as many as 2 percent of clinical cases attributed to pertussis. There is no cross immunity between these organisms. Adenoviruses and other viral agents have been identified in pertussis-like syndromes. The occurrence of such infections confuses evaluation of efficacy of pertussis vaccine unless precise and definitive laboratory diagnosis is undertaken.

Schedules for Immunization. Tables 4-2, 4-3 and 4-4 present the recommended schedules for immunization.

Special Circumstances. Intimate exposure to pertussis or an epidemic may warrant additional DPT or pertussis adsorbed vaccine. For children 6 years of age or under, the full 0.5 ml dose should be employed. For those older than 6 years, a 0.25 ml dose of either vaccine may be used.

In areas of high endemicity or during epidemics, it may be desirable to initiate immunization earlier than generally recommended. Often the vaccine (DPT or pertussis, adsorbed) is begun at 4 to 6 weeks of age, and the older regimen of three doses 1 month apart is employed. Rarely, in severe epidemics affecting very young infants, pertussis immunization can be initiated in the first few days or weeks of life, but this is not recommended as a routine procedure.

A special problem exists in children with neurologic diseases. Protection against pertussis must be provided, but at the same time CNS toxicity of pertussis vaccine must be avoided. Most experts advise using pertussis adsorbed vaccine alone and dividing the needed 12 protective units among multiple small doses. One such regimen would consist of 0.1 ml (approximately 1 protective unit) doses given monthly until 12 protective units are administered. Other practitioners divide the 0.5 ml dose in half and give a total of six injections.

In children with reactions to pertussis vaccine, if the reaction has been local or systemic without CNS symptoms, pertussis vaccine is separated from DPT and the above procedure is followed. *When any CNS symptom follows administration of pertussis vaccine, further pertussis vaccine should not be given.*

Adverse Effects of Immunization. Both local and systemic adverse effects have been associated with administration of pertussis vaccine. Local reactions are frequent and consist of pain, induration, heat, and redness in any combination. As many as 70 percent of recipients in some series have experienced local toxicity. In the rare instances, tissue damage is severe enough to result in development of a "cyst" or "sterile abscess" that may drain.

Systemic reactions occur with variable frequency. Fever is common, and CNS complications have occurred. Unfortunately, the true incidence of these complications is clouded by the changes made in the formulation of the vaccine and by the variability in recognition and reporting of such incidents. Most experts believe CNS complications are rare: in the United States, on the order of one in 100,000 doses. Others have reported frequencies as high as one in 6000 immunizations. There appear to be no reliable indicators of susceptibility. The World Health Organization and English experts claim that a family history of CNS disorders or a personal history of convulsive disorder predisposes an individual to this complication; American experts report no connection between these factors.

For the past decade, considerable controversy has raged in England concerning the risk to benefit ratio for pertussis vaccine. Studies in the 1950's suggested a significant reaction rate for such disorders as febrile convulsions and encephalopathy. A more recent review by an Expert Committee (Morbidity and Mortality Weekly Reports, 1977) revealed no cases of permanent brain damage in 80,000 doses of DTP. In Scotland not a single case of severe brain damage was detected from 1961 to 1975, a period during which 180,000 children received pertussis vaccine in Glasgow.

Other adverse reactions reported in association with pertussis immunization include sudden death, angioneurotic edema, gastrointestinal symptoms, rashes, persistent and uncontrollable screaming, collapse and pallor, and hypersensitivity angiitis. All experts agree that pertussis vaccine is among the most toxic of products used in immunization; they disagree on extent and frequency of toxic reactions.

Passive Immunization. A hyperimmune pertussis globulin is available commercially. There is no convincing evidence that it is effective, either for prophylaxis or therapy. The author does not recommend its use.

Prophylaxis is probably more readily achieved with erythromycin. Once the paroxysmal stage of the disease begins, there is no specific therapy, although antimicrobials may reduce environmental spread of the organisms.

Poliomyelitis Immunization

Rationale for Immunization. Infantile paralysis, or paralytic poliomyelitis, is largely a disease of the past. Most cases of polio in the United States in the recent past have either been imported from other countries or are related to vaccine virus.

The relative safety and efficacy of inactivated vs. attenuated poliovirus vaccines has become a topic of recent concern among scientists, laymen, and politicians. On the one hand, live attentuated vaccine provides both intestinal and systemic immunity but may result rarely in clinical poliomyelitis. On the other hand, inactivated virus vaccine is unassociated with the risk of vaccine-induced polio but does not provide protection against poliovirus replication in the gastrointestinal tract. In the United States, prior to attenuated vaccine availability, and in Finland and Sweden, where only inactivated vaccines have been used, polio has been reduced 80 to 90 percent from prevaccination incidence. Proponents of the live vaccine point to several factors: (1) the inability of inactivated vaccine to restrict gastrointestinal tract multiplication and, therefore, the potential for spread of wild poliovirus, (2) the necessity for repetitive boosters to maintain inactivated vaccine-derived immunity, (3) the failure of inactivated vaccine to always prevent polio in the recipient (more than 30 percent of the cases of paralytic polio in some epidemics occurred despite three or

four doses of inactivated vaccine), and (4) the lesser practicality of a four-dose primary immunization schedule and the need for booster doses to maintain immunity.

Concerns over liability following paralytic polio associated with attenuated poliovirus vaccine have heightened this controversy. The immunization strategy for polio is subtly changing and inactivated vaccine has become a choice for some physicians and patients. The major advisory bodies and a recent special committee of the Institute of Medicine still recommend live vaccine but have become permissive in their recommendations towards inactivated vaccine. This section includes information concerning inactivated vaccine and its use.

Immunizing Antigens

Inactivated Poliovirus Vaccine (IPV). Currently only Connaught Laboratories in Canada manufactures IPV. It is released in the United States through Elkins-Sinn, Inc., 2 Esterbrook Lane, Cherry Hill, New Jersey 08802. The vaccine contains formalin-inactivated polioviruses types 1, 2 and 3, grown in monkey kidney tissue culture. The currently available IPV is more potent than the vaccines used in the 1950's and 1960's. IPV contains trace amounts of formalin, preservatives, and possibly tissue-culture fluid proteins and antibiotics.

Attentuated, Live Poliovirus Vaccine. Oral poliovirus vaccine (OPV) consists of a mixture of the three polioviruses, types 1, 2, and 3, grown either in monkey kidney tissue culture or human fetal-diploid tissue culture. Usually the dose of type 2 poliovirus is adjusted, so as not to overshadow types 1 and 3 on ingestion. The vaccine contains some elements of the tissue culture system, albeit greatly diluted. Monovalent OPV containing the single types alone is usually reserved for use in epidemics and is stockpiled nationally for this purpose. Some physicians prefer monovalent regimens for immunization.

Immunity. There are two known phases of poliovirus immunity: a topical, mucosal phase, and a systemic one. It appears that the secretory IgA antipoliovirus antibody is a significant factor in topical, mucosal immunity. The presence of this antibody in the pharynx, and possibly in the intestinal mucosa as well, serves to neutralize poliovirus and either prevent or limit infection. Other factors also may be involved; the presence of serum antibody correlates directly with immunity and is probably solely responsible for protection from systemic disease.

Systemic immunity is conferred on recipients of both IPV and OPV and also follows recovery from the natural disease. Local immunity has been demonstrated only following successful OPV immunization. Thus it is possible for wild poliovirus to establish and replicate in the gastrointestinal tract of IPV recipients, despite the presence of serum antibody and the lack of symptoms.

Poliovirus immunity is type specific. Following the natural disease, it is lifelong. Thus far OPV seems associated with prolonged immunity (greater than 18 years), perhaps for a lifetime. There is disagreement among experts as to the longevity of immunity derived from IPV. Salk maintains that immunity is very long-lived, particularly using the newer, more potent IPV. Others suggest that booster doses may be necessary every 2 to 4 years.

Schedules for Immunization. Tables 4–2, 4–3, and 4–4 give the recommended schedules for immunization with OPV.

IPV is not manufactured in the United States, and there are no formal recommendations for its use. During the period in which it was the only preparation available, three doses of 1.0 ml each were injected at monthly intervals in infancy; booster doses were given 1 year later, prior to school entry, and were advocated every 2 to 4 years thereafter. If IPV is reintroduced in the United States, dosage and schedules will need to be provided.

Special Circumstances. Breast feeding, once thought to inhibit OPV immunization, is no longer considered in the scheduling.

Pregnancy does not contraindicate OPV administration, but OPV should be given during pregnancy only if the exposure risk is present. Otherwise it is best to administer OPV after delivery.

In epidemics, monovalent vaccine of the type causing the epidemic should be administered to all individuals at risk, regardless of their immunization status.

If a fully immunized individual is traveling to an area endemic for polio or is otherwise subject to increased exposure, a single dose of OPV should be administered.

Any individual suspected of immunodeficiency should not receive poliovirus vaccine containing live virus.

For individuals who have an uncertain polio immunization history, who have been partially immunized with OPV, or who have received only IPV, a single dose of OPV or two doses 8 weeks apart may be indicated.

In epidemic regions it may be desirable to immunize newborns to ensure early protection. The American Academy of Pediatrics advises use of type 1 vaccine in the newborn, as this is the prevalent epidemic type. Of course if other types predominate, epidemic-specific vaccine should be used. This use of monovalent vaccine should not be substituted for full trivalent schedules.

Primary Immunization of Adults. In this context, adults are those who have reached their eighteenth birthday or older. There is an increased risk of paralytic disease in adults given OPV, therefore OPV is *contraindicated* for routine use. TOPV may be used if:

The individual was immunized with OPV prior to age 18 and needs an "insurance" dose because of imminent exposure (for example, foreign travel).

There is no time to give the full series of IPV prior to the expected exposure.

Polio is endemic or epidemic in the community.

The adult elects to receive it after all of the risks are explained and IPV is offered.

Two oral doses of TOPV 8 weeks apart followed by a booster in 8 to 12 months may be utilized.

Adults may be immunized safely with IPV. Consult the manufacturer's brochure for dose and schedule.

The dilemma in regard to use of TOPV in adults is compounded by the fact that contacts of infants who are given TOPV may develop paralytic polio from fecal-oral contamination. This places some susceptible patients and other household and community contacts at risk. It is unclear at present as to how rigorous efforts must be to determine susceptibility, nor is it certain what should be done if such susceptibility is suspected. The optimal course, with present knowledge, would be to give IPV to the adult contacts for a full series before initiating TOPV in the infant.

Adverse Effects of Vaccines. Poliomyelitis due to attenuated poliovirus vaccine, either in persons vaccinated or in their contacts, has been the major cause of paralytic disease in the United States in recent years. The best incidence figures place the risk at 0.06 instances of paralysis per million doses distributed for recipients of OPV, and at 0.14 per million doses in contacts.

Other adverse effects have not been consistently noted. OPV is administered during an age period when many infections and other processes occur that can be confused with OPV etiology. The fact that OPV administration coincides with the occurrence of a specific disease does not establish a relationship.

Persons with immunodeficiency are at increased risk of attentuated poliovirus–associated disease. A number of instances of severe infection have been recorded in such individuals. Therefore, OPV should not be administered to a person with immunodeficiency.

Measles (Rubeola)

Background and Rationale for Active Immunization. In 1962 almost 500,000 cases of measles were reported in the United States alone; in 1972 fewer than 40,000 cases were reported. In the same period encephalitis and deaths from measles also declined dramatically. A resurgence of measles, although not to prevaccine proportions, has occurred in recent years, owing to the failure to provide vaccine to enough of our children. In 1977 a major outbreak (by modern standards) involving more than 50,000 reported cases of measles occurred.

Effective, long-lasting immunity is afforded the recipients of attentuated (live) measles virus vaccine (LMV). The untoward effects of inactivated (killed) measles virus vaccine (KMV) have caused it to be removed from the market.

Live Measles Virus Vaccine (LMV). Though the original LMV developed by Enders, the Edmonston strain, was an effective antigen, its side effects made it unacceptable and it was replaced by the Schwartz strain of further-attenuated vaccine. Both have been replaced by the Moraten strain developed by Merck, Sharp, and Dohme. Its properties resemble those of the Schwartz strain, and it is considered a further-attenuated measles virus (FAMV).

LMV is supplied in lyophilized form for reconstitution just prior to immunization. The manufacturers' directions should be followed explicitly in the storage, reconstitution, and administration of LMV. The virus is fragile and may be rendered inactive if any of the proper steps is omitted or changed. Heating the vaccine, adding improper diluent, using glass syringes, and mixing with immune globulin result in inactivation of the virus.

LMV has been added to mumps virus and rubella virus in varying combinations (see below).

Killed Measles Virus Vaccine (KMV). This is no longer available or used as described here because more than 600,000 children have received it, and its adverse effects are still being observed. KMV was prepared by inactivating live virus grown in tissues derived from monkeys or from chick eggs and adding an adjuvant. It was administered alone or prior to LMV. The usual series consisted of two or three doses, with subsequent boosters of KMV or a dose of LMV. Inactivated vaccine resulted in antibody production in recipients, with short-lived immunity. After a variable period, usually 6 months or longer, recipients of KMV became susceptible to atypical reactions to either attenuated or wild virus. Subsequent LMV administration was associated with local reactions (heat, induration, pain, and rash at the site of inoculation) and, occasionally, with systemic reactions (fever, regional adenopathy, headache, malaise).

Exposure to wild virus results in a bizarre disease with an atypical eruption (atypical distribution, with peripheral accentuation and onset of the rash, vesicles, petechiae, and purpura), severe systemic symptoms (fever, headache, lethargy, uncoordination), and specific tissue symptoms (pneumonia, serositis, and pleural, peritoneal, and CNS symptoms). Extremely high antibody titers and a skin reaction thought to be either a CMI (delayed hypersensitivity type) or an Arthus (antibody-antigen complex type) reaction were noted. This syndrome is termed "atypical measles" and has now been observed as long as 17 years after receipt of KMV.

Immunity. Recovery from measles virus infection is probably independent of antibody synthesis. Hypogammaglobulinemic individuals with intact cell-mediated immunity have a normal course of measles virus infection. Immunity to measles on subsequent exposure, on the other hand, is directly correlated with the presence of antibody. Other factors, notably cell-mediated immunity, may be important, but antibody alone seems sufficient. Administration of antibody can protect an individual completely on exposure to wild virus.

Natural measles immunity is lifelong. Immunity following LMV immunization is believed to be equal to that seen after the natural disease. However, observation of LMV recipients has been possible only for 17 years. During that interval, individuals with demonstrable antibody after LMV have been protected against wild virus exposure. The FAMV vaccine has a shorter history: only 14 years have elapsed since its first use, but immunity has been sustained during this period, despite low antibody levels.

Measles has occurred in vaccine recipients and is usually due to one of the following factors:

1. *Administration of LMV prior to 15 months of age*. LMV was originally recommended for infants 12 months of age and younger; it is now known that LMV may be ineffective owing to persistent maternally derived immunity, even in the absence of detectable serum antibody in the infant. If, in addition, the LMV was given with MIG before 1 year of age, the risk of immunization failure is increased. As many as 35 percent of infants given LMV at 9 months of age may not be immunized. The data conflict on the efficacy of immunization at 12 months of age. Some studies have shown a failure rate of 15 to 22 percent at 12 months of age; others have shown as little as 3 to 5 percent failure, the minimum achievable.

2. *Use of impotent vaccine*. For a host of reasons (improper storage, dilution, or administration), LMV may be inactivated prior to administration.

3. *The "natural" failure rate*. LMV does not successfully immunize all recipients; 3 to 5 percent may not respond despite adequate vaccine and administration technique.

4. Continuing studies by Cherry and others suggest that some failures may be "true" vaccine failures. Thus far, this seems to be rare.

5. *Prior KMV vaccine recipients* of killed measles virus vaccine may develop a severe form of measles upon exposure to wild virus (see Adverse Effects).

Schedules for Active Immunization. Tables 4–2, 4–3, and 4–4 present the recom-

mended schedule for immunization. Certain precautions are advisable in LMV use:

Whenever feasible, a tuberculin test should be performed prior to LMV administration. There is a theoretic risk of exacerbating silent tuberculosis. If prior tuberculin testing is not feasible, simultaneous testing can be substituted. In community vaccination campaigns or in clinical circumstances in which only a single opportunity for contact exists, the prior tuberculin test may have to be eliminated for practical reasons.

Illnesses, particularly febrile illnesses, contra-indicate LMV administration.

Any defect in cell-mediated immunity is a contraindication to LMV administration.

Pregnancy contraindicates LMV use.

LMV should not be given for 2 or 3 months following immune serum globulin (ISG) administration. Measles neutralizing antibody in ISG can counteract effective immunization.

Skin testing with a 1:100 dilution of LMV prepared in egg-derived tissue culture should be performed before administering the vaccine to egg-sensitive individuals.

Special Circumstances. Since children previously given KMV may experience adverse reactions to LMV and are susceptible to atypical measles on exposure to wild virus, the situation should be discussed with the parents and consent for further use of measles vaccine should be obtained. The recommendation is to immunize such children with a single subcutaneous dose of FAMV. Local reactions occur in 10 to 50 percent of children (heat, induration, and tenderness), and systemic symptoms occur in 3 to 10 percent.

If an unimmunized child is exposed to natural measles and is promptly brought to a physician's attention, LMV administration may prevent measles. This protection occurs because LMV has a shorter incubation period than natural measles (7 days as opposed to 11 days).

Children who received their original LMV prior to 12 months of age should be given a second dose of LMV after 15 months of age, since protection from the first dose is uncertain. Considerable confusion exists at present as to the necessity for reimmunizing children who previously received their LMV at 12 months of age. Since the data are conflicting and the risk appears small, routine reimmunization is *not* recommended. If exposure risk to natural disease is high, then reimmunization may be warranted.

In measles epidemics, with high risk of

exposure in infants, one may wish to immunize infants between 6 and 15 months of age with LMV without simultaneous measles immune globulin (MIG). It must be appreciated that some infants will not be immunized but will be protected by natural transplacental immunity. All infants who are under 15 months of age when immunized during epidemic conditions must receive a second dose of LMV at or after 15 months of age.

For individuals who cannot be given LMV due to risks associated with their underlying disease, condition, or age, the use of preventive amounts of MIG on exposure must be considered.

Adverse Effects of LMV. The usual fever and rash in association with LMV have been described. LMV has resulted in disseminated disease and death in individuals with depressed immune function involving absent or diminished cell-mediated immunity. Although a variety of acute CNS disorders have occurred within 30 days of LMV administration, none has definitely been attributed to LMV and a few have been identified as caused by other viruses.

Subacute sclerosing panencephalitis, the slow measles-virus infection of the central nervous system, has been described following LMV at an extremely low incidence, considerably less than that associated with wild virus infection.

Theoretically, tuberculosis can be exacerbated by LMV administration. Several instances of tuberculous meningitis were described within 30 days of LMV administration. However, direct evidence for worsening of tuberculosis secondary to LMV is lacking. Treated tuberculosis is not a contraindication to measles vaccine.

Although a potential problem, egg-sensitive children deliberately immunized with the vaccine virus grown from chick embryo tissue culture have not reacted unusually, although a skin test to the vaccine prior to immunization as already described is a wise precaution.

Passive Immunity. Immune serum globulin (ISG) contains a variable amount of measles antibody; MIG has been adjusted to contain 4000 measles virus–neutralizing units per milliliter. Use of the calibrated product, MIG, results in more certain dosage and effect. MIG or ISG may be used to prevent or modify measles in an exposed, susceptible individual. The usual dose is 0.25 ml per kg of body weight. Protection of children suspect-ed or know to have CMI defects may require 20 to 30 ml ISG on exposure.

Rubella (German Measles)

Background and Rationale for Active Immunization. Rubella is a mild viral disease of childhood and early adult life, with few complications. However, as many as 15 to 20 percent of adults have escaped childhood infection and are susceptible to rubella. Among women of childbearing age this susceptibility can result in infection during critical periods in fetal development. Rubella viremia and subsequent placental and fetal infection result in the congenital rubella syndrome.

Immunization of all children has been the goal in the nearly 10 years of rubella vaccine usage. Field experience has led to some modifications of the original premises as follows:

1. The premise that approximately 15 percent of women of childbearing age are susceptible is correct, but very few are at risk since they must be not only infected but also infected exactly at certain stages of pregnancy for fetal involvement with rubella virus to occur.

2. Despite adequate immunization of as many as 95 percent of a given population, the remaining susceptibles are *not* protected. Rubella infection has occurred among the non-immune with an attack rate identical to that observed in virgin populations.

3. Rubella vaccine does have a number of attributes either not appreciated or not known during the initial trials. The vaccine results in virus spread in the recipient such that 75 percent of vaccinees will have virus, in low titer, recoverable from the throat. No convincing evidence for communicability has been noted. Immunity is not persistent, as was thought during the investigative trials. Rubella vaccine–induced antibody decreases after vaccination to a degree that permits reinfection in as many as 75 percent of the recipients. Such reinfection has been asymptomatic and unassociated with detectable viremia.

Rubella vaccine has been associated with some side effects not described during the initial trials. A painful and persistent neuropathy involving the nerves of either the arms or the legs occurs in a small proportion of vaccinees. Symptoms of arthritis and arthralgia appeared in greater numbers of children than predicted from the field trials. Canine kidney adapted rubella virus vaccine was associated with a larger number of side effects than the original duck embryo grown vaccine, and the dog kidney product has been withdrawn from the market.

4. Rubella infection of the fetus can result from vaccine virus.

The long-term immunity of rubella immunization is still uncertain, but its wide-scale use seems prudent at present and is recommended by all expert committees.

Immunizing Antigens. The original vaccine candidate strain HPV-77 has been passaged in duck embryo tissue culture. Rubella vaccine is a biological that contains live virus, and all of the usual precautions in storage, maintenance, and administration should be observed.

Immunity. It is likely that cell-mediated immunity is responsible for recovery from and immunity to rubella. Antibody plays a role, but infection has been noted in individuals with detectable titer. Recurrent infection with rubella virus is difficult to document in the absence of specific viral diagnostic tests for each episode.

Infants with congenital rubella demonstrate persistent or chronic infection with the agent despite high levels of serum antibodies. It is suspected that persistent rubella virus infection results from direct viral infection of lymphocytes, rendering them unresponsive to rubella antigens. With recovery from lymphocyte infection, cell-mediated immunity is restored and the virus is eradicated.

The fetus is susceptible to rubella virus and initially offers no defense. With persistence of the virus, an immune response characterized by specific IgM antibody develops. Thus the neonate with congenital rubella has both virus and antibody present.

A syndrome analogous to subacute sclerosing panencephalitis has been observed following congenital rubella.

Schedules for Immunization. Tables 4–2, 4–3, and 4–4 present the recommended immunization schedules.

Special Circumstances. Exposure to rubella cannot be "treated" by rubella vaccination; vaccine may be given in the hope that no disease will occur and for protection in case of future exposure.

Primary Immunizaton for Females at or Beyond Menarche. In this strategy, only those whose potential offspring are at risk receive the vaccine. All female children just prior to menarche and all females in the child-bearing years who lack rubella antibody are candidates.

For all postmenarchal females the following conditions must be met: (1) A serum antibody titer from a reliable laboratory must demonstrate absence of rubella antibody. (2) The candidate must not be pregnant. (3) Measures to prevent pregnancy must be taken for at least 2 months following immunization. (4) Full knowledge of the risks of immunization if pregnancy occurs within 2 months must be available to and understood by the recipient (and parents). (5) The recipient (and parents) should be aware of the possible occurrence of arthralgia and arthritis following immunization. The actual immunization procedures does not differ from that for children.

In certain closed or limited population groups, such as colleges, institutions, and military camps, it may be desirable to immunize exposed individuals in an attempt to limit or halt an epidemic. All precautions related to postmenarchal females should be observed. Other adverse effects include infrequent instances of thrombocytopenia, rash, or lymphadenopathy.

Passive Immunization. Specific rubella immune globulin is not available. Different lots of ISG vary markedly in rubella antibody content, which may prevent rash but not infection.

There is no convincing evidence that ISG can protect an exposed, susceptible pregnant woman from rubella or her fetus from congenital rubella. Inapparent infection may occur with virus transmission to the fetus following ISG administration.

Mumps

Background and Rationale for Active Immunization. Though mumps is usually a mild disease in preteenagers, it can be severe in adults. Mumps causes orchitis in almost 20 percent of postpubertal males. This is a painful, incapacitating disease, although sterility, a feared consequence, is extremely rare.

Mumps causes meningoencephalitis and is suspected of being one cause of juvenile diabetes mellitus. Unilateral deafness and nephritis have also been described.

Live mumps virus, isolated from Dr. Maurice Hilleman's daughter, Jeryl Lynn, was attenuated by passage in chick embryo tissue culture. The emergence of a combined vaccine (measles, mumps, and rubella) allowed for easy immunization of the 15-month-old patient, leading to the common practice of using this vaccine routinely for all infants, despite earlier reservations about its use.

Immunizing Antigen. Live mumps virus vaccine, grown in chick embryo tissue culture, is a derivative of the Jeryl Lynn isolate and protects 95 percent of recipients with minimal adverse effects.

Immunity. Mumps virus induces cell-mediated immunity, and mumps virus antigens injected intradermally result in a delayed-type response. Durable immunity follows natural disease; instances of two or more episodes of ''mumps'' may be related to other viral agents which can produce parotitis.

Schedules for Immunization. Tables 4-2, 4-3, and 4-4 present recommended immunization schedules.

Primary Immunization in Prepubertal Males and Adult Males. If desired, mumps virus vaccine can be administered to prepubertal and adult males. A history of mumps can be deceptive, as other viruses occasionally produce parotitis. Failure to recall having mumps is no guarantee that a person has not been infected; 30 percent of childhood mumps are asymptomatic. The author believes that any prepubertal boy can be given live mumps vaccine. Adult males can be tested for mumps antibody; approximately 15 percent will be susceptible.

Special Circumstances. Live mumps virus vacine, after exposure to mumps, does not protect against the current exposure, but, if no disease ensues, offers protection against subsequent exposures.

Adverse Effects of Vaccine. No significant adverse effects have been attributed to live mumps virus vaccine.

Passive Immunization. A specific mumps immune globulin is commerically available but is of unproved efficacy and is not recommended.

Combined Vaccines

The most commonly employed combinations of vaccine products include:

DTP — Diphtheria, tetanus and pertussis.

DT (Pediatric) — Full dosage of both diphtheria and tetanus toxoids, intended for use solely before the seventh birthday.

Td (Adult) — Full dose of tetanus and reduced amounts of diphtheria toxoid. In-

tended for use solely in individuals age 7 or older.

MMR — Measles, mumps and rubella viruses. Intended for simultaneous, primary immunization at any age, but usually in infancy or childhood.

MuR — Mumps virus and rubella virus. Intended for those already immune to measles (rubeola).

MR — Measles and rubella virus. Intended for use in individuals in whom mumps virus immunization is not desirable.

All of these combinations are manufacturers' formulations, rigorously tested for stability, efficacy, and safety. *Ad hoc* combinations have also been utilized, but great care must be exercised. The following caveats should be observed:

Different, single vaccines should not be combined into a single injection. Physical incompatibilities may exist that could result in inactivation or alteration of the active component.

Efficacy for the separate, simultaneous administration of different, single vaccines must have been demonstrated before they are used in clinical practice.

Cumulative side effects must be taken into account whenever two or more products are administered simultaneously.

Never do anything in combination specifically contraindicated, or not specifically recommended. For example, do not mix a globulin (antibody) with a vaccine (antigen) unless that combination is specifically recommended.

Avoid sequences of viral vaccines with short intervals between the separate formulations. Such sequences may result in inhibition of the immune response of the subsequent vaccines.

Some ''combinations'' that have been successfully employed include: DPT and TOPV; DPT, TOPV and MMR (limited data); MMR and TOPV, third and fourth doses.

ACTIVE AND PASSIVE IMMUNIZATIONS OCCASIONALLY OR INFREQUENTLY USED

Cholera. Currently available cholera vaccines are of limited value. On occasion they are required for foreign travel, and individuals older than 6 months of age must receive them. The American Academy of Pediatrics Redbook provides specific dosage recommendations.

Plague. Plague vaccine is recommended only for those traveling to or residing in areas where plague is occurring and domestic rats are known to be infected. For specific dosage recommendations and for those few children who will require this immunization, consult the American Academy of Pediatrics Redbook.

Typhoid. Routine typhoid vaccination is no longer recommended for persons living in the United States. Selective immunization can be given to persons with imminent exposure to a documented typhoid carrier, and to persons traveling to areas where there is an increased risk of exposure to typhoid. Typhoid vaccine should not be used in areas of natural disaster or for persons attending such rural activities as summer camps.

Children less than 10 years old should receive 0.25 ml of typhoid vaccine subcutaneously twice, separated by 4 or more weeks. Children over 10 years old should receive 0.5 ml of vaccine on the same schedule. Booster doses should be given at least every 3 years with continued exposure.

Yellow Fever. Yellow fever vaccine is administered only in public health facilities in the United States and is used exclusively for individuals traveling to areas of the world that are endemic for yellow fever. A single subcutaneous injection of 0.5 ml of vaccine constitutes primary immunization.

Meningococcal Vaccine. Approximately 3000 to 6000 cases of meningococcal infection occur each year in all age groups, and epidemics are noted approximately every 10 years. In the continental United States sera groups B and C produce the majority of disease though recently other groups appear to be emerging as responsible for disease.

There are two polysaccharide vaccines available, consisting of capsular material from meningococci types A and C. The vaccines are specific to each type and do not provide any cross-protection. These vaccines are highly antigenic for individuals older than 2 years of age. Like other polysaccharide bacterial vaccines, they fail to stimulate significant antibody in young infants and cannot be used under 2 years of age. Selective use of the vaccines include travelers to epidemic areas and household contacts in conjunction with antimicrobial prophylaxis.

Pneumococcal Vaccine. Pneumococci produce significant clinical illness in children. Although there are more than 80 types of pneumococci, only a few types account for more than 80 percent of all infections. A few children have a condition in which pneumococci cause serious, or even life-threatening, disease. Examples include congenital asplenia, surgically splenectomized patients, and sicklemia in which infarction of the spleen produces so-called autosplenectomy, the nephrotic syndrome, and certain B cell immunodeficiencies that predispose to pneumococcal sepsis. In recent years, emergence of partially or totally penicillin-resistant pneumococci has been described abroad. This has spurred efforts at active immunization.

Pneumovac (Merck, Sharp and Dohme) consists of 50 mcg each of 14 types of pneumococcal capsular polysaccharides. The vaccine is administered as a single dose of 0.5 ml, intramuscularly or subcutaneously. The polysaccharide is suspended in isotonic saline and contains 0.25 percent phenol as a preservative. The vaccine appears to be effective in children older than 2 years of age. The only trial reported thus far in children indicated that vaccination produced a statistically significant decrease in the mortality rate from serious pneumococcal infections in children with sicklemia. Local reactions are the primary side effect and are generally mild.

Children with asplenia, sickle cell disease, and nephrotic syndrome should be immunized when older than 2 years of age. At the present time, there are no other indications in children for the use of pneumococcal vaccine.

Influenza Immunization. Children with severe cardiopulmonary disease should be immunized against influenza because of their high risk for morbidity and mortality. There is a difference of opinion concerning immunizing the child with uncomplicated asthma, inasmuch as many allergists feel that such children are no more susceptible to complications from influenza than are normal children. On the other hand, others contend that children with asthma fare poorly with influenza infection and should receive routine immunization.

Influenza virus vaccine varies in its specific composition from year to year as judged by the currently epidemic strains. Some useful generalizations can be made about influenza vaccine, however. Influenza vaccine consists of inactivated influenza A and B viruses representative of currently prevalent strains. In general, all vaccines prepared are bivalent, that is, they contain both A and B antigens. Each dose of vaccine will contain a specified amount of antigen distributed between the two types of A and B virus strains prevalent. Specific dosage recommendations will vary from year to year, and the recommendations of the American Academy of Pediatrics and the Center for Disease Control should be consulted for specific usage.

Two types of vaccine are available for clinical use. First is a whole virus preparation that includes capsid antigens of the virus. The second type of vaccine is "split-virus," which contains antigens produced by chemically disrupting the influenza virion. At the present time only split product influenza vaccines are recommended for persons less than 18 years old because of their heightened reactivity when they receive whole virus vaccine.

Infrequent side effects of influenza immunization include:

1. Systemic reaction — fever, malaise, myalgia — which may persist for one or two days.

2. An immediate hypersensitivity reaction, presumably on an allergic basis. These reactions are very uncommon. When the practitioner is confronted with a history of egg allergy, several courses are possible. If the risk from influenza is small, the vaccine should not be administered. If the risk is significant, an intradermal skin test with a 1:100 dilution of the vaccine to be used should be employed. If there is no immediate reaction, the vaccine can be safely administered. With an immediate reaction, it is best to forego immunization in that child. An alternative method of prophylaxis exists in the use of Amantadine (see Glezen, 1977).

3. The Guillain-Barré syndrome, which can result in permanent residual muscle weakness (5 to 10 percent) or death (5 percent), was observed in some patients after swine influenza immunization in 1976. It is not clear whether there is an increased risk of this complication associated with all influenza products, but it seems prudent to warn patients or parents of this possibility before influenza immunizations.

Rabies. Immunoprophylaxis against rabies for animal bites is an extremely complicated subject. Both hyperimmune rabies globulin and duck embryo rabies vaccine are currently available for immunoprophylaxis. For specific indications and dosage recommendations, refer to the standard sources of the American Academy of Pediatrics and the Center for Disease Control.

Our approach to this problem might be considerably simplified if the newly developed diploid rabies vaccine were introduced into the American market. This vaccine has been tested extensively abroad and has distinct advantages: (1) safety from neural paralytic complications and (2) increased antigenicity, when compared with duck embryo vaccine. It is anticipated that this product will be licensed shortly, and specific recommendations for its use will be promulgated.

ACTIVE AND PASSIVE IMMUNIZATIONS OF THE FUTURE

Varicella Virus Vaccine. A live virus vaccine using an attenuated strain of varicella virus has been developed and tested in Japan. The virus has been attenuated by multiple passage in a variety of subhuman and human diploid cell lines. The results of Japanese investigations thus far permit the following conclusions: (1) Seroconversion occurs at the 98 percent level, and antibody has persisted for at least 2 years. (2) Side effects have been minimal. (3) Children with malignancy have been given the vaccine without significant side effects. Fever and mild rash of brief duration have been noted in a few children with lymphatic malignancies. (4) No instances of zoster recrudescence in vaccinated children have yet been detected.

The use of vaccines of the herpes group, including varicella vaccine, has been the subject of intense debate in the United States. This debate is occasioned by the capacity of this group of viruses to become "latent," i.e., to remain within central nervous system tissue in a nondetectable state, only to emerge subsequently and produce clinical symptoms. Because of the concerns over this biologic property of the virus, varicella virus vaccine will be developed only slowly in the United States.

Haemophilus Influenzae Vaccine. This vaccine consists of extracted capsular polysaccharides of the type B *H. influenzae*. All human work thus far has been done with this polysaccharide vaccine. An improved protein polysaccharide antigen is being tested in animals but has not reached the human testing stage.

From data accumulated in Finland, Brazil, and North Carolina, it appears that the following conclusions are warranted: (1) Infants less than 18 months of age respond poorly or not at all to this antigen. (2) Antibody production in infants immunized at an early age is not increased by booster doses. (3) Individuals older than 18 months of age are protected against disease due to H. influenza Type B.

Some trials are underway to study antibody production and efficacy of the current vaccine. Most experts agree that a new approach must be developed, particularly for young infants to protect them against this organism.

Diploid Rubella Vaccine. A new attenuated-virus vaccine, grown in human diploid cells and labeled Wistar RA 27/3, has been developed. This vaccine has been licensed and used extensively abroad and will soon be available in the United States.

In comparison to the current duck embryo vaccine, RA 27/3 produces quantitatively higher antibody responses, will boost antibody titers in previous recipients of duck embryo vaccines, and has fewer side effects. Seroconversion rates of 95 to 100 percent have been reported.

Respiratory Virus Vaccines. Vaccines against important respiratory agents in children other than influenza have met with dismal failures thus far. Although inactivated vaccines have been developed that stimulate the appropriate antibody responses, they have failed to protect, and in a few instances have increased morbidity and mortality from the agent. The current approach is to try to develop attenuated live virus vaccines. Thus far, these experimental vaccines have caused significant illness in young children to whom they were administered.

PASSIVE IMMUNIZATION

Immune serum globulin pooled from a large number of adults is indicated in measles prophylaxis, protection from hepatitis A, replacement of IgG in IgG-deficiency states, and protection against minimal exposure hepatitis B. Replacement therapy in immunodeficient states is discussed in Chapter 7; measles immunoprophylaxis is discussed earlier in this chapter.

Hepatitis A. Individuals exposed to active excreters of hepatitis A virus may be afforded protection against overt disease by the prompt administration of immune serum globulin. In pediatric practice this usually is limited to household contacts or exposure that simulates household contacts, such as occurs in nursery schools or institutional living facilities. Immune serum globulin is administered intramuscularly in a dose of 0.02 to 0.04 ml per kg of body weight as a single injection.

With continuous exposure, such as occurs among attendants in residential facilities, one might wish to use 0.06 ml per kg of body weight, repeated once every 5 to 6 months.

Hepatitis B. Immune serum globulin can also be used in cases of minimal exposure to hepatitis B virus. Such minimal exposure would occur in situations where a needle contaminated with hepatitis B–containing blood scratches the skin of an uninfected susceptible individual. In order to attempt to prevent hepatitis B in such circumstances, 0.12 ml per kg of body weight of immune serum globulin can be given. Alternatively, one may wish to use hepatitis B immune serum globulin, a product containing much larger amounts of hepatitis B antibody. If hepatitis B immune globulin is to be used, it should be used in a dose of 0.06 ml per kg of body weight, up to 5 ml for an adult.

There are many practitioners who use specific immune globulins or immune serum globulin in circumstances in which there is little or no demonstration of its efficacy. We have already discussed the inadequacy of ISG in the prophylaxis of rubella infection during pregnancy.

Some individuals use immune serum globulin in large doses in an effort to prevent varicella. Very young infants exposed to varicella usually experience a mild disease but, on occasion, may have very severe disease. In such circumstances it would be preferable to use zoster immune globulin, which has a higher level of antibody. However, ZIG is not readily available, and large doses of ISG are at times substituted. There is limited data concerning the efficacy of ISG in these circumstances, and the reader is advised to consult standard sources of recommendations for its use.

Unwarranted use of passive immunization with ISG include its use in burns, in specific bacterial infections for which antibody offers no protection, for treatment of recurrent Herpes simplex infections, and in the management of allergic asthma. Chapter 7 discusses use of gamma globulin in greater detail.

Other uses of globulins have included attempts to prevent pertussis in susceptible individuals by using pertussis immune globulin. Similarly, mumps immune globulin has been used in an effort to prevent mumps orchitis in postpubescent males. Neither use has proved efficacious, and in some trials no effect at all has been demonstrated. The author does not recommend the use of specific immune globulins of ISG in either pertussis prophylaxis or therapy or in prevention of mumps orchitis.

Types of Immunologically Mediated Adverse Reactions. Adverse effects following passive immunization are either direct effects of the immunizing products, which vary from local irritation to severe infection of such target organs as the central nervous system, or indirect "allergic" affects. Type I reactions may occur in individuals hypersensitive to a component of the immunizing agent or the vaccine. For example, erythema multiforme following vaccinia vaccination is thought to result from hypersensitivity to some component of the virus. Type I reactions also occur to egg protein, antibiotics, or some other component in the formulation to which the individual is sensitive.

References

This chapter has not given extensive references since much of the information is readily available in a variety of sources. Presented here for the reader seeking additional information are a few general references and a selection of specific references related to individual topics in the chapter.

GENERAL

American Academy of Pediatrics. *Report of the Committee on Infectious Diseases* ("Redbook"), 18th ed. Evanston. Illinois, 1977.

Benenson, A. S. (ed.): *Control of Communicable Diseases in Man,* 12th ed. American Public Health Association, Washington, D.C., 1975.

Fulginiti, V. A.: Active and passive immunization in the control of infectious diseases. *In* Stiehm, R., and Fulginiti, V.: *Immunologic Disorders in Infants and Children,* 2nd ed. Philadelphia, W.B. Saunders Co., 1980.

Krugman, S., Ward, R., and Katz, S.: *Infectious Diseases of Children,* 6th ed. pp. 481–514. C. V. Mosley Co., St. Louis, 1977.

DIPHTHERIA

Brooks, G. F.: Diphtheria in the United States. J. Infect. Dis. *129*:172, 1974.

Center for Disease Control. Diphtheria Surveillance, Report #12, July 1978. Atlanta, United States Department of Health, Education and Welfare.

Morbidity and Mortality Weekly Reports, Diphtheria and Tetanus Toxoids and Pertussis Vaccines, *26*:401, Dec. 9, 1977.

Nelson, L. A., et al.: Immunity to diphtheria in an urban population. Pediatrics *61*:703, 1978.

TETANUS

Blake, P. A., et al.: Serologic therapy of tetanus in the United States. J.A.M.A. *235*:42, 1976.

Morbidity and Mortality Weekly Reports. Diphtheria and Tetanus Toxoids and Pertussis Vaccines, *26*:401, Dec. 9, 1977.

Trinca, J. C.: Antibody response to successive booster doses of tetanus toxoid in adults. Infect. Immun. *10*:1, 1974.

Weinstein, L.: Tetanus. N. Engl. J. Med. *289*:1293, 1973.

PERTUSSIS

Morbidity and Mortality Weekly Reports. Diphtheria and Tetanus Toxoids and Pertussis Vaccines, *26*:401, Dec. 9, 1977.

Griffith, A. H.: Reactions after pertussis vaccine, Br. Med. J. *1*:809, 1978.

Kendrick, P. L.: Can whooping cough be eradicated? J. Infect. Dis. *132*:707, 1975.

Linnemann, C. C., Jr., et al.: Use of pertussis vaccine in an epidemic involving hospital staff. Lancet *2*:540, 1975.

Stewart, G. T.: Vaccination against whooping cough — Efficacy versus Risks. Lancet *1*:234, 1977.

POLIOVIRUS VACCINES

American Academy of Pediatrics, Committee on Infectious Diseases. Poliovirus Immunization Re-examined, News & Comment, 27(12 Suppl.), 1976.

Morbidity and Mortality Weekly Reports. Poliomyelitis Prevention, *26*:329, 1977.

Nightingale, E.: Recommendations for a national policy on poliomyelitis vaccination. N. Engl. J. Med. *297*:249, 1977.

Salk, J., and Salk, D.: Control of influenza and poliomyelitis with killed virus vaccines. Science *195*:834, 1977.

MEASLES

American Academy of Pediatrics, Committee on Infectious Diseases. Measles Vaccine Recommendations, News & Comment, June 1977.

Cherry, J., et al.: Urban measles in the vaccine era: A clinical, epidemiologic and serologic study. J. Pediatr. *81*:217, 1972.

Krugman, S.: Present status of measles and rubella immunization in the United States. A medical progress report. J. Pediatr. *90*:1, 1977.

Morbidity and Mortality Weekly Reports. Measles Vaccine, *25*:359, 1976.

Morbidity and Mortality Weekly Reports. SSPE & Measles, *26*:309, 1978.

Wilkins, J., and Wehrle, P.: Evidence for reinstatement of infants 12–14 months of age into routine immunization programs. Am. J. Dis. Child. *132*:164, 1978.

RUBELLA

Harstmann, D.: Controlling rubella: problems and perspectives. Ann. Intern. Med. *83*:412, 1975.

Krugman, S.: Present status of measles and rubella immunization in the United States. A medical progress report. J. Pediatr. *90*:1, 1977.

Morbidity and Mortality Weekly Reports. Rubella Vaccine, *26*:385, 1977.

Modlin, J. F., et al.: Risk of congenital anomaly after inadvertent rubella vaccination of pregnant women. N. Engl. J. Med. *294*:972, 1976.

Weible, R. E., et al.: Long-term follow-up for immunity after monovalent or combined live measles, mumps and rubella virus vaccines. Pediatrics *56*:380, 1975.

MUMPS

Biedel, C. W.: Recurrent mumps parotitis following natural infection and immunization. Am. J. Dis. Child. *132*:678, 1978.

Modin, J. F., et al.: Current status of mumps in the United States, J. Infect. Dis. *132*:106, 1975.

Morbidity and Mortality Weekly Reports. Mumps Vaccine, *26*:393, 1977.

Weible, R. E., et al.: Long-term follow-up for immunity after monovalent or combined live measles, mumps and rubella virus vaccines. Pediatrics *56*:380, 1975.

CHOLERA

Morbidity and Mortality Weekly Reports. Cholera Vaccine, *27*:173, 1978.

PLAGUE

Morbidity and Mortality Weekly Reports. Plague Vaccine, *27*:256, 1978.

TYPHOID

Morbidity and Mortality Weekly Reports. Typhoid Vaccination Following Natural Disasters, *26*:127, 1977.

Morbidity and Mortality Weekly Reports. Typhoid Vaccine, *27*:231, 1978.

YELLOW FEVER

Morbidity and Mortality Weekly Reports. Yellow Fever Vaccine, *27*:268, 1978.

PNEUMOCOCCAL VACCINE

Arnman, A. J., et al.: Polyvalent pneumococcal polysaccharide immunization of patients with sickle-cell anemia and patients with splenectomy. N. Engl. J. Med. *297*:897, 1977.

Morbidity and Mortality Weekly Reports. Pneumococcal Polysaccharide Vaccine, *27*:25, 1978.

MENINGOCOCCAL VACCINE

Morbidity and Mortality Weekly Reports. Meningococcal Polysaccharide Vaccines, *27*:327, 1978.

HEMOPHILUS INFLUENZAE VACCINE

Makela, P. H., et al.: Polysaccharide vaccines of group A *Neisseria meningitidis* and *Hemophilus influenzae* type B: A field trial in Finland. J. Infect. Dis. *136*:S43, 1977.

Parke, J. C., et al.: Interim report of a controlled field trial of immunization with capsular polysaccharides of *Hemophilus influenzae* type B and group C *Neisseria meningitidis* in Mecklenburg County. North Carolina. J. Infect. Dis. *136*:S51, 1977.

INFLUENZAE VACCINE

Glezen, W. P.: Influenza prophylaxis for children. Am. J. Dis. Child. *131*:628, 1977.

Morbidity and Mortality Weekly Reports. Follow-up Guillain-Barré Syndrome—United States, *26*:52, 1977.

Morbidity and Mortality Weekly Reports. Influenza Vaccine, *27*:351, 1978.

Salk, J. and Salk, D.: Control of influenza and poliomyelitis with killed virus vaccines. Science *195*:834, 1977.

Summary of clinical trials of influenza vaccine. J. Infect. Dis. *134*:100, 1976.

Summary of clinical trials of influenza vaccine, II. J. Infect. Dis. *134*:633, 1976.

RABIES VIRUS VACCINES

Bahmanyar, M., et al.: Successful protection of humans exposed to rabies infection. J.A.M.A. *236*:2751, 1976.

Nicholson, K. G.: Immunization with a human diploid cell strain of rabies virus vaccine: Two year results. J. Infect. Dis. *137*:77, 1978.

VARICELLA VACCINE

Asono, Y., et al.: Protection against varicella in family contacts by immediate inoculation with live varicella vaccine. Pediatrics *59*:3, 1977.

Brunel, P.: Protection against varicella. Pediatrics *59*:1, 1977.

Hans D. Ochs, M.D.
Clifton T. Furukawa, M.D.

5

Host Defense Mechanisms

Clinical observations, animal experiments, and laboratory studies have identified an intricate defense system that prevents invasion and destruction of the host by microorganisms. Disorders of these systems may lead to undue susceptibility to infections, to collagen-vascular diseases, or to allergic manifestations. This chapter will discuss the complement system, phagocytes, and nonspecific defense mechanisms. The physiology of B and T lymphocytes has been described in Chapter 1.

COMPLEMENT

During the late nineteenth century, the bactericidal activity of fresh serum was noted to consist of at least two components: a heat-stable "specific" factor (antibody) and a heat-labile "nonspecific" component (complement). The multicomponent nature and the molecular basis of the complement system were recognized after specific functional and histochemical assays became available (Müller-Eberhard, 1975). The classic complement cascade consists of nine components which either are activated by specific enzymes or become part of a multimolecular complex. Recently, the presence of an "alternative" pathway was confirmed that bypasses the early complement components by activating C3 directly (Gewurz and Lint, 1977).

The nomenclature of this complex system has recently been simplified by assigning each component of the classic pathway a number in the order of its discovery. The sequence of activation for the early components is C1, 4, 2, 3; the later components are activated in the numerically proper sequence C5, 6, 7, 8, 9. C1 is a macromolecule consisting of three distinct subunits (C1q, C1r, C1s). Activated components are designated by a bar above the symbol (e.g., $\overline{C1}$). If a component is split by the enzymatic activity of another component, the small fragment is usually (C2 is an exception) indicated by the letter "a" (e.g., C3a), and the larger component that participates in the complex formation is designated by the letter "b" (e.g., C3b).

Components of the alternative (properdin) pathway are designated by capital letters: B (factor B), formerly known as C3 proactivator (C3PA) or glycine-rich-B-globulin (GBG); D (factor D), also known as C3PA-convertase or pro-GBGase; P indicates properdin. Activation of these components is indicated by a bar ($\overline{B}$, $\overline{D}$, $\overline{P}$).

Methods of evaluating the complement system and measuring individual complement-compounds are described in Chapter 8.

Classic Complement Pathway (Fig. 5–1). The early acting components (C1–C5) are activated enzymatically: each activated component will transform the following component to an active enzyme, resulting in a cascade-like pattern. The classic complement pathway can be activated by soluble or insoluble antigen-antibody complexes or by aggregated immunoglobulins. During activation, C1 (via the C1q molecule) is fixed to the Fc region of IgM or IgG (subclasses IgG1, IgG2, IgG3 but not IgG4). Other substances such as C-reactive protein, plasmin, trypsin-like enzymes, DNA, and staphylococcal protein A also may fix C1q and activate the classic complement pathway or its individual components.

Activated $\overline{C1}$ (C1-esterase) splits C4 and C2 into two fragments each: a major fragment that represents the activated component (C4b, C2a) and a smaller piece which can be detected in the fluid face (C4a, C2b). This reaction forms the complex, $\overline{C42}$, which also is designated C3-convertase.

When C3 is activated by $\overline{C42}$, a small fragment, C3a, is split off. The larger fragment, C3b, forms the complex $\overline{C423b}$, which becomes firmly bound to the cell membrane. This enzymatically active complex $\overline{C423b}$ splits C5 into a small polypeptide C5a and a larger fragment (C5b), which either is bound to the cell membrane at a site distinct from $\overline{C423b}$ or is released into the fluid face.

During the "membrane attack" sequence, C5b binds the next two complement components to form a complex $\overline{C5b67}$. This complex also can react with the membrane of unsensitized cells and cause "reactive" or "deviated" lysis. The trimolecular complex $\overline{C5b67}$ can bind one molecule of C8 and up to six molecules of C9. This larger complex of $\overline{C5b6789}$ has a molecular weight of approximately one million and can produce structural membrane damage if bound to the cell wall, leading to cell lysis.

Alternative Complement Pathway (Fig. 5–1). Characteristically, the alternative complement pathway can be activated *in vitro* by nonimmune means (lipopolysaccharides, inulin, or zymosan) and by human IgA and possibly IgE (see Chapter 9). Not all steps involved in activation of the alternative pathway are known. Activation of factor D results in cleavage activa-

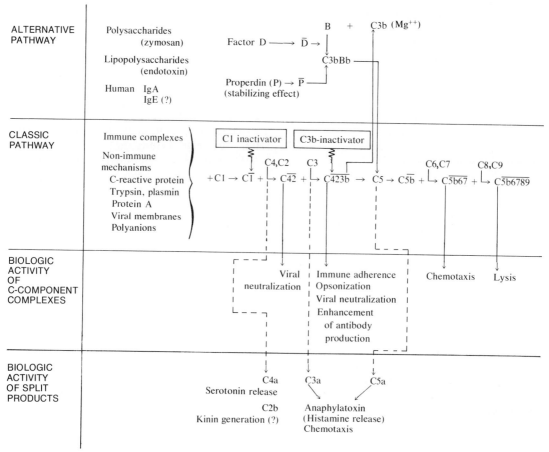

FIGURE 5–1. Sequence of activation of the classic and alternative complement pathway.

tion of factor B in the presence of Mg^{++} and C3b to form the complex C3bBb and increase the stability of the convertase. Thus the alternative pathway can be activated by C3b (which may have been generated by the classic complement pathway), which in turn may stimulate the generation of more C3b through an amplification "loop." This loop can be interrupted by C3b inactivator (C3b-INA), which not only limits the availability of C3b as an initiator of the feedback loop but also inactivates the $\bar{P}$-stabilized C3- and C5-convertases. A significant activation of C3 and C5 can be achieved through the alternative complement pathway to allow completion of the "membrane attack" sequence without the need to activate the early complement components.

Control Mechanisms. Uncontrolled activation of the complement system is prevented by a number of inhibitors. $\bar{C1}$ esterase inhibitor (C1 inactivator) inhibits the enzymatic activity of $\bar{C1}$ by forming an irreversible complex with its subunit $\bar{C1s}$. Deficiency of this inhibitor results in hereditary angioneurotic edema (Chapter 33).

C3b inactivator (C3b-INA), another control protein of complement activation, attacks C3b in the fluid phase and on the surface of cells. The split products are unable to function in the $\overline{C423}$ complex or in the C3b dependent activation loop of the alternative pathway.

Biologic Effects of Complement. The complement system plays an important role in host defense against infections. Activation of complement produces inflammation, attracts phagocytes, localizes infective agents, and contributes to the lysis and killing of microorganisms or virus-infected cells. Deficiencies of most C components have been observed in man and are frequently associated with unusual susceptibility to infections or connective tissue diseases (see Chapter 8).

Anaphylatoxins and Chemotactic Factors. Cleavage of C3 and C5 generates small polypeptides, C3a and C5a. These fragments bind to mast cells and stimulate the release of histamine. This mechanism is IgE-independent, and histamine activity can be blocked with antihistamines. The histamine released enhances capillary permeability and produces edema and contractions of smooth muscles. These two peptides are chemically and biologically distinct; tissue rendered unresponsive to

C3a will still be stimulated by C5a and vice versa, indicating that different receptors are involved. Complement-derived chemotactic factors are important mediators of leukocyte accumulation· in vivo. It was once thought that the polypeptide C3a and the complex $\overline{C567}$ possessed significant chemotactic activity. However, experimental evidence suggests that C5a is the major source of chemotactic activity supplied by the complement system. C5-deficient mice, which have normal levels of C3, show markedly defective accumulation of neutrophils in vivo when challenged with inflammatory agents. C6-deficient rabbits, which are unable to form $\overline{C567}$, produce normal amounts of chemotactic activity when their serum is activated in vitro. Injection of C5a (but not of C3a) produces substantial local granulocyte accumulation (Snyderman and Pike, 1977).

Opsonization and Immune Adherence. Opsonins are serum factors that interact with microorganisms and other particles to facilitate their ingestion by phagocytic cells. The two most important opsonins are the heat stable IgG (specific antibody), and the heat-labile complement component C3b. During activation of the classic or alternative complement pathway, C3b is deposited on the surface of a particle or microorganism. The C3b-coated particle may be recognized by the phagocytic cell and bound to C3b receptors which have been demonstrated on the plasma membranes of mononuclear and polymorphonuclear phagocytes (Griffin, 1977). There is experimental evidence that particles (microorganisms) coated with C3b may be bound to phagocytic cells, but to be ingested, may require in addition specific antibodies.

The complement system has been shown to be important for the ingestion of encapsulated pneumococci, staphylococci, gram-negative bacilli, and possibly *Candida albicans*.

Viral Neutralization. *In vitro* neutralization of enveloped viruses (e.g., vesicular stomatitis virus, vaccinia virus, herpes simplex virus, Newcastle disease virus) is greatly enhanced if the early complement components (C1, C4, C2, C3) are present in addition to small amounts of (early) antibodies. In contrast, the late acting components C5 to C9 are not required for C-dependent viral neutralization. The contribution of the complement system to viral neutralization may be of significance in the early phase of a viral infection, especially if the host is nonimmune or has only limited antibody levels (Leddy et al., 1977).

Immune Lysis. The molecular events of complement action have been studied in detail, using a model system consisting of sheep red blood cells (SRBC) as target cells, rabbit antibody to SRBC and guinea pig serum as a complement source. During the first phase of C-activation, the complex $C\overline{423b}$ is formed, which initiates the "attack sequence" that is finalized in the large complex, $C\overline{5b6789}$. This complex interacts with the surface of the target cell, leading to its lysis or killing. Antibody-dependent complement-mediated killing of nucleated cells is initiated by the same mechanism; however, different cell types seem to be variably susceptible to this killing mechanism.

Serum Bactericidal Activity and Complement. Antibody-sensitized bacteria are killed by complement in a way analogous to the lysis of red cells and nucleated cells. The fact that C4-deficient guinea pig serum kills *E. coli* after a prolonged latent period and at a slow rate (even in the absence of antibody) indicates that activation of the alternative complement pathway may trigger complement-mediated bactericidal activity, especially against gram-negative organisms. While the relative contribution of the two complement pathways to bactericidal action has not been precisely determined, it is undisputed that in both modes of C-activation, the bactericidal activity is directly related to the action of the terminal C components (C5 to C9). Furthermore, at least *in vitro,* the classic pathway — which requires antibody and the entire C-sequence — provides a potent bactericidal system. In contrast to gram-negative bacteria, most gram-positive organisms and the mycobacteria are not susceptible to complement action. This may be related to the thicker wall of the gram-positive bacteria (15 to 80 mμm) as compared to the much thinner cell wall of gram-negative species (7.5 to 10mμm). The lipid-rich cell wall of mycobacteria may be responsible for their resistance to complement.

Complement and Antibody Formation. Two observations have focused on the importance of complement for the induction of the immune response: (1) B lym- phocytes have surface receptors for C3b and (2) C3 and complement fixing immune complexes accumulate within germinal centers and lymphoid follicles. Furthermore, if mice are complement-depleted by the C-activating cobra venom factor (CoF), the antibody response to T-dependent antigens is markedly suppressed (Pepys, 1976). Antibody production to T-independent antigens is unaffected. The T cell-dependent antibody classes (IgG, IgA, IgE) are more affected than the T-independent class (IgM). Treatment with CoF inhibits follicular localization of aggregated IgG or antigen-antibody complexes in lymph nodes of treated mice. Additional evidence of the importance of C4 in normal antibody responses has been demonstrated in C4-deficient guinea pigs who show a markedly depressed primary and secondary antibody response to bacteriophage ϕX 174, characterized by a low titer, lack of amplification, and the formation of only IgM antibody. If these animals are treated with normal guinea pig serum during the primary phage immunization or if the antigen dose is increased or given in complete Freund's adjuvant, a normal antibody response to this antigen is observed (Ochs et al., 1978). Such observations suggest that complement is required to fix antigen-antibody complexes within the follicles and germinal centers. B cells are known to traffic through these areas and binding of the complexes to B cells may be facilitated by their C3 receptor sites.

PHAGOCYTES

Phagocytic cells migrate out of capillaries into the tissue if attracted by invading organisms (chemotaxis). After being coated with opsonins, the offending microorganisms attach to the membranes of phagocytes before being ingested, killed, and digested (Fig. 5–2). Laboratory tests to evaluate leukocyte function are listed in Table 5–1.

Chemotaxis. Chemotaxis is nonrandom locomotion of cells in which the direction is determined by environmental substances. Defects of leukocyte chemotaxis can cause inadequate inflammatory response, resulting in undue susceptibility to infection. Impaired chemotaxis has been described in a variety of conditions; of particular interest in allergy are those patients with defects of

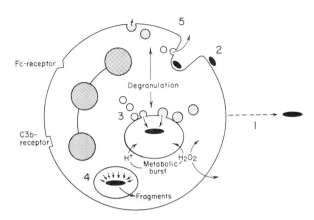

FIGURE 5-2. The neutrophil response: (1) chemotaxis, (2) phagocytosis, (3) intracellular killing, (4) digestion, and (5) extracellular enzyme release. (Modified and reproduced by permission from Beeson and McDermott, *Textbook of Medicine.* 14th ed. Philadelphia, W. B. Saunders, 1975, p. 1475.)

chemotaxis associated with eczema, high IgE levels, and other conditions related to allergic disease.

A simple *in vivo* method for determining chemotaxis is the Rebuck skin window technique. The skin is scraped to a point just short of bleeding then cover slips are applied and removed over specified time intervals. These slips are stained, and the cell type and numbers enumerated. This technique includes such refinements as placing small collecting chambers on the skin instead of cover slips, thereby permitting studies of chemotactic factors.

In the *in vitro* determination of chemotaxis, cells are separated and placed in "chambers" (Boyden chambers) divided by a filter, and chemotactic factors are placed on the opposite side of the filter. The number of cells that pass through the filter during incubation is determined either by visual counting or by radiolabeling. Chemotactic factors include C5a, lymphocyte-derived chemotactic factor (LDCF), products from clot formation (fibrin, plasminogen activator), kallikrein, transfer factor, a factor from polymorphonuclear leukocytes, eosinophil chemotactic factor of anaphylaxis (ECF-A), histamine, bacterial factors, certain proteins, collagen peptides, and N-formyl-methionyl peptide (which is similar to bacterial chemotactic factors). C5a and bacterial factors are employed most commonly to study neutrophil and monocyte chemotaxis. LDCF is used when studying monocyte chemotaxis. Filters with a pore size of 3, 5, or 8 microns are most frequently used. In humans, the association between high serum IgE levels and recurrent infections (Buckley et al., 1972) appears to be due to defective chemotaxis (Clark et al., 1973). Chemotactic defects are not due to high serum IgE levels per se, but may be due to the release of histamine which ele-

vates intracellular cyclic AMP levels and decreases cell mobility.

Chemotactic defects occur in patients with Job's syndrome of "cold" abscesses (Hill et al., 1974), and Wiskott-Aldrich syndrome (Altman et al., 1974). Patients with eczema, extremely high serum IgE levels, and recurrent infections may have defective polymorphonuclear leukocyte chemotaxis (Hill and Quie, 1974). In atopic dermatitis (AD), infected eczema is associated with defective polymorphonuclear leukocyte chemotaxis (Hanifin and Rogge, 1977), though this defect is not present when patients are not infected (Furukawa and Altman, 1978). Furthermore, AD patients may have defective monocyte chemotaxis (Snyderman and Pike, 1977) that is unrelated to eczema, high IgE levels, or susceptibility to

TABLE 5-1 LEUKOCYTE FUNCTION TESTS

Chemotaxis
  Rebuck window
  Boyden chamber: 1. microscopic evaluations
                     2. ^{51}Cr labeling of granulocytes
  Agar plate method

Phagocytosis
  Phagocytic index, using baker's yeast or latex particles
  Iodination

Hexose monophosphate shunt activity
  ^{14}C-1-glucose oxidation
  Oxygen consumption
  NBT reduction: quantitative histochemical

Miscellaneous
  Bacterial killing test
  Myeloperoxidase determination
  Leukocyte deformability

infection (Furukawa and Altman, 1978). Defective chemotactic responsiveness may be amenable to treatment by removal of offending allergic factors (Fontan et al., 1976), the use of immunostimulants such as levamisole, or the use of chemoattractants such as N-formyl-methionyl peptides linked to specific antibody (Isturiz et al., 1978) or linked to antibiotics (Altman and Furukawa, unpublished).

Ingestion. Only opsonized microorganisms can be attached to and ingested by phagocytes. The particles are incorporated into a phagocytic vacuole lined by the invaginated cell membrane. The phagocytic vacuole and adjacent granules fuse, and the contents of the granules pass into the vacuole. The phagocytic process is associated with a burst of metabolic activity, with increased oxygen and glucose consumption and lactic acid production. The most striking metabolic change initiated by phagocytosis is the increase in glucose-C1 oxidation, a measure of hexose monophosphate shunt activity. This metabolic activity is detected by the nitroblue tetrazolium test, in which the NBT changes from a yellow to a blue color, and releases measurable light (chemiluminescence).

Intracellular Killing. Many antimicrobial activities occur in phagocytic vacuoles. Their acidic pH may kill directly certain acid-sensitive bacteria, e.g., pneumococci. Lysozyme, a basic protein present in the granules, hydrolizes the bacterial cell wall polysaccharide. Granular cationic proteins released into the phagocytic vacuole attach to the surface of the ingested organisms and alter their metabolism. The neutrophil oxygen-dependent microbicidal system has been studied in depth. During the respiratory burst, hydrogen peroxide, superoxide anions, hydroxyl radicals, and singlet molecular oxygen are formed (Klebanoff, 1975) and may kill ingested organisms directly. The most potent antimicrobial system, however, consists of myeloperoxidase, H_2O_2, and an oxidizable cofactor such as halides (Klebanoff and Harmon, 1972). Myeloperoxidase is present at a high concentration in human granulocytes and is released into the phagocytic vacuole. H_2O_2 is catalyzed by oxidases within the phagocytes or may be formed by certain microorganisms which lack a catalase, such as pneumococci, streptococci, and lactobacilli.

The importance of this system is supported by several types of evidence: (1) the discovery of a correlation between the virulence of certain microorganisms and their ability to destroy hydrogen peroxide, (2) the finding of defective antimicrobial activity in neutrophils that lack myeloperoxidase or are unable to produce hydrogen peroxide (chronic granulomatous disease of childhood), and (3) the fact that these latter neutrophils can kill microbes that accumulate hydrogen peroxide within the phagocytic vesicle by their own oxygen metabolism (catalase-negative bacteria).

Macrophage Function. The role of macrophages in the immune response is complex and versatile (reviewed in Möller, 1978). After leaving the vascular space, they become either fixed or wandering macrophages. They are attracted by chemotactic factors (e.g., C5a, bacterial chemotactic factors), and have the capability to ingest and kill microorganisms, secrete bactericidal material, and internalize antigen — which they either dispose of or process and present to other cells active in the immune system. Indeed, macrophage-bound antigen is more immunogenic than soluble antigen. The capability of macrophages to phagocytose large particles is enhanced if the particles are opsonized by specific immunoglobulins or C3b. Macrophages produce and secrete lysozyme, which is bactericidal to some gram-positive organisms and may enhance the complement-mediated bacteriolysis of gram-negative organisms. *In vitro* studies have demonstrated that macrophages contain a substance that increases neovascularization and might influence the development of chronic inflammation during an immune response. Macrophages have receptors for Fc, C3b and for a number of lymphokines.

The susceptibility to infections in newborn infants and steroid-treated patients may be explained in part by macrophage dysfunction. The diminished antibody response of newborn animals can quickly be brought to adult standards if nonimmune adult monocytes are administered intraperitoneally.

These findings indicate that macrophages act both as phagocytes and to some extent as regulators of lymphocyte function. They may induce thymic differentiation, ingest antigens and process them for lymphocytes, and potentiate the antibody response to T cell-dependent antigens.

NONSPECIFIC FACTORS IN IMMUNITY

Most living organisms possess a number of "nonspecific" host response factors. These include mechanical barriers and systems for elimination, secretion, inflammation, and metabolism. Failure of any of these can lead to host destruction. The skin, mucous membranes, gastrointestinal tract, and respiratory tree serve to maintain homeostasis, ingest vital material, discharge waste material, and protect the host. Disruption of this anatomic integrity will result in disease or death.

Skin. The itching from atopic dermatitis leads to scratching. The resultant excoriation allows penetration of infectious organisms, which is further enhanced by an alteration in normal protective microbiologic flora, and decreased cutaneous secretions of oils, acids, and enzymes. Infections may be further enhanced by defective specific host defenses, as in chemotactic responsiveness, microbial killing, or decreased humoral immunity.

Mucous Membranes and Gastrointestinal Tract. Mucins, which are glycoproteins and glycolipids, have a structure resembling epithelial surfaces. They serve as an anatomic barrier and, because of their structure, are attacked by organisms mistaking the mucins for epithelial cells. At the "portal of entry," mucins in saliva decrease bacterial adherence to epithelial cells, and promote a nonspecific "washing" effect. Once within the gastrointestinal tract, foreign substances are subjected to mechanical removal by peristalsis, gastric acidity, and pepsin digestion. "Normal" bacterial flora is promoted by factors such as lysozyme (which can lyse certain bacteria with the help of IgA and complement), bile salts, and specific antibodies. The normal flora protects the host by competitively inhibiting the colonization with potentially harmful organisms (Walker, 1976).

Nonliving foreign antigens similarly are excluded by the same protective mechanisms. A defective mucous membrane or other alteration in gastrointestinal defense permits allergic sensitization. For instance, achlorhydria predisposes to the development of antibodies against bovine serum albumin (Kraft et al., 1967). Allergy to food may result from deficiency in secretory IgA. It has been suggested that gastrointestinal allergy may result because the IgE system, which evolved selectively to resist intestinal parasites, inadvertently produces antibodies to food antigens.

Respiratory Tree. Upper airway mucous membranes humidify the air and remove the majority of potentially dangerous substances that are over 10 μm in size. In addition, highly soluble gases such as sulfur dioxide are removed in the upper airway.

As inspired air reaches the bronchioles, the cross-sectional area available for the volume of air increases dramatically, from 2.5 cm^2 at the trachea to 180 cm^2 at the terminal bronchioles. Consequently, flow rate decreases sufficiently to allow sedimentation of particles above 2 μm size, and diffusion of particles below 1 μm size. For this reason, the optimal particle size for alveolar deposition is between 1 and 2 μm (Newhouse et al., 1976).

Once deposition of particles occurs, a host response begins, depending on the site of deposition and the nature of the particle. Irritant substances such as carbon cause coughing or vagally mediated bronchoconstriction. Mucus and ciliated epithelia function together to transport foreign material up the respiratory tree. Material not removed by these mechanisms can be removed by phagocytosis and efflux via lymphatics of blood vessels.

Proper function of the mucociliary transport system depends on several critical factors: the cilia, mucus production, and the ratio of the fluid "sol" to the more viscous surface "gel." The cilia normally beat at a frequency of 1200 per minute, producing a cephalad wave of mucus. The cilia beat within the sol layer, but must just touch the gel layer during the effector stroke. A dysfunction or destruction of cilia, a decrease in mucus production, or a change in the critical sol to gel ratio results in ineffective mucociliary transport (Denton et al., 1968). A defect of ciliary function may be responsible for Kartagener's syndrome and some types of bronchiectasis (Chapter 48).

Metabolic and Nutritional Factors. Proper protein, carbohydrate, and lipid intake and metabolism are necessary for optimal immune responses. Enzymatic pathways must have correct pH and adequate substrate (e.g., including not only sodium, potassium, and calcium, but also magnesium, iron, zinc, and other trace elements and vitamins). Although most nutri-

tional factors provide substrate for more specific reactions, there is a possibility that the immunoglobulins and the viable cells in breast milk play a more definitive immune role in infants (Chapter 2).

References

Altman, L. C., Snyderman, R., and Blaese, R. M.: Abnormalities of chemotactic lymphokine synthesis and mononuclear leukocyte chemotaxis in Wiskott-Aldrich syndrome. J. Clin. Invest. 54:486, 1974.

Buckley, R. H., Wray, B. B., and Belmaker, E. Z.: Extreme hyperimmunoglobulinemia E and undue susceptibility to infection. Pediatrics 49:59, 1972.

Clark, R. A., Root, R. K., Kimball, H. R., and Kirkpatrick, C. H.: Defective neutrophil chemotaxis and cellular immunity in a child with recurrent infections. Ann. Intern. Med. 78:515, 1973.

Denton, R., Forsman, W., Hwang, S. H., Litt, M., and Miller, C. E.: Viscoelasticity of mucus: its role in ciliary transport of pulmonary secretions. Am. Rev. Respir. Dis. 98:380, 1968.

Fontan, G., Lorente, F., Garcia Rodriguez, M. C., and Ojeda, J. A.: Defective neutrophil chemotaxis and hyperimmunoglobulinemia E — A reversible defect? Acta Paediatr. Scand. 65:509, 1976.

Furukawa, C. T., and Altman, L. C.: Defective monocyte and polymorphonuclear leukocyte chemotaxis in atopic disease. J. Allergy Clin. Immunol. 61:288, 1978.

Gewurz, H., and Lint, T. F.: Alternative modes and pathways of complement activation. In Good, R. A., and Day, S. B. (eds.) Biological Amplifications Systems in Immunology (Comprehensive Immunology, Vol. 2). New York, Plenum Publishing Corp., 1977, pp. 17–45.

Griffin, F. M., Jr.: Opsonization. In Good, R. A., and Day, S. B. (eds.) Biological Amplifications Systems in Immunology (Comprehensive Immunology, Vol. 2). New York, Plenum Publishing Corp., 1977, pp. 85–113

Hanifin, J. M., and Rogge, J. L.: Staphylococcal infections in patients with atopic dermatitis. Arch. Dermatol. 113:1383, 1977.

Hill, H. R., and Quie, P. G.: Raised serum IgE levels and defective neutrophil chemotaxis in three children with eczema and recurrent bacterial infections. Lancet 1:183, 1974.

Hill, H. R., Ochs, H. D., Quie, P. G., Clark, R. A., Pabst, H. F., Klebanoff, S. J., and Wedgwood, R. J.: Defect in neu-

trophil granulocyte chemotaxis in Job's syndrome of recurrent "cold" staphylococcal abscesses. Lancet 2:617, 1974.

Isturiz, M. A., Sandberg, A. L., Schiffman, E., Wahl, S. M., and Notkins, A. L.: Chemotactic antibody. Science 200:554, 1978.

Klebanoff, S. J.: Antimicrobial mechanisms in neutrophilic polymorphonuclear leukocytes. Semin. Hematol. 12:117, 1975.

Klebanoff, S. J., and Harmon, C. B.: Role of myeloperoxidase-mediated antimicrobial systems in intact leukocytes. J. Reticuloendothel. Soc., 12:170, 1972.

Kraft, S. C., Rothberg, R. M., Knauer, C. M., Svoboda, A. C., Jr., Monroe, L. S., and Farr, R. S.: Gastric acid output and circulating antibovine serum albumin in adults. Clin. Exp. Immunol. 2:321, 1967.

Leddy, J. P., Simons, R. L., and Douglas, R. G.: Effect of selective complement deficiency on the rate of neutralization of enveloped viruses by human sera. J. Immunol. 118:28, 1977.

Möller, G. (ed.): Role of macrophages in the immune response. Immunol. Rev. 40:1, 1978.

Müller-Eberhard, H. J.: Complement. Ann. Rev. Biochem. 44:697, 1975.

Newhouse, M., Sanchis, J., and Bienenstock, J.: Lung defense mechanisms. N. Engl. J. Med. 295:990 and 1045, 1976.

Ochs, H. D., Jackson, C. G., Heller, S. R., Wedgwood, R. J.: Defective antibody response to a T-dependent antigen in C4 deficient guinea pigs and its correction by addition of C4. Fed. Proc. 37:1477, 1978 (abstract).

Pepys, M. B.: Role of complement in the induction of immunological responses. Transplant. Rev. 32:93, 1976.

Snyderman, R., and Pike, M.,: Biologic aspects of leukocyte chemotaxis. In Good, R. A., and Day, S. B. (eds.): Biological Amplifications Systems in Immunology (Comprehensive Immunology; Vol. 2). New York, Plenum Publishing Corp., 1977, pp. 159–181.

Walker, W. A.: Host defense mechanisms in the gastrointestinal tract. Pediatrics 57:901, 1976.

William T. Kniker, M.D.

6

Disorders of Antibody and Cell-Mediated Immunity

All the immune systems of the body have one chief purpose: maintaining the internal milieu free from foreign matter. Before discussing abnormalities of the immune system, a brief review of the mechanisms that enable the immune system to accomplish its task is useful.

NORMAL IMMUNE FUNCTION

Surveillance Against Foreign Human Cells. Certain lymphocytes are able to recognize foreignness of cellular antigens. Even without prior sensitization, T lymphocytes respond to foreign histocompatability antigens on genetically dissimilar cells. Following sensitization, surveillance mechanisms operate in detection of "foreign" tumor-associated antigens, virus-associated antigens, and autoantigens on the surface of autochthonus (self) cells.

Defense Against Other Potentially Injurious Cells and Agents. While T and B lymphocytes may deal directly with potentially injurious agents, their main contribution to defense is by augmentation of the phagocytic system. In cell-mediated immunity (CMI), the responding T lymphocyte produces many soluble mediators called *lymphokines*. It is the lymphokines that bring about the typical delayed inflammatory reaction (see Fig. 6–1):

Skin reactive factor (SRF) causes erythe-ma and increased vascular permeability, tending to dilute antigen in a pool of edema.

Chemotactic factors for macrophages (MCF) and *PMN's* attract leukocytes to the area.

Macrophage inhibition factor (MIF) inhibits outward migration of accumulated macrophages, and *macrophage aggregation factor* (MAF) coalesces the cells. *Leukocyte inhibition factor* (LIF) immobilizes and traps peripheral blood leukocytes, including PMN's.

Macrophage resistance factor and other postulated factors increase size, metabolic functions and general resistance of macrophages, turning them into "activated" macrophages.

The B lymphocyte system also augments phagocytic defense (see Fig. 6–1). Various mechanisms include:

Secretion of antibody that aggregates particulate antigens and precipitates soluble antigen.

Attachment of cytophilic antibodies to receptors on macrophage or PMN cell membranes provides a means by which these cells can capture specific antigens.

Both specific antibody and complement (C3b) on the surface of particulate antigens promote phagocytosis by opsonization and by immune adherence (attach-

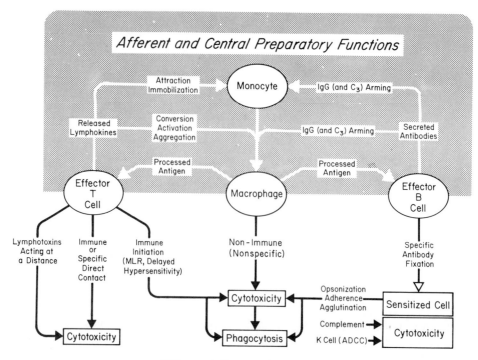

FIGURE 6-1. Pathways of defense—Interrelationship of specific (immune) and nonspecific factors.

ment of human erythrocytes to activated C3b with formation of erythrocyte-antigen clumps).

Antibody-antigen reactions at surfaces of mast cells (IgE-mediated) and platelets (IgG-mediated) lead to immobilization of antigens by edema and thrombosis.

Immobilization of antigen by edema secondary to immune activation of C3a and C5a, "anaphylatoxins" that cause mast cells to release mediators of inflammation that alter vascular permeability.

Attraction of PMN's and macrophages by C5a and C567, complement-derived chemotactic factors, and by other chemotactic factors released from mast cells.

A particularly important part of host defense is the killing of potentially injurious cells and microorganisms. A variety of protective mechanisms can be activated so that some or all operate in such situations as cancer, infection, transplantation reactions, maternofetal interactions, and autoimmune disorders. Immune mechanisms by which target cells are destroyed include (see Fig. 6-1):

Fixation of antibodies directed against

antigens on target cell membranes followed by:

IgM or IgG-dependent cell lysis via the classic complement pathway, and IgA-dependent lysis involving the alternative complement pathway.

or

Antibody-dependent cell-mediated cytotoxicity (ADCC) in which the Fc portion of cell-bound IgG activates a mononuclear cell to kill the target cell by direct contact. This killer (K) cell appears to be a lymphocyte with receptors for IgG, but without other receptors typical of a T cell or B cell.

Lymphocytes (predominantly T cells) sensitized to membrane-associated antigens on target cells, which exhibit:

Cytotoxicity by direct contact with target cell,

or

Indirect cytotoxicity, mediated by elaboration of soluble lymphokines: (1) Lymphotoxin—cytotoxic for some but not all target cells. (2) Proliferation inhibition factor (PIF) and cloning inhibition factor (CIF), which can inhibit proliferation of target cells.

Macrophage killing of target cells, with or without phagocytosis: (1) "Nonspecific" low-level activity. (2) Immunologically augmented activity, secondary to lymphokines (the activated macrophage) or cytophilic IgG and C3b (the "armed" macrophage).

Maintenance of Homeostasis. Older and injured cells, molecular aggregates, and inflammatory debris are promptly and continuously cleansed from the blood by the monocyte-phagocytic system (MPS). Immune mechanisms aid in removal of exogenous agents, including microbial products, cell membranes, and tissue structures. Normal individuals have antibodies to many soluble and cellular autoantigens. The levels of such antibodies usually are low, partly because there is a prevailing environment of great antigen excess. Most of the time such autoantibodies do not appear to be injurious. In fact they may enhance the removal of cells or tissues that have been altered by infection, trauma, or chemical injury. Autoantibody serves as a molecular carrier for endogenous substances, e.g., insulin and thyroglobulin. An autoantibody to gamma globulin, such as rheumatoid factor, may modulate immunologically-induced reactions by binding antibody molecules before they can complex with antigen to perpetuate inflammation.

REGULATION OF IMMUNITY

Our understanding of immune function has been greatly broadened by recent recognition of the crucial roles played by regulators and modulators of immunity. These developments are of particular interest because they make it possible to understand the pathogenetic mechanisms operating in a number of diseases and thus open the door to new therapies, discussed in later sections.

The interrelationships of some immune regulators are shown in Figures 6–1 and 6–2. The degree and quality of immune response to an antigen depend upon the interaction of regulators operating at different levels of control.

First Level of Control: Initiation of the Immune Response to an Antigen. For a lymphocyte to become immunized, two "signals" are required. The antigen itself usually provides the first signal. Generally,

the signal is more effective if the antigen has been processed and delivered by a macrophage and if the antigen is of a relatively large molecular weight or is aggregated or particulate. Antigen alone may not produce a positive signal and may, instead, induce immune tolerance, this is particularly likely when the antigen is small, nonaggregated, or not processed by a macrophage prior to lymphocyte contact.

The second signal to the lymphocyte membrane may come from several sources (Grossi et al., 1978). T cells produce "helper" factors that permit sensitization and antibody production by B cells. They also release lymphokines such as blastogenic factor (BF), which induces blast formation in normal lymphocytes, and potentiating factor (PF), which enhaces ongoing transformation in antigen-stimulated cultures. In some instances, second signals may be provided by macrophage factors, B cell products, or complement components, especially C3b. Some second signals may be "negative," halting the further development of an immune response. One example is the use of specific IgG to stimulate re-

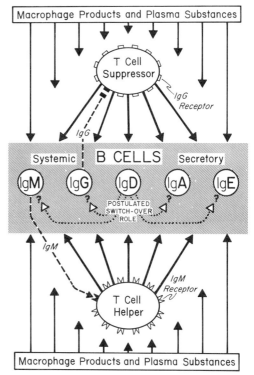

FIGURE 6–2. Cells and products involved in B cell regulation.

ceptors on T suppressor cells that prevent sensitization to the antigen. This mechanism is exemplified clinically by the use of RhoGAM to prevent maternal sensitization to Rh antigen and exemplified experimentally in animals by prevention of sensitization to graft or tumor antigens (the enhancement phenomenon). Suppressor T cell–derived lymphokines that inhibit antibody production by B cells have been demonstrated in animals and man (see Chapter 1).

Second Level of Control: Magnitude and Quality of the Immune Response. A wide variety of enhancing and inhibitory factors, whose functions overlap considerably, regulate the magnitude and quality of the immune response (see Fig. 6–2). The three key cells involved in immune responses (the macrophage, the T lymphocyte, and the B lymphocyte) modulate each other's functions. Various plasma factors also modulate lymphocyte functions. One well-documented example is immune regulatory alpha globulin (IRA), which has been shown to inhibit lymphocyte blastogenesis, primary sensitization by antigen, and the production of antibody by B cells (Namba and Waksman, 1976).

Regulation may be limited to a specific antigen-immune responding system or may be on a wider basis, involving a particular subpopulation of lymphocytes (e.g., B cells producing one class of immunoglobulins) or all B lymphocytes or all T lymphocytes. As long as the antigenic stimulus continues, the thrust of regulation tends to be positive in the direction of a heightened response. Modulators may perpetuate the response by stimulating each other in a circular fashion (see Fig. 6–1). For example, if T lymphocytes respond to a given antigen, macrophages are brought in to phagocytize the antigen (cell-mediated immunity). The macrophages in turn digest and process the antigen, presenting immunogenic antigen to more lymphocytes, which continue and magnify the ongoing CMI response. Once the antigenic stimulus wanes, the thrust of regulation is negative so that immune responses are turned off. High levels of specific IgG antibody serve this role.

Third Level of Control: Participation of Phagocytes and Sensitized Lymphocytes. The ability of any cell to function depends upon internal energy mechanisms, themselves modulated by external signals

acting on the cell membrane. The relative levels of the nucleotides, cyclic adenosine monophosphate (cAMP) and cyclic guanosine monophosphate (cGMP), appear to be particularly critical in this process.

When cAMP is relatively high, compared to cGMP, lymphocytes are at rest: they do not proliferate, release lymphokines, secrete antibodies, or kill cells. Phagocytic leukocytes do not move, phagocytize, or digest previously ingested material. Mast cells and basophils do not release mediators of inflammation.

When cAMP is low, relative to GMP, lymphocytes divide, release lymphokines, secrete antibodies, and kill target cells. Phagocytic leukocytes migrate, respond to chemotaxis, phagocytize and digest particles. Basophils and mast cells release stored mediators (e.g., histamine) and manufacture and release other mediators (e.g., SRS-A).

Many endogenous and exogenous substances act as "first signals" upon cell membranes to regulate the function of immune cells. Agents that *raise* cAMP relative to cGMP include: beta-adrenergic agents, corticosteroids, estrogens, prostaglandins of the E series, glucose (hyperglycemia), and histamine. Agents that *lower* cAMP relative to cGMP include: alpha-adrenergic agents, cholinergic agents, insulin (hypoglycemia), prostaglandins of the F series, and ascorbic acid.

DEVELOPMENT OF IMMUNE COMPETENCE

At birth, immunologic parameters characteristic of fetal life are present (Stites et al., 1975; Lawton and Cooper, 1973.) Studies in mice and preliminary studies in man demonstrate the presence of lymphocyte populations with unique genetic markers and absence of function; these are soon replaced by functioning T and B lymphocytes bearing different genetic markers. The total peripheral blood lymphocyte (PBL) count in neonates is approximately 5000 per mm^3, twice the number found in older children and adults. The number of T lymphocytes (1000 to 3000 per mm^3) is about the same as that found in later ages. The increased newborn PBL count is partially accounted for by the B lymphocyte number (1000 to 2000 per mm^3), which is far greater than the number (200 to 600 per mm³) seen in older children. In neonatal blood, increased EAC-rosetting lymphocytes and increased blastogenic response to pokeweed mitogen, relative to PHA, have been observed; both findings are compatible with high numbers of B lymphocytes at birth. Reports on the proportion of newborn lymphocytes demonstrating surface immunoglobulins (SIG) for individual immunoglobulin classes are sparse and inconclusive.

Newborns, particularly premature infants, are known to have decreased resistance to infection, especially that caused by staphylococci, streptococci, *B. pertussis*, gram-negative bacilli, and certain respiratory tract viruses. Although the basic components of the immune system are present, many factors have been postulated to account for the neonate's susceptibility to infections (Miller, 1973; see also Chapter 2):

General Factors

1. Germinal centers and plasma cells in lymphoid tissues are absent.
2. Primary response to antigens is delayed, in part owing to competition between many new antigens and in part to the immaturity of cellular enzyme systems.
3. Immediate or delayed skin test reactions cannot be demonstrated, perhaps reflecting absence of mediators or vascular responses necessary for appropriate tissue inflammation.
4. Levels of opsonins, including IgM antibodies and certain complement components, are relatively low.
5. Nonspecific chemical bactericidal substances such as macrophage-associated lysozyme and protective substances in secretions are at suboptimal levels.

Phagocytic Leukocytes.

1. Energy metabolism, chemotactic responsiveness, phagocytosis, and microbicidal capacity are sluggish.
2. Total hemolytic complement activity as well as levels of individual components (e.g., C5) may be low, so there may be less complement-derived mediator activation and less edema formation, decreased chemotaxis, and poorer immune adherence and opsonization.

Specific Immune Systems

1. No locally produced IgA or IgE in secretions.

2. No maternally-derived IgM.
3. Sluggish metabolic activity of macrophages, which slows initiation of immune response.
4. Suppression of primary antibody responses to some antigens by presence of maternal specific IgG.

By 3 to 4 months of age, the infant has made vigorous immune responses to countless antigens. Lymphocyte numbers and *in vitro* functional parameters are not far from those observed in adults. In the cortical regions of lymphoid tissues, large germinal centers reflect the intensity of immune responses taking place. In the first year or so of life, the infant remains quite susceptible to infections by mycobacteria, pathogenic fungi, and certain enveloped viruses. During the same period, the child continues to show relatively poor immediate and delayed skin reactivity to locally administered antigens, although sensitization to the antigens can readily be demonstrated by *in vitro* techniques. As the child matures, immunoglobulin levels steadily rise; "adult" levels are reached for IgM by 4 to 5 years of age, for IgG by 6 to 9, and for IgE and IgA sometime during adolescence. During later childhood, all lymphoid structures tend to increase in mass; enlargement of the adenoids and tonsils is physiologically normal in the elementary school years. Upon entering adolescence, the child is at his lifetime peak in overall immune function as well as in relative mass of lymphoid structures.

VARIETIES OF IMMUNE DISORDERS

Immune competence is difficult to define. Presumably, we are competent when our body defense forces recognize and neutralize all injurious agents that would disturb our internal environment. Presently, physicians can recognize those relatively rare cases of *severe* immune deficiency in which extremely low immune globulin levels or lack of cell-mediated immunity is associated with chronic illness and early death. However, it is becoming increasingly apparent that mild and subtle forms of immune deficiency are common. Transient periods of deficiency probably are a common occurrence, associated, for example, with some generalized viral infections, steroid therapy, or pregnancy. Unrecognized immune deficiencies that persist may be associated with a wide variety of disorders. Considering the complexity of the immune system, there are countless possibilities for dysfunction or absence of any of the cell populations, membrane receptors, or mediators of inflammation involved in immune defenses.

The expression of immune deficiency disorders (IDD) is variable, depending upon age. In childhood the male to female ratio is 4:1; while in adults, in whom acquired and secondary deficiency conditions predominate, there is no male preponderance. The age on onset is variable. In general, innate or congenital disorders appear in early childhood; the more severe the deficiency, e.g., grossly deficient numbers of lymphocytes or phagocytes, the more likely disease becomes manifest in early infancy. Most cases of IDD become evident in childhood; about a third first appear in adults. The most common problem by far is recurrent pyogenic infections, usually with a history of frequent courses of antibiotic therapy. Since many forms of IDD are not recognized, the true incidence of IDD is not known. IDD associated primarily with antibody deficiency accounts for approximately 70 percent of cases, combined T and B lymphocyte disorders for 10 to 25 percent and deficiencies primarily of T lymphocyte function account for 5 to 10 percent of IDD. Disorders of phagocytes (numbers or function) and complement deficiencies account for less than 2 percent of the total.

Primary or Congenital Immune Deficiency Disorders

Table 6-1 lists selected disorders of T lymphocyte and B lymphocyte function and is based on a recent classification prepared by the World Health Organization. For B lymphocyte defects it can be seen that some disorders are associated with a paucity of B cells while other syndromes are characterized by normal or increased numbers of B cells, implying that B cell *function* is abnormal or that suppressor substances are inhibiting activities of essentially normal B cells (Cooper at al., 1975). Associated inheritance patterns also are noted in Table 6-1. For many of the disorders, the pattern is variable or unknown.

The chapter briefly reviews important features of the more common forms of IDD in order to emphasize the clinical findings associated with various levels of dysfunction, and to encourage recognition of impaired immune function, rather than emphasizing the diagnosis of specific syndromes.

DISORDERS MAINLY AFFECTING B CELLS

Antibody Deficiencies for Selected Antigens with Normal Levels of Immunoglobulins. B cell disorders that are particularly difficult to recognize are those in which affected patients cannot make antibodies specific for antigens of one or more microorganisms, even though normal levels of B cells, plasma cells, and immunoglobulins for each of the five classes are present. Patients unable to make antibodies against a particular microorganism may lack the appropriate Ir gene. There is no ready explanation for those other rare individuals whose immunoglobulins are devoid of detectable antibody activity against any tested antigen.

Selective Immunoglobulin Class Deficiencies. Selective IgA deficiency in serum (under 5 mg per ml) and secretions is the commonest form of IDD that is diagnosed; it is found in approximately one of 500 randomly selected "normal" Caucasians and in over 1 percent of children with recurrent infections. There is a strong family association, often with autosomal dominant or recessive inheritance. In some patients, B cells containing IgA are lacking; in others, plasma cells contain but are unable to secrete IgA. About half of such IgA-deficient individuals have recurrent sinopulmonary infections and manifest other conditions such as allergy (Ostergaard, 1977), neurologic disorders, ataxia telangiectasia, chronic bowel disease, and congenital rubella syndrome. IgE levels may be increased or may be low. Autoantibodies against various tissues and immunoglobulins are common. Development of anti-IgA antibodies following gamma globulin or plasma therapy leads to the risk of anaphylactic reactions with subsequent administration of serum protein products or blood transfusions.

Selective deficiencies of IgM or IgG have been described; both are much less common than is IgA deficiency. With absence

TABLE 6–1 LYMPHOCYTE DEFECTS AND GENETIC ASPECTS OF SELECTED PRIMARY IMMUNODEFICIENCY SYNDROMES

Disorder	Affected Lymphocyte Populations				Mode of Inheritance
	T Cells		B Cells		
	Stage 1*	Stage 2*	Stage 1	Stage 2	
Disorders apparently affecting stem cells					
Reticular dysgenesis	yes	yes	yes	yes	unknown
SCID† (thymic alymphoplasia)	yes	yes	(yes)‡	(yes)	X-linked
SCID (Swiss type)	yes	yes	(yes)	(yes)	autosomal recessive
SCID with ADA deficiency	yes	yes	(yes)	(yes)	autosomal recessive
SCID with ectodermal dysplasia & dwarfism	yes	yes	yes	yes	? autosomal recessive
SCID (sporadic)	yes	yes	yes	yes	unknown
Disorders mainly affecting B cells					
Congenital hypogammaglobulinemia (Bruton type)	no	no	yes	yes§	X-linked
Congenital hypogammaglobulinemia	no	no	yes	yes	auto recessive
Common variable immunodeficiency	no	(no)	no	yes§	? autosomal recessive
IgA deficiency	no	(no)	no	no§	variable
IgM deficiency	no	no	no	?	unknown
IgG subclass deficiency	no	no	no	?	X-linked
Immunodeficiency with elevated IgM	no	no	no	(yes)	X-linked
X-linked immunodeficiency with normal globulin count or hyperglobulinemia	no	no	(no)	(yes)	X-linked
Hypogammaglobulinemia with thymoma	no	no	no	yes§	unknown
Disorders mainly affecting T cells					
Thymus hypoplasia (Nezelof's syndrome)	yes	yes	(no)	(no)	variable
DiGeorge's syndrome	yes	yes	no	no	variable
Nucleoside phosphorylase deficiency	yes	yes	no	no	? autosomal recessive
Chronic mucocutaneous candidiasis with endocrinopathy	no	yes	no	no	? autosomal recessive
Complex immunodeficiencies					
Wiskott-Aldrich syndrome	yes	yes	no	(yes)	X-linked
Ataxia-telangiectasia	(yes)	yes	no	(yes)	autosomal recessive
Hyper-IgE syndrome	no	yes	no	no	unknown
Cartilage-hair hypoplasia	?	yes	no	(no)	autosomal recessive

*Indicates first or second stages of lymphoid cell differentiation.

†SCID = severe combined immunodeficiency.

‡Statements enclosed in parentheses indicate defects that are variable in severity or expression.

§Recent evidence indicates the presence of excessive suppressor cell activity.

(Courtesy of Dr. D. E. Thor, M.D., Ph.D., Dept. of Microbiology, University of Texas Health Science Center at San Antonio.)

of IgM, there is a reduction of antibodies to polysaccharide antigens (e.g., blood groups), and reduced opsonization and complement activation. Children with IgM or IgG deficiency are susceptible to bacterial respiratory infections and systemic bacterial infections. In some such children, deficiency of selected IgG subclasses may produce a similar clinical picture.

Dysgammaglobulinemias. Some IDD are difficult to classify. Normal numbers of T and B lymphocytes are present but one or more (but not all) immunoglobulin classes are absent, reduced, or elevated. Included in this heterogeneous group is common variable hypogammaglobulinemia, which accounts for the largest number of overall B cell disorders. The onset is usually in older children and adults, and there is a familial tendency for IDD and hypersensitivity diseases. In many cases, immunodeficiency appears to be related to T cell suppression of immunoglobulin synthesis. In others, plasma cell secretory function is defective.

Another example of dysgammaglobulinemia is X-linked immunodeficiency with hyper-IgM. As in common variable immunodeficiency and other examples of this category, B cells representing each of the immunoglobulin classes are normal in number. However, serum IgG and IgA levels are low while IgM is high. Neutropenia and autoimmune phenomena are sometimes present. Plasma cells contain only IgM or sometimes IgD as well, suggesting that there is a block in the postulated "switchover" from primary IgM antibody to secondary IgG and IgA antibody production.

Hypogammaglobulinemia (Deficiency of All Immunoglobulin Classes). The most serious B cell disorders are those in which there is virtually no detectable immunoglobulin of any class in the serum. The condition formerly was called "agammaglobulinemia"; however, hypogammaglobulinemia is the preferred term since trace amounts of immunoglobulins are present. Most cases have X-linked recessive inheritance (Bruton's type) although some are autosomal recessive. Rheumatoid arthritis or other forms of collagen vascular disease occur in 40 percent of cases and lymphoreticular malignancy in 5 to 10 percent. In lymphoid tissues, germinal centers and plasma cells are absent. Surface immunoglobulins (SIG) are absent or sparse on B cells, while variable numbers of mononuclear cells with C3 and Fc receptors can be found. Maternal antibody protects infants until about 6 months of age, when recurrent bacterial infections ensue.

Transient hypogammaglobulinemia of infancy may be a mild, self-limited example of agammaglobulinemia. B cell numbers are normal in serum and lymphoid organs. There is a delay in fully initiating gamma globulin production, but serious infections usually do not occur. The hypogammaglobulinemia resolves in a few months up to 3 years or more, but, generally, serum levels of all immunoglobulins become normal by the age of 2 years.

DEFICIENCIES PRIMARILY OF T LYMPHOCYTE FUNCTION

Inability to Respond to Certain Antigens, with CMI Largely Intact. At one end of the spectrum there are individuals who genetically are incapable of mounting an immune response to certain mycobacteria, pathogenetic fungi, or tumor-associated antigens. This leads to chronic or even fatal disease, despite the presence of an otherwise basically "normal" T lymphocyte system. Other individuals have an isolated defect in CMI. A noteworthy example is chronic mucocutaneous candidiasis (CMC), often associated with inability of lymphocytes to initiate blastogenesis or

to manufacture MIF in response specifically to fungal antigens, so that a protective delayed hypersensitivity reaction does not develop. In other cases, T cell function seems intact but phagocytes, especially macrophages, are defective in candidicidal capacity. These may be other associated problems such as deficiency in serum candicidal factor, selective IgA deficiency, and endocrinopathies involving thyroid, parathyroid, or adrenal glands.

Congenital Aplasia of the Thymus (DiGeorge Syndrome). In the DiGeorge syndrome, T lymphocytes usually are absent but B lymphocytes are normal in numbers and function. Faulty coalescence of the third and fourth branchial pouches in fetal life lead to hypoplasia of the thymus and the parathyroid glands. Associated congenital defects include a peculiar facies with hypertelorism, malformed ears, and micrognathia and defects of the heart and aortic arch. An early clue for the pediatrician is the appearance of neonatal tetany. Life-threatening infections with bacteria, viruses, and fungi begin early in infancy and early death is to be expected. In manner of presentation, there is great clinical similarity between thymic aplasia and severe combined immunodeficiency (see below). IgE levels sometimes are high in disorders of T cell deficiency (e.g., thymic aplasia, Nezelof syndrome, and Wiskott-Aldrich syndrome).

DEFICIENCES IN BOTH T AND B LYMPHOCYTE FUNCTION

Deficiencies Involving Stem Cells. The most serious immune deficiency occurs when bone marrow stem cells do not mature into functional lymphocytes and phagocytic cells. This calamitous situation is termed severe combined immune deficiency (SCID). Older terms meaning SCID include Swiss-type lymphopenic agammaglobulinemia and thymic alymphoplasia. There are many genetic mechanisms: X-linked recessive (Gitlin type), autosomal recessive, as well as sporadic and multifactorial. In some children with SCID, there are few or no circulating lymphocytes, and cells bearing T or B markers are uncommon. In other patients, numbers of T cells and B cells are in the normal range, but effective CMI is lacking and immunoglobulin levels of most or all classes are extremely low or absent.

Occasionally there is neutropenia, thrombocytopenia or abnormal phagocytic function. The thymus is small and dysplastic, containing few lymphocytes. Chronic and recurrent infections begin early in infancy with a progressive downhill course leading to death within the first year from viral, bacterial, fungal, or *Pneumocystis carinii* infections. If a child with SCID is born, it is imperative that *cord blood* from subsequent newborns in the family be tested for numbers of lymphocytes and capacity for lymphocyte blastogenic response to mitogens *in vitro*. If the lymphocyte count is low or the blastogenic responsiveness is nil, the newborn with probable SCID should be isolated and a search begun for a donor of immunocompetent tissue.

Approximately half of all patients with SCID lack the enzyme adenosine deaminase (ADA), normally found on the membranes of blood cells and tissue cells. ADA deficiency leads to the buildup of adenosine in cells, possibly reducing lymphocyte and phagocyte function. Recently, a deficiency in nucleoside phosphorylase, another enzyme in the purine pathway, has been found in some SCID patients having normal ADA activity. SCID also has been associated with the cartilage-hair syndrome. A variant of SCID may be the Nezelof syndrome, in which there is greatly reduced function of T and B lymphocytes; in some cases reduced antibody levels are secondary to absent T cell helper activity. It is noteworthy that the killer lymphocyte of the ADCC, (antibody-dependent cell-mediated cytotoxicity) reaction is absent in SCID but is present in most other IDD, suggesting that the K cell may represent yet another cell line derived from the stem cell.

Complex or Mixed Disorders. Children with hyperglobulinemia E (including Job's syndrome and the Buckley syndrome), usually have recurrent staphlococcal abscesses involving skin, lungs, and bones. Infections with other virulent microorganisms may occur as well. Serum levels of IgE are extremely high, often over 1,000 IU/ml, presumably owing to the absence of a T cell suppressor for the B cells producing immunoglobulins of the IgE class. Many patients have a dermatosis that resembles but is not identical to atopic dermatitis. CMI is impaired, and an inhibitor of chemotaxis for PMN's and monocytes may be present, or there may be defective

phagocyte microbicidal function (Church et al., 1976).

The Wiskott-Aldrich syndrome is an X-linked recessive disorder consisting of a triad of eczema, thrombocytopenia with bleeding, and recurrent pyogenic infections of the middle ear as well as of other sites. Isohemagglutinins (antibodies to blood group antigens A and B) are absent, since there is deficient IgM synthesis and poor antibody response to polysaccharide antigens. IgA or IgE may be deficient, although IgE levels may be high. With advancing age, progressive loss of CMI leads to frequent life-threatening infections.

Ataxia-telangiectasia is an autosomal recessive disorder often associated with immunodeficiency. Telangiectasias of the conjunctivae and ears may be seen in infancy, but progressive cerebellar ataxia may not appear until the child's early school years. Half of the patients with this disorder have immune deficiency, most commonly deficiency of secretory IgA and, at times, IgE as well. CMI deficiency frequently coexists. Chronic sinopulmonary disease and gastrointestinal disorders are associated phenomena. Lymphoreticular malignancies develop in 15 percent of the cases.

Secondary and Acquired Functional Aberrations of Immune Function

IMMUNE DYSFUNCTION SECONDARY TO A PRIMARY DISEASE OR CLINICAL DISORDER

Acquired and secondary deficiencies in defense are common. Indeed, there are times in everyone's life when immune capabilities fall below usual levels. Various causes of acquired immune dysfunction are listed in Table 6–2. There may be dysfunction of the lymphocyte system, the phagocyte system, or both. Immune deficiencies follow metabolic aberrations such as severe malnutrition, chronic diarrhea, malabsorption and protein-losing enteropathy, severe burns, uncontrolled diabetes mellitus, generalized dermatoses, nephrotic syndrome, iron deficiency anemia, and uremia.

Depressed immune function regularly occurs in the progressive or terminal phase of bacterial, viral, and fungal infections, as well as diseases such as cancer and leukemia-lymphomas. During the progressing stages of these disorders, antigen-antibody complexes and free antigen block effector

TABLE 6–2   CAUSES OF SECONDARY OR ACQUIRED IMMUNE DEFICIENCY DISORDERS
INVOLVING LYMPHOCYTES AND PHAGOCYTES

Metabolic Aberrations	Associated With Replicating Antigens*	Administration of Immunosuppressive Agents	Other
Malnutrition	Bacterial sepsis	Corticosteroids	SURGICAL
Chronic diarrhea, malabsorption,	Disseminated virus infection	X-irradiation	Thymectomy
			Splenectomy
enteropathy	Disseminated mycoses	Immune suppressive drugs	Thoracic duct drainage
Severe Burns			
Generalized dermatoses	Cancer, including leukemia-lymphoma	Anti-leukocyte globulin (ALG)	
			DISORDERS
Diabetes mellitus			Myotonia-dystrophy
Nephrotic syndrome			Autoimmune disorders†
Uremia			"Allergic" disorders†
Iron deficiency anemia			

*In advancing disease, free antigen and antigen-antibody complexes may cause immune paralysis (effector tolerance).

†In many cases both the "hypersensitivity" disease and the reduced immune function may be manifestations of an underlying etiologic process.

cell function, neutralize antibodies, and bring about immune paralysis. Soluble factors made by the infectious agents or abnormal host cells also can inhibit phagocytic, chemotactic, and cytotoxic functions. This blockade of effector antibodies, lymphocytes, and phagocytes impairs a maximal immune response of the intensely stimulated host.

The administration of anti-inflammatory or immunosuppressant agents such as corticosteroids, X-irradiation, immune suppressive drugs, and antilymphocyte antibodies (ALG, ALS) may impair function of both the T and B lymphocyte systems. Immune dysfunction also is associated with a variety of disorders of lymphoid function. Some of these are diseases involving lymphoreticular tissues, such as sarcoidosis, myotonia-dystrophy, autoimmune and collagen vascular diseases, and allergic disease.

Individuals with atopic disease may have an increased incidence of respiratory and skin infection and demonstrable evidence of immune dysfunction (Dahl et al., 1976; Furukawa and Altman, 1978; Hill and Quie, 1974; Rogge and Hanafin, 1976; Snyderman et al., 1977; Hill et al., 1976a). In those with atopic dermatitis, recurrent candidiasis or pyoderma has been associated with high IgE levels (decreased T suppressor activity?); impaired chemotaxis for PMN's and macrophages; decreased motile, phagocytic and microbicidal functions of phagocytes, and in vitro and in vivo evidence of depressed T lymphocyte function. Similar findings also have been observed in respiratory allergy, particularly asthma, with improved immune function following the use of transfer factor (Khan et al., 1978) and adjuvants (e.g., levamisole) in vivo and thymosin in vitro (Byrom et al., 1978). In some of these cases it appears that the immune dysfunction is concurrent with or secondary to the atopic disorder, remission of the allergic manifestations often being associated with normalization of the previously disturbed immune functions (Hill et al., 1976b; Rogge and Hanafin, 1976; Uehara & Ofuji, 1977). Our own studies of atopic individuals with the Rebuck skin window technique support such observations. Decreased tissue accumulations of monocytes and conversion into macrophages occurs in 24-hour skin windows in about half of individuals with atopic disease. In the majority of tested individuals with seasonal respiratory allergy, the skin window findings had become normal when subjects were studied out of season, when asymptomatic.

Other acquired immune deficiencies follow surgical procedures or nonsurgical loss of lymphoid tissues. Loss of T cell function and CMI occurs after thymectomy or chronic drainage of lymph from the thoracic duct. Increased susceptibility to sepsis and meningitis, particularly by the pneumococcus, the meningococcus, H influenzae, and E. coli occurs after splenectomy. A decrease in the clearance rate of bacteria from the blood reflects a critical loss of phagocytic function. Primary immune responses to bacteria also may be decreased, especially in infants. The occurrence of sudden overwhelming infection depends not only on age (babies are more prone than older children) but on the condition leading to the splenectomy. The incidence of infection following splenectomy for trauma is less than 1 percent but it may be as high as 20 percent if the splenectomy was required for autoimmune or hematologic disorders.

IMMUNE DISORDERS ASSOCIATED WITH DERANGED IMMUNE REGULATORY FUNCTION

Abnormal regulation of immunity is increasingly being recognized as a cause of immune deficiency (Table 6–3). Of the recognized examples, most concern the B lymphocyte system, with resultant excessive or diminished production of antibodies (Waldmann, 1977). Hyperglobulinemia involving several or all immunoglobulin classes follows excessive "helper" regulatory activity. A macrophage-derived regulator seems responsible for hypergammaglobulinemia seen in sarcoidosis. It is not clear whether such a mechanism explains the hyperglobulinemia found in other conditions in which there is intense lymphoreticular stimulation. Sézary syndrome is a leukemia of T lymphocytes in which the cells secrete large quantities of a T helper substance that stimulates polyclonal immunoglobulin synthesis.

Decreased T cell suppressor activity also is associated with the overproduction of immunoglobulins. NZB B/W mice appear normal at birth but develop a disease resembling systemic lupus erythematosus (SLE) within several months. At the time that hyperglobulinemia and autoantibodies are developing, a concurrent loss of T cell suppressor activity is observed. Loss of T cell suppressor activity, the appearance of autoantibodies, and manifestations of SLE can be prevented by injections of a soluble immune regulatory substance (SIRS) extracted from spleens of normal mice. Decreased T suppressor function also is observed in humans with SLE, along with other evidence of CMI deficiency. In the hyper-IgE syndrome, the elevated IgE levels may be due to the absence of T cell suppressor activity for the B cell line that produces IgE.

Other instances of apparent regulator dysfunction are reflected by low levels of antibodies and by hypogammaglobulinemia. Most of these are associated with elevated levels of a suppressor material, generally T cell derived. In some cases of common variable hypogammaglobulinemia, T cell suppressors to various immunoglobulin classes reduce production of those immu-

TABLE 6–3 REPORTED ABERRATIONS OF REGULATORY FUNCTION IN IMMUNE DISORDERS

Regulatory Derangement	Condition or Disorder	Immunoglobulin Abnormalities
Increased helper activity	Sarcoidosis*	Hyperglobulinemia
	Sézary syndrome* (T cell leukemia)	Hyperglobulinemia
Decreased suppressor activity	Systemic lupus* erythematosus	Hyperglobulinemia, including autoantibodies
	Hypogammaglobulinemia* (some cases)	Autoantibodies
	Hyper-IgE syndrome	Elevated IgE class
Increased suppressor activity	Common variable hypogammaglobulinemia* (some cases)	Reduced or absent immune globulins, some classes
	Selective IgA or IgM deficiency	Absent serum and secretory IgA or IgM
	Multiple myeloma*	Most classes of immune globulins reduced
	Hypogammaglobulinemia (some cases)	All classes of immune globulins absent or reduced
Decreased helper activity	Nezelof Syndrome; some cases of SCID	Absent or reduced immune globulins, some or all classes

*Apparently *acquired,* in contrast to congenital or innate.

noglobulins, while other classes are spared. A suppressor of the B cell line producing IgA accounts for some cases of selective IgA deficiency; a similar mechanism may operate in selective IgM deficiency. Multiple myeloma is a cancer involving one clone (rarely multiple) of B lymphocytes. Although the serum level of the monoclonal abnormal immunoglobulin is enormous, serum levels of all other immunoglobulins are quite low. Such hypogammaglobulinemia apparently is secondary to suppression of B cells by a macrophage suppressor, probably in response to the excessive levels of myeloma immunoglobulin. In some individuals with hypogammaglobulinemia, a T cell or macrophage-derived suppressor seems to be operative; numbers of lymphocytes bearing B cell markers often are normal. This may occur following infectious mononucleosis, in which T cell suppression of EB virus–infected B cells does not turn off. Low or negligible levels of all immunoglobulin classes has also been found owing to insufficient T lymphocyte helper activity (as opposed to increased suppressor activity) in Nezelof's syndrome. Some individuals with ataxia telangiectasia have decreased lymphocyte blastogenesis to mitogens and antigens due to a suppressor of lymphocyte function.

EVALUATION OF PATIENTS WITH SUSPECTED IMMUNE DEFICIENCY DISORDERS

Because the field of allergy and immunology is so complex and is expanding so rapidly, the physician dealing with patients who have problems related to immune response can easily feel overwhelmed. His resources are particularly taxed when the possibility of IDD is raised. There is a bewildering array of diagnostic tests and therapeutic approaches, only some of which may be available to him. Furthermore, *most* examples of IDD probably have not yet been delineated and classified. To make the best of this situation, the primary physician must:

1. Appreciate the clinical clues that suggest the possibility of IDD.

2. Understand the general diagnostic principles.

3. Carry out appropriate screening tests in his office and local supporting laboratories.

4. Obtain expert consultation for patients who have any evidence of significant IDD.

Clues that Suggest IDD

The occurrence of unusual infections — unusual in frequency, severity, or in nature of infectious agent — is the most important clue suggesting immune deficiency. The physician deals with infections in so many forms that it may be difficult to recognize that a particular patient is having more trouble than is to be expected. In the preschool years, normal children may be expected to have as many as ten upper respiratory infections or episodes of gastroenteritis each year. In those first five years, occasional bouts of otitis media, lower respiratory tract infection, and pyoderma are not unusual. During the elementary school years, a half dozen acute infections of one sort or another are common annually.

Infections that should raise suspicion of immune deficiency include those that fall into one or more of the following categories:

Recurrent respiratory infections that lead to the use of antimicrobial therapy every month or so

Severe bacterial infections, such as pneumonia, sepsis, or meningitis

Chronic purulent otitis media

Chronic or recurrent pneumonia; bronchiectasis

Refractory or recurrent pyoderma

Chronic conjuctivitis

Chronic monilial (*Candida albicans*) infection

Pneumocystis carinii pneumonia

Any infection of unusual severity that is slow to heal

Aside from infection, other clues that can indicate an immune deficiency state include:

Chronic or recurrent gastrointestinal disease — diarrhea, malabsorption or protein-losing enteropathy

Failure to thrive

Chronic signs of systemic illness, such as pallor, irritability, apathy, and weakness

Paucity of lymph nodes, tonsils, and adenoids

Hepatosplenomegaly or lymphadenopathy

Disseminated vaccinial disease after smallpox vaccination; disseminated infection after BCG vaccine

Unusual prolonged skin rashes, or alopecia

Hematologic aberrations involving erythrocytes, leukocytes, or platelets

Hypersensitivity disorders may be another indication of an immune deficiency state. Atopic disease, collagen vascular disease, or other autoimmune disease seems a paradoxical consideration for immune deficiency. However, as indicated above, this concurrence is not uncommon, and some immunologists feel that most, if not all, hypersensitivity reactions are associated with some defect in immune competence that sets the stage for the hypersensitivity response.

CLINICAL CHARACTERISTICS OF DYSFUNCTION IN SYSTEMS OF DEFENSE

In evaluating a child for immune deficiency, it is not necessary to be cognizant of the diagnostic criteria for *all* known immune deficiency states. On the other hand, the physician should be familiar with the clinical and laboratory findings that are associated with deficiency in each of the major defense systems. This approach is useful for two reasons: (1) most children evaluated with be found to have normal function in each of the systems, which will rule out the diagnosis of immune deficiency, and (2) among those patients in whom abnormalities in immune function will be demonstrated, few will be easily categorized according to accepted classifications of immunodeficiency states. Therefore, it is better to characterize the patient in terms of measurable levels of immune parameters and according to the degree of abnormality in different immune functions.

Characteristics of B Cell and Antibody Deficiencies. Antibody deficiency syndromes are characterized by chronic or recurrent pyogenic infections with virulent extracellular bacteria such as gram-positive cocci (staphylococci, streptococci, pneumococci) and *H. influenzae*. Chronic sinopulmonary disease is common. There are few problems with viral, fungal, or saprophytic infections. Growth usually is unimpaired and affected children frequently survive to adulthood. In some affected individuals, B cell receptors or numbers of B cells are reduced, cortical germinal centers are scarce in lymphoid structures, and there is a paucity of adenoidal, tonsillar, or other lymphoid tissues.

Many of these same findings are characteristic of deficiencies in complement components or in deficiences of PMN numbers or function (Chapter 8). Because the clinical manifestations are so similar, deficiency in antibody, PMN's, and complement function may be considered conveniently for diagnostic purposes in one category, the *APC group* (discussed subsequently).

Characteristics of T Cell and Macrophage Deficiencies. Affected children have recurrent infections with low-grade or opportunistic infectious agents such as mycobacteria, fungi, and enveloped viruses and saprophytes such as *Pneumocystis carinii*. Live virus vaccination may lead to disseminated infection and death. Serious systemic manifestations such as growth retardation, wasting, malabsorption and diarrhea are common. Children surviving beyond infancy have a 10 to 15 percent chance of developing malignancy of the lymphoreticular system. There may be anergy to delayed cutaneous hypersensitivity testing with common antigens. If CMI deficiency is profound, the child is susceptible to the usually fatal graft-versus-host (GVH) disease, if given fresh blood or blood products like plasma, which may contain small numbers of lymphocytes, or allogeneic bone marrow.

Because macrophages are essential to the development of delayed hypersensitivity reactions and are intimately involved in immune sensitization, surveillance, and destruction of target cells, it is not surprising that deficiencies in macrophage number or function closely resemble the findings typical of T cell deficiency. Accordingly it is useful to consider deficiencies involving T cells or macrophages in the same category, the *CMI group*.

History in Patients With Suspected IDD

Once the possibility of IDD is raised, a careful and systematic history can go a long way in predicting the nature of disordered function and the diagnostic tests to be considered first. In taking the history, establishing the nature of infections is of paramount importance, obtaining details of (a) involved sites, (b) age of onset, (c) frequency and chronicity, and (d) types of microorganisms involved.

Characteristics of APC Infections. APC infections are characterized by pyoderma, abscesses, otitis, sinusitis, pneumonia, meningitis, and sepsis. They may not appear in the first several months of life, when maternal IgG affords passive protection. Recurrent infections at various levels of the respiratory tract are particularly common; chronic otitis in older children and adults strongly suggests APC deficiency. Offending organisms are virulent bacteria such as pneumococci, *S. aureus,* and *H. influenzae.*

Characteristics of CMI Deficiency. Infections associated with CMI deficiency may begin in early infancy, since there is no passive protection. In this group, infectious agents are of low pathogenicity, often having an intracellular macrophagic phase. Enveloped viruses (e.g., herpes and vaccinia), *Candida albicans* and other fungi, mycobacteria, and intracellular invaders such as the protozoan, *Pneumocystis carinii,* also are problems.

Other Findings Suggestive of IDD. A history of *other* findings suggestive of IDD should also be obtained:

1. Prolonged or recurrent fever
2. Atopic disease
3. Autoimmune phenomena, including arthritis and anemia
4. Malnutrition, edema, chronic diarrhea and malabsorption
5. Neuromuscular: neonatal tetany (?DiGeorge syndrome), difficulties in gait (?ataxia telangiectasia)
6. Bleeding or purpura (?SCID, ?Wiskott-Aldrich syndrome)
7. Surgical removal of lymphoid organs (tonsils, adenoids, appendix and spleen); obtain histologic slides, if possible
8. Immunizations: types given, date of initial series, boosters (Live virus vaccine success indicates competent CMI)
9. Immunosuppressive drugs, irradiation (when? why?)
10. Malignancy (T cell immunodeficiency: increased risk of cancer)
11. Previous therapy with immunologically active material: gamma globulin, transfer factor, blood or plasma

The family history is very important for clues to unusual disease and pattern of inheritance. For the immediate family members and close relatives obtain history of incidence of unusual infection, early deaths, IDD, autoimmune disease, and malignancy.

Physical Examination

Any child with suspected IDD deserves a complete physical examination. Certain parts of the examination are of special significance:

1. *Growth parameters and general health*: In APC deficiencies there is generally normal growth and healthy appearance. Children with CMI deficiency often fail to thrive; they may appear chronically ill.
2. *Respiratory infection:* Chronic or recurrent otitis media (unusual in adults), sinusitis, and lower respiratory tract infections (common in APC, but not in CMI deficiency).
3. *Tonsils, adenoids, lymph nodes:* These may be hypoplastic in APC and CMI deficiencies. Particularly sparse in SCID. Hyperplastic in complement-polymorph deficiencies.
4. *Liver and spleen:* Descriptions for lymphoid structures (number 3) apply.
5. *Skin:* Scars of healed infection may be seen following bacterial abscesses in APC deficiency and after infections by fungi or viruses in CMI deficiency. Active pyoderma in APC but not CMI disorders. Candida infections in CMI but not APC deficiency. Eczema in Wiskott-Aldrich and Hyper-IgE syndromes. Petechiae or purpura in SCID and the Wiskott-Aldrich syndrome as well as autoimmune disease.
6. *Mucous membranes:* Dilated vessels in ataxia telangiectasia (conjunctivae). Ulcerated infections at gingival margins evident in neutropenic states.
7. *Congenital defects:* Facial and cardiovascular — DiGeorge syndrome. Children with short limbed dwarfism and fine hair (cartilage-hair syndrome) — SCID. Partial albinism — Chédiak-Higashi syndrome.
8. *Cerebellar ataxia:* Ataxia telangiectasia (preschool age).

Procedures Useful for the Evaluation of Immune Function in the Office and Local Laboratory

Principles in the Evaluation of a Patient with Possible Deficiency in Defense

Assess the competence of each system of defense—T cells, B cells, and phagocyte-complement system (Tables 6–4 and 6–5).

Measure both the serum or blood concentration and the function of each factor. (It is not sufficient to determine that serum levels of immunoglobulins are normal; specific antibody activity to a variety of antigens also must be measured.)

Carry out simpler tests first; reserve complex and expensive tests for appropriate indication.

Evidence of a defect in any defense system is an indication for evaluation of all systems, since *multiple deficiencies are the rule*.

If tests suggest significant deficiency, refer patient for consultation with immunologists for specialized laboratory tests to complete the workup and to plan rational management.

General and Nonimmunologic Studies

Radiologic

1. Films to detect infection or inflammation: chest, sinuses, mastoids, or long bones
2. Films with soft tissue technique to determine mass of lymphoid structures
   a. Lateral view of nasopharynx for adenoids
   b. Lateral and PA of chest for thymus in early infancy (the thymus can be detected only half the time in normal newborns)
   c. Chest film for enlarged hilar nodes, pneumonia, granulomatous infection, and lymphomas

Appropriate Cultures. Culture and identify pathogens responsible for serious or repeated infection. Infections with certain organisms suggest specific immune deficiencies; identifying the pathogen also permits the clinician to measure the level of specific antibody and T cell immunity which should be present in an individual infected with that particular agent.

Hematologic. Measure hemoglobin, he-

TABLE 6–4 SCREENING TESTS FOR EVALUATION OF THE B CELL (ANTIBODY) SYSTEM

Serum level of immunoglobulins by class
  IgG, IgA, IgM: radial immunodiffusion
  IgE: radioimmunoassay (PRIST)

Level of specific antibodies
  Natural: isohemagglutinins (IgM)
      antistreptococcal (IgG)

  Following immunization:
      Routine: diphtheria and tetanus, polio, rubeola, rubella
      Special: typhoid-parathyphoid influenza

  To infecting agents: bacterial, viral, or fungal

  Associated with hypersensitivity disorders:
      Allergens: skin tests or RAST
      Autoantigens: ANA, RF; Coombs' test; organ-specific antibodies as appropriate

---

matocrit, and do a *complete* white blood count
1. The total white blood cell (WBC) and differential count: calculate absolute leukocyte counts.

TABLE 6–5 SCREENING TESTS FOR EVALUATION OF THE T CELL–MACROPHAGE (CMI) SYSTEM

Level of Mononuclear Cells in Blood
  Absolute lymphocyte count
  Absolute monocyte count

Delayed Cutaneous Hypersensitivity to Battery of Recall Antigens
  Candida
  Tricophyton
  Streptococci
  Tetanus toxoid
  Diphtheria toxoid
  Mumps
  Tuberculin
  Histoplasmin
  Coccidiodin
  Phytohemagglutinin (PHA) [experimental]

Rebuck Skin Window—24 Hours
  Relative numbers of mononuclear cells
  Relative conversion of monocytes to macrophages

Lymphocyte Blastogenic Response In Vitro
  Mitogens—PHA, conconavalin A, pokeweed mitogen (PWM)
  Selected antigens
  Mixed leucocyte reaction (MLR)

2. Determine the absolute lymphocyte count: Total peripheral blood lymphocytes (PBL) consistently under 2000 per mm^3 in the preschool years are suggestive of immune deficiency; PBL under 1500 per mm^3 suggest some degree of deficiency, while values under 1000 per mm^3 reflect serious immune deficiency.

3. Absolute PMN counts under 1000 per mm^3 are below the normal range. PMN levels that are maintained below 500 per mm^3 indicate a significant degree of neutropenia often associated with increased risk of infection.

4. Examine the blood smear meticulously. Blastoid or "atypical" lymphocytes are seen with viral infections of lymphocytes (as in infectious mononucleosis), lymphoma-leukemia, or intense stimulation of PBL *in vivo* by potent, often disseminated antigens. PMN's and monocytes with inclusions could indicate Chédiak-Higashi disease or cytoplasmic inclusion disease. Howell-Jolly bodies are seen in the absence of splenic function.

5. Increased numbers of eosinophils are seen with atopy, parasitism, or the hyper-IgE syndrome; increases in both eosinophils and monocytes may occur with hypogammaglobulinemic states.

6. Platelets are decreased in Wiskott-Aldrich syndrome and some forms of SCID.

Evaluation of the B Lymphocyte (Antibody) System

Regardless of where he or she practices, the primary physician can carry out a variety of studies to determine whether or not the patient makes adequate levels of protective antibodies (see Table 6–4). There are two elements to the screening: measurement of serum levels for each of the immunoglobulin classes and determination of specific antibody activity to several different and unrelated antigens.

Serum Levels of Immunoglobulins by Class. Every clinical laboratory has the capacity to quantitate serum levels of immunoglobulins. Today, the radial immunodiffusion technique of Mancini is most widely used in quantitation of IgG, IgA, and IgM. This technique can give false values in patients whose sera contain antibodies to serum proteins of the animals whose antiserum was used to prepare the test plates. This phenomenon is most commonly seen in selective IgA deficiency patients whose serum contain antibodies to goat serum proteins. In those instances, the precipitin ring that develops in the assay does not indicate IgA in the patient's serum, but rather reflects the complexing of the patient's IgG antibodies with goat gamma globulin antigen. *When immunoglobulin levels on a particular serum are reported, they should be related specifically to values normal for age.* A table of age-related normal values can be found on p. 32, Chapter 2.

Serum IgE should be measured in any diagnostic workup for IDD; greatly elevated levels are associated with atopy, the hyper-IgE syndrome, and CMI deficiency (Buckley and Fiscus, 1975). The PRIST radioimmunoassay for total serum IgE now is readily available.

Determination of Functional Immunoglobulin (Specific Antibody) Activity. To assess the B cell system, it is necessary to demonstrate adequate levels of antibody to a variety of antigens (see Table 6–4). When a patient suffers recurrent infections from a particular microorganism, it is especially important to determine whether or not specific antibodies have been made to its antigens. A bacteriologist can help in setting up the required serological studies.

"Natural" Antibodies to Ubiquitous Antigens. Isohemagglutinins are predominantly IgM antibodies specific for blood group A and group B antigens. Antibody production is stimulated by cross-reacting substances in foods and microorganisms, and titers should be greater than 1:8 in all children over the age of two. The test is readily available in any blood bank. Patients who do not respond to complex polysaccharide antigens (e.g., Wiskott-Aldrich syndrome) have abnormally low isohemagglutinin titers.

Antibodies to streptococcal antigens are mostly of the IgG class. Streptozym or ASO titers are readily available. ASO titers of 12 units or greater are usually present by one year of age. Many laboratories do not routinely measure titers below 50 (lower levels are not useful for diagnosis of recent streptococcal infection) and must be instructed to adjust the sensitivity of the test.

Antibodies Formed in Response to Immunization. Immunization with diphtheria, tetanus, polio, rubeola and rubella agents is routinely employed in children. By making inquiry at a local laboratory or the local or state health department, the physician can learn where sera can be sent for determination of antibody titers to several of these immunogens. If it is considered useful to determine whether the child can mount an immune response *de novo,* the serologic response to influenza vaccine or to a series of typhoid-paratyphoid immunogen injections can be measured by many local and regional laboratories. *If there is a question of immune deficiency, live virus vaccine should not be used.*

In a child who has received diphtheria toxoid, the Schick test is both simple and useful. A positive test — erythema and induration at 4 to 6 days — indicates that the patient could not neutralize the injected toxin and is deficient in antitoxin antibody. Unfortunately, it has become difficult to obtain the diphtheria toxin required for the Schick test.

Antibodies Associated with Hypersensitivity Disorders

Detection of autoantibodies may be of use in the workup of patients for IDD, particularly if manifestations of autoimmune or collagen vascular disorders are present. Tests for antinuclear antibodies (ANA), rheumatoid factor (RF), and hemolytic antibody (Coomb's test, direct and indirect) are especially useful.

In any child with atopic disease, determination of the level and specificities of IgE type antibodies may be informative.

Evaluation of the T Lymphocyte–Macrophage (CMI) System

As with the B cell system, assessment of the T lymphocyte system should include measure of the *level* of immune reactants (blood lymphocytes) as well as several of the *functions* associated with CMI, such as delayed hypersensitivity, macrophage activation, and lymphocyte blastogenesis (see Table 6–5). If screening tests are essentially normal, it is unlikely that a child has a serious degree of T cell deficiency.

Absolute PBL Count. Upon multiplying the total white blood cell count by the percentage of lymphocytes (differential count) the absolute count of peripheral blood lymphocytes (PBL) is obtained. Beyond infancy, 50 to 80 percent of blood lymphocytes are T cells, which should number 1000 to 3000 mm^3 at any age. Accordingly, when the PBL count itself is below 1000 per mm^3, T cell numbers are definitely decreased and their function very likely decreased.

Skin Tests for Delayed Cutaneous Hypersensitivity (DCH). The skin test for DCH to antigens to which the patient is likely to have been sensitized is the single most useful indicator for competence of the T lymphocyte–macrophage system. For the skin reaction to be positive, virtually all components of the CMI reaction must be present and functioning properly: there must be adequate numbers of circulating T lymphocytes sensitized to recognize introduced antigen; these lymphocytes must localize in the skin at the antigen site and release a variety of soluble mediators that initiate inflammation and attract, immobilize, and activate sufficient numbers of macrophages. Nonspecific mediators of inflammation and dermal vessels must be capable of supporting the prolonged inflammatory response.

Various commonly encountered antigens useful for testing for DCH are listed below. The aqueous antigens are administered in separate sites, each in a volume of 0.1 ml intradermally, using a tuberculin syringe and a 26 gauge needle, bevel up. Induration (erythema is less reliable) should be measured in two dimensions, at 24 and at 48 hours. An average diameter of 4 mm or more is considered to be a positive DCH reaction; the larger the area of induration, the more intense is the degree of CMI.

It is desirable to make two earlier readings as well. Ten to 20 minutes after injection, wheal and flare reactions that are unusually large, as compared to other test sites, indicate the presence of skin-sensitizing (IgE?) antibody to the antigen. At 5 or 6 hours, induration and erythema may reflect an Arthus reaction, the precipitation of circulating antibody with antigen diffusing into dermal venules. A 6-hour reading is of utmost importance and must be related to the 24-hour reading. If the latter is smaller than the 6 hour reading, a true delayed hypersensitivity reaction may not have occurred. On the other hand, if the 24- or 48-hour readings are larger than the 6-hour reading, it is reasonably certain that CMI for the antigen exists.

Antigens appropriate for DCH testing elicit reactions in over half of normal older children and adults and include:

Candida albicans - Dermatophytin "O." Start with 10 PNU/ml (or 1:100 dilution); if negative, try 100 PNU/ml (or 1:10).

Tricophyton. Start with 50 PNU/ml (or 1:100); if negative, try 500 PNU/ml (or 1:10).

Streptokinase-streptodornase (SKSD), marketed as Varidase (Lederle). The lyophilized material is reconstituted with 5 ml sterile water and aliquots of the concentrated stock solution can be kept frozen. Fresh skin test material should be prepared from this stock every 2 or 3 weeks. Diluting 0.1 ml of the stock solution in 10 ml sterile saline gives a final concentration of 40 SK units/ml. If negative, try a two to five times stronger concentration.

Tetanus fluid toxoid can be obtained from several suppliers: one source provides 1.5 ml vials at a concentration of 15 LF/ml. No dilution is required; test with 0.1 ml volume. Diphtheria toxoid also can be used. Since both diphtheria and tetanus toxoids are routinely used for immunization after 2 months of age, these are excellent skin test antigens in infancy and throughout childhood. By 1 year of age, 80 to 100 percent of normal infants show positive DCH reactions to the toxoids.

Mumps skin test material. Positive DCH responses to this antigen often are not related to mumps viral antigen, but to egg protein or uncharacterized contaminants. Mumps skin test antigen is not available at the present time.

Special microbial antigens. Tuberculin, histoplasmin, and coccidioidin are often listed as useful for DCH testing. Tuberculin, in fact, is the commonest antigen used in DCH testing for CMI competence. These antigens are especially useful in certain regions of the country where the majority of the adult population is skin test positive: the southwestern states and California — coccidioidin; the Ohio and Mississippi River drainage basin states — histoplasmin; and the southeastern and central states, having a high incidence of atypical mycobacterial infection — tuberculin.

There is little data that enable confident assessment of the degree of competence of CMI in a child tested for DCH with a battery of antigens. Virtually all adults will be positive to one or more antigens at 24 or 48 hours, while infants of a few months of age are positive to none. By a year of age, a normal child should be positive to at least one antigen, if an adequate number of antigens (at least four or five) are tested.

Recently we have evaluated a disposable plastic device that simultaneously applies a standardized battery of seven recall antigens and a glycerin buffer control to eight different sites. In adults, use of the Multitest* applicator to inoculate antigens has proved to be rapid, relatively painless, and reproducible (Anderson, et al., 1978). When available, the Multitest System holds promise for utility and convenience in DCH testing of children.

To assess competence of CMI, DCH testing also has been used two other ways: (1) If a child has a chronic infection with a specific organism (e.g., *Candida albicans*), DCH testing attains particular value. A negative DCH reaction in the face of the persisting antigenic stimulus is a clear indication of CMI deficiency, regardless of what positive reactions there are to other antigens. Testing should be initiated with *low* antigen concentration since, in a non-immunodeficient individual with infection, sensitization may be high, and a DCH reaction to concentrated antigen can be extreme. (2) In young infants, DCH skin testing to multiple antigens will not be informative. To circumvent this limitation, phytohemagglutinin (PHA), a mitogen that stimulates all T lymphocytes, can be injected intradermally in a dose of 1 to 10 μg. Infants with intact CMI manifest a DCH reaction similar to that induced by antigen, while infants with deficient CMI may not. At this time, the intradermal administration of PHA for DCH testing is experimental, however, since PHA is potentially sensitizing.

Rebuck Skin Window. Rebuck and Crowley introduced this technique over 20 years ago as a means of studying leukocyte function *in vivo.* Circular areas of skin, approximately 3 to 5 mm in size, are gently abraded with a surgical blade or a rotating Dermabrador wheel. A drop of saline or antigen solution is applied to the moist abraded site, followed by placement of a circular cover slip, kept in place by tape. Serum protein components soon coat the cover slip and leukocytes exuded from the blood stick to the glass. At various times, cover slips can be removed and replaced; after the cover slips are stained, numbers and types of exuded leukocytes can be counted. We have found the technique to be promising as a screening tool for IDD (Anderson and Kniker, 1974). In normal individuals, cover slips left in place for 4 hours demonstrate hundreds of exuded leukocytes, of which over 90 percent are PMN's. Lymphocytes, monocytes or eosin-

---

*Lincoln Laboratories.

ophils generally account for no more than 2 or 3 percent each. In individuals with neutropenia or defective PMN motility or chemotaxis, PMN numbers and percentages are below 90 percent, and other leukocyte types become more numerous. When a solution of allergens to which the patient is sensitive is placed on abraded skin sites, accumulation of eosinophils in excess of 4 to 5 percent of total cells strongly suggest atopic disease and IgE sensitization.

The picture changes greatly between 4 and 24 hours. In normal individuals at 24 hours, hundreds to thousands of leukocytes are present, many of which are diffusely scattered in sheets while some are aggregated in densely staining clumps, often rich in basophils and frequently eosinophils. In the sheets, more than half of the leukocytes are mononuclear. Most of these (56 percent of total WBC with a range of 25 to 87) are macrophages, distinguished by irregular margins and large cytoplasmic vacuoles. Monocytes are fewer in number and lymphocytes account for less than 5 percent of the leukocytes. Less than 3 percent of the cells found in sheets are eosinophils; however, numbers may be elevated if there is atopic disease.

About half of the individuals with deranged immune function (T cell deficiency, B cell deficiency, mixed immune deficiency, chronic pyodermas, recurrent respiratory infections, autoimmune disorders, atopic disease) demonstrate abnormal findings on the 24-hour skin window cover slips. The most significant abnormal finding is diminished numbers of macrophages (<25 percent of WBC) in the cellular sheets, apparently related to defective conversion of monocytes into macrophages. Low numbers of monocytes, and absence of clumps containing basophils and eosinophils also are abnormal findings. The clinical utility of the skin window in the assay of immune competence is under continued study. Because the technique is relatively simple, we anticipate that it will have considerable value as a screening procedure.

Lymphocyte Proliferation or Blastogenesis in vitro. An important parameter of lymphocyte function is the ability to divide at a rapid rate in response to stimulation. With a microscope, one can examine a large number of lymphocytes from a culture and calculate the percentage that have become blastoid preparatory to mitosis. This technique is tedious and is not in clinical use. Instead, lymphocyte transformation or blastogenesis is measured by a radiobioassay method. When lympho-

cytes are cultured *in vitro*, those that become blastoid before cell division incorporate increased amounts of protein, amino acids, and nucleic acids. The degree of lymphocyte transformation is proportional to the rate of incorporation of radioactive thymidine (to make DNA) or radioactive uridine (to make RNA). The degree of lymphocyte response is calculated by comparing the amount of incorporated radiolabeled material (e.g., thymidine) in resting, unstimulated cells to that incorporated in lymphocytes stimulated by mitogens or antigens. The results are expressed either as resting or stimulated absolute counts per minute (CPM) or as a stimulation index (SI) or blastogenic index (BI). The index is derived by dividing the stimulated CPM by the background or resting CPM.

Most of the time, the BI is a satisfactory means of quantifying lymphocyte blastogenesis following stimulating agents. However, when the background or "unstimulated count" is higher than usual (as when PBL are stimulated *in vivo* by infections or neoplastic processes), the BI may be relatively low, even though the absolute CPM in stimulated lymphocytes are in the normal or expected range. Thus, a low BI does not rule out normal lymphocyte responsiveness to a stimulating agent if the resting count is elevated unduly.

The most convenient method of measuring lymphocyte proliferation is to incubate heparinized whole blood with dilutions of stimulating agents in growth medium. Using microtiter plastic plates and automatic harvesting apparatus, only a few milliliters of blood are required to test the patient's cells against several mitogens and antigens. Factors in plasma that suppress or block lymphocyte responsiveness can be recognized if present. The more common approach is more cumbersome: heparinized blood is fractionated on a density gradient so that mononuclear cell suspensions, rich in lymphocytes, can be studied. Almost 10 to 25 ml of blood are required for the desired tests. Cells are washed free of plasma; fetal calf serum, homologous human serum, or human serum albumin is substituted to serve as protein nutrient during culture. Although this technique cannot recognize plasma factors that affect lymphocyte function, it does permit a more precise analysis of lymphocyte blastogenic functions by various kinds of stimulating agents:

Stimulation by Mitogens. To assay lymphocyte blastogenesis, stimulation by mitogens is most commonly employed. Some mitogens such as PHA and concanavalin A (ConA) stimulate T lymphocytes exclusively, while others, such as pokeweed mitogen (PWM) and endotoxin, stimulate both T and B lymphocytes in man. Peak stimulation is apparent after 3 or 4 days of culture. Because the majority of lymphocytes are stimulated at the optimal concentration of a mitogen, BI scores of 50 to several hundred are usual. These *in vitro* tests of lymphocyte function are so sensitive, they may remain in the normal range when a patient has developed anergy to DCH testing *in vivo*. When lymphocyte transformation to mitogens is diminished or absent, a serious abnormality in T lymphocyte function is likely.

Stimulation by Antigens. Antigens that are soluble, particulate, or bound to cell membranes can be used to stimulate specifically sensitized lymphocytes *in vitro*. In a sensitized individual, only 1 to 5 percent of lymphocytes respond, so that the incorporation of thymidine, peaking at 5 to 7 days of culture, is relatively small in relation to that following mitogen stimulation. A BI in excess of 2.5 or 3.0 is generally considered positive for specific CMI after antigen stimulation, and a BI of 10 or more is considered unequivocally positive. In assaying CMI, selection of an antigen to which the patient is known to have had contact is of particular value. For instance in a patient with chronic mucocutaneous candiasis, absent lymphocyte blastogenesis to candida antigens is a definite indication of deficient CMI.

Mixed Lymphocyte Reaction. A particularly useful application of lymphocyte transformation is the mixed lymphocyte reaction (MLR) available in any center performing tissue transplantation. In this test, the lymphocytes of one individual are incubated with lymphocytes from another individual for 3 to 4 days and the amount of incorporation of thymidine measured. The lymphocytes are stimulated by histocompatibility (HLA) antigens scattered on the surface of the allogeneic lymphocytes (Bodmer, 1975). In usual practice, the test is a "one-way" MLR in which the "foreign" human cells are pretreated with the metabolic poison mitomycin, so that the only cells capable of making a blastogenic response are those from the studied patient. Inability to recognize and respond to allogeneic cells in the MLR is clear evidence of serious CMI deficiency. It is emphasized that deficient CMI can be manifested by ab-

sent or decreased lymphocyte blastogenesis in the MLR or after antigen stimulation, even though lymphocyte transformation *in vitro* appears to be normal following the relatively stronger stimulation by mitogens.

INTERPRETATION OF RESULTS AND DISPOSITION OF PATIENT

Determining Whether or Not Immune Deficiency Is Present. Having considered the possibility of immune deficiency in a given child and carried out screening tests for T cell function, B cell function, and complement-phagocyte function (see Chapter 8), the physician must collate the data and interpret the results. If all the screening tests of immune function are within normal limits, it is highly unlikely that any serious primary or secondary immune deficiency disease is present. Subtle immune dysfunctions not recognizable by available techniques no doubt exist in some individuals studied, who will continue to have bothersome infections and other problems for an indefinite period. The majority of children whose tests of immune function prove normal, however, fortunately will respond to vigorous management of their underlying disease (e.g., allergic rhinitis) or will outgrow their annoying susceptibility for infection.

What to Do When There Is Evidence of Immune Deficiency. In some children screened for IDD, one or more of the tests will be abnormal, frequently inducing consternation as to appropriate subsequent action. The first move should be to repeat any tests or procedures considered abnormal, to ensure that the results are bona fide. If abnormalities in immune function are substantiated, immune therapy *should not yet be started* since all therapeutic modalities including administration of gamma globulin are potentially harmful and their premature use can obscure the diagnostic workup, which is *still incomplete*.

Evidence of dysfunction in any immune system is an automatic indication for thorough, comprehensive evaluation of all immune systems. Because deficiencies tend to be multiple, it is imperative that all immune functions be examined to recognize all abnormalities present. An investigation of this magnitude generally is beyond the capabilities of the primary physician and the local laboratory resources. The primary physician should now obtain consultation from a specialist familiar with immune deficiency disorders and who has sophisticated laboratory resources available.

The Clinical Immunologist and the Secondary or Tertiary Referral Center. The majority of practicing allergists–clinical immunologists are particularly competent in the area of atopic disease, as well as in related pulmonary and dermatologic disorders. Although they frequently are knowledgeable about immune deficiency disease, it is only the clinical immunologists at major medical centers who are likely to have available most or all of the advanced and sophisticated procedures described in the following section. Their expertise can provide the referring physician with the critical information needed to establish the proper diagnosis and help design the most appropriate plan of therapy.

Advanced Procedures in Immunology Laboratories to Characterize IDD

Once there is evidence of immune dysfunction and the child has been referred for definitive studies, a variety of tests and procedures are available in a secondary or tertiary level medical center (see Table 6–6). The clinical immunologist will recommend some but generally not all of the procedures described here. These procedures are described briefly for general information. Tests designed to measure complement and phagocyte functions are considered in Chapter 8.

Advanced Procedures to Further Test the B Cell System. The first four procedures listed involve quantitative measurement of B cells or their products *in vitro;* the final three tests are miscellaneous measures of *in vivo* B cell–plasma cell dynamics (see Table 6–6).

Enumeration of B Lymphocytes. With serum immunoglobulin deficiency, it is useful to know whether a particular class of B cells is deficient in number or whether all B lymphocytes are decreased. B cells are identified by the presence of membrane-bound immunoglobulins, using immunofluorescent antibody reagents specific for single immunoglobulin classes. B cells recognized by SIG (surface immunoglobulin) markers account for 10 to 20 per cent of PBL, except in early infancy when the percentage is higher. Ranges for B cells of each immunoglobulin class have not yet been defined. Approximate normal values are about 7 percent for IgM bearing cells, 7 percent for IgD (many positive lymphocytes also contain IgM), and 1 to 2 percent for IgG and IgA each. B lymphocytes can be distinguished from other cells by receptors that specifically bind the Epstein-Barr virus and by heterologous antihuman B lymphocyte antisera. Neither of these techniques is routine.

B lymphocytes previously were counted by incubating peripheral blood mononuclear cells with sheep erythrocytes sensitized by rabbit hemolysin (IgG) and mammalian complement (C3). Because B cells have receptors both for aggregated IgG (Fc receptor) and for the third component of complement (C3 receptor), clusters of coated erythrocytes form around B lymphocytes (EAC rosettes). This method of counting B cells leads to falsely

---

TABLE 6–6   ADVANCED PROCEDURES USED TO CHARACTERIZE THE IMMUNE SYSTEM

B Cell System	T Cell System
IN VITRO QUANTITATION	IN VITRO LYMPHOCYTE STUDIES
Enumeration of B cells	Enumeration of T cells
Measurement of secretory immunoglobulin levels	Measurement of lymphokine production
Immunoelectrophoretic study of immunoglobulins	Assay of cytotoxicity against target cells
Search for abnormalities in helper and suppressor regulatory factors	Assay of helper and suppressor regulatory functions
MISCELLANEOUS	MISCELLANEOUS
Biopsy of lymphoid tissue	Induction of delayed hypersensitivity by DNCB
Measurement of antibody response to new antigen	Placement of allograft (not recommended)
Tests for increased catabolism of immune globulins	Lymph node biopsy

high values, since monocytes and PMN's also have Fc and C3 receptors and therefore form EAC rosettes as well. In children and adults, the normal range for EAC rosetting lymphocytes is 15 to 35 percent.

Secretory Immunoglobulin Levels. Patients with deficiency of IgA, the predominant secretory immunoglobulin, lack IgA both in serum and secretions, so that the diagnosis is readily made on analysis of serum alone. Rarely, however, a patient with a normal serum IgA level may lack secretory IgA or secretory component, a protein that links two IgA molecules into a dimer resistant to digestion. While any secretion can be studied, tears are easy to obtain in disposable capillary tubes. Tearing can be induced readily by placing a crystal of salt in the conjunctival sac. Absolute concentrations of immunoglobulins cannot be determined due to dilution; proportions of immunoglobulin classes to each other are more meaningful. In our laboratory, levels of IgA were found to be 5–10 times higher than those of IgG and IgM in tears (Anderson, et al., 1977). In some individuals, it is helpful to measure levels of secretory antibody to specific antigens, such as infectious agents or foods.

Immunoglobulin Subclasses Measured by Immunoelectrophoresis. A given immunoglobulin class can be divided into subclasses by virtue of differences in distinctive chemical groups on the Fc portion of the heavy chain, associated with differences in electrophoretic mobility, binding to cell receptors, and activation of enzymes. While the total level of IgG, IgM, or IgA may appear to be in the normal range, one or more subclasses may be deficient. This can be demonstrated by analyzing the position and length of the immunoglobulin precipitin arcs on immunoelectrophoretic slides.

Abnormalities in Regulation of B Lymphocyte Function. Some cases of antibody deficiency are secondary to faulty regulation of essentially normal B cells (see Table 6–3). There may be excessive "suppressor" activity from T cells or factors in the serum, or there may be deficient "helper" activity by T cells or macrophages. Recognition of such aberrations in regulation requires a complex lymphocyte culture system. Measuring the emergence of plasma cells or secretion of immunoglobulins after culturing lymphocytes stimulated by pokeweed mitogen has been especially helpful.

Biopsy of Lymphoid Tissue. With evidence of antibody or B cell deficiency, it may be helpful to obtain a lymph node biopsy to examine the cortex for presence of germinal centers that contain plasma cells and lymphocytes exhibiting cytoplasmic immunoglobulins. It is preferable to obtain such a biopsy about a week after antigenic stimulation, e.g., 0.5 cc of typhoid-paratyphoid vaccine administered in the thigh followed by excision of a proximal inguinal node if the latter becomes enlarged.

Rectal mucosa can be biopsied by a simple suction technique, allowing the analysis of lymphoid tissue, germinal centers, plasma cells, and immunoglobulin-containing mononuclear cells in the lamina propria. This biopsy procedure carries an element of risk, since it may serve as a portal of entry for infection.

Measurement of Antibody Response to a New Immunogen. This is a useful technique, especially to study immune competence related to a particular pathogen or chemical substance. For instance, patients with Wiskott-Aldrich syndrome tend to respond poorly to polysaccharide antigens, exemplified by blood group substances, dextran polymers, meningococcal vaccine (currently experimental), or pneumococcal vaccine. A bacteriophage virus, ϕX, is available to serve as a neoantigen.

Increased Loss of Gamma Globulins with Protein Loss. Hypogammaglobulinemia occasionally may follow chronic loss of protein from the gastrointestinal tract or a metabolic disorder that increases the rate of catabolism of immunoglobulins. Such processes can be recognized by demonstration of abnormally high rates of protein ($51C_r$ serum albumin) loss from the gut or by serum protein turnover studies, using radiolabeled immune globulins.

Advanced Procedures to Further Test the T Cell–Macrophage System. The first four procedures concern quantitation of T lymphocytes or measurement of some aspect of T lymphocyte function *in vitro*. The last three tests are miscellaneous measures of T cell–macrophage dynamics.

Enumeration of T Cells. When deficiency in T lymphocyte function is suggested by screening tests, it is useful to quantitate the number of T cells in the PBL, since they are reduced in many CMI disorders. T cells are counted by sedimenting mononuclear cells from whole blood and incubating the cell suspension with sheep erythrocytes in the cold. The erythrocytes attach to receptors on T lymphocyte membranes; the resulting cell clusters are called E rosettes. After infancy, using this technique, 50 to 85 percent of PBL are found to be T lymphocytes. Absolute numbers of T cells may be calculated by multiplying percent T cells by total lymphocytes per mm^3 blood.

Measurement of Lymphokine Production. When T lymphocytes (and probably B lymphocytes as well) are stimulated by mitogens, soluble antigens, or foreign cells, their response includes blastoid transformation as well as the production and release of soluble factors (lymphokines). The lymphokine most commonly measured in individuals with presumed CMI deficiency is MIF (macrophage inhibition factor). When skin DCH is adequate, lympokine production and lymphocyte transformation usually are normal. However, in cases in which skin DCH is absent and lymphocyte transformation to a particular stimulus is present, there may be deficient production of one or more lymphokines. As an example, in some patients with chronic mucocandidiasis, lymphocyte transformation is normal but MIF production is absent and there is skin test anergy to candida antigen.

Assay of T cell Killer Function (Direct Cytotoxicity). When incubated with animal or human target cells (e.g., a tumor cell line) some T cells, called killer lymphocytes, destroy the target cells on direct contact. This phenomenon has been observed in tumor and transplantation immunology. It deserves wider study in the assay of CMI competence, particularly since some patients with common variable hypogammaglobulinemia, the Wiskott-Aldrich syndrome, aplastic anemia, and malignancy have defective activity.

Assay of Helper and Suppressor Regulatory Functions. Recent studies have clearly demonstrated that immune dysfunction may be caused by overproduction or underproduction of factors that regulate the immune and protective functions of other lymphocytes and macrophages (see Waldmann, 1977). Unfortunately, the technique for measurement of T lymphocyte–derived helper and suppressor factors is available in relatively few centers. Wider application of these measurements undoubtedly would enhance our understanding of the pathogenesis of many immune deficiency disorders.

Induction of Delayed Hypersensitivity by DNCB. If a battery of commonly encountered antigens does not elicit a positive DCH response, a defect in CMI is probable. It may be desirable to attempt sensitization with a potent immunogen, such as 2,4-dinitrochlorobenzene (DNCB). About 95 percent of normal individuals can be sensitized by application of 0.1 to 0.2 ml of DNCB, 2 to 10 percent in acetone, freshly made up. The solution is applied to a small skin site and allowed to dry by evaporation in 5 to 10 minutes. After 14 days, a different area can be challenged with a weaker 0.02 to 0.1 percent DNCB solution, applied in a similar fashion. Erythema and induration 24 to 48 hours later are typical of a contactant-induced DCH reaction. Sometimes a normal individual will experience a typical DCH reaction at the site of initial sensitization a week or so after the sensitization, reflecting a response to residual antigen from the sensitizing application. A vigorous DCH response precludes the carrying out of the challenge step.

DNCB must be used with great care. It is such a powerful contactant that physicians and nurses who work with it readily become sensitized and may experience skin reactions or burns if technique is not meticulous. Some tested patients develop ulcerations and burns at test sites. Because of this risk, some immunologists do not use DNCB sensitization, preferring to employ a more innocuous neoantigen, such as hemocyanin (KLH), to induce CMI.

Rejection of Allograft. An immunologically competent recipient rejects a skin allograft in the second or third week. Before rejection is final, a biopsy of the graft — including its margin — permits identification of the infiltrating cells and the nature of the inflammatory reaction. There is relatively little justification for this procedure currently, since other tests such as the MLC *in vitro* test provide comparable information, without risk of infection or sensitization to histocompatibility antigens.

Lymph Node Biopsy. Examining the architecture of a lymph node may be of help, using some of the same criteria described for study of the B lymphocyte system. If there is lymphopenia or serious derangement of T cell function, lymphocyte accumulations in the paracortical and medullary regions may be sparse. These pathologic findings roughly parallel deficiency in CMI function and numbers of circulating T cells.

References

Special acknowledgment is made for the liberal use of information contained in teaching outlines provided by J. A. Bellanti, Georgetown University; M. Blaese, National Cancer Institute; R. H. Buckley, Duke Univeristy; and C. T. Anderson, R. Keightley, W. T. Kniker, and M. Michels, University of Texas Health Science Center at San Antonio.

Anderson, C. T., and Kniker, W. T.: Modified skin window technique in assessment of immunological functions. Fed. Proc. *33*(1):727, 1974.

Anderson, C. T., Thorne, G. C., Jr., Shoemaker, J. G., and Kniker, W. T.: Immunoglobulins in childrens' tears. Presented at 1st Congress of Allergy and Immunology, New York, March. 1977. Manuscript accepted for 1980 publication.

Anderson, C. T., Roumiantzeff, M., and Kniker, W. T.: The multitest system for assay of delayed cutaneous hypersensitivity (DCH) to ubiquitous antigens. Ann. Allergy, *43*:73, 1979.

Bodmer, W. F.: Summary of the W. H. O. 6th International Transplant Congress. Nature *256*:695, 1975.

Buckley, R. H., and Fiscus, S. A.: Serum IgD and IgE concentrations in immunodeficiency disease. J. Clin. Invest. *55*:157, 1975.

Byrom, N. A., Caballero, F., Campbell, M., Chooi, M., Lane, A. M., Hugh-Jones, K., Timlin, D. M., and Hobbs, J. R.: T-cell depletion and *in vitro* thymosin inducibility in asthmatic children. Clin. Exp. Immunol. *31*:490, 1978.

Church, J. A., Frenkel, L. D., Wright, D. G.,and Bellanti, J. A.: T lymphocyte dysfunction, hyperimmunoglobulinemia E, recurrent bacterial infections, and defective neutrophil chemotaxis in a Negro child. J. Pediatr. *88*(6):982, 1976.

Cooper, M. D., Keightley, R. G., and Lawton, A. R. III: Defective T and B cells in primary immunodeficiencies in membrane receptors of lymphocytes. Seligman, H., Pruedhomme, J. K., and Kourilsky, F. M. (eds): International Symposium on Membrane Receptors of Lymphocytes. Amsterdam, North Holland Publishing Company, 1975, pp. 431–442.

Dahl, M. V., Greene, W. H., Jr., and Quie, P. G.: Infection, dermatitis, increased IgE, and impaired neutrophil chemotaxis. Arch. Dermatol. *112*:1387, 1976.

Furukawa, C. T., and Altman, L. C.: Defective monocyte and polymorphonuclear leukocyte chemotaxis in atopic disease. J. Allergy Clin. Immunol. *61*(5):288, 1978.

Grossi, C. E., Webb, S. R., Zicca, A., Lydyard, P. M., Moretta, L., Mingari, M. C., and Copper, M. D.: Morphological and histochemical analyses of two human T-cell subpopulations bearing receptors for IgM or IgG. J. Exp. Med. *147*:1405, 1978.

Hill, H. R., and Quie, P. G.: Raised serum-IgE levels and defective neutrophil chemotaxis in three children with eczema and recurrent bacterial infections. Lancet *1*:183, 1974.

Hill, H. R., Williams, P. B., Krueger, G. G., and Janis, B.: Recurrent staphylococcal abscesses associated with defective neutrophil chemotaxis and allergic rhinitis. Ann. Int. Med. *85*:39, 1976b.

Hill, H. R., Estensen, R. D., Hogan, N. A., and Quie, P. G.: Severe staphylococcal disease associated with allergic manifestations, hyperimmunoglobulinemia E, and defective neutrophil chemotaxis. J. Lab. Clin. Med. *88*(5):796, 1976a.

Khan, A., Sellars, W., Grater, W., Graham, M., Pflanzer, J., Antonetti, A., Bailey, J., and Hill, N. O.: The usefulness of transfer factor in asthma associated with frequent infections. Ann. Allergy *40*(4):229, 1978.

Lawton, A. R., and Cooper, M. D.: Development of immunity. *In* Steihm, E. R., and Fulginti, V. A. (eds.): *Immunologic Disorders in Infants and Children*. Philadelphia, W. B. Saunders Co., 1973, Chapter 3, pp. 28–41.

Miller, M. E.: The immunodeficiencies of immaturity. *In* Steihm, E. R., and Fulginti, V. A. (eds.): *Immunologic Disorders in Infants and Children*. Philadelphia, W. B. Saunders Co., 1973, Chapter 11, pp. 168–183.

Namba, Y., and Waksman, B. H.: On soluble mediators of immunologic regulation. Cell. Immunol. *21*:161, 1976.

Ostergaard, P. A.: IgA levels, bacterial carrier rate, and the development of bronchial asthma in children. Acta Pathol. Microbiol. Scand. (C) *85*(3):187, 1977.

Rogge, J. L., and Hanifin, J. M.: Immunodeficiencies in severe atopic dermatitis. Arch. Dermatol. *112*:1391, 1976.

Snyderman, R., Rogers, E., and Buckley, R. H.: Abnormalities of leukotaxis in atopic dermatitis. J. Allergy Clin. Immun. *60*(2):121, 1977.

Stites, D. P., Caldwell, J., Carr, M. C., and Fudenberg, H.H.: Ontogeny of immunity in humans. Clin. Immunol. and Immunopathol. *4*:519, 1975.

Uehara, M., and Ofuji, S.: Suppressed cell-mediated immunity associated with eczematous inflammation. Acta Dermat. *57*:137, 1977.

Waldmann, T. A.: Disorders of suppressor cells in the pathogenesis of immunodeficiency, autoimmune and allergic diseases: Human disease associated with disorders of an immunological breaking system. Ann. Allergy *39*:79, 1977.

GENERAL

Alexander, J. W., and Good, R. A.: *Fundamentals of Clinical Immunology*. Philadelphia, W. B. Saunders Co., 1977.

Bellanti, J. A.: *Immunology II*. Philadelphia, W. B. Saunders Co., 1978.

Bergsma, D., Good, R. A., and Finstad, J. (eds.): *Immunodeficiency in Man and Animals*. National Foundation March of Dimes Original Article Series, Sinauer Assoc., 1975.

Fudenberg, H. H., Stiles, D. P., Caldwell, J. L., and Wells, J. V.: *Basic and Clinical Immunology*, 2nd ed. Los Altos, Lange, 1978.

Goldman, A. S., and Goldblum, R. M.: *Defects in Host Resistance*. Chapel Hill, N. C., Health Sciences Consortium, 1977.

Hong, R.: Immunologic assessment of the immunodeficient. J. Allergy Clin. Immunol., *60*(1):83, 1977.

Pediatric Annals, *5*(6), June 1976: Doughaday, C. C., and Douglas, S. D.: Phagocytes. pp. 11–25. Harris, M. D.: Neonatal host-defense mechanisms. pp. 86–93. Henley, W. T.: The immunoglobulins. pp. 30–39. Papageorgiou, P. S.: Cell mediated immunity. pp. 40–71.

Rose, N. R., and Friedman, H.: *Manual of Clinical Immunology*. Washington, D. C., Am. Soc. for Microbiology, 1976.

Stiehm, E. R., and Fulginiti, V. A. (eds.): *Immunologic Disorders in Infants and Children*, 2nd ed. Philadelphia, W. B. Saunders Co., 1980.

Warren, S. L.: A systematic approach to the evaluation of immunological disease patterns. Ann. Allergy *36*:180, 1976.

E. Richard Stiehm, M.D.

7

Therapy of Immunodeficiency

PRINCIPLES OF THERAPY

Prevention

Measures to prevent immune deficiency diseases include vaccination to prevent congenital rubella, genetic counseling, and prenatal diagnosis with interruption of pregnancy. Unfortunately, even maximum use of the limited preventive measures now available would have a negligible effect on the prevalence of immunodeficiency disease. Nevertheless, rubella vaccination programs should result in the disappearance of immunodeficiency secondary to congenital rubella; genetic counseling is of value when the genetic pattern is established; and amniocentesis may reveal certain immunodeficiencies.

Patients with a hereditary immunodeficiency should be counseled about the risks of occurrence in their offspring. Parents who have a child with an autosomal recessive or X-linked immunodeficiency can be counseled about the likelihood of further children having a similar problem. Amniocentesis can predict the sex of the child and can aid in counseling, particularly in X-linked disorders. Further, the adenosine deaminase deficiency variant of combined immunodeficiency can be diagnosed by amniocentesis (by assay of the enzyme in cultured amniotic cells), and therapeutic abortion can be offered (Hirschhorn et al., 1975).

Immunoglobulin and complement levels should be obtained on the immediate family of patients with antibody or complement deficiencies to determine if there is a familial pattern. In disorders (e.g., chronic granulomatous disease) for which tests for heterozygosity are available, parents, children and siblings of the affected person should be tested. If other family members have suggestive histories, they also should be studied. Newborn siblings of an affected patient should be followed carefully from birth for manifestations of a similar disorder.

Neonatal Management

If a previous sibling has had *severe combined immunodeficiency* and the mother is again pregnant, planning before the delivery is imperative. If a prenatal diagnosis of immunodeficiency is made with reasonable certainty, cesarean section should be considered, especially if a difficult labor is anticipated, to minimize bacterial and fungal contamination associated with vaginal delivery. At birth, blood should be obtained for blood count, immunoglobulin assays, B and T cell enumeration, phytohemagglutinin- and mixed leukocyte culture stimulation assays, and chromosome and HLA studies for chimerism. The newborn with suspected immunodeficiency should be placed in a sterile Isolette and maintained on reverse isolation until immunologic status is clarified. A chest x-ray study for thymic size should then be done.

95

In the rare case in which immunodeficiency is diagnosed at birth, the immunodeficient newborn should be placed in a sterile Isolette with reverse isolation or in a laminar flow isolator and all food and liquid should be sterilized. Gastrointestinal sterilization (with nonabsorbable antibiotics) and prophylaxis for *Pneumocystis carinii* infection (with sulfamethoxazole-trimethoprim) also is recommended.

General Care

Patients with immunodeficiency require extraordinary amounts of care to maintain general health and nutrition, to prevent emotional problems related to their illness, and to manage their numerous infectious episodes. There are no special dietary considerations. Patients should be protected from unnecessary exposure to infection. They should sleep in their own beds, preferably have rooms of their own, and be kept away from individuals with respiratory or other infections.

On the other hand, many patients with immunodeficiency have a normal life span on gamma globulin or other therapy, and parents must be given a perspective of the particular disease affecting their child to avoid overprotection. In most instances, it is appropriate to encourage the child to play outdoors and with other children in small groups, as well as to attend nursery and regular school. The aim is to teach the child to live with his disease, in a near-normal fashion much like the child with diabetes. Killed vaccines (diphtheria-pertussis-tetanus, inactivated poliomyelitis, pneumococcal, and, when they become commercially available, *H. influenzae* and meningococcal vaccine) should be given if there is evidence of any antibody synthesis. Tuberculin testing should be done every two years. The teeth should be kept in good repair.

Complications of chronic infection such as mastoiditis, sinusitis, chronic bronchitis, and bronchiectasis should be managed as in other patients. Patients with chronic pulmonary disease should have pulmonary function tests performed at regular intervals and have a home treatment plan of postural drainage and inhalation therapy similar to that used in cystic fibrosis. Special attention must be directed toward such problems as hearing loss, the need for tutors to make up for school absences, and financial help for the family.

Special Precautions

Patients with suspected or proven T-cell immunodeficiencies should not be given whole blood transfusions because of the possibility of a graft-versus-host reaction from heterologous lymphocytes. If transfusion is necessary, old blood (over two weeks old) should be used, and it should be irradiated with 3000 rads prior to administration. Tonsillectomy and adenoidectomy should be performed only with strict indications. Splenectomy, except in unusual circumstances, is contraindicated, because the addition of a phagocytic defect (absence of the spleen) to the already existing immunodeficiency may result in sudden overwhelming sepsis. Corticosteroids and other immunosuppressive agents are contraindicated; only under extreme conditions is their use warranted.

Vaccines. Live attenuated vaccines (smallpox, poliomyelitis, measles, mumps, rubella, BCG) should be avoided in all patients with severe antibody or cellular immunodeficiencies because of the risk of vaccine-induced infection. (We have successfully given live virus vaccines to patients with selective IgA deficiency, mucocutaneous candidiasis with intact cellular immunity to other antigens, and phagocytic and complement immunodeficiencies). The risk from smallpox vaccination is especially great, and cellular immunodeficiencies initially were diagnosed in many infants as a result of progressive vaccine. Paralytic poliomyelitis and prolonged virus shedding from the gastrointestinal tract are recognized complications of oral poliovirus vaccination in children with immunodeficiency. Parents, siblings, and other household members also should not be given smallpox or live poliomyelitis vaccines because of the risk of spread to the patient.

Antibiotics. Antibiotics are lifesaving in the treatment of the infectious episodes of patients with immunodeficiency. Prior to their availability, most patients with immunodeficiencies probably died from their initial infection. The choice of specific antibiotic and dosage is identical to those for normal subjects. Because immunodeficient patients may succumb rapidly to infection, any fever or other manifestation of infection is assumed to be secondary to bacterial infection, and antibiotic treatment is begun immediately. Throat, blood, and other cultures as appropriate are obtained prior to therapy; these will be especially important if the infection does not respond promptly to the initial antibiotic chosen. In general, immunodeficient patients should be "overtreated" for infectious episodes, even if this necessitates frequent antibiotics and occasional "unnecessary" hospitalization. If the infection does not respond to antibiotics, the physician should consider the possibility of fungal, mycobacterial, viral, or protozoal (*Pneumocystis carinii*) infection. Since certain of these infections can be treated only with special drugs (for example, pentamidine or trimethoprim-sulfamethoxazole for *Pneumocystis carinii* infection), specific microbiologic diagnosis is imperative.

Continuous "prophylactic" use of antibiotics is often of benefit, especially in disorders characterized by rapid overwhelming infections (e.g., immunodeficiency with thrombocytopenia and eczema or Wiskott-Aldrich syndrome) and in antibody immunodeficiencies when recurrent infections occur despite optimal gamma globulin therapy. In these instances, oral penicillin, ampicillin, or dicloxacillin, using 0.5 to 1.0 gm per day in divided doses, is recommended. If diarrhea or vomiting results, dosage is lowered, or other drugs are used. The continuous use of antibiotics in the antibody immunodeficiencies is not an adequate substitute for gamma globulin therapy, but can be used in its place in patients in whom gamma globulin therapy is refused on religious grounds.

TREATMENT OF ANTIBODY IMMUNODEFICIENCIES

Gamma Globulin

Human immune serum globulin (gamma globulin) is prepared from pooled human serum by Cohn's alcohol fractionation procedure (thus deriving its alternative name of Cohn Fraction II). This removes most other serum proteins and hepatitis viruses, providing a safe product for intramuscular injection. It is reconstituted as a sterile 16.5 percent solution (165 mg per ml) and assayed for poliomyelitis antibodies. Gamma globulin is 95 percent IgG globulin, but trace quantities of IgM and IgA globulins and other serum proteins are present. The IgM and IgA globulins are therapeutically insignificant because of their rapid half-lives (about 7 days) and their presence in low concentrations.

Gamma globulin is the mainstay in the treatment of most antibody immunodeficiencies. Treatment is lifelong except in transient hypogammaglobulinemia of infancy. However, in selective IgA deficiency, gamma globulin therapy is contraindicated. These patients rarely are seriously ill and are readily sensitized to the IgA in gamma globulin; the resulting anti-IgA antibodies may cause an anaphylactic reaction to IgA in blood, plasma, or subsequent gamma globulin injection.

Gamma globulin therapy allows many patients to be symptom-free, similar to the well controlled diabetic on insulin therapy. Others given gamma globulin remain chronically ill or have a progressive downhill course; often these patients have other immunologic or hematologic deficits. Gamma globulin is not of value in the treatment of cellular immunodeficiencies, and it is of only limited value in combined antibody and cellular immunodeficiencies.

The usual dose of gamma globulin for antibody immunodeficiency is 100 mg per kg of body weight per month, about equivalent to 0.6 ml per kg per month of commercially available preparations. A double or triple dose is given at the onset of therapy, often over a 3 to 5 day period. The maximum dose should not exceed 20 or 30 ml per week. The total gamma globulin dose should be given at multiple sites in order to avoid more than 5 ml at any one site (10 ml in a large adult). The buttocks are preferred sites, but the anterior thighs can be used. Tenderness, sterile abscesses, fibrosis, and sciatic nerve injury may result from these injections. The danger of sciatic nerve injury is especially great in a small, malnourished infant with inadequate muscle and fat in the gluteal regions. Intramuscular gamma globulin should not be given to patients with thrombocytopenia, because of the risk of hematoma.

Injections are initially given at monthly intervals. If the patient continues to have infection or if a characteristic symptom recurs at the end of the injection period (such as cough, conjunctivitis, diarrhea, arthralgia, or purulent nasal discharge), the interval between doses is decreased to 3 or 2 weeks. Older patients often report that they can tell when their gamma globulin level is low and they need another injection. During acute infections gamma globulin catabolism increases, so extra injections of gamma globulin are necessary.

Since no specific serum level of IgG must be maintained, serial immunoglobulin assays are unnecessary in assessing the effectiveness of treatment. The maximum increase of the serum IgG level after a standard gamma globulin dose will vary between patients and dosages used because of different rates of absorption, local proteolysis at the injection site, and distribution within the tissues. An intramuscular injection of 100 mg of gamma globulin per kg of body weight usually raises the serum level of IgG only 100 mg per dl (Stiehm et al., 1966). Thus, a recent gamma globulin injection usually does not obscure the diagnosis of hypogammaglobulinemia.

Gamma globulin is approved only for intramuscular use. It aggregates *in vitro* to large molecular weight complexes (9.5S to 40S) which are strongly anticomplementary. These aggregates probably are responsible for the occasional systemic reaction to gamma globulin and are a major reason that the usual commercial gamma globulin preparations cannot be used intravenously. However, special intravenous preparations are available in other countries and may be marketed in the United States in the future (see next section). Small intradermal injections of gamma globulin are not of value, except perhaps as a placebo.

Although gamma globulin is one of the safest biological products available, rare anaphylactic reactions to intramuscular injections have been reported (Ellis and Henney, 1969). The symptoms include anxiety, nausea, vomiting, malaise, flushing, facial swelling, cyanosis, and loss of consciousness. Immediate treatment with epinephrine and antihistamines is indicated. Individuals who experience such an anaphylactic reaction should be given gamma globulin from a different manufacturer when therapy is resumed. A skin test with the new gamma globulin lot should be done prior to injection (Ellis and Henney, 1969).

Immunologically normal patients given gamma globulin (or plasma) may develop antibodies to a genetic gamma globulin type different from their own (usually anti-Gm antibodies). Stiehm and Fudenberg (1965) noted anti-Gm antibodies in normal children given single gamma globulin injections and hypogammaglobulinemic children given repeated injections. Patients with severe antibody immunodeficiency do not develop such antibodies. Patients with antibodies to IgA may have a reaction to gamma globulin as a result of the IgA in the gamma globulin (Vyas et al., 1968).

Exogenous gamma globulin may inhibit the endogenous synthesis of gamma globulin. In immunodeficiency with hyper-IgM, intramuscular IgG results in diminution of IgM levels, suggesting feedback inhibition of endogenous IgM synthesis (Stiehm and Fudenberg, 1966).

We have noted depressed IgG levels that returned to normal when gamma globulin injections were stopped. In a few patients given gamma globulin from early infancy, late side effects to gamma globulin injections have not been noted; several patients have had continuous gamma globulin therapy for 10 or more years without apparent adverse effects.

Intravenous Gamma Globulin

There are several theoretic advantages to the administration of gamma globulin by the intravenous route. These include ease of administering large doses, more rapid action, no loss in the tissues due to proteolysis, and avoidance of painful intramuscular injections.

Gamma globulin for intravenous use has been prepared by eliminating high molecular weight complexes and their resultant anticomplementary activity. An intravenous gamma globulin prepared with sulfhydryl agents and iodoacetamide is under clinical trial in the United States and appears to be safe and effective. This preparation is not yet licensed for use in the United States but is available in certain European countries.

Plasma

Plasma infusions can be used to administer IgG, IgM, and IgA by the intravenous route to patients with antibody immunodeficiencies (Stiehm et al., 1966; Buckley, 1972). In addition to supplying large quantities of undenatured gamma globulin, plasma supplies complement components and other proteins of possible importance in host resistance to infection. Plasma infusions may be of particular benefit in immunodeficiency with thrombocytopenia and eczema (Stiehm and McIntosh, 1967), common variable immunodeficiency with diarrhea (Binder and Reynolds, 1967), and ataxia-telangiectasia (Ammann et al., 1969). A trial of plasma therapy is indicated in patients who continue to have severe infection or diarrhea despite intramuscular gamma globulin injections. Buckley (1972) reported several patients who responded better to plasma therapy than to intramuscular gamma globulin.

Since plasma therapy may result in serum hepatitis, the plasma from a single hepatitis-free donor, usually a relative, is used. This is collected by plasmapheresis, aliquoted in plasma bags, and frozen prior to use; the freezing destroys lymphocytes that may cause graft-versus-host disease. A minor cross-match of the donor plasma with the patient's red cells must be negative for the plasma to be given. Plasma contains about 10 mg of IgG, 1 mg of IgM, and 2 mg of IgA globulin per ml. The usual dose of plasma is 20 ml per kg of body weight, per month. Larger doses may be given if plasma is removed concomitantly from the recipient by plasmapheresis. Patients may develop tingling and paresthesias of the lips and a slight tightening of the chest during plasma infusions; these have not been severe enough to warrant terminating the infusion. Such reactions often can be minimized by pretreating the patient with 600 mg of aspirin.

Plasma infusions may sensitize the recipient to gamma globulin and other donor plasma proteins that have different genetic markers than the recipient. Plasma infusions also can result in the development of anti-IgA antibodies in patients who lack IgA. Plasma from normal donors should not be given to patients who have anti-IgA antibodies because of the possibility of febrile or anaphylactic reactions (Schmidt et al., 1969). In such individuals, however, plasma from donors with selective IgA deficiency can be used (Vyas et al., 1975).

TREATMENT OF CELLULAR IMMUNODEFICIENCY

Unlike the treatment of antibody immunodeficiencies, in almost all of which gamma globulin is indicated and is reasonably effective, treatment of cellular immunodeficiencies varies considerably depending on the disorder and usually is only moderately helpful at best. Furthermore, many of the cellular immunodeficiencies have associated antibody defects (e.g., Wiskott-Aldrich syndrome, ataxia-telangiectasia, cellular immunodeficiency with abnormal immunoglobulin synthesis [Nezelof syndrome]). In these circumstances, replacement gamma globulin or plasma is given in addition to treatment aimed at the cellular immunodeficiency. It is emphasized that patients with Wiskott-Aldrich syndrome cannot be given gamma globulin by intramuscular injection, because of thrombocytopenia and the risk of inducing bleeding.

The ideal in treatment of cellular immunodeficiency is restoration of cellular immunity. Transplantation of immunocompetent tissue has accomplished this in many patients with severe combined immunodeficiency, thymic aplasia, and the Wiskott-Aldrich syndrome. However, this is not a feasible approach in most patients because of a lack of suitable donor. Consequently, other forms of partial immune restoration are utilized.

Also in contrast to antibody-deficiency syndromes — which can be treated with gamma globulin by the primary care physician — the various treatment modalities potentially available for cellular immunodeficiency require specialized procedures, materials, and medical expertise available only at medical centers. It is recognized that the primary care physician is not likely to be involved directly with these procedures. However, modes of therapy for treatment of cellular immunodeficiency will be reviewed to provide a perspective on therapy that may be available for the occasional patient encountered in practice who may require such therapy.

Levamisole. Levamisole, an antihelmintic agent known to enhance cell-mediated immunity by nonspecific stimulation of T lymphocytes and macrophages, has been used in several patients with cellular immunodeficiency. Despite some restoration of immune function (Lieberman and Hsu, 1976), preliminary results in Wiskott-Aldrich syndrome, mucocutaneous candidiasis, and ataxia telangiectasia indicate that this is not a promising approach in severe cellular immunodeficiency (Stiehm and Gatti, unpublished observations).

Transfer Factor. Transfer factor has been used in a variety of cellular immunodeficiencies with limited success. Transfer factor (TF) is a dialyzable extract of immune leukocytes that can transfer delayed hypersensitivity from a skin test–positive donor to a skin test–negative recipient (Lawrence, 1969). Concomitantly there may be the acquisition of lymphocyte responsiveness to a specific antigen, with lymphocyte transformation and mediator production. The exact mechanism of action of TF is uncertain. There is no risk of graft-versus-host disease with its use. TF is a nonantigenic, low molecular weight (5000 to 10,000 daltons) nucleopeptide that is heterogenous in column chromatography. It is prepared from isolated peripheral blood leukocytes obtained by leukopheresis. The dialysate is checked for pyrogenicity and reconstituted in 1 ml saline for subcutaneous injection. It also can be lyophilized and stored for years. TF is not commercially available and each center using it prepares its own.

While transfer factor is nonantigenic, local reactions and mild constitutional symptoms are common; whether the rare serious side effects reported (nephrotic syndrome, monoclonal gammopathy, hemolytic anemia, malignancy) are coincidental or a result of the transfer factor is not established (Hitzig and Grob, 1974).

In some cases of Wiskott-Aldrich syndrome treated with transfer factor, a decrease in infections and in eczema, and a lessening of the thrombocytopenia for up to 6 months from a single treatment has been reported (Spitler et al., 1972). Repeat injections of transfer factor were necessary when skin tests became negative. Some patients with mucocutaneous candidiasis have benefited from TF injections, particularly when concomitant antifungal therapy was used to reduce the load of fungal antigens (Schulkind et al., 1972). An occasional patient with combined immunodeficiency also may show clinical improvement (Strauss and Hake, 1974). Several patients with combined deficiency have been given TF in conjunction with fetal thymus transplant, but the extent to which TF contributed to the success of the procedures is unclear (Ammann et al., 1973; Rachelefsky et al., 1975).

Transplantation of Fetal Thymus. Fetal thymus transplantation (either into the subcutaneous tissue or into the peritoneum) from a fetus of less than 16 weeks' gestation has restored cellular immunity in several patients with thymic aplasia (Cleveland et al., 1968; August et al., 1970), combined immunodeficiency (Rachelefsky et al., 1975), and cellular immunodeficiency with immunoglobulins (Ammann et al., 1973). In thymic aplasia, implantation of fetal thymus results in rapid (within days) immunologic reconstitution and appears to be permanent, and lymphoid chimerism is absent. Some factor in the fetal thymus appears to activate the patient's own thymic precursor cells (Wara and Ammann, 1976). In combined immunodeficiency, fetal thymus transplantation results in slow reconstitution of T cell immunity, mild graft-versus-host manifestations, and lymphoid chimerism derived from the implanted thymocytes. Transfer factor has been given concurrently with fetal thymus. In cellular immunodeficiency with immunoglobulins (Nezelof syndrome), fetal thymus transplantation results in slow restoration of T cell immunity without chimerism but the effect wanes after several months. The timing and the temporary reconstitution distinguishes this from the reconstitution in thymic aplasia. Fetal thymic tissue often is difficult to obtain; intact fetuses are available only following hysterotomies or prostaglandin-induced abortions, or at laparotomy for the removal of an unruptured tubal pregnancy.

Thymosin. While several thymus gland extracts have been studied *in vitro,* only thymosin has been evaluated as a therapeutic agent in man. Thymosin is a low molecular weight protein, free of lipid and carbohydrate, extracted from the thymus glands of calves (Goldstein et al., 1966). Thymosin converts null cells to T cells in certain patients with T cell immunodeficiency. Some recipients develop increased lymphocyte proliferative responses to antigens and conversion of negative skin tests to antigens which they had had previous contact with. Several patients with the Nezelof syndrome and one patient with the Wiskott-Aldrich syndrome have had some clinical improvement after weekly injections of thymosin (Wara et al., 1975; Goldstein et al., 1976). Reports of its effect in mucocutaneous candidiasis are encouraging. Thymosin is not available commercially, and supplies are extremely limited.

Transplantation of Cultured Thymic Epithelium. Transplantation of cultured thymic epithelium has been utilized in combined immunodeficiency when a suitable bone marrow donor has not been available (Hong et al., 1978). Thymic fragments removed from normal subjects undergoing heart surgery are held for several weeks in tissue culture, during which time most of the lymphoid cells die while the epithelial elements persist. The cultured thymic tissue is implanted intraperitoneally or intramuscularly; following this procedure increased immunoglobulin levels, antibody production, and restoration of T cell numbers and lymphocyte proliferative responses to antigens may occur, in association with moderate to marked clinical improvement. This procedure may become the treatment of choice in certain T cell immunodeficiencies.

Transplantation of Fetal Liver. Transplantation of fetal liver is another alternative in patients with combined immunodeficiency when a bone marrow donor is not available. Fetal liver is a source of stem cells and can reconstitute lethally irradiated

mice both immunologically and hematologically. Although earlier attempts with human fetal liver cells were unsuccessful, Keightley et al. (1975) and Buckley et al. (1976) have reported successful reconstitution in combined immunodeficiency using large numbers (8.4×10^7 to 3.0×10^8 cells) of fresh liver cells from fetuses of less than 10 weeks' gestation. One of the three recipients has survived at least 3 years. Another successful reconstitution utilized both fetal liver and thymus (Ackeret et al., 1976). Graft-versus-host reactions and chimerism have been observed in some cases of transplantation with fetal liver.

Transplantation of Bone Marrow. Transplantation of bone marrow from an HLA-identical, mixed leukocyte culture (MLC) nonreactive sibling is the treatment of choice for patients with combined immunodeficiency and Wiskott-Aldrich syndrome. It has restored health to at least 30 infants throughout the world since the initial transplantation was performed in 1969 (Biggar et al., 1975). Dramatic and permanent (up to 9 years) restoration of both cellular and antibody functions ensues with evidence of engraftment. Some degree of graft-versus-host reaction is the rule; such reactions vary in severity and some patients have succumbed from infection during this period. The graft-versus-host reaction usually is self-limited, and following its disappearance, the child is restored to a state of relative good health.

Because each sibling of the patient has only a 1 in 4 chance of being HLA and MLC identical, most patients will not have a potential donor. When a sibling donor is not available, parents and relatives should be examined for HLA and MLC identity. A few transplantations have been performed utilizing MLC-identical nonsibling family donors (Geha et al., 1976), and unrelated donors (Horowitz et al., 1975).

Bone marrow transplantation for combined immunodeficiency is available in many major medical centers. If transplantation is contemplated, the parents and all siblings should be HLA typed, and if any are identical to the patient, MLC cultures should be done. All MLC-identical matches should be confirmed by repeat testing. The MLC-identical donor is hospitalized at the time of transplantation, and the marrow is obtained under general anesthesia. The marrow is enumerated, filtered, and injected intravenously or intraperitoneally (Thomas and Storb, 1970). Prophylactic chemotherapy for *Pneumocystis carinii* infection is used before and throughout. Immunosuppression is unnecessary if there is a complete lack of cellular immunity, as in combined immunodeficiency; immunosuppression of the recipient otherwise is necessary to achieve engraftment (Parkman et al., 1978).

When a sibling donor is unavailable, mixed leukocyte typing is done on parents and relatives. If a MLC-identical donor is still not found, unrelated donors of the same HLA type can be tested for MLC identity. An unrelated but MLC-identical marrow transplant is probably preferable to a fetal liver, a fetal thymus, or a cultured thymic epithelium transplant.

Special Therapeutic Considerations in Specific Cellular Immunodeficiency

Combined Immunodeficiency. One child with combined immunodeficiency with adenosine deaminase (ADA) deficiency had partial restoration of immune function and clinical improvement following transfusions with normal red blood cells containing adequate amounts of adenosine deaminase (Polmar et al., 1976). Other ADA-deficient children have had no clinical benefit from such transfusions (Schmalsteig et al., 1977).

One child has been kept in strict reverse isolation since birth and has survived 5 years (Williamson et al., 1977). This approach generally is impractical.

Wiskott-Aldrich Syndrome. These patients may need platelet transfusions to abort severe bleeding episodes. Continuous antibiotic therapy usually is indicated to prevent sudden overwhelming infection. Splenectomy may be of value in decreasing the risk of bleeding; it also increases the risk of infection so that continuous antibiotics must be used concomitantly (Lum et al., 1978). Bone marrow transplantation should be attempted if an HLA-matched sibling donor is available (Parkman et al., 1978).

Mucocutaneous Candidiasis. These patients have a limited immunologic defect against *Candida albicans* and a few related fungi. Although attempts to reconstitute their immunity (e.g., administration of transfer factor or thymosin, thymus transplantation) have had limited success in a few patients, the mainstay of management is oral, topical, and intravenous antifungal drugs (Edwards et al., 1978). Mycostatin and gentian violet are used on the oral mucosa; nystatin, haloprogin, and miconazole are used topically. Amphotericin and miconazole are used intravenously, the latter reserved for episodes when the skin or mucous membranes are particularly severely affected. Nail involvement is refractory to antifungal therapy; avulsion of the nails may be necessary. Pulmonary complications may develop and shorten the life span; otherwise, most patients are not severely affected and lead a nearly normal life.

DiGeorge Syndrome (Thymic Aplasia). These patients present at birth with congenital tetany, secondary to hypoparathyroidism. Many have congenital heart disease. Calcium and vitamin D therapy is necessary to reverse the tetany, and heart surgery may be necessary to correct the circulatory defect. In many instances the cellular immune defect is not complete (partial DiGeorge syndrome) and spontaneous recovery ensues (Pabst et al., 1976). Serial immune studies are indicated to decide if fetal thymic transplantation is indicated.

TREATMENT OF PHAGOCYTIC DISORDERS

The most important aspect of therapy in these disorders is the optimal use of antibiotics. Bactericidal antibiotics should be used promptly to treat even mild infections, after appropriate cultures are obtained. Prompt and complete surgical drainage is essential when abscesses occur.

Continuous treatment with antibiotics may be important in keeping patients infection-free. In chronic granulomatous disease, continuous sulfisoxazole may be particularly valuable because it can increase bactericidal activity of phagocytes (Johnson et al., 1975). We have used continuous sulfamethoxazole-trimethoprim with favorable results in the hyper-IgE immunodeficiency syndrome described by Buckley et al. (1972).

Granulocyte infusions are of value in the management of infection crises, but because they have a short half-life and are difficult to procure, infusions are not used as a routine form of treatment. Nevertheless, they may be lifesaving in severe refractory infection (Raubitschek et al., 1973).

Granulocytes for infusions are obtained from donors by continuous flow centrifugation or filtration of blood through special nylon fiber filters, which allow selective removal of granulocytes and return the rest of the blood to the donor (Boggs, 1974). The use of compatible leukocytes of the same HLA type is not imperative but does result in fewer reactions and longer granulocyte survival in the recipient. The separated granulocytes must be given within 3 to 4 hours of procurement; repeated courses of therapy generally are necessary.

Bone marrow transplantation has been performed in one patient with chronic granulomatous disease and offers the possibility of permanent cure (Westminster Hospital, 1977).

Anemia is a constant feature of many of these disorders, particularly chronic granulomatous disease (CGD). Red cells of many children with CGD possess the rare Kell system phenotype K_o. As a result of previous transfusions, they may develop anti-K and be sensitized to all blood except K_o red cells.

Drugs that alter leukocyte metabolism have not been of proven clinical benefit. Methylene blue and glucose oxidase attached to latex particles improve *in vitro* granulocyte function but are not clinically useful.

Vitamin C enhances the chemotaxis of normal granulocytes, probably by increasing the intracellular levels of cyclic guanosine 3', 5'-monophosphate (cyclic GMP) and will improve the *in vitro* bactericidal capacity of the granulocytes from patients with the Chediak-Higashi syndrome (Boxer et al., 1976). Therapeutic studies of vitamin C in Chediak-Higashi syndrome are promising.

Antihistamines also may enhance phagocytic chemotaxis under some circumstances. Hill and Quie (1974) found that patients with elevated IgE have defective chemotaxis secondary to high levels of intracellular histamine, which in turn affects immune function. Histamine may modify levels of cyclic AMP and cyclic GMP and may alter chemotaxis, but the extent to which this occurs is of uncertain clinical significance. Other drugs that influence cyclic AMP may prove to be of benefit in chemotactic disorders.

THERAPY OF OPSONIC (COMPLEMENT) DISORDERS

The therapy of opsonic deficiencies, other than supportive therapy, consists of plasma infusions in order to replace the missing complement component(s). Since complement components have short half-lives (less than 10 days), frequent plasma infusions are necessary. Miller and Nilsson (1970) have treated infants with C5 dysfunction successfully in this fashion. However, since susceptibility to infection is only minimally increased in most of these disorders, periodic plasma infusions rarely are indicated. Opsonic deficit in newborns, particularly in prematures (Forman and Stiehm, 1969), is responsive to plasma infusions. The usual dose of plasma is 10 to 20 ml per kg of body weight.

References

Ackeret, C., Pluss, H. J., and Hitzig, W. H.: Hereditary severe combined immunodeficiency and adenosine deaminase deficiency. Pediatr. Res. *10*:67, 1976.

Ammann, A. J., Good, R. A., Bier, D., and Fudenberg, H. H.: Long-term plasma infusions in a patient with ataxia-telangiectasia and deficient IgA and IgE. Pediatrics *44*:672, 1969.

Ammann, A. J., Wara, D. W., Salmon, S., and Perkins, H. L.: Thymus transplantation: Permanent reconstitution of cellular immunity in a patient with sex-linked combined immunodeficiency. N. Engl. J. Med. *289*:5, 1973.

August, C. S., Levey, R. H., Berkel, A. I., and Rosen, F. S.: Establishment of immunological competence in a child with congenital thymic aplasia by a graft of fetal thymus. Lancet *1*:1080, 1970.

Biggar, W. D., Park, B. H., and Good, R. A.: Compatible bone marrow transplantation and immunologic reconstitution of combined immunodeficiency disease. In Bergsma,

D., Good, R. A. and Finstad, J.: *Immunodeficiency in Man and Animals*. New York, Sinauer, 1975, pp. 385–390.

Binder, H. J., and Reynolds, R. D.: Control of diarrhea in secondary hypogammaglobulinemia by fresh plasma infusions. N. Engl. J. Med. 277:802, 1967.

Boggs, D. P.: Transfusions of neutrophils as prevention or treatment of infection in patients with neutropenia. N. Engl. J. Med. 290:1055, 1974.

Boxer, L. A., Watanabe, A. M., Rister, M., Besch, H. R., Jr., Allen, J., and Baehner, R. L.: Correction of leukocyte function in Chediak-Higashi syndrome by ascorbate. N. Engl. J. Med. 293:1041, 1976.

Buckley, R. H.: Plasma therapy in immunodeficiency diseases. Am. J. Dis. Child. 124:376, 1972.

Buckley, R. H., Wray, B. B., and Belmaker, E. Z.: Extreme hyperimmunoglobulinemia E and undue susceptibility to infection. Pediatrics 49:59, 1972.

Buckley, R. H., Whisnant, J. K., Schiff, R. I., Gilbertsen, R. B., Huang, A. T., and Platt, M. S.: Correction of severe combined immunodeficiency by fetal liver cells. N. Engl. J. Med. 294:1076, 1976.

Cleveland, W. W., Fogel, B. J., Brown, W. T., and Kay, H. E. M.: Foetal thymic transplant in a case of DiGeorge's syndrome. Lancet 2:1211, 1968.

Edwards, J. E., Jr., Fischer, T. J., Lehrer, R. I., Stiehm, E. R., and Young, L. E.: Severe candidal infections: Clinical perspectives, immune defense mechanisms, and current concepts of therapy. Ann. Int. Med. 88:91, 1978.

Ellis, E. R., and Henney, C. S.: Adverse reactions following administration of human gamma-globulin. J. Allerg. 43:45, 1969.

Forman, M. L., and Stiehm, E. R.: Impaired opsonic activity but normal phagocytosis in low-birth-weight infants. New Engl. J. Med. 281:926, 1969.

Goldstein, A. L., Slater, F. D., and White, A.: Preparation, assay, and partial purification of a thymic lymphocytopoietic factor (thymosin). Proc. Natl. Acad. Sci. U.S.A. 56:1010, 1966.

Goldstein, A. L., Cohen, G. H., Rossio, J. L., Thurman, G. B., and Ulrich, J. T.: Use of thymosin in the treatment of primary immunodeficiency diseases and cancer. Med. Clin. North Am. 60:591, 1976.

Hill, H. R., and Quie, P. G.: Raised serum-IgE levels and defective neutrophil chemotaxis in three children with eczema and recurrent bacterial infections. Lancet 1:183, 1974.

Hirschhorn, R., Beratis, N., Rosen, F. S., Parkman, R., Stern, R., and Polmar, S.: Adenosine-deaminase deficiency in a child diagnosed prenatally. Lancet 1:73, 1975.

Hitzig, W. H., and Grob, P. J.: Therapeutic uses of transfer factor. Prog. Clin. Immunol. 2:69, 1976.

Hong, R., Schulte-Wissermann, H., Horowitz, S., Borzy, M., and Finlay, J.: Cultured thymic epithelium (CTE) in severe combined immunodeficiency. Transplant Proc 10:201, 1978.

Horowitz, S. D., Groshong, T., Bach, F. H., Hong, R., and Yunis, E. J.: Treatment of severe combined immunodeficiency with bone marrow from an unrelated mixed-leukocyte-culture-non-reactive donor. Lancet 2:431, 1975.

Johnston, R. B., Jr., Wilfert, C. M., Buckley, R. H., Webb, L. S., DeChatelet, L. R., and McCall, C. E.: Enhanced bactericidal activity of phagocytes from patients with chronic granulomatous disease in the presence of sulphisoxazole. Lancet 1:824, 1975.

Keightley, R. G., Lawton, A. R., and Cooper, M. D.: Successful fetal liver transplantation in a child with severe combined immunodeficiency. Lancet 2:850, 1975.

Lawrence, H. S.: Transfer factor. Adv. Immunol. 11:195, 1969.

Lieberman, R., and Hsu, M.: Levamisole-mediated restoration of cellular immunity in peripheral blood lymphocytes of patients with immunodeficiency diseases. Clin. Immunol. Immunopathol. 5:142, 1976.

Lum, L. G., Tubergen, D. G., and Blaese, R. M.: Splenectomy and prophylactic antibiotics in the management of the Wiskott-Aldrich syndrome. Pediatr. Research 12:483, 1978 (abstract).

Miller, M. E., and Nilsson, U. R.: A familial deficiency of the phagocytosis-enhancing activity of serum related to a dys-

function of the fifth component of complement. N. Engl. J. Med. 282:354, 1970.

Pabst, H. F., Wright, W. C., LeRiche, J., and Stiehm, E. R.: Partial DiGeorge syndrome with substantial cell-mediated immunity. Am. J. Dis. Child. 130:316, 1976.

Parkman, R., Rappaport, J., Geha, R., Belli, J., Cassady, R., Levey, R., Nathan, D. G., and Rosen, F. S.: Complete correction of the Wiskott-Aldrich syndrome by allogeneic bone-marrow transplantation. N. Engl. J. Med. 298:921, 1978.

Polmar, S. H., Stern, R. C., Schwartz, A. L., Wetzler, E. M., Chase, P. A., and Hirschhorn, R.: Enzyme replacement therapy for adenosine-deaminase deficiency and severe combined immunodeficiency. N. Engl. J. Med., 295:1337, 1976.

Rachelefsky, G. S., Stiehm, E. R., Ammann, A. J., Cederbaum, S. C., Opelz, G., and Terasaki, P. I.: T-cell reconstitution by thymus transplantation and transfer factor in severe combined immunodeficiency. Pediatrics 54:114, 1975.

Raubitschek, A. A., Levin, A. S., Stites, D. P., Shaw, E. B., and Fudenberg, H. H.: Normal granulocyte infusion therapy for aspergillosis in chronic granulomatous disease. Pediatrics 51:230, 1973.

Schmalsteig, F. C., Goldblum, R. M., Mills, G. C., May, L. T., and Goldman, A. S.: Effect of RBC transfusions on adenosine-deaminase (ADA) deficient severe combined immunodeficiency. Pediatr. Research 11:493, 1977 (abstract).

Schmidt, A. D., Taswell, H. F., and Gleich, G. T.: Anaphylactic transfusion reactions associated with anti-IgA antibody. N. Engl. J. Med. 280:188, 1969.

Schulkind, M. L., Adler, W. M., Altemeier, W. A., and Ayoub, E. M.: Transfer factor in the treatment of a case of chronic mucocutaneous moniliasis. Cell Immunol. 3:606, 1972.

Spitler, L. E., Levin, A. S., Stites, D. P., Fudenberg, H. H., Pirofsky, B., August, C. S., Stiehm, E. R., Hitzig, W. H., and Gatti, R. A.: The Wiskott-Aldrich syndrome: Results of transfer factor therapy. J. Clin. Invest., 51:3216, 1972.

Stiehm, E. R., and Fudenberg, H. H.: Antibodies to gamma globulin in infants and children exposed to isologous gamma globulin. Pediatrics 35:229, 1965.

Stiehm, E. R., and Fudenberg, H. H.: Clinical and immunologic features of dysgammaglobulinemia type I. Report of a case diagnosed in the first year of life. Am. J. Med. 40:805, 1966.

Stiehm, E. R., Vaerman, J. P., and Fudenberg, H. H.: Plasma infusions in immunologic deficiency states: Metabolic and therapeutic studies. Blood 28:918, 1966.

Stiehm, E. R., and McIntosh, R. M.: Wiskott-Aldrich syndrome: Review and report of a large family. Clin. Exp. Immunol. 2:179, 1967.

Strauss, R. G., and Hake, D. A.: Combined immunodeficiency disease with response to transfer factor. J. Pediatr. 85:680, 1974.

Thomas, E. D., and Storb, R.: Technique for human marrow grafting. Blood 36:507, 1970.

Vyas, G. N., Perkins, H. A., and Fudenberg, H. H.: Anaphylactoid transfusion reactions associated with anti-IgA. Lancet 2:344, 1968.

Vyas, G. H., Perkins, H. A., Yaug, Y. M., and Basantani, G. K.: Healthy blood donors with selective absence of immunoglobulin A: Prevention of anaphylactic transfusion reactions caused by antibodies to IgA. J. Lab. Clin. Med. 85:838, 1975.

Wara, D. W., Goldstein, A. L., Doyle, W., and Ammann, A. J.: Thymosin activity in patients with cellular immunodeficiency. N. Engl. J. Med. 292:70, 1975.

Wara, D. W., and Ammann, A. J.: Thymic cells and humoral factors as therapeutic agents. Pediatrics 57:643, 196.

Westminster Hospital's Bone Marrow Transplant Team: Bone-marrow transplant from an unrelated donor for chronic granulomatous disease. Lancet 1:210, 1977.

Williamson, A. P., Montgomery, J. R., South, M. A., and Wilson, R.: A special report: Four-year study of a boy with combined immunodeficiency maintained in strict reverse isolation from birth. Pediatr. Res. 11:63, 1977.

James M. Corry, M.D.
Richard B. Johnston, Jr., M.D.

8

Disorders of Complement and Phagocyte Function

The immune response in host defense acts as an integrated system involving humoral and cellular components. Although the important initial event is the formation of specific antibody and sensitized T cells, complement and phagocytic cells are subsequently required to remove the infectious agent. That antibody and cell-mediated immunity alone are ineffective in host protection is evidenced by the various clinical problems that are seen when defects occur in the complement or phagocytic systems.

COMPLEMENT

The complement system and its biologic activities have been described in Chapter 5. The clinical manifestations of various deficiency states attest to the importance of the complement system in host defense against infection and in the practice of medicine. Defects in the complement system can be hereditary or acquired and can involve either the classic or alternative complement pathways.

Hereditary Defects of the Complement System

Complete or almost complete deficiencies of each of the components of the classic pathway except C9 have been described as hereditary disorders (Table 8–1). C2 deficiency has been reported in almost 100 individuals, while reports of congenital deficiencies of the other components are rare, involving fewer than 10 patients for each component. However, these reports have appeared only in recent years, and the true incidence of these defects remains to be determined.

Deficiency of the C1 subcomponent C1q has been reported in association with severe combined immunodeficiency diseases and hypogammaglobulinemia. Restoration of C1q levels occurred in four patients following bone marrow transplantation used to restore lymphocyte function. However, selective complete deficiency of C1q also has been described in a healthy boy. C1r deficiency has been reported in association with autoimmune diseases, including systemic lupus erythematosus (SLE), an SLE-like syndrome, and chronic nephritis.

Two patients with SLE were discovered to lack C4. Neither had any increase in incidence or severity of infections. Inheritance conformed to an autosomal recessive pattern, with heterozygous family members having approximately half-normal C4 levels, a pattern referred to as autosomal codominant. In these persons, as in most individuals heterozygous for genes coding for a complement protein, the remaining intact gene functions normally. In one individual, genetic studies showed that the C4 gene

TABLE 8–1 HEREDITARY DEFICIENCIES OF COMPLEMENT SYSTEM

Deficient Component	Inheritance*	Associated Clinical Findings†
C1q	AR, ?XLR	SCID, hypogammaglobulinemia
C1r	?ACD	CGN, SLE syndrome
C1s	?	SLE
C1 INA	AD	Angioedema, SLE
C4	ACD	SLE syndrome
C2	ACD	SLE syndrome, MPGN, H-S purpura, dermatomyositis, septicemia
C3	ACD	Septicemia, meningitis, pneumonia
C5	ACD	Pyogenic infections, SLE
C5 (dysfunction)	?AD	Pyoderma, septicemia, Leiner's disease
C6	ACD	Gonococcal and meningococcal infections
C7	ACD	Raynaud's phenomenon, sclerodactyly, ankylosing spondylitis, meningococcal infection
C8	ACD	Disseminated gonococcal infection, SLE syndrome
C3b INA	?ACD	Pyogenic infections

*AR = autosomal recessive; XLR = X-linked recessive; ACD = autosomal codominant; AD = autosomal dominant; ? = mode of inheritance unproved.

†SCID = severe combined immunodeficiency disease; CGN = chronic glomerulonephritis; SLE = systemic lupus erythematosus; MPGN = membranoproliferative glomerulonephritis; H-S = Henoch-Schönlein.

was located on chromosome six, which also carries the genes that code for antigens of the major histocompatibility complex (MHC) (see Chapter 3). Certain MHC antigens in this family were inherited with the C4 gene, indicating linkage between the C4 gene and genes for histocompatibility antigens.

C2 deficiency is the most commonly reported hereditary complement deficiency. The majority of patients with C2 deficiency are otherwise normal. Some have had an increased incidence of autoimmune disease, including anaphylactoid purpura, dermatomyositis, discoid lupus, SLE, and glomerulonephritis (Day et al., 1973). Heterozygous family members have half-normal C2 levels and may have an increased incidence of SLE or juvenile rheumatoid arthritis (JRA) (Glass et al., 1976). These patients are the exception to the general finding that patients heterozygous for a deficient complement protein are healthy. The half-normal level of a complement component in heterozygous individuals usually allows completely normal complement functions as studied in vitro.

The reason for the association of complement deficiencies with autoimmune disease is unclear. Various (not mutually exclusive) explanations have been hypothesized, but they remain entirely speculative. For example, there may be an increased incidence of clinically inapparent viral infections in complement-deficient patients owing to defective virus neutralization, with a resultant increased incidence of autoimmune disease. It also is possible that reduced systemic clearance of immune complexes, a process that requires complement, may predispose to development of autoimmune disease. Finally, immune response genes have been suggested as important in permitting autoimmune disease to occur. If the defective complement genes are closely linked to these immune response genes, there may be a linked genetic transmission of complement deficiencies and abnormal immune functions that predisposes to autoimmune disease.

A few patients with homozygous C2 deficiency have had recurrent infections, including pneumococcal bacteremia (Newman et al., 1978). Freedom from infection in most patients with C2 deficiency is presumed to be due to a normally functioning alternative pathway. However, many C2-deficient patients have had approximately half-normal levels of factor B. Thus, the alternative pathway may not serve to fully protect these individuals from infections.

C3 is the major component responsible for effective enhancement of phagocytosis (opsonization) of infectious agents. Conversion of C3 to C3b through either the classic or the alternative pathway, and fixation of C3b to the microorganism results in binding and subsequent ingestion of the organism. Since fixation of C3 is crucial for enhancement of phagocytosis, it is not surprising that patients with absent C3 have recurrent infections. All but one of the individuals described with C3 deficiency have had severe recurrent infections with extracellular pyogenic bacteria, manifested as meningitis, pneumonia, or septicemia (Alper et al., 1972). The heterozygotes have not demonstrated an abnormality in handling infectious agents.

Several infants have been described with a syndrome similar to Leiner's disease, including severe seborrheic dermatitis, diarrhea, and recurrent infections with gram negative organisms and *Staphylococcus aureus* (Miller et al., 1968). Despite normal levels of C5 protein and normal hemolytic activity of the complement system in these patients, C5 present in their sera appears to function abnormally. This is manifested as defective enhancement of phagocytosis of yeast and defective generation of chemotactic activity. Their clinical symptoms and the phagocytic defect are improved with infusions of normal plasma or pure C5 but not C5-deficient sera. The structure of dysfunctional C5 appears to be normal, but its activity declines more rapidly on storage when compared to normal C5.

The absence of C5 was first described in two sisters: one with SLE and superficial infections, the other healthy. The increased susceptibility to infections is presumably due to the lack of the C5-derived chemotactic factor, C5a.

Several patients with C6 deficiency have had neisserial infections; one patient had two episodes of gonococcal arthritis and others had recurrent meningococcal meningitis or meningococcemia. Their sera lacked bactericidal activity against several bacteria, including *Neisseria*. However, opsonization of these same bacteria was normal. Preparing bacteria for effective phagocytosis is the most important function of the complement system in response to infection and undoubtedly protects against most organisms. Killing of organisms by the complement system is evidently not as important in bacterial defense. Neisseria may represent an important exception to this rule.

C7 deficiency has been reported in patients with autoimmune diseases or recurrent meningococcemia. One patient with C7 deficiency, however, is reported to be healthy. C8 deficiency has been described associated with SLE or prolonged disseminated gonococcal infections.

Only two cases involving a genetically determined defect in the alternative pathway have been reported (Alper et al., 1970). Both resulted from decrease or absence of C3b inactivator, the function of which is to remove C3b attached to any surface (see Chapter 5). Without removal of C3b, the enzyme responsible for activating C3 through the alternative pathway, C3bBb, continues to destroy C3. The result is a deficiency of C3 and extreme susceptibility to bacterial infections, including pneumonia, septicemia, and recurrent meningitis. Infusions of plasma or purified C3b inactivator have restored serum C3 levels and opsonization of bacteria.

More extensive reviews of congenital defects of the complement system can be found in Spitzer, 1977; Johnston and Stroud, 1977; and Agnello, 1978.

Acquired Defects of the Complement System

Numerous disease states are associated with a partial decrease in one or more complement components (Table 8–2). C1 inactivator (C1 INA) deficiency, which results in hereditary angioedema, occurs on a genetic basis, as discussed in Chapter 33. An acquired deficiency of C1 INA has been described in several patients with lymphoproliferative diseases. Episodic angioedema was present in all.

The serum concentration of the early-acting components of the classic pathway (C1, C4, C2, and C3) are frequently decreased in SLE as a consequence of activation of C1q by immune complexes. Treat-

TABLE 8–2 ACQUIRED DEFECTS OF THE COMPLEMENT SYSTEM

Deficient Component	Underlying Mechanism	Associated Clinical Findings*
C4, C2	C1 INA deficiency	Lymphoproliferative diseases
C1, C4, C2, C3	Immune complexes	SLE, leprosy, SBE, VJS, mononucleosis, dengue fever, hepatitis, AGN, dermatitis herpetiformis, celiac disease
C3	Decreased synthesis	Thermal injury, malnutrition
C3	Nephritic factor	MPGN, lipodystrophy
Factor B, P; C3, C5	Normal physiologic state	Neonates
Alternative pathway function	Decreased synthesis of components	Sickle cell anemia

*SLE = systemic lupus erythematosus; SBE = subacute bacterial endocarditis; VJS = ventricular jugular shunt; AGN = acute glomerulonephritis; MPGN = membranoproliferative glomerulonephritis.

ment restores component levels to normal, and serum C3 concentrations serve as a sensitive means of following activity of the disease. An interesting SLE-like syndrome with recurrent urticaria, angioedema with laryngeal edema, and arthralgia, but with negative titers of antinuclear antibody has been described in several patients. Unlike patients with typical SLE, these individuals have had persistently decreased C1q and C3.

Hypocomplementemia involving the early-reacting components has been described in leprosy, subacute bacterial endocarditis, ventriculojugular shunts, malaria, infectious mononucleosis, dengue hemorrhagic fever, viral hepatitis, acute glomerulonephritis, dermatitis herpetiformis, and celiac disease. All of these disorders involve immune complexes, which activate the classic pathway, with reduction in C1, C4, C2 and C3.

Both malnutrition and burns can result in hypocomplementemia, reflected in low C3 levels. The mechanism is not known but may involve excessive loss or decreased synthesis.

Patients with membranoproliferative glomerulonephritis have long been known to have depressed levels of C3. In the last several years, these patients have been found to have a serum protein termed "C3 nephritic factor," which promotes the cleavage of C3 (Spitzer, 1969). The cleavage takes place through the alternative pathway, the alternative pathway C3-cleaving enzyme (C3bBb) being protected by C3 nephritic factor from inactivation. Accumulating evidence indicates this factor may be IgG. Recently, two reports of transplacental transport of nephritic factor have appeared in which the infants had transient hypocomplementemia. Many patients with nephritic factor and hypocomplementemia also have partial lipodystrophy. These patients sometimes develop renal disease, and at least one patient had recurrent bacterial infections. The relationship of hypocomplementemia to glomerulonephritis is unclear. A recent hypothesis suggests that hypocomplementemia predisposes to increased infections, which result in glomerulonephritis.

Abnormal opsonization of pneumococci, described in sickle cell anemia, appears to involve the alternative pathway. Other assays of alternative pathway activity have also been abnormal in some patients with sickle cell disease (Johnston et al., 1973). Such a defect may help explain these patients' known susceptibility to pneumococcal disease.

Neonates have long been noted to have an increased susceptibility to infection. Along with other defects in their immune system, analysis of cord blood has shown levels of C3, factor B, and early components of the classic pathway that are about two-thirds the adult values.

Recently, adverse reactions to radiocontrast media have been shown to be mediated through the alternative pathway. The dye directly activates C3 and C5 through the alternative pathway, resulting in production of the anaphylatoxins C3a and C5a. Binding of these peptides to mast cells results in degranulation and the symptoms of anaphylaxis in susceptible individuals.

When to Suspect Defects in the Complement System

Defects in the complement system should be suspected in several clinical situations.

1. *Autoimmune diseases* such as SLE, anaphylactoid purpura, dermatomyositis, chronic nephritis, and ankylosing spondylitis, *particularly if the clinical and laboratory findings are not completely typical.* This occurs most frequently with congenital deficiencies of C1r, C1s, C4, C2, C5, C7, and C8. It is important to make the diagnosis of a complement deficiency since the prognosis, associated problems, and risk to other family members may differ from those of the usual patient.

2. *Recurrent severe infections with extracellular pyogenic organisms* occur with C3 or C3b INA deficiency. These infections resemble those in hypogammaglobulinemia. Meningitis and septicemia are particularly common. Recurrent pneumococcal septicemia should support the possibility of C2 deficiency.

3. *Severe or recurrent skin and respiratory tract infections* should make one consider a defect in chemotaxis resulting from C5 deficiency or dysfunction.

4. *Recurrent gonococcal or meningococcal infections,* even beginning in adulthood, should raise the possibility of deficiency of a late-acting component (C6, C7, or C8).

As mentioned, complement abnormalities occur as secondary phenomena in many disease states. Determination of the individual component values listed in Table 8–2, may be of value in diagnosis of these diseases. Low levels of the early components C4, C2, C3 may be due to activation by immune complexes, while low C3 levels in a patient with chronic renal disease suggests membranoproliferative glomerulonephritis.

Evaluation of Complement System

Whole Complement Titer (CH50). When the clinician suspects that a patient with "collagen disease" or recurrent infections has a complement deficiency, blood should be drawn for determination of the whole complement titer (CH50). The blood must be carefully handled by separating the serum from the clot and freezing the serum at −70° C *within one hour.* The assay (available in most hospital laboratories) tests the capacity of serum to lyse antibody-coated sheep erythrocytes, which requires all nine components of the classic pathway. The assay easily identifies all homozygous complement-deficient patients, since the capacity of their serum is invariably zero. Therefore, a normal CH50 eliminates deficiency of the *classic* pathway as a cause of recurrent infections. Once a patient is identified by a zero CH50 result, his family members should also be investigated. Other homozygous relatives will have a zero CH50 test result. Heterozygous family members (with half normal levels of the defective component) will have a normal CH50 and no clinical abnormalities. Therefore, to pinpoint the exact defect in the patient, and thereafter in the heterozygous relatives, the individual complement components, through C9, should be determined in the patient's serum. Certain medical centers and some commercial laboratories can perform these determinations; serum should be prepared as for CH50 testing. Family members will require genetic counseling appropriate for an autosomal recessive disorder. Parents of the patient have a one in four chance of producing another affected child.

Patients with autoimmune diseases should be managed similarly, remembering that patients heterozygous for C2 deficiency may have clinical disease (JRA or SLE) and a normal CH50. The level of C2 in their serum must be measured to make this diagnosis.

Alternative Pathway Function. In general, as mentioned, patients with recurrent infections and a normal CH50 do not have an abnormality of the complement system that can explain their problem. However, if a cause for the patient's infections cannot be found and the clinician remains suspicious, an abnormality of the alternative pathway should be considered. Determinations of alternative pathway function are not commercially available but can be performed at many medical centers.

C3 Level. The level of the crucial component C3 is determined by radial immunodiffusion using specific antibody and is available at most hospital laboratories. As mentioned before, C3 levels are frequently low in diseases associated with immune complexes, membranoproliferative glomerulonephritis, and obviously, hereditary C3 deficiency.

PHAGOCYTE FUNCTION

Effective phagocytic function comprises an orderly sequence of events resulting in destruction of the invading microorganism. *Chemotaxis* is the initial response of the phagocyte and leads to contact with the organism. Upon contact, if the organism has been properly opsonized, *ingestion* occurs, moving the organism into the cell's interior. At the same time, the cell consumes oxygen and converts it to toxic by-products required for killing most microorganisms. Intracellular granules fuse with the phagocytic vacuole as it forms, and *intracellular killing* begins. Any break in this sequence — chemotaxis, ingestion, and killing — impairs the host's ability to resist infection.

Primary Cellular Defects of Chemotaxis

Several defects of chemotaxis result from primary abnormalities of the phagocyte cell itself (Table 8–3). *Chediak-Higashi syndrome* (CHS) is a genetically determined, probably autosomal recessive disease, characterized by recurrent infections; partial loss of pigment in the skin, iris, and retina; photophobia; nystagmus; and giant granules in most granule-containing cells (Blume and Wolff, 1972). Most patients develop an "accelerated phase" with a lymphoma-like illness consisting of pancytopenia, lymphadenopathy, and hepatosplenomegaly. The majority of patients die of infection or hemorrhage in their first decade. An analogous syndrome occurs in several animal species.

The loss of pigmentation, "partial albinism," is among the most constant features and may be present at birth. The depigmentation may be subtle and appear only as a silver hue of the hair. Melanin is not lost but is aggregated in large granules rather than distributed homogenously in the cell. Abnormally large granules are present in many other cells, including all neutrophils, eosinophils, and basophils, and a variable number of lymphocytes, but the granules do not appear in platelets or erythrocytes. Recognition of depigmentation and abnormal granules in patients with frequent infections has usually led to the diagnosis.

Information on infections is scant. However, in four carefully studied patients, 29 pyogenic infections were documented. *Staphylococcus aureus,* group A β-hemolytic streptococci, and *H. influenzae* organisms were the most common pathogens. Sites of infection included the lungs, skin, subcutaneous tissue, and upper respiratory tract (including otitis media and sinusitis). All infections responded to appropriate doses of antibiotics.

The patient with CHS suffers several defects in the granulocytic function that predispose him to pyogenic infections. Neutropenia may be profound. The granulocytes have impaired chemotactic ability and move sluggishly to the site of infection. Characteristically, peripheral leukocytosis fails to occur even with severe infections. Once granulocytes are at the site of infection, ingestion of the organisms appears normal. Degranulation of lysosomes into the phagocytic vacuole is impaired, however. The levels of lysosomal enzymes are normal, as is phagocytosis-associated oxidative metabolism, including nitroblue tetrazolium (NBT) reduction. There is a mild defect in phagocytic killing of bacteria, similar to the defect found in carriers of chronic granulomatous disease (CGD), who do not have increased infections. This bactericidal defect most likely results from the slow release of lysosomal enzymes into the phagocytic vacuoles containing bacteria. Recurrent infections appear to be due to the neutropenia and the chemotactic defect.

Recent evidence indicates that the impaired chemotaxis and degranulation of leukocytes in CHS may be due to a defect in function of intracellular structures termed *microtubules*. The functions of microtubules, which serve as a cell skeleton, are regulated by the cyclic nucleotides, cAMP and cGMP. Addition of cGMP, or of cholingeric agents which increase cGMP, to leukocytes from CHS patients *in vitro* improves their chemotaxis, degranulation, and bactericidal activity. Ascorbate — known to increase intracellular cGMP levels —was fed to one infant with CHS. The result was normalization of *in vitro* chemotaxis, degranulation, and bactericidal activity; the neutropenia and abnormal granules were unchanged (Boxer et al., 1976).

The *lazy leukocyte syndrome* involves the combination of severe neutropenia with normal numbers and types of cells in the marrow, abnormal neutrophil chemotaxis into "skin windows," and defective neutrophil chemotaxis *in vitro* (Miller et al., 1971). The clinical picture consists of recurrent gingivitis, stomatitis, otitis media, furunculosis, and pneumonia. Phagocytosis and bactericidal activity are normal. The ability of neutrophils to squeeze through narrow spaces (deform) is decreased, which is a possible explanation for the functional abnormalities. Other syndromes of defective chemotaxis, some of them familial, have been reported (Table 8–3).

Defective function of actin (an important part of the contractile elements of the phagocytic cell and required for chemotaxis

TABLE 8–3 CELLULAR DEFECTS OF CHEMOTAXIS

Primary
  Chediak-Higashi syndrome
  Lazy leukocyte syndrome
  Familial defect with normal motility
  Actin dysfunction

Secondary
  Hyperimmunoglobulinemia E
  Diabetes mellitus
  Rheumatoid arthritis
  Other

and ingestion) has been described in a patient with defective chemotaxis and severe recurrent infections (Boxer et al., 1974).

Secondary Cellular Defects of Chemotaxis

Another group of chemotactic disorders consists of conditions in which the cellular abnormality presumably results from an underlying disease state in cells other than leukocytes (Table 8–3). The patient's cells function abnormally *in vitro* even though their serum has no detrimental effect on the chemotaxis of normal cells.

A number of patients have been reported who have shown decreased neutrophil chemotaxis and *hyperimmunoglobulinemia E* in association with a variety of clinical syndromes and increased susceptibility to infection. These include several patients with mucocutaneous candidiasis.

A combination of chronic dermatitis, usually eczematous, and recurrent staphylococcal abscesses has been associated with elevated IgE and depressed chemotaxis (Hill and Quie, 1974). These patients include those with "Job's syndrome." The same syndrome with ichthyosis rather than eczema has been described. Several patients have had urticaria or allergic rhinitis. Other infections have included furunculosis, cellulitis, pneumonia, empyema, otitis media and, occasionally, a deep abscess or septicemia. *S. aureus* has been the most common pathogen. The syndrome of elevated IgE, pyoderma, subcutaneous abscesses, and depressed cell-mediated immunity also could be related since chemotaxis is occasionally abnormal in these patients (Buckley et al., 1972). The chemotactic defect in these hyper-IgE syndromes may not be persistent. In addition, patients with atopic dermatitis without elevated IgE have been reported to have chemotactic defects.

In these syndromes it is unlikely that the defect in chemotaxis is directly due to the hyperimmunoglobulinemia E. On the other hand, histamine release from IgE-coated basophils could be responsible. Histamine inhibits chemotaxis of normal neutrophils *in vitro*, perhaps because it elevates intracellular cAMP. Treatment of some of these patients' neutrophils *in vitro* with the H_2

antihistamine, burimamide, produced a significant improvement in chemotaxis.

Patients with *diabetes mellitus* have been reported to have abnormal chemotaxis and ingestion. The chemotactic defect can be corrected *in vitro* by the addition of insulin (Mowat and Baum, 1971a). Insulin deficiency could theoretically result in defective neutrophil function through potassium or glucose deficiency. The significance of the relationship between the phagocyte dysfunction and infections in diabetes is unclear.

Patients with *rheumatoid arthritis* have been reported with abnormal chemotaxis (Mowat and Baum, 1971b). Phagocytosis of rheumatoid complexes may contribute to the impairment. Other conditions which may involve secondary cellular defects in chemotaxis include acrodermatitis enteropathica; hypophosphatemia due to parenteral hyperalimentation; mannosidosis; Down's syndrome; alcoholism; cancer; malnutrition; bone marrow transplantation; corticosteroid therapy; burns, and the neonatal state.

Chemotactic Defects Attributable to Serum

Defective chemotaxis may be due to an abnormality of serum or plasma, either from a deficiency or from inhibitory activity (Table 8–4). *Abnormalities of chemotactic factor production* include the *complement deficiencies,* specifically C3 and C5, previously discussed.

Direct inhibitors of chemotactic factors have been found in the sera of patients with glomerulonephritis, cirrhosis, Hodgkin's disease, lepromatous leprosy, and sar-

TABLE 8–4   SERUM DEFECTS OF CHEMOTAXIS

Complement Deficiencies

Circulating Inhibitors
  Glomerulonephritis
  Cirrhosis
  Hodgkin's disease
  Lepromatous leprosy
  Sarcoidosis
  Elevated IgA
  Wiskott-Aldrich syndrome

TABLE 8–5   DEFECTS OF INGESTION

Neutropenia

Splenic Hypofunction

Intrinsic Cellular Abnormalities
  Actin dysfunction
  Hypophosphatemia

coidosis. Similar inhibitors are present in normal sera but at much lower levels. Thus, chronic inflammation may stimulate increased production of what may be a normal control mechanism.

Decreased chemotaxis has been associated with *elevated serum IgA* in several patients. The serum of one such girl with eczema, persistent purulent rhinitis, staphylococcal conjunctivitis and pyoderma, and recurrent pneumonia had a direct inhibitory effect on neutrophil chemotaxis. Four siblings with recurrent bacterial infections, elevated IgA, and a chemotactic defect have also been reported. Circulating IgA-associated inhibitors of chemotaxis have been found in patients with alcoholic liver disease. A role for IgA in these cases is suggested by the finding that isolated IgA myeloma protein inhibits neutrophil chemotaxis *in vitro.*

Depressed monocyte chemotaxis toward a lymphocyte-derived chemotactic factor and C5a was reported in the Wiskott-Aldrich syndrome (Altman et al., 1974). Supranormal levels of this chemotactic factor found in the patients' plasma were felt to deactivate the patients' cells for chemotaxis. A similar increase in serum chemotactic factors may occur in some patients with renal disease. Defects of chemotaxis are reviewed in greater detail in Snyderman (1977) and Johnston and McPhail (in press).

Defects of Ingestion

Defects of ingestion by neutrophils will also result in recurrent infections (Table 8–5). A striking abnormality in ingestion occurs when serum opsonization is defective owing to reduced concentrations of antibody or C3. *Neutropenia* is a well known cause of recurrent infections (Howard et al., 1977). Since the extent of phagocytosis is decreased, the basic defect might be considered one of ingestion. *S. aureus* is the most common pathogen involved but Pseudomonas organisms and *E. coli* are almost as frequent. The most frequent infections are pneumonia, otitis media, and abscesses. Neither meningitis nor serious viral or fungal infections have been reported in patients with isolated neutropenia.

Splenic hypofunction — whether due to congenital absence, surgical removal, or the sludging of erythrocytes in sickle cell disease — might be considered a defect of ingestion, since a large mass of phagocytic cells is actually or functionally absent. The clinical picture contrasts with neutropenia, in that superficial infections are rare, since neutrophil function at the periphery is normal; but septicemia and meningitis are relatively common, since bloodstream filtering by splenic macrophages does not occur. Pyogenic bacteria, especially the pneumococcus, are the usual infecting organisms (Johnston, 1974).

Intrinsic cellular abnormalities can also result in abnormal ingestion. An infant with defective neutrophil actin function and recurrent bacterial infections has been mentioned previously (Boxer et al., 1974). *S. aureus* was repeatedly cultured from skin lesions. Both chemotaxis and ingestion were abnormal. Along with its importance in chemotaxis, actin, as a component of microfilaments, is involved in the process of ingestion.

Defects in both chemotaxis and ingestion have been reported in patients with pyoderma gangrenosum or with hypophosphatemia secondary to parenteral hyperalimentation. Since defects in chemotaxis and ingestion often occur together, it has been suggested that the two functions are linked. The contractile system of the cell is involved in both processes, the rearrangement of microfilaments being responsible for migration of the cell and internalization of bound organisms.

Defects of Microbicidal Activity

Killing of the intracellular organism after normal chemotaxis and ingestion is the final step in phagocytic function. Defects in

TABLE 8–6 DEFECTS OF MICROBICIDAL ACTIVITY

Chronic granulomatous disease

Glucose-6-phosphate dehydrogenase deficiency

Myeloperoxidase deficiency

Abnormality of neutrophil granules

Other

this microbicidal activity can have profound effects on host defense (Table 8–6).

The term *chronic granulomatous disease* (CGD) has been applied to a syndrome of recurrent purulent infections of the skin, lymph nodes, liver, and lungs, associated with an inability of patients' phagocytes to kill fungi or bacteria that do not produce hydrogen peroxide. Recent evidence suggests that the syndrome can be caused by various molecular defects.

The most characteristic clinical abnormalities reflect the involvement of the reticuloendothelial system. Lymphadenopathy has been described in all but a few infants and children with a milder form of the disease. Hepatomegaly, splenomegaly, and hepatic or perihepatic abscesses are common. All of these findings reflect the accumulation of bacteria or fungi by phagocytic cells that cannot kill them (Johnston and Newman, 1977).

The second major group of signs reflects the inability of circulating phagocytes to kill invading bacteria at the site of penetration. These include pneumonitis, subcutaneous abscesses, furunculosis, osteomyelitis, perianal abscess, conjunctivitis, and ulcerative stomatitis. These serious infections are generally localized, but septicemia or meningitis may occur if defenses are overwhelmed.

Other features, which are less easily explained, include eczematoid or seborrheic dermatitis, often present on eyelids, external nares, or around the mouth; persistent diarrhea; and rhinitis. The onset of CGD has been heralded by dermatitis or lymphadenitis in most of the cases reported. Less common manifestations include esophagitis, recurrent otitis media, arthritis, pericarditis, cystitis, recurrent urinary tract infections, persistent vomiting due to gastric obstructions, and chorioretinal lesions.

The majority of patients manifest the disease in the first year of life — some in the first week. There have been 60 reported deaths, 45 before age 7 and 51 before age 12. However, with milder forms of disease, survival into the fourth decade has been reported. Pulmonary disease was the cause of death in the majority, although septicemia and meningitis have been lethal in several patients.

Except for studies of phagocyte function, laboratory findings reflect only chronic infection. Biopsy and autopsy material from infected sites show granulomas and histiocytes containing pigmented lipid. Most patients have abnormalities on chest radiographs. This primarily represents the high incidence of acute pneumonia, although some children have had pulmonary fibrosis or striking pulmonary infiltrates.

Infecting organisms are predominantly staphylococci and enteric bacteria. Aspergillus and Candida also have been common pathogens. *Salmonella* was the most common cause of septicemia or meningitis. The absence of *H. influenzae,* pneumococcus, and streptococcus correlates with the ability of CGD phagocytes to kill these catalase-negative, peroxide-producing organisms *in vitro.* Tuberculosis and disseminated BCG infection have occurred.

X-linked and autosomal recessive modes of inheritance for CGD have been demonstrated. The existence of different "varieties" of CGD in addition to those represented by different modes of inheritance seems likely. Patients with similar defects but a milder course have been described. Separation of these cases will require identification of a precise molecular defect.

Cells from patients with CGD do not undergo the normal phagocytosis-associated increase in oxygen consumption and conversion to microbicidal metabolites, including superoxide anion and H_2O_2. Presumably the basic molecular defect of CGD is deficient activity of an enzyme responsible for conversion of oxygen to bactericidal species. NADH oxidase, NADPH oxidase, and glutathione peroxidase have each been proposed as the defective enzyme, but none has been clearly proven as such.

Recent evidence suggests that in some patients the phagocytes possess normal oxidative enzyme activity but have an abnormal system for triggering this activity (Weening et al., 1976). Several patients have been reported to carry the rare null Kell blood group phenotype (Marsh and Kimball, 1977). Their neutrophils also lack an antigen, K_X, present in normal individuals. This highly significant association raises the possibility that the absence of a membrane structure on CGD neutrophils is involved in their abnormal function.

Deficiency of glucose-6-phosphate dehydrogenase involving leukocytes as well as erythrocytes could be considered a variant of CGD. At least it represents the first enzyme defect shown clearly to cause the CGD syndrome. When G-6-PD levels are less than 1 per cent of normal, the patient suffers a clinical syndrome that mimics CGD but is milder.

In *primary myeloperoxidase (MPO) deficiency,* peroxidase activity is absent from both neutrophils and monocytes. Patients are not generally abnormally susceptible to disease. However, one patient with disseminated candidiasis and two with severe acne vulgaris have been reported. MPO deficiency may also occur as a secondary phenomenon in association with leukemia, anemia, psoriasis, and neuronal storage disease. Functionally, the MPO-deficient leukocytes have impaired microbicidal activity that is not as severe as that in CGD. Microbicidal mechanisms independent of myeloperoxidase appear to protect effectively against infections.

Impaired bactericidal activity has been associated in a few instances with an *abnormality of neutrophil granules.* Unfortunately, the defect in these patients has not been well defined. Bactericidal defects have also been reported in Felty's syndrome, leukocyte alkaline phosphatase deficiency, neutrophil pyruvate kinase deficiency, and leukemia. The biochemical basis for the killing defects associated with these disorders is not known. Defects of both ingestion and microbicidal activity are reviewed in greater detail in Johnston and McPhail (in press).

When to Suspect a Defect of Phagocyte Function

The pattern of infections seen in 22 patients with an isolated defect of chemotaxis

TABLE 8–7 INFECTIONS IN 22 PATIENTS WITH AN APPARENT ISOLATED DEFECT OF CHEMOTAXIS

Infection	Patients Involved*
Subcutaneous abscess	14
Furunculosis	13
Pneumonia	13
Sinusitis or persistent rhinitis	9
Recurrent otitis media	8
Impetigo	7
Recurrent conjunctivitis	5
Stomatitis	3
Deep abscess	3
Septicemia	3
Cellulitis	2
Mastoiditis	2
Bronchiectasis	1
Septic arthritis	1

*Number of patients who sustained that infection on at least one occasion. (From Johnston, R. B., Jr. and McPhail, L. C.: The patient with impaired phagocyte function. *In* Nahmias, A. J., and O'Reilly, R. J. (eds.): Immunology of Human Infection. New York, Plenum, In press.)

is shown in Table 8–7. These infections characteristically occur at the interface between the host and microbial world, where a small inoculum can become significant if the neutrophil response is delayed or absent. Thus, patients should be investigated for abnormalities of chemotaxis if recurrent infections of the skin, subcutaneous tissue, or respiratory tract are present. As shown in the table, recurrent furunculosis, subcutaneous abscesses, sinusitis, otitis media, and pneumonia have been most common, with deep abscesses or septicemia being unusual. Particular attention should be given to patients who exhibit these infections and have hyperimmunoglobulinemia E, eczema, or elevated IgA.

Neutropenia predisposes to a pattern of infections similar to that seen in patients with chemotactic defects. Patients with overwhelming septicemia, especially from pneumococcus, may have actual asplenia or functional asplenia (similar to the asplenia in sickle cell disease). To date, other defects of ingestion have not been diagnosed often enough to allow their characterization.

Marked lymphadenopathy with suppuration, dermatitis, hepatic abscesses, perianal abscesses, and recurrent pneumonia suggests an ability of phagocytes to ingest but not to kill microorganisms. The prototypic disorder presenting these clinical findings is chronic granulomatous disease (osteomyelitis, ulcerative stomatitis, septicemia, meningitis, persistent diarrhea, and rhinitis also occur commonly in this disorder). The other defects of microbicidal activity, e.g., glucose-6-phosphate dehydrogenase deficiency, have a similar clinical pattern, but infections are less severe.

Evaluation of Phagocyte Function

When the history and physical examination suggest a disorder of phagocyte function, evaluation should begin with total and differential leukocyte counts, hematocrit, and red and white blood cell morphology. Neutropenia and Chediak-Higashi syndrome, in which granulocytes and monocytes contain abnormal granules, can be diagnosed by this simple procedure. The presence of abnormal erythrocyte morphology or Howell-Jolly bodies in erythrocytes suggests the presence of splenic hypofunction. A sickle cell preparation should be ordered on patients with anemia and recurrent pneumococcal infections.

Evaluation of leukocyte chemotaxis *in vitro* requires a complicated technique that is often difficult to obtain. However, a Rebuck inflammatory skin window provides a screening test for chemotactic disorders that can be performed in the office (Rebuck and Crowley, 1955). Patients whose results in the screening test are abnormal should be referred to a medical center where chemotaxis can be evaluated in a standardized *in vitro* assay.

Patients suspected of a disorder of microbicidal activity should have a nitroblue tetrazolium (NBT) test performed on their leukocytes. This test is available at many hospitals and serves as an effective screening test for chronic granulomatous disease and G-6-PD deficiency in that a normal reaction in this test requires the leukocytes to convert oxygen to superoxide anion and other microbicidal products. Testing for myeloperoxidase is done in hematology-oncology laboratories as a means of differentiating certain leukemias. If available, this is a suitable screening test for myeloperoxidase deficiency.

If results of any screening procedures are abnormal, further studies to fully define the defects should be performed at immunology centers where the required laboratory procedures are available. In most cases complete therapy is not available, but supportive therapy can be very effective in reducing the frequency of infections (see Chapter 7).

References

Agnello, V.: Complement deficiency states. Medicine 57:1, 1978.

Alper, C. A., Abramson, N., Johnston, R. B., Jr., Jandl, J. H., and Rosen, F. S.: Studies in vivo and in vitro on an abnormality in the metabolism of C3 in a patient with increased susceptibility to infection. J. Clin. Invest. 49:1975, 1970.

Alper, C. A., Colten, H. R., Rosen, F. S., Rabson, A. R., Macnab, G. M., and Gear, J. S. S.: Homozygous deficiency of C3 in a patient with repeated infections. Lancet 2:1179, 1972.

Altman, L. C., Synderman, R., and Blaese, R. M.: Abnormalities of chemotactic lymphokine synthesis and mononuclear leukocyte chemotaxis in Wiskott-Aldrich syndrome. J. Clin. Invest. 54:486, 1974.

Blume, R. S., and Wolff, S. M.: The Chediak-Higashi syndrome: Studies in four patients and a review of the literature. Medicine 51:247, 1972.

Boxer, L. A., Hedley-White, E. T., and Stossel, T. P.: Neutrophil actin dysfunction and abnormal neutrophil behavior. N. Engl. J. Med. 291:1093, 1974.

Boxer, L. A., Watanabe, A. M., Rister, M., Besch, H. R., Allen, J., and Baehner, R. L.: Correction of leukocyte function in Chediak-Higashi syndrome by ascorbate. N. Engl. J. Med. 295:1041, 1976.

Buckley, R. H., Wray, B. B., and Belmaker, E. Z.: Extreme hyperimmunoglobulinemia E and undue susceptibility to infection. Pediatrics 49:59, 1972.

Day, N. K., Geiger, H., McLean, R., Michael, A., and Good, R. A.: C2 deficiency: Development of lupus erythematosus. J. Clin. Invest. 52:1601, 1973.

Glass, D., Gibson, D. J., Carpenter, C. B., and Schur, P. H.: Hereditary C2 deficiency: HLA gene complex associations with recombinant events. J. Immunol. 116:1734, 1976.

Hill, H. R., and Quie, P. G.: Raised serum IgE levels and defective neutrophil chemotaxis in three children with eczema and recurrent bacterial infections. Lancet 1:183, 1974.

Howard, M. W., Strauss, R. G., and Johnston, R. B., Jr.: Infections in patients with neutropenia. Am. J. Dis. Child. 131:788, 1977.

Johnston, R. B., Jr., Newman, S. L., and Struth, A. G.: An abnormality of the alternative pathway of complement activation in sickle cell disease. N. Engl. J. Med. 288:803, 1973.

Johnston, R. B., Jr.: Increased susceptibility to infection in sickle cell disease: Review of occurrence and possible causes. South. Med. J. 67:1342, 1974.

Johnston, R. B., Jr., and Newman, S. L.: Chronic granulomatous disease. Pediatr. Clin. North Am. 24:365, 1977.

Johnston, R. B., Jr., and Stroud, R. M.: Complement and host defense against infection. J. Pediatr. 90:169, 1977.

Johnston, R. B., Jr., and McPhail, L. C.: The patient with impaired phagocyte function. In Nahmias, A. J., and O'Reilly, R. J. (eds.): Immunology of Human Infection. New York, Plenum. In press.

Marsh, W. L., and Kimball, L. F.: The Kell blood group, Kx antigen, and chronic granulomatous disease. Mayo Clin. Proc. 52:150, 1977.

Miller, M. E., Seals, J., Kaye, R., and Levitsky, L. C.: A familial, plasma associated defect of phagocytosis. A new cause of recurrent bacterial infections. Lancet 2:60, 1968.

Miller, M. E., Oski, F. A., and Harris, M. B.: Lazy leukocyte syndrome: A new disorder of neutrophil function. Lancet 1:665, 1971.

Mowat, A. G., and Baum, J.: Chemotaxis of polymorphonuclear leukocytes from patients with diabetes mellitus. N. Engl. J. Med. 284:621, 1971a.

Mowat, A. G., and Baum, J.: Chemotaxis of polymorphonuclear leukocytes from patients with rheumatoid arthritis. J. Clin. Invest. 50:2541, 1971b.

Newman, S. L., Vogler, L. B., Feigin, R. D., and Johnston, R. B., Jr.: Recurrent septicemia associated with congenital deficiency of C2 and partial deficiency of factor B and the alternative complement pathway. N. Engl. J. Med.: 299: 290, 1978.

Rebuck, J. W., and Crowley, J. H.: A method of studying leukocyte functions in vitro Ann. N. Y. Acad. Sci. 59:757, 1955.

Snyderman, R., and Pike, M.: Disorders of leukocyte chemotaxis. Pediatr. Clin. North Am. 24:377, 1977.

Spitzer, R. E., Vallota, E. H., Forristal, J., Sudora, E., Stitzel, A., Davis, N. C., and West, C. D.: Serum C3 lytic system in patients with glomerulonephritis. Science 164:436, 1969.

Spitzer, R. E.: The complement system. Pediatr. Clin. North Am. 24:341, 1977.

Weening, R. S., Roos, D., Weemaes, C. M. R., Homan-Müller, J. W. T., and van Schaik, M. L. J.: Defective inifiation of the metabolic stimulation in phagocytizing granulocytes: A new congenital defect. J. Lab. Clin. Med., 88:757, 1976.

Rebecca H. Buckley, M.D.

9

IgE Antibody in Health and Disease

As recently as 1963, Stanworth wrote that skin-sensitizing antibodies represented an elusive subject and nebulous concept to most immunologists. Many crucial discoveries since then not only have firmly established that the substances responsible for skin-sensitizing activity are "true" antibodies, but also have documented that most skin-sensitizing antibodies belong to a unique immunoglobulin class.

DEFINITION AND SYNONYMS

Skin-sensitizing antibodies are defined as antibodies that exhibit a high affinity for membrane receptors on basophils and mast cells of members of the same or closely related species. Although it is clear that the majority of such molecules belong to the IgE class of immunoglobulins, there also is evidence in animals and man that some skin-sensitizing antibodies may belong to the IgG class. The interaction of antigen with two or more basophil or mast cell–bound antibodies results in the release of chemical mediators that cause a variety of biologic effects. When antigen is injected into the skin, the mediators released from dermal mast cells cause vasodilatation, pruritus, and increased capillary permeability — resulting in an immediate wheal and flare reaction. Synonyms for skin-sensitizing antibodies include reaginic anti-

bodies, atopic reagin, anaphylactic antibodies, and homocytotropic antibodies. The reasons for the diverse names will become apparent in the succeeding sections, but primarily the names reflect the various levels of understanding of the functions of these antibodies at the times the terms came into use.

HISTORICAL BACKGROUND

Prausnitz in 1921 clearly demonstrated the feasibility of transferring immediate wheal and flare skin test reactivity to himself by the intracutaneous injection of serum from his fish-sensitive patient, Küstner. In spite of that, scientists were puzzled for the next four decades over the fact that sera from allergic subjects lacked activity in the classic *in vitro* immunological reactions of precipitation, agglutination, complement fixation, and guinea pig passive cutaneous anaphylaxis (PCA). This peculiar reactivity in the sera of patients with hay fever and asthma was termed "atopic reagin" by Coca and Grove in 1925 (reviewed in Stanworth, 1963).

Not until the early 1960's did the notion evolve that antibodies of different immunoglobulin classes might have different biologic properties. In 1963, Ovary et al. demonstrated that the fraction of 7S antibody protein in immune guinea pig serum capable of passively transferring both cutaneous and systemic anaphylaxis to normal guinea pigs was of γ_1 electrophoretic mobility, whereas the fraction causing complement fixation was of γ_2 mobility. From these and many other subsequent experimental studies, it became apparent that the serum fraction carrying the ability to sensitize members of the same or closely related species for anaphylactic reactions differed from the fraction demonstrating serological reactivity in *in vitro* immunological tests.

This was confusing to most immunologists because, prior to that time, investigations with human sera in guinea pig passive and systemic anaphylaxis experiments had shown a good correlation between the presence of guinea pig anaphylactic reactivity and the presence of precipitating and agglutinating activity in a given serum. Consequently, antibodies of the latter type were mistakenly thought for several years to be the same as those responsible for human anaphylaxis.

Although it had been shown repeatedly that sera from allergic individuals did not give positive PCA reactions in guinea pigs, a number of investigators observed in the mind-1960's that such sera would give strongly positive reactions in monkey PCA experiments (Buckley and Metzgar, 1965). Thereafter, the terms "homocytotropic" and "heterocytotropic" came into usage, the former referring to antibodies capable of transferring skin sensitization or anaphylaxis to members of the same or closely related species, and the latter to those capable of transferring similar reactivity across species to lower animals. It was quickly determined that only IgG antibodies were heterocytotropic and that such antibodies were not reactive in nonhuman primate PCA studies, but the immunoglobulin identity of homocytotropic antibodies was more difficult to establish. Reports in the early 1960's linked the latter activity to the IgA class of immunoglobulins.

In 1966, the Ishizakas isolated a fraction from allergic human serum that did not contain detectable amounts of IgA or the other known immunoglobulin classes, yet contained reaginic activity that could be removed by absorption of the fraction with antibodies to human immunoglobulin light chains (see Ishizaka and Ishizaka, 1975).

Immunization of rabbits with this fraction (which contained only minute amounts of protein) yielded an antiserum that, when absorbed with immunoglobulins of the other known classes, could remove all reaginic activity from the original fraction. By chance a year later, Johansson and his coworkers identified a myeloma protein, which they termed ND (IgND), that had antigenic characteristics different from any of the four known immunoglobulin classes (reviewed in Bennich and Johansson, 1971; Bennich et al., 1976). This protein subsequently was shown to have antigenic identity with the protein found by the Ishizakas to carry reaginic activity. The World Health Organization officially designated this unique immunoglobulin class "IgE."

IgE SKIN-SENSITIZING ANTIBODIES

Sites of IgE Production

IgE-producing plasma cells are found predominantly in paragut and pararespiratory lymphoid tissues and in regional lymph nodes (Table 9–1). In addition, germinal centers of tonsils, adenoids, and bronchial and mesenteric lymph nodes contain IgE-producing cells. By contrast, few plasma cells containing IgE are found in the spleen or in subcutaneous lymph nodes. Thus, the distribution of IgE-producing plasma cells is similar to the distribution of plasma cells that produce IgA (Bloch, 1976). This fact and the fact that many allergens that cause allergic symptoms are inhaled or ingested have raised the question whether IgE-producing lymphoid tissue may represent a distinct local immune system. Although this possibility remains, since IgE has been detected in nasal washings, colostrum and saliva, no conclusive evidence for selective local production has been presented thus far. In addition, a structure analogous to secretory piece has not been found on IgE molecules in external secretions.

Peculiarities of Antigens That Induce IgE Formation

Antigens that induce most IgE-antibody responses are widespread in nature and in-

TABLE 9–1 DISTRIBUTION OF IgE-FORMING CELLS IN
LYMPHOID TISSUES

Lymphoid Tissues	Human		Monkey	
	PLASMA CELLS	GERMINAL CENTER	PLASMA CELLS	GERMINAL CENTER
Tonsil	+~+++	+~++	+	++
Adenoid	+~+++	+~++		
Bronchial and peritoneal	++	(+)*	++	(+)
Subcutaneous lymph nodes	±~+	−	±	−
Spleen	±~+	−	+~++	±
Respiratory mucosa	+	−	+	−
Intestinal mucosa	+~++	−	+~++	(+)†
Lung	−	−	−	−
Blood	−	−	Not done	
Bone marrow	−	−	Not done	

*Results in parentheses were negative in some cases.
† + in Peyer's patches.

(From Ishizaka T., and Ishizaka, K.: Biology of immunoglobulin E. Progr. Allergy *19*:60–121, 1975. Used with permission.)

nocuous to most nonallergic subjects. The major categories of antigens include pollen, food, mold, insect, animal, and parasitic antigens; these will be discussed in detail in Chapters 16 and 17. Many other antigens are known to elicit vigorous immune responses of other types but do not selectively stimulate IgE production. Antigens that stimulate IgE-antibody production usually are protein in nature and are of medium size, most ranging from around 20,000 to 40,000 daltons in molecular weight (King, 1976). Major antigenic components have been purified from a few of these agents, including ragweed, rye and Timothy grasses, cat dander, codfish, and ascaris, but thus far no common or unique structures have been identified to account for their tendency to stimulate IgE antibody synthesis. Certain types of adjuvants, such as aluminum hydroxide gel or killed *Bordetella pertussis* organisms, also facilitate an IgE-antibody response, for unknown reasons (Tada, 1975; Ishizaka, 1976).

Physicochemical Characteristics of IgE

The availability of myeloma proteins of the IgE class has enabled extensive characterization of the physicochemical properties of IgE (Bennich and Johansson, 1971; Bennich et al., 1976). IgE myeloma proteins

consist of four polypeptide chains, two identical heavy (epsilon) chains and two identical light chains, which may be of either the kappa or lambda type (Fig. 9–1). IgE antibodies are considerably heavier than IgG antibodies, having a molecular weight of around 190,000 and a sedimentation coefficient of 8.0 S. The molecule also differs from IgG in the content of carbohydrate, which represents 12 percent of IgE's total weight. The estimated molecular weight of each heavy chain is 72,300 and of each light chain, 22,500.

When IgE is treated with enzymes such as papain and pepsin, it can be cleaved into smaller fragments the same way molecules of the other immunoglobulin classes can be (Fig. 9–1) (Bennich and Johansson, 1971; Bennich et al., 1976). If papain is used, three fragments result, one termed Fc (or *crystallizable fragment*) and the other two Fab (or antigen-binding fragments). Pepsin digestion, on the other hand, results in destruction of the carboxyl-terminal two-thirds of the Fc portion, yielding one large fragment called $F(ab')_2$. Use of these enzymatic probes has allowed analysis of the antigenic characteristics of various segments of the molecule. From such studies it has been learned that the Fc fragment has two different immunoglobulin class-specific antigenic determinants. These are termed E_1 and E_2, with E_2 residing on the

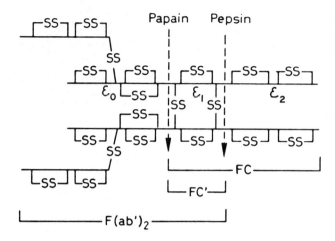

FIGURE 9–1. Structure of immunoglobulin IgE and sites of action of enzymes, as drawn by Ishizaka and Ishizaka (Prog. Allergy, *19*:60, 1975) from the data of Bennich and von Bahr-Lindström (Progress in Immunology, Amsterdam, North-Holland, 1974). (Used with permission.) There are three major antigenic determinants on each of the epsilon chains. Proceeding from right to left, the class-specific E_2 determinant is probably associated with the C terminal portion of the Fc fragment, not included in the F(ab')$_2$ fragment; the E_1 determinant is present on the Fc' segment; and the E_0 (or idiotypic) determinant is in the Fd or N terminal segment.

carboxyl-terminal ends of the epsilon chains and E_1 on the adjacent heavy chain segment in the amino-terminal third of the Fc fragment, designated Fc' (Fig. 9–1). In addition, a third antigenic determinant is present in the Fab fragment on the Fd portion of the epsilon chain; this is the idiotypic, or E_0 antigenic determinant. The E_0 determinant has been different for each IgE myeloma protein studied (thus the term "idiotypic") and should differ for all IgE molecules having different hypervariable regions. The remainder of the Fab fragment is composed of a light chain.

Each IgE molecule contains 40 half-cysteine residues, or 20 disulfide bonds (Bennich and Johansson, 1971). Sixteen of these are intrachain bonds, 12 on the epsilon chains and four on the light chains. Two others link the epsilon chains within the Fc' region, and the remaining two connect the light chains to the Fc portions of the heavy chains at the hinge region. The amino acid sequence of the epsilon chains as well as locations of the intrachain disulfide bonds have been determined, and five domains on the epsilon chain, two in the Fd portion and three in the Fc portion, have been defined (Bennich et al., 1976). By using varying concentrations of sulfhydryl bond-reducing agents such as dithiothreitol, it has been possible to selectively cleave certain disulfide bonds and study the effects of disruption of these bonds on the biologic activity of the molecule. The effects will be mentioned in the following discussion of the biologic properties.

Biologic Properties of IgE

IgE exists in serum and other body fluids in minute concentrations, significantly lower than those of the other four immunoglobulin classes. Waldmann et al. (1976) found the geometric mean serum concentration for normal individuals to be 96 ng/ml. Metabolic studies done by those investigators demonstrated the low concentration to be due to both a low total body synthetic rate and a very short serum half-life (2.7 days). As will be discussed, however, other biologic characteristics of IgE more than compensate for its low availability, since devastating effects on human health can result upon interaction of antigen with just a few strategically located IgE molecules.

General Characteristics. Before discussing its affinity for basophil and mast cell membrane receptors — the most prominent biologic characteristic of IgE — it is important to note IgE's similarities and dissimilarities to other immunoglobulin classes (Ishizaka and Ishizaka, 1975; Spiegelberg, 1974). IgE antibodies in serum are heat-labile, losing their capacity to passively sensitize normal skin, blood basophils, or lung mast cells following heating at 56°C for from 2 to 4 hours (Table 9–2). Treatment of IgE molecules with sulfhydryl bond reducing agents, such as 2-mercaptoethanol or dithiothreitol, similarly will affect their ability to sensitize. In addition, IgE antibodies, like antibodies of the IgA, IgM, and IgD classes, fail to cross the

TABLE 9–2 PROPERTIES OF HOMOCYTOTROPIC ANTIBODIES*

Properties	IgG Type				IgE Type						
	HUMAN	GUINEA PIG*	MOUSE	RAT	HUMAN	MONKEY	DOG	RABBIT	GUINEA PIG	RAT	MOUSE
Sedimentation coefficient	6.5	6.5	6.5	6.5	8.0	8.0	8.0	8.0	8.0	8.0	8.0
Heat lability	–	±	±	–	+	+	+	±	+	+	+
Sulfhydryl lability	–	±	±	–	+	+	+	+	+	+	+
Optimal latent period	4 to 6 hours	3 to 6 hours	1 to 2 hours	3 hours	1 day	1 to 2 days	2 days	3 days	6 days	3 days	3 days

*Properties of guinea pig antibody in this table are IgG 1a antibody. Guinea pig has IgG 1b antibody whose optimal latent period is 16 hours. The IgG 1b antibody is heat-stable but susceptible to reduction-alkylation treatment.

(From Ishizaka, T., and Ishizaka, K.: Biology of immunoglobulin E. Prog. Allergy *19*:60–121, 1975. Used with permission.)

TABLE 9–3   IMMUNOLOGIC PROPERTIES OF IgE

Reactions	Minimum Concentration of Antibody, μg N/ml	Activity
In vitro		
Agglutination	10^{-2}	+
C fixation (classic)	>800*	−
C fixation (alternative)	80*	+
In vivo		
PK in human	4×10^{-5}	+
PCA in monkey	10^{-3}	+
PCA in guinea pig	>100	−

*Aggregated IgE.

(From Ishizaka, T., and Ishizaka, K.: Biology of immunoglobulin E. Progr. Allergy *19*:60–121, 1975. Used with permission.)

placenta from the mother to the fetus. They are incapable of mediating guinea pig PCA even when concentrated manyfold more than they occur *in vivo* (Table 9–3) (Ishizaka and Ishizaka, 1975). Although highly concentrated preparations are able to agglutinate erythrocytes coated with ragweed antigen, it is doubtful that agglutination is an important biologic function of IgE antibodies, since concentrations of the magnitude required to demonstrate this effect are not achieved in the natural state. The ability of IgE molecules to fix complement was investigated by using nonspecifically aggregated IgE myeloma protein and its enzymatically produced fragments. High concentrations of aggregated IgE are unable to activate the complement system by the classic pathway but can do so by the alternative pathway. Aggregated Fc fragments also are capable of activating the alternative pathway, whereas F(ab')₂ fragments are less active (see Table 9–3).

Cell Membrane Affinity. The most important biologic property of IgE antibody molecules is their extremely high binding affinity for membrane receptors on homologous basophils and mast cells. Using ¹²⁵I-labeled anti-IgE and ¹²⁵I-labeled IgE myeloma proteins, Ishizaka and his coworkers were able to show that IgE binds only to primate basophils and mast cells. In contrast, similar studies with radiolabeled human IgG or anti-IgG showed that IgG molecules attach to membrane receptors on primate monocytes and neutrophils. Equilibrium constants of the binding affinities of these two types of immunoglobulins for their respective cell membrane receptors were found to be 10^{-9}/M for IgE and 10^{-5}/M for IgG (Ishizaka and Ishizaka, 1975). Despite the high avidity of IgE for its receptor, it is well known that a minimum latent period of about 4 hours exists before skin sensitization occurs in passive transfer experiments, and full sensitization is not accomplished until around 24 hours. The extremely high avidity of IgE for basophils and mast cells allows these molecules to persist in tissues far longer than in serum. Although there are reports that passively transferred IgE antibodies may persist for weeks or even months, the half-life of radiolabeled IgE injected into human skin is between 12.5 and 18 days (Ishizaka and Ishizaka, 1975).

The structural portion of IgE that binds to basophil and mast cell membrane receptors has been identified through experimental attempts to block passive sensitization by pretreatment with fragments of the molecule (Ishizaka and Ishizaka, 1975). These studies have shown that only Fc fragments are capable of such binding, Moreover, failure of Fc' fragments to block indicates that the carboxyl-terminal two-thirds of the Fc fragment contains the structures essential for binding to these receptors. Further evidence in support of the latter conclusion was obtained by Bennich and Dorrington (reviewed in Bennich et al., 1976), who demonstrated that the long-recognized heat lability of IgE is due to irreversible conformational changes in the Fc fragment, resulting in loss of its affinity for mast cell and basophil receptors. No such conformational changes were seen with the Fc' or F(ab')$_2$ fragments. Finally, reduction-alkylation studies using dithiothreitol showed that cleavage of intra-epsilon chain disulfide bonds located at the junction of the hinge and Fd portions also resulted in loss of affinity of IgE molecules for their natural cell receptors (Ishizaka and Ishizaka, 1975). Since these bonds are remote from the carboxyl-terminal two-thirds of the FC portion, it is postulated that their cleavage must have a secondary effect on the conformation of the Fc portion.

Role in Allergic Reactions. It is entirely possible that IgE antibodies would be essentially functionless molecules if they did not have the capacity to bind to homologous basophils or mast cells. With this capacity, they are able to trigger one of the body's most potent biologic amplification systems upon interaction with antigen to cause "explosive" reactions. These reactions are caused by the sudden release of a variety of chemical mediators from blood basophils or tissue mast cells or both sub-

sequent to interaction of antigen with very few molecules of cell-bound IgE (Fig. 9-2). These cells are major sources of blood and tissue histamine and also produce at least six other substances that mediate IgE-associated hypersensitivity reactions (Austen et al., 1976). These mediators (see Chapter 11) include histamine, slow-reacting substance of anaphylaxis (SRS-A), eosinophil chemotactic factor of anaphylaxis (ECF-A), basophil kallikrein of anaphylaxis (BK-A), platelet activating factor (PAF), neutrophil chemotactic factor (NCF), and heparin. These substances, depending upon the extent and sites of their release, may produce a wide variety of allergic reactions clinically and experimentally. They include active and passive systemic anaphylaxis, active and passive local anaphylaxis (as in the direct immediate skin test, the Prausnitz-Küstner reaction, or homologous PCA reactions), asthma, allergic rhinitis, urticaria, and angioedema.

The events that initiate generation and/or release of these chemical mediators most likely take place on and in the basophil and mast cell membranes. In the usual situation in which IgE antibodies are involved, bridging of two membrane-attached antibody molecules appears to be required in order to initiate the series of biochemical events that leads to basophil or mast cell degranulation and mediator release (Ishizaka and Ishizaka, 1975; Austen et al., 1976). Conroy et al. (1977) have reported that the number of IgE molecules bound to the surfaces of blood basophils ranged from 4000 to 100,000 per cell for normal individuals and from 100,000 to 500,000 per cell for allergic individuals. Since these molecules most likely have many diverse specificities, the chance is remote that two IgE molecules having the same antigen specificity would occupy adjacent Fc receptors on the cell membrane. It is known, however, that minute amounts of allergen (10^{-8} to 10^{-10}M) can trigger leukocyte histamine release or induce wheal and flare skin reactions in sensitive individuals. These considerations are difficult to reconcile with the bridging hypothesis, unless one assumes that IgE molecules bound to cell surface Fc receptors are constantly moving and that antigen may bind to one IgE antibody and be carried with it by normal receptor movement until another IgE molecule with the same

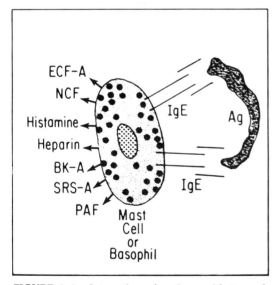

FIGURE 9-2. Interaction of antigen with two adjacent IgE molecules attached to Fc receptors on a basophil or mast cell, resulting in the release (or generation and release) of seven known primary mediators of IgE-mediated hypersensitivity reactions. Degranulation occurs concomitantly. ECF-A = eosinophilic chemotactic factor of anaphylaxis; NCF = neutrophil chemotactic factor; BK-A = basophil kallikrein of anaphylaxis; SRS-A = slow-reacting substance of anaphylaxis; PAF = platelet activating factor.

antigen specificity is encountered, at which time the bridging would occur. The mechanism whereby bridging triggers basophils and mast cells to release mediators is as yet unknown, but the step is known to be energy- and calcium-dependent and to be modulated by the intracellular concentrations of cyclic nucleotides (Austen et al., 1976). It has been postulated that a membrane-associated enzyme, possibly a serine esterase, is activated either by the local disturbance of membrane structure or by receptor interaction that occurs as a result of bridging of the two IgE molecules. Alternately, it is conceivable that bridged immunoglobulin molecules may have enough (hypothetical) binding sites collectively for such an enzyme that they could induce its activation. Further study is needed to clarify the local events that trigger mediator release.

Possible Beneficial Roles. Augmented IgE biosynthesis is associated with the atopic diseases; certain bacterial, fungal, and parasitic diseases; and a number of the primary immunodeficiency diseases (see Buckley and Becker, 1978). Studies in rats experimentally infested with *Nippostrongylus braziliensis* or *Schistosoma mansoni* have implicated important roles for IgE antibodies in host defense against these parasites. It is well known that IgE antibody-antigen reactions result in the influx of eosinophils into the local site. Recently, Butterworth et al. (1977) demonstrated antibody-dependent eosinophil cytotoxicity against ^{51}Cr-labeled schistosomula that appears to be mediated by IgG antibody and is inhibited by antigen-antibody complexes. In addition, there is evidence that IgE antibodies can interact with membrane receptors on macrophages to increase the binding of these cells to *Schistosoma mansoni* schistosomula and enhance the lethal effect of IgG antibody-dependent macrophage-mediated cytotoxicity (Capron et al., 1977). The predominant production of both IgA and IgE immunoglobulins by plasma cells in lymphoid tissues adjacent to mucosal surfaces suggests that, if IgE antibodies do have a protective role, it would be as a mediator of local immunity (Bloch, 1976). Although there is no firm evidence for either a local protective action of IgE antibodies or for a collaborative interaction between

IgA and IgE antibodies in man, it does not seem likely that IgE would have survived in evolution on the basis of its harmful properties from a teleological standpoint. In addition to the above roles, it also has been postulated that vasoactive substances released following the interaction of antigen with mast cell or basophil-fixed IgE antibodies may alter vascular permeability so as to facilitate the passage of other components of the immune system into sites where they are needed.

IgG SKIN-SENSITIZING ANTIBODIES

Although IgG skin-sensitizing antibodies exist in several lower species including guinea pigs, mice, and rats (Bloch and Ohman, 1971), such antibodies have been difficult to demonstrate in man. Several early reports described reaginic activity in apparently pure IgG fractions. Such reports were received with skepticism, however, and the skin-sensitizing activity in these fractions was attributed to contamination by small amounts of IgE. However, recent investigations in two laboratories provide convincing evidence for the existence of IgG homocytotropic antibodies in man (Parish, 1973; Bryant et al., 1975). It is not likely that such antibodies constitute a frequent clinical problem, however, since this type of skin-sensitizing activity could not be found in any of the sera obtained from 149 patients highly sensitive to a variety of allergens (Nelson and Branch, 1977). All such sera did contain IgE antibody to appropriate antigens.

Physicochemical Characteristics of IgG. Little is known about the physicochemical characteristics of human IgG skin-sensitizing antibodies except those characteristics generally known for IgG antibodies in general. All IgG homocytotropic antibodies identified in all species had molecular weights of approximately 150,000 daltons and sedimentation coefficients of 6.5 S, both of which are lower than the values for IgE (see Table 9–2). Like IgE, IgG antibodies are four-chain monomers, with both inter- and intrachain disulfide bonds. The IgG skin-sensitizing antibodies of several lower species have been characterized: in the guinea pig they have been found in the IgG1a and 1b classes; in the mouse they are IgG1; and in the rat they are IgGa (Bloch and Ohman, 1971). Parish (1973) coined the term "short-term sensitizing" antibody, or IgG S-T S, for human IgG skin-sensitizing antibodies. There has been considerable interest in the possibility that human IgG skin-sensitizing antibodies might belong to a particular IgG subclass. Vijay and Perelmutter (1977) found that IgG4 (but no other IgG subclass) myeloma protein was capable of blocking passive sensitization of monkey skin and human basophils by IgE antibody, evidence which strongly supports such a hypothesis. Moreover, anti-IgG4 antiserum caused histamine release from human basophils sensitized by IgG4.

Biologic Properties of IgG. In order for IgG antibodies to function as skin-sensitizing antibodies, they must have the capacity to bind to basophils and mast cells. Direct evidence that some IgG molecules possess this property derives from autoradiographic studies of basophils and from the demonstration of histamine release upon treatment with anti-IgG (see Ishizaka and Ishizaka, 1975) or anti-IgG4 (Vijay and Perelmutter, 1977). As noted earlier, the equilibrium constant for the binding affinity of IgG to neutrophils and monocytes has been estimated at 10^{-5}/M. Since so few IgG molecules have the capacity to bind to basophils and mast cells, its binding affinity for these cell types has not been determined. Nevertheless, it is likely that the affinity is far lower than that of IgE antibodies, since studies following the disappearance rate of radiolabeled IgG injected into human skin have estimated a half-life of only 2 days, in contrast to the much longer tissue half-life of IgE (reviewed by Ishizaka and Ishizaka, 1975). The optimal sensitization (or latent) period for all IgG homocytotropic antibodies studied thus far has been much shorter than that for IgE, with the times ranging from 1 to 2 hours in the mouse, up to 4 to 6 hours for man (see Table 9–2) (Bloch and Ohman, 1971; Parish, 1973).

Other biologic properties that distinguish IgG skin-sensitizing antibodies from those of the IgE class include the failure of reduction-alkylation or heating at 56°C for 2 to 4 hours to effect the binding of IgG homocytotropic antibodies to basophils and mast cells in all species except the guinea pig (see Table 9–2) (Bloch and Ohman, 1971).

Parish (1973) used these observations to establish the IgG nature of skin-sensitizing antibodies present in sera from persons who had immediate wheal and flare skin reactions to milk proteins or to bacterial antigens but who did not have demonstrable IgE antibodies to these antigens. The skin-sensitizing activity was demonstrated by passive sensitization of monkey skin with both heated (56°C for up to 6 hours) and unheated serum, injecting the sera 24, 4, and 1.5 hours prior to antigen challenge. Sera from these patients showed greater reactions at the sites sensitized for only 1.5 hours than at sites sensitized for 4 hours and none at those injected 24 hours earlier. Moreover, there was no difference between the sites injected with heated and unheated sera or by sera reduced with 2-mercaptoethanol.

Parish (1973) also reported that many of the sera with S-T S antibody contained precipitins. Reactions observed at 1.5 to 2.5 hours appeared to be distinguishable from Arthus reactions by virtue of the fact that no latent period is required for passive Arthus reactions. Moreover, S-T S activity was demonstrable in monkeys depleted of neutrophils and in those with greatly reduced levels of serum complement, both of which are needed for Arthus reactions.

The antigens to which IgG homocytotropic antibodies are directed appear to be more restricted than those which induce IgE antibody responses, since there have been few documented examples of IgG S-T S antibodies against pollen allergens. Parish (1973) found IgG homocytotropic antibodies in sera from patients with serum sickness from horse globulin, from those with severe local reactions to tetanus toxoid, from some with cutaneous vasculitis due to streptococcal infection, and from some patients with pulmonary disorders. Finally, Bryant et al. (1975) found serum IgG skin-sensitizing antibodies that were not removed by anti-IgE antibodies nor inactivated by heating or reduction-alkylation in asthmatic patients with positive bronchial provocation tests to antigens from the house dust mite, *Dermatophagoides pteronyssinus*.

METHODS OF MEASURING SKIN-SENSITIZING ANTIBODIES

Skin-sensitizing antibodies may be detected by immediate skin testing procedures which involve mediator release *in vivo*, *in vitro* histamine release from peripheral leukocytes, and radioimmunoassays. Details of skin testing and indications for the various tests are given in Chapter 21; only general principles are described here.

Immediate Skin Testing

Direct Testing. This test for skin-sensitizing antibodies is both the oldest and the most sensitive technique available (Stanworth, 1963; Ishizaka and Ishizaka, 1975). Allergen injected into the epidermis or placed on the abraded skin of an allergic patient interacts with IgE molecules attached to skin mast cells and induces release of histamine (see Fig. 9–2), which causes a wheal and flare reaction within 5 to 15 minutes. This test detects skin-sensitizing antibodies on tissue mast cells that may be relevant to the patient's allergy. The major limitation of this test is that it provides only a rough estimate of the amount of the particular IgE antibody detected, for two reasons: (1) it is not a primary binding assay; therefore, results are dependent on releasability of mediators from recipient mast cells and (2) the amount of IgE detected is quantifiable only in terms of the least amount of antigen required to elicit a wheal and flare reaction.

Passive Transfer Tests. Most commonly these studies have been done by injecting a 1:10 or higher dilution of serum from an allergic individual into the skin of a nonsensitized human, as described originally by Prausnitz and Küstner in 1921 (Stanworth, 1963). This procedure thus is usually referred to as the "P-K test." After allowing time for donor IgE to bind optimally to the recipient's skin mast cells (usually 24 hours), antigen is injected into the site sensitized earlier by serum, as well as into an unsensitized site as a control. Buffer alone is injected into another sensitized site as an additional control. A wheal and flare reaction developing within 5 to 15 minutes at

only the antigen-injected sensitized site indicates that IgE antibodies to that antigen were present in the donor serum. The test can be used to quantify the amount of IgE antibodies to that antigen by sensitizing with serial dilutions of donor serum. Although the procedure does detect mast cell–fixed IgE, it is not as sensitive as direct skin testing. It also is unlikely that the distribution or relative density of the IgE molecules in question is the same on the recipient's mast cells as on the donor's, since the recipient's own IgE molecules occupy many of the receptor sites. In the past this procedure was used frequently to test for IgE antibodies in sera from patients with generalized dermatitis, dermatographia, or histories of anaphylactic reactions to drugs or insect stings. Since the procedure carries the risk of transmitting hepatitis virus, it is now used primarily as an investigative tool and has been essentially replaced, for clinical purposes, by the radioimmunoassays described subsequently.

Nonhuman primates also can be used as recipients of IgE passive transfer tests (Buckley and Metzgar, 1965). Skin sensitization of anesthetized monkeys is done in exactly the same manner as for the P-K test, and a similar latent period of 24 to 48 hours is allowed to elapse before antigen challenge is given. The procedure differs from the P-K test in the latter aspect, however, in that antigen is usually given intravenously, along with a colloidal blue dye. When antigen reacts with IgE molecules on mast cells at the previously sensitized skin site, mediators are released, resulting in increased vascular permeability, and bluing occurs at the sites due to leakage of dye from the intravascular space (Fig. 9–3). This procedure is called *passive cutaneous anaphylaxis* (PCA), since a local anaphylactic reaction occurs at the passively sensitized skin site. In principle, it measures the same reaction as the P-K test. The P-K assay, however, is at least 100-fold more sensitive than the monkey PCA procedure in detecting and quantifying IgE antibodies in donor serum (Ishizaka and Ishizaka, 1975). The PCA procedure is an investigative tool primarily and has been the principal assay used for detecting IgG short term skin-sensitizing (S-T S) antibodies.

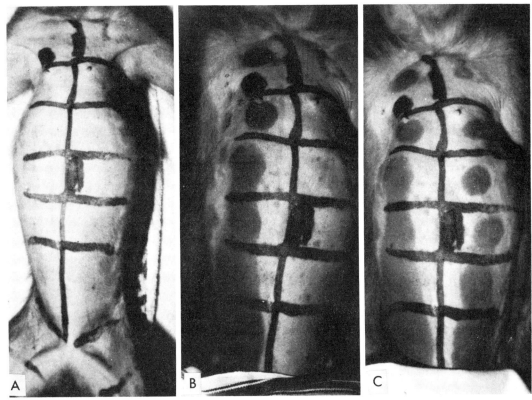

FIGURE 9–3. Monkey PCA. *A*, Anesthetized monkey 48 hours following passive sensitization of abdominal skin sites with dilutions of sera from a ragweed-sensitive donor (left half) and from a grass-sensitive donor (right half). *B*, Five minutes after intravenous injection of crude ragweed extract and Evans' blue dye. Positive reactions occur only at sites sensitized with serum from the ragweed-sensitive donor. *C*, Same monkey as in *A* and *B*, approximately 5 minutes after challenge with crude grass extract and saline. Sites sensitized with serum from grass sensitive donor are now positive. (From Buckley and Metzgar, J. Allergy Clin. Immunol. *36*:382, 1965; used with permission.)

Mediator Release Procedures

Leukocyte Mediator Release. This assay detects IgE antibodies on peripheral blood basophils of allergic subjects by quantifying the amount of one or more of the primary chemical mediators released as a consequence of antigen and basophil-fixed IgE antibody interaction. It also can be used to detect IgE antibodies in the sera of allergic donors by preincubating those sera with basophils from nonsensitized subjects. The test is performed by separating leukocytes from heparinized blood by dextran sedimentation and suspending them in a buffer containing Ca^{++} and Mg^{++}. Varying quantities of allergen are added to tubes containing fixed numbers of cells, and the tubes are incubated at 37°C for 1 hour. The mediators released into the supernatants can be quantified by a variety of methods,

including a bioassay for SRS-A that measures the contraction of guinea pig ileum in the presence of atropine and antihistamines; a secondary mediator release assay for PAF which measures ^3H serotonin released from radiolabeled platelets; a chemotaxis assay for ECF-A; and either a spectrofluorometric or a radioenzyme assay for histamine (Austen et al., 1976). The assay also can be used to detect serum blocking antibodies by adding heat-inactivated test sera to a parallel set of tubes. In most studies designed to detect IgE, only histamine has been measured because the other assays are more difficult to perform. The quantity of histamine released per tube is expressed as a percentage of the total histamine available in the cells and as a function of the dose of allergen added. The amount of allergen needed to cause 50 percent histamine release is usually between

10^{-4} and 10^{-6} μg/ml (King, 1976). The same limitations apply to this method that apply to skin testing: (1) it does not measure primary binding of antigen to antibody, (2) the results in the direct assay are dependent upon the releasability of the chemical mediators from the subject's basophils, and (3) the amount of IgE detected in the direct assay is quantifiable only in terms of the least amount of antigen needed for 50 per histamine (or other mediator) release. Some quantification of serum IgE antibody titers can, however, be achieved by diluting a test serum serially prior to incubation with nonsensitized basophils. Results of leukocyte histamine release assays generally have correlated with results of skin tests, although the latter tests are more sensitive. Because of the technical difficulty in performing mediator release tests, they are used primarily for investigational purposes. They have been particularly well suited for this, since they provide more quantifiable data than does skin testing. This type of assay also can be used to quantify IgG-blocking antibody titers in patients undergoing immunotherapy. It may also be used to identify loss of cell sensitivity during immunotherapy and to study pharmacologic modulation of mediator release (Austen et al., 1976).

Mediator Release from Tissues. The same methods for detecting mediator release may be employed to determine mast cell–fixed IgE present in small tissue fragments. Tests have been performed with chopped human or monkey lung, with skin slices, and with nasal polyps (Austen et al., 1976). These procedures, which are used strictly as investigational tools, have the same limitations as basophil assays.

Radioimmunoassays

Radioimmunoassays have advantages over skin tests or mediator release tests in that they are performed *in vitro* and do not require either sensitized cells or tissues. They measure binding of antigen and IgE antibody directly rather than indirectly through mediator release. In general, however, these tests are less sensitive than are skin tests. The types of radioimmunoassays employed in IgE measurements can be divided into those that involve competitive binding and those that employ noncompetitive binding (Wide, 1971).

Competitive Binding Assays. In these assays, antibody to IgE is allowed to react with radiolabeled purified IgE protein in antigen excess (Wide, 1971). Known quantities of unlabeled IgE or unknown quantities in test samples are added to the mixtures; these molecules displace radiolabeled IgE from its binding with antibody so that less labeled IgE is bound. In solid phase assays, which employ either Sephadex beads, microcrystalline cellulose, or filter paper discs, antibody-bound IgE is separated from nonbound IgE by washing the solid phase material to remove nonspecifically bound IgE. In double antibody radioimmunoassays, anti-IgE in solution reacts with radiolabeled and unlabeled IgE in the same manner as for the solid phase assay (Fig. 9–4). By employing a second antibody directed against the anti-IgE antibody, bound IgE is precipitated from solution and is removed by centrifugation. The quantity of bound IgE from unknown samples is determined by reading from a calibration curve established by plotting known concentrations of unlabeled IgE added against the percentage of counts per minute detected in the solid phase material or precipitate as compared to the counts per minute in tubes containing no unlabeled IgE. The two best known versions of this test are the radioimmunosorbent test, or RIST (Wide, 1971), and the double antibody radioimmunoassay (Gleich et al, 1971), both of which have been used to measure IgE concentrations in serum and body fluids. The RIST assay does not measure IgE concentrations reliably below 20 I.U./ml* however, and gives falsely high values for IgE in secretions. (An improved version of this test, the paper RIST, is described in the following section.) The double antibody assay does not have these limitations. Neither assay permits measurement of specific IgE *antibodies*.

Noncompetitive Binding Assays. In these procedures, either antigen or anti-IgE antibody is covalently coupled to a solid material. Antigen is allowed to interact with antibodies to it or anti-IgE is permitted to react with known or unknown quantities of

---

*I.U. = International Unit. One International Unit is equivalent to 2.4 ng (reviewed in Orgel, 1975).

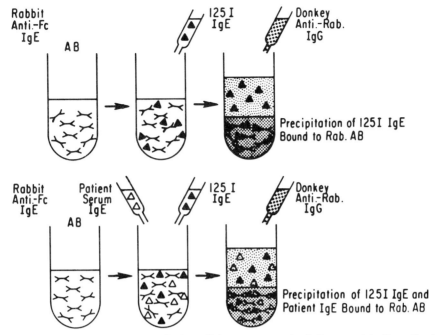

FIGURE 9–4. Principle of the double antibody radioimmunoassay for IgE, as used in the author's laboratory (Buckley and Fiscus, J. Clin. Invest., 55:157, 1975). This is one type of competitive binding assay. The more IgE in the test sample, the fewer counts detected in the precipitate.

IgE (Wide, 1971). Either cellulose or other types of particles (Fig. 9–5), filter paper discs (Fig. 9–6), or plastic tubes or dishes may be used as the solid phase material. After incubation, the solid phase material is washed, and radiolabeled, immunospecifically purified anti-IgE antibody is added. After a second wash, the solid phase material is analyzed for its radioactivity. If antigen is used for coupling, the more antigen-specific IgE antibody present in the standard or test sample, the greater the radioactivity finally associated with the solid material. A version of this test is widely known as the radioallergosorbent test, or RAST (Figs. 9–5 and 9–6). RAST results are usually expressed in terms of percent of total counts of radiolabeled anti-IgE antibody added bound, or in units of an arbitrary scoring system based on the counts per minute bound by a known high-titered positive serum. This assay is useful in detecting and semi-quantifying IgE antibodies to various allergens and for measuring the potency of various allergenic extracts. Allergen potency can be measured by varying the amount of standard and test allergen extracts coupled to the solid phase material (referred to as the direct RAST) or by measuring the degree that the allergen inhibits the binding

of IgE antibodies in a known allergic serum to solid-phase antigen (RAST inhibition).

In the situation where anti-IgE is coupled to the solid phase, the more IgE present in the standard or test sample, the greater the radioactivity ultimately associated with the solid phase. A standard curve can be constructed by plotting the counts bound against known quantities of IgE added. This method forms the basis for the well-known paper disc radioimmunosorbent test (PRIST), a sensitive, accurate, and easily performed method for measuring total IgE in serum or other body fluids.

Enzyme-linked Immunoassays (ELISA)

These assays are similar in principle and application to radioimmunoassays except that the anti-IgE antibody used in the final phase is coupled to an enzyme rather than being radiolabeled (Weltman, et al., 1976). The amount of enzyme-linked anti-IgE antibody reacting with the solid phase material is detected and quantified by measuring the intensity of color that results from adding the enzyme's substrate. Though this technique is still in the development stage, it will have

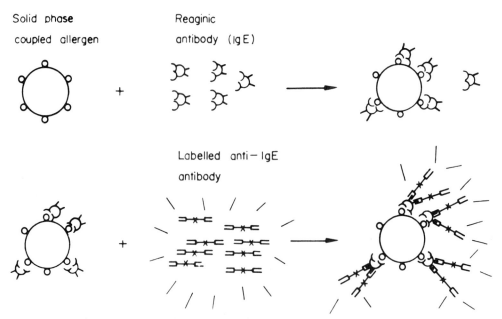

FIGURE 9–5. Principle of the radioallergosorbent test (RAST) for detecting and quantifying IgE antibodies to allergens. In this example of a noncompetitive binding assay, the solid phase material is a cellulose particle. (From Wide, in Kirkham and Hunter, Radioimmunoassay methods. Edinburgh, Churchill Livingstone, 1971, used with permission.)

obvious advantages over radioimmunoassays: it will be far safer because it does not involve radioactivity, and it does not require an expensive gamma counter.

ONTOGENY OF IgE BIOSYNTHESIS

Fetal IgE Synthesis.   Miller et al. (1973) demonstrated that the human fetus is capable

of synthesizing IgE as early as 11 weeks *in utero*. Synthesis of IgE may occur by 11 weeks in fetal lung and liver and by 21 weeks in fetal spleen. Even though the capacity for IgE synthesis develops very early, the fetal synthesizing rate is low in most instances, as evidenced by low cord serum IgE concentrations (mean = 2 I.U. per ml) and the fact that injection of anti-IgE antibody into the skin of neonates does not cause an immediate

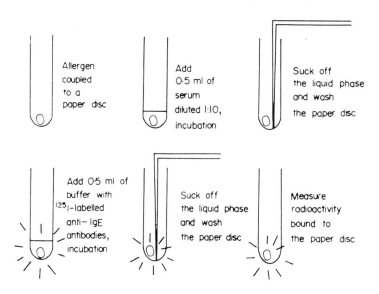

FIGURE 9–6. The RAST assay using a filter paper disc as the solid phase material. If anti-IgE had been coupled to the disc instead of allergen, the schematic would illustrate the paper radioimmunosorbent, or PRIST, test for total IgE.

wheal and flare reaction. The latter is not due to a paucity of skin mast cells, however, since both premature and full-term newborns have been shown to be capable of developing wheal and flare reactions when they served as recipients in P-K tests (Orgel, 1975). The low rate of IgE synthesis in fetal and neonatal life correlates well with the known freedom of infants from IgE-mediated diseases up to 2 to 3 months of age.

IgE in Normal Infants and Children. In 114 apparently nonallergic, healthy infants, the serum IgE concentration 2 S.D. above the geometric mean was 1.5 I.U./ml at birth but increased to 20 I.U. by 1 year of age (Kjellman, 1976). In 93 nonallergic children it was 40 I.U. at age 2 and peaked at 140 I.U. at age 10 years, gradually declining thereafter. IgE concentrations reported in this study were lower overall than those in a study by Gerrard et al. (1974), possibly because the patients in the latter study were unselected and because Kjellman employed the noncompetitive binding PRIST assay, which generally gives lower IgE values. Nevertheless, a similar trend was seen in both studies. Geometric mean serum IgE concentrations reached adult levels by 4 years of age and then increased gradually until a maximum level was reached between 10 and 12 years of age. They then dropped sharply, to reach adult levels again by age 14 (Fig. 9–7). Adult normal values have varied widely between laboratories because of different methods, standards, nomenclature, sample sizes, and statistical analyses employed in deriving the normative data. Published mean IgE values for normal adults have ranged from 15 to

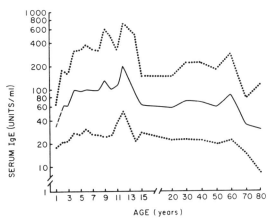

FIGURE 9–7. Serum IgE concentrations in members of 80 families. The solid line represents the geometric mean and the dotted line the anti-log of the mean log ± 1 S.D. of the $\log_{10}$ of the data. (From Gerrard et al., J. Pediatr. 85:660, 1974, as modified by Orgel, Pediatr. Clin. North Am. 22:17, 1975; used with permission.)

100 I.U./ml. In the author's laboratory, in which a double antibody radioimmunoassay is employed (Gleich et al., 1971), the normal geometric mean is 55 I.U./ml and the 95 percent confidence interval is 5–621 I.U./ml.

IgE and IgA in Atopic Infants and Children. In 34 infants whose IgE was followed serially throughout the first year of life, every child who developed a serum IgE concentration greater than 20 I.U./ml by 1 year of age had evidence of atopic disease by 2 years of age (Table 9–4) (Orgel, 1975). An initial IgE 1 S.D. above the mean in the first year of life in 114 infants appeared predictive of allergy in that 75 percent of those with elevated IgE had developed atopic or probably atop-

TABLE 9–4 CORRELATION BETWEEN SERUM IgE LEVEL AT 1 YEAR OF AGE AND SYMPTOMS AND SIGNS OF ATOPIC DISEASE MANIFESTED BY 2 YEARS OF AGE

Serum IgE I.U./ml by 1 Year of Age	n	Symptoms or Signs of Atopic Disease by 2 Years of Age		
		DEFINITE	POSSIBLE	DEFINITE AND POSSIBLE
<10	17	2 (12%)	4	6 (35%)
10 to 20	5	1 (20%)	1	2 (40%)
20.1 to 100	6	5 (83%)	1	6 (100%)
>100	6	3 (50%)	3	6 (100%)
Total	34	11	9	20

(From Orgel, H. A.: Genetic and developmental aspects of IgE. Pediatr. Clin. North Am., 22:17–32, 1975. Used with permission.)

ic disease 18 months later, as compared to only 6.4 percent of those with normal serum IgE levels (Kjellman, 1976). A similar trend occurred in 93 children from 2 to 14 years of age, in whom 41.7 percent of those with elevated IgE values (>1 S.D. above mean) had obvious or probable atopy 18 months later, compared to only 5 percent of those with normal initial IgE values. Thus, serum IgE concentrations appear useful in predicting future atopy in infants and may be especially useful in evaluating the likelihood of atopy in offspring of atopic parents.

Some investigators have reported transient or persistent (non-statistically significant) deficiencies of serum IgA in infants who later develop allergic symptoms (Taylor et al., 1973). Since both IgA and IgE are produced predominantly in paragut and pararespiratory lymphoid tissues (Ishizaka and Ishizaka, 1975; Bloch, 1976) these authors have suggested that IgA deficiency may contribute to increased mucous membrane permeability to antigens, leading to stimulation of increased IgE production and consequently a greater likelihood of developing the atopic state. Recent evidence by Platts-Mills et al. (1976), however, suggests that the opposite is true; that is, individuals predisposed to make increased IgE antibodies have a normal or even increased ability to produce allergen-specific IgA antibodies.

GENETIC CONTROL OF IgE BIOSYNTHESIS

Since the diseases with which increased IgE production are associated have long been recognized for their heritable nature, there is reason to believe that genetic factors regulate IgE biosynthesis. As with the mode of inheritance of the atopic diseases, however, studies done in animals and man to date indicate that control of IgE biosynthesis appears to be multifactorial, with at least two genetic loci implicated (Levine, 1974; Orgel, 1975; Tada, 1975; Watanabe et al., 1976). One of these controls the level of IgE antibody production and appears to be unassociated with the major histocompatibility complex (MHC) (Levine, 1974; Watanabe, 1976). The other controls immune recognition of allergens and may be linked to the MHC (Levine, 1974).

Genetic Influence on Overall Level of IgE Production

IgE Production in Mice. When various mouse strains were immunized with multiple antigens, all were found to produce IgE antibodies to one or more antigens, but only certain strains exhibited high or moderate reaginic antibody responses (Levine, 1974). The differences noted in these studies pertained only to the IgE response, regardless of the antigen or dose administered. Breeding experiments demonstrated that the genetic control for high or low IgE response in these strains was not linked to the MHC. Recent studies by Watanabe et al. (1976) and Chiorazzi et al. (1977) in IgE "non-responder" mice of the SJL strain and "low responder" AKR strain have shown that such animals can be converted to IGE "responders" by elimination of suppressor T cell activity through irradiation or the use of cyclophosphamide. The augmented IgE production in such mice in turn could be terminated by transferring syngeneic normal thymocytes or spleen cells (Watanabe et al., 1976; Chiorazzi et al., 1977). These findings were interpreted as demonstrating that poor IgE antibody formation in untreated SJL and AKR strain mice is not based on a genetic inability to develop IgE responses but rather is a manifestation of a genetic capability to actively inhibit IgE antibody synthesis. It is possible, therefore, that high IgE "responder" mice and humans who manufacture large amounts of IgE antibodies represent states of a genetically controlled insufficiency of suppressor T cells, the activity of which is directed towards IgE-producing B cells.

Human IgE Production. In several studies of serum IgE concentrations in unselected populations of adults, the distribution of values appears to be multimodal. The explanation for this is not clear, but the multimodality likely is due to a combination of genetic and environmental influences. Twin studies (Orgel, 1975) provide strong evidence for an appreciable genetic effect on basal serum IgE concentrations. The effect appears greater in monozygous twin children than in monozygous twin adults. Those studies also demonstrated that nongenetic factors also may contribute to variability in IgE levels, making it more difficult to analyze the genetic mechanisms. Three separate population studies suggest that serum levels of IgE in man are controlled by two alleles at a single locus (reviewed by Gerrard et al., 1978). Marsh et al. (1974) hypothesized from their data that high levels of IgE are inherited as a recessive trait. Gerrard et al. (1978) present evidence for a single major regulatory locus for serum IgE concentrations, the locus having two alleles, a dominant allele designated "RE" and a recessive allele, "re." Persons who are re/re homozygotes maintain persistently high levels of IgE, whereas heterozygotes or RE/RE homozygotes have normal or low levels. The gene frequency of re was found to be 0.489 by Gerrard et al. (1978), and the displacement was 1.67 S.D. Whether this locus is analogous to that described above for mice, determining "high" and "low" IgE responder types, and whether the genetic control is by suppressor T cells remain to be demonstrated.

Immune Response (Ir) Genes That Control IgE Antibody Synthesis

Ir Genes in Mice. It is well established that genes controlling immune responsiveness to synthetic branched polypeptides in mice are linked to the H-2 complex (reviewed in Orgel, 1975). In studies designed to investigate whether reaginic antibody responses are regulated by genes within the MHC, Levine and Vaz (reviewed in Levine, 1974) found clear-cut differences among inbred mouse strains in reaginic antibody responsiveness to repeated minute (0.1 μg) doses of benzylpenicilloyl-bovine γ globulin. This difference in responsiveness correlated with the H-2 genotype of the strain. It should be noted, however, that the differences among strains were demonstrable only with repeated low-dose immunization. In addition, the differences extended to general immune responsiveness to the particular antigen, rather being unique to reagin production, in contrast to the strain differences in overall IgE responsiveness discussed before.

Ir Genes in Man. A number of studies have addressed the question of whether genes analogous to the Ir genes in mice exist for man (Levine, 1974; Orgel, 1975). Levine (1974) and his coworkers examined seven families with a high familial incidence of ragweed hay fever and showed that the occurrence of hay fever and intense immediate skin sensitivity to ragweed antigen E were highly correlated with a particular HLA haplotype in successive generations of allergic families. The associated haplotype varied from family to family, however, and was different for each of the seven families studied. Studies of IgE antibodies to antigen E revealed that the presence of these antibodies also correlated with the hay fever–IgE antibody–associated haplotype. Since some family members with the haplotype in question failed to manifest either hay fever or skin reactivity to ragweed antigen E, whereas none of those lacking the haplotype had hay fever or antigen E reactivity, Levine and his associates concluded that the presence of an Ir gene linked to a particular HLA A and B locus haplotype within a family is necessary but not sufficient for the development of an intense IgE immune response to antigen E and clinical hay fever (Levine, 1974). Similar findings were reported by Blumenthal et al. (reviewed by Orgel, 1975), who studied a very large family through three generations and found that sensitivity to ragweed antigen E was associated with the HLA A2, B 12 haplotype. In contrast to these studies, Marsh et al. (1974) were unable to confirm a within-family haplotype association for ragweed hay fever and skin sensitivity to antigen E. However, in populations of unrelated, highly allergic individuals, Marsh and his coworkers did report a significant correlation between skin sensitivity to the ragweed antigen RA5 and the presence of the HLA B7 cross-reacting group of antigens. As in the studies of Levine (1974), the presence of IgG antibodies to Ra5 was found only in those able to produce IgE antibodies to RA5.

It can be seen from these studies that the evidence for Ir genes controlling IgE antibody responses in man is, though highly suggestive, still controversial. Finally, it seems probable that multiple other genetic factors interact to influence the expression of IgE-mediated disease in a given individual (Levine, 1974; Orgel, 1975).

T CELL REGULATION OF IgE BIOSYNTHESIS

Rodent Studies

Until recently, little was known of immunoregulatory mechanisms controlling IgE antibody formation. Important observations bearing on this were made by Tada and his associates in 1971 when they demonstrated enhancement of ongoing IgE antibody production in the rat by treating the animals with small doses of antithymocyte serum, whole body irradiation, and adult thymectomy and splenectomy, or by administering various immunosuppressive drugs before or shortly after immunization (Tada, 1975). Further studies revealed that administration of carrier-specific T lymphocytes inhibited ongoing hapten-specific homocytotropic antibody formation. The augmentation of ongoing homocytotropic antibody production by immunosuppressive manipulations was surprising and paradoxical, since these workers had shown earlier that priming of carrier-specific T helper cells was necessary for production of homocytotropic antibody by hapten-specific antibody-forming B cells. IgE synthesis thus appears to require T helper cells for initiation, while also under active T suppressor cell control. Since those initial studies, the mechanism(s) of T cell regulation of IgE formation has been investigated extensively by various investigators (reviewed by Tada, 1975; and Ishizaka, 1976). Information as to how thymocytes could be both inhibitory and facilitating has come from further work by Tada and his coworkers (reviewed by Tada, 1975), who found an antigen-specific T cell factor derived from mechanically disrupted rat thymocytes that had a negative regulatory effect on IgE antibody synthesis. This factor was characterized as a nonimmunoglobulin protein that eluted in gel exclusion chromatography in fractions ranging from 35,000 to 60,000 daltons and that migrated in the alpha and beta globulin regions on electrophoresis. Recent evidence obtained by Tada (1975) indicates that the action of the antigen-specific inhibitory factor from T cells is on T helper cells, suppressing their function, rather than on B cells. Soluble enhancing factors have been isolated from both rat and rabbit T lymphocytes and characterized as proteins with molecular weight between 100,000 and 200,000 daltons (reviewed by Tada, 1975; and Ishizaka, 1976). Finally, it appears likely that IgE synthesis may be regulated by non–antigen-specific T suppressor cells as well (Tada, 1975).

Immunodeficiency Disorders Characterized by Excessive IgE Production

Patients with partial deficiencies in their thymic-dependent systems could have sufficient numbers of T helper cells for initiation of IgE antibody formation but an inadequate number of T suppressor cells, resulting in augmented IgE biosynthesis. The most convincing evidence to date suggesting an association between impaired thymus-dependent immunity and excessive IgE production in man derives primarily from associations found in patients with certain types of immunodeficiency diseases (Buckley and Fiscus, 1975).

The regular association of increased IgE biosynthesis with a particular immunodeficiency disorder was first noted in patients with the Wiskott-Aldrich syndrome (reviewed in Buckley and Becker, 1978). Later, the author and her associates (Buckley et al., 1972) described two adolescent boys with lifelong histories of severe recurrent staphylococcal abscesses involving the skin, lungs, and joints, who had exceptionally high serum IgE concentrations but normal concentrations of other immunoglobulins. In 1972, Polmar et al. reported that an infant with DiGeorge's syndrome consistently had an elevated serum IgE concentration, and in 1973 Kikkawa et al. first described a high serum IgE concentration in an infant with a variant of thymic alymphoplasia (the so-called Nezelof syndrome) (reviewed in Buckley and Becker, 1978). In other studies in the author's laboratory (Buckley and Fiscus, 1975), concentrations of IgE were measured in sera from 165 patients with a variety of well-defined primary immunodeficiency disorders. IgE concentrations were significantly lower than normal in patients who had marked deficiencies in all three major immunoglobulin classes, such as those with transient hypogammaglobulinemia of infancy, severe combined immunodeficiency disease, and x-linked and non-x-linked agammaglobulinemia. In addition, IgE concentrations were depressed in patients with x-linked immunodeficiency with hyper IgM and in those with ataxia telangiectasia. In contrast, IgE values were significantly elevated in patients with the Wiskott-Aldrich syndrome, with the Nezelof syndrome, with selective IgA deficiency, and with hyper-IgE syndrome. Except for the patients with selective IgA deficiency, all immunodeficiency patients with excessive IgE production in this and other reports have had impaired but not absent cell-mediated immunity (reviewed in Buckley and Becker, 1978).

In Vitro Studies of Human IgE Biosynthesis

Study of IgE biosynthesis *in vitro* has been difficult owing to the extremely small quantities made even in laboratory animals with augmented IgE synthesis or in human disease states characterized by greater than normal production. Some success has been gained recently by using cultured human mononuclear cells and a double antibody radioimmunoassay to measure IgE synthesized and secreted into the supernatant fluid (Buckley and Becker, 1978). These studies demonstrated that IgE can be detected in the supernatants of cells cultured for from 4 to 7 days. IgE synthesis by peripheral blood mononuclear cells from 10 normal controls

was slightly augmented by the addition of pokeweed mitogen. In contrast, synthesis was greatest in unstimulated cultures of peripheral blood mononuclear cells from patients with a variety of disorders characterized by elevated serum IgE. The results suggest that peripheral blood IgE-producing B cells from patients with elevated serum IgE already are maximally stimulated and cannot be further stimulated by the addition of a polyclonal B cell activator. IgE biosynthesis by unstimulated cultured peripheral blood mononuclear cells from patients with a variety of disorders characterized by elevated serum IgE ranged from 5- to 13-fold higher than in unstimulated cultures from normal controls. Co-cultures of patients' mononuclear cells with those of normal controls revealed an average of 87 percent inhibition of IgE biosynthesis from that expected from the individual culture data, indicating the presence of cells in normal mononuclear cell populations that can inhibit IgE biosynthesis by the patients' cells. In contrast, there was no significant inhibition of IgM or IgG synthesis in these same co-cultures, suggesting that the suppression is specific for IgE. These studies are consistent with the hypothesis that patients who have diseases characterized by greater than normal serum IgE concentrations may have a deficiency of suppressor cells that regulate IgE biosynthesis in normal individuals.

References

Austen, K. F., Wasserman, S. I., and Goetzl, E. J.: Mast cell–derived mediators: Structural and functional diversity and regulation of expression. *In* Johansson, S. G. O., Strandberg, K., and Uvnas. B. (eds.): *Molecular and Biological Aspects of the Acute Allergic Reaction.* New York, Plenum Press, 1976, pp. 293–320.

Bennich, H., and Bahr-Lindström, H. V.: Structure of immunoglobulin E (IgE). *In* Brent, L., and Holborow, J. (eds.): *Progress in Immunology II,* Vol. 1. Amsterdam, North-Holland, 1974, pp. 49–58.

Bennich, H., and Johansson, S. G. O.: Structure and function of human immunoglobulin E. Adv. Immunol. *13*:1, 1971.

Bennich, H., Johansson, S. G. O., Bahr-Lindström, H., and Karlsson, T.: Function and structure of immunoglobulin E (IgE). *In* Johannson, S. G. O., Strandberg, K., and Uvnas, B. (eds.): *Molecular and Biological Aspects of the Acute Allergic Reaction.* New York, Plenum Press, 1976, pp. 175–197.

Bloch, K. J.: The special relationship of IgA and IgE antibodies to mucosal surfaces. *In* Bouheys, A. (ed.): *Lung Cells in Disease.* Amsterdam, North-Holland, 1976, pp. 183–196.

Bloch, K. J., and Ohman, J. L.: The stable homocytotropic antibodies of guinea pig, mouse and rat. Some indirect evidence for the *in vitro* interaction of homocytotropic antibodies of two different rat immunoglobulin classes at a common

receptor on target cells. *In* Austen, K. F., and Becker, E. L. (eds.): *Biochemistry of the Acute Allergic Reactions.* Oxford, Blackwell Scientific Publications, Ltd., 1971, pp. 45–64.

Bryant, D. H., Burns, M. W., and Lazarus, L.: Identification of IgG antibody as a carrier of reaginic activity in asthmatic patients. J. Allergy Clin. Immunol. *56*:417, 1975.

Buckley, R. H., and Becker, W. G.: Abnormalities in the regulation of human IgE synthesis. Immunol. Rev. *41*:288, 1978.

Buckley, R. H., and Fiscus, S. A.: Serum IgD and IgE concentrations in immunodeficiency diseases. J. Clin. Invest. *55*:157, 1975.

Buckley, R. H., and Metzgar, R. S.: The use of nonhuman primates for studies of reagin. J. Allergy Clin. Immunol. *36*:382, 1965.

Buckley, R. H., Wray, B. B., and Belmaker, E. Z.: Extreme hyperimmunoglobulinemia E and undue susceptibility to infection. Pediatrics *49*:59, 1972.

Butterworth, A. E., Remold, H. G., Houba, U., David, J. R., Franks, D., David, P. H., and Sturrock, R. F.: Antibody-dependent eosinophil-mediated damage to ^{51}Cr-labelled schistosomula of *Schistosoma mansoni:* Mediation by IgG and inhibition by antigen-antibody complexes. J. Immunol. *118*:2230, 1977.

Capron, A., Dessaint, J. P., Joseph, M., Torpier, G., Capron,

M., Rousseaux, R., Santoro, F., and Bazin, H.: IgE and cells in schistosomiasis. Am. J. Trop. Med. Hyg. 26:39, 1977.

Chiorazzi, N., Fox, D. A., and Katz, D. H.: Hapten-specific IgE antibodies in mice. VII. Conversion of IgE "non-responder" strains to IgE "responders" by elimination of suppressor T cell activity. J. Immunol. 118:48, 1977.

Conroy, M. C., Adkinson, N. F., Jr., and Lichtenstein, L. M.: Measurement of IgE on human basophils: Relation to serum IgE and anti-IgE-induced histamine release. J. Immunol. 118:1317, 1977.

Gerrard, J. W., Horne, S., Vickers, P., Mackenzie, J. W. A., Goluboff, N., Garson, J. Z., and Maningas, C. S.: Serum IgE levels in parents and children. J. Pediatr. 85:660, 1974.

Gerrard, J. W., Rao, D. C., and Morton, N. E.: A genetic study of immunoglobulin E. Am. J. Hum. Genet. 30:46, 1978.

Gleich, G. J., Averbeck, A. K., and Swedlund, H. A.: Measurement of IgE in normal and allergic serum by radioimmunoassay. J. Lab. Clin. Med. 77:690, 1971.

Ishizaka, K.: Cellular events in the IgE antibody response. Adv. Immunol. 23:1, 1976.

Ishizaka, T., and Ishizaka, K.: Biology of immunoglobulin E. Molecular basis of reaginic hypersensitivity. Prog. Allergy 19:60, 1975.

King, T. P.: Chemical and biologic properties of some atopic allergens. Adv. Immunol. 23:77, 1976.

Kjellman, N.-I. M.: Predictive value of high IgE levels in children. Acta Paediatr. Scand. 65:465, 1976.

Levine, B. B.: Genetics of atopic allergy and reagin production. In Brostoff, J. (ed.): Clinical Immunology-Allergy in Paediatric Medicine. Oxford, Blackwell Scientific Publications, Ltd., 1974, pp. 49–68.

Marsh, D. G., Bias, W. B., and Ishizaka, K.: Genetic control of basal serum immunoglobulin E level and its effect on specific reaginic sensitivity. Proc. Natl. Acad. Sci. 71:3588, 1974.

Miller, D. L., Hirvonin, T., and Gitlin, D.: Synthesis of IgE by the human conceptus. J. Allergy Clin. Immunol. 52:182, 1973.

Nelson, H. S., and Branch, L. B.: Incidence of IgG short-term sensitizing antibodies in an allergic population. J. Allergy Clin. Immunol. 60:266, 1977.

Orgel, H. A.: Genetic and developmental aspects of IgE. Pediatr. Clin. North Am. 22:17, 1975.

Ovary, Z., Benacerraf, B., and Bloch, K. J.: Properties of guinea pig 7S antibodies. II. Identification of antibodies involved in passive cutaneous and systemic anaphylaxis. J. Exper. Med. 117:951, 1963.

Parish, W. E.: Reaginic and non-reaginic antibody reactions on anaphylactic participating cells. In Goodfriend, L., Sehon, A. H., and Orange, R. P. (eds.): Mechanisms of Allergy: Reagin-mediated Hypersensitivity. New York, Marcel Dekker, Inc., 1973, pp. 197–219.

Platts-Mills, T. A. E., Von Maur, R. K., Ishizaka, K., Norman, P. S., and Lichtenstein, L. M.: IgA and IgG anti-ragweed antibodies in nasal secretions. Quantitative measurements of antibodies and correlation with inhibition of histamine release. J. Clin. Invest. 57:1041, 1976.

Spiegelberg, H. L.: Biological activities of immunoglobulins of different classes and subclasses. Adv. Immunol. 19:259, 1974.

Stanworth, D. R.: Reaginic antibodies. Adv. Immunol. 3:181, 1963.

Tada, T.: Regulation of reaginic antibody formation in animals. Progr. Allergy, 19:122, 1975.

Taylor, B., Norman, A. P., Orgel, H. A., Stokes, C. R., Turner, M. W., and Soothill, J. F.: Transient IgA deficiency and pathogenesis of infantile atopy. Lancet 2:111, 1973.

Vijay, H. M., and Perelmutter, L.: Inhibition of reagin-mediated PCA reactions in monkeys and histamine release from human leukocytes by human IgG4 subclass. Int. Arch. Allergy Appl. Immunol. 53:78, 1977.

Waldmann, T. A., Iio, A., Ogawa, M., McIntyre, O. R. and Strober, W.: The metabolism of IgE. Studies in normal individuals and in a patient with IgE myeloma. J. Immunol. 117:1139, 1976.

Watanabe, N., Kojima, S., and Ovary, Z.: Suppression of IgE antibody production in SJL mice. I. Nonspecific suppressor T cells. J. Exp. Med. 143:833, 1976.

Weltman, J. K., Frackelton, A. R., Szaro, R. P., and Rotman, B.: A galactosidase immunosorbent test for human immunoglobulin E. J. Allergy Clin. Immunol. 58:426, 1976.

Wide, L.: Solid phase antigen-antibody systems. In Kirkham, K. E., and Hunter, W. M. (eds.): Radioimmunoassay Methods. Edinburgh, Churchill Livingstone, 1971, pp. 405–412.

Wide, L.: Clinical significance of measurement of reaginic (IgE) antibody by RAST. In Brostoff, J. (ed.): Clinical Immunology-Allergy in Paediatric Medicine. Oxford, Blackwell Scientific Publications, Ltd., 1974, pp. 93–105.

Douglas C. Heiner, M.D.

10

Non-IgE Antibody in Disease

If there is a lesson to be learned from recent developments in immunology as they relate to allergic diseases, it is that IgE responses, though important, are rarely isolated occurrences. Indeed, a simple IgE response is the exception rather than the rule. Similarly, even though many manifestations of allergic disease relate to the presence of IgE antibodies, there are instances of classic clinical allergy in which IgE antibodies cannot be demonstrated. Von Pirquet initially used the term *allergy* to describe an altered immunologic responsiveness to a foreign substance. Common usage has since defined the term as unusual responses not seen in the majority of individuals exposed to comparable amounts of the foreign substance in question. A few writers and many physicians, nevertheless, tend to restrict the term to indicate only those conditions that are IgE-mediated. It has become clear, however, that antibody responses of other classes as well as cell-mediated immune responses frequently accompany IgE-mediated responses, modify the intensity and duration of illness, and contribute to the clinical manifestations observed. In addition, a variety of hypersensitivity reactions mediated by immunologic mechanisms that do not involve IgE antibody are of clinical importance. Thus, the importance of recognizing non-IgE tissue-damaging antibodies, and delineating the manner in which they can participate in untoward clinical responses is self-evident. In this chapter, several kinds of humoral immune responses that have been observed to occur with or without the concomitant involvement of IgE will be considered. Attention also will be given to certain immunoregulatory mechanisms that are important to consider in IgE-mediated as well as non-IgE-mediated hypersensitivity responses.

The classification of allergic responses by Gell and Coombs into four major categories has been helpful over the years in the study and understanding of hypersensitivity disorders. As originally stated, it is an oversimplification of the situation actually encountered in the laboratory or observed in the patient. Nevertheless, within the context of this admonition, there is some utility for this classification. Briefly, tissue damage is considered in four general categories (Coombs and Gell, 1975):

Type I. Anaphylactic reactions due to IgE antibodies attached to specific receptors on basophils or mast cells are the classic example. Antibody that, on contact with antigen, triggers the release of chemical mediators from the cells, results in a local or systemic anaphylactic response. It is now recognized that IgE-mediated reactions may manifest themselves rapidly, and/or evolve over a few hours. Considerations involving non-IgE antibodies are discussed on p. 138.

Type II. Cytotoxic reactions in which the basic mechanism involves antibody directed towards a cell component or an antigen affixed to the cell. Damage to the cell can then result from the action of complement or mononuclear cells that are focused onto the cell surface by the antibody.

Type III. Antigen-antibody complex-induced tissue injury, usually due to microprecipitates in or around small blood vessels or basement membranes. The greatest damage usually is caused by immune complexes of a million daltons or more molecular weight formed at equivalence or slight antigen excess, which are capable of activating complement.

Type IV. Delayed type (cell-mediated) tissue damage, classically due to the triggering of sensitized T lymphocytes (bearing antigen-specific receptors on the cell surface) which, on contact with antigen, release lymphokines. Cell-mediated cytotoxicity ensues.

HOMOCYTOTROPIC IgG ANTIBODY

It has long been known that there are two distinct types of cytotropic antibody response in rodents involving antibodies with an affinity for mediator-releasing cells (Becker, 1971). Homocytotropic antibodies adhere to specific cells in animals of the same species. The cells that possess receptors for the immunoglobulin are considered to be sensitized when a critical density of specific antibody has accumulated on the cell surface, so that on exposure to small or moderate amounts of antigen, chemical mediators are released and an allergic response ensues.

IgE antibodies are the classic homocytotropic antibodies (see Chapter 9). They are denatured by heating at 56° C, after which they no longer bind to cellular receptors; they require a latent period of several hours or days following injection into a recipient's skin before maximal passive cutaneous anaphylactic (PCA) responses occur; they persist at the local site for several days or weeks; and the PCA response (Prausnitz-Küstner response in humans) can be blocked by prior addition of purified E-myeloma protein or abrogated by specific removal of IgE from the donor serum before passive transfer. A second type of homocytotropic antibody also passively sensitizes recipient skin for PCA reactions. These antibodies, however, are heat stable at 56° C; they do not require a prolonged latent period for maximal expression; and passive sensitization usually lasts less than 36 hours. Maximal responses can be obtained within a few hours or less of passive sensitization. Sensitizing activity of rodent serum is abrogated by specific removal of IgG1 before it is used for passive transfer.

Several investigators have performed experiments that suggest that human IgG antibodies also may be homocytotropic and contribute to allergic responses (Parish, 1970; Bryant, 1975; Vijay and Perelmutter, 1977; Gwynn et al., 1978). In these instances, the characteristics of the IgG antibody are similar to those of rodent IgG1 antibody in that the homocytotropic property is stable at 56° C, only a few minutes to an hour are required for maximal fixation to cell receptors, passive sensitization persists only for hours rather than days, and the effect can be abrogated by specific removal of the antibodies using anti-IgG. In the opinion of some investigators, the IgG4-subclass of human antibodies specifically is responsible for this short-term sensitizing homocytotropic antibody activity. Gwynn et al. (1978) reported that elevated concentrations of both IgG4 and IgE were commonly seen in atopic dermatitis and that it was rare to find only one of these two immunoglobulin classes elevated in subjects with this disorder. They noted a correlation in asthmatic subjects between clinical responsiveness to disodium chromoglycate and high levels of IgE but not high levels of IgG4. They reportedly observed a pattern of elevation of IgE alone in certain types of allergic disorders, combined elevations of IgE and IgG4 antibodies in other types, and isolated elevations of IgG4 in asthmatic patients who were not responsive to disodium chromoglycate therapy. Further studies will be required to determine the consistency and clinical relevance of these observations.

ANTITISSUE OR ANTICELL ANTIBODIES

Antibodies reactive with a number of different cell types or tissues have been associated with tissue damage. A classic example is Coombs-positive hemolytic anemia, in which antibody-coated red blood cells have a markedly shortened life span. In an analogous manner, anti-platelet antibodies may cause thrombocytopenia and purpura, and antibodies to polymorphonuclear leukocytes can result in neutropenia. Anti–basement membrane antibodies are important in both the renal and pulmonary manifestations of Goodpasture's syndrome. Antiskin antibodies probably participate in the production of dermatitis herpetiformis, pemphigus, and bullous pemphigoid. Antibodies to gastric parietal cells are common in pernicious anemia. Antinuclear and anti-DNA antibodies are prevalent in disseminated lupus erythematosus (Gell, Coombs and Lachman, 1975; Bach, 1978). Many other examples have been cited. Not all antitissue antibodies have been shown convincingly to be tissue-damaging, but some, particularly those involving cells of the hematologic system, have been shown to possess this capability.

ANTIGEN-ANTIBODY COMPLEXES

Disseminated lupus erythematosus is one disease that has long been known to be associated with the presence of antigen–non-IgE-antibody complexes, both in the serum and in deposits in the renal glomeruli. Serum sickness is another example of a disease in which antigen-antibody complexes of non-IgE type appear to play a central pathogenetic role. In this instance, a single dose of antigen produces a series of immunologic changes that result in vasculitis and multisystem disease. Symptoms accompany antibody production and the accumulation of circulating antigen-antibody complexes. After the complexes have been eliminated, symptoms decline and pathologic lesions regress. It is of interest that an IgE response frequently precedes or accompanies the appearance of antigen-antibody complexes and may contribute to the clinical manifestations of the disease process. Indeed, it may well be that an IgE-mediated increase in vascular permeability contributes to the actual deposition of antigen-antibody complexes in vessel walls and the subsequent production of vasculitis (Kniker and Cochrane, 1968; Benveniste et al., 1972, 1976).

It appears that IgE responses may constitute an integral part of many antigen-antibody complex diseases, two examples of which are hepatitis B infection and allergic bronchopulmonary aspergillosis. Since the advent of techniques that permit the detection of circulating antigen-antibody complexes, evidence has accumulated that circulating complexes are common in many diseases. It is of particular interest that immune complexes have been reported in serum in a high proportion of atopic subjects who are undergoing hyposensitization (Cano et al., 1977). Circulating immune complexes also have been reported to occur regularly in normal infants following the ingestion of cow milk, perhaps resulting from maternal IgG antibodies passed to the infant via breast milk (Delire et al., 1978). It is likely that formation of immune complexes is a common, perhaps daily, occurrence in the blood and interstitial fluids of most humans. Many of these appear to have little or no pathogenetic significance, which underscores the need for laboratory tests that can discriminate between pathologic and innocuous immune complexes.

The nature of the antigen-antibody complexes formed and the way in which the body handles them are probably critical determinants in whether or not symptoms or other manifestations of disease result. As alluded to above, circulating complexes that are in slight antigen excess and larger than 1 million daltons are particularly likely to cause tissue damage. Benveniste et al. (1976) suggest that the development of glomerular lesions in acute serum sickness depends on the simultaneous presence of circulating immune complexes of a particular size and a critical degree of IgE-induced basophil degranulation with mediator release. Sherzer and Ward (1978) have shown that pulmonary damage from immune complexes administered intratracheally to rats depends on a critical ratio of antigen to antibody in the complexes, those preformed at antigen-antibody equivalence being most injurious. Other studies suggest that immune complex binding to lymphocyte receptors for Fc and complement can modulate lymphocyte proliferation and function. For example, altering the ratio of antigen to antibody in complexes can either stimulate or depress antigen-induced lymphocyte reactivity (Eisen and Karush, 1964; Banks, 1973, Kontiainen and Mitchison, 1975; Askonas, 1976).

Another disease of interest is gliadin-induced celiac disease. Non-IgE antibodies to gliadin and circulating immune complexes are much more prominent than in control populations. Delayed (6 to 8 hour, Arthus-like) skin responses to gliadin also have been reported to be common. *In vitro* cell-mediated immune responsiveness to gliadin frequently is observed. Thus, a combination of two or more types of pathologic immune response may be important in the genesis of celiac disease.

In the author's laboratory "mid-normal" amounts of IgE antibody to alpha gliadin were present in all 15 subjects with biopsy-confirmed gluten-related celiac disease. In other words, none of the subjects studied had either the high or the low levels of specific IgE antibodies seen in other populations. One can speculate that high levels of specific IgE antibodies would favor an immediate-type reaction to wheat that would preclude the development of celiac disease, and that low levels would be unable to induce any reaction, whereas intermediate levels may facilitate the deposition of antigen-antibody complexes in a host genetically programmed to produce non-IgE antibodies to gliadin.

Antigen-antibody complexes also may play an important role in immunoregulatory mechanisms in that they can suppress *in vitro* antibody production by spleen cells, possibly by acting on antigen receptors (Diener and Feldmann, 1972).

COMPLEMENT-FIXING ANTIBODIES

It is clear that transient inflammation can result from the reaction of antigen with IgE antibodies without activating complement. However, any antigen-antibody reaction that activates complement may induce allergic symptoms through release of chemical mediators (see Chapter 11). Antitissue antibodies, anti–blood cell antibodies, antigen-antibody complexes (whether circulating or deposited in blood vessels or glomeruli), and many autoantibodies are capable of activating complement. Although complement is principally activated by IgG

and IgM antibodies, antibodies of other classes or substances that are not antibody-dependent, such as endotoxin, yeasts, polysaccharides, and radiopaque contrast material, may activate complement by the alternative pathway (see Chapter 5).

INTERRELATIONS BETWEEN ANTIBODIES OF DIFFERENT IMMUNOGLOBULIN CLASSES

As indicated before, the usual immune response to antigen contact involves antibodies of several, and frequently of all, immunoglobulin classes. Many interrelationships between different types of antibodies, and between antibodies and cells, may be important in tissue injury. Research has only begun to unravel these interactions. Some antibodies may be additive in causing tissue damage, whereas some directed at the same antigen may have opposing actions and modify the reaction. Antibodies may act to inhibit or to enhance antibody synthesis. Antibodies of all immunoglobulin classes probably play important interrelated roles in a vast immunoregulatory network (Jerne, 1974).

An example of additive antibody effects is seen in the activation of complement by both IgG and IgM antibodies. Under most circumstances, IgM antibodies appear earlier in immunologic responses and persist for a shorter time. Both, however, activate the classic complement pathway following reaction with antigen, assisting in the neutralization or killing and removal of macromolecules and microorganisms. IgG ordinarily has a higher affinity for monovalent haptens than does IgM. However, at a molecular level, IgM activates complement more efficiently than does IgG. IgM also is more effective as a hemagglutinin or bacterial agglutinin. IgM is larger and can form more bonds with multivalent antigens than IgG. Thus IgM and IgG reinforce each other, and the two acting together may be much more effective than either alone. It is likely that the tissue-damaging effects of IgG and IgM antibodies also are additive. Examples include the anti-DNA antibodies that may participate in the pathogenesis of disseminated lupus erythematosus, IgG and IgM rheumatoid factors in the joints of patients with rheumatoid arthritis, and mixed IgM-IgG cryoglobulins in some forms of cryoglobulinemia.

There is evidence, on the other hand, that the presence of IgG antibodies under certain circumstances may ameliorate or block the tissue-injuring effects of other immunoglobulins such as IgE. For example, allergy injection therapy for IgE-mediated disease such as hay fever, stimulates the production of IgG "blocking" antibodies which may combine with antigen, restricting its access to the circulation and its potential for producing anaphylaxis. It also may bind to antigen and prevent its combination with mast cell–fixed IgE at the target organ, and may inhibit IgE antibody synthesis by suppressing IgE-producing B cells or by stimulating antigen-specific suppressor T cells.

IMMUNOREGULATORY EFFECTS OF ANTIBODY

The ability of specific antibodies to regulate the synthesis of tissue-damaging antibodies is used clinically to prevent Rh sensitization of D-negative mothers. Anti-D antibody (RhoGAM) administered during late pregnancy or at delivery binds to D-positive infant cells, facilitating their removal and preventing maternal sensitization (Freda et al., 1964). A small amount of passively administered antibody given at the proper time inhibits the formation of large amounts of maternal anti-D antibody, permitting subsequent pregnancies to proceed to term without the development of erythroblastosis.

As the concentration of IgG increases, so does its catabolic rate (Morell et al., 1970). This is another autoregulatory mechanism by which antibody influences its own concentration. These regulatory mechanisms appear to create cycles of antibody production, which in turn serves as an important regulatory factor of immune responses (Weigle, 1975).

Jerne (1974) has proposed a provocative theory of immune regulation involving a network of antibody molecules in which each specific antibody has a unique antigenic structure or idiotype specificity which itself elicits and reacts with anti-idiotype antibodies within the system. When a critical concentration of anti-idiotype antibodies is reached, antigen-specific humoral and cellular immune responses are turned off. Anti-allotypic antibodies, on the other hand, may turn off class-specific immune responses. Antibodies of high affinity are more immunosuppressive than antibodies of low affinity. In general, IgG antibodies are more suppressive than IgM antibodies. Passively administered antibodies, and presumably naturally occurring antibodies, have less inhibitory effect on secondary immune responses than on primary responses.

It has been demonstrated that identical idiotype specificities exist on B and T lymphocytes of the same individual, suggesting that both of these cell types participate in the network. Both T and B lymphocyte responses have been demonstrated to be directed toward idiotypes present on an animal's own immunoglobulin molecule. Anti-idiotypic antibodies passively administered will suppress T and B lymphocyte function when the lymphocyte possesses the corresponding idiotype. Anti-idiotype T cells also can suppress the production of antibodies carrying the corresponding idiotype just as can auto-anti-idiotypic antibodies. Mixed lymphocyte, graft-versus-host, and lymphocyte cytotoxicity reactions — all of which can cause tissue damage — are inhibited either by anti-idiotypic antibodies directed towards antibody and lymphocyte idiotypes or by anti-allotypic antibodies directed towards histocompatibility antigens. Thus anti-idiotype antibodies are now known to play an important regulatory role in the immune system. A possible result of their deficiency could be the overproduction of specific antibodies seen in certain immunodeficiency disorders with immunoglobulins of restricted heterogenicity, also the oligoclonal CSF gammapathies seen in multiple sclerosis and subacute sclerosing panencephalitis (SSPE), and the benign and malignant gammapathies of old age, including myelomas and lymphomas.

A special role for IgD in immunoregulation has been proposed. IgD is a prominent lymphocyte surface immunoglobulin (Rowe et al., 1973; Fu et al., 1974). Vitetta and Uhr (1975) suggested that lymphocyte surface IgD may play an important role in determining whether an active immune response with antibody formation will ensue following contact of early B cells with antigen or whether, in the absence of surface IgD, immunologic tolerance will result. The addition of anti-IgD under experimental conditions has been shown to inhibit the production of other immunoglobulins. Indeed there appears to be a natural sequence of immunoglobulin production by B cells, and the presence of one immunoglobulin on early B cell surfaces may be of fundamental importance to the subsequent production of other immunoglobulins as well as to the overall immune response (see review by Möller, 1977).

Preliminary observations in our laboratory revealed a striking inverse relationship between serum concentrations of IgD and IgE in over half of a population of allergic patients examined (Tamura et al., 1978). When serial specimens from the same person were studied over a period of months or years, total IgE and IgD levels frequently followed a mirror image pattern of change. When either total or specific IgD antibodies were found to increase, there was a striking tendency toward a decrease in the corresponding total or specific IgE, suggesting the possibility of an immunoregulatory effect of one immunoglobulin class on the other. This reciprocal relationship between IgE and IgD was not always found, however.

In some patients, there was a similar inverse relationship between IgD and IgM. Reciprocal relationships between IgD and IgA or between IgD and IgG, on the other hand, were not found. Other observations in our laboratory indicate that IgE responses to antigen exposure or to viral infections occur rapidly and peak at 7 to 14 days, concomitant with or before IgM peak responses. IgD responses, as measured by peak increases either in total immunoglobulin or in specific IgD antibody, occur 40 to 50 days after an antigen exposure such as a bee sting or a specific viral infection. The data are consistent with the idea that IgD antibody serves as a signal for turning off antibody production of IgE or IgM or both. Further studies, however, will be needed to elucidate the precise role of circulating IgD in immunoregulation.

INTERRELATIONSHIPS BETWEEN ANTIBODIES AND LYMPHOCYTES THAT MAY CONTRIBUTE TO TISSUE DAMAGE

There are many ways in which antibodies and lymphocytes cooperate to produce a particular immune response. For example, in kidney graft rejection, antibodies may act with lymphocytes to destroy histoincompatible donor kidney cells. The reaction has been termed antibody-dependent cell-mediated cytotoxicity (ADCC), and the antibodies have been called lymphocyte-dependent antibodies (LDA). Such antibodies can also sensitize mononuclear cells (K, or killer cells) from unimmunized subjects and cause them to destroy target cells. Complement is not required, the antibodies are not cytophilic, and their action can be inhibited by immune complexes. These antibodies usually are of the IgG variety and only low concentrations are needed. Antibody-dependent lymphocyte cytotoxicity may be particularly important in immune defenses against malignant cells that arise as the result of cellular mutation or transformation. It also may be a particularly important defense mechanism in children with thymic deficiencies and in certain other types of immunodeficiency diseases.

INTERRELATIONSHIPS BETWEEN NON-IgE ANTIBODIES AND NONLYMPHOID CELLS

IgG or IgM antibody, acting with complement, may cause cell lysis by a mechanism independent of lymphocytes. These "cytotoxic" antibodies often are important in hyperacute renal graft rejection. Such tissue damage requires a higher level of antibody than that of antibody-dependent cell-mediated cytotoxicity. Cytotoxic antibodies may play a role in other hypersensitivity phenomena. For instance, antiplatelet antibody plays an important pathogenetic role in many cases of thrombocytopenia in newborn infants. In these cases, maternal IgG antiplatelet antibody induces the disease, which clears spontaneously as the maternal antibodies disappear from the infants' circulation. Antibodies to polymorphonuclear leukocytes, produced after many blood transfusions, may cause neutropenia in some subjects. Antineutrophil antibodies also are seen in systemic lupus erythematosus and other autoimmune disorders, in which they may contribute to neutropenia. Anti–red cell antibodies are a common cause of hemolytic anemia. Such reactions may be drug-induced (Ackroyd, 1975) or idiopathic. A wide variety of tissue-damaging autoantibodies to nonhematologic tissues are noted in Table 10–1.

Antibodies, particularly those of the IgG class, may affix to nonlymphoid cells by means of Fc receptors and impart to these cells such properties as antigen recognition, complement-related chemotaxis, and opsonic activity leading to enhanced phagocytosis. Both polymorphonuclear leukocytes and monocytes possess surface membrane IgG receptors and may be passively sensitized to specific soluble or cellular antigens. Fc-receptor bearing leukocytes thus can be involved in antibody-dependent tissue-damaging reactions.

NON-IgE ANTIBODIES IN TISSUE DAMAGE

One method of implicating antibodies in the pathogenesis of tissue damage is to demonstrate antigen-induced tissue damage following passive transfer of antibodies to an otherwise unaffected recipient. Nature performs this experiment in newborn infants who receive transplacental IgG anti–red cell antibodies from the mother. Unfortunately, in most situations, such a clear-cut cause and effect cannot be demonstrated because of the complexity of immune responses that ordinarily follow contact with antigen. Celiac disease illustrates this important problem.

Celiac Disease. For many years, celiac disease was considered to result from the toxic action of incompletely digested peptides of wheat gliadin. A deficient intestinal mucosal peptidase was postulated and in some instances demonstrated. The probability that a primary peptidase deficiency causes the disease appears unlikely, however, since all enzymatic deficiencies identified to date have proved to be transient, disappearing once the patient was in remission on a strict gluten-free diet. On the other hand, increased levels of non-IgE antibodies to wheat gliadin (Taylor et al., 1961; Heiner et al., 1962) have been found in many celiac subjects. In addition, antireticulin antibodies have been reported which are thought to cross-react with constituents of wheat gluten (Seah et al., 1973; Alp and Wright, 1971), and Arthus-like skin responses to gluten digests have been observed (Baker and Read, 1976). A variety of antibodies to foods other than wheat antigens also have been described (Carswell and Ferguson, 1972). Both elevated (Asquith et al., 1969) and reduced (Crabbe and Heremans, 1966) levels of serum and secretory IgA are common, as are deficiencies in IgM production (Hobbs and Hepner, 1968).

A B cell surface antigen, GSE Ag, separate from HLA antigens (Mann et al., 1976), and the HLA antigens, B8 and DW3, are commonly associated with this disease (Falchuk et al., 1972; Keuning et al., 1976). The GSE lymphocyte surface antigen occurs much more frequently together with HLA B8 or DW3 in subjects with gluten-sensitive enteropathy than in controls. These findings attest to strong genetic influences in the pathogenesis of celiac disease and suggest that a mechanism involving specific immune responses may be operative.

Activation of serum complement following the administration of wheat gluten to celiac subjects in remission has been reported (Mohammed et al., 1976), the presence of both local (Shiner and Ballard, 1972) and circulating antigen-antibody complexes (Doe et al., 1973; Mohammed et al., 1976) prior to the institution of a wheat-free diet has been recorded, and lymphocyte-mediated immune responses to gluten have been demonstrated in patients with celiac disease (Ferguson et al., 1975; Sikora et al., 1976; Holmes et al., 1976; Ashkenazi et al., 1978). Studies of jejunal mucosal biopsies in patients with celiac disease have shown an increased number of lymphocytes and plasma cells, and IgA and IgM antibody production to wheat gliadin is increased following oral challenge with wheat or gluten fractions. Cultures of jejunal mucosal biopsies from patients in relapse show inhibition of normal maturation of epithelial cells, and brush border enzyme

TABLE 10–1 NON-IgE ANTIBODIES AND RELATED IMMUNOLOGIC FINDINGS THAT MAY HELP IN DIAGNOSIS AND MANAGEMENT OF SELECTED DISEASES

Disease	Finding
Non-IgE allergic bronchial asthma	Negative scratch and prick skin tests Positive intradermal skin tests Heat-stable, short-term sensitizing antibody Positive bronchial challenge Negative IgE studies
Extrinsic allergic alveolitis	Serum precipitins to offending antigen, e.g., to *Micropolyspora faeni* in farmer's lung, to pigeon serum or droppings in pigeon-breeder's lung. Cell-mediated immunity to offending antigen.
Allergic bronchopulmonary aspergillosis	Dual skin reactions (15 minute and 8 hour) Precipitins to one or several *A. fumigatus* antigens in low to moderate titer. Elevated total IgE, IgE antibodies
Aspergilloma	Serum precipitins to multiple *A. fumigatus* antigens in relatively high titer. Normal total and antibody IgE
Systemic lupus erythematosus	LE cell formation Antinuclear antibodies in serum including anti-DNA Serum DNA–anti-DNA immune complexes Decreased serum C3, C4, CH50 Granular deposits of Ig, C, sometimes DNA in glomerular basement membrane (GBM) False positive reaction for syphilis
Post-streptococcal glomerulonephritis	Elevated serum ASO titer Decreased serum C3, C4, CH50
Hypocomplementemic membranoproliferative nephritis	Decreased serum C3, not C4 Alpha$_2$D and C3 NeF in serum Granular C3 deposits in GBM
Subacute bacterial endocarditis (SBE)	Serum immune complexes Decreased serum C3, CH50 Positive blood cultures
Rheumatoid arthritis	Rheumatoid factor in serum, joint fluid Decreased synovial fluid C3 Complexes of IgG and rheumatoid factor in synovium, joint fluid
Rheumatic fever	Anti-myocardial sarcolemmal antibodies Elevated antistreptolysin, antistreptokinase, and antihyaluronidase titers
Sjögren's syndrome	Antibodies to salivary and lacrimal gland periductal epithelium Positive rheumatoid factor Antithyroglobulin and antinuclear antibodies common
Goodpasture's syndrome	Linear deposits of immunoglobulin on renal GBM, pulmonary epithelial basement membranes Serum antibodies to glomerular and pulmonary basement membranes
Celiac disease	Chronic jejunal inflammatory changes clear on gluten-free diet, reappear on challenge High titer of non-IgE serum antibodies to alpha gliadin Arthus-like skin responses to gluten *In vitro* induction of LIF lymphokine by gliadin
Milk-induced enteropathy	Jejunal inflammatory changes clear on milk-free diet, reappear on challenge Excessive loss of ^{51}Cr-tagged red blood cells or albumin clears with milk-free diet, returns on challenge

TABLE 10–1 NON-IgE ANTIBODIES AND RELATED IMMUNOLOGIC FINDINGS THAT MAY HELP IN DIAGNOSIS AND MANAGEMENT OF SELECTED DISEASES *(Continued)*

Disease	Finding
Milk-induced pulmonary hemosiderosis in children	Serum precipitins in high titer to cow milk antigens Positive intradermal skin tests with cow milk antigens
Autoimmune hemolytic anemia	Positive direct Coombs test (IgG, IgM antibody and/or complement on red blood cell) Positive indirect Coombs test (serum antibody to autologous red blood cells)
Erythroblastosis fetalis	Positive direct Coombs test on cord or neonatal cells Positive indirect Coombs using mother's serum, infant's red cells
Dermatitis herpetiformis	Granular IgA and C3 along dermal-epidermal junctions
Pemphigus vulgaris	IgG antibodies to epithelial intercellular cement Complement (C3) deposition along with the antibodies
Bullous pemphigoid	Linear deposits IgG on epithelial basement membranes
Pernicious anemia	Antibodies to intrinsic factor Antibodies to gastric parietal cells
Hashimoto's thyroiditis	Antibodies to thyroglobulin in high titer Antibodies to thyroid microsomes
Graves' disease	Long-acting thyroid stimulator antibodies (LATS) Low levels of antithyroglobulin
Addison's disease	Anti-adrenal mitochondrial antibodies Anti-thyroglobulin, anti–gastric parietal cell, and anti–intrinsic factor antibodies

production when wheat gluten is added (Katz and Falchuk, 1975). Although this provides a good *in vitro* model of gluten-induced tissue damage, it does not establish an immunologic mediated mechanism. It opens the door, however, to critical tests which might implicate specific immunologic mechanisms.

Only rarely, if at all, do many of these findings occur in normal subjects. Thus it is clear that in celiac patients there are many exaggerated immune responses to the ingestion of wheat gliadin which may be disease specific. It would not be surprising if one or several participated in causing the jejunal mucosal damage in celiac disease, but it is not clear which is (are) responsible for it.

Other Disorders of Immune Response. A similar discussion is pertinent to many disorders which are associated with aberrant immune responses. Since responses to provoking antigens are complex and include the development of various kinds of antibodies, investigators and practitioners alike should observe caution in ascribing the etiology or pathogenesis of a hypersensitivity disorder to a single mech-

anism simply because of the presence of a particular antibody. Even allergic reactions that appear clinically to be solely IgE-mediated usually occur in the presence of antibodies of various immunoglobulin classes as well as sensitized lymphocytes, all of which may play important pathogenetic roles in specific instances.

Tests to Identify Non-IgE-Mediated Tissue Damage. A thorough discussion of laboratory procedures designed to identify non-IgE-mediated tissue damage and follow its progress is beyond the scope of this chapter. Such procedures, in fact, are multiplying at such a rapid pace that what is optimal this year may be out of date next year. One must utilize wisely the facilities and personnel available, relying largely on laboratories where there is experience and skill in performing the procedure and knowledge concerning interpretation of results. A partial listing of procedures that may be of assistance in the diagnosis and management of selected disorders is given in Table 10–1. A brief general description of some of these procedures follows.

Fluorescence microscopy is used to identify antibodies directed towards specific autologous antigens. Antinuclear antibodies are identified routinely by fluorescence microscopy, as are linear and lumpy deposits of immunoglobulin and complement, for example, in renal glomeruli in Goodpasture's syndrome and lupus erythematosus, respectively.

Fluorescence microscopy helps considerably in studying specific antibody responses in subjects with a variety of dermatologic diseases, e.g., complement-fixing IgG antibodies to epithelial intercellular cement in pemphigus vulgaris; linear deposits of IgG antibodies to epithelial basement membrane in bullous pemphigoid; and granular accumulations of IgA and C3 along dermal-epidermal junctions in dermatitis herpetiformis. It also has facilitated greater understanding of gastrointestinal disturbances such as celiac disease, milk-induced enteropathy, Crohn's disease, and ulcerative colitis. The technique is widely used in detecting autoantibodies in disorders such as Hashimoto's thyroiditis, hyperthyroidism, Addison's disease, and certain types of diabetes. In spite of its limitations, which include the need for subjective interpretation and a lack of precise quantitation, this technique will continue to be used in the foreseeable future to detect non-IgE tissue-reactive antibodies.

Immune electron microscopy is a specialized technique which, like fluorescence microscopy, will permit identification of tissue-binding antibodies according to specific immunoglobulin class. Its greater resolving power will permit localization of antibodies not only to specific cell types but also to certain organelles, providing a more detailed picture of their potential pathogenetic role than would be otherwise possible. This procedure is too specialized and expensive to be used for routine investigative studies in more than a few centers or in any but the most provocative circumstances. Electron microscopy also is of value in searching for viruses which, if found, might be implicated in tissue damage, either directly or in consort with antibodies.

Cell and organ cultures offer promise of insight into the nature of immunologic responses at the cellular and tissue levels. Cultures of lymphocytes and of jejunal mucosal biopsies are examples. It is possible to quantitate intrinsic antibody production according to immunoglobulin class, to observe and test for tissue-binding antibodies produced elsewhere, and to observe the effects of added antigen, antibody, lymphoid cells, lymphokines, other chemical mediators, and hormones on *in vitro* enzyme or antibody synthesis and on tissue integrity. The use of this technique in sorting out relevant pathogenetic mechanisms is highly promising.

Tests for complement activation or depletion have provided presumptive evidence for the involvement of non-IgE antibodies in many instances of tissue injury. The lowering of serum C3 and C4, which accompanies disease activity in disseminated lupus erythematosus, is an example. Oral administration of cow milk to milk-sensitive children and of wheat gluten to celiac subjects has been reported to cause activation of complement and to decrease levels of serum complement components. Most such studies do not provide proof of pathogenetic involvement of complement-fixing antibodies, but they do suggest their presence indirectly.

Tests for circulating antigen-antibody complexes are developing at a rapid pace. At present, however, it may be advantageous to study patients by at least two different techniques as a check on both the sensitivity and reproducibility of the tests being used. The C1q deviation and binding assays and Raji cell tests commonly are successful. Each depends on complexes that activate the complement system, and each has the potential drawback of false positive results, it there is non-specific aggregation of immunoglobulins or the generation of C3b by improper serum handling. Searches for cryoprecipitins, lowered total complement (CH50) or C3 or C4, and the presence of rheumatoid factor are other techniques of value. These and other procedures and their clinical applications have been ably summarized by Kohler (1978) and by Zubler and Lambert (1978).

Radioimmunoassays provide a sensitive technique for measuring specific antibodies of each immunoglobulin class as well as for measurements of specific antigen, antigen-antibody complexes, chemical mediators of allergic responses, and thymic hormones. Allergists and pediatricians are perhaps most aware of the availability of radioimmunoassays to measure specific antibodies of the IgE class (RAST). Modifications of RAST have been used with some success to measure antibodies of other immunoglobulin classes, and it is possible to measure specific antibodies of any of the five immunoglobulin classes or of their subclasses by appropriate radioimmunoassay procedures. The double antibody procedure currently is the most reliable for measuring IgG and IgA antibodies. IgE and IgD antibodies are measured best by the RAST procedure or a modification thereof. Neither has yet emerged as superior for quantitating specific IgM antibodies, but time will sort out the advantages and disadvantages of various procedures.

Radioimmunoassays have the decided advantage of providing a sensitive quantitative measurement of antibodies when low concentrations are present. They also permit quantitative studies concerning the timing and magnitude of humoral immune responses following specific antigen challenge or during the course of specific diseases. Like most other tests, they do not in themselves prove that the antibody identified is responsible for a specific symptom or tissue injury.

Immunodiffusion in gel permits simple demonstration and identification of precipitating antibodies. Radial immunodiffusion provides the simplest quantitation of total IgG, IgA, and IgM concentrations. When precipitating antibodies are observed by double immunodiffusion, one can be certain that a high concentration of antibody is present, usually of the IgG class but occasionally IgA or IgM. Neither radial nor double immunodiffusion is sufficiently sensitive to reflect accurately total or antigen-specific IgD or IgE in the serum of children. Caution must be exercised to prove that observed precipitates are indeed antigen-antibody reactions rather than nonspecific protein or polysaccharide aggregates. The experienced worker can do this through ensuring the quality of his reagents and the proper use of standards and controls. One should also remember that many subjects have antibodies of the IgG, IgM, or IgA variety that frequently are demonstrable by other techniques but are not detected by the relatively insensitive precipitin technique.

Radioimmunodiffusion adds sensitivity to the versatility of double immunodiffusion. New approaches employing radiolabeled, highly purified antigen or isolated specific antibody have promise of increasing the sensitivity of immunodiffusion to a degree comparable to radioimmunoassays. This will permit identification of minute amounts of specific antigen or of specific antibody according to immunoglobulin class. However, such procedures still lack the quantitative precision and reproducibility of properly performed radioimmunoassays.

Passive transfer tests. Human IgG heat-stable antibodies that cause passive cutaneous anaphylactic (PCA) reactions have been demonstrated by tests both in experimental animals and man. Positive immediate skin tests in humans ordinarily indicate that IgE antibodies are present, but in some instances IgG antibodies have been incriminated. There is some evidence that intradermal tests may provide a more reliable indicator of short-term skin sensitizing IgG antibodies than do scratch or prick tests. Preheating serum to 56° C for one half-hour abrogates IgE but not IgG responses in a passive recipient. Also, if serum is injected intradermally 2 days before antigen challenge, IgE but not IgG antibodies will yield positive results since IgG antibodies rarely remain fixed to mast cells for more than 36 hours. Because of the possibility of passive transfer of hepatitis viruses during passive transfer tests between human subjects, most passive sensitization tests are done on monkeys. Perhaps the most convincing method of proving the immunoglobulin class of an antibody involved in PCA or other physiologic responses involves the removal of individual immunoglobulins using specific anti – heavy chain antisera and then demonstrating that removal of only the incriminated immunoglobulin abrogates the untoward response.

Additional tests to detect non-IgE antibodies have been used, with varying degrees of success, in relating the findings to clinical symptoms and tissue injury. Many of these are discussed in other chapters of this book. Immunoassays of lymphokines, complement components and derivatives, of circulating immune complexes, and of chemical mediators of inflammation hold considerable promise in providing much-needed simple tests to quantitate the various types of immune responses which occur in patients.

References

Ackroyd, J. F.: Immunological mechanisms in drug hypersensitivity. In Gell, P. G. H., Coombs, R. R. H., and Lachmann, P. G. (eds.): *Clinical Aspects of Immunology,* 3rd ed. Oxford, Blackwell Scientific Publications, Ltd., 1975, pp. 913–961.

Alp, M. H., and Wright, R.: Autoantibodies to reticulin in patients with idiopathic steatorrhea, coeliac disease, and Crohn's disease, and their relation to immunoglobulins and dietary antibodies. Lancet 2:682, 1971.

Ashkenazi, A., Idar, D., Handzel, Z. T., Ofarim, M., and Levin, S.: An in-vitro immunological assay for diagnosis of coeliac disease. Lancet 1:627, 1978.

Asquith, P., Thompson, R. A., and Cooke, W. T.: Serum immunoglobulins in adult coeliac disease. Lancet 2:129, 1969.

Askonas, B. A., McMichael, A. J., and Roux, M. E.: Clonal dominance and the preservation of clonal memory cells mediated by antigen-antibody. Immunology 31:541, 1976.

Bach, J. F.: Pathology of immune complexes and systemic lupus erythematosus. In *Immunology.* New York, John Wiley and Sons, 1978, Chapter 28, pp. 699–730.

Baker, P. G., and Read, A. E.: Positive skin reactions in coeliac disease. Q. J. Med. 180:603, 1976.

Banks, K. L.: The effect of antibody on antigen-induced lymphocyte transformation. J. Immunol. 110:709, 1973.

Becker, E. L.: Nature and classification of immediate-type-allergic reactions. Adv. Immunol. 13:267, 1971.

Benveniste, J., Egido, J., and Gutierrez-Millet, V.: Evidence for the involvement of the IgE-basophil system in acute serum sickness. Clin. Exp. Immunol. 26:449, 1976.

Benveniste, J., Henson, P., and Cockrane, C. G.: Leukocyte-dependent histamine release from rabbit platelets; the role of IgE, basophil, and a platelet-activation factor. J. Exp. Med. 136:1356, 1972.

Bryant, D. H., Burns, M. W., and Lazarus, L.: Identification of IgG antibody as a carrier of reaginic activity in asthmatic patients. J. Allergy Clin. Immunol. 56:417, 1975.

Cano, P. O., Chow, M., Jerry, L. M., and Sladowski, J. P.: Circulating immune complexes in patients with atopic allergy. Clin. Allergy 7:167, 1977.

Carswell, F., and Ferguson, A.: Food antibodies in serum — a screening test for celiac disease. Arch. Dis. Child. 47:594, 1972.

Coombs, R. R. A., and Gell, P. G. H.: Classification of allergic reactions responsible for clinical hypersensitivity and disease. In Gell, P. G. H., Coombs, R. R. A., and Lachmann, P. G. (eds.): *Clinical Aspects of Immunology,* 3rd ed. Oxford, Blackwell Scientific Publications, 1975, Chapter 25, pp. 761–782.

Crabbe, P. A., and Heremans, J. F.: Lack of gamma A globulin in serum of patients with steatorrhea. Gut 7:119, 1966.

Diener, E., and Felmann, M.: Relationship between antigen and antibody induced suppression of immunity. Transplant. Rev. 8:76, 1972.

Delire, M., Cambiaso, C. L., and Misson, P. L.: Circulating immune complexes in infants fed on cow's milk. Nature 272:632, 1978.

Doe, W. F., Booth, C. C., and Brown, D. L.: Evidence for complement-binding immune complexes in adult celiac disease, Crohn's disease, and ulcerative colitis. Lancet 1:402, 1973.

Eisen, H. N., and Karush, F.: Immune tolerance and an extracellular regulatory role for bivalent antibody. Nature 202:677, 1964.

Falchuk, Z. M., Rogentine, G. N., and Strober, W.: Predominance of histocompatibility antigen HL-A8 in patients with gluten-sensitive enteropathy. J. Clin. Invest. 51:1602, 1972.

Ferguson, A., MacDonald, T. T., McClure, J. P., and Holden, R. J.: Cell mediated immunity to gliadin within the small intestinal mucosa in coeliac disease. Lancet 1:895, 1975.

Freda, V. J., Gorman, J. G., and Pollack, W.: Successful prevention of experimental sensitization in man with an anti-Rh gamma globulin antibody preparation. Transfusion 4:26, 1964.

Fu, S. M., Winchester, R. J., and Kunkel, H. G., Occurrence of surface IgM, IgD, and free light chains on human lymphocytes. J. Exp. Med. 139:451, 1974.

Gell, P. G. H., Coombs, R. R. A., and Lachmann, P. G. (eds.): *Clinical Aspects of Immunology,* 3rd ed. Oxford, Blackwell Scientific Publications, 1975.

Gwynn, C. M., Morrison-Smith, J., Leon, G. L., and Stanworth, D. R.: Role of IgG4 subclass in childhood allergy. Lancet 1:910, 1978.

Heiner, D. C., Lahey, M. E., Wilson, J. F., Gerrard, J. W., Shwachman, H., and Khaw, K. T.: Precipitins to antigens of wheat and cow's milk in celiac disease. J. Pediatr. 61:813, 1962.

Hobbs, J. R., and Hepner, G. W.: Deficiency of gamma M globulin in coeliac disease. Lancet 1:217, 1968.

Holmes, G. K., Asquith, P., Cooke, W. T.: Cell mediated immunity to gluten fraction III in adult coeliac disease. Clin. Exper. Immunol. 24:259, 1976.

Jerne, N. K.: Towards a network theory of the immune system. Ann. Immunol. Inst. Pasteur 125C:373, 1974.

Katz, A. J., and Falchuk, Z. M.: Current concepts in gluten-sensitive enteropathy. Ped. Clin. No. Amer. 22:767, 1975.

Keuning, J. J., Peña, A. S., vanLeeuwan, A., vanHooff, J. P., and vanRood, J. J.: HLA-DW3 associated with coeliac disease. Lancet 1:506, 1976.

Kniker, W. T., and Cochrane, C. G.: The localization of circulating immune complexes in experimental serum sickness. The role of vasoactive amines and hydrodynamic forces. J. Exp. Med. 127:119, 1968.

Kohler, P. F.: Immune complexes and allergic disease. In Middleton, E., Jr. et al. (ed.): *Allergy Principles and Practice,* Vol. I. St. Louis, C. V. Mosby Co., Chap. 10, pp. 155–176.

Kontiainen, S., and Mitchison, N. A.: Blocking antigen-antibody complexes on the T-lymphocyte activation during in vitro incubation before adoptive transfer. Immunology 28:523, 1975

Mann, D. L., Katz, S. I., Nelson, D. L., Abelson, L. D., and Strober, W.: Specific B-cell antigen associated with gluten sensitive enteropathy and dermatitis herpetiformis, Lancet 1:110, 1976.

Mohammed, I., Holoborow, E. J., Fry, L., Thompson, B. R., Hoffbrand, A. V., and Stewart, J. S.: Multiple immune complexes and hypocomplementemia in dermatitis herpetiformis and coeliac disease. Lancet 2:487, 1976.

Möller, G. (ed.): Immunoglobulin D: structure, synthesis, membrane representation and function. Immunol. Rev. Vol. 37, 1977.

Morell, A., Terry, W. D., Waldmann, T. A.: Metabolic properties of IgG subclasses in man. J. Clin. Invest. 49:673, 1970.

Parish, W. E.: Short-term anaphylactic IgG antibodies in human sera. Lancet 2:591, 1970.

Rowe, D. S., Hug, K., Forni, L., and Pernis, B.: Immunoglobulin D as a surface lymphocyte receptor. J. Exp. Med. *138*:965, 1973.

Seah, P. P., Fry, L., Holborow, E. J., Rossiter, M. A., Doe, W. F., Magalhaes, A. F., and Hoffbrand, A. V.: Antireticulin antibody: Incidence and diagnostic significance. Gut *14*:311, 1973.

Scherzer, H., and Ward, P. A.: Lung injury produced by immune complexes of varying composition. J. Immunol. *121*:947, 1978.

Shiner, M., and Ballard, J.: Antigen-antibody reactions in jejunal mucosa in childhood coeliac disease after gluten challenge. Lancet *1*:1202, 1972.

Sikora, K., Anand, B. S., Truelove, S. C., Ciclitira, P. J., and Offord, R. E.: Stimulation of lymphocytes from patients with coeliac disease by a subfraction of gluten. Lancet *2*:389, 1976.

Tamura, H., Tateno, K., and Heiner, D. C.: Reciprocal relationships between serum levels of IgE and IgD. J. Allergy Clin. Immunol. *61*:178, 1978.

Taylor, K. B., Truelove, S. C., Thompson, D. L., et al.: An immunological study of coeliac disease and idiopathic steatorrhea. Serological reactions to gluten and milk proteins. Brit. Med. J., *2*:1727, 1961.

Vijay, H. M., and Perelmutter, L.: Inhibition of reagin-mediated PCA reactions in monkeys and histamine release from human leukocytes by human IgG4 subclass. Int. Arch. Allergy Appl. Immunol., *53*:78, 1977.

Vitetta, E. S., and Uhr, J. W.: Immunoglobulin receptors revisited. Science, 189:964, 1975.

Weigle, W. O., Cyclical production of antibody as a regulatory mechanism in the immune response. Adv. Immunol. *21*:87, 1975.

Williams, C. A., and Chase, M. W.: *Methods in Immunology and Immunochemistry*, Vol. 5. New York, Academic Press, Inc., 1976, pp. 424–451.

Zubler, R. H., and Lambert, P. H.: Detection of immune complexes in human diseases. Prog. Allergy 24:1, 1978.

11

Robert C. Strunk, M.D.
William E. Berger, M.D.

Chemical Mediators of Inflammation

The interaction between antigen and antibody or sensitized lymphocyte serves to stimulate release or activation of numerous low molecular weight compounds. These substances, termed humoral or chemical mediators, are responsible for inflammatory responses associated with immune reactions and play a major role in the production of tissue damage observed in various human diseases, as well as in the protective inflammatory responses involved in host defense against bacteria, viruses, and other foreign substances. Pharmacologic alteration of the action of mediators of inflammation is an important therapeutic tool, and an appreciation of the nature and action of these mediators is of particular importance to physicians who treat allergic diseases.

In this discussion, mediators will be considered as *primary* or *secondary* mediators. In general, primary mediators are released early in the inflammatory response and participate in the early phases of the reaction. Secondary mediators usually are released as a result of the events in the primary reaction and often modulate or prolong inflammation produced in the primary phase.

Much of the information concerning involvement of mediators in the human inflammatory response has been obtained from *in vitro* studies and from animal models of disease states. Where appropriate studies have been possible in humans,

much of the indirect evidence that these mediators are involved in the pathogenesis of human disease has been shown to be correct.

Although mediators will be considered individually, it is important to recognize that these mediators act in a system in which there is often extensive mediator interaction. In addition, a given mediator may elicit different responses in different tissues.

PRIMARY MEDIATORS

Histamine. Histamine is a low molecular weight substance formed from the amino acid L-histidine by the action of histidine decarboxylase. A major portion of histamine stored in the body is in circulating basophils and tissue fixed mast cells, where it is present in granules in a biologically active form (Austen, 1971). Release from the granules occurs after the cells are activated. Once released, histamine is rapidly degraded by oxidative deamination and is eliminated by renal excretion. In addition to the basophil–mast cell pool, histamine is present in small quantities in plasma and body fluids and in several tissues unassociated with mast cells, where histamine turnover occurs rapidly.

Histamine is one of the few mediators that can be measured by a specific chemical assay. Although several assays have been used, the recently developed enzymatic isotropic assay is the most sensitive and thus preferred (Beaven et al., 1972).

The mechanism of the release of histamine from mast cells and basophils has been studied extensively using *in vitro* systems (Plaut and Lichtenstein, 1978). The most widely studied system has been antigen-induced histamine release from basophils (peripheral blood) or mast cells (chopped human lung fragments) sensitized with IgE antibody. Following the interaction of antigen and IgE antibody at the cell surface, a series of biochemical events are triggered that result in the release of histamine from the intracellular granules. These events require energy (an intact glycolytic pathway and/or oxidative phosphorylation), extracellular calcium, and the presence of an intact cytoskeleton. Histamine release is modulated by the levels of two intracellular hormones, cyclic adenosine monophosphate (cAMP), and cyclic guanosine monophosphate (cGMP). In gen-

eral, release is enhanced by decreased levels of cAMP and increased levels of cGMP and, conversely, is diminished by increased levels of cAMP.

Histamine acts on cells and tissues through two distinct receptors, type-1 and type-2 (H_1 and H_2), which are defined pharmacologically by the antagonistic activity of specific antihistamines (Black et al., 1972). Stimulation of these receptors produces different effects in different tissues (Table 11–1). Within single cells the stimulation of these different receptors results in functions that can be either antagonistic or synergistic. For example, activation of H_1 receptors in sensitized lung fragments results in increased intracellular levels of cGMP, enhancing antigen-induced release of mediators from the cells, whereas activation of H_2 receptors increases intracellular levels of cAMP, decreasing mediator release. On the other hand, stimulation of both H_1 and H_2 receptors in guinea pig brain increases cAMP levels. In general, the inflammatory effects of histamine are

TABLE 11–1 COMPARISON OF HISTAMINE ACTION MEDIATED BY H_1 AND H_2 RECEPTORS

	Actions Observed	
	H_1 Receptor	H_2 Receptor
Guinea pig	Slow atrioventricular node conduction time, possibly inducing arrhythmias	Stimulate sinoatrial node leading to an elevated heart rate
	Contract ileum	Increase cardiac inotropic effects
	Contract bronchial smooth muscle	Limit severity of anaphylactic actions *in vivo*
Sheep		Relax tracheal muscle
Rat		Relax uterine muscle
Human	Contract bronchial smooth muscle	Stimulate gastric acid secretion
	Increase in vascular permeability — possibly synergistic with H_2 vascular receptor	Anti-inflammatory effects Inhibition of release of histamine from basophils Inhibition of the capacity of lymphocytes to kill lymphocytes and to produce lymphokines after antigen challenge Inhibition of delayed-type hypersensitivity skin responses *in vivo*

mediated through the H_1 receptors and anti-inflammatory effects through H_2 receptors.

The participation of histamine in human allergic inflammatory responses is supported by numerous studies, although the entire role of this agent in various disorders has not been entirely clarified. Evidence for the participation of histamine in human allergy includes: (1) Histamine levels in tears of patients with vernal conjunctivitis are elevated when compared to levels in tears of normal subjects (Abelson et al., 1977). (2) Elevated plasma histamine levels are found in several clinical settings — during anaphylaxis, during exacerbations of asthma (Simon et al., 1977), in several types of acute urticarial reactions, after aspirin challenge in aspirin-intolerant asthmatics (Stevenson et al., 1976), and following trauma to a mastocytoma. (3) Intravenous infusion of histamine produces a significant decrease in static lung compliance in normal subjects (Laitinen et al., 1976). (4) Increased levels of histamine are found in the sputum of extrinsic asthmatics and patients with chronic bronchitis (Turnbull et al., 1977).

In addition to its role in the production of inflammation, histamine presumably serves various normal regulatory functions. Proposed physiologic roles for histamine include regulation of normal microvascular circulation, enhancement of normal host defense by removal of toxic products of tissue damage, and promotion of tissue growth and repair (Beaven, 1976).

Histamine action can be modified *in vivo* by metabolism of extracellular histamine by histaminase present in plasma, by blocking the action of histamine on histamine receptors on cells, or by decreasing histamine release. Antihistamines in common clinical use, such as chlorpheniramine, block the actions of histamine on H_1 receptors but do not effect H_2 receptors or alter histamine release. They reduce, but do not eliminate, many of the manifestations of reactions that result in the release of histamine, e.g., IgE-mediated reactions. Their ineffectiveness in many instances may be due to an inability to compete successfully with large amounts of histamine, the participation of H_2 receptors in mediating the clinical response, or the action of other mediators not affected by the antihistamines.

Eosinophil Chemotactic Factor of Anaphylaxis (ECF-A). Several eosinophil chemotactic factors have been described. ECF-A, which is released from human mast cells and basophils by reactions which induce histamine release, is thought to be the most important (Austen and Orange, 1975). As implied by its name, this mediator attracts eosinophils potently and relatively selectively. It is a small molecule with a molecular weight of approximately 500 daltons. Similar to histamine, it is present in mast cell granules in an active, preformed state, but unlike histamine, it is found in circulating basophils only after activation of the cells. Although certain proteolytic enzymes can inactivate ECF-A, how it is inactivated or metabolized *in vivo* is not yet known. ECF-A is measured by bioassay, a test performed by only a few laboratories.

Chemotactic responsiveness of eosinophils diminishes (deactivation) after incubation with a constant concentration (i.e., not a gradient) of ECF-A for periods as short as 2 minutes (Wasserman et al., 1975*b*). Other activities of eosinophils are unaffected by exposure to ECF-A. This chemotactic deactivation may permit accumulation of eosinophils in tissues.

Participation of ECF-A in human disease is suggested by the presence of eosinophils in allergic exudates. Other agents, such as histamine, C5a and lymphocyte products, may participate along with ECF-A in attracting eosinophils to sites of inflammation. Elevated blood levels of ECF-A have been detected in experimental cold urticaria and anaphylaxis in the human (Soter et al., 1976).

Slow Reacting Substance of Anaphylaxis (SRS-A). SRS-A is a sulfur-containing acidic ester with a molecular weight of less than 500 daltons. Its structure has not been fully elucidated, but a recently synthesized compound, designated as Leukotreine C, appears to possess activities identical to those of SRS-A. A quantitative bioassay measures prolonged contraction of antihistamine-treated guinea pig ileum (Austen and Orange, 1975).

SRS-A is produced by mast cells and basophils, but unlike histamine is not preformed prior to cell stimulation. SRS-A can be detected intracellularly within minutes after an antigen-antibody reaction on the cell surface. It is distributed throughout the cytoplasm immediately before release. SRS-A can be detected intracellularly but is not released from the cell if a relatively small amount of antigen is used for challenge.

The ratio of SRS-A to the other mediators of immediate hypersensitivity in inflammatory fluids varies from tissue to tissue and with time after the antigen-antibody reaction. The release of preformed mediators, such as histamine, from sensitized lung fragments is more rapid than the release of mediators that are synthesized following the stimulus. Thus in the first 3 to 4 minutes after antigen exposure there is more histamine released than SRS-A. However, by 5 minutes there is twice as much SRS-A as histamine, and by 30 minutes there is six times more SRS-A than histamine. In contrast to the lung, where the ratio of total amount SRS-A to histamine released is approximately 5:1, nasal polyps release more histamine than SRS-A (Brocklehurst, 1975).

The biologic activities of SRS-A are similar to those of histamine, but can be separated from histamine by pretreatment with antihistamines, which inhibit histamine but not SRS-A. SRS-A is a potent contractor of bronchial smooth muscle. Intracutaneous injection of SRS-A increases vascular permeability. Intravenous administration of SRS-A to guinea pigs decreases pulmonary compliance and increases pulmonary resistance. Atropine and other anticholinergic drugs block the increased resistance, but not the changes in compliance and vascular permeability. Histamine and SRS-A appear to act synergistically on certain smooth muscles. The most prominent example is histamine-induced bronchiolar muscle constriction, which is potentiated markedly by SRS-A.

In addition to release from cells and tissue fragments *in vitro,* SRS-A release has been demonstrated in the perfusate of lung removed at surgery from two pollen-sensitive individuals following lung perfusion with the appropriate pollen. It is possible that SRS-A mediates much of the prolonged bronchospasm of asthma.

SRS-A is inactivated by arylsulfatase B, which is present in eosinophils and several other cell types (Wasserman et al., 1975a). Muscle contractions caused by SRS-A can be terminated by epinephrine. When this short-lived bronchodilator or other bronchodilators are metabolized or washed away, contraction from SRS-A returns. Pharmacologic agents that inhibit SRS-A are currently being developed.

Platelet Activating Factor (PAF). PAF is a small phospholipid with a molecular weight of approximately 300 to 500 daltons. It promotes rabbit platelet aggregation and facilitates release of intracellular serotonin and other agents (Henson, 1970). The aggregated platelets appear to promote coagulation. PAF is released from peripheral blood leukocytes of rabbits and humans by IgE-mediated reactions and probably originates in basophils. PAF is degraded by phospholipase D, which is secreted by eosinophils. Although PAF appears to play an important role in the initiation of antigen-induced anaphylaxis in the rabbit (Henson and Pinckard, 1977), its significance in human disease is unclear.

Neutrophil Chemotactic Factor of Anaphylaxis (NCF-A). NCF-A recently has been described by several investigators. It is released from human peripheral basophils and lung fragments and from purified rat mast cells by IgE-dependent mechanisms. It is also present in serum following bronchial challenges of ragweed-sensitive asthmatic patients with ragweed extract, and the level of serum activity correlates with the degree of bronchospasm (Atkins et al., 1978). It appears to be a large protein. Whether NCF-A plays a significant role in the pathogenesis of the inflammatory response is unknown. It may account for the presence of neutrophils late in the course of IgE-mediated reactions (Austen and Orange, 1975).

Kinins. Kinins are polypeptides with numerous roles in inflammation (Kaplan and Austen, 1975). Two major types of kinins have been identified: *bradykinin,* a 9–amino acid peptide formed in the plasma, and *tissue kinins,* which are larger (10 to 11 amino acids). All kinins are present as precursor substances, known as kininogens (Table 11–2). The formation of kinins from kininogens in plasma is dependent on the action of enzymes (kallikreins) on the kininogens. Kallikreins must in turn be acti-

TABLE 11–2 MECHANISM OF ACTIVATION OF THE PLASMA KININ SYSTEM

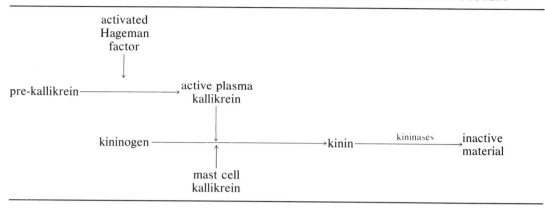

vated from their precursors, pre-kallikreins, before this action can occur. The activation of kallikrein from pre-kallikrein is mediated by Hageman factor activated during clotting. Kallikrein-like substances that can activate kininogens are released from mast cells and basophils by reactions that induce histamine release. Kinins are rapidly inactivated by kininases located in the plasma and tissues (Table 11–2).

The various biologic actions of kinins (Cochrane, 1976) include: (1) contraction of certain smooth muscles, e.g., bronchiolar constriction in man, (2) vasodilation, (3) increase in vascular permeability, (4) pain, redness, and edema of skin, (5) increase in secretion of sweat and salivary glands, and (6) vasodepressor activities. Generally, tissue kinins are less active than plasma bradykinin in causing smooth muscle contraction, but are more potent as permeability factors and have a more potent action on the cardiovascular system.

Kinins may play a role in producing symptoms of hay fever, angioedema, and asthma. Kinins have been found in nasal secretions of allergic individuals following local instillation of pollens, and in skin after antigen injection. Some patients with cold urticaria have increased serum levels of bradykinin, and kinins often can be found in the urticarial lesions. Increased levels of kinins have been found in the blood of patients with asthma or carcinoid syndrome, while decreased kininogen levels have been found during acute anaphylaxis in humans. Since kinins are present in blister fluid after burns, activation of bradykinin has been suggested as an important mediator in other inflammatory states. Kinins may also play a role in inflammation in both gouty and rheumatoid arthritis.

SECONDARY MEDIATORS

Prostaglandins. The prostaglandins (PG's) are a family of naturally occurring 20-carbon unsaturated hydroxyl aliphatic acids with wide biologic activity (Hyman et al., 1978). In most organ systems, arachidonic acid is the precursor of PG's. The synthetic sequence is initiated when arachidonic acid is cleaved from cell membrane phospholipids by phospholipases. The release of arachidonic acid is the rate limiting step in PG formation. PG formation is enhanced during inflammation, which increases release of phospholipases into tissue fluid and damages cell membranes, making phospholipid more accessible. PG synthetase, found abundantly in all tissues, converts the newly formed arachidonic acid to prostaglandins of various types; these are released rapidly into the circulation. The lungs play a major role in both the synthesis and the inactivation of PGs, because they contain large amounts of both PG synthetase and PG-inactivating enzymes. Increased systemic levels of PGs are associated with diminished functional lung tissue and may be responsible for some of the systemic manifestations of lung diseases (Kadowitz et al., 1975).

PG's have diverse tissue effects and act through various specific tissue receptors. In general, PG's decrease pain threshold, dilate and increase permeability of capillaries, and contract smooth muscle. Their specific effects on the lungs depend on the the type of PG: PGE_1 and PGE_2 cause dilation of smooth muscle, while $PGF_{2\alpha}$ causes constriction. The vasodilating effects of PGE are particularly prominent in the presence of increased tone produced by hypoxia or by stimulation with other vasoactive agents. PG's also have indirect effects on smooth muscle since they control release of mediators from pulmonary mast cells by influencing their intracellular levels of cAMP and cGMP. PGE_1 and PGE_2 stimulate cAMP formation to inhibit mediator release, whereas $PGF_{2\alpha}$ increases cGMP to increase mediator release. Consequently, the amount, as well as type of PG found at a particular tissue site probably influences the resulting clinical symptoms (Hyman et al., 1978). PG's potentiate the pain produced by bradykinin and also histaminic actions on certain tissues (Eakins and Bhattacherjee, 1977).

Asthmatic patients have elevated levels of both serum PGE_1 and $PGF_{2\alpha}$, and a greater amount of $PGF_{2\alpha}$ relative to PGE_1 when compared to normal individuals (Nemoto et al., 1976). When given by aerosol, $PGF_{2\alpha}$ induces bronchoconstriction. Aerosolized PGE may produce bronchodilatation, but the aerosol solution is irritating and its clinical usefulness is limited (Piper, 1977).

Several methods of altering PG activity have been identified. Nonsteroid antiinflammatory drugs, such as aspirin and indomethacin, are inhibitors of PG synthetase and prevent the formation of PG's. These drugs can be used to alter tissue and circulating levels. Steroids inhibit the release of arachidonic acid, thus decreasing the amount of substrate available for prostaglandin formation. Postulated mechanisms of this steroid action include decreasing susceptibility of cell membranes to the activity of phospholipases, or directly inhibiting release of these enzymes during the inflammatory reaction (Hong and Levine, 1976; Lewis and Piper, 1975).

Mediators of the Autonomic Nervous System. The autonomic nervous system regulates activities of structures that are not under voluntary control and that, as a rule, function below the level of consciousness. Thus, respiration, circulation, digestion, body temperature, metabolism, sweating, and secretions of certain endocrine glands are regulated, in part or entirely, by the autonomic nervous system and its central nervous system connections. Actions of the sympathetic and parasympathetic systems tend to be antagonistic to each other, and this dual antagonism is considered of prime physiologic importance (Koelle, 1975).

The *parasympathetic system* is organized mainly for discrete and localized discharge of acetylcholine at the postganglionic terminal portion of the system. Localization of the effects of parasympathetic stimulation also are ensured by the exceedingly rapid inactivation of acetylcholine by cholinesterases. The parasympathetic system is concerned primarily with the conservation and restoration of energy rather than with its expenditure. For example, parasympathetic activity slows heart rate, lowers blood pressure, stimulates gastrointestinal movement and secretion, aids in absorption of nutrients, and protects the retina from excessive light exposure. Parasympathetic fibers, via the vagus nerve, supply the secretory tissue and smooth muscle of the respiratory tract and play an important role in regulating airway smooth muscle tone in normal subjects. Interference with vagal tone, either by cutting the vagus nerve or by administering atropine, causes bronchodilatation. Conversely, activation of irritant or cough receptors in large airways of asthmatic patients causes bronchoconstriction, which is mediated by vagal efferent nerve activity. Acetylcholine released at nerve endings in the respiratory tract also may influence the actions of other drugs at the level of the smooth muscle, either potentiating or inhibiting their action.

Acetylcholine and the parasympathetic nervous system may play a role in the pathogenesis of cholinergic urticaria, a condition in which small wheals surrounded by a prominent flare appear after exercise, hot showers, sweating, or anxiety (Kaplan, 1977). These patients have a hypersensitivity to cholinergic mediators, and the characteristic lesion can be reproduced by intradermal injection of methacholine. The exact mechanism of formation of the lesions is unknown. The intense itching that occurs with these lesions may be related to histamine release, but this has been demonstrated in only a small number of patients whose symptoms were particularly severe (Kaplan et al., 1975).

The three naturally occurring catecholamines, dopamine, norepinephrine and epinephrine, are the chemical transmitters of the *sympathetic nervous system*. They are synthesized in specialized neuroendocrine cells that are widely distributed throughout the body. Dopamine is an important neurotransmitter in basal ganglia of the central nervous system and in the peripheral autonomic ganglia. Norepinephrine is the neurotransmitter at postganglionic sympathetic nerve terminals, whereas epinephrine is the major hormone of the adrenal medulla and is the major "systemic" humoral agent. In addition to continuous activity in any given organ, the entire sympathoadrenal system can discharge as a unit. This occurs especially during rage and fright, when sympathetically innervated structures over the entire body are affected simultaneously. Many of the local effects in the rage and fright reaction result from adrenal medullary secretion of epinephrine into the systemic circulation.

Norepinephrine, epinephrine, and other adrenergic agents can cause either excitation or inhibition of smooth muscle, depending on the site and the type of adrenergic receptor present in the tissue. Two major types of adrenergic receptors, alpha and beta, have been defined. In addition, there are at least two subpopulations of beta receptors (beta$_1$ and beta$_2$), which mediate somewhat different physiologic functions. Although the specific response of stimulation of adrenergic receptors varies with the tissue, alpha receptors generally mediate excitatory responses and beta receptors generally mediate inhibitory responses. For example, alpha receptors mediate contraction of the iris ciliary muscle, whereas beta receptors mediate relaxation.

Sympathomimetic agents are widely used as bronchodilators in the treatment of asthma. Although the role the sympathetic nervous system plays in the maintenance of normal bronchial smooth muscle tone is not completely clear, sympathomimetic activity is believed to be important in regulating airway patency. Human bronchial smooth muscle does not appear to have sympathetic innervation, so that if the prominent beta receptors in the human bronchi play any role in the normal respiratory function, they must be activated by circulating catecholamines, especially epinephrine. It has been suggested that the underlying basis of asthma and other atopic disorders may be a derangement in beta receptor function (see Chapter 14).

Stimulation of beta adrenergic receptors on the surface of cells activates adenylate cyclase and enhances the formation of cAMP. In *in vitro* studies, elevated levels of cAMP inhibit the release of mediators from mast cells, lysosomal enzymes from neutrophils and monocyte-macrophages, and lymphokines from lymphocytes. It is uncertain to what extent these anti-inflammatory effects of beta adrenergic stimulation are important clinically.

Lymphokines. When sensitized lymphocytes interact with antigen, a number of soluble substances are released that possess a variety of biologic actions important in the process of cell-mediated immunity. These lymphocyte-derived mediators collectively are known as lymphokines (Waksman, 1971), and serve as an amplification system, acting, for example, to recruit and activate inflammatory cells and to keep them at the site of inflammation, predisposing to intimate contact between various cells. This is a necessary part of "cellular immunity."

Relatively few of these lymphocyte mediators have been purified sufficiently for simple detection, and the total number involved in cellular immunity has yet to be determined. The best known and understood lymphokine is migration inhibition factor (MIF), a protein that acts upon macrophages to inhibit their migration, possibly by increasing aggregation and cell adherence. The clumping together of cells may physically impede subsequent migration from the area of inflammation. Other actions of lymphokines include nonspecifically lysing cells in an area of inflammation; enhancing migration of macrophages, PMN's, eosinophils, and basophils (Lett-Brown et al., 1976); increasing vascular permeability; stimulating mast cells to release histamine; inducing transformation of normal, nonsensitized, lymphocytes; and activating osteoblasts to decalcify bone.

Thus, lymphokines play important roles

in the development of cellular immune reactions. Their amplification of an initially small reaction may be critical to the successful host inflammatory response to a particular antigen.

Neutrophil-derived Mediators. PMN's contain enzymes that play various roles in the inflammatory process. The best known of these are the bactericidal and digestive functions that occur when enzymes stored in lysosomal granules are released into phagocytic vacuoles within the cells. In addition, enzymes stored in granules are released extracellularly during phagocytosis and when PMN's contact immune complexes or tissue-bound IgG. Biologic properties of PMN-derived extracellular enzymes include: antibacterial activity; conversion of the precursor complement proteins, C1s, C4, C3 and C5, to their active, split products, which have chemotactic and other activities (Venge and Olsson, 1975); inactivation of chemotactic activity of the chemotactic fragments after prolonged contact (Venge and Olsson, 1975); and, degradation of various tissue constituents. The activation of the complement components is by direct action of proteolytic enzymes and is independent of either major pathway of complement activation. A recent study described two separate protease systems stored in separate intracellular granules, one responsible for the activation and the other for the degradation of chemotactic factors. These granules are released sequentially during phagocytosis, with the activators appearing earlier (Wright and Gallin, 1977). The activators function only at neutral pH, while the inactivators function at both neutral and acid pH.

Contact of phagocytic cells with antigen-antibody complexes or tissue-bound IgG also can induce phagocytic cells to release products of oxidative metabolism, e.g., superoxide anion and hydrogen peroxide. These metabolites are highly toxic and have the capacity to induce oxidative tissue damage at sites of inflammation (see Chapters 8 and 5).

Mediators Generated During Complement Activation. The complement system, acting as a primary humoral mediator of antigen-antibody reactions, consists of a series of chemically and immunologically distinct serum proteins that possess many effector functions. Two distinct and independent mechanisms for complement activation, termed the "classic" and "alternative" pathways, both result in activation of components C3 and C5 through C9. The by-products of the activation of these "terminal" components are responsible for the majority of the biological activities of the complement system, which are extremely important to the immunologic modulation of the inflammatory host response. The complete complement system and the role of the various activating agents is detailed in Chapter 5.

Some of the by-products of complement activation enhance the inflammatory process both directly, through actions on the vascular system and cellular components of inflammation, and indirectly, by stimulating the release of other soluble mediators. An example of these dual roles is represented by the low molecular weight fragments split from C3 (C3a) and C5 (C5a) during their activation. Both fragments are anaphylatoxins, releasing histamine from tissue mast cells. Injection of C3a intradermally is followed by a typical wheal and flare reaction (Wuepper et al., 1972). C5a has chemotactic activity primarily for PMN's (Fernandez et al., 1978), but it also attracts monocytes, eosinophils and basophils (Lett-Brown et al., 1976). In addition, these compounds stimulate PMN's to release lysosomal enzymes.

Other soluble products released during complement activation include a fragment of C2 with kinin-like activity; a fragment of C3 distinct from C3a that stimulates leukocytosis by mobilization of PMN's from bone marrow; the trimolecular complex, $\overline{C567}$, which can be formed in the fluid phase and has chemotactic activity; and the split product of activation of factor B (Ba) of the alternative pathway, which has chemotactic activity (Hamuro et al., 1978). The generation of the C2-kinin during classic pathway activation is dependent on the presence of activated plasmin and is thought to be responsible for the clinical manifestations of hereditary angioneurotic edema, a disease due to genetic deficiency of the inhibitor of the first component of complement (see Chapter 33).

Thus, the complement system, through its

intermediate products, can stimulate chemotaxis and activation of several types of cells and induce smooth muscle contraction. During homeostasis the system is kept in check by several inhibitors that inactivate the complement components and by the inherent lability of several of the activated complement intermediates.

THE CHEMICAL MEDIATOR SYSTEM — A PERSPECTIVE

Information about the mediators of inflammation has accumulated rapidly in the last 10 to 15 years. New mediators are still being described, and studies are under way to define their role in the inflammatory process. Examples of these new mediators are high molecular weight heparin and the intermediate weight eosinophil chemotactic factors, both released from mast cells during IgE-mediated reactions. Heparin is known to inhibit the functions of the first component of complement (C1) and the C3-converting enzyme formed during activation of the alternative complement pathway. These observations suggest that heparin may modulate the inflammatory process. The intermediate molecular weight eosinophil chemotactic factors may provide a more continuous gradient for the attraction of eosinophils than would occur with the single low molecular weight ECF-A alone. Other new mediators generated during the activation of neutrophils and lymphocytes are being defined. In addition to the study of the structure and function of individual mediators, there is more to be learned about the mechanisms of their release and about the interaction of individual mediators, which modulate the release and functions of the other mediators.

In the past several years, general understanding of the inflammatory process has been advanced by the recognition that individual components of the response interact extensively, in addition to having their own individual actions. It has become clear that various defense systems are intimately interwoven and that these various systems rarely act in isolation (Ratnoff, 1976). Although these interactions are highly complex and often difficult to elucidate, further understanding of these interactions undoubtedly will stimulate new pharmacologic approaches to the alteration of inflammatory responses.

Although the classic Gell and Coombs classification of immunologic reactions has provided a useful framework for the early study of the role of mediators in immune reactions, it is probably overly simplistic, however, considering the overlap of the various types of immunologic reactions and mediator systems that occur during host responses to foreign agents. For example, the fact that mediators released from mast cells played a major role in the pathogenesis of type I hypersensitivity reactions was recognized long ago. More recently, activation products of the complement system, C3a and C5a, and lymphokines also have been shown to stimulate mast cells to release mediators. Thus it is probable that mast cell–derived mediators are involved in all four types of inflammatory reactions as classified by Gell and Coombs. In addition, mediators from mast cells derived from mastocytomas participate in reactions that are initiated by nonimmunologic tissue injury or by direct mechanical, cold, or chemical stimulation of tissue not associated with injury. It is likely that similar mechanisms operate in normal mast cells. Similar considerations apply to the participation and interactions of various cell types in the inflammatory response. Although one cell type generally predominates in any given type of inflammatory response, all cell types probably are involved directly or indirectly in every type of response. For example, in type I hypersensitivity, eosinophils, neutrophils and platelets are activated by various mast cell mediators and all three cell types are involved in the production of the ultimate reaction.

It should be obvious that the system of soluble mediators is varied and complex. The wide-ranging interactions provide an efficient mechanism for response to various stimuli. The responses are as vigorous when the system is initiated by various hypersensitivity states as during clearance of invading microorganisms. Modulation of these responses by altering actions of the individual components or by interfering with interactions between the various components of the system provides a useful pharmacologic approach to therapy of a wide variety of diseases.

References

Abelson, M. B., Soter, N. A., Simon, M. A., Dohlman, J., and Allansmith, M. R.: Histamine in human tears. Am. J. Ophthalmol. 83:417, 1977.

Atkins, P. C., Norman, M. E., and Zweiman, B.: Antigen-induced neutrophil chemotactic activity in man. Correlation with bronchospasm and inhibition by disodium cromoglycate. J. Allergy Clin. Immunol. 62:149, 1978.

Austen, K. F.: Histamine and other mediators of allergic reactions. In Samter, M.: Immunological Diseases. Boston, Little, Brown & Co., 1971, pp. 332–335.

Austen, K. F., and Orange, R. P.: Bronchial asthma: The possible role of the chemical mediators of immediate hypersensitivity in the pathogenesis of subacute chronic disease. Am. Rev. Respir. Dis. 112:423, 1975.

Beaven, M. A., Jacobsen, S., and Horakova, Z.: Modification of an enzymatic isotropic assay of histamine and its application to measurement of histamine in tissues, serum, and urine. Clin. Chim. Acta 37:91, 1972.

Beaven, M. A.: Histamine N. Engl. J. Med. 294:30, 1976.

Black, J. W., Duncan, W. A., Durant, C. J., Ganellin, C. R., and Parsons, E. M.: Definition and antagonism of histamine H_2-receptors. Nature 236:385, 1972.

Brocklehurst, W. E.: Pharmacological mediators of hypersensitivity reactions. In Gell, P. G. H., Coombs, R. R. A., and Lachmann, P. J. (eds.): Clinical Aspects of Immunology, 2nd Ed., Philadelphia, J. B. Lippincott Co., 1975, pp. 821–857.

Cochrane, C. G.: The Hageman factor pathways of kinin formation, clotting, and fibrinolysis. In Beers, R. F., and Bassett, E. G. (eds.): Role of Immunological Factors in Infections, Allergic, and Autoimmune Processes. New York, Raven Press, 1976, pp. 237–246.

Eakins, K. E., and Bhattacherjee, P.: Histamine, prostaglandins and ocular inflammation. Exp. Eye Res. 24:299, 1977.

Fernandez, H. N., Henson, P. M., Otani, A., and Hugli, T. E.: Chemotactic response to human C3a and C5a anaphylatoxins. I. Evaluation of C3a and C5a leukotaxis in vitro and under simulated in vivo conditions. J. Immunol. 120:109, 1978.

Hamuro, J., Hadding, U., and Bitter-Suermann, D.: Fragments Ba and Bb derived from guinea pig factor B of the properdin system: Purification, characterization, and biological activities. J. Immunol. 120:438, 1978.

Henson, P. M., and Pinckard, R. N.: Basophil-derived platelet-activating factor (PAF) as an in vivo mediator of acute allergic reactions: Demonstration of specific desensitization of platelets to PAF during IgE-induced anaphylaxis in the rabbit. J. Immunol. 119:2179, 1977.

Henson, P. M.: Release of vasoactive amines from rabbit platelets induced by sensitized mononuclear leukocytes and antigen. J. Exp. Med. 131:287, 1970.

Hong, S. L., and Levine, L.: Inhibition of arachidonic acid release from cells as the biochemical action of anti-inflammatory corticosteroids. Proc. Natl. Acad. Sci., USA 73:1730, 1976.

Hyman, A. L., Spannhake, E. W., and Kadowitz, P. J.: Prostaglandins and the lung. Am. Rev. Respir. Dis. 117:111, 1978.

Kadowitz, P. J., Joiner, P. D., and Hyman, A. L.: Physiological and pharmacological roles of prostaglandins. Annu. Rev. Pharmacol. 15:285, 1975.

Kaplan, A. P., Gray, L., Shaff, R. E., Horakova, Z., and Beaven, M. A.: In vivo studies of mediator release in cold urticaria and cholinergic urticaria. J. Allergy Clin. Immunol. 55:394, 1975.

Kaplan, A. P.: Mediators of urticaria and angioedema. J. Allergy Clin. Immunol. 60:324, 1977.

Kaplan, A. P., and Austen, K. F.: Activation and control mechanisms of Hageman factor–dependent pathways of coagulation, fibrinolysis, and kinin generation and their contribution to the inflammatory response. J. Allergy Clin. Immunol. 56:491, 1975.

Koelle, G. B.: Neurohumoral transmission and the autonomic nervous system. In Goodman, L. S., and Gilman, A. (eds.): The Pharmacological Basis of Therapeutics. New York, Macmillan Publishing Co., Inc., 1975. pp. 404–444.

Laitinen, L. A., Empey, D. W., Poppius, H., Lemen, R. J., Gold, W. M., and Nadel, J. A.: Effects of intravenous histamine on static lung compliance and airway resistance in normal man. Am. Rev. Respir. Dis. 114:291, 1976.

Lett-Brown, M. A., Boetcher, D. A., and Leonard, E. J.: Chemotactic responses of normal human basophils to C5a and to lymphocyte-derived chemotactic factor. J. Immunol. 117:246, 1976.

Lewis, G. P., and Piper, P. J.: Inhibition of release of prostaglandins as an explanation of some of the actions of anti-inflammatory corticosteroids. Nature 254:308, 1975.

Nemoto, T., Aoki, H., Aiko, I., Yamada, K., Kondo, T., Kobayashi, S., and Inagawa, T.: Serum prostaglandin levels in asthmatic patients. J. Allergy Clin. Immunol. 57:89, 1976.

Piper, P. J.: Anaphylaxis and the release of active substances in lungs. J. Pharmacol. Ther. (B) 3:75, 1977.

Plaut, M., and Lichtenstein, L. M.: Cellular and chemical basis of the allergic inflammatory response. Component parts and control mechanisms. In Middleton, E., Reed, C. E., and Ellis, E. F. (eds.): Allergy, Principles and Practice. St. Louis, C. V. Mosby and Co., 1978, pp. 115–138.

Ratnoff, O. D.: Mediators of inflammation. J. Allergy Clin. Immunol. 58:438, 1976.

Simon, R. A., Stevenson, D. D., Arroyave, C. M., and Tan, E. M.: The relationship of plasma histamine to the activity of bronchial asthma. J. Allergy Clin. Immunol. 60:312, 1977.

Soter, N. A., Wasserman, S. I., and Austen, K. F.: Cold urticaria: Release into the circulation of histamine and ECF-A during cold challenge. N. Engl. J. Med. 294:687, 1976.

Stevenson, D. D., Arroyave, C. M., Bhat, K. N., and Tan, E. M.: Oral ASA challenges in asthmatic patients: A study of plasma histamine. Clin. Allergy 6:493, 1976.

Turnbull, L. S., Turnbull, L. W., Leitch, A. G., Crofton, J. W., and Kay, A. B.: Mediators of immediate-type hypersensitivity in sputum from patients with chronic bronchitis and asthma. Lancet 2:526, 1977.

Venge, P., and Olsson, I.: Cationic proteins of human granulocytes. VI. Effects on the complement system and mediation of chemotactic activity. J. Immunol. 115:1505, 1975.

Waksman, B. H.: Delayed (cellular) hypersensitivity. In Samter, M. (ed.): Immunological Diseases. Boston, Little, Brown & Co., 1971, pp. 220–252.

Wasserman, S. I., Goetzl, E. J., and Austen, K. F.: Inactivation of slow reacting substance of anaphylaxis by human eosinophil arylsulfatase. J. Immunol. 114:645, 1975a.

Wasserman, S. I., Whitmer, D., Goetzl, E. J., and Austen, K. F.: Chemotactic deactivation of human eosinophils by eosinophil chemotactic factor of anaphylaxis. Proc. Soc. Exp. Biol. Med. 148:301, 1975b.

Wright, D. G., and Gallin, J. I.: A functional differentiation of human neutrophil granules: Generation of C5a by a specific (secondary) granule product and inactivation of C5a by azurophil (primary) granule products. J. Immunol. 119:1068, 1977.

Wuepper, K. D., Bokisch, V. A., Müller-Eberhard, H. J., and Stoughton, R. B.: Cutaneous responses to human C3 anaphylatoxin in man. Clin. Exp. Immunol. 11:13, 1972.

12

Abraham H. Eisen, M.D.

Eosinophils

In 1879, Paul Ehrlich described distinctive cells with large, brightly staining granules in smears of peripheral blood. He named the cells "eosinophils" for their affinity for the acid stain eosin (Ehrlich, 1879). It was soon noted that the number of eosinophils was increased in patients with allergic disorders, especially those with eczema and late onset asthma, also in patients with drug reactions, parasitic infestations, certain collagen vascular diseases, and in patients with some malignancies. Rarely, patients with recurrent pulmonary infiltrates or obscure gastrointestinal abnormalities also had tissue and/or peripheral eosinophilia. Despite one hundred years of clinical observation, the precise mechanism(s) of inducing eosinophilia and the function(s) of these cells still are unknown.

DESCRIPTION

Under the light microscope, the eosinophil appears as a white blood cell granulocyte 12 to 17 microns in diameter, with a bilobed (occasionally trilobed) nucleus. The cytoplasm contains large, refractile granules that stain orange with eosin. In common with other mature granulocytes, the nucleus does not contain a nucleolus, indicating that production of ribosomal RNA has ceased.

When viewed under the electronmicroscope, three types of granules are apparent. The predominant type of granule has an electron dense core and a less dense matrix. There is reversal of this usual staining pattern when the cells are stained for peroxidase, which localizes in the matrix. Under very high magnification, the core is seen to be composed of a crystalline substructure with a cubic lattice of 40 angstroms. A second type of granule is smaller and is bound by a membrane. This granule contains acid phosphatase and aryl sulfatase. The third type of granule is large, often with no limiting membrane, and the electron dense material has a sunburst appearance. Other enzymes associated with the granules in man and other species include cathepsin, ribonuclease, sulfatase, beta glucuronidase, and alkaline phosphatase. Antihistaminic and antibradykinin substances and a plasminogen have been described but have never been localized, and their presence in eosinophils is not uniformly accepted.

KINETICS

Eosinophils in man originate from a stem cell (myeloblast); there is evidence that this stem cell is different from those that give rise to the neutrophil and basophil. Once the myelocyte stage is reached, the cell is committed to the eosinophil line and contains enzymes specific for eosinophils in the rough endoplasmic reticulum, Golgi cisternae, and immature granules. The normal life cycle is from bone marrow to blood to tissue. The blood to tissue ratio in man is 1:100, suggesting that the eosinophils are not primarily blood cells but appear there en route to the tissues. The blood half-life of the eosinophil has been estimated to be 4.5 to 5 hours (Herion et al., 1970). However, in a recent study, eosinophils from hypereosinophilic patients were radio-labeled with chromium 51 and reinjected into the patients: there was an initial fall followed by an increase in radioactivity peaking at 6 to 24 hours, and then a slow decline with a half-life of 44 hours (Dale et al., 1976). This study showed that eosinophils recirculate and that the short half-life initially described may reflect only part of the circulation pattern. The tissue half-life and the precise mechanism of destruction are not known. Tracer studies suggest that loss of eosinophils occurs in a random fashion, probably in the gastrointestinal tract and perhaps in the uterus. Eosinophils have an affinity for estrogenic compounds and are present in increased amounts in the rat uterus during estrus. After estrus, the cells undergo lysis and are phagocytosed (Ross and Klebanoff, 1966).

The number of peripheral blood eosinophils varies with a circadian rhythm, and the total eosinophil count (TEC) varies inversely with the concentration of 17-hydroxycorticosteroids. Thus, eosinophil counts normally are low at 9:30 a.m. and high in the early hours of the morning.

CHEMOTAXIS

Normally, eosinophils exhibit random motion, but they can respond by direct movement to a chemotactic stimulus. There are a number of factors that are chemotactic for eosinophils:

Eosinophil Chemotactic Factor of Complement (ECF-C). When complement is activated, either through the classic or alternative pathway, the activated components C5a and C5b67, are chemotactic for both eosinophils and polymorphonuclear leukocytes (Ward, 1969).

Eosinophil Chemotactic Factor of Anaphylaxis (ECF-A). When lung tissue *in vitro* or *in vivo* is sensitized actively or passively with IgE (for guinea pig gamma$_1$ globulin) and the tissue is challenged with specific antigen, the lung tissue will release ECF-A. This material is preformed and released from mast cells and basophils (Kay et al., 1971). It has a molecular weight of 500

daltons; its release is modulated by cyclic AMP, with enhancement of release when cyclic AMP decreases. Cation (calcium) and intact glycolytic pathways are required for release. ECF-A acts synergistically with C5a. Recently, eosinophil chemotactic substances with molecular weights varying between 1500 and 2500 daltons have been described in rat mast cell granules. It has been suggested that the release by the mast cell of several chemotactic factors differing in size and charge stabilizes the chemotactic gradient and sustains a constant influx of eosinophils (Boswell et al., 1978).

Lymphokine Chemotactic Factors. Lymphocytes, under certain conditions, will release soluble factors chemotactic for eosinophils. In one study, animals were sensitized with o-chlorobenzoyl bovine gamma globulin (OCB gamma globulin). The lymphocytes from these animals were then incubated with OCB gamma globulin followed by a second incubation with guinea pig antibovine gamma globulin–bovine gamma globulin complexes. The supernatant from this mixture was chemotactic specifically for eosinophils (Cohen and Ward, 1971). In another experiment, lymphocytes from animals infected with *Schistosoma mansoni* were incubated with a soluble extract of *S. mansoni*. The supernatant from this mixture was chemotactic for eosinophils. The active material had a molecular weight of 2400 to 5600 daltons and was heat stable (Colley, 1973).

Spontaneous Eosinophil Chemotactic Activity (SECA). Sera from some patients with rheumatoid arthritis, vasculitis, and acute nephritis have chemotactic properties. The serum factor is heat stable and possibly related to C5a.

FUNCTION

The precise function or functions of eosinophils are not known. In general, eosinophils behave like polymorphonuclear leukocytes (PMN's) in terms of motility and phagocytosis.

Motility. The eosinophil and PMN can move at comparable speeds, although initial reports suggested that the eosinophil was more sluggish.

Phagocytosis. Eosinophils phagocytose zymosan particles, coated red blood cells, gram-positive and gram-negative bacteria, mycoplasma, and mast cell granules, and have a particular avidity for immune complexes in which the antibody is IgE. Phagocytosis occurs in the conventional way with pinocytosis and progressive engulfment of the particle into a membrane-limited vacuole (phagosome). Degranulation occurs shortly after the phagosome vacuole is completed; the granule membranes coalesce with the phagosome membrane and discharge their enzyme contents into the vacuole. Sometimes the matrix of the granule is seen to surround the particle, while the core remains intact. With respect to bacterial killing, the eosinophil has a myeloperoxidase hydrogen peroxide–halide system, with production of superoxide and singlet oxygen. Resting iodination in eosinophils is higher than in PMN's. After phagocytosis, PMN's have a three- to fourfold increase in iodination, whereas eosinophils show no such increase. The eosinophil has a resting level of oxidative metabolism higher than that of PMN's, with a higher hexose monophosphate and reduced nicotinamide adenine dinucleotide phosphate (NADPH) oxidase activity. In addition, inhibition of myeloperoxidase in PMN's inhibits bacterial killing, whereas it enhances killing power in eosinophils. Thus, while there are similarities between eosinophils and PMN's, there are sufficient differences to suggest that phagocytosis and killing of bacteria are not primary functions of eosinophils (Bujak and Root, 1974).

Recent studies on the interaction between eosinophils and parasites are of particular interest with regard to the function of eosinophils. The parasite presents a large, non-phagocytosable object to the eosinophil. Eosinophils possess receptors for the Fc portion of IgG (MacKenzie et al., 1977) and adhere to parasites through IgG antibody directed towards antigens on the parasite membrane. The initial response of the eosinophil after adherence to the parasite membrane is degranulation, with formation of large cytoplasmic vacuoles. Peroxidase is discharged into the vacuole. The vacuole becomes connected to the basal membrane adherent to the parasite surface, and the peroxidase eventually is secreted directly onto the surface of the parasite (McLaren et al., 1977). As a result of adherence and enzyme activity, there are changes in the permeability of the parasite membrane as measured by chromium 51 release and methylene blue uptake. The precise mechanism of damage, if any, to the parasitic membrane, however, is not understood.

Human eosinophils also can be shown to adhere to non-phagocytosable sepharose beads treated with serum. Adherence to the beads depends on the C3 component of serum and not on IgG. Further, the release of aryl sulfatase and other eosinophil-specific enzymes is dependent on C3. Enzyme release requires magnesium and occurs in sera deficient in C2, C4, C5, and C6, suggesting a requirement for the activation of the complement through the alternative pathway (Metcalfe et al., 1977). Thus, eosinophils encountering a non-phagocytosable surface that can activate the alternative pathway will adhere to that surface and release granule-associated enzymes. Once the immune response is activated, adherence will be enhanced by the presence of specific antibody.

Studies of Eosinophil Function

Probes into eosinophil function fall into three major categories, namely, clinical observations, animal models, and immunochemical analysis of eosinophil subcellular components.

Clinical Observations. Eosinophils are intimately associated with the immune system. They always are present in the thymus, thoracic duct, and lymph nodes. Immature eosinophils sometimes are seen in the thymus, suggesting that the thymus may be a site of maturation and proliferation for eosinophils. Elevated numbers of eosinophils are seen in the peripheral blood of the most profoundly immunodeficient patients, e.g., patients with severe combined immunodeficiency. In chronic benign hypereosinophilic states, suppression of eosinophilia (and presumably the inflammatory process), usually with steroid therapy, is associated with clinical improvement. In the progressive fatal hypereosinophilic states, there is no response to treatment and there is evidence to suggest that tissue damage is mediated by mature eosinophils. In general, clinical evidence can be interpreted in two ways — the eosinophil mediates tissue damage or the eosinophil is protective to the patient.

Animal Models. There are several methods of inducing eosinophilia in laboratory animals. Repeated intravenous (not subcutaneous or intraperitoneal) injection of *Trichinella* larvae results in impaction of the larvae in small vessels, followed by an inflammatory reaction with large mononuclear cells. Eosinophilia begins the third day after injections commence, and peaks on the sixth day (Basten et al., 1970). Repeated injection of foreign protein also will lead to local or systemic eosinophilia (Spiers, 1955). Immune complexes administered intraperitoneally lead to peritoneal eosinophilia, and when guinea pigs are passively sensitized with gamma$_1$ globulin antibody and then are injected with the corresponding antigen, blood eosinophilia results. All antibodies that sensitize for passive cutaneous anaphylaxis or systemic anaphylaxis mediate blood and local eosinophilia upon injection of the antigen (Parish, 1970).

It has been claimed that histamine can induce local eosinophilia, but there is controversy on this point (Eidinger et al., 1964). Cellular immune mechanisms may play a role in eosinophilia. The inductive phase of eosinophilia is thought to be dependent on T lymphocytes, based on the following observations: antilymphocyte serum interferes with the development of eosinophilia following an appropriate stimulus. Thymectomized mice do not respond to appropriate stimuli with eosinophilia, and adult mice that are thymectomized, lethally irradiated, and reconstituted with bone marrow do not respond with eosinophilia until grafted with a thymus (Basten and Beeson, 1970). The proliferative phase of eosinophilia can be blocked with either methotrexate or cyclophosphamide (Boyer et al., 1970).

When eosinophils are injected into rabbits, antisera to eosinophil surface membrane antigens are produced. Such antieosinophilic sera (AES) may partially cross-react with polymorphonuclear leukocytes, although they are more cytotoxic to eosinophils. AES injected into guinea pigs markedly reduces the number of eosinophils in peripheral blood and peritoneum, and produces a milder decrease in the bone marrow, spleen, and duodenum (Gleich et al., 1975). AES decreases granuloma formation in lungs of animals infected with *S. mansoni* and abolishes partial immunity to *S. mansoni,* suggesting that eosinophils play an important role in the resistance to parasites (Mahmoud et al., 1975).

Immunochemical Analysis of Eosinophils and Eosinophil Granules. The electron dense portion of the eosinophil granule contains a protein that is highly basic by virtue of its high arginine content. Since this basic protein constitutes the major protein component of the granule, it is termed *major basic protein* (MBP). The precise function of MBP is not clear. It has weak antibacterial activity, precipitates with desoxyribonucleic acid, neutralizes heparin (heparin is acidic), and activates papain. It does not increase vascular permeability or contract guinea pig ileum, and there is no appreciable antihistamine activity (Gleich et al., 1974).

Charcot-Leyden crystals (CLC) have been observed for many years in pulmonary secretions from patients with eosinophilia. CLC is a protein different from MBP, with a higher molecular weight and a different amino acid sequence. The function, if any, of CLC is unknown (Gleich et al., 1976).

Disruption of eosinophils from allergic patients releases a supernatant that can inhibit IgE-mediated histamine release from peripheral leukocytes. The inhibitory factor (eosinophil-derived inhibitor or EDI) is preformed and is released in small amounts without stimulation, suggesting that a secretory process is involved in its release. It has been hypothesized that eosinophils recognize specific antigen through membrane-associated IgE antibody, avidly phagocytose antigen-IgE-antibody complexes, and release EDI as a result of phagocytosis (Hubscher, 1975). The eosinophil enzyme, aryl sulfatase, is capable of inactivating slow reactive substance of anaphylaxis (Wasserman et al., 1975), and histaminase contained by eosinophils inactivates histamine (Zeiger et al., 1976). These observations suggest that the role of the eosinophil is to modulate the allergic inflammatory reaction.

Just as the clinical data on the eosinophil can be viewed in two ways, so the laboratory data lends itself to two interpretations. In the first, the eosinophil's main function is to modify allergic inflammation and prevent tissue damage. In the second, the eosinophil is a primary effector (killer) cell, directed towards foreign antigens (parasites) and equipped to neutralize and/or phagocytose the invading organism. If the second interpretation is correct, the presence of eosinophils in allergic reactions may be only incidental to the release of chemotactic factors.

References

Basten, A., and Beeson, P. B.: Mechanism of eosinophilia. II. Role of the lymphocyte. J. Exp. Med. *131*:1288, 1970.

Basten, A., Boyer, M. H., and Beeson, P. B.: Mechanism of eosinophilia I. Factors affecting the eosinophil response of rats to *Trichinella spiralis*. J. Exp. Med. *131*:1271, 1970.

Boswell, R. N., Austen, K. F., and Goetzl, E. J.: Intermediate molecular weight eosinophil chemotactic factors in rat peritoneal mast cells: Immunologic release, granule association, and demonstration of structural heterogeneity. J. Immunol. *120*:15, 1978.

Boyer, M. H., Basten, A., and Beeson, P. B.: Mechanism of eosinophilia. III. Suppression of eosinophilia by agents known to modify immune responses. Blood *36*:458, 1970.

Bujak, J. S., and Root, R. K.: The role of peroxidase in the bactericidal activity of human blood eosinophils. Blood *43*:727, 1974.

Cohen, S., and Ward, P. A.: In vitro and in vivo activity of a lymphocyte and immune complex–dependent chemotactic factor for eosinophils. J. Exp. Med. *133*:133, 1971.

Colley, D. G.: Eosinophils and immune mechanisms. I. Eosinophil stimulation promotor (ESP): A lymphokine induced by specific antigen or PHA. J. Immunol. *110*:1419, 1973.

Dale, D. C., Hubert, R. T., and Fauci, A.: Eosinophil kinetics in the hyper-eosinophilic syndrome. J. Lab. Clin. Med. *87*:487, 1976.

Ehrlich, P.: Uber die specifischen Granulationen des Blutes. Archiv fur Anatomie und Physiologie. 571–579 (abstract), 1879.

Eidinger, D., Wilkinson, R., and Rose, D.: A study of the cellular responses in immune reactions utilizing the skin window technique. J. Allergy *35*:77, 1964.

Gleich, G. J., Leogering, D. A., Kueppers, F., Bajaj, S. P., and Mann, K. G.: Physiochemical and biological properties of the major basic protein from guinea pig eosinophil granules. J. Exp. Med. *140*:313, 1974.

Gleich, G. J., Leogering, D. A., Mann, K. G., and Maldonado, J. E.: Comparative properties of the Charcot-Leyden crystal protein and the major basic protein from human eosinophils. J. Clin. Invest. *57*:633, 1976.

Gleich, G. J., Leogering, D. A., and Olson, G. M.: Reactivity of rabbit antiserum to guinea pig eosinophils. J. Immunol. *115*:950, 1975.

Herion, J. C., Glasser, R. M., Walker, R. I., and Palmer, J. G.: Eosinophil kinetics in two patients with eosinophilia. Blood *36*:361, 1970.

Hubscher, T.: Role of the eosinophil in the allergic reactions. I. EDI — An eosinophil-derived inhibitor of histamine release. J. Immunol. *114*:1379, 1975*a*.

Hubscher, T.: Role of the eosinophil in the allergic reactions. II. Release of prostaglandins from human eosinophilic leukocytes. J. Immunol. *114*:1389, 1975*b*.

Kay, A. B., Stechschulte, D. J., and Austen, K. F.: An eosinophil leukocyte chemotactic factor of anaphylaxis. J. Exp. Med. *133*:602, 1971.

MacKenzie, C. D., Ramalho-Pinto, F. J., McLaren, D. J., and Smithers, S. R.: Antibody-mediated adherence of rat eosinophils to schistosomula of *Schistoma mansoni* in vitro. J. Exp. Immunol. *30*:97, 1977.

Mahmoud, A. A. F., Warren, K. S., and Peters, P. A.: A role for the eosinophil in acquired resistance to *Schistosoma mansoni* infection as determined by antieosinophil serum. J. Exp. Med. *142*:805, 1975.

McLaren, D. J., MacKenzie, C. D., and Ramalho-Pinto, F. J.: Ultra-structural observations on the *in vitro* interaction between rat eosinophils and some parasitic helminths (*Schistosoma mansoni, Trichinella spiralis* and *Nippostrongylus brasiliensis*). Clin. Exp. Immunol. *30*:105, 1977.

Metcalfe, D. D., Gadek, J. E., Raphael, G. D., Frank, M.D., Kaplan, A. P., and Kaliner, M.: Human eosinophil adherence to serum-treated sepharose: Granule-associated enzyme release and requirement for activation of the alternative complement pathway. J. Immunol. *119*:1744, 1977.

Parish, W. E.: Investigation on eosinophilia. The influence of histamine, antigen-antibody complexes containing gamma-1 or gamma-2 globulins, foreign bodies (phagocytosis) and disrupted mast cells. Br. J. Dermatol. *82*:42, 1970.

Ross, R., and Klebanoff, S. J.: The eosinophilic leukocyte. Fine structure studies in the uterus during the estrous cycle. J. Exp. Med. *124*:653, 1966.

Spiers, R. S.: Physiological approaches to an understanding of the function of eosinophils and basophils. Ann. N.Y. Acad. Sci. *59*:706, 1955.

Ward, P. A.: Chemotaxis of human eosinophils. Am. J. of Pathol. *54*:121, 1969.

Wasserman, S. I., Geotzl, E. J., and Austen, K. F.: Inactivation of slow reacting substance of anaphylaxis by human eosinophil arylsulfatase. J. Immunol. *114*:645, 1975.

Zeiger, R. S., Yurdin, D. L., and Colten, H. R.: Histamine metabolism. II. Cellular and subcellular localization of the catabolic enzymes, histaminase and histamine methyl transferase, in human leukocytes. J. Allergy Clin. Immunol. *58*:172, 1976.

Raymond G. Slavin, M.D.
Laurie J. Smith, M.D.

13

Epidemiologic Considerations in Atopic Disease

As defined in the Preface to this book, an allergic disease is considered to be "a complex of signs and symptoms in which immune events are thought frequently to play a major role." The atopic disorders represent a subgroup of allergic diseases in which there is a familial tendency, and which often coexist in the same individual. Epidemiologic and clinical studies firmly support an association between the propensity to produce IgE antibody and the atopic diseases — bronchial asthma, seasonal and perennial allergic rhinitis, and atopic dermatitis. Although IgE antibody frequently is elevated in these diseases, its involvement is not universal. Even when present, its role in the pathogenesis of a particular atopic disease often is unclear. Thus, while there is an association between IgE antibody and the atopic diseases, the heritability of the atopic diseases and the genetics of IgE production appear to be separate.

EPIDEMIOLOGIC STUDIES

A major aim of epidemiologic studies is to define and characterize etiologic factors responsible for disease. The most commonly used investigative technique is to examine the incidence, prevalence, and mortality in contrasting populations and to attempt to relate any differences to the factors that distinguish one population from another. A literature search reveals enormous variations in reported incidence, prevalence, and prognosis of atopic disorders. Some understanding of the reasons for this is necessary in order to appreciate the difficulties encountered in comparing findings of different studies.

Differences in the Definition of "Atopic." Some or all of several characteristics of the atopic state have been required in some studies but few of these in others. These include history of atopic disease, associated or concomitant atopic disorders in the same patient, evidence of skin-sensitizing antibody, elevated serum IgE, and radioimmunoassay (RAST) demonstration of specific IgE. Demonstration of skin-sensitizing or, specifically, IgE antibody, has been a requisite of some studies but not of others.

Differences in the Definition of the Particular Disease Entity. This uncertainty is especially true of bronchial asthma. Some investigators have relied upon a history of asthma, others have relied on the presence of wheezing at the time of examination, and still others have demanded objective pulmonary function evidence of obstructive airway disease.

Differences in Patient Population Selection. Studies vary enormously in the composition of the study groups with respect to such factors as sex, age, race, and socioeconomic status.

Differences in Methodology Used. Some studies are retrospective; others prospective. Data collection may be by questionnaire, personal interview, physical examination, or by physiologic tests (e.g., pulmonary function tests, in asthma). Questionnaires present inherent problems since fallibility of memory generally results in underestimation of cumulative prevalence rates.

GENERAL EPIDEMIOLOGIC CONSIDERATIONS

Despite the problems encountered, it is possible to make certain observations on the epidemiology of atopic diseases. Each disease is considered separately later in this chapter, but first a few general comments concerning several epidemiologic factors are presented.

Prevalence. The prevalence and incidence of allergic respiratory disease, i.e., hay fever and asthma, vary considerably in different parts of the world. As discussed, comparison of studies is difficult because of differences in definition, methodology, and whether data refer to current or past problems.

Family History. Studies performed in Iowa by Smith (1975) revealed that 87 percent of children who developed an allergic disorder before 10 years of age had a close relative with an allergic disorder. It was found that 16 percent of girls and 28 percent of boys born into households in which someone already had an allergic respiratory disorder had developed asthma or allergic rhinitis by age 20, compared to 0.08 percent of girls and 1.5 percent of boys born into households in which neither disease was present. Family epidemiologic studies support a connection between "intrinsic," or nonallergic, asthma and "extrinsic" or allergic, asthma: 66 percent of adults with intrinsic asthma had a positive family history of a respiratory allergic disorder compared with 26 percent in the general population (Smith, 1978). In general, familial associations are found for the atopic diseases themselves, irrespective of the presence or absence of IgE antibody. In addition, however, there are familial associations between the atopic diseases and the propensity to develop IgE antibody, as well as familial associations in the ability to make IgE antibody per se.

Coexistence of Atopic Diseases. The grouping of allergic rhinitis, bronchial asthma, and atopic dermatitis rests on solid clinical and epidemiologic grounds. In one study, 78 percent of patients with allergic asthma had allergic nasal symptoms, while 38 percent of patients with allergic rhinitis had asthma (Smith, 1965). The frequency of atopic dermatitis in patients with asthma or allergic rhinitis ranges from 6 to 63 percent. In children with atopic dermatitis, the risk of developing allergic rhinitis and/or asthma is five to ten times greater than in the population at large.

Age. The atopic diseases generally begin early in childhood, but they can arise at any age. The majority of patients with allergic asthma develop symptoms before 20 years of age and most before the age of 10 years. Atopic dermatitis begins in infancy or early childhood, whereas seasonal allergic rhinitis tends to develop somewhat later, largely as a result of the time required for sufficient exposure to develop sensitization to pollen and other seasonal allergens. Perennial allergic rhinitis, on the other hand, may develop earlier, probably as a result of earlier intense exposure to perennial allergens. Table 13–1 shows the onset and estimated incidence of the various atopic diseases at different ages.

Sex. Boys develop asthma and atopic dermatitis twice as often as girls do before the age of 10 years. Girls "catch up," at least in asthma, in the teens and twenties.

Race. There are notable examples of racial differences in susceptibility to atopic disease, particularly with respect to bronchial asthma. An example is Tokyo-Yokohama asthma — presumably due to sensitivity to petrochemical fumes — which affected large numbers of American servicemen but only a small proportion of the local Japanese population.

Environmental vs. Genetic Factors. A major influence on the prevalence of allergic disease is the amount and nature of allergens in different environments. Some apparent racial differences in fact appear to be due to differences in environmental influences. Smith (1975), for example, has shown an increased incidence of asthma in

TABLE 13–1 ONSET AND INCIDENCE OF ATOPIC DISEASE

Disease	Incidence (percent)	Age Factors
Asthma	Children: 1–11	Onset between 0 and 10 yrs: 8–63%*
	Adults: 2–7	Onset between 10 and 50 yrs: 24–72%
Allergic rhinitis	Children: 2–9 ⎫ Adults: 4–20 ⎭	Not known
Atopic dermatitis	General population: 1–3	60 percent by age 6

*Extracted from Gregg, I.: Epidemiology (Table 11.4). In Clark, J. T. H. and Godfrey, S. (eds.): Asthma. London, Chapman and Hall, 1977, Chapter 11.

black and Asian children born in Great Britain compared with children of these races in their countries of origin. There also is an apparent correlation between the prevalence of asthma and urbanization and increased socioeconomic status.

The increased prevalence of asthma in immigrants compared to the same group in their native country speaks against great racial differences in susceptibility. Studies on twins generally show that prevalence of atopic disease is only slightly higher in monozygotic than in dizygotic twins and that, in both, concordance is less than 50 percent. Concordance of asthma in dizygotic twins is similar to that in ordinary sibships (Lubs, 1971). Thus, the marked tendency of asthma and allergic rhinitis to occur in families may not be entirely genetic. Genetic factors may predispose to allergic disorders, but environmental factors are critical determinants in their development. Unexplained, however, is why among patients with similar genetic makeup and apparently similar environmental exposure, allergic symptoms develop early in life in some, and much later or not at all in others.

Natural History. Use of medications, environmental control measures, and immunotherapy all have led to some alterations in the natural history of atopic diseases. This point is discussed in later sections on the specific diseases.

Immune Factors — IgE Antibody. The family history of atopic disease seems paramount in the predisposition of an individual to developing an atopic disease. The mode of inheritance seems more complicated than the original belief, which was that inheritance depended on a single dominant or recessive gene with variable penetrance. Most investigators feel that the familial tendency to allergic disease results from multiple factors, or polygenic inheritance, dependent on the interaction of several genes at more than one locus. There seems to be an association between HLA haplotype, Ir genes, and the ability to form IgE and IgG antibody to ragweed antigen E (see also Chapter 3). Current information suggests that independent genetic factors influence (1) the immune responses to specific antigens, (2) the ability to form IgE antibody specifically, and (3) the level of IgE; however, these factors frequently coexist with end-organ hyperirritability e.g., of the skin or respiratory tract (see also Chapter 14). In addition to a tendency to form IgE antibody, the IgE antibody response is more persistent in patients with atopic disorders. In groups given diphtheria toxoid, positive immediate skin tests persisted only in "atopic" individuals (Kuhns and Pappenheimer, 1952).

The tendency to develop IgE antibody and to have elevated IgE levels may be related to a predisposition for asthma. In a study of small children who experienced episodes of wheezing with an upper respiratory infection, increased serum IgE was found in 44 percent of those who had a wheezing episode for the first time and in whom asthma was later diagnosed, in contrast to only 7 percent of those in whom asthma was not diagnosed (Foucard, 1974).

Several studies indicate that individuals with atopic disease tend to differ from nonatopic individuals in sensitivity to antigenic stimulation. This increased potential for sensitization relates specifically to the route by which the allergen is introduced. If an antigen is injected intradermally, subcutaneously, or intramuscularly, the degree of sensitization as manifested by development of skin-sensitizing antibody is similar between atopic and nonatopic individuals. With intranasal application of a protein antigen or an artificial polysaccharide, however, immediate type hypersensitivity is induced more readily in atopic subjects. This increased respiratory tract "mucosal sensitivity" to antigenic stimulation seems to be true for the gastrointestinal tract as well. The alimentary tract is an especially important route of sensitization early in life. Evidence of IgE antibody to food allergens is more frequently found early in life, with antibody to inhalant allergens found at various ages. It is tempting to speculate that severe respiratory tract infection, an especially important precipitant of asthma, changes the bronchial mucosa and renders it more permeable to various antigens.

A low serum IgA in 3-month-old infants was shown in one study to be associated with a significantly greater degree of atopic disease later in life (Taylor et al., 1973). It is postulated that a defect in the protective mechanism mediated by secretory mucosal IgA during early infancy results in a failure to exclude or eliminate antigens in the gastrointestinal tract and possibly the respiratory tract. This is thought to lead to increased mucosal entry of antigens during the IgA deficient period, resulting in an enhanced stimulation of the IgE system. Some investigators have claimed that exclusion of potent antigens such as cow milk during this critical "immunodeficient" period results in a significant decrease in the development of allergic disease in genetically predisposed individuals (see Chapter 25). Others have not found any effect of such exclusion, nor evidence of IgA deficiency in atopic individuals.

Nonimmune Factors. The pathogenesis of the atopic diseases involves complex interactions between the immune response, autonomic regulatory mechanisms, and other, poorly understood factors. As discussed in detail in Chapter 14, many of the manifestations of atopic diseases cannot be explained solely on the basis of IgE antibody-mediated mechanisms. There is evidence that the autonomic nervous system plays an important regulatory role in

the atopic diseases and that an "imbalance" in autonomic regulation relates to the pathogenesis of these disorders. Blockade of beta adrenergic receptors has been postulated as an underlying defect in the atopic patient. This abnormality has been demonstrated in asthmatic patients and patients with atopic dermatitis in whom there is no demonstrable "allergic" (i.e., IgE antibody-mediated) component. Of considerable importance in all atopic diseases are infectious, irritant, emotional, and other nonimmune precipitating or aggravating factors, such as cold air, air pollutants, cigarette smoke, and other contact irritants, and exercise and weather changes (particularly in asthma).

EPIDEMIOLOGIC CONSIDERATIONS IN ALLERGIC RHINITIS

Seasonal allergic rhinitis lends itself easily to characterization (see Chapter 39). A history of seasonal nasal symptoms with demonstration of skin-sensitizing or IgE antibody to allergens appropriate to the seasonal symptoms are characteristics that can be obtained without difficulty even in large populations under study. Perennial allergic rhinitis may be more difficult to identify. Evidence of IgE antibody in this population often is less clearly related to causation of the disease. Up to 75 percent of asymptomatic normal subjects have been shown to have skin-sensitizing antibody to at least one allergen on intradermal screening (Lindblad and Farr, 1961). Assessing by history a causal relationship between perennial symptoms and positive skin tests is difficult to achieve in studies using questionnaires and interviews by relatively unskilled persons. In most surveys, a history of seasonal rhinitis has been obtained more commonly than of perennial rhinitis, but it is not clear to what extent milder perennial allergic nasal symptoms have been ignored.

The frequency of allergic rhinitis in childhood is not known with certainty: reports range from an incidence of 0.5 percent to over 20 percent. The incidence is lower in the very young and increases progressively with age. Fewer than 2.9 percent of children age 4 years or younger are reported as having allergic rhinitis (Broder et al., 1974).

In all age groups the incidence of allergic rhinitis usually is cited as between 8 to 10 percent of the general population in the United States. Most studies of university student populations give figures considerably higher than that, ranging from 12 to 21 percent. A study of twelfth graders revealed a prevalence of 21 percent for seasonal allergic rhinitis and approximately 9 percent for patients with perennial symptoms (Freeman and Johnson, 1964).

Males and females appear to have equal incidence of allergic rhinitis at any age. Racial factors contributing to incidence of allergic rhinitis in varying populations are difficult to interpret, as lower reported incidences in European, African, and Asian populations may be attributable to differences in study design. Foreign students attending an American university had an incidence of allergic rhinitis comparable to that of American students. It is not certain whether this reflects a true incidence of allergic rhinitis in a foreign student population when studied in similar manner to American populations or whether the environment in the United States — with ragweed pollen abundant, for example — evoked symptoms in a population susceptible to a potent allergen that would have been avoided if they had remained at home. An increased incidence of skin-sensitizing antibodies and symptoms of allergic rhinitis has been reported in higher socioeconomic groups, but whether changes in socioeconomic status or other paraphenomena are responsible for this is not clear.

Family history of atopic disease in patients with allergic rhinitis ranges as high as 87 percent. In general, the risk for a child developing allergic rhinitis increases when one parent has an atopic disorder and may be 50 percent or greater when both parents have atopic disease (Smith, 1978).

Allergic rhinitis tends to develop in childhood, persist into adulthood, and decline in old age. Reports of spontaneous remissions vary but suggest that 15 to 25 percent of cases remit when followed over 5 to 7 years; symptoms in an approximately equal number of persons appear to increase in the same period, however. A variety of studies are available showing the effect of immunotherapy on allergic rhinitis. Treat-

ment success, meaning amelioration of symptoms, ranges from 43 to 100 percent in groups receiving immunotherapy, while successful responses range from 10 to 56 percent in placebo-treated groups. The best responses to immunotherapy have been observed in patients with seasonal allergic rhinitis treated with high dose-specific antigens for at least 3 to 5 years. The subsequent duration of symptom amelioration is not known, however. It is evident that immunotherapy has an impact on the morbidity of allergic rhinitis, and there is reason to believe it has a significant effect on the ultimate course as well. Although there have been suggestions that immunotherapy for allergic rhinitis may prevent the development of asthma, evidence is weak, and many studies indicate that onset of asthma precedes onset of allergic rhinitis. In several studies, less than 10 percent of children with asthma had allergic rhinitis for more than a year before asthma began.

EPIDEMIOLOGIC CONSIDERATIONS IN BRONCHIAL ASTHMA

Studies on the epidemiology of asthma represent a bewildering array of differing populations, differing sampling methods, differing survey methods, and differing definitions of asthma. An exact definition of asthma has defied groups of experts for years, and presently asthma is defined only in a descriptive manner. This undoubtedly is due to the heterogeneity of factors that influence the disease, and the lack of an identifiable etiologic factor uniformly present in every asthmatic patient. As a result, there are enormous variations in criteria for diagnosis of asthma. Compounding the problem is the wide variation in severity of airway obstruction in asthmatic patients, insensitivity of methods for detecting airway obstruction, and the frequent lack of awareness of symptoms and signs of asthma. As a result, the true incidence and prevalence of asthma tends to be underestimated, and figures on prognosis tend to be overly optimistic.

Although asthma occurs in patients with allergic rhinitis and atopic dermatitis, it seems to have a separate pattern of inheritance. Nonallergic and allergic asthmatics have similar family histories for asthma although relatives of allergic asthmatics have a higher incidence of allergic rhinitis. In various surveys, the incidence of allergic rhinitis in patients with asthma is as high as 67 percent, generally being far more common in extrinsic than intrinsic asthmatics. In addition, from 6 to 63 percent of asthmatic patients have been reported to have had eczema. McNicol and Williams (1973) found that children with wheezy bronchitis and children with moderate to severe asthma had a similar incidence of allergic rhinitis and of positive skin tests to allergens, both higher than in control subjects. In addition, these authors found eczema to be more common in the more severe asthmatics.

The reported prevalence of asthma varies from less than 3 percent to over 11 percent, depending upon criteria for patient inclusion. The high figure of 11 percent from Williams and McNicol (1969) includes the total of children who had an unequivocal diagnosis of repeated wheezing and continued to have wheezing at age 10 years (3.7 percent) together with the group who had more than five episodes of wheezing, but whose asthma had ceased by age 10 (7.7 percent). The report excluded an additional group of school children with a history of fewer than five episodes of wheezing associated with infection. Had they been included, there would be an overall prevalence of 18 to 19 percent. Broder et al. (1974) in a study in Tecumseh, Michigan, also reported similar figures in children under age 15, with a cumulative incidence of asthma of 8 percent in boys and 4.8 percent in girls. Some European studies have placed the incidence of childhood asthma between 0.5 and 5 percent. In spite of the wide range in reported series, the figure for cumulative prevalence of asthma in childhood generally is stated as being between 5 and 7 percent. The reasons for this variability have been discussed. However, even this range of 5 to 7 percent probably substantially underestimates the true incidence of hyperactive airway disease in children. Children who may have exercised-induced bronchoconstriction and/or bronchoobstruction, mainly with upper respiratory infections, often are not identified as asthmatic in population surveys by questionnaire.

Most studies reveal a male to female ratio between 1.5 and 3.3 to 1, with this difference tending to equalize in adolescence. After adolescence, the incidence of asthma tends to be higher in females. Although various hypotheses have been advanced, the reason for differences in incidence according to sex is unclear. The greater frequency of upper respiratory infection in young boys compared to girls is of interest in this regard, however, since viral respiratory tract infection can both initiate and aggravate asthmatic symptoms.

Asthma tends to develop (or at least tends to be diagnosed) at an earlier age than does allergic rhinitis. Many surveys show that at least a third of all asthma begins before the age of 10 years. The vast majority of childhood asthma develops before age 8 years, and half before age 3 years. There is a tendency for asthma to begin at an earlier age in patients prone to develop IgE antibody. Rackemann and Edwards (1952) reported that 74 percent of patients with asthma whose disease began prior to age 15 years were allergic, whereas of those in whom it began after age 45 years, only 32 percent were allergic.

In nearly every study of the natural history of asthma, significant spontaneous improvement in asthma is reported by age 10 to 14 years, improvement rates ranging from 26 to 78 percent. Generally, children who had fewer episodes of asthma beginning after age 3 years tended to "outgrow" their asthma by age 10 years. Early onset asthma (before age 3 years) and severe asthma tended to persist. Unfortunately, most long-term studies of the natural history of asthma have relied upon survey information, which tends to grossly underestimate the persistence of bronchial obstruction, hence the frequent and (in the authors' opinion) erroneous conclusion that childhood asthma generally is outgrown. More recent studies using pulmonary function tests suggest that at least some degree of asthma tends to persist, and that it may be relatively uncommon to remain completely free from this disease (Chapter 45).

Because of the heterogeneous nature of asthma and the multiple factors capable of precipitating an attack, the role of immunotherapy in asthma is difficult to assess. A search of the literature reveals nearly equal numbers of reports either supporting or denying efficacy of immunotherapy in asthma. Assessment of severity of asthma and perceptions of need for medications are subjective criteria in a disease noted for discrepancy between objective pulmonary abnormalities and patient (and often physician) assessment of degree of obstruction. However, these criteria were most often used to grade response to immunotherapy in asthma. A conclusion concerning overall efficacy of immunotherapy in asthma and its influence on the natural history of the disease is difficult to reach.

In 1973, 1912 deaths due to asthma were reported in the United States, of which 250 occurred in individuals between 5 and 34 years of age (Speizer, 1976). Asthma is a disorder in which mortality is not strikingly high, but in which morbidity takes an excessive toll.

EPIDEMIOLOGIC CONSIDERATIONS IN ATOPIC DERMATITIS

The prevalence of atopic dermatitis as judged by history is difficult to assess. In the mild form, atopic dermatitis may be forgotten or ignored. In older children, other skin conditions may be confused with it. Its incidence is estimated at from 1 to 3 percent of the general population. In populations in which asthma is uncommon, eczema also is uncommon. The sex distribution is approximately the same as in asthma, i.e., twice as common early in life in boys as in girls. The proportion of patients with atopic dermatitis who subsequently develop bronchial asthma ranges from 20 to 60 percent, whereas figures for subsequent development of allergic rhinitis range from 30 to 45 percent. Thus, in patients with atopic dermatitis, the risk of developing atopic disease of the upper and/or lower respiratory tract is 5 to 10 times greater than in the population at large.

Atopic dermatitis generally begins in infancy or early childhood. It rarely is expressed before 5 weeks of age. Cutaneous autonomic dysfunction in the form of increased vasoconstriction and xerosis generally is found. Serum IgE levels frequently are elevated and IgE antibodies to foods are present in 43 to 72 percent of patients.

The incidence of IgE antibodies to inhalant allergens also is high, but the contribution of environmental allergens to the pathogenesis of atopic dermatitis seems minimal (see Chapter 31).

Spontaneous resolution of the condition occurs in about two thirds of patients by the age of 6 years. Those patients who persist generally have mild disease, but unfortunately, there are numerous exceptions, who have severe disease. Although antiallergic therapy in some cases may modify the disease, there is no evidence that symptomatic treatment or specific antiallergic therapy shortens the duration of disease.

OTHER ALLERGIC DISEASE STATES

While appropriate studies firmly support a familial or genetic association between bronchial asthma, allergic rhinitis, and atopic dermatitis, the evidence for such an association with other conditions is vague. Urticaria or hives varies in frequency from 2.9 to 14 percent in patients with atopic diseases; in the general population, it occurs in from 3.2 to 12.8 percent.

Some examples of insect sensitivity, such as that due to the Hymenoptera group, or drug sensitivity, as in the case of penicillin, are mediated by IgE antibody. Examination of patients with these sensitivities reveals that the incidence of allergy is only slightly higher in patients with atopic diseases than in nonatopic patients. However, the severity of allergic reactions to these materials tends to be greater in atopic patients.

CONCLUSION

It is evident from this perspective that while a good deal of information is accumulating regarding the etiology and pathogenesis of atopic disease, much work remains to be done. The various atopic disease states become manifest in different generations, in different ways, and at different ages. The basic question of *why* an individual develops a particular disease at a particular time in his life remains unanswered. Once developed, the diseases tend to persist, a point many physicians do not know or do not appreciate.

There is a critical need for studies that might lead to a better understanding of the pathogenesis of the atopic diseases. More prospective studies are necessary to elucidate the natural history and to determine factors responsible for the initiation and persistence of this group of diseases. Environmental factors have been extensively studied, often to the neglect of host factors. Atopic diseases constitute a public health problem involving millions of patients and hundreds of millions of dollars in health care costs. Evidence points to an increase in the number of patients affected and in the complexity of diseases associated with technologically advanced society and demands an intense attack on the pathogenesis of atopic and other allergic disorders. Accurate epidemiologic studies should help in this attack.

References

Broder, I., Barlow, P. P., and Horton, R. J. M.: Epidemiology of asthma and allergic rhinitis in a total community: Tecumseh, Michigan. J. Allergy Clin. Immunol. 54:100, 1974.

Foucard, T.: A follow-up study of children with asthmatoid bronchitis. Act. Paediatr. Scand. 63:129, 1974.

Freeman, G. L., and Johnson, S.: Allergic diseases in adolescents. II. Changes in allergic manifestations during adolescence. Am. J. Dis. Child. 107:560, 1964.

Kuhns, W. J., and Pappenheimer, A. M., Jr.: Immunochemical study of antitoxin products in normal and allergic individuals hyperimmunized with diptheria toxoid: Relationship of skin sensitivity to presence of circulating nonprecipitating antitoxin. J. Exp. Med. 95:363, 1952.

Lindblad, J. H., and Farr, R. S.: The incidence of positive intradermal reactions and the demonstration of skin sensitizing antibody to extracts to ragweed and dust on humans without history of rhinitis or asthma. J. Allergy 32:392, 1961.

Lubs, M. L.: Allergy in 7,000 twin pairs. Acta Allergol. 26:249, 1971.

McNicol, K. N., and Williams, H. B.: Spectrum of asthma in childhood. I. Clinical and physiological components. II. Allergic components. Br. Med. J. 4:7, 1973.

National Health Survey, Public Health Service, Rockville, Md. Series 10, No. 84, September 1973.

Rackemann, F. M., and Edwards, M. C.: Asthma in Children. N. Engl. J. Med. 246:815, 1952.

Smith, J. M.: Epidemiology and natural history of asthma, allergic rhinitis and atopic dermatitis. In Middleton, E. J., Reed, C. E., and Ellis, E. F. (eds.): Allergy: Principles and Practice. St. Louis, C. V. Mosby, 1978, Chap. 35.

Smith, J. M.: Studies of the prevalence of asthma in childhood. Allergol. Immunopathol. 3:127, 1975.

Smith, J. M., and Knowler, L.: Epidemiology of asthma and allergic rhinitis. I. In a rural area. II. In a university-centered community. Am. Rev. Respir. Dis. 92:16, 1965.

Speizer, F. B.: Epidemiology, prevalence and mortality in asthma. In Weiss, E. B., and Segal, M. S. (eds.): Bronchial Asthma. Mechanisms and Therapeutics. Boston, Little, Brown and Co., 1976, Chap. 4.

Taylor, B., Norman, A. P., Orgel, H. A., Stokes, C. R., Turner, M. W., and Soothill, J. F.: Transient IgA deficiency and the pathogenesis of infantile atopy. Lancet 2:111, 1973.

Williams, H. B., and McNicol, K. N.: Prevalence, natural history and relationship of wheezy bronchitis and asthma in children. An epidemiological study. Br. Med. J. 4:321, 1969.

GENERAL

Cohen, C.: Genetic aspects of allergy. Med. Clin. North Am. 58:25, 1974.

Gregg, I.: Epidemiology. In Clark, J. T. H., and Godfrey, S. (eds.): Asthma. London, Chapman & Hall, 1977.

Stiffler, W. C.: Conference on infantile eczema. J. Pediatr. 66:166, 1966.

Andor Szentivanyi, M.D.
Joseph F. Williams, Ph.D.

14

The Constitutional Basis of Atopic Disease

Atopic derm, while not perfection,
At least points in the right direction
It says that here's a skin disease
More common in families that *sneeze*
   and *wheeze,*
That are *stigmatized* to varying degrees
By *other abnormalities.* *

Only a minority of the population shows some form of atopic disease despite that, by and large, identical conditions of antigen exposure must be presumed to exist for all members of the same population. The nature of the constitutional basis of atopy, that is, of the underlying determinant for the development of atopic disease, is as yet unexplained.

Many theories of the constitutional basis of atopy have been proposed since Coca and Cooke's (1923) original definition. Only two general ideas, however, have survived: the perception of atopy as a primary disorder of the immune system with sequelae in the various effector tissues; a concept of atopy as a primary autonomic imbalance, essentially beta adrenergic in character, with sequelae in effector cells *including* those engaged in the production of antibodies. This autonomic imbalance is perceived *as caused not by some disorder of the au-*

tonomic nervous system itself, but by a de-*fective functioning of its effector cells* (Szentivanyi, 1968*a*).

These two concepts are not mutually exclusive. In fact, they may be interdependent. Although the immune features of atopic disease can be understood within the framework of a basic adrenergic disorder of various effector cells, many, if not most, of the nonimmune features of atopic conditions are not readily explicable on the basis of a primary immune abnormality.

THE ORIGINAL CONCEPT OF ATOPY

It had long been known that hay fever and asthma often occurred together in the same individual and that both conditions showed a marked familial tendency. Similarly, it had been recognized that acute and chronic urticaria as well as gastrointestinal manifestations of idiosyncrasy to a specific food were more common in patients with these diseases than in the general population, and a relation to infantile eczema (prurigo Besnier, neurodermatitis) also was observed. Eczema was found to occur more frequently in the children of patients with hay fever or asthma, and individuals who had had eczema in infancy showed an unusual incidence of hay fever and asthma later in life.

---

*From Sulzberger, M. B.: Atopic dermatitis: A semantic ballad. In Baer, R. L. (ed.): *Atopic Dermatitis.* Philadelphia, J. B. Lippincott Company, 1955, p. 41.

These diseases were, therefore, considered together by Cooke and Vander Veer (1916) as a special group of diseases of human sensitization with a hereditary background, and they concluded that such "sensitized individuals transmit to their offspring not their own specific sensitization, but an unusual capacity for developing bioplastic reactivities to any foreign proteins." With further progress in determining additional characteristics of "human sensitization" in contrast to those of experimental anaphylaxis in laboratory animals, Coca and Cooke (1923) concluded that a clear distinction must be made between two types of hypersensitivity manifestations: the "anaphylactic" type of allergic response to abnormal substances and the "atopic" type of response to substances that are generally innocuous. As they stated:

This latter sub-group evidently needs a special term by which it may be conveniently designated and this need is satisfactorily met with the word atopy, which was kindly suggested by Professor Edward D. Perry of Columbia University. The Greek word ἀτοπία from which the term was derived, was used in the sense of a strange disease. However, it is not, on that account, necessary to include under the term all strange diseases; the use of the term can be restricted to the hay fever and asthma group.

To these, Wise and Sulzberger then added neurodermatitis under the new designation of "atopic dermatitis." Based on the close association of this condition with other atopic manifestations, Wise and Sulzberger (1933) concluded that the skin lesions of this disorder were the cutaneous analog of hay fever and asthma, and suggested that the name "atopic dermatitis" replace "disseminated neurodermatitis."

Several characteristics of the atopic state emerged from these early concepts: atopy was felt to be a hereditary manifestation, subject to a dominant gene, a peculiarly human disorder with a reacting serum element different from classic antibodies and reminiscent of the Wasserman reagin (hence the name, "atopic reagin"). Atopic antibodies, furthermore, seemed to occur only in man, many times without any demonstrable prior exposure to incitant substances and induced by agents that often

appeared to be nonantigenic ("atopens" of Grove and Coca, 1925).

Over the years, most of these postulated differences between atopy and anaphylaxis gradually could be eliminated. Thus, antibody essentially identical to atopic reagin was found in various animal species (Ishizaka, 1976). Moreover, atopic disease was shown to occur in animals (Patterson, 1969). Some of the other distinctions between anaphylaxis and atopy also were amenable to various alternative explanations, indicating that these conditions may not be separated by wide and irreconcilable differences as it was believed by the originators of the concept of atopy. Nevertheless, some differences remained and other important new differences emerged, making it imperative that a concept of atopy be reformulated.

A REFORMULATION OF THE CONCEPT OF ATOPY

In the past two decades, it has become increasingly evident that in addition to some of the remaining immunologic differences between anaphylaxis and atopic allergy, there are critically important nonimmune differences between the immediate hypersensitivities of the atopic and nonatopic type. Thus, it appears that in anaphylaxis we are dealing with a normal (physiologic) antibody response to an unnatural exposure to antigen, whereas in atopic allergy an "abnormal" antibody response to natural antigenic exposure seems to be involved. Anaphylactic reactivity of the sensitized individual depends on the release of an amount of pharmacologic mediator sufficient to be toxic for most members of the same species. *In contrast, individuals with atopic disease possess a quantitatively and qualitatively abnormal reactivity to otherwise nontoxic concentrations of endogenously released or exogenously administered pharmacologic mediators.* Furthermore, the quantitative change consistently is in the direction of a decreased response when beta adrenergic agents are the agonists, and consistently in the direction of an increased response when any one of the other mediators is involved.

Another essential difference between the atopic and nonatopic varieties of immedi-

ate hypersensitivities is the major contributory role played by infection in atopy, whereas infection has not been shown to be causally related to anaphylactic allergy — anaphylaxis, the Arthus reaction, or serum sickness. Moreover, *atopic conditions can be precipitated by a number of totally unrelated stimuli,* whereas anaphylaxis can be brought about only by the specific antigen. Finally, the latter conditions may be produced artifically, but *atopic disease with its spontaneous pattern of familial occurrence, cannot be induced at will.* Acute human pulmonary anaphylaxis, which can include asthmatic features, for example, has never been reported to lead to the development of bronchial asthma or other atopic disease (Szentivanyi and Fishel, 1966).

As has been repeatedly described (Szentivanyi, 1968a and 1968b; Szentivanyi and Fishel, 1976; Szentivanyi et al., 1979; Szentivanyi and Fitzpatrick, 1979), in our reformulation of the original concept of atopy, *the essential difference between immediate hypersensitivities of the nonatopic and atopic varieties is that the former conditions are mediated by normal immune and pharmacologic mechanisms, whereas atopy is based on abnormal immune and pharmacologic mechanisms. This difference between anaphylaxis and atopy we regard as fundamental. In this view, furthermore, it is the altered pharmacologic reactivity that is considered as the uniformly present, single atopic characteristic of pathognomonic significance.* Attention, therefore, will first be focused on the pharmacologic mediation of immediate hypersensitivities as this problem relates to the constitutional basis of atopy.

THE PHARMACOLOGIC MEDIATORS OF IMMEDIATE HYPERSENSITIVITIES

The currently established pharmacologic mediators of immediate hypersensitivities include amines, peptides, and lipid substances (Szentivanyi and Fitzpatrick, 1979; also see Chapter 11). The primary pharmacologic mediators, i.e., mediators that may be released "directly" by interaction of antigen with cell-fixed antibody, include histamine, SRS-A, ECF-A, PAF, BK-A, and

NCF.* The catecholamines, acetylcholine, and bradykinin are generally considered secondary mediators because they are mostly released indirectly, as a consequence of primary mediator release. Serotonin and dopamine as well as the prostaglandins of the E_1, E_2, and $F_{2\alpha}$ classes may serve as primary mediators when the immune injury involves cell types with which these substances are associated or as secondary mediators when they are released by a primary mediator.

Special mention should be made of the catecholamines since almost all the primary mediators release, or are capable of releasing, these amines. They are, therefore, at least potential participants in immediate hypersensitivities of both the nonatopic and atopic varieties. Although in this capacity — in contrast to the other mediators — they usually have no untoward effect, under certain conditions (i.e., atopy) their entry into the reaction may be harmful. Of further importance is the fact that in many tissues of most species, the catecholamines are the principal natural antagonists of both the primary and secondary mediators, and thus play a major role in determining the nature of ultimate reactivity of the effector cells to these substances released by immune or other mechanisms (Szentivanyi and Fitzpatrick, 1979).

THE PHARMACOLOGIC MEDIATORS OF IMMEDIATE HYPERSENSITIVITIES AS THE NATURAL CHEMICAL ORGANIZERS OF NEURAL ACTION

The discovery that a major group of hypersensitivities is mediated by pharmacologically active substances was a revolutionary advance in the history of allergy. It supplied the long awaited explanation for the elusive fact that the symptoms of immediate hypersensitivities are wholly unrelated to the physicochemical or biologic properties of the offending antigen. As various naturally occurring pharmacologically active agents were shown to mediate hypersensitivity responses, neurophysiologic

*SRS-A = slow reacting substance of anaphylaxis; ECF-A = eosinophil chemotactic factor of anaphylaxis; PAF = platelet aggregating factor; BK-A = bradykinin of anaphylaxis; NCF = neutrophil chemotactic factor.

research proceeded to demonstrate that impulse transmission from one neuron to another is accomplished through chemical transmitter substances. These two parallel processes of chemical identification ultimately converged in the common recognition that many, if not most, of the pharmacologic mediators of hypersensitivity reactions also are the physiologic (chemical) transmitters, or, in a broader sense, chemical organizers of neural integration.

Emergence of Pharmacologic Mediation in Allergy

Histamine became the first to be suspected as a possible mediator as early as 1911 by Sir Henry Dale; by 1919 he was capable of concluding that histamine was the long sought "anaphylatoxin" that had been hypothesized from work on guinea pig anaphylaxis. This was complemented by the description and experimental analysis of the so-called "triple response" by Sir Thomas Lewis. As early as 1927, Lewis recognized that this response, which occurs after injury to the skin by physical, thermal, or chemical agents, is similar to the reaction resulting from intradermal injection of histamine and to the phenomenon of human urticaria. In the succeeding two decades, as the result of a series of investigations by various workers, histamine gained wide acceptance as a mediator of certain hypersensitive manifestations.

The immune release of acetylcholine was demonstrated subsequently in animal anaphylaxis, and later in some human allergic reactions (Szentivanyi and Fishel, 1966). In the middle fifties a third amine-mediator, serotonin, was implicated in animal anaphylaxis. By that time, it was established that these three amines release or are capable of releasing their principal amine-antagonists, the catecholamines, and that the latter can similarly mobilize each of the preceding three agents. This led to the realization of the conspicuous fact that *the entire class of naturally occurring, physiologically important biogenic amines participates, either primarily or secondarily, in the pharmacologic mediation of the allergic response.*

The dawn of the antihistaminic era broke in the 1930's, and the availability of antihistamines unmasked the existence of still another mediator, SRS-A. The appreciation that neither histamine nor highly purified SRS-A is chemotactic for homologous eosinophils led to the discovery of ECF-A, a third mast cell–connected mediator of immediate hypersensitivities. Similarly, the use of antihistamines and other specific antagonists as analytic tools cleared the way for the recognition that still other mediators, such as bradykinin and the prostaglandins, are released by antigen-antibody reactions.

Emergence of Chemical Transmission in Neurophysiology

In 1921, Otto Loewi presented the first evidence that transmission of the nerve impulse at the junctional gaps of the autonomic nervous system is accomplished by humoral substances. These substances were designated "Vagusstoffe" and "Acceleransstoffe," corresponding respectively to the substances released from vagal and sympathetic terminals. Vagusstoffe later was shown to be identical with acetylcholine, and Acceleransstoffe with norepinephrine (Bennett, 1972; Hubbard, 1973; Krnjević, 1974).

Peripheral Nervous System. From these works, the emerging picture of chemical transmission in the autonomic, or in the efferent peripheral nervous system in general, can be summarized as follows: the efferent fibers of the peripheral nervous system can be divided into two classes, cholinergic (release acetylcholine from their terminals) and adrenergic (release norepinephrine from their nerve endings). Patterned after the "two-unit" organizational principle of the mammalian nervous system, the term "cholinergic" implies transmission from the first to the second neuron through acetylcholine, whereas the term "adrenergic" implies transmission through norepinephrine.

In addition, a network of nonadrenergic and noncholinergic inhibitory neurons represents a third neural component of the autonomic nervous system. ATP has been postulated to be the inhibitory transmitter released from these neurons, and since the effect of stimulation of these nerves on smooth muscle can be reproduced by exogenous purine nucleotides and nucleosides, these neurons have been termed, *purinergic* (Burnstock, 1972, 1975). Existence of this system has been shown most satisfactorily in the gastrointestinal tract, but presence of purinergic inhibitory nerves also has been postulated in the lung and trachea, the blood vessels, and the urogenital system (Coburn and Tomita, 1973; Burnstock, 1976).

Central Nervous System. In the central nervous system, this "two-unit" arrangement as a basic structural principle is preserved, and the mechanism by which a nerve impulse is transmitted across the junctional gap between one neuron and the next is fundamentally the same. Thus, central transmitters are liberated in the same way from synaptic vesicles or cytoplasmic storage granules in the presynaptic terminals and act in the same manner as transmitters at peripheral junctions. Furthermore, synaptic regions of both central and peripheral neurons are electrically inexcitable (Grundfest, 1957). These considerations led to the conclusion that transmission of the nerve impulse must be mediated chemically at all central as well as peripheral junctions (Eccles, 1973).

There is strong circumstantial evidence that acetylcholine serves as a major transmitter in the central nervous system. However, not all central neurons transmit impulses by liberation of acetylcholine, and the three catecholamines (epinephrine, norepinephrine, and dopamine), histamine, serotonin, and the prostaglandins also have been implicated in central transmission or in some form of modulation of the nerve impulse in the central nervous system. In the peripheral nervous system the existence of tryptaminergic neurons in which serotonin functions as a neurotransmitter has been demonstrated in invertebrates (Szentivanyi et al., 1979), and evidence is accumulating that histamine, the prostaglandins, and the plasma kinins exert an important modulatory influence on autonomic control (Szentivanyi, 1979).

THE RECEPTOR AS THE PHARMACOLOGICALLY SPECIFIC EFFECTOR-CELL COMPONENT OF MEDIATOR ACTION

The pharmacologic mediators elicit their characteristic effect through the activation of certain cells that are their specific effectors. These cells, called "effector cells," are further defined as cells that are endowed with receptive substances ("receptors") possessing sites with a steric configuration complementary to the mediator in question. The released or administered mediator combines with the complementary receptor-site, thereby initiating a chain of biochemical reactions that culminates in the observable biologic response. From the standpoint of specificity of action, the strategically important component of the effector cell is the receptor. Most receptors have not been isolated and purified, and despite irrefutable evidence for their existence (Szentivanyi & Fitzpatrick, 1979), their properties are thus still largely conjectural.

The Adrenergic Receptors

The receptor concept implies two distinct functions: recognition of specific pharmacologically active molecules, such as catecholamines, and activation of biologic processes through, for example, changes in ion permeability or of enzyme activity.

Pharmacologic Classification of Adrenergic Receptors. Because the exact nature of the various adrenergic receptors has not been known, receptors conventionally have been described by the effector response resulting from their activation and/or by the absence of this response resulting from their selective blockade. Classified on this basis, there are two principal types of adrenergic receptors, termed, for convenience, alpha and beta (Ahlquist, 1948). Over the years, this dualistic receptor classification has been validated and extended. Thus, at least two major types of beta receptors have been delineated. One type, termed β_1 receptors, have relatively high affinity for norepinephrine, which is generally equipotent with epinephrine, and a third to a quarter as potent as isoproterenol. A second type of beta receptor, termed β_2, is found in vascular, bronchial, and uterine smooth muscle, and also appears to mediate the metabolic effects of catecholamines in skeletal muscle and liver. Beta$_2$ receptors have much higher affinity for isoproterenol than norepinephrine (about 100 times).

"Interconversion" of Adrenergic Receptors. The large body of pharmacologic evidence serving the basis of the dualistic re-

ceptor classification concept created an illusion that α and β adrenergic receptors are functionally and morphologically separate, static membrane structures. In the past few years a more dynamic image of these receptors, with considerable molecular plasticity, has emerged, beginning with the finding that the beta receptors of the frog heart could be converted to an alpha receptor by cold (Kunos and Szentivanyi, 1968). This and subsequent observations

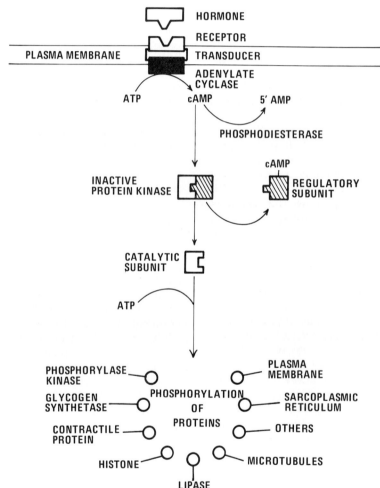

FIGURE 14–1. Diagrammatic conceptualization of cAMP as a "second messenger." Certain hormones or catecholamines ("first messengers") interact with specific receptor sites on the exterior surface of the cell, causing activation of adenylate cyclase on the interior surface. This increases cAMP synthesis and accumulation within the cell. cAMP then functions as an intracellular mediator, a "second messenger," of hormonal action by modifying enzyme activities and permeability barriers through the activation of a class of enzymes known as protein kinases. These enzymes consist of at least two subunits, one catalytic, the other regulatory or inhibitory; when the two are complexed, the enzymes are inactive. Activation occurs when cAMP complexes with the inhibitory subunit, allowing the catalytic subunit to perform its function, which is the phosphorylation of many different proteins. It is believed that this sets in motion a cascade of biochemical reactions that produce the extracellular alterations of metabolic, genetic, electrochemical, and mechanical activities that may be regulated by cAMP. Conversely, protein kinase is inactivated when the enzyme's inhibitor subunit recombines with its catalytic subunit. This occurs when the concentration of cAMP is no longer high enough to provide for complex formation with the inhibitor subunit. (From Szentivanyi, A., Krzanowski, J. J., and Polson, J. B.: The autonomic nervous system: Structure, function, and altered effector responses. *In* Middleton, E., Reed, C. E., and Ellis, E. F. (eds.): Allergy — Principles and Practice. St. Louis, The C. V. Mosby Co., 1978, by permission.)

were interpreted to indicate that alpha and beta receptors may represent different conformations of a metabolically controlled single receptor, rather than separate and independent molecular entities; this will be discussed in more detail later. Here we would only add that, while from the pharmacologic standpoint the dualistic receptor classification has been and continues to be an extremely useful concept, from the physiologic viewpoint there is no need for two adrenergic receptors (Ahlquist, 1977).

The Adenylate Cyclase Coupled Beta Adrenergic Receptors. The enzyme adenylate cyclase is stimulated by catecholamines in virtually all tissues in which beta receptors can be demonstrated by pharmacologic means. The beta adrenergic receptors appear to exist as lipoproteins located in membrane fractions in close proximity to the catalytic unit of adenylate cyclase. However, the receptor binding sites and the adenylate cyclase can be uncoupled from each other and even recoupled (Kunos, 1978), hence they probably are separate entities (Lefkowitz, 1974).

Biochemical Consequences of Adrenergic Stimulation. Little is known about the biochemical consequences of alpha adrenergic stimulation. Much more is known about the events that occur subsequent to beta receptor occupancy.

The beta adrenergic receptor, when occupied by a catecholamine, indirectly activates the enzyme adenylate cyclase. This activation involves a component of the cell membrane, which is interposed between the receptor and the enzyme, and which has been termed the transducer (Fig. 14–1). The transducer's activation of adenylate cyclase is modulated by several substances, the chief of which is guanosine triphosphate (GTP), a chemical analog of ATP and also the chemical precursor of cyclic GMP (see later). By an unknown mechanism, GTP sensitizes the receptor-transducer–adenylate cyclase system to catecholamine action (Wolfe et al., 1977).

Adenylate cyclase (formerly called adenyl cyclase), has been detected in nearly every mammalian cell in which it has been sought, and with few exceptions, has been found to be associated with the cell membrane. In the presence of magnesium ions, the adrenergically activated adenylate cyclase catalyzes the formation of a cyclic nucleotide from ATP, and one mole of

pyrophosphate per mole of ATP utilized. This cyclic nucleotide, adenosine-3′,5′-monophosphate (cyclic AMP), then functions as an intracellular mediator, a "second messenger," of catecholamine or hormonal action by modifying enzyme activities and permeability barriers (Figure 14–1 and Table 14–1) through the activation of a class of enzymes known as protein kinases (Fitzpatrick and Szentivanyi, 1977).

Regulation of the intracellular concentration of cyclic AMP is a function shared with adenylate cyclase by one or more specific cyclic adenosine-3′,5′-monophosphate phosphodiesterases. This enzyme hydrolyses the 3′-phosphate ester bond of cyclic AMP to yield 5′-AMP. It requires a divalent cation for catalytic activity (usually Mg^{++}), seems to be ubiquitous, and may exist in the cell in either (or both) a soluble or a particulate form (Weiss and Hait, 1977; Polson, Krzanowski, Fitzpatrick, and Szentivanyi, 1978).

TABLE 14–1 REGULATORY EFFECTS OF CYCLIC NUCLEOTIDES

Regulated Activity	Cyclic AMP	Cyclic GMP
Cardiac muscle contraction	Enhancement	Inhibition
Smooth muscle contraction	Inhibition	Enhancement
Lysosomal enzyme release	Inhibition	Enhancement
Lymphocyte cytotoxicity	Inhibition	Enhancement
Release of histamine, SRS-A	Inhibition	Enhancement
Glycogen storage	Glycogenolysis	Enhancement
Triglyceride storage	Lipolysis	?
Salivary amylase secretion	Enhancement	Enhancement
Ganglionic post-synaptic membrane polarization	Enhancement	Diminution
Cell-mediated bone resorption	Enhancement	?
Collecting tubule water permeability	Enhancement	?

Note: Cyclic AMP accumulations modulate a variety of important cellular events, as indicated by this partial list. Thus, modification of cellular cyclic AMP synthesis or inactivation by certain drugs, hormones, and catecholamines can produce a variety of effects depending on the target cells involved. Much less is known about the biologic function of cyclic GMP; however, it has been proposed that cyclic GMP may promote effects opposite to cyclic AMP in bidirectionally controlled systems.

Cholinergic Receptors

As with the adrenergic receptors, the exact nature of cholinergic receptors is unknown, and they too are described by the effector response resulting from their activation.

Pharmacologic Classification of Cholinergic Receptors. There are at least three types of cholinergic receptors: atropine-sensitive (muscarinic), tetraethylammonium-sensitive (nicotinic), and curare-sensitive (nicotinic). They correspond to the cholinergic receptor of the postganglionic cholinergic, synaptic, and neuromuscular (striated muscle) junctions, respectively. Nevertheless, the possibility that acetylcholine has only one receptor has not been excluded. Thus, the apparent differences in susceptibility to various cholinergic blocking agents may not reflect qualitative but rather quantitative differences that rest on nonreceptor factors such as those controlling the accessibility of acetylcholine or that of its blocking agent to the receptor site.

The Cholinergic Receptor Protein. From extensive studies on purified receptors from fish electric organ, it has been adduced that the cholinergic receptors are proteins, but not enzymes, and have a molecular weight of 42,000. The receptor is most probably a lipoprotein with four subunits, and in its membrane environment it is positioned in close proximity to the enzyme acetylcholinesterase (Cohen and Changeux, 1975).

Cholinergic Activity and Cyclic GMP. Under a variety of experimental conditons, cholinergic stimulation leads to the intracellular accumulation of cyclic 3′5′-guanosine monophosphate (cyclic GMP). This substance is similar to cyclic AMP except that the purine base guanine replaces the adenine ring of the latter. Besides cyclic AMP, cyclic GMP is the only cyclic nucleotide that is known with certainty to occur in nature. It has been detected in all mammalian tissues investigated so far (Posternak, 1974), and in most tissues, its levels are generally at least tenfold lower than those of cyclic AMP (Polson, Krzanowski, and Szentivanyi, 1976; Krzanowski, Polson, and Szentivanyi, 1976; Krzanowski, Polson, Goldman, Ebel, and Szentivanyi, 1979). A specific enzyme system, guanylate cyclase, catalyzes the synthesis of cyclic GMP from guanosine triphosphate (GTP), and hormones or other agents that activate adenylate cyclase do not stimulate (in physiologic concentrations) guanylate cyclase.

The two cyclic nucleotides, cyclic AMP and cyclic GMP, have been shown to exert opposing effects (Goldberg and Haddox, 1978), with a reciprocal counterregulatory interplay similar to that of the adrenergic and cholinergic divisions of the autonomic nervous system. It is possible, therefore, that cyclic GMP will prove to be a biochemical intermediate of cholinergic action (Table 14–1).

ALTERED AUTONOMIC EFFECTOR RESPONSES

There are three types of effector cells in the autonomic nervous system: neurons, smooth muscle, and exocrine gland cells. In addition to these classic autonomic effector cells, the humoral neurotransmitters including those of the pharmacologic mediators of allergic reactions act or are capable of acting on lymphocytes, leucocytes, macrophages, mast cells, eosinophils, and platelets, that is, on cells of major immunologic interest (Szentivanyi and Fitzpatrick, 1978).

As noted previously, the mechanism of atopy appears to involve a qualitatively and quantitatively abnormal reactivity to the pharmacologic mediators that may be related also to the immune peculiarities in atopy as well. Since the nature of this abnormal reactivity in atopy is not known, in the ensuing discussions conditions are described in which similar abnormal responses can be produced surgically or chemically. Analysis of these conditions and the basis of the experimentally-induced abnormal reactivity, therefore, may facilitate an understanding of the basis of the abnormal reactivity in atopy.

Inhibition of the Specific Enzyme Which Normally Inactivates the Mediator

Although enhancement or prolongation of effector response to any of the mediators may be obtained by inhibition of its specific catabolizing enzyme, some distinction must be made between acetylcholine and the other mediators. Thus, suppression of cholinesterase activity results in a rather consistent enhancement of acetylcholine action, regardless of the species and effector responses tested or which of the anticholinesterases is employed (Szentivanyi and Fishel, 1965). In contrast, results of similar procedures concerning catecholamines, histamine, and serotonin vary with all of these factors. This disparity might in part be attributed to the several different and competing degradative pathways available for each of the latter amines. Selective blockade of one of them may be compensated by an increase in the catabolic contribution of the alternative pathways. Furthermore, the relative importance of noncatabolic processes in inactivating some of the latter mediators seems to be greater than is the case with acetylcholine (Szentivanyi, Krzanowski, and Polson, 1978).

Surgically or Pharmacologically Induced "Denervation Supersensitivity"

Small amounts of neurotransmitters are released continually by the nerve terminals during the resting state of the neuron, and in much greater amounts following the arrival of an impulse (Hubbard, 1973). Apparently *the function of the resting secretion, which is too small to activate the effector cell, is to keep the sensitivity of the effector at a low level (Simpson, 1974). When the effector cell is deprived of this resting secretion, it acquires within a few days a hypersensitivity to its specific neurotransmitter.* For example, surgical interruption of the final neuron results in degeneration of the distal portion of the axon and cessation of its resting secretion. In the case of an adrenergic nerve ending, this results in a hypersensitivity to catecholamines in the succeeding effector cell. *In many instances, a hypersensitivity of the effector ensues also to other natural neurohumors (serotonin, histamine) and to a number of similar as well as unrelated chemicals* (Cannon and Rosenblueth, 1949). When acetylcholine is used as test substance and the striated muscle as an indicator tissue, the order of magnitude of the level of sensitivity so produced is within the range of 20 to 200 times that of the normal level. Under appropriate conditions of testing, the increase in the level of sensitivity may reach 100,000 (Thesleff, 1960). A less pronounced hypersensitivity develops after the penultimate neuron, i.e., the presynaptic neuron, is cut. In this case, the effector is deprived only of the transmitter released by the incoming impulses. Regeneration of the neuron or local application of the transmitter restores the normal level of sensitivity (Trendelenburg, 1966).

Denervation hypersensitivity also can be produced by pharmacologic means. Drugs having as their main effect the interruption of impulse transmission at any point and which are allowed to act for an extended period, can produce a hypersensitivity essentially identical with that caused by surgical denervation. In general, it would appear that any natural constituent or foreign substance capable of blocking the synthesis, storage, release, or action of the transmitter, and thereby depriving the effector cell of its specific controlling agent, can produce a denervation supersensitivity (Emmelin, 1961).

While the effects of denervation have been adequately described in a number of effector tissues, it is only recently that the process of supersensitivity has been studied as it relates to the β adrenergic receptor–adenylate cyclase system. It is important, therefore, that increased postjunctional responsiveness to catecholamines — as judged by the increase in cyclic AMP production — has been demonstrated in several tissues after surgical, chemical, or environmental reduction of their adrenergic input, including chemical or pharmacologic depletion of norepinephrine stores in terminals of central neurons.

Within the past 4 years, evidence has begun to accumulate in several adrenergic effector systems indicating an important role of changes in receptor density in the development of hyperresponsiveness to catecholamines. Specifically, in all effector tissues thus far examined, increased beta adrenergic responsiveness as reflected by enhanced cyclic AMP synthesis has been accompanied by an increase in the concentration of β adrenergic receptors. Furthermore, this increase in the number of receptors, brought about by the prolonged absence of the mediator, does not require the synthesis of new receptors (Wolfe, Harden and Molinoff, 1977).

Depletion of Nonjunctional
Mediator Stores

It is implicit in the foregoing concept of denervation supersensitivity that the lacking transmitter is normally derived from a store (i.e., synaptic vesicles) that stands in a junctional relationship with the effector cell. However, an alteration in sensitivity of the effector to a mediator can also be produced when the action of the mediator is preceded by depletion of its specific, though nonjunctional, stores. Although available information does not permit a detailed comparison between this altered reactivity and that produced by denervation, it seems that, in contrast to denervation, this hypersensitivity develops more rapidly, is short-lived, and is limited to the mediator whose tissue stores were previously depleted (Szentivanyi, Krzanowski and Polson, 1978).

Selective Blockade of One of Two
Antagonistic Sets of Receptors
Specifically Activated by the Same
Mediator

If at the time of action of a mediator there is a shift in the relative availability of its two functionally antagonistic sets of specific receptors, the normal response to that mediator will be quantitatively or qualitatively altered. For instance, in the tracheobronchial tract, the normal balance between the alpha adrenergic and beta adrenergic receptor systems appears to favor a beta adrenergic response of the smooth musculature to epinephrine. If, however, the beta adrenergic receptors are blocked by dichloroisoproterenol, bronchoconstriction occurs instead of the usual relaxation, exemplifying a qualitatively abnormal response to the mediator. In certain segments of the vascular system, where the normal receptor distribution seems to favor adrenergic alpha contracting effects, the same pharmacologic beta blockade results in a qualitatively normal but quantitatively enhanced response to epinephrine, i.e., exaggerated vasoconstriction of the small cutaneous vessels.

In the foregoing examples, the two antagonistic receptors may be components of the same target cell. Similar considerations apply to those situations in which the two receptors are associated with two different cell systems that have a common function with respect to the organism as a whole. For instance, hyperglycemia to epinephrine is the net result of a combination of adrenergic effects: (1) hepatic glycogenolysis leading to the release of free glucose into the extracellular space and (2) a simultaneous reduction of glucose uptake by the muscle and other extrahepatic cells. In the mouse, hepatic glycogenolysis appears to be an alpha adrenergic function. When the beta receptors of the mouse are blocked by dichloroisoproterenol, the blood sugar level fails to rise following epinephrine administration and this occurs despite increased hepatic glycogenolysis (Szentivanyi, Fishel and Talmage, 1963). This illustrates a quantitatively and qualitatively abnormal response to a mediator produced by the selective blockade of one of its receptors.

Selective blockade of one receptor system, however, can modify the effector cell response not only to the specific activator of the receptor affected but also to unrelated mediators. An example is the dichloroisoproterenol-induced hypersensitivity of mice to both histamine and serotonin. Within a certain dose range, this beta adrenergic blockade can increase the normal sensitivity of mice to histamine and serotonin about fifty- and ten-fold, respectively (Fishel, Szentivanyi and Talmage, 1964). This nonspecificity is similar to pharmacologic or surgical denervation of the salivary glands. Normally, the secretion of these glands is stimulated by both adrenergic and cholinergic impulses. When the cholinergic receptors of the cat's submaxillary gland cells are blocked for an extended time by chronic atropinization, they become hypersensitive to epinephrine and to a number of other sympathomimetics as well as to adrenergic nerve stimulation. The same hypersensitivity to adrenergic agents arises following section of the chorda (Emmelin, 1961).

Desensitization and Resensitization of
Receptors

Development of catecholamine-induced adrenergic subsensitivity has been shown to occur *in vitro* in erythrocytes, leukocytes, lymphocytes, macrophages, and fat cells, and in several cultured cell lines such as cultured fibroblasts, glioma cells, and astrocytoma cells. Although the precise molecular mechanism of catecholamine-induced desensitization to adrenergic stimuli is as yet not understood, it is known that: (1) both *in vivo* and *in vitro* desensitization is accompanied by a reduction in the number of β-adrenergic receptors in the effector tissue in question; (2) decreases in catecholamine-stimulated adenylate cyclase activity and in the density of β-adrenergic receptors are of similar magnitude; (3) alterations in receptor concentration and adrenergic responsiveness are independent of protein synthesis; (4) receptor occupancy alone, or in combination with elevated cyclic AMP levels is not sufficient to cause loss of adrenergic responsiveness or a decrease in the density of β adrenergic receptors; and (5) adenylate cyclase must be present for desensitization to occur (Perkins, 1975; Wolfe, Harden and Molinoff, 1977; and Kunos, 1978). These considerations led to the suggestion that desensitization of the β adrenergic receptor–adenylate cyclase system involves "inactivation" and, under appropriate circumstances, subsequent "reactivation" of existing and not newly formed receptor molecules.

Without knowing more about the molecular nature of the difference between the inactive versus the functional or active configuration of adrenergic receptors, it will still be instructive to glance at at least one of the factors that may be involved in the process of recovery of adrenergic responsiveness, i.e., in the resensitization of the receptors. In this connection, it will be recalled that guanosine triphosphate (GTP) serves not only as a precursor for cyclic GMP, but also as a modulator of the transducer's activation of adenylate cyclase. Guanine nucleotides modulate both basal and catecholamine-sensitive adenylate cyclase activity in a variety of systems. The naturally occurring nucleotide, GTP, increases the efficacy of catecholamines for the stimulation of adenylate cyclase activity, whereas the synthetic analogue, 5′-guanylimidodiphosphate (GMPPNP), increases both the efficacy and the potency of catecholamines for the same. It is be-

lieved that these nucleotides bind to a regulatory site that can affect either the interaction of the catecholamine with the receptor or the coupling of activated receptors to the catalytic subunit of adenylate cyclase (Schramm, 1975; Rodbell et al., 1975).

With this in mind, the recent observations of Murkherjee and Lefkowitz (1976) are pertinent. They described the phenomenon of catecholamine-induced desensitization in a purified membrane preparation from frog erythrocytes. In this cell-free system, the desensitized β adrenergic receptors were rapidly resensitized by exposure of the membranes to guanine nucleotides. Although the effect was most clearly seen with GTP and GMPPNP, the sensitivity of the membrane receptors was also restored by exposure to ATP. It was suggested that nucleotides induce a conformational change in adenylate cyclase that leads in turn to a conformational change in β adrenergic receptors and to the resultant reappearance of sensitivity to catecholamines. Another feature of the role of guanine nucleotides in the regulation of receptor behavior will be discussed below.

It is to be noted also that repeated efforts in our laboratory to increase the sensitivity of various laboratory species to the pharmacologic mediators of immediate hypersensitivities by desensitization of the adrenergic receptors have entirely failed. This is in sharp contrast to the consistent success of the pharmacologic blockade of the β adrenergic receptors to produce such hypersensitivity. It seems, therefore, that induction of hypersensitivity to the pharmacologic mediators requires the selective and not indiscriminate blockade of the adrenergic receptors.

The Phenomenon of Receptor "Interconversion"

The original observation on the effect of temperature shifting the balance of the adrenergic receptors of the frog heart (Kunos and Szentivanyi, 1968) has been extended to include similar "shifts" under a number of conditions associated with low metabolic activity, including hibernation in frogs, low ambient temperatures, low rates of contraction, hypoxia, muscarinic cholinergic stimulation, some metabolic inhibitors, myocardial ischemia, adrenalectomy, and hypothyroidism (Ahlquist, 1977; Nickerson and Kunos, 1977). Current interpretation of these observations favors a true "interconversion" of α- and β-adrenergic receptors over the coexistence of active and nonfunctional receptors inactivated or activated by changes in temperature, hormonal level and other metabolic conditions, respectively.

Two mechanisms of receptor interconversion have been suggested. One speculation is that α and β receptors may represent allosteric configurations of the same structure. Since, furthermore, allosteric enzymes can be influenced by compounds unrelated to the specific substrate, allosteric adrenergic receptors could be appropriately influenced by the postulated modulator substance that has been reported to alter the balance of α- and β-adrenergic vascular responses in skeletal muscle (Szentivanyi, Kunos and Juhasz-Nagy, 1970), or by hormones. The other approach focuses on the physical state of membrane lipids, which is known to be temperature-dependent and can profoundly influence many membrane-associated processes. Indeed, there is evidence that membrane lipids have an essential role in the coupling between β adrenergic binding sites and adenylate cyclase; and discontinuities in the Arrhenius plots of catechol-activated adenylate cyclases were found at temperatures similar to the critical temperature for changes in adrenergic receptor properties. Binding of GTP to a regulatory site, which has been implicated above in the catecholamine-induced activation of adenylate cyclase, was proposed to be the temperature-sensitive event since GTP analogs abolished the break in the Arrhenius plot (Kunos, 1978).

The receptor interconversion phenomenon also includes the histamine receptors. The receptor system for histamine that mediates the contraction of guinea pig intestine is usually regarded as being of a classic H_1 type. When the temperature of the preparation is reduced to 15° C from 37° C, it is found that the H_2 blocking agent metiamide becomes active in this preparation, while the conventional H_1 antihistamines become either less potent or cease to be competitive reversible antagonists (Cook, Kenakin and Krueger, 1977). Thus, receptor interconversion is probably a general feature of receptor behavior, and we expect that it will be shown to occur in all receptor systems of the pharmacologic mediators of immediate hypersensitivities.

Hormonal Deprivation and Overdosage

Whether due to receptor interconversion, another mechanism, or both, the reactivity of the autonomic effector cell to pharmacologic mediators may depend on the hormonal balance within the body.

Glucocorticoids. The most striking illustration of this dependence is the effect of bilateral adrenalectomy in various laboratory species. Adrenalectomy increases the sensitivity to a variety of stressful stimuli and to pharmacologic mediators including histamine, serotonin, bradykinin, and some of the prostaglandins. For instance, cats without adrenals are 13 to 60 times as sensitive to histamine as intact animals, and in adrenalectomized mice the corresponding figure for serotonin is about 30. Since, in most reported studies, response after medullectomy or total sympathectomy has not been tested, it is not possible to assess the relative role of catecholamine versus corticosteroid deficit in these conditions. Nevertheless, in general, the sympathectomized animal occupies an intermediate position between the normal and the adrenalectomized.

Although there are several possible mechanisms by which steroid deprivation could induce hypersensitivity to pharmacologic mediators, it is interesting that a recent study showed that the properties of adrenergic receptors mediating glycogen phosphorylase activation in rat liver shift from α- to β and in muscle from β- to α. It is not known which metabolic process is critical for the change in receptor properties and how is it affected by steroids, but the observed changes appear to be opposite to what may be expected from the association of low metabolic rate with α adrenergic receptors in the heart. This may be owing to different effector tissues, but the possibility that adrenalectomy may have activated the pituitary-thyroid axis could have contributed to the observed changes (Chan and Exton, 1977).

Thyroid Hormones. The reciprocal relationship between corticosteroids and thyroid function is well known. Hyperthyroidism causes a temporary state of cortical deficiency, whereas hypothyroidism results in a temporary accumulation of corticosteroids in tissues. Thus, it is not surprising that thyroxin and triiodothyronine have been shown to sensitize laboratory animals to histamine and serotonin. In addition, thyroid hormones may influence sensitivity to the pharmacologic mediators through their direct effect on adrenergic receptors. Recent *in vitro* binding studies with ^{3}H-dihyroalprenolol suggest that changes in adrenergic reactivity in altered thyroid states may be associated with parallel changes in the number of adrenergic binding sites (Williams et al., 1977).

Estrogen. Estrogen pretreatment has been recently shown to shift adrenergic receptor behavior from beta to alpha as judged by the effect of isoproterenol on rat tail temperature. Normally, isoproterenol induces a marked, rapid increase in tail temperature, an effect that is specifically blocked by propranolol. After 15 weeks of treatment with ethynyl estradiol, this effect is completely abolished. Similarly, estrogen pretreatment reduces the positive chronotropic action of isoproterenol (Ahlquist, 1977).

Insulin. Excess amounts of insulin are also known to increase the sensitivity of some laboratory species to histamine and serotonin. The mechanism of this sensitizing effect is not known, but might be related to the physiologic action of this hormone, since an increased peripheral uptake of glucose occurs in pertussis sensitization and in pharmacologic beta-adrenergic blockade, i.e., in conditions in which hypersensitivity to these mediators has been demonstrated (Szentivanyi, Fishel and Talmage, 1963). Also, alloxan diabetes restores the normal resistance of pertussis-sensitized and beta adrenergically blocked mice to pharmacologic mediators (Fishel and Szentivanyi, 1963); no such sensitization can be produced in inbred mice with the so-called "obese-hyperglycemic" syndrome (Townley, Trapani, and Szentivanyi, 1967). Another congruent observation involves the development of profound changes in the adrenergic receptor quality in human diabetes (Szentivanyi and Pek, 1973). In this condition, the noradrenergic reactions of blood vessels normally sensitive only to α

adrenergic antagonists, can be inhibited by β-blocking agents. This β-sensitive constriction, previously found in alloxan diabetic rabbits (Cseuz, Wenger, Kunos and Szentivanyi, 1973) appears to be now an inherent characteristic of diabetic blood vessels, whether the diabetes has been alloxan-induced or spontaneously developed (Szentivanyi, Takacs and Botos, 1978; Vertesi, Szentivanyi and Szigeti, 1978).

Reflexly and Centrally Induced Hypothalamic Imbalance

There are two reciprocally antagonistic divisions in the hypothalamus: the anterior hypothalamus, which mediates mainly cholinergic responses, and the posterior hypothalamus, in which stimulation results largely in adrenergic responses (Hess, 1954). A balance between these antagonistic divisions is thought to be important in maintaining normal autonomic functions, e.g., blood pressure.

It is possible to produce imbalance of the hypothalamus through the sino-aortic baroreceptors reflexly (Gellhorn, 1957), by applying histamine, acetylcholine, or catecholamines directly on hypothalamic structures, by the electrolytic removal or electrical stimulation of one of the divisions of the hypothalamus, and by many other stimuli (Filipp, Szentivanyi and Mess, 1952; Filipp and Szentivanyi, 1956, 1957; Szentivanyi and Filipp, 1956, 1958; Szentivanyi and Szekely, 1956, 1957a, 1957b, 1958).

The reflexly or locally induced hypothalamic imbalance leads not only to an increased excitability of one hypothalamic division but to simultaneous inhibition of the antagonistic division. Consequently, the action of either a parasympathomimetic stimulus (acetylcholine, histamine) or a sympathomimetic stimulus (catecholamines) may be reduced by a counteracting imbalance induced in the hypothalamus. If, therefore, at the time of action of an exogenously administered or endogenously released pharmacologic mediator the hypothalamus is already in a state of imbalance for any reason, the capacity of the hypothalamus to counteract and control the stimuli will be markedly reduced. In this way the action of the mediator may be profoundly modified both quantitatively and qualitatively even to the complete reversal of its usual pharmacologic activity.

Conclusions

The foregoing procedures used for altering autonomic effector responses were discussed separately and in succession as though the resultant conditions were mechanistically distinct entities. In reality, there is no clear borderline between them, and each contains elements shared by the others. Because of the interrelated effects of the various mediators in autonomic regulation, the altered responsiveness in each of these conditions can be explained on the basis of an imbalance of autonomic regulation at the level of the autonomic effector cell or at the level of its mediator-specific receptors. Implicit in this conclusion is the realization that *manifestations of autonomic imbalance, localized or systemic, need not imply the presence of a neural lesion, that is, a functional and/or organic disorder of any part of the central or peripheral autonomic or somatic nervous systems. Rather it may be due entirely to the abnormal reactivity of the effector cell to neural input or to stimulation by any of the pharmacologic mediators*. In this context, an "autonomic effector cell" is determined by the presence of specific receptors for the chemical organizers of autonomic action, and may be located within or outside the anatomically defined nervous system. There are various mechanisms by which effector cell or tissue hypersensitivity to one or several pharmacologic mediators could occur. However, as indicated in foregoing sections, in any such situations, *it is not the excessive presence but the prolonged lack of the mediator that is likely to result in the development of a chronic effector hypersensitivity*. These conclusions have important bearing on our perception of the nature of the constitutional basis of atopy.

DEVELOPMENT OF THE BETA ADRENERGIC APPROACH TO THE STUDY OF THE CONSTITUTIONAL BASIS OF ATOPY

Authentic atopy cannot be produced at will in animals or humans — neither induced directly nor transferred passively. In addition to anaphylaxis, there are a number of animal models simulating human atopy as well as isolated systems suitable for studying segmented areas of atopic reactivity. As such, they are useful for the analysis of some of the individual events (i.e., mediator release) in the human reaction. Nevertheless, these *in vivo* and *in vitro* models are anaphylactic variants and represent immunologically and pharmacologically normal reactivities. Therefore, they cannot be used for the study of the constitutional abnormality in atopy.

The Two Experimental Models for the Study of the Constitutional Basis of Atopy

Our long search for a laboratory model was guided by the premise that, if it is to be meaningful, the model must be able to imitate not only the immunologic but also the pharmacologic abnormality of the atopic state. As discussed in preceding sections, the latter is manifested against substances which, in mammalian physiology, serve as the natural chemical organizers of autonomic action. It seemed likely, therefore, that an abnormal reactivity to these agents could be most effectively produced through some alteration of normal autonomic regulation significant enough to result in an autonomic imbalance.

The first model: the hypothalamically "imbalanced" anaphylactic guinea pig. With Prof. G. Filipp, the senior author's (A.S.) first attempts to establish a more meaningful experimental counterpart of the atopic state were made in the years of 1952 to 1958 by studying hypothalamically "imbalanced" anaphylactic guinea pigs (Filipp, Szentivanyi and Mess, 1952; Filipp and Szentivanyi, 1956, 1957; Szentivanyi and Filipp, 1956, 1958; Szentivanyi and Szekely, 1956, 1957a, 1957b, 1958).

Briefly, by electrolytic removal of one hypothalamic division or electric stimulation of the antagonistic division, it was possible to profoundly alter the anaphylactic reactivity of guinea pigs both immunologically and pharmacologically. Both from the immunologic and pharmacologic standpoints, the conditions so produced more closely approximated those of the human atopic state than does anaphylaxis. Nevertheless, it was felt that the artificiality of such surgically-induced hypothalamic imbalance is far removed from that natural setting (involving various inherited or acquired factors or both) which may surround the development of an atopic state. In order to imitate more closely those naturally occurring conditions, some of which (i.e., infection) may conceivably serve as a developmental background for atopy, it was felt that the *Bordetella pertussis*-induced hypersensitive state may be a more appropriate model.

The second model: the Bordetella pertussis-induced hypersensitive state of mice and rats. Injection of living or killed *Bordetella pertussis* organisms into certain strains of mice and rats modifies the normal responses of these animals to a number of various stimuli. The possible applicability of the results of these investigations to atopy is implied by the following principal features of the *B. pertussis*–induced altered responsiveness: (1) Hypersensitivity to endogenously released or exogenously administered histamine, serotonin, bradykinin, and, at least in two strains, to acetylcholine. (2) Hypersensitivity to less specific stimuli such as cold, changes in atmospheric pressure, respiratory irritants. (3) In contrast with these increased sensitivities, a reduced sensitivity to catecholamines and, concerning some metabolic parameters, a reversal of normal adrenergic activity. (4) Enhanced antibody formation in general (adjuvant activity), and facilitated production in quantity of antibodies not ordinarily induced by antigenic stimulation. These antibodies exhibit many of the features peculiar to atopic reagin and are thought to represent its animal counterpart. (5) Presence of a marked eosinophilia.

The major advance in these experiments, paving the way for a meaningful analogy to atopic disorders, has been the finding that hypersensitivity of the pertussis-sensitized mouse to pharmacologic mediators may be due to an acquired autonomic imbalance caused primarily by a reduced functioning of the beta receptors or of some of the reactions between receptor activation and adrenergic end-response. In particular, the deprivation of the normal beta adrenergic inhibition of peripheral (extrahepatic) uptake of glucose appears to be instrumental in the production of the hypersensitivity to the various pharmacologic mediators. In addition, this increased rate of entry of glucose may well be the biochemical explanation for the pertussis-induced alterations of the immune response.

Principal Tenets of the Beta Adrenergic Theory of Atopic Disorders

The above considerations as well as conclusions of the two consecutive series of model experiments have culminated in the postulation of the beta adrenergic theory of atopic disorders (Szentivanyi, 1968a). *This theory regards these disorders, i.e., perennial and seasonal allergic rhinitis, bronchial asthma, and atopic dermatitis, not as "immunologic diseases," but as unique patterns of altered reactivities to a broad spectrum of immunologic, psychic, infectious, chemical, and physical stimuli. This view gives to the antigen-antibody interaction the same role as that of a broad category of nonspecific stimuli which function only to trigger the same defective homeostatic mechanism in the various effector cells of the biochemical reaction sequence of immediate hypersensitivities.*

Activation of the same defective mechanism by such a broad spectrum of unrelated triggers is believed to be made possible by the unusual character of the pharmacologic mediators as a biologically distinct class of natural substances. As discussed earlier, these mediators, when viewed from the standpoint of their probable physiologic function, are the chemical organizers of autonomic action, that is, of homeostatic control. Consequently, regardless of the immunologic or nonimmunologic nature of the triggering event, its chemical realization would be expected to be brought about by essentially the same mediators.

Homeostatic adjustment to these influences requires, among others, mobilization of the adrenergic neurotransmitters and their balanced (uninhibited) interaction with their effector systems. The theory postulates that *the constitutional basis of atopy lies in the reduced functioning of the beta adrenergic effector system, irrespective of what the triggering event may chemically be in a particular case (e.g., immunologic, infectious, psychic). In this situation, the adrenergic neurotransmitters are released in the face of a relatively unresponsive beta effector system, and the resultant autonomic imbalance deprives the effector tissues of their normal counterregulatory adjustment. This constellation of mediators and effectors leads then to a unique pattern of quantitatively and qualitatively altered reactivity to the chemical organizers of autonomic action, mostly in response to trivial trauma.*

The most critical component of this malfunctioning effector system, is the adenylate cyclase–coupled beta adrenergic receptor or, more specifically, the receptor-transducer-adenylate cyclase complex. It follows, therefore, that the fundamental abnormality common to all atopic persons may lie in an inherited or acquired lesion of this complex resulting in its defective functioning. This reduced responsiveness to catecholamines could reflect alterations at any of a number of sites, including (a) changes in the affinity of catecholamines and their receptor sites, (b) decreases in the concentration of beta receptors, (c) "interconversion" of adrenergic receptors from beta to alpha, (d) alterations in the efficiency of coupling of activated receptors to the catalytic units of adenylate cyclase, and (e) reductions in the concentration of adenylate cyclase. Alternatively, the postulated lesion may occur at a point beyond the cAMP generation step in the biochemical sequence leading to the adrenergic end-response, in a cAMP-related pathway, in a complementary interacting or modulating system such as that provided by the prostaglandins, or in an intracellular messenger system with counterregulatory potential such as that connected with cyclic GMP. Nevertheless, *the currently available evidence seems to favor the possibility that the postulated lesion lies at an early point of the adrenergic reaction sequence involving either a reduction in beta receptor concentration or mechanisms similar to those that may occur in receptor interconversions.*

Progression of the disease process from a subclinical to a clinical form conceivably requires the operation of a preparatory and a triggering factor. The preparatory factor involves the postulated abnormality and it may be familial (presumably hereditary) or acquired in nature, but in either case, it must set the stage for the development of a functional imbalance. On the other hand, the triggering event must be appropriate to result in an increase in the rate of firing of adrenergic neurons, in the release of catecholamines from extraneuronal stores or in any conceivable mediator constellations appropriate to make the latent abnormality clinically manifest. However, the preparatory and triggering factors need not be separate or unrelated entities. Infection (probably viral), for example, could serve in both capacities.

With the exception of nonnucleated erythrocytes, the adenylate cyclase system has been found to be present in all animal cells examined to date. Its ubiquitous character suggests, therefore, that *the ultimate clinical manifestation of the fundamentally same atopic abnormality will be determined by the type of cell primarily involved, that is, by the effector cell system which harbors primarily the postulated abnormality* (cells of bronchial tissue versus those of nasal mucosa, skin, and circulating cells of blood).

THE SIGNIFICANT FACTS TO BE ACCOUNTED FOR BY ANY THEORY OF THE CONSTITUTIONAL BASIS OF ATOPY

Ideally, an examination of evidence supporting the hypothesis just described should proceed following a clear and valid definition or characterization of these disease states themselves. The latter may be defined on the basis of their established cause, functional or morphologic characteristics, or clinical manifestations. When attempting to take this approach, however, we are confronted with presently unsolvable difficulties.

For instance, the cause of asthma is not known, and no single manifestation or combination of criteria permits its precise definition at present. The term "asthma" rarely is used with the same connotation or defined in the same way by different authorities. Even greater are the difficulties faced with considering atopic dermatitis as an entity.

Nevertheless, it is possible to assemble the most consistently prominent, common characteristics of atopic disorders, and such a combination of features may be used as an analytical guide to their constitutional basis. Thus, any interpretation of the constitutional basis of atopy must account for the following significant facts surrounding these conditions:

1. The altered reactivity to the chemical organizers of autonomic action
2. The primary clinical involvement of one effector tissue (the concept of the "shock organ")
3. The immunologic abnormality
4. Close association with infection
5. Eosinophilia of common occurrence
6. Increased tolerance to beta adrenergic stimulation
7. Eminent therapeutic effectiveness of agents which are capable of restoring normal beta adrenergic action
8. Susceptibility to a variety of unrelated precipitating factors.

Once we have accepted that these are indeed the cardinal features of the atopic state with pathognomonic potential, it will be necessary to further ask (1) is it possible, and (2) is there any need, to explain all these characteristics by one single primary mechanism? It is the fundamental assumption of the beta adrenergic approach to the constitutional basis of atopy that both of these questions may be answered in the affirmative.

THE ALTERED REACTIVITY TO THE CHEMICAL ORGANIZERS OF AUTONOMIC ACTION

The immunologic concept postulates that the constitutional abnormality in atopy is due to the development and actions of IgE antibody. However, there are numerous features of the atopic state not in accord with a strictly immunologically based perception of atopy. For instance, atopic disorders have been recorded in both agammaglobulinemic and otherwise normal individuals who have no detectable reaginic antibody. Conversely, the postulated causative factor, the reagin, can be shown to be present in individuals who never had in the past or at the time of testing any evidence of atopic disease or of clinical allergy to the corresponding allergen. Similarly, a high degree of skin reactivity (implying the presence of reagin) can, and frequently does, remain when clinically sensitive patients become asymptomatic as a result of specific hyposensitization (Szentivanyi and Fishel, 1966). Moreover, when the reagin is found in atopic disorders, reagins present may be directed against antigens that never elicited any clinical manifestations, while the

patient's history may clearly point to an offending substance to which reaginic antibody is undetectable. There are additional observations which appear irreconcilable with an immunologic basis of atopy.

Unusual Predilection for Certain "Shock Organs" in Atopy. An example of this is the unusual predilection for certain "shock organs" in atopy: the bronchial tree in asthma, the nasal mucosa in allergic rhinitis, and the skin in atopic dermatitis. Although a selective involvement of the immune apparatus in the shock tissue in question could be postulated, it is difficult even on this basis to explain the observation that an individual with one form of these disorders frequently develops another, and it is a common occurrence for there to be an alternation in the focus from one shock organ to another, i.e., from atopic dermatitis to asthma (Takino and Takino, 1956; Pearlman and Szentivanyi, 1968). Moreover, given an individual with any of the atopic disorders, the symptomatology characteristic to that particular disorder can be reproduced by the exogenous administration of otherwise harmless amounts of pharmacologic mediators (Samter, 1933; Curry and Leard, 1948; Curry and Lowell, 1948; Nakamura, 1954; Tiffeneau, 1957; Olivier, 1958; Scherbel and Harrison, 1959; Duchaine and Spapen, 1959; Hajos, 1962; deVries et al., 1962; Melon and Lecomte, 1962). For example, in asthmatics, the injection of pharmacologic mediators (acetylcholine, histamine, serotonin) induces wheezing, but not hives, while in individuals suffering from chronic urticaria it induces hives, but not wheezing (Weiss et al., 1929, 1932; Rose, 1940, 1947; Curry, 1946, 1947; Rose et al., 1950; Graham and Wolf, 1950; Morgan, 1943; Melon and Lecomte, 1958). The same applies to atopic dermatitis (Baer, 1955).

It will be recalled that in atopic dermatitis perhaps the best-known clinical peculiarity is the presence of certain well-delineated sites of predilection, that is, the favored involvement of the skin of the face, the neck, the antecubital, and the popliteal flexural regions. It was found that these sites of predilection are identical with histamine flush regions. When histamine is injected hypodermically, the characteristic flush appears in these sites of predilection, together with an increase in skin temperature in these areas. This phenomenon applies whether or not the patient has active atopic dermatitis at the time of testing (Williams, 1938). Furthermore, the amounts of pharmacologic mediators needed to reproduce the characteristic symptomatology in individuals with various atopic manifestations is sometimes on the order of several thousand fold less than that required to produce any demonstrable changes in nonatopic persons (Mathe et al., 1973).

Quantitatively Increased and Qualitatively Altered Pharmacologic Reactivities in Atopy. Not only do atopic individuals exhibit a quantitatively striking hyperreactivity to the pharmacologic mediators of immediate hypersensitivities confined to autonomic effector cells corresponding to the shock organ of the particular atopic disorder, but an exquisite degree of such hypersensitivity can persist for years after the atopic individual becomes asymptomatic (Szentivanyi and Fitzpatrick, 1979). In addition, relatives of atopic individuals with no disorder of this kind may show some degree of hypersensitivity to the pharmacologic mediators (Nakamura, 1954; Takino and Takino, 1956).

Signs of a qualitatively abnormal responsiveness also can be found in atopy. An outstanding example of this is the so-called "delayed blanch" reaction to acetylcholine (Lobitz and Campbell, 1953). This phenomenon refers to a local blanching, i.e., to an abnormal vasoconstrictor effect of intradermally injected acetylcholine, instead of its usual vasodilatory effect producing an erythematous response. This abnormal response to acetylcholine, first described in atopic dermatitis (Lobitz et al., 1957; Davis and Lawler, 1958; Reed and Kierland, 1958; Kalz and Fekete, 1960), also has been reported to be present in a high percentage of asthmatic and hay fever patients who do not suffer from atopic dermatitis (West et al., 1962). Of further interest is the lacking flare portion of the triple response in patients with atopic dermatitis, when histamine is injected intradermally. This is reminiscent of the situation seen following section and/or degeneration of the peripheral sensory nerve, when the flare component no longer is obtained.

Atopics also exhibit dermographism, increased sino-aortic reflex activity, a flat glucose tolerance curve and tendencies toward hypoglycemia and hypotension, increased blood levels of cholesterol, an increased potassium-calcium quotient, abnormal vascular reactions, i.e., signs which have been interpreted to indicate a malfunction of the autonomic effector cells of some kind. This autonomic instability may be present even before the atopic disease becomes manifest (Rothlin and Bircher, 1952). Furthermore, the influence of psychic stimuli on atopic disorders is well known.

The Altered Reactivity to the Chemical Organizers of Autonomic Action as the Uniformly Present, Single Atopic Characteristics of Pathognomonic Significance. The foregoing facts and considerations are not easily reconcilable with the immunologic concept as an all-inclusive view of the nature of the constitutional abnormality in atopic disease. To account for both the immunologic and nonimmunologic aspects of atopy, a second concept had to be invoked, which has been discussed above. Because of the essential identity of the pharmacologic mediators of immediate hypersensitivities and the chemical organizers of normal autonomic action, and because of their interrelated effects, these two concepts may not necessarily be mutually exclusive. In fact, to some extent, they may even be interdependent. The immunologic injury may contribute to the development of an autonomic imbalance, and conversely, the autonomic imbalance may be operative in determining the characteristics of the antibody response (Szentivanyi, 1968a).

In yet another way, atopy may constitute an etiologically and pathomechanistically heterogeneous group of diseases and the two concepts may cover different categories of atopic persons; therefore, both concepts, when limied to the corresponding category, could be entirely valid. The obvious inference of such a conclusion would be that the nature of the constitutional background itself is heterogeneous. In other words, one may suppose that there are atopic individuals wherein the underlying constitutional abnormality is the excessive production of reagin, whereas, there are other individuals in whom the postulated adrenergic abnormality is the primary constitutional factor.

However, the altered responsiveness to the chemical organizers of autonomic action is one single characteristic that seems to be shared by such a high percentage of atopics that, for all practical purposes, it could be regarded as being uniformly present. The uniform presence of one, single characteristic feature in an otherwise heterogeneous group of diseases must of necessity indicate its primary pathognomonic significance. This implies that any acceptable definition of atopic disease must be able to account for that single characteristic of pathognomonic significance and also that it is both possible and necessary to explain the various features of atopy through the postulation of a single primary mechanism. For this and other reasons (see later), the *beta adrenergic theory defines atopic diseases not as immunologic diseases, but as manifestations of altered effector reactivities to the chemical organizers of autonomic action.*

As shown by the animal model experiments below, the cause of the altered effector reactivity in atopy may lie in the reduced functioning of some of the beta adrenergic mechanisms involved in the regulation of such responses.

Sensitization by Pertussis and Beta Adrenergic Blocking Agents to the Pharmacologic Mediators. Whole cells of *Bordetella pertussis,* or their purified component, which is responsible for the histamine sensitizing activity, the so-called "histamine sensitizing factor" (HSF), have been shown to produce hypersensitivity to endogenously released or exogenously administered histamine, serotonin, bradykinin, SRS-A, $PGF_{2\alpha}$, and, at least in two mouse strains, to acetylcholine. In contrast, a reduced sensitivity to catecholamines and, concerning some metabolic parameters, a reversal of the normal beta adrenergic response may be produced both by whole pertussis cells and by HSF. Using the latter, inhibition of some beta adrenergic responses can also be demonstrated *in vitro* (see later). It is believed, therefore, that the histamine and other pharmacologic hypersensitivities are due to a blockade of some of the beta adrenergic receptors produced by the HSF component of the bacterial cell.

Indeed, the evidence is unequivocal that pharmacologic blockade of the beta adrenergic receptors is capable of inducing a hypersensitivity to histamine, serotonin, acetylcholine, bradykinin, slow-reacting substance of anaphylaxis, and $PGF_{2\alpha}$, regardless of whether these agents were released (formed) endogenously or administered exogenously.

All laboratory species tested thus far were shown to be susceptible to sensitization by beta blockade with any of the available specific beta$_2$ blockers. Although within the same species there are substantial strain differences in susceptibility, a combination of beta blockade and of various procedures conceivably resulting in additive blockade of beta or simultaneous stimulation of alpha, could invariably break strain-resistance to sensitization (Townley, Trapani and Szentivanyi, 1967). Conversely, protection of susceptible strains was obtained through interventions known to protect beta receptors against development of a blockade, or to bypass or eliminate an already established one.

Sensitization by beta blockade is still effective after pithing of the spinal cord and cutting of the cervical vagus nerves. Structure-activity comparisons designed to characterize the structural requirements for sensitization by beta blocking agents showed that their sensitizing activity is specific; that is, it is due to their ability to inhibit the beta pharmacologic actions of catecholamines (Katsh, Halkias and Szentivanyi, 1969). In contrast to this consistent success of beta adrenergic blockade to produce histamine hypersensitivity, repeated efforts to increase the sensitivity of various laboratory species to histamine by the simultaneous desensitization of both alpha and beta adrenergic receptors have entirely failed. Induction of hypersensitivity to the pharmacologic mediators requires, therefore, selective blockade of beta adrenergic receptors (Szentivanyi and Fitzpatrick, 1979). Even within the beta adrenergic receptor range, there is further specificity required for sensitization to histamine, inasmuch as the cardioselective beta$_1$ blocking agent, practolol, is devoid of sensitizing activity. Furthermore, since the postulated role of cyclic AMP is that of an intracellular mediator of beta adrenergic mechanisms, it is important to note that a significantly reduced cyclic AMP synthesis to adrenergic stimulation was found in various tissues and cell systems of the pertussis-sensitized mouse (Ortez, Klein and Szentivanyi, 1970; Klein, Szentivanyi and Fishel, 1974; Ortez, Seshachalam and Szentivanyi, 1975; Szentivanyi, Polson and Krzanowski, 1979).

A natural bridge between the foregoing discussion and the beta adrenergic interpretation of the atopic abnormality has now been provided by the finding that histamine sensitivity, epinephrine-induced changes in blood sugar, and isoproterenol-induced alteration in heart rate are influenced by pertussis immunization; immunization of normal healthy children remarkably increases histamine sensitivity and, concurrently, markedly diminishes epinephrine-induced hyperglycemia and isoproterenol-induced change in heart rate. Thus, humans also can be sensitized to histamine by pertussis vaccination and the hypersensitive state so produced is accompanied by manifestations of defective adrenergic mechanisms (Sen, Arora, Gupta and Sanyal, 1974).

Mice sensitized to pertussis and exposed to ragweed pollen experimentally by aerosolization or naturally in the late summer when ragweed pollen is in the air develop anaphylactic sensitivity to pollen (Chang and Gottshall, 1974). The pertussis vaccination–induced adrenergic lesion, therefore, may provide the type of natural developmental background that appears to operate in a spontaneously acquired atopic state.

Finally, reactivity of the sensitized guinea pig to inhalational antigen-challenge can be markedly enhanced when, prior to aerosol exposure to the specific antigen, the animal is blocked beta adrenergically by a specific pharmacologic blocking agent (Townley, Trapani and Szentivanyi, 1967). The foregoing finding may add yet another conceptual bridge to similar observations described below in human asthmatics.

Effect of Beta Adrenergic Blocking Agents in Atopy. Beta adrenergic blockade has been shown to enhance bronchial reactivity to inhaled allergens, or to methacholine in patients with seasonal allergic rhinitis and without a previous history of bronchial asthma. By progressively increasing doses of the beta blocker, an acute airway obstruction could be produced that seemed to reach an intensity that may be found in patients with bronchial asthma (Reed and Townley, 1978). Administration of beta blockers also has been reported (McNeill, 1964; McNeill and Ingram, 1966; Meier, Lydtin and Zollner, 1966) to aggravate already existent asthmatic conditions and to cause precipitous and prolonged falls in forced expiratory volume in one second ($FEV_{1.0}$).

Blockade of beta receptors was found to increase significantly the bronchial sensitivity of asthmatic subjects to methacholine, whereas no such effect was detectable in normal human subjects as judged by the change in $FEV_{1.0}$ (Zaid and Beall, 1966). However, by using a more specific and sensitive measurement of airway resistance, the whole-body plethysmograph method, a 50 to 100 percent increase in airway resistance has been observed also in normal subjects in the first 30 minutes after the administration of a beta blocker (Besterman and Friedlander, 1965; Besterman, 1966; McNeill and Ingram, 1966). It is important to note that in the latter experiments, beta blockade was capable of producing airway obstruction even without any simultaneous respiratory provocation such as exposure to histamine or methacholine. Conversely, production of alpha adrenergic blockade has been reported to ameliorate asthmatic attacks as well as to reduce the observed hypersensitivity to exogenously administered histamine and cholinergic agents (Curry, Fuchs and Leard, 1950; Goodman and Nickerson, 1950).

In atopic dermatitis, the only available information on the effect of a pharmacologically established beta adrenergic blockade has to do with the analysis of the acetylcholine-induced sweat gland response in atopic and nonatopic subjects. This study was prompted by the finding that the response of the sweat gland to intradermal injection of acetylcholine is abnormally increased in patients with atopic dermatitis both in terms of threshold sensitivity as well as total sweat production. When these observations were repeated with or without propranolol in healthy individuals, in patients with nonatopic dermatoses, and in patients with atopic dermatitis, it was found that beta blockade enhanced the sweat response to acetylcholine in the first two groups, but not in the third. This was interpreted to mean that patients with atopic dermatitis already have an "endogenous" beta blockade resulting in a baseline sweat response to acetylcholine that is maximally enhanced, so that propranolol cannot produce a further increase in acetylcholine reactivity (Hemels, 1970).

The Evidence Against Cholinergic Overactivity as the Constitutional Basis of Atopy. In the past two decades, Nadel (1977), Gold (1978), and their associates have accumulated evidence indicating that stimulation of rapidly adapting epithelial nerve receptors of the airways by mechanical, chemical, and pharmacologic stimuli, reflexly increases the output of acetylcholine by the vagus nerves, causing a reflex bronchoconstriction. In particular, it was shown that although histamine is capable of constricting airway smooth muscles directly, most of its bronchoconstrictor effect *in vivo* is indirect, and due to this reflex mechanism. This is accomplished both by direct stimulation of these epithelial receptors and also by decreasing their firing threshold to other introduced stimuli. Thus, when histamine is injected into dog bronchial arteries, most of the airway constriction can be abolished by atropine. In otherwise healthy subjects, viral upper respiratory tract infections, through damage to the bronchial epithelium, cause transient bronchial hyperreactivity to inhaled histamine and citric acid, a phenomenon that also is abolished by anticholinergic drugs. On the basis of these and similar observations as well as the fact that bronchial hyperreactivity is associated with a decrease in cough threshold, these workers suggested that airway epithelial damage with sensitization of airway nerve endings causes exaggerated cough and bronchomotor responses. With this background, Nadel, Gold, and their associates, further postulated that bronchial asthma is a constellation involving two ingredients: release of pharmacologic mediators, and sensitization of airway epithelial nerve receptors providing a positive feedback system for increasing bronchomotor tone.

This mechanism in fact probably contributes to the bronchial obstructive process in asthma. The altered pharmacologic reactivity in atopy, however, is not restricted to airway epithelial effectors, but it is a universal trait. In fact, as explained earlier, the altered pharmacologic reactivity is the uniformly present, single atopic characteristic, which by its very nature must be explained in any theory attempting to elucidate the constitutional basis of atopy. For the reasons below, cholinergic overactivity cannot serve in this capacity.

Using spontaneously breathing, unanesthetized guinea pigs, it has been found that the vagal reflex component in histamine bronchoconstriction is small and probably a consequence rather than a cause of the constriction. In histamine-sensitive and histamine-insensitive strains of guinea pigs it has been demonstrated that the ease of *in vivo* histamine-induced reduction in lung compliance in the guinea pig is inversely related to its *in vitro* tracheal sensitivity to isoproterenol, revealing the primary homeostatic importance of the tracheobronchial beta adrenergic receptors rather than that of cholinergic control, in determining the sensitivity of this effector tissue to histamine (Holgate and Warner, 1960; Douglas et al., 1973, 1976).

Furthermore, no reproducible evidence of elevated levels of acetylcholine in tissues or body fluids of atopic individuals is available. This, in fact, is not surprising when the issue of cholinergic overactivity is examined in the broader biologic context of the general nature of cholinergic versus adrenergic control. Thus, the sympathetic system is distributed to effectors throughout the body, whereas the parasympathetic distribution is much more limited. For instance, sympathetic postganglionic fibers also innervate smooth muscles and glands of somatic (nonvisceral) regions; no comparable distribution has been established for the parasympathetic division. Moreover, the sympathetic fibers ramify to a much greater extent, and their preganglionic terminals make contact with a large number of postganglionic neurons. In general, the ratio of preganglionic to postganglionic axons may be about 1:20 or more. In addition, there is an overlapping of synaptic innervation so that one ganglion cell is supplied by several preganglionic fibers. By contrast, the parasympathetics are more discrete in the action, i.e., there is closer to a 1:1 relation between pre- and postganglionic neurons (Szentivanyi, Krzanowski and Polson, 1978). Also, the parasympathetic nervous system has no reinforcing mechanism comparable to that of the adrenal medulla for the sympathetic division.

Usually, when any part of the sympathetic nervous system is stimulated, the entire system, or at least major portions of it, are stimulated at the same time, a phenomenon called mass discharge. Norepinephrine and epinephrine, therefore, are almost always released by the adrenal medulla at the same time that the different tissues are being stimulated directly by the sympathetic nerves. The two means of stimulation support each other and either can actually substitute for the other. Without any stimulation, however, the normal resting rate of secretion by the adrenal medulla is sufficient to maintain blood pressure almost to normal even if all direct sympathetic pathways to the cardiovascular system are removed. Another important value of the adrenal medulla is the capability of catecholamines to stimulate structures of the body that are not innervated by sympathetic fibers. In contrast, the characteristics of parasympathetic reflexes are discrete. For instance, they usually act only on the heart to increase or decrease its activity, or frequently cause secretion only in the mouth or, in other instances, secretion only by the stomach glands.

Acetylcholine (ACh), i.e., the cholinergic transmitter released by parasympathetic fibers, is almost instantaneously destroyed in the junctional clefts by an unusual enzyme, acetylcholinesterase (true cholinesterase, AChE). The principal evidence for this is the decay time of the end-plate current, which is more rapid than diffusion of ACh out of a synaptic cleft would allow. Also, the most recent preparation of AChE hydrolyzed 960 nmoles ACh per mg of protein per hour, thus placing it among the enzymes having the highest turnover number that is known (Szentivanyi, Krzanowski and Polson, 1978). This powerful destructive capacity is reinforced by a battery of butyryl cholinesterases ("pseudo" or nonspecific cholinesterases) which destroy most of whatever acetylcholine may have escaped into the blood stream. Thus, it is doubtful whether acetylcholine can reach noninnervated cells or is present in the extracellular space in regulatory concentrations for cells with immunologic significance such as the antigen-sensitive lymphocytes (see later). There is no comparable system of rapid destruction for the catecholamines, a fact which accounts in part for the widespread nature of sympathetic action.

Another way to determine whether we are dealing with a primary cholinergic overactivity in atopy is to examine whether there is any evidence for an enhanced guanylate cyclase activity in cells obtained from patients with atopic disease. This is all the more necessary, since as mentioned earlier, cholinergic and alpha adrenergic agents activate guanylate cyclase, and markedly reduced adenylate cyclase-cyclic AMP responses to beta adrenergic stimulation have been shown to be present in atopic individuals.

Under these circumstances, it is highly significant that the available evidence shows not an enhanced but a reduced cholinergic responsiveness in lymphocytes of atopic individuals. Thus, it was found that in normal subjects alpha adrenergic stimulations with norepinephrine plus propranolol, and cholinergic stimulation with acetylcholine evoked significant increases in cyclic GMP formation. In contrast, the lymphocytic guanylate cyclase activity did not show a significant response to the same agents in patients with acute asthma, but the normal guanylate cyclase responsiveness was found to be partially restored in patients in remission (Haddock, Patel, Alston and Kerr, 1975). Similarly, Lang, Goel and Grieco (1978), in their study (described later) on adrenergic and cholinergic responses of peripheral lymphocytes in the "active" E rosette assay, demonstrated not only a subsensitivity of T lymphocytes to beta adrenergic but also to cholinergic stimulation in patients with bronchial asthma. In the same experiments, phenylephrine, an alpha adrenergic agonist, showed no difference between the normal and asthmatic groups in enhancing the "active" E rosette formation. A subsensitive beta adrenergic and cholinergic system with a normal alpha adrenergic effector system may produce a state of relatively enhanced alpha adrenergic activity, a circumstance which may explain some of the findings showing that by giving alpha receptor blockers one can restore beta adrenergic responsiveness toward normal in lymphocytes of asthmatics (Logsdon et al., 1973; Alston, Patel and Kerr, 1974).

There are additionally at least three major arguments against cholinergic overactivity as the primary mechanism of atopy. First, neither pulmonary sympathectomy nor pulmonary vagotomy produces any lasting improvement in bronchial asthma. Second, as shown previously, *it is never the excessive presence of a neurohumor, but if anything, it is its prolonged lack that is likely to result in the development of chronic effector hypersensitivities.* Consequently, it is inconceivable that cholinergic overactivity could produce a hypersensitivity to acetylcholine or similar mediators of immediate hypersensitivities. On the contrary, cholinergic overactivity would be expected to lead to desensitization of the cholinergic receptors, as has been extensively demonstrated in numerous preparations such as the skeletal muscles of the frog, the hearts of vertebrates and invertebrates, the

Renshaw cells, the neurons of molluscks, etc. (Michelson and Danilov, 1971). Finally, if the atopic state were to be due to cholinergic overactivity, then anticholinergic agents should have a far more demonstrable therapeutic effect than what we are able to observe in asthma, let alone the other atopic conditions where they are useless.

THE IMMUNE ABNORMALITY

From what has been and will continue to be discussed about the role of IgE antibody in atopy, it follows that involvement of IgE antibody is not a required characteristic of an atopic disorder despite their frequent association. The nature of this relationship is not known, but its interpretation in the beta adrenergic approach requires a prior understanding of some aspects of the reactivities of the antigen-sensitive lymphocytes as they relate to cyclic nucleotides in normal as well as in atopic states.

Normal Reactivities of Antigen-Sensitive Lymphocytes and Their Relation to Cyclic Nucleotides

Antigen-sensitive lymphocytes are of two types, T (thymus-derived) and B (bone marrow–derived) cells (see Chapter 1). Lymphocytes and thymocytes contain both cyclic AMP and cyclic GMP and possess the enzymes catalyzing their synthesis as well as destruction providing the same possibilities for regulation of cellular function that are inherent in other cells.

Intracellular levels of cyclic AMP in human peripheral lymphocytes can be increased up to several-fold by beta adrenergic agents, prostaglandins, and various glucocorticoids. Parallel with their cyclic AMP increasing effects, these agents all inhibit the proliferation of lymphocytes (Parker, Sullivan and Wedner, 1974). This antiproliferative effect of beta adrenergically–induced cyclic AMP accumulation in lymphocytes correlates well with extensive similar observations on nonlymphocytic normal as well as transformed cells in tissue culture and other preparations indicating that cyclic AMP is an inhibitor of cell proliferation in a variety of cell systems (Pastan et al., 1975; Anderson and Pastan, 1975; MacManus et al., 1975).

In addition to the antiproliferative effect exhibited by catecholamines acting through β-adrenergic receptors, there exists a proliferation-augmenting action resulting from an α-adrenergic mechanism. Analysis of this mechanism showed that α-adrenergic stimulation increases lymphocytic glucose uptake and utilization, and glycogen accumulation, and that norepinephrine acting through this α-adrenergic mechanism directly stimulates adenosine triphosphatases (ATPases) in lymphocytic plasma membranes. The relationship of cyclic nucleotides to these transport-linked enzymes remains unclear at this time, and while such action of norepinephrine has been linked to cyclic GMP in vas deferens and in platelets, so far this association has not been reported in lymphocytes, nor has a direct link of cyclic GMP to membrane ATPases been established (Hadden, 1977).

Agents that increase cyclic GMP in lymphocytes, such as acetylcholine, also augment proliferation of these cells. This action of acetylcholine involves an atropine-sensitive muscarinic receptor mechanism. To date it has not been possible to show that acetylcholine exerts any positive influence on calcium influx or transport of nutrients into lymphocytes, indicating that the proliferation-promoting action of acetylcholine is directly linked to cyclic GMP and may not involve transport-related mechanisms. Increase in lymphocytic cyclic GMP, through inhibition of cyclic GMP phosphodiesterase by imidazole, also augments mitogen-induced human lymphocyte proliferation.

Another naturally occurring substance shown to act on lymphocytes is insulin. Insulin was found to increase glucose uptake in lymphocytes and to augment lymphocyte proliferation in response to mitogen and allogeneic stimulation. The mechanism of this insulin action on lymphocytes has not been studied in detail, but it has been shown in other cells that insulin inhibits intracellular accumulation of cyclic AMP through inhibition of adenylate cyclase or stimulation of cyclic AMP phosphodiesterase or both. Insulin action also has been linked to cyclic GMP accumulation in fibroblasts, fat, and liver cells (Goldberg, 1974; Goldberg and Haddox, 1977), and at least one laboratory found two- to three-fold increases in cyclic GMP in lymphocytes following exposure to insulin (Hadden, 1977).

For all the complexities involved in the regulation of lymphocyte proliferation by cyclic nucleotides, including the many controversial aspects, other recent reviews should be consulted (Parker et al., 1974; Pastan et al., 1975; MacManus et al., 1975; Hadden, 1977; Watson, 1977; Strom and Carpenter, 1977; Szentivanyi et al., 1979). For our purposes it will suffice to state that α-adrenergic, β-adrenergic, and cholinergic mechanisms as well as their biochemical correlates, the cyclic nucleotides, could conceivably have a major controlling influence on the proliferation of lymphocytes. This control appears to be bidirectional inasmuch as *cholinergic and α-adrenergic influences enhance whereas beta adrenergic effects inhibit lymphocyte proliferation. The bidirectional character of this regulation, however, may be more apparent than real, since, as previously mentioned, we have no clear understanding of the regulatory potential of acetylcholine outside the junctional cleft. Therefore, the presence of the aforementioned muscarinic acetylcholine receptor on lymphocytes may or may not have physiologic significance. Thus, it is possible that homeostatic regulation of circulating lymphocytes is essentially adrenergic in character.* The significance of this problem lies in the fact that the *primum movens* in the induction of the immune response is the replication of cells selected by the antigen from a large number of preexisting clones of lymphocytes. Replication is needed to generate the necessary mass of cells with specificity for antigen, and thereby convert a preexisting potential into the quantitative reality of antibody production. Any malfunctioning in this highly critical replication step would be expected to result in an abnormal antibody response.

The Illuminating Lawfulness of a Biologic Paradox. A full appreciation of the significance of these considerations requires a closer definition of the general role of cyclic AMP in cell function and that of the primary biologic mission of the lymphocyte. A generalized interpretation of all the available evidence indicates that *cyclic 3',5'-adenosine monophosphate participates in those biologic processes that involve the promotion of pre-programmed events consistent with the differentiated phenotype, i.e., the functions for which that cell type is developed* (e.g., for the liver, glucose production from glycogen;

for the adrenal gland, steroid production; for fat tissue, lipolysis). As to the lymphocyte, its mature, circulating form is a resting cell (restricted "G_1"), the biology of which, among other responses, is dominated by clonal proliferation on exposure to antigen. *The lymphocyte, then, appears to be an exception to almost all other cells in that its dominant response appears to be antagonized rather than promoted by cyclic AMP. In fact, cyclic AMP appears to participate as an inhibitory regulator of the functions of virtually every cell involved in the expression of the immune response,* including the B and T lymphocyte, macrophage, polymorphonuclear and basophilic leukocyte, mast cell and platelet. *From the standpoint of autonomic control, therefore, it is the beta adrenergically activated cyclic AMP system that represents the most important restrictive influence on the functions of cells responsible for the organization of the immune response.* A reduced functioning of this restrictive mechanism, therefore, would be expected to result in an abnormally exaggerated antibody response.

Abnormal Reactivities of Antigen-Sensitive Lymphocytes and Their Relation to Adrenergic Mechanisms

Many atopic individuals react with an abnormal antibody response to natural exposures to antigen. The nature of this abnormality is not known, but it involves the production of an antibody, the so-called reagin, skin-sensitizing antibody, or immunoglobulin E (IgE) possessing distinct physicochemical and biologic properties. Increased IgE levels occur in about 40 percent to 60 percent of patients with "extrinsic" asthma, whereas in "intrinsic" asthma normal IgE values are regularly found. In isolated hay fever, usually a smaller fraction of patients have elevated IgE, and their mean values are lower than in asthmatics (Johansson and Foucard, 1978). Patients with atopic dermatitis frequently have high serum IgE levels, but as in asthma and rhinitis, patients with atopic dermatitis can be divided into two groups: one with elevated and one with normal or even low IgE levels (Öhman and Johansson, 1974). It is not clear how to relate an elevated level (serum and/or tissue) of IgE to the cutaneous manifestation of atopic dermatitis, since it is unlikely that an IgE-mediated wheal and flare contributes substantially to the genesis of an eczematous disease (Rasmussen and Provost, 1978).

Furthermore, IgE levels in hypo- and agammaglobulinemia are extremely low or undetectable (McLaughlan et al., 1974; Stites et al., 1972) despite that eczematous dermatitis clinically indistinguishable from atopic dermatitis is known to occur in X-linked agammaglobulinemia (Peterson et al., 1962). Conversely, reaginic antibody to specific antigen can be shown to be present in individuals who never had in the past or at the time of testing any evidence of atopic allergy whatsoever (Rackemann and Simon, 1935; Grow and Herman, 1936; Lamson and Rogers, 1936; Efron et al., 1940; Efron and Boatner, 1942; Szentivanyi et al., 1952; Lindblad and Farr, 1961; Farr, 1963). Often, when the reaginic antibody is found in atopic disorders, there is no correspondence between the particular reaginic antibody present and those antigens (or nonantigenic stimuli for that matter) that appear to be responsible for eliciting the clinical symptoms of the disorder (Bonifazi et al., 1978). Finally, enhanced IgE production occurs in many nonatopic diseases without the presence of any other atopic feature (Johansson and Foucard, 1978; Buckley, 1978).

For these reasons, *the ability to develop IgE antibody and to develop atopic disease must be considered as characteristics independent of one another. Likewise, the altered reactivity of atopic individuals to the chemical organizers of autonomic action present uniformly, and their capacity to produce IgE antibody not always present, appear to be independent variables* (Muranaka et al., 1974). Thus, the difference between high and low IgE producers may be related to genetic information at a step irrelevant to autonomic imbalance. *On the other hand, probably at a different step of biologic control, the postulated adrenergic lesion in atopy could conceivably enhance IgE production* by mechanisms described earlier and continued to be discussed below.

Pertussis-Induced Alterations of Antibody Formation and Adrenergic Mechanisms. Available evidence indicates that the purified HSF of the *B. pertussis* cell, which is responsible for the histamine sensitizing activity, is either identical with or inseparable by a wide variety of procedures from the factor possessing the immunologic adjuvant activity. It also is known that pertussis vaccine produces a striking increase in the rate of formation of lymphocytes in thymus, spleen, and lymph nodes (Fichtelius and Hassler, 1958; Morse, 1978) and has an accelerating effect on the growth of murine lymphomas (Floersheim, 1967; Hirano et al., 1967). Pertussis-vaccinated mice rendered lymphocytopenic by x-radiation, or by hydrocortisone, still have lymphocytosis. The ability of pertussis vaccine to promote lymphocytosis closely resembles its capacity to produce pharmacologic hypersensitivity, and can be reproduced by purified HSF preparations. Hyperplasia of lymphoid tissue also has been produced by chronic administration of pharmacologic beta adrenergic blocking agents. This is consistent with the potent inhibition of lymphocyte division by beta adrenergic agonists, described earlier.

Thus, both pertussis and pharmacologic beta blockade induce proliferation of lymphoid elements, that is, of cells mainly associated with antibody formation and inhibit a biochemical system known to reduce lymphoid cell proliferation. In addition, pertussis induces accelerated and prolonged multiplication of antibody-forming spleen cells in mice immunized with sheep red blood cells (Finger, Emmerling and Schmidt, 1967), and pertussis and pharmacologic beta adrenergic blockade both markedly inhibit the adenylate cyclase–cyclic AMP system in murine spleens *in vivo* and under *in vitro* conditions (Ortez, Seschachalam and Szentivanyi, 1975).

An important factor affecting the rate of mitosis, at least in mammalian cells studied in detail, is the energy supply of the cell. This in turn seems to depend primarily on the intracellular availability of glucose derivatives. Agents capable of stimulating or inhibiting particular rate-limiting reactions in the intermediary metabolism of carbohydrates also are capable of influencing mitotic activity (Bullough, 1962). Insulin and alpha adrenergic activation, which stimulate the peripheral (extrahepatic) uptake of glucose, also increase the rate of mitosis. Conversely, beta adrenergic stimulation, which inhibits the peripheral uptake of glucose, also inhibits mitosis. The rate-limiting factor of mitosis may, therefore, be the rate of entry of glucose into the cell. In the beta adrenergically blocked (propranolol) mouse, a striking increase in the normal rate of entry of glucose into several extrahepatic tissues was found, and the spleen, a prominent lymphoid tissue, was among them (Fishel and Szentivanyi, 1963). Thus, beta adrenergic blockade conceivably could induce proliferation of the immuno-competent cells by preparing them to meet the high energy requirements of increased mitotic activity through the elimination of the normal beta adrenergic inhibition of glucose uptake.

Since in most areas of adrenergic activity the alpha and beta receptor systems are functionally associated with antagonistic responses, one would expect that alpha-blockade would suppress mitotic activity in immunocompetent cells. Such a postulate is all the more tempting since the most specific alpha-blockers, the haloalkylamines, are chemically related to the nitrogen mustards and similar immunosuppressive agents; like the latter, the tertiary amine cyclizes to form a reactive ethylenimonium intermediate, the formation of which appears to be critical for specific blocking activity at the alpha-site. Similarly, formation of the ethylenimonium ion constitutes the initial reaction of the nitrogen mustards. Without establishing it conclusively, some data do in fact suggest that beta adrenergic blockers are able to imitate the pertussis-enhancement of reaginic antibody formation (Reed et al., 1972), whereas a partial suppression of the same can be accomplished by alpha adrenergic blockade (Pieroni and Levine, 1967).

Applicability of the Pertussis Model to the Immune Abnormality in Atopy. A natural bridge between the foregoing discussion and the possible beta adrenergic contribution to the immune abnormality in atopy has now been provided by some recent experiments. Results of these studies indicate that a macromolecular component of pertussis cultures is able to alter cyclic AMP metabolism in human lymphocytes *in vitro*. There is a reduction in the response of lymphocytes to agents that normally raise their cyclic AMP levels, including isoproterenol, and PGE_1. With purified pertussis fractions, the lymphocytosis-producing activity in intact mice and the cyclic AMP inhibitory activity in isolated human lymphocytes seem to correlate closely.

Furthermore, in recent experiments, a protein of approximately 70,000 MW has been isolated from *B. pertussis* culture supernatant fluids that appears to be essentially homogeneous by immunologic, physical, and electron microscopic criteria. *This single molecular entity has both lymphocytosis-producing and histamine-sensitizing activities, and, in addition, causes hypoglycemia and refractoriness to epinephrine-induced hyperglycemia* (Morse, 1978).

Beta Adrenergically Subsensitive Lymphocytes and Impairment of T Cell Function in Atopy. Evidence has been provided by several laboratories for the presence of a beta adrenergic abnormality in peripheral blood lymphocytes obtained from asthmatic individuals. Such cells were shown to have a substantially reduced susceptibility to adrenergic activation as measured by the amount of cyclic AMP synthesized in response to beta adrenergic agonists. The abnormality also was demonstrable in unstimulated cells inasmuch as they exhibited a decreased baseline cyclic AMP content. In most cases, the reduced responsiveness to adrenergic activation correlated well with the severity and chronicity of asthmatic symptoms, and therefore, the possibility was raised that such manifestations of adrenergic subsensitivity are drug- and not disease-induced, and are due to desensitization of adrenergic receptors. This will be discussed later, and here we shall only state that the correlation with the severity of asthma may only partially imply tachyphylactic causation since the abnormality may be clearly manifest also in the absence of adrenergic medication.

The clearest example of this is provided by the lymphocytes of patients with atopic dermatitis uncomplicated by asthma or other atopic disorder, since in this condition no adrenergic medication is employed. In view of the results of a largely overlooked abstract of Parker and Eisen (1972) reporting a substantially diminished cyclic AMP response to adrenergic stimulation in leukocytic suspensions of patients with atopic dermatitis, Reed, Busse and Lee (1976) reinvestigated this problem on purified lymphocytes and polymorphonuclear leukocytes of blood. They found that these cells, isolated from patients with atopic dermatitis, show a markedly diminished glycogenolysis, a substantial loss of inhibition of lysosomal enzyme release, and a significantly decreased rise in the intracellular level of cyclic AMP upon incubation with beta adrenergic agonists, while these responses to PGE_1 remained normal.

The magnitude and duration of IgE antibody responses appear to be determined by multiple negative and positive regulatory signals derived from T cells in addition to the direct antigenic stimulation of B cells (Waldmann, 1977). Consequently, a reduction in the number or function of regulatory T cells that are normally involved in terminating IgE responses could explain the high IgE levels observed in certain disease states that are known to have abnormalities of T cell function.

This raises the possibility that the high IgE levels in some atopic individuals may be indicative of a defective T cell function, as appears to be the case in other disease states. Indeed, there is considerable evidence for a regulatory immune defect in atopic dermatitis. Such patients have frequent bacterial and severe viral skin infections (notably herpes simplex and vaccinia) and exhibit decreased delayed-type hypersensitivity to a variety of antigens including tuberculin, tetanus toxoid, staphylococcal, and streptococcal antigens. In evaluating the phytohemagglutinin skin test response in 50 patients with no known immunodeficiency, responses were absent in only three, two of whom had atopic dermatitis. Anergy to candida and streptococcal antigens has been observed in six of ten children with atopic dermatitis, and lymph node morphology in two atopic dermatitis patients disclosed normal germinal centers, but deficient thymic-dependent cortical areas. Also, eczema, a consistent component of the Wiskott-Aldrich syndrome, is occasionally seen in ataxia telangiectasia and in X-linked hypogammaglobulinemia, and appears to be associated with recently described defects in chemotaxis and phagocytic capacity. Although less consistently, similar findings also have been reported in patients with bronchial asthma and allergic rhinitis (Buckley, 1978).

These observations, taken together with the high IgE levels, do indeed suggest that in some cases defective T cell function may be a part of the atopic disease. Furthermore, in the framework of the beta adrenergic theory, these defective T cell functions in some individuals may be manifestations of the underlying beta adrenergic abnormality of the same cells.

Such a possibility has been considerably strengthened by recent observations in both mouse and human systems that T cells are more susceptible to beta adrenergic stimulation of cyclic AMP synthesis than are the B lymphocytes (Teh and Paetku, 1976; Niaudet et al., 1976). Furthermore, it is now generally agreed that one of the mechanisms whereby cyclic AMP exerts its regulatory effect on B cell function is indirectly via its effect on T lymphocytes (Katz and Fauci, 1978). A reduced adrenergic sensitivity of the latter would then be expected to have critical consequences on T cell function and antibody formation.

It is significant, therefore, that Lang, Goel and Grieco (1978) have showed that the normal inhibitory activity of beta adrenergic stimulation on "active" E rosette formation is markedly reduced in asymptomatic adult asthmatics. This marked beta adrenergic subsensitivity of T lymphocytes occurred, furthermore, in the face of a normal absolute number of baseline "active" E rosettes, a finding recently confirmed in asthmatic children by another laboratory (Hsieh, 1976).

CLOSE ASSOCIATION WITH INFECTION

The beta adrenergic approach to atopy also offers an explanation for the nature of the close relation between infection and the atopic state, whether the role of infection is immunologic, pharmacodynamic, or both. In addition to the HSF of pertussis, there are numerous bacterial as well as viral agents and/or their products that can be shown to cause profound disturbances in autonomic regulation by altering the quality and quantity of autonomic effector responses (Szentivanyi and Fishel, 1965; Szentivanyi, 1968a, 1971). Of these, in the bacterial category, the endotoxins deserve special consideration. Although they generally are considered to be produced only by gram-negative microorganisms, materials with similar properties may be found in gram-positive bacteria and in a variety of plant and animal tissues as well. Therefore, endotoxins and substances with similar pharmacodynamic activity are likely to participate in many of the infections associated with atopy. Endotoxins not only are potent releasers of the pharmacologic mediators but also are potent sensitizers of the adrenergic effector cells (in an alpha position) to the catecholamines so released, in some systems potentiating vasoconstrictor responses to epinephrine, for example, 100-fold. Such endotoxin-induced hypersensitivity to the vasoconstrictive effects of catecholamines can be of sufficient magnitude that "preparation" of an animal or tissue by an injection of endotoxin can lead to the induction of a profound hemorrhagic necrosis in the site subsequently injected with epinephrine. In contrast, 200-fold doses of epinephrine in animals not pretreated with endotoxin, does not induce tissue destruction.

At the receptor level, such endotoxin-induced alterations in responses to catecholamines could be explained by a hypersensitivity of the alpha or by a functional deficiency of the beta receptor system. Lesions grossly resembling the endotoxin-induced "epinephrine-lesion" already described may be produced in the skin of both guinea pigs and rabbits following the injection of a mixture of beta blocker and epinephrine. Conversely, the local Shwartzman reaction is inhibited by alpha but not by beta blockade. Also the generalized form of this reaction can be inhibited by alpha blockers as well as by making the test animal epinephrine-tolerant.

The principal pathology of the generalized Shwartzman phenomenon is the bilateral cortical necrosis of kidneys. Development of this lesion appears to be related to an alteration in plasma fibrinogen, i.e., to the appearance of the so-called "heparin-precipitable fibrinogen" (HPF), with subsequent deposition of this material in glomerular capillary loops, causing obstruction and resulting in renal necrosis. In accord with this, inhibition of the generalized Shwartzman reaction by epinephrine tolerance was found to be related to prevention of development of the HPF in the plasma.

While it is not known whether endotoxins produce a similar adrenergic lesion on vascular smooth muscle of the atopic patient, it is difficult to ignore the tempting analogy between these animal findings and the occurrence of fibrinoid degeneration of pulmonary connective tissue and blood vessel walls in human asthma (Szentivanyi and Fishel, 1966). Furthermore, the functional associations of adrenergic receptors of vascular smooth muscle seem to parallel those of bronchial smooth muscle within the same species.

It is not surprising, therefore, that endotoxin sensitization of human bronchial smooth muscle to α-adrenergic agonists has, in fact, been reported (Simonsson et al., 1972). Phenylephrine-induced contractions were enhanced two to ten times in normal lung and a thousand times in lung from a patient with chronic bronchitis. Endotoxin also causes a decrease in cyclic AMP of the tissue.

Against this bacterial background, more recent studies increasingly emphasize the role of viral infection in respiratory atopic disease — primarily in asthma. There is a close association between asthma (or asthmatic symptoms) and respiratory syncytial virus, especially in children under 3 years of age. Infections with parainfluenza or coronavirus also are relatively important. In older children and adults, rhinovirus and influenza virus predominate. Study of rhinovirus infection, which seems to be associated with the majority of infection-related asthma exacerbations, suggests, however, that only a few rhinovirus serotypes are associated with asthmogenicity. This selectivity is another finding that is difficult to reconcile with the concept that asthma is due to sensitization by epithelial damage of rapidly-adapting sensory receptors in the bronchial epithelium by the virus (Nadel, 1977; Gold, 1978), and raises the question of other mechanisms related to the biochemical properties of the virus and to the autonomic effectors including the anti-inflammatory cells.

Considerations of an autonomic imbalance due to a beta-adrenergic deficit consistently have emphasized (Szentivanyi, 1968a; Szentivanyi and Fishel, 1976; Szentivanyi et al., 1979; Szentivanyi and Fitzpatrick, 1979) that infection — both of bacterial and viral varieties — produces the same type of damage in autonomic effector cells that has been described for the HSF of pertussis and endotoxin above. In one longitudinal study, Minor et al., (1974) found that simple colonization of the respiratory tract by viruses was not sufficient to provoke asthma: such attacks occurred only when the infection produced symptoms of fever, malaise, cough, or coryza. The dominant role of fever in these episodes immediately suggests the profound involvement of adrenergic effector mechanisms.

Additional support for this view comes from studies showing that killed influenza virus vaccine, which has no local inflammatory activity, increases the sensitivity of asthmatics to aerosolized methacholine, and that during respiratory infections that provoked an attack of asthma, the responsiveness of peripheral lymphocytes and granulocytes to beta adrenergic activation is reduced more than usual. In the studies of Busse (1977), this additional reduction in beta adrenergic responsiveness during upper respiratory infections was shown to apply both to the cyclic AMP synthesizing as well as the lysosomal enzyme-releasing properties of granulocytes. Also, it has been repeatedly observed that patients with chronic bronchitis, with no previous history of asthma, may experience frank asthmatic attacks during therapy with a beta blocker instituted for some unrelated reason. Finally, an example of cyclic AMP-mediated beta adrenergic receptor interconversion has been observed after virus transformation of a cultured cell line (Sheppard, 1977).

EOSINOPHILIA OF COMMON OCCURRENCE

A peculiar distinction of eosinophils is their conspicuous association with atopic disorders. Such association may be a consistent finding, even when the patient shows no sensitivity to inhaled allergens by skin test or inhalation challenge, as in so-called intrinsic asthma. However, the nature of this association and their role in atopic events remain to be clarified and will not be discussed here in detail.

Of the catecholamines, both epinephrine and isoproterenol produce eosinopenia, whereas norepinephrine has no such effect. The eosinopenic effect of catechols is blocked by dichloroisoproterenol and by propranolol but not by dibenamine. These operations define eosinopenia as a beta adrenergic action of catecholamines. Consequently, an impairment of beta adrenergic mechanisms would be expected to eliminate one of the important suppressing influences in the homeostatic control of eosinophils and possibly result in eosinophilia. In line with this reasoning are two important findings: (a) comparison of the effect of epinephrine on circulating eosinophils of normal and asthmatic subjects shows a significantly reduced eosinopenic response in asthmatic patients (Reed et al., 1970), and (b) deficiency in magnesium, that is a deficiency in the essential catalyst of the beta adrenergic activation of adenyl cyclase, has been shown to induce eosinophilia in rats (Hungerford & Karson, 1960).

INCREASED TOLERANCE TO BETA ADRENERGIC STIMULATION

It is widely recognized that with increasing severity of asthma, a marked resistance to the bronchial and to many of the systemic activities of epinephrine may develop and in status asthmaticus the majority of patients are "epinephrine-fast." In fact, this feature of status asthmaticus is so conspicuous that the condition is sometimes defined as persistent severe refractory asthma which is epinephrine-resistant. Mechanical obstruction cannot adequately account for the phenomenon, since in many cases the bronchodilator activity of theophylline derivatives is retained, and there are cases of epinephrine-fastness without evidence of substantial obstruction (Hansen and Werner, 1967). Restoration of epinephrine-responsiveness by correction of respiratory acidosis does not establish a causal relationship, since no consistent correlation can be found to exist between epinephrine-fastness and acidosis.

On the other hand, the types of biochemical defects in the cyclic AMP-mediated control mechanisms postulated by the beta adrenergic theory can explain easily the phenomenon of epinephrine-fastness. Consequently, in the wake of the early presentations of the beta adrenergic theory this possibility received major interest and gained more experimental support by observations of reduced asthmatic responsiveness to catecholamines as measured by various systemic parameters of adrenergic reactivity (Cookson and Reed, 1963; Inoue, 1967; Fireman et al., 1970; Bernstein et al., 1972, 1973; Kirkpatrick and Keller, 1967; Lockey et al., 1967; Makino et al., 1970; Maselli et al., 1970; Middleton and Finke, 1968; Schwartz and White, 1973). These studies showed less rise in blood sugar, free fatty acids, lactate, pyruvate, pulse rate, and urinary and plasma cyclic AMP levels as well as a higher diastolic pressure and reduced eosinopenic response following beta adrenergic stimulation in asthmatic patients. Reduction in adrenergic responsiveness correlated well with the severity of the disease and with the degree of pharmacologic hypersensitivity as judged by exposure to acetylcholine (Makino et al., 1970).

Although they are highly compatible with the beta adrenergic theory, interpretation of these results is handicapped by the inherent limitations of *in vivo* studies involving complex homeostatic regulations. It is, therefore, of major importance that the same pattern of reduced adrenergic responsiveness is demonstrable in *in vitro* preparations of isolated cells derived from asthmatic individuals. In such studies, leukocytes and lymphocytes from asthmatic donors exhibit a reduced cyclic AMP response to beta adrenergic agents but a completely intact response to prostaglandin E_1, suggesting that the biochemical defect may in fact be at the level of the beta adrenergic receptor (Coffey et al., 1972; Falliers et al., 1971; Logsdon et al., 1972, 1973; Parker and Smith, 1973; Parker, Baumann and Huber, 1973; Parker, Huber and Baumann, 1973; Alston et al., 1974; Haddock et al., 1975; Williams and Lefkowitz, 1978). Moreover, in these studies a clear demonstrability of the biochemical lesion depended on the severity of the disease. This is reminiscent of clinical observations on the developmental pattern of epinephrine-fastness, and is in line with one of the basic tenets of the beta adrenergic theory, namely, that it is only when a continuing series of adaptive responses is demanded of the adrenergically incapacitated asthmatic tissues that the postulated defect becomes readily manifest (Szentivanyi, 1968 a).

Observations that manifestations of adrenergic subsensitivity in asthma can be simulated, at least in part, in nonasthmatic individuals by pretreatment with adrenergic medication raised the question whether the autonomic abnormalities observed in asthma may be due not to the disease itself, but rather to medication taken by asthmatic patients (Nelson et al., 1975; Morris et al., 1977; Kalister et al., 1977; Greenacre et al., 1978). While there is no question that drug-induced adrenergic desensitization may contribute in many situations to the overall adrenergic subsensitivity, adrenergic subsensitivity can be shown to be a fundamental characteristic of atopy for the following reasons.

Beta adrenergic subsensitivity is demonstrable also without concurrent medications, long after medication has been discontinued, and in atopic conditions in which adrenergic medication never has been involved (Parker and Eisen, 1972; Busse & Lee, 1976). Disease-induced (atopic) beta adrenergic malfunction in the lymphocyte is manifested not only in reduced responsiveness of the cyclic AMP system to adrenergic stimulation, but also in a reduced responsiveness of the cyclic GMP system to cholinergic stimulation. In contrast, in adrenergically desensitized but otherwise normal individuals, even at the height of adrenergic subsensitivity, no impairment of the lymphocytic guanylate cyclase–cyclic GMP system can be demonstrated.

Disease-induced and drug-induced patterns of behavior of cyclic nucleotides also differ with respect to their responses to histamine in the H_2-position. As is known, release of granulocyte lysosomal enzymes is inhibited not only by beta adrenergic agonists, but also by histamine, and in both cases through increasing the granulocytic cyclic AMP concentration. This effect of histamine is an H_2-response inasmuch as it can be blocked by metiamide but not by chlorpheniramine. Both in terms of enzyme released and cyclic AMP synthesis, responsiveness of granulocytes to beta adrenergic agonists as well as histamine is markedly reduced in asthma as well as in atopic dermatitis. On the other hand, in adrenergically desensitized normal individuals, there is a complete dissociation between the adrenergic and histaminic responses of granulocytes; the former are reduced and the latter are unimpaired. Similarly, in disease-induced adrenergic subsensitivity of lymphocytes, normal sensitivity can be restored by the *in vitro* treatment of the preparations with alpha adrenergic blocking agents, whereas no such reversal can be achieved in drug-induced adrenergic subsensitivity. Thus, in disease-induced adrenergic subsensitivity we are primarily dealing with an authentic imbalance produced by receptor interconversion or some other mechanism, whereas in drug-induced adrenergic subsensitivity, whatever else is operative in the mechanism of desensitization, an indiscriminate blockade of the adrenergic receptors clearly is present.

The foregoing evidence raises the question

of how do cyclic nucleotide abnormalities in lymphocytes compare with pulmonary behavior in asthmatics? Although a definitive answer to this question is not yet possible, recent observations from our laboratory on lung tissue from patients undergoing thoracotomy for known or suspected pulmonary malignancy indicate that patients with a history of asthma or reversible airways obstruction show a reduced capacity to synthesize cyclic AMP to beta adrenergic activation. Furthermore, this adrenergic lesion appears to lie in an early phase of the sequence of reactions leading to beta adrenergic activation, since no alterations in the phosphodiesterase-catalyzed cyclic AMP and cyclic GMP breakdowns occurred in the pulmonary tissues of patients with reversible airways obstruction (Krzanowski, Polson, Goldman, Ebel and Szentivanyi, 1979; Polson, Krzanowski, Goldman and Szentivanyi, 1979).

Similar findings now are available in patients with atopic dermatitis, which could be summarized as follows: (1) *in vitro* studies of epidermis show that catecholamines fail to evoke the normal beta adrenergic inhibition of mitosis of basal cells of patients with atopic dermatitis (Carr et al., 1973); (2) lymphocytes and polymorphonuclear leukocytes obtained from such patients respond with a decreased cyclic AMP rise to beta adrenergic agonists, but with a normal rise to other activators of the cyclic AMP system (Parker and Eisen, 1972; Busse and Lee, 1976); (3) beta adrenergic stimulation of lymphocytic glycogenolysis and inhibition of lysosomal enzyme release from granulocytes after zymosan exposure is significantly reduced in patients with atopic dermatitis (Busse and Lee, 1976); and (4) lymphocytes isolated from patients with atopic dermatitis respond with a low to normal increase of cyclic GMP to cholinergic stimulation (Szentivanyi, Williams, Szentivanyi and Polson, 1977). In contrast, activities of cutaneous adenylate cyclase, cyclic AMP-phosphodiesterase, and protein kinase appear to be normal (Mier and Urselmann, 1970; Mier and van den Hurk, 1972; Holla et al., 1972). Such combination of findings could be interpreted most easily to mean that in the adrenergic reaction sequence, in atopic dermatitis, the step responsible for the diminished beta adrenergic response lies antecedent to the catalytic site of adenylate cyclase

and must involve either a defective binding of catecholamines or a defective transfer of the adrenergic signal between the beta receptor and the catalytic site of the enzyme. Thus, the nature of the adrenergic abnormality in asthma and atopic dermatitis does in fact appear to be similar.

EMINENT THERAPEUTIC EFFECTIVENESS OF AGENTS THAT ARE CAPABLE OF RESTORING NORMAL BETA ADRENERGIC ACTION

From the foregoing evidence it seems that the existence of the phenomenon of epinephrine-fastness may itself be an excellent argument for the beta adrenergic theory. The potential strength of this argument will become more evident with consideration of the pharmacodynamics of those drugs or procedures which are still relatively effective in this condition. These drugs or therapeutic interventions are capable of restoring normal adrenergic action apparently either by (a) bypassing the biochemical site of the postulated beta adrenergic lesion or (b) sensitizing the beta receptors, i.e., lowering the receptor threshold to catecholamine action.

Aminophylline or other methylxanthines would seem to be representatives of the first category of drugs. These agents are potent inhibitors of phosphodiesterase, which is the enzyme responsible for the destruction of cyclic AMP. Since current evidence places this point beyond the receptor-activation step, it is possible that the effectiveness of these drugs in epinephrine-fast individuals and other asthmatic persons is due to their capability of producing adrenergic action by a bypass of the site of the postulated beta adrenergic lesion. Indeed, in animal models of beta adrenergic block, methylxanthines still are capable of their normal pharmacologic activities and can reverse or amelioriate effects of blockade (Townley, Trapani, and Szentivanyi, 1967; Blumenthal and Brody, 1956; Polson et al., 1978, 1979).

The glucocorticoids can be regarded as representatives of the second category of drugs. Their mechanism of action in asthma is unexplained, especially when small maintenance doses are involved that do not inhibit IgE production or possess significant anti-inflammatory activity. Even in massive doses, however, their bronchodilatory action is insignificant (Hackney and Szentivanyi, 1975, 1976), and in the absence of concurrent sympathomimetic therapy, their effectiveness is limited (Rebuck and Read, 1971). However, in such situations the inclusion of small amounts of beta adrenergic agents may produce a dramatic improvement suggesting that glucocorticoids may influence the adrenergic responsiveness of asthmatic tissues. Indeed, from animal experiments the corticosteroids are known to support the normality of the effector cell responses to catecholamines, and it is well established that in the absence of glucocorticoids the receptor-threshold for catecholamines may be raised occasionally to the point of complete unresponsiveness (Ramey and Goldstein, 1957). Therefore, corticosteroid deprivation can simulate clinically either an indiscriminate or a selective adrenergic blockade, depending on the types of effector responses tested (Ramey and Goldstein, 1957; Fishel, Szentivanyi and Talmage, 1964). Conversely, even a pharmacologically established beta adrenergic blockade in an intact animal, i.e., in an organism in which normal concentrations of steroids must be presumed to have been present, can be overcome with an excess amount of glucocorticoid administered exogenously (Szentivanyi, Fishel and Talmage, 1963). In addition, massive doses of corticosteroids can increase beta adrenergic responsiveness *in vitro* in human tracheal muscle preparations exposed to propranolol (Townley et al., 1970, 1972). These findings may indicate that the glucocorticoids are capable of sensitizing the adrenergic effector cells to the action of catecholamines. It is of further importance that neither the anti-inflammatory nor the catechol-potentiating activities of the steroid molecule are separable from its glucocorticoid properties (Bush, 1962). Results of other *in vitro* studies on leukocytes and lymphocytes obtained from asthmatic and normal donors (Coffey et al., 1972; Logsdon et al., 1972; Parker et al., 1973) also suggest the possibility that the beneficial effects of steroids in epinephrine-fast and other asthmatic individuals are due to their action on the beta adrenergic receptors.

A similar explanation may apply to the previously mentioned restoration of epinephrine responsiveness in asthmatic patients by administration of sodium lactate or bicarbonate, the mechanism of which cannot be attributed to the correction of respiratory acidosis since many of these cases show normal or alkaline pH (Turiaf et al., 1961, 1962; Tsuchiya and Bukantz, 1965). Effectiveness of these procedures is more easily explicable by sensitization of the adrenergic receptors to catecholamines or by interconversion of adrenergic receptors from alpha to beta (Williams and Lefkowitz, 1978).

As far as the drug therapy of atopic dermatitis is concerned, there are two series of recent observations which are of importance in the context of this discussion. First, beta adrenergic subsensitivity of lymphocytes from patients with atopic dermatitis can be restored to normal by glucocorticoids (Busse & Lee, 1976). Second, caffeine-hydrocortisone creams have been shown to be more effective than plain hydrocortisone creams in improving lichenification and excoriation in patients with atopic dermatitis (Kaplan et al., 1976, 1977, 1978). Caffeine is a methylxanthine, and as such could be expected to increase epidermal cyclic AMP by inhibiting epidermal cyclic AMP phosphodiesterase, and therefore, to bypass the biochemical site of the postulated beta adrenergic lesion.

SUSCEPTIBILITY TO A VARIETY OF UNRELATED PRECIPITATING FACTORS

In addition to the antigen-antibody interaction, asthma, and in some cases, other atopic disorders, is known to be triggered by a large variety of stimuli such as infection, various synthetic and natural chemicals, conditioned reflexes, psychic stimuli, changes in atmospheric pressure, inhalation of cold air, nonantigenic dusts, fumes, and other irritants. Any molecular interpretation of a susceptibility to such a large variety of unrelated stimuli would appear to necessitate the postulate that the atopic lesion, i.e., the primary constitutional abnormality, be connected with a final common pathway operating through a messenger system of unusually broad biologic activity.

The adenylate cyclase–cyclic AMP system is the first known messenger system capable of responding to a wide variety of neurohumoral and hormonal agents subserving homeostasis. This unusually broad reactive capacity of the system may be explained by the current hypothetical model of the enzyme. In this model, adenylate cyclase, linked to the receptor through the transducer coupling unit, is pictured as a single protein extending from one side of the cell membrane to the other and being composed of two functional subunits. One is a regulatory subunit facing the extracellular space, whereas the other is a catalytic subunit, the active center of which is in contact with the cell interior. The neurohumor or hormone, through the receptor-transducer unit, interacts with the regulatory subunit, bringing into motion a sequence of reactions described above. From a cybernetic point of view, cyclic AMP may represent a common target molecule in a set of intracellular signals involved in the transduction of environmental information. Interestingly, a cybernetic software model of the data relevant to atopy and incorporating the cyclic

AMP system has recently been presented by Mier and Cotton (1976).

Thus, the cyclic AMP system would ideally fit the requirement for a biologically unusually broad homeostatic messenger system. *The atopic constellation, however, poses another requirement for the qualification of the likely messenger-candidate. The latter must be a biochemical control system which, normally, in response to beta adrenergic activation, promotes the dominant function of the classic autonomic effector cells (i.e., smooth muscle, exocrine gland, and nerve cells), but in response to the same stimulation, inhibits the dominant functions of the cells responsible for the organization of the immune response (i.e., lymphocytes, macrophages, mast cells, etc.). Only a homeostatic control system with this unique behavioral dichotomy can provide a concordant base for the present or future understanding of atopy.*

References

Ahlquist, R. P.: A study of the adrenotropic receptors. Amer. J. Physiol. 153:586, 1948.

Ahlquist, R. P.: Adrenoceptor sensitivity in disease as assessed through response to temperature alteration. Fed. Proc. 36:2572, 1977.

Alston, W. C., Patel, K. R., and Kerr, J. W.: Response of leukocyte adenyl cyclase to isoprenaline and effect of alpha-blocking drugs in extrinsic bronchial asthma. Br. Med. J. 1:90, 1974.

Anderson, W. B., and Pastan, I. H.: Altered adenylate cyclase activity: Its role in growth regulation and malignant transformation of fibroblasts. Adv. Cyclic Nucleotide Res., 5:681, 1975.

Baer, R. L.: *Atopic Dermatitis*. New York University Press, New York, 1955.

Bennett, M. R.: *Autonomic Neuromuscular Transmission*. London, Cambridge University Press, 1972.

Bernstein, R. A., Linarelli, L., Facktor, M. A., Friday, G. A., Drash, A., and Fireman, P.: Decreased urinary cyclic 3′,5′-adenosine monophosphate (cAMP) after epinephrine in asthmatic patients. J. Allergy Clin. Immunol. 49:86, 1972.

Bernstein, R. A., Linarelli, L., Friday, G. A., Drash, A., and Fireman, P.: Effect of ephedrine sulfate on urinary cyclic adenosine monophosphate (cAMP) in normals. J. Allergy Clin. Immunol. 51:89, 1973.

Besterman, E. M. M.: Discussion to the paper of McNeill, R. S., and Ingram, C. G. Effect of propranolol on ventilatory function. Am. J. Cardiol. 18:473, 1966.

Besterman, E. M. M., and Friedlander, D. H.: Clinical experiences with propranolol. Postgraduate Med. J. 41:526, 1965.

Blumenthal, M., and Brody, T. M.: Studies on the mechanism of smooth muscle relaxation. J. Allergy 36:205, 1965.

Bonifazi, E., Garofalo, L., Monterisi, A and Meneghini, C. L.: Food allergy in atopic dermatitis: Experimental observations. Acta Dermatovener. 58:349, 1978.

Buckley, R. H.: Immunologic deficiency and allergic disease. *In* Middleton, E., Reed, C. E., and Ellis, E. F. (eds): *Allergy—Principles and Practice*. St. Louis, C. V. Mosby Co., 1978.

Bullough, W. A.: The control of mitotic activity in adult mammalian tissues. Biol. Rev. 37:307, 1962.

Burnstock, G.: Purinergic nerves. Pharmacol. Rev., 24:509, 1972.

Burnstock, G.: Purinergic transmission. *In* Iversen, L. L., Iversen, S. C., and Snyder, S. H. (ed.): *Handbook of Psychopharmacology: Synaptic Modulators*. Vol. 5, New York, Plenum Press, 1975.

Bush, I. E.: Chemical and biological factors in the activity of adrenocortical steroids. Parmacol. Rev. 14:317, 1962.

Busse, W. W.: Decreased granulocyte response to isoproterenol in asthma during upper respiratory infections. Am. Rev. Respir. Dis. 115:783, 1977.

Busse, W. W., and Lee, T. P.: Decreased adrenergic responses in lymphocytes and granulocytes in atopic eczema. J. Allergy Clin. Immunol. 58:586, 1976.

Cannon, W. B., and Rosenblueth, A.: *The Supersensitivity of Denervated Structures*. Macmillan Co., New York, 1949.

Carr, R. H., Busse, W. W., and Reed, C. E.: Failure of catecholamines to inhibit epidermal mitosis *in vitro*. J. Allergy Clin. Immunol. 51:255, 1973.

Chan, T. M., and Exton, J. H.: Enhanced β-adrenergic activation of glycogen phosphorylase in hepatocytes from adrenalectomized rats. Fed. Proc. 36:608, 1977.

Chang, I. C., and Gottshall, R. Y.: Sensitization to ragweed pollen in *Bordetella pertussis*-infected or vaccine-injected mice. J. Allergy Clin. Immunol. 54:20, 1974.

Coca, A. F., and Cooke, R. A.: On the classification of the phenomena of hypersensitiveness. J. Immunol. 8:163, 1923.

Coffey, R. G., Logsdon, P. J., and Middleton, E.: Effects of glucocorticosteroids on leukocyte adenyl cyclase and ATPase of asthmatic and normal children. J. Allergy Clin. Immunol. 49:87, 1972 (Abstract).

Cohen, J. B., and Changeux, J.-P: The cholinergic receptor protein in its membrane environment. Ann. Rev. Pharmacol. 15:83, 1975.

Cook, D. A., Kenakin, T. P., and Krueger, C. A.: Alterations in temperature and histamine receptor function. Fed. Proc. 36:2584, 1977.

Cooke, R. A., and Vander Veer, A., Jr.: Human sensitization. J. Immunol. 1:201, 1916.

Cookson, D. U., and Reed, C. E.: A comparison of the effects of isoproterenol in the normal and asthmatic subject. Am. Rev. Respir. Dis. 88:636, 1963.

Cseuz, R., Wenger, T. L., Kunos, G., and Szentivanyi, M.: Changes of adrenergic reaction pattern in experimental diabetes mellitus. Endocrinology 93:752, 1973.

Curry, J. J.: The action of histamine on the respiratory tract in normal and asthmatic subjects. J. Clin. Invest. 25:785, 1946.

Curry, J. J.: Comparative action of acetyl-beta-methyl choline and histamine on the respiratory tract in normals, patients with hay fever, and subjects with bronchial asthma. J. Clin. Invest. 26:430, 1947.

Curry, J. J., Fuchs, J. E., and Leard, S. E.: The effect of dihydroergocornine on the pulmonary response to methacholine and histamine in subjects with bronchial asthma. J. Clin. Invest. 29:439, 1950.

Curry, J. J., and Leard, S. E.: The action of pilocarpine on the lungs in normal and asthmatic subjects. J. Lab. Clin. Med. 33:585, 1948.

Curry, J. J., and Lowell, F. C.: Measurement of vital capacity in asthmatic subjects receiving histamine and acetyl-beta-methyl choline. A clinical study. J. Allergy 19:1948.

Davis, M. J., and Lawler, J. C.: Observations on the delayed blanch phenomenon in atopic subjects. J. Invest. Dermatol. 30:127, 1958.

de Vries, K., Goei, J. T., Booy-Noord, H., and Orie, N. G. M.: Changes during 24 hours in the lung function and histamine hyperreactivity of the bronchial tree in asthmatic and bronchitic patients. Int. Arch. Allergy 20:93, 1962.

Douglas, J. S., Brink, C., and Bouhuys, A.:Actions of histamine and other drugs on guinea pig airway smooth muscle. Lung Cells in Disease. Amsterdam, 1976, Elsevier/North Holland Biomedical Press, pp. 245–259.

Douglas, J. S., Dennia, M. W., Ridgway, P., and Bouhuys, A.: Airway constriction in guinea pigs: Interaction of histamine and autonomic drugs. J. Pharmacol., Exp. Ther. 184:169, 1973.

Duchaine, J., and Spapen, R.: Modifications de la sensibilité pulmonaire à l'acétylcholine et de la sensibilité pulmonaire allergenique par les derives de l'hydrocortisone. Acta allergologica 14:23, 1959.

Eccles, J. C.: The Understanding of the Brain. New York, McGraw-Hill Book Co., 1973.

Efron, B. G., and Boatner, C. H.: Studies with antigens; significance of reactions to intracutaneous tests performed with solutions of purified extracts of ragweed pollens. J. Invest. Dermatol. 5:49, 1942.

Efron, B. G., Boatner, C. H., and Pabst, M. R.: Studies with antigens; significance of scratch test reactions to purified house dust extracts. J. Invest. Dermatol. 3:401, 1940.

Emmelin, N.: Supersensitivity following "pharmacological denervation." Pharmacol. Rev. 13:16, 1961.

Eppinger, H., and Hess, L.: Zur Pathologie des vegetativen Nervensystem. Z. Klin. Med. 67:345, 1909.

Falliers, C. J., de A. Cardoso, R. R., Bane, H. N., Coffey, R., and Middleton, E.: Discordant allergic manifestations in monozygotic twins: Genetic identity versus clinical, physiologic, and biochemical differences. J. Allergy 47:207, 1971.

Farr, R. S.: Some comments regarding the allergic state and the initiation of antibody synthesis. Arch. of Environmental Health 6:92, 1963.

Fichtelius, K. E., and Hassler, O.: Influence of pertussis vaccine on the lymphocyte production in adrenolectomized rats. Acta Pathol. Microbiol. Scand. 42:189, 1958.

Filipp, G., and Szentivanyi, A.: Experimentelle Data zur regulativen Rolle des Neuroendokriniums in experimenteller Anaphylaxie. I. Relazioni e Communicazioni, 299–305, Rome, Il Pensiero Scientifico, 1956.

Filipp, G., and Szentivanyi, A.: Die Wirkung von Hypothalamusläsionen auf den anaphylaktischen Schock des Meerschweinchens. Allergie und Asthmaforschung, Bd. 1, 23–28, 1957.

Filipp, G., Szentivanyi, A., and Mess, B.: Anaphylaxis and the nervous system. Acta. Med. Hung., Tomus III, Fasciculus 2., 163–175, 1952.

Finger, H., Emmerling, P., and Schmidt, H.: Accelerated and prolongated multiplication of antibody-forming spleen cells by Bordetella pertussis in mice immunized with sheep red blood cells. Experientia 23:591, 1967.

Fireman, P., Palm, C. R., Friday, G. A., and Drash, A. L.: Metabolic responses to epinephrine in asthmatic, eczematous, and normal subjects. J. Allergy 45:117, 1970 (Abstract).

Fishel, C. W., Halkias, D. G., Klein, T. W., and Szentivanyi, A.: Characteristics of cells present in peritoneal fluids of mice injected intraperitoneally with Bordetella pertussis. Infect. Immunol. 13:263, 1976.

Fishel, C. W., and Szentivanyi, A.: The absence of adrenaline-induced hyperglycemia in pertussis-sensitized mice and its relation to histamine and serotonin hypersensitivity. J. Allergy 34:439, 1963.

Fishel, C. W., Szentivanyi, A., and Talmage, D. W.: Sensitization and desensitization of mice to histamine and serotonin by neurohumors. J. Immunol. 89:8, 1962.

Fishel, C. W., Szentivanyi, A., and Talmage, D. W.: Adrenergic factors in Bordetella pertussis-induced histamine and serotonin hypersensitivity of mice. In Landy, M., and Braun, W. (eds.): Bacterial Endotoxins. New Brunswick, NJ, Rutgers University Press, 1964, pp. 474–481.

Fitzpatrick, D. F., and Szentivanyi, A.: Stimulation of calcium uptake into aortic microsomes by cyclic AMP and cyclic AMP-dependent protein kinase. Naunyn-Schmiedeberg's Arch. Pharmacol. 298:255, 1977.

Floersheim, G. L.: Facilitation of tumor growth by Bacillus pertussis. Nature 216:1235, 1967.

Gold, W. M.: Anticholinergic drugs. In Middleton, E., Reed, C. E., and Ellis, E. F. (eds.): Allergy – Principles and Practice. St. Louis, C. V. Mosby Co., 1978.

Goldberg, N. D.: Cyclic nucleotides and cell function. Hosp. Practice 9:127, 1974.

Goldberg, N. D., and Haddox, M. K.: Cyclic GMP metabolism and involvement in biological regulation. Ann. Rev. Biochem. 46:823, 1977.

Goodman, L. S., and Nickerson, M.: Clinical applications of adrenergic blockade: A critical appraisal. Med. Clin. North America 34:379, 1950.

Graham, D. T., and Wolf, S.: Pathogenesis of urticaria: Experimental study of life situations, emotions and cutaneous vascular reactions. J.A.M.A., 143:1396, 1950.

Greenacre, J. K., Schofield, P., and Conolly, M. E.: Desensitization of the β-adrenoceptor of lymphocytes from normal subjects and asthmatic patients in vitro. Br. J. Clin. Pharmacol. 5:199, 1978.

Grove, E. F., and Coca, A. F.: Studies in specific hypersensitiveness. XV. On the nature of the atopens of pollens, house dust, horse dander and green pea. J. Immunol. 10:471, 1925.

Grow, M. H., and Herman, N. B.: Intracutaneous tests in normal individuals. J. Allergy 7:108, 1936.

Grundfest, H.: Electrical inexcitability of synapses and some consequences in the central nervous system. Physiol. Rev. 37:337, 1957.

Hackney, J. F., and Szentivanyi, A.: The unique action of glucocorticoid succinates on respiratory smooth muscle in vitro. Pharmacologist 17:271, 1975 (Abstract).

Hackney, J. F., and Szentivanyi, A.: The action of non-glucocorticoid steroid succinates on guinea pig trachealis muscle in vitro. Pharmacologist 18:182, 1976. (Abstract)

Hadden, J. W.: Cyclic nucleotides in lymphocyte proliferation and differentiation. In Hadden, J. W., Coffey, R. G., and Spreafico, F. (eds.): Immunopharmacology. New York, Plenum Press, 1977.

Haddock, A. M., Patel, K. R., Alston, W. C., and Kerr, J. W.: Response of lymphocyte guanyl cyclase to propranolol, noradrenaline, thymoxamine, and acetylcholine in extrinsic bronchial asthma. Br. Med. J., 2:357, 1975.

Hajos, M. K.: Clinical studies on the role of serotonin in bronchial asthma. Acta allergologica, 17:358, 1962.

Hansen, K., and Werner, M.: Lehrbuch der klinischen Allergie. Georg Thieme Verlag, Stuttgard, 1967.

Hemels, H. G. W. M.: The effect of propranolol on the acetylcholine-induced sweat response in atopic and nonatopic subjects. Br. J. Dermatol. 83:312, 1970.

Hess, W. R.: *Diencephalon, Autonomic and Extrapyramidal Functions.* Grune & Stratton, Inc., 1954.

Hirano, M., Sinkovics, J. G., Schullenberger, C. C., and Howe, C. D.: Murine lymphoma: Augmented growth in mice with pertussis vaccine-induced lymphomatosis. Science, 158:1061, 1967.

Holgate, J. A., and Warner, B. T.: Evaluation of antagonists of histamine, 5-hydroxytryptamine, and acetylcholine in the guinea pig. Br. J. Pharmacol. 15:561, 1960.

Holla, S. W. J., Hollman, E. P. M. J., Mier, P. D., v. d. Staak, W. J. B. M., Urselmann, E., and Warndorff, J. A.: Adenosine 3',5'-cyclic monophosphate phosphodiesterase in skin. II. Levels in atopic dermatitis. Br. J. Dermatol. 86:147, 1972.

Hsieh, K.: Study of E rosettes, serum IgE, and eosinophilia in asthmatic children. Ann. Allergy 37:383, 1976.

Hubbard, J. I.: Microphysiology of vertebrate neuromuscular transmission. Physiol. Rev. 53:674, 1973.

Hungerford, G., and Karson, E. F.: The eosinophilia of magnesium deficiency. Blood 16:1642, 1960.

Inoue, S.: Effects of epinephrine on asthmatic children. Effects of epinephrine on blood glucose, pulmonary function, and heart rate of children with asthma of varying severity. J. Allergy 40:337, 1967.

Ishizaka, K.: Cellular events in the IgE antibody response. Adv. Immunol. 23:1, 1976.

Johansson, S. G. O., and Foucard, T.: IgE in immunity and disease. *In* Middleton, E., Reed, C. E., and Ellis, E. F. (eds.): *Allergy – Principles and Practice.* St. Louis, C. V. Mosby Co., 1978.

Kaliner, M., and Austen, K. F.: Immunologic release of chemical mediators from human tissues. Ann. Rev. Pharmacol. 15:177, 1975.

Kalisker, A., Nelson, H. E., and Middleton, E., Jr.: Drug-induced changes of adenylate cyclase activity in cells from asthmatic and nonasthmatic subjects. J. Allergy Clin. Immunol. 60:259, 1977.

Kalz, F., and Fekete, Z.: Studies on the mechanism of the white response and delayed blanch phenomenon in atopic subjects by means of coomassie blue. J. Invest. Dermatol., 35:135, 1960.

Kaplan, R. J., Daman, L., Rosenberg, E. W., and Feigenbaum, S.: Treatment of atopic dermatitis with topically applied caffeine — a follow-up report. Arch. Dermatol. 113:107, 1977.

Kaplan, R. J., Daman, L., Rosenberg, E. W., and Feigenbaum, S.: Topical use of caffeine with hydrocortisone in the treatment of atopic dermatitis. Arch. Dermatol. 114:60, 1978.

Kaplan, R. J., Daman, L., Shereff, R., Rosenberg, E. W., and Robinson, H.: Treatment of atopic dermatitis with topically applied caffeine. Arch. Dermatol. 112:880, 1976.

Katsh, S., Halkias, D. G., and Szentivanyi, A.: Analysis of the structural requirements for the histamine-sensitizing activity of beta adrenergic blocking agents. J. Allergy 43:171, 1969 (Abstract).

Katz, P., and Fauci, A. S.: Activation of human B lymphocytes VII. The regulatory effect of cyclic adenosine monophosphate on human B cell activation. J. Allergy Clin. Immunol. 61:334, 1978.

Kirkpatrick, C. H., and Keller, C.: Impaired responsiveness to epinephrine in asthma. An. Rev. Respir. Dis. 96:692, 1967.

Klein, T. W., Szentivanyi, A., and Fishel, C. W.: Effects of serotonin on platelets of normal and *B. pertussis*-injected mice. Proc. Soc. Exp. Biol. Med. 147:681, 1974.

Krnjevic, K.: Chemical nature of synaptic transmission in vertebrates. Physiol. Rev. 54:418, 1974.

Krzanowski, J. J., Polson, J. B., Goldman, A. L., Ebel, T. A., and Szentivanyi, A.: Reduced adenosine 3',5'-cyclic monophosphate levels in patients with reversible obstructive airways disease. Clin. Exp. Pharmacol. Physiol. 6:111, 1979.

Krzanowski, J. J., Polson, J. B., and Szentivanyi, A.: Pulmonary patterns of adenosine-3'5'-cyclic monophosphate accumulations in response to adrenergic or histamine stimulation in *Bordetella pertussis*-sensitized mice. Biochem. Pharmacol. 25:1631, 1976.

Kunos, G.: Adrenoceptors. Ann. Rev. Pharmacol. 18:291, 1978.

Kunos, G., and Szentivanyi, M.: Evidence favouring the exis-

tence of a single adrenergic receptor. Nature 217:1077, 1968.

Lamson, R. W., and Rogers, E. L.: Skin hypersensitivity to molds. J. Allergy 7:582, 1936.

Lang, P., Goel, Z., and Grieco, M. H.: Subsensitivity of T lymphocytes to sympathomimetic and cholinergic stimulation in bronchial asthma. J. Allergy Clin. Immunol. 61:248, 1978.

Lefkowitz, R. J.: Molecular pharmacology of beta-adrenergic receptors — A status report. Biochem. Pharmacol. 23:2069, 1974.

Lindblad, J. H., and Farr, R. S.: The incidence of positive intradermal reactions and the demonstration of the skin sensitizing antibody to extracts of ragweed and dust in humans without history of rhinitis or asthma. J. Allergy 32:392, 1961.

Lobitz, W. C., and Campbell, C. J.: Physiological studies in atopic dermatitis (disseminated neurodermatitis); local cutaneous response to intradermally injected acetylcholine and epinephrine. A.M.A. Arch. Derm. 67:575, 1953.

Lobitz, W. C., Heller, M. L., and Dobson, R. L.: Physiologic studies in atopic dermatitis (disseminated neurodermatitis). II. The effect of denervation on the "delayed blanch phenomenon." A.M.A. Archiv. Derm. 75:228, 1957.

Lockey, S. D., Glennon, J. A., and Reed, C. E.: Comparison of some metabolic responses in normal and asthmatic subjects to epinephrine and glucagon. J. Allergy 40:349, 1967.

Logsdon, P. J., Carnright, D. V., Middleton, E., and Coffey, R. G.: The effect of phentolamine on adenylate cyclase and on isoproterenol stimulation in leukocytes from asthmatic and nonasthmatic subjects. J. Allergy Clin. Immunol. 52:148, 1973.

Logsdon, P. J., Middleton, E., and Coffey, R. G.: Stimulation of leukocyte adenyl cyclase by hydrocortisone and isoproterenol in asthmatic and nonasthmatic subjects. J. Allergy Clin. Immunol. 50:45, 1972.

MacManus, J. P., Whitfield, J. F., Boynton, A. L., and Rixon, B. H.: Role of cyclic nucleotides and calcium in the positive control of cell proliferation. Adv. Cyclic Nucleotide Res. 5:719, 1975.

Makino, S., Oulette, J. J., Reed, C. E., and Fishel, C. W.: Correlation between increased bronchial response to acetylcholine and diminished metabolic and eosinopenic responses to epinephrine in asthma. J. Allergy, 46:178, 1970.

Maselli, R., Meltzer, E. O., and Ellis, E. F.: Pharmacologic effects of epinephrine in asthmatic children. J. Allergy 45:117, 1970 (Abstract).

Mathe, A. A., Hedquist, P., Holmgren, A., and Svanborg, N.: Bronchial hyperreactivity to prostaglandin F$_{2\alpha}$ and histamine in patients with asthma. Br. Med. J. 1:193, 1973.

McLaughlan, P., Stanworth, D. R., Webster, A. D. B., and Asherson, G. L.: Serum IgE in immune deficiency disorders. Clin. Exp. Immunol. 16:375, 1974.

McNeill, R. S.: Effect of a beta-adrenergic blocking agent, propranolol on asthmatics. Lancet 2:1101, 1964.

McNeill, R. S., and Ingram, C. G.: Effect of propranolol on ventilatory function. Am. J. Cardiol. 18:473, 1966.

Meier, J., Lydtin, H., and Zollner, N.: Über die Wirkung von adrenergen B-Rezeptorenblockern auf ventilatorische Funktionen bei obstruktiven Lungenkrankheiten. Dtsch. med. Wschr. 91:145, 1966.

Mélon, J., and Lecomte, J.: Action de l'histamine et d'un liberateur d'histamine neis au contact de la muquense nasale. Acta allergologica 22:43, 1958.

Mélon, J., and Lecomte, J.: Étude comparée des effets de la bradykinine et des réactions anaphylactiques locales chez l'homme. Int. Arch. Allergy 21:89, 1962.

Michelson, M. J., and Danilov, A. F.: Cholinergic transmissions. *In* Bacq, Z. M. (ed.): *Fundamentals of Biochemical Pharmacology.* Oxford, Pergamon Press, 1971.

Middleton, E., and Finke, S. R.: Metabolic response to epinephrine in bronchial asthma. J. Allergy 42:288, 1968.

Mier, P. D., and Cotton, D. W. K.: *The Molecular Biology of Skin.* Oxford, Blackwell Scientific Publications, 1976.

Mier, P. D., and Urselmann, E.: The adenyl cyclase of skin. II. Adenyl cyclase levels in atopic dermatitis. Br. J. Dermatol. 83:364, 1970.

Mier, P. D., and van den Hurk, J.: Cyclic 3',5' adenosine

monophosphate-dependent protein kinase of skin. Br. J. Dermatol., *87*:571, 1972.

Minor, T., Dick, E. C., DeMeo, A. N., Ouellete, J. J., Cohen, M., and Reed, C. E.: Viruses as precipitants of asthmatic attacks in children. J.A.M.A. *227*:292, 1974.

Morgan, J. K.: Observations on cholinogenic urticaria. J. Invest. Dermatol., *21*:173, 1953.

Morris, H. G., Rusnak, S. A., and Barzens, K.: Leukocyte cyclic adenosine monophosphate in asthmatic children: Effects of adrenergic therapy. Clin. Pharmacol. Ther. *22*:352, 1977.

Morse, S. I.: Influence of microbial products on allergic reactions. *In* Middleton, E., Reed, C. E., and Ellis, E. F. (eds.): *Allergy—Principles and Practice*. St. Louis, C. V. Mosby Co., 1978.

Mukherjee, C., and Lefkowitz, R. J.: Desensitization of β-adrenergic receptors in a cell-free system: Resensitization by guanosine 5'-(β,γ-immino) triphosphate and other purine nucleotides. Proc. Natl. Acad. Sci., USA *73*:1494, 1976.

Muranaka, M., Suzuki, S., Miyamoto, T., Takeda, K., Okumura, H., and Makino, S.: Bronchial reactivities to acetylcholine and IgE levels in asthmatic subjects after long-term remissions. J. Allergy Clin. Immunol. *54*:32, 1974.

Nadel, J. A.: The parasympathetic system and its role in asthma. Adv. Asthma Allergy *4*:15, 1977.

Nakamura, K.: *Allergy and Anaphylaxis*. Tokyo, Nippon Medical School, 1954.

Nelson, H. S., Black, J. W., and Branch, L. B.: Subsensitivity to epinephrine following the administration of epinephrine and ephedrine to normal individuals. J. Allergy Clin. Immunol. *55*:299, 1975.

Niaudet, P., Beaurain, G., and Bach, M. A.: Differences in effect of isoproterenol stimulation on levels of cyclic AMP in human B and T lymphocytes. Eur. J. Immunol. *6*:834, 1976.

Nickerson, M., and Kunos, G.: Discussion of evidence regarding induced changes in adrenoceptors. Fed. Proc. *36*:2580, 1977.

O'Brien, R. D., Thompson, W. R., and Gibson, R. E.: *Neurochemistry of Cholinergic Receptors*. ed. by E. deRobertis and J. Schacht, New York, Raven, 1974, pp. 49–62.

Öhman, S., and Johansson, S. G. O.: Immunologlobulins in atopic dermatitis with special reference to IgE. Acta Derm. Venereol. *54*:193, 1974.

Olivier, H. R.: Sensibilité du poumon asthmatique à l'acétylcholine. Int. Arch. Allergy *12*:262, 1958.

Ortez, R. A., Klein, T. W., and Szentivanyi, A.: Impairment of the adenyl cyclase system in spleens of mice sensitized bacterially or by beta pharmacological blockade. J. Allergy *45*:111, 1970 (Abstract).

Ortez, R. A., Seshachalam, D., and Szentivanyi, A.: Alterations in adenyl cyclase activity and glucose utilization of *Bordetella pertussis* sensitized mouse spleen. Biochem. Pharmacol. *24*:1297, 1975.

Parker, C. W., Baumann, M. L., and Huber, M. G.: Alterations in cyclic AMP metabolism in human bronchial asthma. II. Leukocyte and lymphocyte responses to prostaglandins. J. Clin. Invest. *52*:1336, 1973.

Parker, C. W., and Eisen, A. Z.: Altered cyclic AMP metabolism in atopic eczema. Clin. Res. *20*:418, 1972 (Abstract).

Parker, C. W., Huber, M. G., and Baumann, M. L.: Alterations in cyclic AMP metabolism in human bronchial asthma. III. Leukocyte and lymphocyte responses to steroids. J. Clin. Invest. *52*:1342, 1973.

Parker, C. W., and Smith, J. W.: Alterations in cyclic adenosine monophosphate metabolism in human bronchial asthma. I. Leukocyte responsiveness to β-adrenergic agents. J. Clin. Invest. *52*:48, 1973.

Parker, C. W., Sullivan, T. J., and Wedner, H. J.: Cyclic AMP and the immune response. Adv. Cyclic Nucleotide Res. *4*:1, 1974.

Pastan, I. H., Johnson, G. S., and Anderson, W. B.: Role of cyclic nucleotides in growth control. Ann. Rev. Biochem. *44*:491, 1975.

Patterson, R.: Laboratory models of reaginic allergy. Prog. Allergy *13*:332, 1969.

Pearlman, D. S., and Szentivanyi, A.: Excessive reactivity of defense mechanisms — Allergy. *In* Cook, R. E. (ed.): *The Biologic Basis of Pediatric Practice*. New York, McGraw-Hill Book Co., Inc., 1968, pp. 536–546.

Perkins, J. P.: Regulation of the responsiveness of cells to catecholamines: Variable expression of the components of the second messenger system. *In* Weiss, B. (ed.): *Cyclic Nucleotides in Disease*. Baltimore, University Park Press, 1975.

Peterson, R. D. A., Page, A. R., and Good, R. A.: Wheal and erythema allergy in patients with agammaglobulinemia. J. Allergy *33*:406, 1962.

Pieroni, R. E., and Levine, L.: Properties of the immunogenic and sensitizing activities of *Bordetella pertussis* in mice. J. Allergy *39*:25, 1967.

Polson, J. B., Krzanowski, J. J., Fitzpatrick, D. F., and Szentivanyi, A.: Studies on the inhibition of phosphodiesterase-catalyzed cyclic AMP and cyclic GMP breakdown and relaxation of canine tracheal smooth muscle. Biochem. Pharmacol. *27*:254, 1978.

Polson, J. B., Krzanowski, J. J., Anderson, W. H., Fitzpatrick, D. F., Hwang, D. P. C., and Szentivanyi, A.: Analysis of the relationship between pharmacological inhibition of cyclic nucleotide phosphodiesterase and relaxation of canine tracheal smooth muscle. Biochem. Pharmacol. *27*:(in press), 1979.

Polson, J. B., Krzanowski, J. J., Goldman, A. L., and Szentivanyi, A.: Inhibition of human pulmonary phosphodiesterase activity by therapeutic levels of theophylline. Clin. Exp. Pharmacol. Physiol. *5*:535, 1978.

Polson, J. B., Krzanowski, J. J., and Szentivanyi, A.: Effects of methacholine, histamine and atropine on pulmonary guanosine-3',5'-monophosphate levels in hypersensitive mice. Naunyn-Schmiedeberg's Arch. Pharmacol. *295*:27, 1976.

Posternak, T.: Cyclic AMP and cyclic GMP. Ann. Rev. Pharmacol. *14*:23, 1974.

Rackemann, F. M., and Simon, F. A.: Technic of intracutaneous tests and results of routine tests in normal persons. J. Allergy *6*:184, 1935.

Ramey, E. R., and Goldstein, M. S.: The adrenal cortex and the sympathetic nervous system. Physiol. Rev. *37*:155, 1957.

Rasmussen, J. E., and Provost, T. T.: Atopic dermatitis. *In* Middleton, E., Reed, C. E., Ellis, E. F. (eds.): *Allergy – Principles and Practice*. St. Louis, C.V. Mosby Co., 1978.

Rebuck, A. S., and Read, J.: Assessment and management of severe asthma. Am. J. Med. *51*:788, 1971.

Reed, C. E., Benner, M., Lockey, S. D., Enta, T., Makino, S., and Carr, R. H.: On the mechanism of the adjuvant effect of *Bordetella pertussis* vaccine. J. Allergy Clin. Immunol. *49*:174, 1972.

Reed, C. E., Busse, W. W., and Lee, T.-P.: Adrenergic mechanisms and the adenyl cyclase system in atopic dermatitis. J. Invest. Dermatol. *67*:333, 1976.

Reed, C. E., Cohen, M., and Enta, T.: Reduced effect of epinephrine on circulatory eosinophils in asthma and after beta-adrenergic blockade of *Bordetella pertussis* vaccine. J. Allergy *46*:90, 1970.

Reed, C. E., and Townley, R. G.: Asthma: Classification and pathogenesis. *In* Middleton, E., Reed, C. E., and Ellis, E. F. (eds.): *Allergy – Principles and Practice*. St. Louis, C.V. Mosby Co., 1978.

Reed, W. B., and Kierland, R. R.: Vascular reactions in chronically inflamed skin. II. Action of epinephrine and phentolamine (regitine); action of acetylcholine and metacholine (mecholyl), and the delayed branch. A.M.A. Arch. Derm. *77*:181, 1958.

Rodbell, M., Lin, M. C., Salomon, Y., Londos, C., Harwood, J. P., Martin, B. R., Rendell, M., and Berman, M.: Role of adenine and guanine nucleotides in the activity and response of adenylate cyclase systems to hormones: Evidence for multisite transition states. Adv. Cyclic Nucleotide Res. *5*:3, 1975.

Rose, B.: Production of symptoms by subcutaneous injection of histamine without increase of the blood histamine. Science 92:454, 1940.

Rose, B.: Role of histamine in anaphylaxis and allergy. Am. J. Med. 3:545, 1947.

Rose, B.: Antihistamine agents in allergy. Ann. N.Y. Acad. Sci. 50:1066, 1950.

Rose, B., Rusted, I., and Fownes, A.: Intravascular catheterization studies of bronchial asthma. I. Histamine levels in arterial and mixed venous blood of asthmatic patients before and during induced attack. J. Clin. Invest. 29:1113, 1950.

Rothlin, E., and Bircher, R.: Allergy, the autonomic nervous system, and ergot alkaloids. Prog. Allergy 3:434, 1952.

Samter, M.: Bronchial asthma and sensitivity to histamine. Ztsch. f. d. ges. exp. Med. 89:24, 1933.

Scherbel, A., and Harrison, J.: Serotonin hypersensitivity in collagen diseases. Bull. Rheumat. Dis. 9:179, 1959.

Schramm, M.: The catecholamine-responsive adenylate cyclase system and its modification by 5'-guanylimidodiphosphate. Adv. Cyclic Nucleotide Res., 5:105, 1975.

Schwartz, H. J., and White, L. W.: Urinary and plasma cyclic AMP responses to epinephrine in asthmatic and normal subjects. J. Allergy Clin. Immunol. 51:88, 1973.

Sen, D. K., Arora, S., Gupta, S., and Sanyal, R. K.: Studies of adrenergic mechanisms in relation to histamine sensitivity in children immunized with Bordetella pertussis vaccine. J. Allergy Clin. Immunol. 54:25, 1974.

Sheppard, J. R.: Catecholamine hormone receptor differences identified on 3T3 and simian virus-transformed 3T3 cells. Proc. Natl. Acad. Sci., USA 74:1091, 1977.

Simonsson, B. G., Svedmyr, N., Skoogh, G.-E., Andersson, R., and Bergh, N. P.: In vivo and in vitro studies on alpha receptors in human airways — potentiation with bacterial endotoxin. Scand. J. Respir. Dis. 53:227, 1972.

Simpson, L. L.: The use of neuropoisons in the study of cholinergic transmission. Ann. Rev. Pharmacol. 14:305, 1974.

Stites, D. P., Ishizaka, K., and Fudenberg, H. H.: Serum IgE concentrations in hypogammaglobulinemia and selective IgA deficiency: Studies on patients and family members. Clin. Exp. Immunol. 10:391, 1972.

Szentivanyi, A.: The beta adrenergic theory of the atopic abnormality in bronchial asthma. J. Allergy 42:203, 1968a.

Szentivanyi, A.: The beta adrenergic theory of bronchial asthma. An alternative to the classical concept. Abstract No. 9, Proceedings of the 24th Annual Congress of the American College of Allergists, Denver, Co., March 25–29, 1968b.

Szentivanyi, A.: Effect of bacterial products and adrenergic blocking agents on allergic reactions. In Samter, M. et al. (ed.): Textbook of Immunological Diseases. Boston, Little, Brown & Co., 1971, pp. 356–374.

Szentivanyi, A.: The conformational flexibility of adrenoceptors and the constitutional basis of atopy. Triangle, 1979. (in press)

Szentivanyi, A., and Filipp, G.: Experimentelle Data zur regulativen Rolle des Neuroendokriniums in experimenteller Anaphylaxie. I. Relazioni e Communicazioni, 229–235, Rome, Il Pansiero Scientifico, 1956.

Szentivanyi, A., and Filipp, G.: Anaphylaxis and the nervous system. Part II. Ann. Allergy, 16:143, 1958.

Szentivanyi, A., Filipp, G., and Legeza, I.: Investigations on tobacco sensitivity. Acta. med. hung., Tomus III, Fasciculus 2., 175–186, 1952.

Szentivanyi, A., and Fishel, C. W.: Effect of bacterial products on responses to the allergic mediators. In Samter, M. (ed.): Immunological Diseases. Boston, Little Brown & Co., 1956, pp. 226–241.

Szentivanyi, A., and Fishel, C. W.: Die Amin-Mediatorstoffe der allergischen Reaktion und die Reaktionsfahiegkeit ihrer Erfolgszellen. In Fillip, G.: Pathogenese und Therapie allergischer Reaktionen. Grundlagenforshung und Klinik. Stuttgart, Germany, Ferdinand Enke Verlag, 1966, pp. 558–683.

Szentivanyi, A., and Fishel, C. W.: The beta adrenergic theory and cyclic AMP-mediated control mechanisms in human asthma. In Weiss, E. B., and Segal, M. S.: Bronchial Asthma: Mechanisms and Therapeutics. Boston, Little Brown & Co., 1976, pp. 137–153.

Szentivanyi, A., Fishel, C. W., and Talmage, D. W.: Adrenaline mediation of histamine and serotonin hyperglycemia in normal mice and the absence of adrenaline-induced hyperglycemia in pertussis-sensitized mice. J. Infect. Dis. 113:86, 1963.

Szentivanyi, A., and Fitzpatrick, D. F.: The altered reactivity of the effector cells to antigenic and pharmacological influences and its relation to cyclic nucleotides. II. Effector reactivities in the efferent loop of the immune response. In Pathomechanismus und Pathogenese allergischer Reaktionen. ed. by G. Filipp, Werk-Verlag, Dr. Edmund Banaschewski, Gräfelfing bei München, 1979.

Szentivanyi, A., Krzanowski, J. J., and Polson, J. B.: The autonomic nervous system: structure, function and altered effector responses. In Middleton, E., Reed, C. E., and Ellis, E. F. (eds.): Allergy—Principles and Practice. St. Louis, C. V. Mosby Co., 1978, pp. 265–300.

Szentivanyi, A., Polson, J. B., and Krzanowski, J. J.: The altered reactivity of the effector cells to antigenic and pharmacological influences and its relation to cyclic nucleotides. I. Effector reactivities in the afferent loop of the immune response. In Pathomechanismus und Pathogenese allergischer Reaktionen. ed. by G. Filipp, Werk-Verlag, Dr. Edmund Banaschewski, Gräfelfing bei München, 1979.

Szentivanyi, A., and Szekely, J.: Effect of injury to and electrical stimulation of hypothalamic areas on the anaphylactic and histamine shock of guinea pig. Ann. Allergy 14:259, 1956.

Szentivanyi, A., and Szekely, J.: Über den Effekt der Schädingung und der elektrischen Reizung der hypothalamischen Gegenden auf den anaphylaktischen und Histamin-Schock des Meerschweinchens. Allergie und Asthmaforschung, Bd. 1, 29–31, 1957a.

Szentivanyi, A., and Szekely, J.: Wirkung der konstanten Reizung hypothalamischer Strukturen durch Tiefenelektroden auf den histaminbedingten und anaphylaktischen Schock des Meerschweinchens. Acta Physiol. Hung., Suppl., Tomus XI, 41–43, 1957b.

Szentivanyi, A., and Szekely, J.: Anaphylaxis and the nervous system. Part IV. Ann. Allergy 16:389, 1958.

Szentivanyi, A., Williams, J. F., Szentivanyi, J., and Polson, J. B.: Beta adrenergic dysfunction and atopic dermatitis. Proceedings of the VI Latin-American Congress of Allergy and Immunology, Guarujá, São Paulo, Brasil, 1977, p. 109.

Szentivanyi, M., Kunos, G., and Juhasz-Nagy, A.: Modulator theory of adrenergic receptor mechanism: Vessels of the dog hindlimb. Amer. J. Physiol. 218:869, 1970.

Szentivanyi, M., and Pek, L.: Characteristic changes of vascular adrenergic reactions in diabetes mellitus. Nature New Biol. 243:276, 1973.

Szentivanyi, M., Takacs, K., and Botos, K.: A new aspect in treatment of diabetic vascular disease. Proc. Seventh Int. Cong. of Pharmacology, Pergamon Press, Ltd., 1978, p. 271.

Takino, M., and Takino, Y.: Allergy and asthma. Maruzen Co., Ltd., Tokyo, Japan, 1956.

Teh, H. S., and Paetkau, V.: Regulation of immune responses. II. The cellular basis of cyclic AMP effects on humoral immunity. Cell. Immunol. 24:220, 1976.

Thesleff, S.: Effects of motor innervation on the chemical sensitivity of skeletal muscle. Physiol. Rev. 40:734, 1960.

Tiffeneau, R.: Examen pulmonaire de l'asthmatique. Déductions diagnostiques, prognostiques et thérapeutiques. Masson et Cie Editeurs, Paris, 1957.

Townley, R. G., Honrath, T., and Guirgis, H. M.: The inhibitory effect of hydrocortisone on the alpha adrenergic responses of human and guinea pig isolated respiratory smooth muscle. J. Allergy Clin. Immunol. 49:88, 1972.

Townley, R. G., Reeb, R., Fitzgibbons, T., and Adolphson, R. L.: The effects of corticosteroids on the beta-adrenergic receptors in bronchial smooth muscle. J. Allergy 45:118, 1970.

Townley, R. G., Trapani, I. L., and Szentivanyi, A.: Sensitization to anaphylaxis and to some of its pharmacological mediators by blockade of beta adrenergic receptors. J. Allergy *39*:177, 1967.

Trendelenburg, U.: Mechanisms of supersensitivity and subsensitivity to sympathomimetic amines. Pharmacol. Rev. *18*:629, 1966.

Tsuchiya, Y., and Bukantz, S. C.: Studies on status asthmaticus in children. I. Capillary blood pH and pCO$_2$ in status asthmaticus. J. Allergy *36*:514, 1965.

Turiaf, J., Georges, R., Basset, G., and Marland, P.: Equilibre acide-base et taux des gaz du sang dans l'asthme. Rev. Tuberc. *26*:238, 1962.

Turiaf, J., Marland, P., Basset, G., and Georges, R.: Intéret de la mesure des gaz du sang pour la sécurité et l'efficacité du traitement de l'état de mal asthmatique grave. In XXIII e Congrès Francais de Médecine. Paris: Masson, 1961.

Vertesi, C., Szentivanyi, M., and Szigeti, K.: Histological evaluation of the therapy in diabetic angiopathy. Proc. Seventh Int. Cong. of Pharmacology, Pergamon Press, Ltd., 1978, p. 271.

Waldmann, T. A.: Disorders of suppressor cells in the pathogenesis of immuno-deficiency, auto-immune and allergic diseases: Human disease associated with disorders of an immunological breaking system. Ann. Allergy *39*:79, 1977.

Watson, J.: Involvement of cyclic nucleotides as intracellular mediators in the induction of antibody synthesis. *In* Hadden, J. W., Coffey, R. G., Spreafico, F. (eds.): *Immunopharmacology*. New York, Plenum, 1977.

Weiss, B., and Hait, W. N.: Selective cyclic nucleotide phosphodiesterase inhibitors as potential therapeutic agents. Ann. Rev. Pharmacol. *17*:441, 1977.

Weiss, S., Robb, G. P., and Blumgart, H. L.: The velocity of blood flow in health and disease as measured by the effect of histamine on the minute vessels. Am. Heart J. *4*:664, 1929.

Weiss, S., Robb, G. P., and Ellis, L. B.: The systemic effects of histamine in man — with special reference to the responses of the cardiovascular system. Arch. Int. Med. *49*:360, 1932.

West, J. R., Johnson, L. A., and Winkelmann, R. K.: Delayed-blanch phenomenon in atopic individuals without dermatitis. A.M.A. Arch. Dermatol. *85*:227, 1962.

Williams, D. H.: Skin temperature reaction to histamine in atopic dermatitis (disseminated neurodermatitis). J. Invest. Dermatol. *1*:119, 1938.

Williams, L. T., and Lefkowitz, R. J.: *Receptor Binding Studies in Adrenergic Pharmacology*. Raven Press, New York, 1978.

Williams, L. T., Lefkowitz, R. J., Watanabe, A. M., Hathaway, D. R., and Besch, H. R., Jr.: Thyroid hormone regulation of β-adrenergic receptor number. J. Biol. Chem. *252*:2787, 1977.

Wise, F., and Sulzberger, M. B.: Editorial remarks in Year Book of Dermatology and Syphilology. Chicago, Year Book Pub., 1933.

Wolfe, B. B., Harden, T. K., and Molinoff, P. B.: *In vitro* study of β-adrenergic receptors. Ann. Rev. Pharmacol. *17*:575, 1977.

Zaid, G., and Beall, G. N.: Bronchial response to beta-adrenergic blockade. N. Engl. J. Med. *275*:580, 1966.

Stanley P. Galant, M.D.

15

Common Food Allergens

Foods are an important cause of adverse reactions in children. The exact incidence of food sensitivity is unknown, but the incidence of milk protein allergy alone in children is estimated to be 2 percent (Halpern et al., 1973). Foods are especially important allergens in infancy, probably because of immaturity of the digestive and immune processes of the gut, which increases the risk of sensitization to ingested materials. Food allergy may appear at any age but most commonly occurs early in life. Sensitivity to foods frequently is lost as the child becomes older but may be life-long, particularly with certain foods such as nuts and fish. It should be noted that not all reactions following food ingestion are truly allergic, i.e., mediated by immune mechanisms. In order to understand the spectrum of reactions and the various mechanisms by which foods may induce these reactions, consideration first will be given to pertinent immunochemistry and pharmacology of foods.

IMMUNOCHEMISTRY OF FOOD ALLERGENS

Certain physicochemical properties of food proteins appear to be major determinants of their allergenicity (Bleumink, 1970). As seen in Table 15–1, food allergens tend to be glycoproteins with a molecular weight between 18,000 and 36,000 daltons (similar in structure to the inhalant allergen, antigen E from ragweed), and most are resistant to heat and proteolytic enzymes. All are capable of eliciting an immediate skin test reaction with a small quantity of allergen, demonstrating an additional characteristic in common — high biologic activity. Generally it is certain components in the food, often representing only a small portion of the total protein content, that are allergenically important. For example, Bleumink found the most allergenic fraction of egg to be ovomucoid in egg white. Aas (1972) characterized a highly allergenic fraction in fish, referred to as allergen M; the bulk of fish muscle is not allergenic. In cow milk, the most important allergenic food in infancy, only five of more than 20 component proteins have special allergic significance. These include the heat-labile proteins, bovine serum albumin (BSA) and bovine gamma globulin (BGG); the partially heat-labile protein, alpha lactalbumin (ALA); and the heat-stable proteins, beta lactoglobulin (BLG) and casein. From a clinical standpoint and from the frequency with which specific IgE antibodies are identified, BLG is the most allergenically important and potent protein fraction. In common with other important food allergens, it is a glycoprotein and has a molecular weight of 36,000 daltons. It is resistant to heating and to the actions of the proteolytic enzymes of the gastrointestinal tract, properties which facilitate its absorption relatively intact.

Interaction with other substances or alteration by other physicochemical action can alter the allergenicity of food proteins. For instance, tomatoes become more allergenic as they ripen, a phenomenon associated with increased carbohydrate incorporation into

TABLE 15–1   IMMUNOCHEMICAL CHARACTERISTICS OF ALLERGENS

	Cod Fish	Tomato	Egg White	Cow Milk	Antigen E
Active component	glycoproteins	glycoproteins	glycoproteins	glycoproteins	glycoproteins
mgm. of component isolated from 100 grams	200	2.5	225	100	40
Skin reactivity (μg) (quantity giving positive skin test)	0.0001	0.15	0.0025	0.10	0.001
Molecular weight (daltons)	18,000	20,000	31,500	36,000	38,000
Stability to:					
heat (100°C)	+ +	+ +	+ +	+ +	–
acid (pH2)	+ +	+ +	+ +	+ +	–
enzymes (proteolytic)	–	+	+	–	+|

(Adapted from Aas, K.: Studies of hypersensitivity to fish. Int. Arch. Allergy *30*:257, 1966, and Bleumink, E.: Food allergy: The chemical nature of the substance eliciting symptoms. World Rev. Nutr. Diet. *12*:505, 1970.)

the protein moiety by N-glycosidic linkage. The allergenicity of BLG can be enhanced by incubation with lactose, which is another process that increases N-glycosidically–bound carbohydrates ("browning reaction"). Thus, clinically, mild heating of milk, particularly in the presence of milk sugar, can enhance allergenicity. It is possible also to develop sensitivity to denatured (cooked) foods, while tolerating the raw form (e.g., fish). On the other hand, the denaturation of foods, by heating for example, frequently reduces the allergenicity of the food. For example, children allergic to heat-labile proteins in cow milk may tolerate boiled milk.

The digestive process may also affect allergenicity. It has been speculated that the delayed onset of symptoms that can follow food ingestion may reflect the time required for formation of important antigenic determinants during digestion. Spies et al. (1970) demonstrated the presence of many new antigenic determinants in milk following exposure to proteolytic enzymes, and Cooke (1947) reported symptoms 2 hours after milk ingestion in a man who exhibited skin-sensitizing antibody to a proteose digest of cow milk whey protein, but not to the intact protein. The frequency with which delayed-onset reactions may reflect sensitivity to partially digested food products is unknown, but the possibility of such a relationship should be considered when attempting to correlate the allergy history with skin test data for food allergy.

Food allergens share antigenic and biologic similarities within botanic families. Important food families are listed in Table 15–2 (Speer, 1973). Although by no means universal, allergy to one member of a plant food family frequently results in a variable degree of allergy to other members of the same family. Thus, a patient allergic to peanut may be allergic to peas and other legumes. Cross-reactivity in animal foods is not as predictable as it is with plant foods. Fish and other seafoods tend to be extremely allergic. Aas studied children with asthma and/or urticaria from bony fish (1966). Approximately 40 percent of the patients tolerated some species of fish, while 60 percent reacted to all species tested, suggesting that fish contain species-specific antigens as well as antigens that may be shared by several species. Thus, sensitivity to fish of one family also may be associated with sensitivity to fish in other families (see Table 15–2). Sensitivity to shellfish (mollusks and crustaceans) generally does not imply sensitivity to bony fish, but dual sensitivities do occur. A less clear relationship exists between sensitivity to one form of animal protein and another in the

TABLE 15–2 FOOD GROUPS OF ALLERGENIC IMPORTANCE†

Plant (families)
Citrus
    oranges, lemons, grapefruit
*Cola nut
    chocolate, cola
Gourd
    melons, cucumbers, squash, pumpkin
*Grass
    corn, wheat, rye, oats, rice
Laurel
    cinnamon, bay leaf
Lily
    onion, garlic, asparagus
Mustard
    cabbage, broccoli, mustard, cauliflower,
    Brussels sprout
Nightshade
    tomato, potato
*Pea
    peanuts, peas, beans including soybean,
    alfalfa, clover, licorice
Pepper
    black pepper
Plum
    plums, peaches, apricots, almonds
Rose
    strawberry, raspberry
Sunflower
    lettuce, artichoke, sunflower

Animal (phylum, family or class as appropriate)
Mollusks
    abalone, clams, oysters,
    scallops, mussels } shellfish
Crustaceans
    shrimp, lobster, crab
*Fish (common families of bony fish)
    flounder, halibut, cod, trout,
    tuna, salmon
*Birds
    turkey, chicken, duck (including egg)
*Mammals
    cow, goat, sheep, pig (including milk)

*Denotes food allergens most frequently found in children by this author.
†(Adapted from Speer, F.: Intolerance to foods. In Speer, F. and Dockhorn, R. J. (eds.): *Allergy and Immunology in Childhood.* Charles C Thomas, Springfield, Ill., 1973, pp. 276–290.)

same animal. Thus, patients allergic to milk usually are not allergic to beef protein or to inhalation of cattle dander. A similar lack of relationship generally is noted between egg protein sensitivity and sensitivity to chicken meat or chicken feathers.

FOODS AS PHARMACOLOGICALLY ACTIVE AGENTS

A variety of foods contain vasoactive amines and other pharmacologically active substances that can induce a wide range of symptoms, particularly of the gastrointestinal tract and central nervous system (Sapeika, 1969). For example, the vasoactive amines, which include epinephrine, norepinephrine, tyramine, dopamine, histamine, and 5-hydroxytryptamine, are found in highest amounts in banana (particularly the peel), but also in tomatoes, avocados, pineapples, cheeses (cheddar and Camembert in particular), and certain wines (Chianti, for instance). Chocolate, which frequently has been reported to precipitate migraine headaches, does not contain tyramine but does possess large amounts of phenylethylamine. Both agents are potent inducers of headaches. Patients who take monamine oxidase inhibitors, which are found in antidepressants and inhibit the catabolism of vasoactive amines, may develop hypertension upon ingestion of foods which contain vasoactive amines. The methylxanthines, caffeine, theobromine, and theophylline are found in numerous foods including coffee, cocoa, tea, cola drinks, Dr. Pepper, Mountain Dew, and chocolate bars. Caffeine in particular causes CNS stimulation, with headache and jitteriness as well as abdominal pain. It has been estimated that a 12 oz. glass of cola contains 55 mgm of caffeine, a cup of coffee 150 mgm of caffeine, and a 4 oz. chocolate bar 200 mgm of theobromine. These quantities of methylxanthines are considered to be pharmacologic concentrations and are capable of producing the clinical side effects mentioned.

Food additives, particularly food colors, flavors, and preservatives, have attracted much attention recently. The food color tartrazine (FD&C Dye #5) the preservative sodium benzoate, and aspirin have been implicated in causing asthma and urticarial syndromes (Juhlin et al., 1972; Stenius and Lemola, 1976). Aggravation of hyperkinesis also has been claimed, but this remains largely unproved (Connors, et al., 1976; Harley, et al., 1978). However, Williams et al. (1978) have found some support for the induction of hyperkinesis by artificial food colors. Allergic (immune) mechanisms probably are not involved. Chinese food that contains large amounts of the food additive monosodium l-glutamate may induce the "Chinese restaurant syndrome," consisting of severe headache, facial pressure, and chest pain. L-glutamate is thought to be an important neurohumoral transmitter. Finally, a mineralocorticoid-like substance in licorice can produce hypertension and myopathy if ingested in large amounts (Sapeika, 1969).

Thus, foods may induce adverse reactions by pharmacologic as well as immunologic mechanisms. In addition, toxins in foods may induce symptomatology with varying degrees of susceptibility to these toxins amongst the populace; and, in the face of lactase or other dissacharridase deficiencies, ingestion of certain foods can induce even life-threatening reactions.

ABSORPTION OF MACROMOLECULES BY THE GUT

Nonimmune Factors. The gut is well prepared to impede the absorption and subsequent penetration of intact macromolecules such as food antigens (Walker, 1976). A low gastric pH and a variety of proteolytic enzymes help to digest antigens. Glycoproteins in the mucus form an effective blanket for the intestinal epithelial surface and decrease macromolecular absorption, which is a prerequisite for mucosal penetration. (Secretory antibodies serve much the same function.) Once antigen enters the epithelial cell (enterocyte), lysosomal enzymes digest the antigen. Those macromolecules that escape these processes are phagocytosed and digested by macrophages in the lamina propria. Variations with age and variations in other factors that influence the completeness of exclusion of intact protein from absorption, as indicated below, probably are important determinants of the risk of sensitization and reaction to foods.

Immune Factors. Walker and Isselbacker (1977) have shown that antibodies secreted into the gut's mucus layer specifically inhibit epithelial cell adherence of the macromolecular antigen to which it is formed. Hindering adherence not only impedes penetration, but also results in more effective digestion of the macromolecule in the gut lumen. Secretory IgA (SIgA) serves this function in man. Its unique polymeric structure renders it resistant to proteolysis, and better able to agglutinate intestinal antigens. Patients who lack IgA have a high incidence of milk-precipitating antibody in the serum, attesting to the importance of SIgA in controlling antigen absorption.

The infant appears to be at increased risk from intact antigen absorption for at least two reasons: (1) a residual premature absorptive mechanism in the gut which results in the capacity to absorb large molecules and (2) a relative secretory (S) IgA deficiency. It is not known when SIgA reaches adult levels, but possibly it may not occur until 6 to 12 months of age. In addition, several reports suggest that the atopic child may have a transient IgA deficiency in early infancy, which corrects between 6 and 12 months (Taylor et al, 1973). Supporting this concept of increased risk of sensitization is the fact that infants fed cow milk before age 3 months have a higher incidence of skin-sensitizing antibody to milk antigens than do older infants (Kletter et al., 1971). Furthermore, there is an indirect relationship between the age of introduction of milk into the diet and the level of circulating antibodies to milk proteins observed. Thus, the effectiveness of the gut as a barrier to absorption of intact protein is an important determinant of the allergenicity of potent food antigens such as cow milk. In diarrheal syndromes or intestinal inflammation in general, there tends to be greater absorption of intact protein thereby increasing the risk of reactivity to foods ingested during that time.

MECHANISMS OF FOOD-INDUCED INFLAMMATION

Immune Injury

Various kinds of food-induced immune injury have been considered by numerous investigators. Most allergic food reactions appear to be due to mediator release (Type I reaction; Gell and Combs, 1968) and only rarely to an immune complex reaction (Type III).

Type I Reactions. A Type I (anaphylactic) reaction is illustrated by the patient who, seconds to minutes following the ingestion of an allergenic food, may develop any or all of these symptoms: urticaria-angioedema, laryngeal edema and bronchospasm, profuse vomiting and diarrhea or shock. IgE antibody has been identified in patients with this type of reaction by a variety of techniques, including skin tests and the radioallergosorbent test (RAST) (Hoffman and Haddad, 1974).

A serum IgG_4 skin-sensitizing antibody to such foods as milk and egg also may be associated with food reactions such as eczema and abdominal pain (Parish, 1970). Unlike IgE, IgG_4 is relatively heat stable and confers passive-cutaneous anaphylaxis (PCA) sensitivity in the monkey for only 4 hours. Foods most commonly associated with anaphylaxis are fish, egg, nuts, peanuts, and cow milk (see Table 15–1), but the list of foods that have been associated with anaphylactic reactions is extensive.

Type III Reactions. Type III reactions involving antigen-antibody complexes, either circulating (serum sickness) or formed locally in the tissues (Arthus reaction) are associated with specific serum precipitating antibodies to food antigens, a depressed C3 (suggesting utilization) after food challenge, and tissue evidence of immune complex deposition at the site of inflammation by immunofluorescent staining. Milk precipitins are found in a few selective disorders thought to be associated with milk hypersensitivity, but also in 1 to 2 percent of the population without clinically apparent milk sensitivity. Their role in producing milk-induced injury remains controversial. Heiner et al. (1962) reported a group of children with chronic respiratory infection, poor growth and development, and iron deficiency anemia with gastrointestinal symptoms. Some had gastrointestinal hemorrhage, while others showed evidence of pulmonary hemosiderosis. (See Chapter 48.) These patients had high levels of milk precipitins with multiple precipitant bands and showed clinical improvement following withdrawal of milk. Matthews and Soothill (1970) demonstrated a reduced serum C3 90 minutes after feeding milk to five infants with milk-induced gastroenteritis, but others have not been able to confirm these observations.

Type IV Reactions. Type IV (delayed-type hypersensitivity) mechanisms have been implicated in celiac disease and in ulcerative colitis. However, evidence for the pathogenetic importance of Type IV mechanisms in these disorders is meager. In celiac disease, positive delayed hypersensitivity skin tests to wheat fractions appear to correlate well with flattened lesions seen in small bowel biopsies. Whether this implies that celiac disease is an "allergic" disease or that the positive skin test is only a result of the disease is not clear.

Frequently, children and adults who have had immediate, anaphylactic-like reactions to foods have positive allergy skin tests to those foods, which can be reproduced also by *in vitro* histamine release techniques (Galant et al., 1973). Patients with symptoms that occur several hours to days after ingesting a particular food, on the other hand, generally do not show positive allergy skin tests, histamine tests, or precipitating antibody to the suspected foods. This suggests that patients with delayed food symptoms are not allergic to the foods, or they are allergic to antigenic determinants formed in digesting the food. It also does not rule out the possibility of a Type III or a Type IV cell-mediated immune mechanism in such instances.

Nonimmune Mechanisms

Pharmacologic Reactions. Foods are capable of causing a spectrum of adverse reactions through nonimmune pathways because of potent pharmacologic constituents. Characteristically, ingestion of sufficient quantities of pharmacologically active foodstuffs will result in symptoms in virtually all individuals, although the threshold of susceptibility may vary considerably. As mentioned earlier, many foods contain vasoactive amines that directly induce headache, abdominal pain, and gastrointestinal dysfunction. These agents also may be capable of activating prostaglandins, particularly in the lung and gut (Collier et al., 1975), with symptoms consequent to the activation of these agents.

Prostaglandin synthesis may be inhibited by food additives such as tartrazine (Szczeklik et al., 1975), which could alter the balance between competing prostaglandins. This, in turn, could induce asthma or urticaria in some individuals. In addition, constituents of certain foods such as strawberries and eggs act as nonimmune histamine releasers and thus probably are capable of inducing symptoms that mimic those of IgE-mediated reactions (Beall, 1964).

Other Nonimmune Reactions. Certain foods may be harmful because they contain substances that some children with specific enzyme deficiencies or other metabolic diseases cannot tolerate. Examples include celiac disease due to a gladian fraction of gluten found in wheat and rye flour; inborn errors of metabolism, such as maple syrup disease and phenylketonuria which interfere with the metabolism of specific amino acids; deficiency of lactase, maltase or sucrase which interferes with sugar digestion; or deficiency of an enzyme important in specific sugar metabolism (galactosemia).

Clinical Syndromes Associated with Food Allergy

Food-induced inflammation is not limited to the gut, and *food allergy* should not be used synonymously with the term *gastrointestinal allergy*. Symptoms attributed to food allergy are legion, but in many instances, such associations have been difficult to document. In some cases, a specific reaction to a food has been established as allergic, and the mechanism has been clearly defined. Cause and effect associations have been established in many instances, but in other cases the associations have been poorly documented. Particularly in highly sensitive individuals, foods also may act as inhalant allergens. Gastrointestinal and other syndromes that may be induced by food allergies are considered in detail in other chapters of this book.

Diagnosis of Allergy to Foods

In approaching the problem of food allergy in children, several points require emphasis: a presumptive diagnosis of Type I sensitivity to foods generally can be made on historical grounds alone. Clinical manifestations of Type I reactivity to foods usually occur within 2 hours of food ingestion, and should be reproducible (Bock et al., 1977). As a practical matter, skin tests or other confirmatory tests frequently are not necessary.

Intradermal skin tests generally are not recommended because of the large number of "false positive" reactions as well as the potential danger of inducing a systemic reaction in inordinately sensitive individuals. Similarly, scratch, prick, or puncture tests (recommended skin testing techniques for food antigens) should be employed with caution. Large local skin test reactions correlate well with clinical sensitivity while small skin test reactions correlate poorly but may be used as a starting point for elimination and challenge to determine whether clinical sensitivity to foods exists. Also, the clinical significance of skin test reactions varies significantly according to the specific food tested. Skin test reactions to peas, for example, are more likely to be more meaningful clinically than skin test reactions to wheat (Aas, 1978). RAST testing also is a useful diagnostic test (Hoffman and Haddad, 1974). Though safer than skin testing, it seldom is more accurate in implicating a particular food and appears less sensitive.

Delayed-onset food sensitivities, i.e., reactions that occur hours to days after food ingestion, seldom are identified by skin testing or RAST since the majority do not appear to be IgE-mediated, at least to native food antigens. Determination of milk precipitins may be useful in the child ingesting milk who has a clinical pattern described by Heiner et al. (1962). Proof of diagnosis also depends upon reproducible demonstration of a cause and effect relationship, by specific *elimination and challenge* (see Chapter 29). It is emphasized, however, that establishment of a reaction to a food does not in itself establish the pathogenetic mechanism involved.

GENERAL THERAPEUTIC CONSIDERATIONS IN FOOD ALLERGY

Specific Therapy. Avoidance of the offending food is the most successful means of treating food allergy as is true with sensitivity to inhalants or other allergens. *In all cases, a nutritionally adequate diet must be ensured* (see Chapters 28 and 29). Parenteral and oral hyposensitization to foods is not effective and can be dangerous.

Pharmacotherapy. Several investigators have attempted to block food-induced mediator release (Type I allergic reactions) by pretreatment with oral cromolyn sodium, administered 30 minutes before food ingestion. Although preliminary studies show promise in preventing gastrointestinal symptoms, asthma, urticaria and eczema in some patients, questions regarding efficacy, drug dosage and time of administration remain unresolved (Danneus et al., 1977). Antihistamines have been used with success in lessening food-induced gastrointestinal or systemic symptoms. Steroid therapy has been helpful in controlling protein-losing enteropathy but is not otherwise recommended.

PREVENTION OF FOOD ALLERGY

The virtues of prophylaxis both with breast milk and other hypoallergenic milks in the potentially atopic child are discussed in Chapter 25. Breast milk is an ideal food for the infant because it provides both immune and nonimmune passive protection, and it is hypoallergenic. However, food proteins ingested by the mother may be secreted in breast milk sufficiently intact to induce sensitization and reactivity in the infant. Donnolly (1930) demonstrated that egg white protein eaten by the mother could be found in her breast milk in low concentration (approximately 1 part per million). Others have reported urticaria or flaring of eczema in breast-fed infants, purportedly related to milk ingested by the mother. Although there is little definitive data on potential food allergens contained in breast milk, observations to date suggest that it may be advisable to recommend that nursing mothers of allergic infants restrict their intake of foods considered to be highly allergenic (especially cow milk, eggs, and perhaps wheat) or other foods specifically incriminated in the child's disorder.

References

Aas, K.: Studies of hypersensitivity to fish. Int. Arch. Allergy *30*:257, 1966.

Aas, K.: *The Biochemical and Immunologic Bases of Bronchial Asthma.* Springfield, Ill., Charles C Thomas, 1972, p. 112 (Allergens of asthma).

Aas, K.: The diagnosis of hypersensitivity to ingested foods. Clinical Allergy *8*:39, 1978.

Beall, G. N.: Urticaria: A review of laboratory and clinical observations. Medicine *43*:131, 1964.

Bleumink, E.: Food allergy: The chemical nature of the substance eliciting symptoms. World Rev. Nutr. Diet. *12*:505, 1970.

Bock, S. A., Buckley, J., Holst, A., and May, C. D.: Proper use of skin tests with food extracts in diagnosis of hypersensitivity to food in children. Clin. Allergy *7*:375, 1977.

Collier, H. O., McDonald-Gibson, W. J., and Saud, A.: Stimulation of biosynthesis by capsaicin, ethanol and tyramine. Lancet *1*:702, 1975.

Cooke, R. A.: *Allergy in Theory and Practice.* Philadelphia, W. B. Saunders Co., 1947, p. 25.

Coombs, R. R. A., and Gell, P. G. H.: *Clinical Aspects of Immunology,* 2nd ed. Oxford, Blackwell Scientific Publications, 1968, p. 575.

Conners, C. K., Goyette, C. H., Southwick, D. A., et al.: Food additives and hyperkinesis. A controlled double-blind experiment. Pediatrics *58*:154, 1976.

Danneus, A., Foucard, T., and Johannson, S. G. O.: The effect of orally administered sodium cromoglycate on symptoms of food allergy. Clin. Allergy *7*:109, 1977.

Donnolly, H. H.: The question of the elimination of foreign protein (egg-white) in women's milk. J. Immunol. *19*:1, 1930.

Galant, S. P., Bullock, J., and Frick, O. L.: An immunological approach to the diagnosis of food sensitivity. Clin. Allergy *3*:363, 1973.

Halpern, S. R., Sellars, W. A., Johnson, R. B., et al.: Development of allergy in children fed soy or cow's milk in the first six months of life. J. Allergy Clin. Immunol. *51*:139, 1973.

Harley, J. P., Roy, R. S., Tomasi, L., et al.: Hyperkinesis and food additives: Testing the Feingold hypothesis. Pediatrics *61*:818, 1978.

Heiner, D. C., Sears, J. W., and Kniker, W. T.: Milk precipitins to cow's milk in chronic respiratory disease. Am. J. Dis. Child. *103*:634, 1962.

Hoffman, D. R., and Haddad, Z. H.: Diagnosis of IgE mediated reactions to food antigens by radioimmunoassay. J. Allergy Clin. Immunol. *54*:165, 1974.

Juhlin, L., Michelson, C., and Zetterstrom, O.: Urticaria and asthma induced by food and drug additives in patients with aspirin hypersensitivity. J. Allergy Clin. Immunol. *50*:92, 1972.

Kletter, B., Gray, I., Freier, S., et al.: Immune response of normal infants to cow's milk. Int. Arch. Allergy Appl. Immunol. *40*:656, 1971.

Matthews, T., and Soothill, J.: Complement activation after milk feeding in children with cow's milk allergy. Lancet *2*:893, 1970.

Parish, W. E.: Short-term anaphylactic IgG antibodies in human sera. Lancet *2*:591, 1970.

Sapeika, N.: *Food Pharmacology.* Springfield, Ill., Charles C Thomas, 1969.

Speer, F.: Intolerance to foods. *In* Speer, F., and Docknorn, R. J. (eds.): *Allergy and Immunology in Childhood.* Charles C Thomas, Springfield, Ill., 1973, pp. 276–290.

Spies, J. R., Stevan, M. A., Stein, W. J., et al.: The chemistry of allergens. XX. New antigens generated by pepsin hydrolysis of bovine milk protein. Allergy *45*:208, 1970.

Stenius, B. S., and Lemola, M.: Hypersensitivity to aspirin and tartrazine in patients with asthma. Clin. Allergy *6*:119, 1976.

Szczeklik, A., Gryglewski, R. J., and Czerniawska, M. G.: Relationship of inhibition of prostaglandin biosynthesis by analgesics to asthma attacks in aspirin-sensitive patients. Br. Med. J. *1*:67, 1975.

Taylor, B., Norman, A. P., Orgel, H. A., et al.: Transient IgA deficiency and pathogenesis of infantile atopy. Lancet *2*:111, 1973.

Walker, A. W.: Host defense mechanisms in the gastrointestinal tract. Pediatrics *57*:901, 1976.

Walker, A. W., and Isselbacker, K. J.: Intestinal antibodies. N. Engl. J. Med. *297*:767, 1977.

Williams, J. I., Douglas, M. C., Tausig, F. T., et al.: Relative effects of drugs and diet on hyperactive behaviors: An experimental study. Pediatrics *61*:811, 1978.

William R. Solomon, M.D. # 16

Common Pollen and Fungus Allergens

FUNGI

Allergy to inhaled fungal allergens, a common factor in childhood allergic rhinitis and asthma, was recognized a half century ago. The clinical impact on respiratory allergy of many widespread, potential offenders still must be determined, however. The overall role of fungus materials in urticaria and eczema is speculative.

Basic Characteristics of Fungi

Fungi comprise a unique group of organisms, which differ fundamentally from plants, animals, actinomycetes, and slime molds (Myxomycetes). Fungi have true nuclei and cell walls of chitin or cellulose. Except for a limited number of unicellular forms, fungi are composed of microscopic strands or "hyphae"; these (Fig. 16–1) proliferate simply (as "molds") or form specialized fleshy structures (e.g., as in mushrooms and sac fungi). In most forms, well-defined septa divide the hyphal strands, and metabolic debris tends to be concentrated in older, more central segments as growth proceeds peripherally.

Specific fungi colonize a variety of substrates. Most allergenic fungi can grow on nonliving organic matter, while other types, i.e., obligate parasites, require a viable host. Both groups need moisture, oxygen,

preformed carbohydrate and occasionally additional growth factors.

Many familiar fungi grow actively at 20° C and may flourish well above or below this level; others require low temperatures, proliferating even under refrigeration. A small group of "thermophilic" fungi grow *only* at temperatures of 50° C or higher,

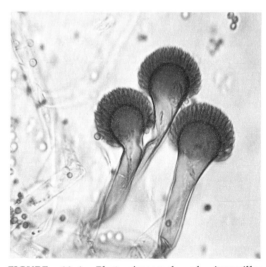

FIGURE 16–1. Photomicrograph of *Aspergillus fumigatus,* a typical filamentous imperfect fungus. Hyphal strands (left) are the basic structural units of these organisms. Spores (conidia) are characteristically borne on specialized hyphae (conidiophores), which, in *Aspergillus* form species, are terminally expanded; three such "vesicles" are shown at the right.

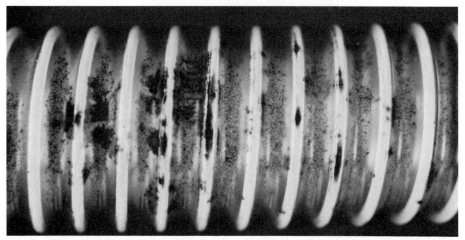

FIGURE 16–2. Fungal growth within the plastic tubing leading to a water-filled spirometer used for ventilatory testing. Airborne dust and droplets of saliva provide the only nutrient source of these organisms. An ample supply of moisture permits fungi to colonize such marginal sites.

while certain types (e.g., *Aspergillus fumigatus*) tolerate this level but also grow well below it. With adequate moisture, many fungi grow actively at 20°C on nutritionally barren substrates (Fig. 16–2) in homes and work environments.

Fungal vegetative strands may be ingestant allergens; however, airborne spores are the major source of inhalant exposure. Spores are specialized reproductive structures that facilitate the spread of fungi and are resistant to harsh environmental conditions. Depending upon the fungus (or even upon a particular growth phase), spores may be asexual (diploid) or sexual (haploid) with dissimilar "mating types." Many fungi may produce both sexual and asexual spores at separate phases of their life cycles. Since these stages may occur separately, the fungi have been described individually and named as if they were separate organisms.

Those types which generate asexual spores (i.e., imperfect fungi) are classified according to the form of their spore-producing organs. However, it is now clear that biologically dissimilar fungi may have imperfect (asexual) stages which are morphologically almost alike. Since the arrangement of the imperfect fungi does not necessarily reflect natural affinities, its taxa are termed *"form* species" and these are grouped in *"form* genera." While the concept of form taxa imparts some order to a large and difficult group, it is clear that members of form genera cannot be expected automatically to contain identical allergens. This limitation often has been overlooked in the past, both by physicians and pharmaceutical suppliers in considering the specificity of fungus extracts labeled with generic names only.

Classes of Fungi

The taxonomy of fungi is based largely upon the morphology, mode of development, and genetic endowment of their spores. Although many species exist, including many which are wholly aquatic, airborne molds constitute the most important source of allergens. They can be classified into five principal groups:

Fungi Imperfecti (Deuteromycetes). This class includes most of the currently recognized fungal allergens and fungi that reproduce asexually. With a few exceptions, these form taxa are saprophytic, and spores ("conidia") are formed on more or less specialized hyphal structures. In one subclass (Sphaeropsidales), spores arise in flask-shaped organs and are extruded in slimy masses which are dispersed by dew and raindrop outwash; prominent representatives of the subclass recognized as being allergenic include *Phoma* species. Another distinctive subclass (Melanconiales) has spore-forming hyphae in cushion-like masses; some members are plant pathogens, but apparently none serve as important allergens. The imperfect fungi bear spores singly or multiply on exposed hyphae except for a tiny group (Mycelia Sterilia), which appear to multiply by vegetative appendages alone. Tenuous attachments permit spores of many taxa to be scoured and dispersed readily by air currents; such "dry spore" dispersal is typical of such common genera as *Alternaria* (Fig. 16–3), *Cladosporium* (formerly *Hormodendrum*), and *Penicillium*. Out of doors, these types are most prevalent during hot, dry, windy diurnal periods. By contrast, many fungi (e.g., species of *Phoma, Fusarium,* and *Cephalosporium*) produce mucinous masses of "slime" spores that become airborne during rainy and humid nocturnal periods.

Although allergists are most familiar with imperfect fungi, there remains substantial uncertainty concerning their clinical role for a variety of reasons: gaps in knowledge of their prevalence in many areas of the country and of the amount of exposure in specific environments or with specific activities, a dearth of information on the intensity of exposure necessary to induce symptoms and unclear antigenic relationships between biologically related genera.

Table 16–1 is an annotated list of imperfect fungi of acknowledged or widely suspected clinical importance.

Downy Mildews (Oömycetes). These relatively primitive fungi include economically important parasites of plants and certain insects. Agricultural exposure to heavily infected crops occasionally provokes allergic respiratory responses.

Sugar and Bread Molds (Zygomycetes). The allergic impact of this class is due largely to members of the order Mucorales including species of *Rhizopus, Mucor,* and *Absidia*. These fungi are prominent saprophytes on diverse biologic debris including food residues and leaf litter. They are ubiquitous in soil, but their level in air usually is low. With seepage of ground water or soiling of furnishing with foods, these organisms may flourish indoors and contribute to the burden of inhaled allergens. Close inspection of infected substrates may disclose the dark, globular reproductive structures (sporangia), each containing myriad spores (sporangiospores). Members of the order

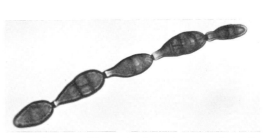

FIGURE 16–3. *Alternaria alternata* spores, borne in characteristic chains. These brown, multiseptate particles are widely abundant in outdoor air and are among the most clinically important fungus allergens.

Mucorales typically have comparatively broad hyphae with few septa.

Ascomycetes (Sac Fungi). Production of sexual spores (ascospores) in a sac-like cell (or "ascus") is a unifying feature of these fungi. Ascospores often are actively launched into air by processes requiring moisture and are notably abundant in humid or rainy weather. Many familiar imperfect fungi, including certain *Aspergillus, Fusarium,* and *Helminthosporium* form species, are asexual states of ascomycetes. Brewer's (baker's) yeast is an additional member of this class. The few ascospore types evaluated as allergens have induced moderate rates of reactivity in exposed atopic subjects (Bruce, 1963).

Basidiomycetes (Mushrooms, Puffballs, Rusts, and Smuts). These fungi resemble ascomycetes in producing sexual spores (among other types), are shot from their points of origin when they have adequate moisture, and are abundant at night and during rainy periods. Characteristic spores, "basidiospores", are formed — most commonly in tetrads — on specialized cells or "basidia". In addition, many parasitic forms (e.g., smuts, bunts, and rusts) produce additional spores during states of development which may involve a succession of hosts. Heavy exposures to spores of rusts and grain smuts in agriculture have produced symptoms of respiratory allergy, but it is not known whether light exposure to these spores will produce symptoms. Asthma has been associated with homes containing spores of the dry rot fungus (*Merulius lacrymans*), suggesting that clinical evaluation of additional basidiospore types is warranted.

Concepts of Fungus Prevalence and Their Limitations

Unlike allergens such as pollens and danders which come from obvious sources, airborne fungi originate largely from inapparent microscopic growth. Consequently, determination of exposure necessitates direct air sampling. Limitations in atmospheric collection techniques have seriously delayed and distorted understanding of this area. Total reliance upon molds that grow on exposed agar media, for example, has limited data to *viable* particles and excluded possibly significant allergens that fail to grow recognizably on mold culture plates. (Selective recovery is a property of all known media, although some, e.g., malt extract agar and Sabouraud's glucose agar, are less restrictive than others.) Prevalence

data also may be biased by collecting particles on greased slides or on open plates of growth media by fallout. Since variations in air speed, direction, and turbulence level affect deposition and the volume of air contributing particles is unknown, the data obtained cannot be readily compared sequentially or from site-to-site. Furthermore, particle fallout on collection surfaces is proportional to particle diameter (or, more specifically, to diameter squared) so that larger particles will predominate in collections (Fig. 16–4). Recent development of techniques, accurate for particles of all sizes, has altered our knowledge of the true abundance of many ascospores and basidiospores as well as of small imperfect fungus spores which previously were unnoticed (see p. 221 and Ogden et al., 1974, for additional detail).

TABLE 16–1   IMPERFECT FUNGI OF SPECIAL INTEREST TO ALLERGISTS

Form Genus and Major Form Species*	SRR†	Noteworthy Characteristics D = dark gray or black colonies ("Dematiaceous")
Alternaria — *A. alternata* = *A. tenuis*	++++	Widespread on vegetation; probably most clinically reactive airborne fungus allergen (D)
Cladosporium (formerly Hormodendrum) — *C. cladosporioides, C. herbarum*	++	Highest outdoor spore levels in most regions. Form species' allergens may differ (D)
Epicoccum — *E. purpurascens*	++	Especially on grains, grasses; produces orange pigments but sporulates poorly on many agar media
Stemphylium — *S. botryosum*	+++	Imperfect form of *Pleospora herbarum*, an ascomycete (D)
Curvularia *(C. lunata)*	+++	Especially in warmer areas (D)
Helminthosporium — *H. solani*	+++	Agriculturally-centered, epidemic at times (D) (*Drechslera* and *Bipolaris* are similar form genera)
Fusarium — *F. roseum, F. nivale*	++	Imperfect forms of several ascomycete genera; colonies produce slime spores and prominent pigments. Ascospores may produce much *Fusarium* growth
Phoma — *P. herbarum*	+++	Sphaeropsid; slime-spored; reactivity said to parallel that to *Alternaria* species
Penicillium (more than a dozen common types)	+	Often perennially present *in* and outdoors; *unrelated* to sensitivity to penicillin.
Aspergillus — *A. flavus, A. fumigatus, A. amstelodami, A. glaucus*, others	++	Indoor and occupational exposures common; *A. fumigatus, A. flavus* also produce allergic aspergillosis

Many airborne fungi possess distinctive morphology that enables identification microscopically. Identification by microscopic examination is applicable especially to the dark-spored imperfect fungi (see Table 16–1), many sexual spores of fleshy fungi, and to rust and smut spores. Though there is no comprehensive guide for identification available, illustrations of a selection of these particles have been published (Gregory, 1973). An extensive set of ascospore drawings (Dennis, 1960) and monographs depicting the spores of imperfect fungus taxa also can be found (Barron, 1968; Barnett, 1972; Ellis, 1971).

The growth of fungi on semisolid media is essential for numerous taxa (e.g., form species of *Penicillium* and *Aspergillus*, yeasts and zygomycetes) with minute, nondescript, spheroidal spores. The interested reader is referred to the publication by Arx (1970) which describes generic identification, also to Barron (1968), Barnett, (1972) Ellis (1971), and to Smith (1960) for technical advice in identifying fungi.

Recoveries in culture considerably understate prevalence as judged by spores in microscopic deposits. In addition, it is clear that many airborne spore types — especially sexual spores of certain fleshy fungi — cannot be identified because they are neither distinctive in form nor capable of growing on available media.

Fungi Outdoors. Since fungi grow principally on leaf surfaces, in plant litter and soil, spore concentrations vary with local cycles of plant growth and are decreased by snow cover. Airborne fungi are prominent throughout the growing season in temperate areas, but peak spore levels occur in

TABLE 16–1 IMPERFECT FUNGI OF SPECIAL INTEREST TO ALLERGISTS (*Continued*)

Form Genus and Major Form Species*	SRR†	Noteworthy Characteristics D = dark gray or black colonies ("Dematiaceous")
(A. niger)	(±)	(Prominent on wood and paper)
Candida — *C. albicans, C. tropicalis*	++	*C. albicans* is a common human gut and orificial saprophyte; uncommon in air
Rhodotorula — *R. glutinis*	+	Prominent during wet weather; acid-tolerant yeast; grows well in indoor fluid reservoirs
Aureobasidium — *A. pullulans*	++	Formerly termed "Pullularia"; common soil, leaf saprophyte. Pleomorphic on agar media (D)
Monilia sitophila	+	Prominently associated with milling and bakery trades; extremely rapid grower
Botrytis — *B. cinerea*	++	Prevalence regionally variable; prominent plant pathogen
Geotrichum — *G. candidum*	+	Vaguely defined form genus; probably asexual forms of basidiomycetes
Sporobolomyces — *S. roseum*	++	Yeast, usually pink, actively discharging spores; suspected autumn allergen in Great Britain
Gliocladium — *G. roseum*	++	Slime-spored; young growth Penicillium-like
Trichoderma — *T. viride*	+	Prominent in soil; rapid grower

*Note that additional form genera including *Cephalosporium, Verticillium, Sporothrix, Pithomyces,* and numerous yeasts are widely encountered but have received little or no clinical evaluation.

†SRR = Estimated relative Skin Reactivity Rate among exposed atopic subjects in North America using available materials.

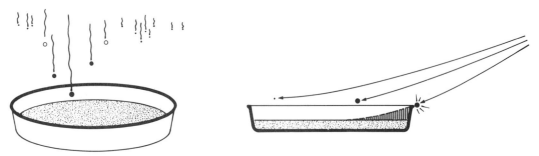

FIGURE 16–4. Problems in particle collection by open culture plates. At left, the markedly greater fallout of larger (than smaller) particles is emphasized using the (unnatural) example of still air. A similar effect is easily observed with normal atmospheric motion (right). Here again, recovery varies with particle size, and in rapidly moving air, deposition may be hindered by the protruding lip of the culture dish.

late summer and autumn, particularly during hot, breezy periods when "dry-spore" forms are especially abundant. Recoveries at these times are dominated by spores of *Alternaria* and *Cladosporium* species, which seem to achieve their highest levels in grassland and cultivated (especially, grain-growing) areas. At night and on rainy days, ascospores and basidiospores reach maximum prevalence along with splash-dispersed spores of imperfect types. Whether respiratory symptoms that worsen during humid and rainy weather reflect exposure to these little studied particles is unknown. Symptoms are induced in fungus-sensitive subjects by many situations and activities that promote fungus exposure. Spore levels are higher close to the ground in natural areas than at rooftop sites. Substantial airborne dispersion of fungus particles occurs when plant growth is disturbed. A hiker traversing any type of vegetation may be exposed to massive numbers of fungal particles. Similar exposure may occur with mowing a lawn or harvesting grain. Composting plant materials pose special hazards for mold-sensitive patients because fungi flourish in them. Fungus-sensitive persons commonly develop symp-toms after exposure to hay, ensilage, mulches, dry soil, commercial peat moss, compost piles, and leaf litter. There is little objective support for the belief that spore levels are specifically increased in the vicinity of lakes and other surface waters.

Fungi Indoors. Fungi in enclosed spaces can produce perennial symptoms. Occupational contact with plant or animal products — especially in humid interiors — is associated with heavy exposure to air-borne fungal antigens. When spores are numerous out of doors, they tend to dominate recoveries made in normally ventilated interiors; fungi originating indoors are more likely to be evident when buildings are closed (e.g., in winter or with central air conditioning in summer), and especially when outdoor levels are low. At these times, dominant recoveries often include *Penicillium, Aspergillus* and *Fusarium* form species and occasionally *Rhodotorula* and other yeasts. This contrasts sharply with the "*Cladosporium-Alternaria*" pattern so typical of outdoor air in northern states in summer (Solomon, 1976).

In winter studies of midwestern homes, correlation between relative humidity and indoor fungus levels has been strong. This association probably reflects both the effect of moisture on fungus growth and also the colonization of humidifying devices by fungi. "Cool-mist" vaporizers are frequently contaminated and emit fungus-laden aerosols (Solomon, 1974); presumably furnace humidifiers may do so also. Pets and active small children foster increased indoor fungus levels by soiling surfaces with food residues and outside dust. It is possible that houseplants may contribute to indoor mold exposure, but current information makes recommendations for total elimination of houseplants difficult to justify.

Reduction of indoor mold spore exposure depends upon meticulous general hygiene, with either elimination or encasing in plastic of fibre and/or foam-filled furnishings. Central air conditioning will permit window closure during warm periods, thus limiting ingress of outdoor particles and reducing relative humidity. At other times, supplementary humidification should be restrained, with levels of 20 to 25 percent relative humidity viewed as adequate. Shower curtains, refrigerator drip trays, and window moldings as well as cold basement and outside walls where water condenses or seeps deserve special concern. If these areas are cleaned with solutions of sodium hypochlorite, Lysol or commercial products such as X14, or zephiran, mold growth is inhibited although microbial regrowth occurs all too quickly. (Zephiran, available as Roccal, is used in a dilution of 1 ounce to 1 gallon of tap water). Specific indoor antifungal agents have not yet been proven safe and effective. Small moldy objects may be decontaminated by placing them in a plastic bag for 12 to 24 hours with a small amount of paraformaldehyde or several milliliters of propylene oxide. Fungus growth in limited spaces also may be attacked by volatilizing paraformaldehyde. These fumes are toxic, however, and treated areas must be completely ventilated before use.

Sampling indoor air by use of open culture dishes ("settling plates") is of dubious value in evaluating obscure symptoms. If this method is used, the physician must be aware of the serious limitation of preferential recovery of large particles by this method, with exclusion of smaller particles (Solomon, 1975). This is especially important since small-spored fungi often predominate in indoor air.

Fungi in Foods. Fungi are important in the production of many foods and industrial chemicals (Smith, 1960). Various yeasts *(Saccharomyces cerevisiae)* are employed in preparation of baked goods, beer, wines and some liquors as well as vinegar and vinegar products — especially processed meats. Most cheeses result from bacterial fermentations but are readily contaminated in storage; in addition, Camembert and blue-veined cheeses (e.g., Roquefort) utilize specific *Penicillium* species. Commercial mushrooms, the spore-producing organs of basidiomycetes *(Agaricus bisporis),* are rarely ingestant allergens. Soy sauce and steak sauces are produced using *Aspergillus oryzae.* Fungi are employed in the early stages of chocolate production. In addition, fungi commonly contaminate stored foodstuffs, even at refrigeration temperatures.

Although massive ingestion of yeast-containing foods (e.g., a wine, cheese and pizza feast) will, at times, provoke respiratory symptoms in young adults, ingested fungi probably are an infrequent cause of prolonged allergic problems. Highly allergic children occasionally may benefit from a trial withdrawal of dietary fungi followed by a diagnostic challenge. Such a diagnostic "mold-free diet" eliminates fresh rolls, coffee cakes, and pizza dough, dried yeast, and foods refrigerated over 72 hours. Fresh fruits and vegetables should be peeled or scrubbed before consumption. Products such as jellies and preserves are acceptable, and commercial breads are allowed. If low-fungus diets are employed for more than a short time, nutritional adequacy must be ensured. Duration should be tailored to individual clinical needs. Often, avoidance of a few foods can provide a great benefit.

Significance of Fungus Sensitivity. Evaluation of sensitivity to fungi is difficult because of their diversity, their uncertain regional distribution and often prolonged periods of exposure. Clinical allergy to fungal allergens *alone* is uncommon. However, there is little doubt that IgE-mediated allergy to fungi is widespread, especially to species of *Alternaria* and other dark-spored imperfect genera. These may be responsible for symptoms throughout most of a local growing season or, at least, at times different from major pollen peaks. Although many additional molds produce positive skin tests, their clinical importance and allergenic similarities, if any, are yet to be fully defined. Determining fungus prevalence in air remains a key to estimating exposure and to setting priorities for clinical evaluation.

POLLENS

Pollen allergy (pollinosis) is the most frequently recognized allergic syndrome. Symptoms are caused by exposure to windborne pollens in subjects allergic to them. They may react with symptoms of seasonal allergic rhinitis (hay fever), asthma, or conjunctivitis. Atopic dermatitis occasionally flares during pollen seasons while pollen-provoked urticaria is usually related to running through fields of pollinating tall grass or ragweed.

Pollen in Reproductive Biology

Pollen grains — common to all flowering plants — serve as vectors for male gametes or reproductive cells. Pollens develop in specialized floral structures (Fig. 16–5), the *anther sacs,* which are lined by a specialized tissue, the *tapetum.* One or more anther sacs with a suitable protective covering, i.e., the anther, is usually borne on a stalk or *filament,* and termed a *stamen.* The total developmental process that provides mature pollen grains for dispersal is termed *anthesis.*

In most flowering plants, *pollination* (i.e., the transport of mature pollen) is effected by one or more animal vectors — generally an insect. However, all of the grasses, many of the trees of temperate regions, and a minority of broad-leafed herbs (or "forbs") have developed adaptations for wind dispersal of pollen (and are termed "anemophilous"). The goal of pollen transport, in either case, is deposition of viable grains on a receptive *stigma,* the terminal and most exposed part of the female floral organ (or "pistil") as shown in Figure 16–5. After this is accomplished, both grain and stigmatic surface release one or more poorly characterized "recognition substances." Aside from their fundamental biologic importance to the plant, many of these substances (e.g., antigen E of short ragweed) appear to be important as clinical allergens. When an exchange of chemical signals occurs between a compatible grain and stigma, it may be followed by *pollen germination.* In this process, a tubular structure emerges from the grain, penetrates the stigma and grows down through the subjacent *style,* finally reaching the *ovary,* the reproductive nexus of the pistil. Gametes are formed during pollen tube development and effect fertilization, producing both an embryo and nutritive *endosperm,* the components of the future seed.

Sources of Windborne Pollen

Floral Similarities Among Wind-pollinated Plants. Since anemophilous plants rely upon random transport of pollen, increasing the number of pollen grains dispersed increases fertilization rates. This goal has been achieved by evolutionary adaptations which have produced a similar floral pattern (see Fig. 16–6) in all wind-

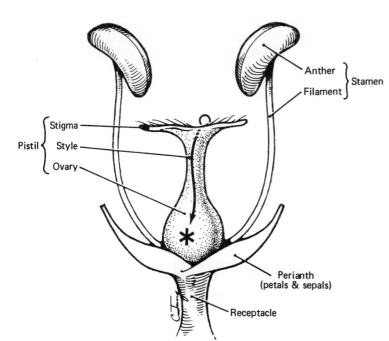

FIGURE 16–5. Structure of a wind-pollinated flower. Note the relatively large anthers, broad stigma, and reduced perianth; no nectaries are present. The arrow indicates the general path of pollen tube growth to effect fertilization (*). Having both male and female organs, this flower is "perfect."

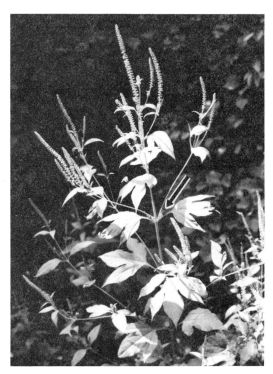

FIGURE 16–6. Giant ragweed, a highly successful wind-pollinated species. Male flowers are produced in crowded terminal spikes, whereas female flowers (arrow) are fewer and occupy the bases of the leaves. The three-lobed leaves are the basis of the Latin name of this plant, *Ambrosia trifida.*

pollinated species. Modifications include: production of numerous, miniature grouped flowers; increased output of pollen per stamen; and reduction or absence of brightly colored parts and of scent (which attracts insects). In addition, anemophilous flowers commonly have relatively expanded stigmas, long anther filaments, and may be *imperfect,* i.e., of two types — with only male or only female parts — in a single floret. (Species having individuals bearing male or female flowers *only* are termed "dioecious".) Most wind-borne grains are relatively smooth-surfaced and are among the smallest of all pollens, with diameters of 15 to 60 microns.

Tree, Grass, and Weed Sources. The heterogeneous group of anemophilous plants associated with pollinosis often is subclassified colloquially into trees, grasses, and weeds. While these terms are useful, certain qualifications deserve emphasis. Trees are woody plants capable of reaching heights of 20 feet or more at maturity.

Members of many plant families share this growth form, and there is no reason to expect allergic similarities among diverse tree pollens. Pollination by tree species usually occurs early in the local growing season and often before leaf expansion is complete. While this schedule probably aids pollen penetration of forest canopies, it means flower buds must form in the autumn and endure the winter, so some losses from cold weather are inevitable. For this reason and because there may be temperature extremes in early spring in colder regions, the period and intensity of airborne pollens vary widely from year to year.

All grasses are wind-pollinated, yet only a few shed sufficient pollen to serve as *clinically* important sources. Pollens from certain grasses are antigenically similar (see p. 231). Peaks of grass pollen prevalence generally occur in the early to mid-summer periods, but may extend throughout a prolonged growing season in warmer regions.

"Weed" pollens generally are those derived from any sources besides trees and grasses. While many such broad-leafed herbs are horticultural pests (i.e., "weeds" in the strict sense), they represent numerous plant families and allergenic specificities. Furthermore, many grasses and trees also display "weediness," i.e., growth where they are unwanted.

Bases of Pollen Recognition

Pollens and Plant Taxonomy. Morphologic characteristics, evident on light microscopy, suffice to distinguish airborne pollens of most major plant groups. In some cases, the source of pollen grains may be identified only to the level of an *Order* (e.g., Graminales, the grass order) while, rarely, individual species may produce distinctive particles or only a single local source may be implicated. Relationships among anemophilous plants and pollens are best examined beginning with the order level. Each order comprises several related *families,* each composed of (one or more) *genera* sharing closer similarities. Each *genus* contains one or more *species,* the narrowest classification level with circumscribed structural traits and mating affinities.

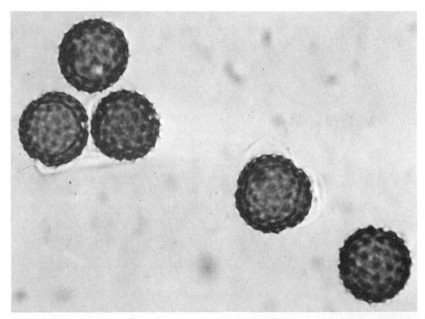

FIGURE 16–7. Photomicrograph of short ragweed pollen stained with fuchsin. Spiny grains, each with three pores, are typical of ragweed and of many additional species of the family Compositae. Several grains show intramural air spaces between the pores.

Fundamentals of Pollen Structure. Typical wind-borne pollen grains are spherical or ovoid structures (Fig. 16–7), often of a faintly yellow hue, which show remarkable grain-to-grain uniformity in structure for single types. An outermost layer, the *exine* is notable for its rigidity, resistance to chemical degradation, and capacity to be stained with certain dyes (e.g., basic fuchsin). The exine may show shallow sculpturing (e.g., spines or undulations) or may be essentially smooth. In addition, most pollen types have apertures in the exine which are round ("pores") or elongate ("furrows"). Within the exine is a continuous wall layer, the *intine,* composed largely of cellulose and enclosing the *protoplast,* with its nuclear material and subcellular organelles.

Criteria for pollen identification center largely on grain size and shape (in aqueous mounting media) as well as the ornamentation and apertural characteristics of the exine. However, the overall width of the transparent intine (as in yews, junipers, and their allies) or discrete thickenings in this layer (as in the birch family) may create distinctive appearances. Even protoplast structures may aid identification, as with the easily observed starch granules of dock and sorrel pollens.

Additional features give a distinctive appearance to certain pollen types such as those airborne as tetrads (e.g., broad leafed cattail) or larger aggregates *(Mimosa).* Grains of pines, spruces, and firs are noteworthy for their two lateral air-filled bladders which add to the buoyancy of these large (> 50 microns) particles. Although salient features of major airborne pollens will be noted (pp. 231–238), the reader is referred to several illustrated references for a systematic approach to identification (Ogden et al., 1974; Kapp, 1969; Hyde and Adams, 1958).

Ecology of Airborne Pollen Prevalence

The overall impact of pollens in human allergic diseases depends on such factors as sources, aerial transport, and allergenicity. The prevalence of pollen grains is affected by the number produced by the plant, the number of plants, and the efficiency of airborne transport; the effect on the individual depends on the person's activities as well as the degree of allergy to the pollen.

In general, pollen emission is fostered by relatively warm, dry conditions. Ragweed pollen shedding, for example, falls off sharply or ceases when the temperature is below 10° C or relative humidity is above 70 percent at "anther" level. Many flowers have mechanisms for storing ripe pollen until conditions are optimal for distribution (Gregory, 1973). Requirements for warm, dry air may explain the general tendency for most pollens to be released during daylight hours. Ragweed can shed in complete darkness, however, and certain grasses may show peak anthesis at night.

The process of pollen release often is complex, although only a few types (e.g., mulberries) actively expel grains from the anthers. In short ragweed, it is a multistage process in which anther protrusion of individual florets is followed by drying, plication, and ultimate cracking of the anther wall and spillage of moist pollen onto leaf surfaces (Bianchi, Schwemmin and Wagner, 1959). The sequence begins before dawn and is abetted by solar warming (and lowered humidity) after sunrise. Deposited grains dry, separate, and become airborne as heat-induced air movement stirs the foliage. Close to source plants, airborne levels are maximal 2 to 3 hours after sunrise, whereas at greater distances, diurnal peaks are delayed, reflecting transport time.

It is difficult to generalize about the effects of weather on pollen transport. Rain washes pollen from the air, and particle removal varies principally with the duration rather than intensity of precipitation. This scouring process, however, may be offset by associated air turbulence and disturbance from impacting raindrops which serve to refloat particles. Rainfall also is accompanied frequently by atmospheric temperature inversions, which tend to concentrate particles close to the ground.

Brisk winds promote pollen transport, but active atmospheric mixing also carries pollen aloft, thereby diluting levels near the ground, to which humans are exposed. During evening hours, atmospheric stability often is restored, and particle-bearing air from higher altitudes moves downward toward the surface.

Determining Pollen and Spore Prevalence

"Gravity" Slides and Plates. Atmospheric variables that affect particle prevalence also can modify the behavior of pollen and spores with respect to sampling devices. These effects are most troublesome with traditional "fallout" techniques using greased microslides (Ogden et al., 1974) or open plates of culture medium. Horizontal surfaces will collect particles, and pollen data have been gathered in this way for decades. In practice, an adhesive-coated, 1-inch by 3-inch glass microslide is exposed for 24 hours in a housing of standard design (Durham, 1946). Particles are deposited from turbulent air flow, and following exposure, particles are identified microscopically using transmitted light. Data are expressed as "particles per unit area" (usually per cm²) of slide surface. Viable recoveries have also been studied by substituting plates of nutrient agar in the standard housing (or Durham sampler) for 12 to 60 minute periods. Colonies are identified after the culture plate has incubated for from 1 to 7 days.

Sampling by fallout is simple and requires inexpensive, readily available materials. Unfortunately, with gravitational techniques, the volume of air from which particles are recovered cannot be determined, and comparisons of particle prevalence on different dates or locations are subject to additional serious uncertainties, since recoveries by gravity slides (and plates) are affected by wind speed, wind direction, and turbulence levels. Furthermore, collections are sparse for all but the most abundant pollens and spores and larger particles are more likely to accumulate than smaller ones. For these reasons, "gravitational" techniques are useful in identifying prominent pollens "qualitatively" but do not yield reliable "quantitative" pollen concentrations.

Volumetric Samplers. "Volumetric" denotes the ability to relate recoveries to unit volumes of air. Recently, two types of mechanical samplers have been introduced that provide particle data in relation to unit volumes of air (Fig. 16–8). These are: (1) impactors, in which an adhesive-coated sampling surface is whirled in a circular path through particle-bearing air, and (2)

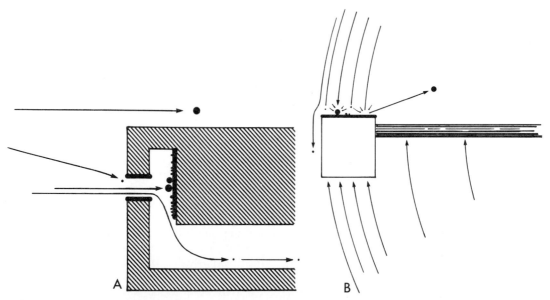

FIGURE 16–8. Collection principles employed by volumetric samplers. *A,* Suction traps (impingers) deposit particles at bends in their internal flow systems. These devices have especially high efficiency for small particles, which readily enter the traps from a moving air stream. *B,* Rotating arm impactors employ rapidly-rotated, adhesive-coated, narrow surfaces to intercept particles. The efficiency of impaction varies predictably with increasing particle size. Bounce-off can occur, and its frequency defines the "adhesive efficiency" of the collecting surface.

suction samplers (spore traps) which aspirate air at fixed rates into flow channels with sharp bends. Particles with too much momentum to allow these shifts in direction strike the walls at predictable points where sampling surfaces are positioned. Both types of devices provide quantitative data on the concentration of particles of any size per unit volume of air. Popular rotating impactors include the rotorod and rotoslide samplers, while the slide (Casella) and drum (Burkard) versions of the Hirst spore trap are widely used to collect microscopic particle deposits. Suction devices that provide volume-related recoveries on agar media include several slit samplers and the Andersen sampler. Detailed information about these devices is available in Ogden et al., 1974 and Solomon and Mathews, 1978.

Use and Abuses of Atmospheric Data

Although it is generally assumed that there is a direct relationship between pollen exposure and allergic symptoms, neither threshold levels nor dose-response effects have been proven. British workers have observed that grass pollen-sensitive patients, with few exceptions, develop symptoms when mean (24 hour, integrated) levels reach 20 grains per meter.[3] Comparable data for ragweed are not available, although a modal value of about 100 grains per meter[3], with considerable intersubject variation in threshold, might be anticipated. In addition, the nasal response appears to be related to recent exposure to other allergens as well as to the intensity of pollen exposure. Previous exposure to pollens to which the patient is allergic appear to "prime" the nasal mucosa to react at lower exposure levels of the same or unrelated pollen allergen (Connell, 1969). For these reasons, one should be skeptical of the value of "pollen counts" in predicting severity of pollen symptoms, especially when counts are derived from gravity samplers. Further, there are marked differences between pollen counts done at rooftop level and ground level, and from place to place within a community. Optimally performed "background" samples may be useful in identifying the major pollens in the air at a give time, but they will not reflect true personal levels of exposure.

Despite these reservations, aeroallergen data provide, at the least, a qualitative view of exposure and an opportunity for correlation retrospectively with clinical events. Annual dates of pollen and mold appearance and disappearance may be estimated and peak periods identified. For relatively abundant pollens and larger fungus spores, even gravity slides allow prevalence trends to be identified, although their correlative value is limited.

In areas where ragweed is prevalent, pollen counts based on gravity slide data often are announced by news media to an eager public. Unfortunately, the limitations of these data are mentioned only rarely, and patients often are perplexed by apparent discrepancies between their symptoms and published exposure levels. In general, such reports, describing periods one or more days previously, are no more informative than trends derived from several previous pollen seasons. Moreover, patients often are needlessly distressed by minor day-to-day variation in published data, viewing these as predictors of serious discomfort. The physician should be aware of these misunderstandings about the significance of pollen counts and should try to educate his patients.

MAJOR POLLEN ALLERGENS AND THEIR SOURCES

Grasses

The grasses (Family Gramineae) are the most abundant, successful, and widely distributed natural grouping of wind-pollinated plants. Grass pollinosis is recognized on all major land masses and is the principal form of pollen allergy in Great Britain, central Europe, and much of Asia. Symptoms provoked by exposure to (flowering) hay fields long ago prompted the term "hay fever," which has now been broadened to connote all forms of seasonal allergic rhinitis.

Although many regions support a profusion of grass species, only a limited number shed sufficient pollen to deserve clinical interest. In North America, Bermuda grass *(Cynodon dactylon),* timothy *(Phleum pratense),* and orchard grass *(Dactylis glomerata)* are probably the most copious pollen producers, although over a dozen species play noteworthy secondary roles.

Grass pollen grains are subspherical bodies with finely pitted surfaces and single pores (Fig. 16–9). Emanations of most species average 28 to 35 microns; however, those of certain grains are larger (e.g., rye, 60 microns, and corn, over 100 microns). Typically, pores are closed by a membrane, derived from the intine, which bears a single fleck of exine substance (the "operculum").

Several characterizable antigens (Groups I, II and III), described from rye grass *(Lolium perenne)* pollen, have been identified also in certain other temperate zone grass pollens but *not* in that of Bermuda grass, which has its own unique sensitizers. A molecular weight of 27,000 has been estimated for rye grass Group I, which constitutes approximately one-third of the extractable pollen protein.

The sedges (Cyperaceae), rushes (Juncaceae), and cattails (Typhaceae) are families of grass-like plants that shed wind-borne pollens in moderate amounts. Whether these agents ever elicit symptoms or have allergens in common with grass pollens remains uncertain.

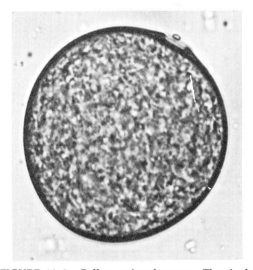

FIGURE 16–9. Pollen grain of a grass. The single pore, with its "operculum" of exine substance, is seen in side view and optical section.

Weeds (Broad-leafed Herbs or "Forbs")

Ragweeds. Members of the ragweed genus *(Ambrosia)* are confined largely to within this range, however, they are the most important source of pollinosis, annually affecting over 5 million persons. Of approximately 40 American ragweeds, less than a dozen are substantial local pollen sources, with "common" or "dwarf" ragweed *(A. artemisiifolia)* and giant ragweed *(A. trifida)* the most widely abundant offenders. Ragweed pollinosis in eastern North America involves these species exclusively, except for contributions from southern ragweed *(A. bidentata)* present in Missouri and surrounding states. To the west, perennial ragweed *(A. psilostachya)* and additional species including perennial slender ragweed *(A. confertiflora)* and annual bur ragweed *(A. acanthocarpa)* are prominent in the Great Plains and Great Basin areas, while canyon ragweed *(A. ambrosioides)*, rabbit bush *(A. deltoidea)*, and burroweed *(A. dumosa)* are ragweeds of southwestern deserts. Several of these species previously were classified in the genus *Franseria* (as "false ragweeds"); however, they appear to be valid ambrosias with respect to both form and pollen allergens. Floral development in most ragweeds is stimulated by decreasing day length, a response that determines their late summer periods of anthesis. As a consequence, peak pollen emission by North American ragweeds proceeds from north to south over a period of several weeks beginning in mid-August. (Several exceptional ragweed species, e.g., burroweed *(A. dumosa)* and rabbit bush *(A. deltoidea),* shed pollen during late spring in arid portions of the southwest and may elicit symptoms at that time.) The northern limit of ragweed growth is defined by the average occurrence of freezing temperatures before flowering can reach a stage resulting in viable seed. Where killing frost ($\sim -3°$ C at night) occurs, its advent terminates pollen dispersion by ragweeds, although anthesis usually has declined to low levels weeks before.

Although some ragweeds are confined largely to remote areas, the more familiar species (e.g., short ragweed) are truly "weedy," serving as prominent pests of cultivated sites. Despite their success, the growth of these types requires disturbance of competing perennial species, and ragweeds can be crowded out over several years by other natural cover (viz., grasses and perennial forbs). Ragweeds readily utilize soils "disturbed" by flowing water, cultivation and winter salting of roads, and, in Michigan, peak (short) ragweed abundance has been identified with cultivated grain fields (Fig. 16–10). Ragweeds obtained competitive advantages also by their rapid seedling growth in spring and by persistence of seed viability, which may exceed 60 years.

Pollen grains of common ragweed species are relatively small (18 to 23 microns) and are covered with short conical spines. Typically, three equally spaced pores are discernible, lying in a single (equatorial) plane. Between the pores, the outer wall layers separate to form shallow air spaces which increase buoyancy and give a mildly trilobate outline to the grains.

The nature of short ragweed pollen allergens has been studied exhaustively, and several active components characterized. Principal interest has centered on antigen E, a two-chain, linear protein (M.W. [molecular weight] 37,800) that appears to carry over 90 per cent of the allergenic potency of whole pollen eluate. Despite this activity, antigen E constitutes less than 0.5 per cent of the solid and less than 6 per cent of the protein ex-

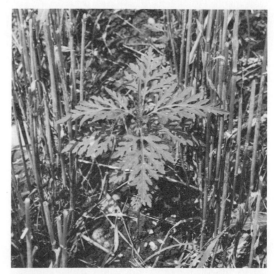

FIGURE 16–10. Young short ragweed plant in grain stubble of a Michigan oatfield. In many areas, agricultural disturbance makes cultivated fields dominant sources of ragweeds and their pollen.

tractable from short ragweed pollen. Although trace amounts of antigen E may be detectable in vegetative organs of short ragweed (e.g., stems and leaves) this material is confined essentially to pollen, where it appears to function as a recognition factor during pollination (see p. 228). Other described allergens include antigens K (M.W. 38,200), Ra3 (M.W. ca 15,000), and Ra5 (M.W. ca 5000), all of which appear to sensitize fewer persons than antigen E; additional components probably remain to be identified.

Ragweeds are members of the large composite family (Compositae), characterized by many small specialized flowers ("florets") which are borne in tight aggregates. While only a few of the composites are anemophilous, many species have pollens that resemble those of ragweeds morphologically and may cross-react antigenically, although human exposure to them may be sporadic. Such cross-reactivity seems to depend on components besides antigen E in most cases (Yunginger and Gleich, 1972). Clinically prominent ragweed relatives include the wind-pollinated marsh elders *(Iva)* — especially burweed marsh elder or "prairie ragweed" *(I. xanthifolia)* and rough marsh elder *(I. ciliata)* of the south-central and Gulf states. Additional *Iva* species — including poverty weed *(I. axillaris)* of the far West and *I. frutescens* of eastern salt marshes — appear to shed relatively little pollen. A similar verdict seems justified in the case of the abundant cockleburs *(Xanthium* species), casting doubt on the importance traditionally assigned to these plants as allergen sources.

The sages, sagebrushes, wormwoods and mugworts of the genus *Artemisia* constitute a second group of clinically important, anemophilous plants within the Compositae. Although herbs of this group are widespread, substantial pollen levels are confined to western regions where common sagebrush *(A. tridentata)* and sand sagebrush *(A. filifolia)* are abundant, and in the Pacific coastal range of *A. californica*. Additional local sources are present especially about the upper Great Lakes and in Tennessee and bordering states. However, the overall importance of artemisias as allergen sources east of the Great Plains seems minor. Although pollens of sages and ragweeds appear to share certain allergens, this similarity apparently is not based on antigen E.

In many areas, small amounts of pollen derived from insect-pollinated composites become airborne. Suspected sources of these particles include asters, sneezeweeds *(Helenium)*, and goldenrods *(Solidago* species) as well as dandelions and their allies. While the impact of their pollens usually is negligible, close respiratory contact with these native composites or with cultivated types including sunflowers, chrysanthemums, dahlias, and marigolds can precipitate symptoms in certain ragweed-sensitive persons. This potential is rarely evident, but probably has contributed to the enduring myth which links late summer hay fever and goldenrods. Antigen E seems absent from canteloupe, banana and watermelon, although these foods clearly provoke pharyngeal pruritus and/or rhinitis in certain ragweed-sensitive subjects.

Chenopodiales. The goosefoot and amaranth families (Chenopodiaceae and Amaranthaceae, respectively,) represent the order Chenopodiales and comprise many anemophilous types that are thought to share (certain) pollen allergens (Weber, Mansfield and Nelson, 1978). Differences in pollen productivity are marked within both families. Russian thistle *(Salsola kali* var. *pestifer)* and burning bush *(Kochia scoparia)* shed copiously over much of central and western North America, while western water hemp *(Acnida tamariscina)* and Palmer's amaranth are prominent in the south central states. In the far west, several "scales" *(Atriplex* species) greasewoods, and carelessweeds contribute pollen of this type, and sugar beet *(Beta vulgaris)* may serve as an allergen source — especially where it is grown for seed. However, pollen shedding by many widely evident species including lamb's quarters *(Chenopodium album)* and redroot pigweed *(Amaranthus retroflexus)* appears limited, and their clinical roles remain doubtful, despite widespread reactivity to the respective extracts.

Goosefoot and amaranth pollens conform to a pattern featuring spherical grains with pitted surfaces and many precisely spaced circular pores (Fig. 16–11). Although grain sizes, pore numbers, and interpore distances can distinguish some types, most observers are content to record a "chenopodamaranth" category, relying upon field observations to implicate specific sources.

Plantains *(Plantago* species). Of the

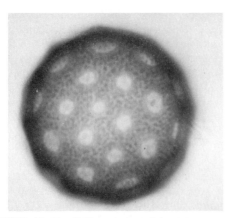

FIGURE 16–11. Pollen grain of lamb's quarters. The "golf-ball" appearance, due to numerous regularly spaced pores, is typical of the goosefoot and amaranth families (Chenopodiaceae and Amaranthaceae, respectively).

several plantains established in North America, only one — narrow leafed or buckhorn plantain (*P. lanceolata*) — commonly known as "English plantain" sheds sufficient pollen to warrant serious clinical attention. The species is a familiar, perennial, rosetting weed of lawns with elongate leaves and conical flower clusters on long central stalks. Plantain grains superficially resemble those of the chenopod-amaranth group but have substantially fewer (usually five to eight) scattered pores — each with an operculum. Pollen shedding by plantains often extends over several months without a well-defined peak. Rates of skin reactivity to plantain pollen are high in many temperate regions, and frank pollinosis has been ascribed to this factor in the Pacific Northwest. However, the relatively low levels prevailing elsewhere suggest that the overall clinical importance of the plantains probably is low.

Sorrels and Docks. Pollens of these wind-pollinated members of the knotweed family (Polygonaceae) are allergenically distinct from other "weed" types and appear during late spring in temperate regions. In North America, red or sheep sorrel (*Rumex acetosella*) is the principal source, and pollen shedding accompanies or precedes anthesis of the early grasses. Sheep sorrel forms large clones of male or female plants in lawns and grasslands and may escape casual observation except when flowering growth is present. Although other *Rumex* species are robust and familiar weeds, their pollen output

is relatively low. Pollen grains typical of the genus show three or four slitlike furrows, each with a central pore, and a protoplast packed with starch granules.

Nettles (*Urtica* Species). Increasing use of high efficiency impactors and spore traps has demonstrated abundant airborne nettle pollen at sites in North America and Great Britain. Typical grains are subspheroidal with three collared pores and are small enough (12 to 17 microns) to appear rarely in gravity slide collections. In North America *U. dioica* var. *procera* appears to be the main source species. However, the classification of the nettles is controversial, and this variably prickly, perennial inhabitant of stream banks and moist meadows has several designations. Nettle pollen is shed in mid- and late summer, with peak levels just preceding the ragweed pollinosis season.

Trees

Single species of anemophilous trees commonly shed pollen, in a given locality, for relatively brief periods. However, the "seasons" of anthesis for several types often evolve concurrently or overlap broadly, imposing intense exposures that involve numerous unrelated pollen allergens. This complexity often makes specific sensitivities difficult to discern and can present a serious barrier to the success of immunotherapy. In temperate regions, wind-pollinated trees are the rule, and source types represent the conifers (Class Gymnospermae) as well as numerous families of more conventional flowering plants (viz., Class Angiospermae). (The "Class" is a taxonomic level which includes one or more Orders (see p. 227), and, in turn, is one component of a "Division." In this case, the Division of flower plants, Spermatophyta, comprises the Classes Gymnospermae and Angiospermae.)

Conifers (Class Gymnospermae). Conifers and their allies dominate the extensive boreal forests of Canada and the contiguous states as well as the southern "pinelands," Appalachian summits, and the slopes of the Cascades and Rockies. Much of the huge pollen output by this group affects remote areas only; however, coniferous trees and shrubs in ornamental plantings are potential exposure sources.

Pollens of the pines *(Pinus)*, spruces *(Picea)*, and firs *(Abies)* as well as the true cedars *(Cedrus)* planted in southern states, the mountain hemlock *(Tsuga mertensiana)* and golden larch *(Pseudolarix amabilis)* of western mountains are large grains bearing two air bladders. The clinical importance of these pollens generally is unproven; overt allergy has been recognized rarely despite their regional abundance. However, instances of pollinosis and of strong positive skin reactivity *do* exist, and these pollens cannot be summarily dismissed as inert.

A second type of conifer grain — spherical, lacking bladders, and showing both a thick intine and a thin exine (which may be shed at anthesis) — is often encountered. Members of the cypress-juniper family (Cupressaceae), the yew family (Taxaceae) and sequoia–bald cypress family (Taxodiaceae) share this form of pollen, and similar grains of larger size are shed by larches *(Larix)* and Douglas fir *(Pseudotsuga taxifolia)*. This group includes acknowledged sensitizers, with the mountain cedars, especially *Juniperus mexicana* (previously designated *Juniperus sabinoides)* serving as major factors in pollinosis. These compact evergreen trees are found from the hills of west Texas and mountains of central Mexico northward at moderate elevations and shed pollen copiously in the period from late December to February. In its range, many regard *J. mexicana* as the most important cause of pollinosis morbidity, while to the north, related *Juniperus* species shed similar pollens in lesser amounts.

There is increasing evidence that pollens of additional junipers (and of related *Cupressus* species) may deserve clinical attention. Skin test surveys have suggested allergenic similarities among species of both genera, including the eastern red cedar *(Juniperus virginiana)*, the incense cedar *(Libocedrus decurrens)* and Port Orford cedar also known as western red cedar *(Chamaecyparis lawsoniana)* of the Pacific Northwest; pollens of cultivated yews *(Taxus media* varieties*)* also may share this activity. Clarification of these relationships holds additional interest due to the widespread use of yews and junipers (especially varieties of *Juniperus sinensis* and *J. horizontalis)* in ornamental plantings about homes and in population centers generally.

Pollen of the bald cypress has not been evaluated as an allergen, and much of it is shed in sparsely settled wetlands. However, a related member of the Taxodiaceae, the "Sugi" cedar *(Cryptomeria japonica)*, is considered an important cause of pollinosis in Japan.

Palm Family (Arecaceae). Members of this large group, which includes a host of economically important species, generally are restricted to frost-free regions. Many species are anemophilous, and pollen shedding by sabal *(Sabal spp.*)*, date *(Phoenix dactylifera)*, coconut *(Cocos nucifera)* and queen *(C. plumosa)* palms can produce moderate atmospheric levels where extensive planting occurs. The date palm has been a suspected minor and highly local source of pollinosis in southern California and Hawaii, but other palms have not been definitely implicated.

Australian Pine or Beefwood Family (Casuarinaceae). Clinical interest in this group of Australasian trees is a result of the widespread introduction of a single species, *Casuarina equisetifolia* in highly populated subtropical areas. The plant is tolerant of dry, sandy soils and highly wind-resistant. In Florida, Hawaii and southern California, it is encountered both as a tall triangular tree or sheared as a hedge or windbreak. A "pinelike" aspect is imparted by reduction of leaves to minute scales which are clustered along innumerable short, slender branchlets. Flowering by this species is uniquely prolonged and sporadic, extending over several months in Florida. The 30- to 35-micron pollen grains have three collared pores and recall those of bayberry and the birch family. Pollen emission may be copious in some areas, and pollinosis seems definitely to result, although its frequency is uncertain.

Willow-Poplar Family (Salicaceae). The numerous North American members of this family represent only two genera: (1) the willows *(Salix spp.)* and (2) poplars and aspens *(Populus spp.)*. Many of the willows rely on insect pollination as well as wind-pollination, and in a given area, sequential shedding by several species creates prolonged "seasons" of quite low intensity. The prevalence (if any) of willow pollinosis is problematical,

---

*Spp. = species.

although skin sensitivity is easily demonstrated.

Separate male and female trees are characteristic of both *Salix* and *Populus* species; however the poplars and aspens are exclusively anemophilous "hay fever plants." In northern states, the quaking *(P. tremuloides)* and big-toothed *(P. grandidentata)* aspens are among the earliest trees to flower; although their pollen output is moderate, most is shed away from population centers. In the eastern states and Great Plains, most poplar pollen probably is derived from eastern cottonwood *(P. deltoides)*. Additional regional sources include the California cottonwood *(P. fremontii)*, the black cottonwood *(P. trichocarpa)* of the Northwest, and the swamp cottonwood of southern river bottoms. Female cottonwoods (and some willows) release wind-borne seeds bearing tufted hairs in early summer. At times, this "cotton" has been indicted falsely as the cause of coexisting hay fever (generally grass pollinosis).

Pollen grains of the willows are relatively small with reticulate surfaces and prominent furrows, while those of the poplars are larger, lack apertures and show a distinctive fragmentation of the thin exine. Despite their family ties, pollen allergens of the willows and poplars also appear to be relatively distinctive.

Walnut-Hickory Family (Juglandaceae). Pollens of the hickories *(Carya spp.)* and walnuts *(Juglans spp.)* are relatively potent sensitizers, and clinical pollinosis may result where they are cultivated extensively or contribute to forest associations. *Carya* species are large trees of eastern and southern states and include the pecans *(C. texana* and *C. illinoensis)*, which are cultivated both for edible nuts and as street trees in warmer regions. Pollen shedding by pecans occurs in March and April, while late spring pollination is typical of the cold-tolerant hickories (e.g., *C. laciniosa, C. ovalis,* and *C. glabra)*. Walnuts, including the black walnut *(J. nigra)*, butternut *(J. cinerea)*, and California walnut *(J. californica)*, also are among the latest flowering spring trees. The 40- to 50-micron, three-pored hickory grains are among the largest wind-borne pollen types; those of walnuts are smaller, flattened spheres with numerous pores restricted to half of each grain's surface.

Birch Family (Betulaceae). In North America, this family includes major pollen producers such as hazelnuts *(Corylus spp.)*, birches *(Betula spp.)* and alders *(Alnus spp.)* as well as the hornbeams or ironwoods *(Carpinus caroliniana)* and *Ostrya virginiana)* with lesser outputs. Hazelnuts and filberts, including cultivated forms, flower from January to April depending on latitude. The alders, including the naturalized European, *(A. glutinosa)*, follow and although widely established in moist locations, are associated with pollinosis mainly in the Pacific Northwest. Several native birches, including the paper birch *(B. papyrifera)* and cherry birch *(B. lenta)* are prominent in eastern states, and paper birch grows widely in western mountains as well. In many areas, varieties of the European white birch *(B. pendula,)* used extensively in ornamental plantings, may serve as factors in pollinosis.

Except for the characteristic four-pored grains of alders, pollens of the Betulaceae typically show three, collared pores. *B. pendula* is considered the principal source of hay fever in Scandinavia, and a heat-stable major allergen (M.W. *ca* 20,000) has been isolated from its pollen. A similar pollen allergen has been reported in emanations of *Alnus glutinosa* and may indicate similarities within the Betulaceae; however intergeneric relationships remain speculative.

Oak Family (Fagaceae). Although this family also includes the beeches *(Fagus spp.)* and remaining chestnuts *(Castanea spp.)*, their pollen output is, at best, modest, leaving the true oaks *(Quercus spp.)* as the proper focus of clinical attention. In many areas, diverse oak species contribute importantly to the airborne pollen load. However, red oak *(Q. rubra)* and eastern white oak *(Q. alba)* are especially prominent in the northeast, while *Q. gambelii* is a scrubby dominant in the southwest and *Q. garryana* is a notable oak pollen source of the Pacific Northwest. Oaks are widely planted, with pin oak *(Q. palustris)* favored in northern states; to the south the evergreen live oak *(Q. virginiana)* and partially evergreen laurel oak *(Q. laurifolia)* are often chosen by urban and residential landscapers. Oaks often have begun to shed pollen in the Gulf States by February and pollination is not complete in some northern areas before early June. Rough-surfaced grains with 3 torn furrows are common to all of the oaks, and attempts to determine their species or groups of origin by light microscopy are not recommended. The degree of cross antigenecity between various oak pollens has not been determined.

Elm Family (Ulmaceae). Although the American elm *(Ulmus americana)* has been decimated by fungus infections, trees surviving in urban "islands" are still a source of pollinosis. In addition, more blight-resistant species — including the slippery elm *(U. fulva)*, the red *(U. serotina)* and scrub *(U. crassifolia)* elms of south central states, as well as the Chinese elm *(U. parvifolia)* — are regionally significant pollen sources. Grains of all elms have a finely undulating surface, (much like a peanut) and five pores in one (equatorial) plane imparting a somewhat pentagonal outline. In northern and eastern states, elms typically reach anthesis in early spring. However, the red (or "September") and scrub (or "cedar") elms flower in late summer, when *some* Chinese elms also shed pollen.

The hackberries *(Celtis spp.)* are a unique group within the Ulmaceae, shedding delicate-appearing, three-pored grains. In North America, *C. occidentalis* is common locally in the east and *C. laevigata* abundant in southern and south-central states, both naturally and in cultivation. Pollen shedding by the latter species occurs in February and March and is an acknowledged cause of pollinosis. Pollen of a related species, *C. tala* has been implicated as a clinical allergen in Argentina.

Ash-Olive Family (Oleaceae). In North America, clinical interest in this large family is focused largely on the ashes *(Fraxinus spp.)*. Among these, the white or American ash *(F. americana)*, Oregon ash *(F. oregona)*, and Arizona ash *(F. velutina)* are regionally important in pollinosis. Additional species and cultivated varieties contribute to local pollen loads, and all typically produce four-furrowed reticulate grains of angular outline.

The olive *(Olea europaea)* is grown in warmer western states and, like the ashes, is widely used in ornamental and sidewalk plantings. Although the olive enjoys substantial insect pollination, wind-borne pollen may be abundant locally; clinical allergy is said to result especially in Arizona and southern California. The olive also is regarded as a major allergenic factor in the Mediterranean basin.

Sycamore or Plane Tree Family (Platanaceae). Although the native sycamore *(Platanus occidentalis)* is locally prominent in eastern river bottom floras, most exposure to sycamore pollen is related to urban plantings of the English plane tree *(P. acerifolia)*. Along with equally smog-resistant ash species, this imported sycamore has been a replacement for the vanishing elms in cities such as Philadelphia, New York, and Washington. In addition, the related *P. orientalis* is a modest pollen source at points of introduction in California. All species shed small reticulate grains with verrucous flecks of exine substance on the three wide furrow membranes. In eastern states, sycamore pollen is airborne in April and May (concurrently with many additional types), making assessment of its clinical impact difficult; skin sensitivity is easily demonstrated, however.

Maple Family (Aceraceae). Maples *(Acer spp.)* are widely prominent in North America and vary from almost exclusive insect pollination, as in the widely planted Norway maple *(Acer platanoides)* to the total wind pollination of box elder *(Acer negundo)*. Between these extremes are familiar species, such as red maple *(A. rubrum)* and sugar maple *(A. saccharum)* of northern and eastern regions and broad-leafed maple *(A. macrophyllum)* of the Pacific coast, with suggested but uncertain clinical significance. In many areas, the flowering of staminate box elders defines the local peak period of maple pollen prevalence. This species is abundant in the Midwest, where it is an aggressive urban weed; in the West, it is often planted for shade or as a windbreak. Pollen grains of maples have three furrows and, at high magnification, display delicate surface striations. Although most are easily identified (to genus), those of box elders are relatively small (ca 25 to 32 microns) and short-furrowed, strongly resembling the pollens of oaks. Box elder anthesis occurs in April and causes substantial pollinosis. Additional species flower sequentially from March to mid-May, producing pollens of uncertain clinical importance. Their allergenic relationships remain to be studied.

Mulberry Family. This family, the Moraceae, includes several genera of variably important anemophilous trees: the mulberries *(Morus spp.)*, the paper mulberry *(Broussonetia papyrifera)* and Osage Orange *(Maclura pomerifera)*. Pollens of the true and paper mulberries are highly sensitizing and copiously produced. Furthermore these two- and three-pored grains are quite small (generally 14 to 20 microns) and have been substantially underestimated in gravity slide samples (see p. 229). *M. rubra* is native to eastern North America, whereas white *(M. alba)* and paper mulberries are naturalized in warmer regions. *Morus alba* currently enjoys special favor as a residential and street tree in the arid Southwest.

Osage Orange is a spiny small tree of the South-central states, attaining special abundance in Oklahoma where it is also cultivated as a hedge. The small, three-pored grains attain moderate levels in air and may be a source of brief symptoms in skin-reactive persons.

Two herbaceous species, hemp *(Cannabis sativa)* and cultivated hops *(Humulus japonica)*, also are generally treated with the Moraceae. The delicate, three-pored pollens of these species are essentially indistinguishable, and both are shed in midsummer. However, hops cultivation is restricted largely to the Pacific Northwest while the natural range of *Cannabis* is Western Iowa and adjacent states. Separate male and female plants are a feature of the latter species, which is now sparsely established in many areas. The celebrated psychotropic components of *Cannabis* are obtained from the female flower clusters and appear to be unassociated with its pollen.

Myrtle Family (Myrtaceae). This largely tropical group includes many insect-pollinated trees which also "spill" pollen into the atmosphere. In California, large plantings of gum trees *(Eucalyptus spp.)* can create notable levels locally; in Florida, widespread planting of bottle-brush *(Melaleuca spp.)* has had a similar result. *Melaleuca,* especially, has received attention as a possible source of pollinosis; however, neither pollen type has been well studied clinically.

POLLEN DISTRIBUTION IN NORTH AMERICA

Table 16–2 summarizes the distribution and seasonal prevalence of wind-borne pollens in portions of North America with distinctive climate and flora. Ten regions, defined for this purpose, are shown in Fig. 16–12. Although sharp boundaries have been drawn, in most cases these "life zones" intermingle over broad transition areas, so that border sites share characteristics of the adjacent ecological areas. Furthermore, individual regions are not uniform in pollen prevalence; however, they provide workable alternatives to more minute, or more inclusive, divisions.

Portions of the Northern Forest region occur in northern New England, Michigan, and Minnesota, as well as at higher elevations in the Appalachians. This zone covers much of eastern and northwestern Canada, as well as the interior of Alaska. However, portions of southern Ontario and Quebec, including their largest cities, are well within the northern reaches of the Eastern Agricultural region. The Eastern Agricultural region was covered originally by deciduous forest but has been cleared and cultivated; its seasonal sequence of tree, grass and finally "weed" (i.e., broad-leafed herbaceous) pollen is typical of temperate regions in general.

A summary of pollen surveys organized by states has been presented by Chang (1972), and an older review (Samter and Durham, 1955), which also treats Mexico and points in the Caribbean may be helpful. The annual Statistical Report of the American Academy of Allergy's Committee on Pollen and Mold may be consulted for additional regionally-based, aeroallergen prevalence data*.

Table 16–2 necessarily is incomplete, since substantial gaps remain in our knowledge of pollen sources and distribution, and many established data must be updated. In most areas, questions of current allergen prevalence can be answered precisely only by a program of local atmospheric sampling. For brevity, many pollens are listed as "types" without indicating their (frequently multiple) source species.

INTERNATIONAL POLLEN EXPOSURE RISKS

Many North Americans experience decreased symptoms of respiratory allergy dur-

---

*Current copies may be obtained from the Executive Office, 411 Wells Street, Milwaukee, Wisconsin 53262.

TABLE 16–2 POLLEN DISTRIBUTION IN THE UNITED STATES

Trees	Grasses	Weeds
Northern Forest		
A brief hectic growing season is typical, with copious shedding of pine, spruce, fir, hemlock, and arbor vitae (*Thuja occidentalis*) pollens from May to early July. In the same period, pollens of alders, birches, hazelnuts, poplars, and aspens may contribute to pollinosis where the forest climax has been disturbed.	Summer levels of grass pollen are relatively low, and often insignificant.	With few late-summer pollen sources, these areas have been traditional refuges for ragweed-sensitive persons.
Eastern Agricultural		
Red cedar — Feb.–April	Sharply defined mid-May to mid-July grass pollen season in north; to the south, a longer season with earlier onset typical.	Sheep (red) sorrel — May–June
Hazelnut — Feb.–April	Importance of various species is difficult to determine; however, acknowledged sources include:	Plantain — May–Oct.
Elm — March–April	Blue grasses (*Poa* ssp.)	Nettles — July–Sept.
Alder — March–May	Orchard grass (*Dactylis glomerata*)	Hemp — July–Sept. (NW)
Maples — March–May	Timothy (*Phleum pratense*)	Western water hemp — July–Sept. (W)
Poplar, aspen — March–May	Red top (*Agrostis alba*)	Russian thistle — July–Sept. (W)
Birch — March–May	In eastern region, increase in:	Kochia — July–Sept.
Ash — March–May	Perennial rye (*Lolium perenne*)	Pigweeds, amaranths — July–Sept.
Paper mulberry — March–May (S)*	Sweet vernal grass (*Anthoxanthum odoratum*)	Sages and mugworts — July–Oct. (L)
Willow — March–July	In southern region, allergenically distinctive Bermuda grass (*Cynodon dactylon*) is dominant.	Short ragweed — Aug.–Oct.
Box elder — April–May (W)		Giant ragweed — Aug.–Oct.
Beech (*Fagus grandifolia*) — April–May (N)		Southern ragweed — Aug.–Oct. (SW)
Sycamore — April–May		Perennial ragweed — Aug.–Oct. (W)
Hackberry — April–May		Burweed marsh elder — Aug.–Oct (S)
Oak — April–June		Rough marsh elder — Aug.–Oct. (S.W)
Mulberry — April–June		
Walnut — April–June		
Hickory — April–June		

Pollens of dogwoods (*Cornus*), sweet gum (*Liquidambar styraciflua*), and black cherry (*Prunus serotina*) prominent locally, but significance uncertain.

Shrubby species including bayberry (*Myrica carolinensis*) and sweet fern (*M. asplenifolia*) are sources in certain sandy eastern areas, but not evaluated clinically.

*Where a pollen type is confined largely to one portion of a region, this is indicated by the following notations: N = north; S = south; E = east; W = west; or L = local.

Table continued on the following page.

TABLE 16-2 POLLEN DISTRIBUTION IN THE UNITED STATES (Continued)

Trees		Grasses	Weeds	

Southeastern Coastal Plain

Trees		Grasses	Weeds	
Pecan, Hickory	March–May (S)	Except for northeastern extremity, zone is dominated by Bermuda grass, which sheds most abundantly from March to September; lesser contributions come from species prominent in the Eastern Agricultural zone.	Sheep (red) sorrel	April–June
Sweet gum	March–May		Plantain	May–Oct.
Maples	March–May		Nettle	July–Sept.
Sycamore	March–June		Sagewort, Mugwort	July–Sept. (L)
Mulberry	March–June		Western water hemp	July–Sept. (W)
Oak	March–May		Russian thistle	July–Sept. (NW)
Walnut	April–May	More typically southern grasses, including Johnson grass (*Holcus halepensis*) and Sudan grass (*Holcus sudanensis*), add small amounts of of wind-borne pollen.	Pigweeds, Amaranths	July–Sept.
Red cedar	Jan.–April		Kochia	July–Oct.
Hackberry	Jan.–May		Short ragweed	Aug.–Oct.
Elm	Feb.–April		Giant ragweed	Aug.–Oct.
Willow	Feb.–May		Southern ragweed	Aug.–Oct. (W)
Poplar	March–April		Rough marsh elder	Aug.–Oct. (W)
Ash	March–May		Burweed marsh elder	Aug.–Oct. (W)
Birch	March–May			

Other, locally abundant tree pollens include those of beech, paper mulberry, the alders, bald cypress (*Taxodium distichum*), the hornbeams (*Carpinus caroliniana* and *Ostrya virginiana*) and, in northern Florida, types characteristic of the Florida Subtropical zone.

Pollen shedding by the pines also is prominent in spring throughout much of region.

Florida Subtropical

Trees		Grasses	Weeds	
Bald cypress	Jan.–March	Grass pollen is airborne throughout the year in subtropical Florida, derived largely from Bermuda grass. Other suspected sources include Johnson grass and Bahia grass (*Paspalum notatum*).	Locally variable levels of short ragweed pollen occur from July–Sept., and Baccharis (*Baccharis spp.*) contribute an apparently related type in coastal areas.	
Oak	Jan.–April			
Palm	Jan.–Dec.			
Melaleuca	April–Jan.		Pollens of chenopods and diverse amaranths are present almost perennially, peaking in late summer.	
Australian pine	Oct.–April			

Additional tree pollens of variable and local occurrence include those of red maple (*Acer rubrum*), citrus (*Citrus sinensis*), pepper tree (*Schinus molle*), and *Eucalyptus* species.

A massive background of pine pollen (especially Jan.–April) cannot be completely ignored.

Central Plains

Mountain cedar	Dec.–March (SW)
Elm	Jan.–April
	Aug.–Sept. (S)
Ash	Jan.–May
Oak	Jan.–May
Poplar	Feb.–April
Box elder	Feb.–April
Willow	Feb.–May
Hackberry	Feb.–May (S)
Sycamore	March–May
Walnut	March–May
Hickory, Pecan	March–May
Mulberry	March–May
Osage orange	April–May (SE)

Although originally this area was the province of long and short grass prairies, contemporary grass pollen levels are no greater than those of other areas.

To the north, the June–July peak and the source species are those of the Eastern Agricultural zone; to the south, a prolonged season is dominated by Bermuda grass.

Additional sources of lesser importance include smooth brome (*Bromus inermis*), fescue (*Festuca elatior*), *Koeleria cristata*, and Johnson grass.

Sheep (red) sorrel	May–July
Atriplex species	June–Aug. (W)
Hemp	July–Sept. (NE)
Russian thistle	July–Sept.
Kochia	July–Sept.
Greasewood	July–Sept. (W)
Smotherweed (*Bassia*)	July–Sept. (NW)
Burweed marsh elder	July–Sept.
Rough marsh elder	July–Oct. (S)
Sagebrush, sages	July–Oct.
Western water hemp	July–Oct.
Short ragweed	Aug.–Oct.
Giant ragweed	Aug.–Oct.
Western ragweed	Aug.–Oct.
Bur ragweeds	Aug.–Oct.

Especially in western extremity of zone, a variety of additional chenopods and amaranths add small quantities of wind-borne pollens.

Rocky Mountain

Mountain cedar, junipers	Jan.–March (SE)
Elm	Feb.–April
Alder	March–April
Ash	March–May
Willow	March–June
Poplar, aspen	April–May
Birch	April–June
Oak	May–June (S)

Although clinical significance unproven, bulk of tree pollen is produced by vast forests of conifers, including pines, spruces, mountain hemlock, Douglas fir, and the sequoias.

Grass pollen levels generally decrease with elevation and are present from May to July.

Major source species are those of adjacent Central Plains region; *Poa sandbergii* also has been implicated.

Pollens of ragweeds and related herbs, chenopods, and amaranths diminish sharply above 5000-foot altitude.

At lower elevations, sources are similar to those of adjacent Central Plains, Great Basin, or Arid Southwestern zones.

Table continued on the following page.

TABLE 16–2 POLLEN DISTRIBUTION IN THE UNITED STATES (Continued)

Trees	Grasses	Weeds
Arid Southwestern		
Mountain cedar — Dec.–March (E)	Grass pollen is airborne in all warm months and is derived predominantly from Bermuda grass; some contributions from other species of southern Central Plains regions.	Burroweed (*Ambrosia dumosa*) — Feb.–June
Elm — Feb.–March		Sagebrush, sages — Feb.–May
— Aug.–Oct.		Rabbit bush — March–May
Arizona cypress — Feb.–March (W)	Salt grass (*Distichlis spicata*) and Canary grass (*Phalaris minor*) may shed sufficiently to warrant some attention.	(*Ambrosia deltoides*)
Ash — Feb.–April		Shadscale — May–Aug.
Poplar — Feb.–April		Greasewood — May–Sept.
Mulberry — Feb.–April		Burweed marsh elder — July–Sept.
Mesquite — Feb.–June		Kochia — July–Oct.
Olive — March–May		Sugar beet — July–Oct. (L)
		Short ragweed — July–Oct.
In irrigated areas, moderate numbers of sycamores, oaks, eucalyptus, pecans, and acacias may be locally important sources.		Slender ragweed — July–Oct.
Additional shrubby types include:		
Creosote bush		Several additional ragweeds as well as representatives of composite genera including *Dicorea, Hymenoclea,* and *Chrysothamnus* shed "ragweed-like" pollen in spring and fall. Pollens of chenopods and amaranths are airborne in most months; derived from drought- and alkali-resistant types (many known locally as "scales" and "creosote bushes"), including species of *Atriplex* (especially *A. canescens* and *A. polycarpa, Eurotia, Suaeda,* and *Amaranthus,* as well as iodine bush (*Allenrolfia occidentalis*).
Palo verde (*Cercidium spp.*)		
Castor bean (*Ricinus communis*)		
Tamarisk (*Tamarix spp.*)		
Great Basin		
Juniper — Feb.–May	Although the overall levels of grass pollen appear relatively low, its sources are varied. To the north, the grasses are largely those of the Central Plains; in the southern section, species of the Arid Southwestern zone predominate.	Sagebrush, sages — June–Nov.
Elm — March–April		Russian thistle — July–Sept.
Poplar — March–April		Kochia — July–Oct.
Willow — March–May		Greasewood — July–Oct.
Sycamore — April–May		Short ragweed — Aug.–Oct.
Box elder — April–May		Bur ragweeds — Aug.–Oct.
		Poverty weed — Aug.–Nov.
		(*Iva axillaris*)

At modest elevations, birches, alders, aspens, and oaks contribute additional tree pollens.

Many anemophilous chenopods and amaranths, native to the Arid Southwestern region, are also prominent in Great Basin, although source strengths are conjectural.

California Lowlands

Mulberry	Jan.–April
Alder	Jan.–April
Ash	Jan.–April
Willow	Jan.–April
Walnut	Jan.–May
Poplar	Feb.–April
Elm	Feb.–April
Oak	Aug.–Oct.
Sycamore	Feb.–May
Birch	Feb.–April
Olive	March–May (S)

Many additional tree species contribute limited quantities of wind-borne pollen, including acacias, coast maple (*Acer macrophyllum*), box elder (*Acer negundo*), *Eucalyptus* species, and pecan.

In much of region, airborne grass pollen, largely from Bermuda grass, is present from early March to November; in extreme north of zone, season is shorter, beginning in April or May.

Many other species are implicated including rye grasses (*Lolium ssp.*), the brome grasses (*Bromus ssp.*), wild oats (*Avena fatua*), and types present in zones to the east.

Nettle	May–Aug. (N.W)
Bur ragweeds	June–Sept. (S.W)
Western ragweed	July–Oct.
Sagebrush, sages	July–Oct.

Wind-borne pollens of chenopods and amaranths are moderately abundant in summer and fall; major sources include Russian thistle, *Atriplex* species, *Bassia hyssopifolia*; also *Amaranthus retroflexus* and *A. palmeri*.

Northwest Coastal

Hazelnut	Jan.–March
Alders	Feb.–April
Willow	Feb.–April
Ash	Feb.–April
Box elder	March–April
Birch	March–May
Poplar, Aspen	March–June
Elm	March–June
Coast maple	April–June
Oak	April–June
Walnut	April–June (L)

Tree pollen levels vary widely according to local topography and, especially, altitude. In forested portions, conifer pollens of several types are abundant.

Ample grass pollens are present from May to August. Major source species appear to be similar to Eastern Agricultural zone; also being investigated are sweet vernal grass (*Anthoxanthum odoratum*) and velvet grass (*Holcus lanatus*).

Species including the rye grasses and tall oatgrass (*Arrhenatherum elatius*) may shed clinically significant pollen.

Plantain	May–Sept.
Sheep (red) sorrel	June–Aug.
Poverty weed	June–Aug. (L)
Nettle	July–Aug.
Russian thistle	July–Sept.
Sagebrush, sages	July–Sept. (L)
Short ragweed	Aug.–Sept. (L)

Although all these contribute allergenic pollen, resulting concentrations are relatively low; much of region remains essentially ragweed-free.

Levels of plantain and sorrel pollens may be higher than in northeastern states, but conclusive comparative data have not been gathered.

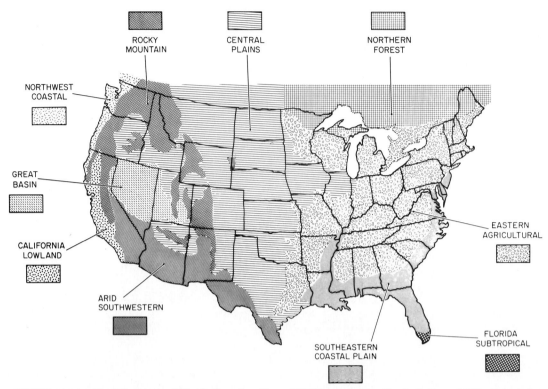

FIGURE 16–12. Floristic zones of North America. (From Middleton, E., Jr., Reed, C. E. and Ellis, E. F. (eds.): *Allergy — Principles and Practice*, Vol. 2. St. Louis, C. V. Mosby Co., 1978.)

ing travel abroad. This improvement commonly reflects the absence of ragweed pollen and lower levels of dark-spored imperfect fungi in most other regions; for certain individuals, differences in dust and dander exposures also may contribute. However, available aerometric data from many areas are too scanty to permit patterns of pollen exposure to be sketched in any detail on a global basis.

Grasses are the most generally distributed sources of pollinosis, although groups of temperate and tropical species appear to differ allergenically. However, cosmopolitan types such as Bermuda grass are encountered widely in both hemispheres, and many taxa (e.g., *Phleum pratense* and *Dactylis glomerata*) are common to Europe and much of eastern North America, with significant pollinosis resulting in both areas.

Significant tree pollinosis may be reawakened in some travelers to Scandinavia by the abundant birch pollen present in spring, or, further south, where native ashes, oaks, mulberries, walnuts and elms occur, as well.

Insect pollination is present almost exclusively among tropical trees, although some, (e.g., certain palms and mesquite) can produce endemic pollinosis. Whether recognized similarities between the temperate floras of eastern Asia and eastern North America also are relevant clinically is uncertain. However, local representatives of genera such as *Fraxinus* are recognized sources of tree pollinosis in Mexico and South America.

Ragweed pollinosis is a familiar clinical problem as far south as central Mexico. However, ragweeds of several species also are variably distributed throughout lowland areas of Central and South America as well as many Caribbean islands, where their clinical impact seems small. In addition, short ragweed *(A. artemisiifolia)* has become established at several Old World sites (Charpin, Surinyach and Frankland, 1975). The most notable of these stations is in the upper Rhône valley of France near the city of Lyon, where typical, late summer pollinosis has been recognized for over a decade. Significant ragweed growth and clinical pollinosis have been evident also in the Krasnodar region of the USSR and recently, at points in several Balkan nations. With these (limited) exceptions, the risk of ragweed pollen exposure at locations away from North America remains negligible.

Even ragweed-free regions often harbor certain herbaceous sources that shed clinically relevant, wind-borne pollens. *Rumex* species (including *R. acetosella)* are widespread in Eurasia and elsewhere, while *Urtica* species shed abundantly in Great Britain and continental Europe. Pellitory *(Parietaria officinalis)*, of the Mediterranean basin, is an allergen source closely allied to the nettles, although possibly differing from them in its pollen allergens. Many chenopods, such as Russian thistle, are widely distributed in warmer portions of the Eastern Hemisphere, and the numerous tropical amaranths have not been evaluated as potential pollen sources. In addition, certain non-ambrosioid composites (e.g., *Parthenium* species) shed moderately in warmer regions and may pose minor problems for travelers with ragweed pollinosis.

REDUCING POLLEN EXPOSURE

Outdoors. Major allergenic pollens (and spores) are so well mixed throughout the lower atmosphere that avoidance measures can only hope to curtail *excessive* exposure. However, this goal seems justifiable and may be reached by attention to "common sense" considerations. Sensitive subjects should recall that just after a prolonged rain, relatively low pollen levels prevail, while extended fair weather promotes dispersion. Exposure hazards associated with auto travel have not been examined minutely, although extended trips *with open windows* seem to augment symptoms and should be limited.

The tendency of ragweeds to colonize cultivated fields and flood plains defines a significant, avoidable hazard, especially during morning hours of peak pollen emission. Repeatedly disturbed vacant lots, unpaved parking areas and construction sites pose similar problems for urban children. Grass-sensitive subjects are well-advised to avoid hiking through old fields during symptomatic periods and to recall that pollens of corn and various grains can provoke "grass pollinosis" on intimate exposure.

Although ambitious programs of urban ragweed eradication have not proven successful (Walzer and Siegel, 1956), ragweeds and other sources around the homes of sensitive persons, should be manually removed or treated annually with herbicides.

Multiple intense tree pollen sensitivities might appropriately lead the prospective home owner to choose a deforested lot over a thickly wooded one. Pollen production by single trees often is great enough to influence symptoms when arboreal sources are close by, and plantings about homes should be chosen accordingly. Many splendid shade trees (e.g., locusts, lindens, mountain ashes, ginkgo, Norway maple) are insect-pollinated or shed minimally, making them especially useful for multiple sensitive subjects. In addition, trees such as mulberries, ashes, and poplars have separately-sexed individuals, making selection of (female) seed-bearers practical.

Indoors. Enclosed spaces offer refuges from aeroallergens, and still, sealed rooms were preferred decades ago in treating pollinosis. However, such therapeutic incarceration is accepted poorly in general, and the value of any indoor avoidance options is limited.

Indoor pollen levels may be reduced effectively by closing windows. Merely forcing particles to turn a corner will prevent many of them from entering a structure. In warm areas, artificial air cooling is the price of closed windows; central air conditioning will substantially reduce indoor particle levels. Particle exclusion by window units is variable, although patients often report benefit from their use. In general, a sealed bedroom, fitted with an air conditioner which is operated only at night, should give optimal protection when a central system is infeasible.

Devices that provide a laminar output of essentially particle-free air can be directed at the head of a sleeping individual creating an allergenically clean microenvironment. Similar (HEPA) filters with high capacity air movers also have been adapted for central installation recently. However, older fibre filters mounted in window openings have been poorly accepted by patients.

Centrally installed electrostatic precipitators are often viewed as a panacea by patients or by their well-motivated parents. In fact, air entering these devices is effectively cleaned of pollen and even smaller particles, although overloading (e.g., due to smoke of one cigar) readily occurs. However, particles derived from factors, including open windows, at *room level* obviously can elicit symptoms uninfluenced by electrostatic cleaners, and measures to nullify pollen, dust, and dander sources should not be relaxed. Also, precipitators lose efficiency as particles accumulate on the collection plates, which must be removed and washed periodically — a requirement that is often overlooked. At best, however, these devices merely complement other effective particle avoidance procedures, adding relatively little to the protection from pollen afforded by central air conditioning. Considering their modest benefits as compared to their high cost and tendency to produce ozone, precipitators probably should be recommended only for carefully chosen clinical problems. A host of free-standing precipitators, air filters, and ion generators also have been marketed as aids for allergic subjects. In general, except (as noted above) for some laminar flow devices, these units have seemed ineffectual, and many impose significant shock or ozone hazards.

The Pollen Refuge Option. To escape one's allergies through a bold geographic move is a popular fantasy among affected persons and their families. Such translocations can be effective, if the offenders are regionally limited and newly encountered allergens are unimportant. Escape often is difficult, however, because of multiple pollen and spore sensitivities, the importance of allergens (e.g., danders, house dust) that travel with the patient or vasomotor, infective, and psychological factors that may actually worsen following relocation. In addition, the so-cial disruption, loss of job seniority, and financial hardships involved emphasize the need for *caution in advising or condoning a major family move*. Where this option is contemplated seriously, trial periods of at least four weeks in the new area (preferably, in more than one season) should be employed before a final decision is implemented. The physician's responsibility to provide regular medication, environmental instruction, and professional liaison for these periods of adjustment is obvious.

Despite the foregoing caveats, temporary travel may be used effectively for pollen avoidance. Ragweed-sensitive subjects have long used trips abroad, ocean cruises, or sojourns on the West Coast or in northern Canada to secure late summer relief. Early in this century, extensive gravity slide data were collected to map North American ragweed "refuges" close to mid-continent population centers, and the resulting patterns are still cited. Unfortunately, changing land use practices have made many of these data obsolete, and their comparative validity was always questionable (see p. 230). Physicians and their patients should be wary, therefore, of communities claiming to be "pollen-free," although many portions of northern New England, and Michigan as well as the southern tip of Florida afford relative relief for the harassed easterner. Highly ragweed-sensitive young persons contemplating several comparable job offers are justified in giving precedence to coastal Pacific Northwest and West Coast opportunities, secondarily considering those in the Southwest and judging Midwestern and East Coast options least desirable. However, the wide distribution of grass and deciduous tree pollens in North America leaves little hope for avoiding these factors in settled areas.

References

Arx, J. A. von: *The Genera of Fungi Sporulating in Pure Culture*. Lehre, J. Cramer., 1970.

Barnett, H. L., and Hunter, B. B.: *Illustrated Genera of Imperfect Fungi*, 3rd ed. Burgess Publ. Co., Minneapolis, 1972.

Barron, G. L.: *The Genera of Hyphomycetes from Soil*. Baltimore, Williams & Wilkins Co., 1968.

Bianchi, D. E., Schwemmin, D. J., and Wagner, W. H., Jr.: Pollen release in common ragweed *(Ambrosia artemisiifolia)*. Bot. Gazette 4:253, 1959.

Bruce, R. A.: Bronchial and skin sensitivity in asthma. Int. Arch. Allergy Appl. Immunol. 22:294, 1963.

Chang, W. W. Y.: Pollen survey. *In* Patterson, R. (ed.): *Allergic Diseases — Diagnosis and Management*. Philadelphia, J. B. Lippincott Co., 1972.

Charpin, J., Surinyach, R., and Frankland, A. W.: *Atlas of European Allergenic Pollens*. Sandoz Editions, 1975.

Connell, J. T.: Quantitative intranasal pollen challenges. III. The priming effect in allergic rhinitis. J. Allergy 43:33, 1969.

Dennis, R. W. G.: *British Cup Fungi and Their Allies*. Dorking, Bartholomew Press, 1960.

Durham, O. C.: The volumetric incidence of airborne allergens. IV. A proposed standard method of gravity sampling, counting and volumetric interpolation of results, J. Allergy *17*:79, 1946.

Ellis, M. B.: *Dematiaceous Hyphomycetes*. Kew, Surrey, Commonwealth Mycol. Instit., 1971.

Gregory, P. H.: *Microbiology of the Atmosphere,* 2nd ed. New York, John Wiley & Sons., 1973.

Hyde, H. A., and Adams, K. F.: *An Atlas of Airborne Pollen Grains*. New York, St. Martin's Press, 1958.

Kapp, R. O.: *How to Know Pollen and Spores*. Dubuque, Iowa, Wm. C. Brown Co., 1969.

Ogden, E. C., Raynor, G. S., Hayes, J. V., Lewis, D. M., and Haines, J. H.: *Manual for Sampling Airborne Pollen*. New York, Hafner Press, 1974.

Samter, M., and Durham, O. C.: *Regional Allergy of the United States, Canada, Mexico and Cuba*. Springfield, Illinois, Charles C Thomas, 1955.

Smith, G.: An *Introduction to Industrial Mycology,* 5th ed. London, Edward Arnold (Pub.) Ltd., 1960.

Solomon, W. R.: Fungus aerosols arising from cold-mist vaporizers. J. Allergy Clin. Immunol. *54*:222, 1974.

Solomon, W. R.: Assessing fungus prevalence in domestic interiors. J. Allergy Clin. Immunol. *56*:235, 1975.

Solomon, W. R.: Volumetric study of winter fungus prevalence in the air of midwestern homes. J. Allergy Clin. Immunol. *57*:46, 1976.

Solomon, W. R., and Mathews, K. P.: Aerobiology and inhalant allergens. *In* Middleton, E., Jr., Reed, C. E., and Ellis, E. F. (eds): *Allergy: Principles and Practice*. St. Louis, C. V. Mosby Co., 1978.

Walzer, M., and Siegel, B. B.: The effectiveness of the ragweed eradication campaigns in New York City. A 9-year study (1946–1954). J. Allergy *27*:113, 1956.

Weber, R. W. Mansfield, L. E., and Nelson, H. S.: Cross-reactivity among weeds of the Amaranth and Chenopod families. J. Allergy Clin. Immunol. *61*:172, 1978.

Yunginger, J. W., and Gleich, G. J.: Measurement of ragweed antigen E by double antibody radioimmunoassay. J. Allergy Clin. Immunol. *50*:326, 1972.

17

Kenneth P. Mathews, M.D.

Other Common Inhalant Allergens

The number of inhalants that act as allergens is large, and their relative importance differs from time to time and place to place. This chapter focuses on those inhalants considered to be of prime importance, especially in the United States and Canada.

HOUSE DUST

Various types of dust frequently precipitate or aggravate respiratory symptoms. Inorganic dusts, such as road dust, often irritate the mucous membranes. Organic dusts may act as irritants or may evoke immunologically mediated responses. Hypersensitivity pneumonitis from organic dusts is considered in Chapter 47. The discussion here is limited to IgE-mediated reactions from dust of household origin.

"House dust" seems so heterogeneous that one may wonder how it could be a distinct allergen. In some instances, in fact, its allergenic properties may be due to its content of animal danders, fungi, or insect debris (see below). House dust also usually contains bacteria, human epidermis, fibrous materials of plant and animal origin, food remnants, and inorganic substances. Yet by the early 1920's house dust allergy was considered a distinct entity caused by a unique (but undefined) allergen(s). The striking immediate skin test reactions to crude extracts in some allergic patients supported

this concept. Some individuals reacted to no other known allergens, while in others with multiple sensitivities, there was no relationship between the skin test reactions to house dust and to the other allergens. Furthermore, patients in one locale react to extracts of house dust collected in many different parts of the world.

Although house dust extracts induce positive immediate skin test reactions in many patients with atopic disorders, this in itself does not prove clinical sensitivity. Up to 50 percent of nonallergic subjects also react positively to intracutaneous injections of house dust, depending upon the concentration of extract used for testing (Lindblad and Farr, 1961). However, prick testing or intracutaneous tests with relatively weak dilutions of house dust extract discriminate better between controls and atopic patients. Furthermore, inhalation of house dust extracts induces bronchospasm in asthmatic patients and nasal reactions in allergic rhinitis patients who are clinically allergic to house dust. In addition, there is a diurnal variation in bronchial responses to house dust, with peak reactivity at 11 p.m. (Gervais et al., 1977). Of considerable interest is the observation of Booij-Nord et al. (1972) that 26 of 55 asthmatic subjects had a late secondary phase of bronchoconstriction, as well as an immediate response, to inhalation of house dust extract. In sensitive subjects house dust allergen induces positive

248

conjunctival tests, leukocyte histamine release (May et al., 1970; Bullock and Frick, 1972; Kawai et al., 1972), skin window eosinophilia (Bullock and Frick, 1972), and positive RAST (Holford-Strevens et al., 1970). Precipitins and lymphocyte transformation with house dust extracts have been observed both in some patients and in normal controls (Romagnani et al., 1973). Worldwide observations leave little doubt that allergy to some substance or substances in house dust is common, particularly in subjects with perennial respiratory allergy. For example, more than 80 percent of 133 asthmatic children in Britain gave positive prick test reactions to house dust extracts (Sarsfield, 1974), and half the pollenosis patients in Holland also reacted to house dust (Voorhorst, 1972). Such observations underscore the enormous importance of identifying the allergen(s) in house dust.

Mites in House Dust

More than 50 years ago mites in infested grains were identified as a cause of asthma. In 1928 Dekker reported that mites in bedding were a major cause of asthma in Germany. In the early 1960's Voorhorst, Spieksma and their associates in Leiden undertook a comprehensive study of house dust mites (Voorhorst et al., 1967; Voorhorst, Spieksma and Varekamp, 1969; Voorhorst, 1972). They as well as Japanese investigators developed semiquantitative techniques for recovering mites from house dust specimens. Since there are more than 50,000 species of mites, the mites in house dust had to be identified and cultured in order to carry out clinical studies.

In Holland, mites were found invariably in house dust specimens; the dominant one was *Dermatophagoides pteronyssinus* (Fig. 17–1). Similar observations soon were reported from Japan, the United Kingdom, Scandinavia, India, South Africa, and many other places. In the United States, however, mites were not identified as frequently, and *D. farinae* (*D. culinae*) proved to be the dominant species of Dermatophagoides (van Bronswijk and Sinha, 1971). A closely related mite, *Euroglyphus maynei*, also has been associated with house dust allergy.

There was a strong correlation between the number of Dermatophagoides in different house dust specimens and the skin test activity of their extracts in house dust–sensitive subjects. Furthermore, inoculating and incubating sterilized dust samples with living *D. pteronyssinus* produced a marked increase in their skin test reactivity which paralleled the number of mites in the preparation (Voorhorst et al., 1967).

Further studies of the house dust mites indicated that warmth and humidity predispose to mite growth. Also, there may be a seasonal variation in prevalence of mites in homes in certain locations. In Leiden the peak counts of *D. pteronyssinus* occurred from August to October — a time at which the largest number of house dust–sensitive patients first presented themselves for treatment. Similar studies in Britain, however, failed to show such pronounced seasonal fluctuations.

The mite content of house dust specimens varies greatly depending on source of material. They predominate in damp houses and mattresses, perhaps in part because human epidermal scales are a preferred substrate for Dermatophagoides. They are rare in hospital dust, baby carriages (Sarsfield, 1974), or on the surfaces of mattresses encased in plastic covers, but uncovered foam rubber mattresses may harbor mites. Sarsfield (1974) has noted that children tend to develop positive skin test reactions to house dust soon after they are transferred to ordinary beds. Lamb skins used in infants' cribs in some parts of the world appear to contain fewer mites than mattresses, and this exposure can be further decreased by periodic vacuuming (Ingham and Ingham, 1976). Programs to reduce the exposure of sensitive persons to house dust are described in Chapter 22; it has been shown that such measures can decrease the mite content of bedroom dust (Sarsfield, 1974).

Much of the evidence relating Dermatophagoides mites to house dust allergy is based on observations that skin test reactivity of house dust and of *D. pteronyssinus* extracts were highly correlated (Voorhorst, Spieksma and Varekamp, 1969). Moreover, Dermatophagoides extracts often produced equivalent skin test reactions at concentrations 10 to 1000 times less than house dust extracts. Extracts of *D. farinae* induced skin test reactions that correlated well with those of both house dust and *D. pteronyssinus*. Employing Prausnitz-Küstner tests, Miyamoto et al. (1968) showed that house dust and *D. farinae* extracts produced almost complete cross-neutralization of each other *in vivo* and *in vitro*.

Mite extracts also have been studied by several other techniques. *Bronchial inhalation challenge tests* with *D. pteronyssinus* or *D. farinae* extracts induced bronchospasm in the large majority of house dust–sensitive asthmatics in much lower concentration than house dust extracts (McAllen, Assem and Mannsell, 1970). *Nasal chal-*

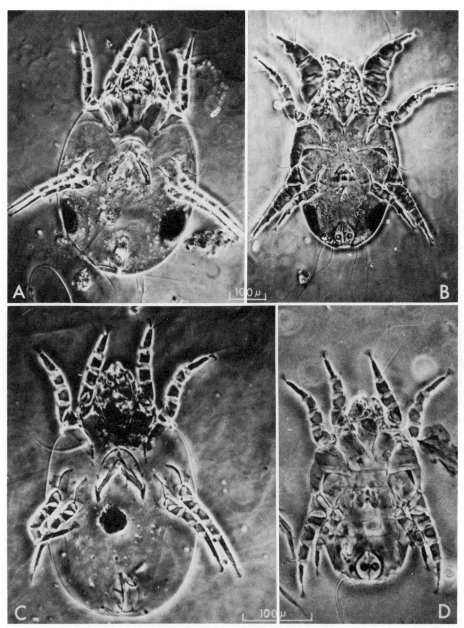

FIGURE 17–1.   *Dermatophagoides farinae,* (A) female, (B) male. *D. pteronyssinus,* (C) female, (D) male. (From van Bronswijk, J. E. M. H., and Sinha, R. N.: Pyroglyphid mites (Acari) and house dust allergy. A review. J. Allergy 47:31, 1971.)

lenge tests with mite extracts induce nasal symptoms in house dust–sensitive subjects. Conjunctival reactions also can be elicited.

Several laboratories have obtained positive RAST with *D. pteronyssinus* and *D. farinae* antigens and sera of house dust–sensitive patients (Holford-Strevens et al., 1970; McAllen, Assem and Mannsell, 1970; Morita et al., 1976). RAST titers with house dust and mite extracts correlated significantly, and each allergen was active in inhibiting the other in RAST inhibition tests. Human lung fragments, passively sensitized with such sera, released histamine *in vitro* with mite extracts (McAllen, Assem and Mannsell, 1970). Extracts of *D. pteronyssinus* or *D. farinae* also induced leukocyte histamine release *in vitro* from the cells of most house dust–sensitive donors both in the United States and Britain (McAllen, Assem and Mannsell, 1970; Bullock and Frick, 1972; Kawai et al., 1972). However, on a weight basis, substantially more dialyzed mite extract than dialyzed house dust extract was required to produce 50 percent histamine release from the leukocytes of dust-sensitive donors living in the Baltimore area. In addition, Kawai et al. found no significant relationship between the amount of mite extract and the amount of house dust extract required to produce 50 percent histamine release among different subjects.

Bullock and Frick (1972) found that *D. pteronyssinus* extract produced a significant accumulation of eosinophils at skin windows in 23 of 24 house dust–sensitive subjects. Some investigators have identified *precipitins* to mite extracts, but they did not correlate well with the patient's disease (Holford-Strevens et al., 1970). Late skin test reactions generally are absent. *D. pteronyssinus* extracts may induce lymphocyte transformation in both atopic and normal subjects (Romagnani et al., 1973). By employing *fractionation* procedures, some investigators have found the capacity to elicit skin test reactions in sensitive persons to reside in similar fractions of both house dust and mite extracts having molecular weights in the range of 10,000–69,000 daltons (Miyamoto, Oshima and Ishizaki, 1969). Others, however, have found the allergens of house dust and *D. farinae* extracts to be dispersed among several fractions.

In summary, much biologic data suggest that Dermatophagoides mites are a major source of house dust allergen in many areas of the world, but they are not the entire source, particularly in geographic areas with low relative humidity. Immunochemical data (discussed in the following section) also would indicate other sources of the house allergen(s) (Berrens, 1970).

Other Possible House Dust Allergens

As mentioned above, the most potent sources of house dust allergen, such as mattress dust, often contain substantial amounts of *human epidermis*. In addition to being a substrate for mite proliferation, it has been claimed that human epidermis itself is an important allergen for man (Voorhorst, 1977). Human epidermal extracts may also produce skin test reactions in subjects allergic to house dust. On the other hand, the *in vitro* release of histamine from leukocytes from house dust–allergic patients by house dust is not inhibited by anti-human epidermal rabbit serum (Kawai et al., 1972). The question whether human epidermis is a significant allergen is unresolved at present.

Degeneration products of vegetable materials, particularly *cotton linters,* have also been thought to be house dust allergens. Cohen, Nelson and Reinarz (1935) stored fresh cotton linters under various conditions for a period of about 8 months. There was a marked increase in capacity of extracts made from these linters to elicit skin test reactions in house dust–sensitive patients. Although at the time the increased allergenicity was attributed to breakdown products from cotton linters, in retrospect it could also have been due to mite growth under some of the conditions of storage employed in this work. A more recent study by Berrens et al. (1975) suggested the possibility that mites and microorganisms may act upon suitable substrates in such a way as to generate the house dust allergen(s). Endotoxins, blood group active substances, and human serum proteins can be detected in house dust but seem unrelated to the house dust allergen(s) (Berrens, 1970). Berrens also observed that fractions that are active in eliciting skin test reactions contain carbohydrates of plant origin.

His biochemical data showing diffuse activity among various glycoproteins oppose the concept that there is a single molecular species that is the unique house dust allergen.

EPIDERMAL ALLERGENS

Type I hypersensitivity to animal danders, such as epidermal scales of cats, dogs and horses, is common and well known. Frequently the allergy becomes obvious to the patient or parent (though some resist recognizing the possibility of an adverse effect from a favorite pet). Children with severe animal allergy, particularly to cats, may experience symptoms in the many households owning pets, even without direct animal contact. Contamination of the home is due not only to epidermal scales but also to saliva in which allergens are present as well (Spain, Gillson and Strauss, 1942). The hair of cats and dogs is a poor source of allergen, whereas allergen extracts from animal pelts or full-thickness skin are highly active.

Cat. In various studies 9 to 36 percent of allergic patients have shown positive immediate skin test reactions to cat epidermis (Fontana, Wittig and Holt, 1963; Ohman, Kendall and Lowell, 1977). However, not all skin test positive subjects have known clinical intolerance to cats, and many with asthma fail to respond to bronchial provocation tests with cat extracts (Aas, 1970). RAST also has been used to assess the presence of IgE antibodies to cat allergen, but again correlations with clinical evaluation are imperfect (Ohman, Kendall and Lowell, 1977). Recent immunochemical studies indicate that the major allergen in cat pelts, cat allergen 1, differs from cat serum proteins, but cat albumin also may serve as a minor allergen (Ohman, Lowell and Bloch, 1974). Variation in allergens among different types of cats has not been thoroughly studied, but some observations suggest that Siamese cats may differ from other types.

Dog. Five to 30 percent of allergic patients give skin test reactions to dog extracts, but, as with cat allergens, some skin test positive individuals deny clinical symptomatology due to dog contact and do not react to provocative tests. As before, however, historical information about lack of symptoms on exposure to domestic animals can be inaccurate when patients rarely are separated from them or are emotionally attached to these pets. Thus a trial period of removal of the pet from the household (followed by thorough cleaning) may be necessary before clinical sensitivity can be properly assessed. Variation in allergic reactivity to different breeds of dogs was shown many years ago by skin tests and passive transfer neutralization test data (Hooker, 1944). More recently these observations have been confirmed using the RAST and RAST inhibition techniques with epidermal extracts from various breeds of dogs (Fagerberg and Wide, 1970). Such data imply the desirability of using mixed extracts from several breeds of dogs for ordinary diagnostic testing purposes. Considering that the epidermal scales are of major allergenic importance, it is not surprising that both long-haired and short-haired breeds of dog can cause allergy.

Horse. Allergy to horses is less of a problem now than it was in the early years of this century not only because there are fewer of these animals in our cities but also because of the less extensive use of horse hair–containing items such as furniture, mattresses, mattings, padding, and felts. Nevertheless, significant exposures continue in rural areas, in persons who ride as a hobby, and with exposure to horse manure. Approximately 10 to 20 percent of allergic patients react to horse allergens on intracutaneous testing, although significant clinical sensitivity appears to be less frequent. In some studies RAST with horse dandruff has correlated well with results of prick tests in children (Leegaard and Roth, 1977). Horse–sensitive patients are said also to react frequently to mule, donkey, and zebra extracts. Of particular practical importance is the relationship between allergy to horse dander and allergy to horse serum. Confirming several earlier immunochemical studies of this problem, RAST data employing fractions of horse dandruff separated by isoelectric focusing, polyacrylamide gel electrophoresis and/or filtration through Sephadex have shown the presence of both horse serum albumin and unique allergens in horse dandruff (Ponterius et al., 1973).

Sera from different patients may contain IgE antibodies to dandruff proteins, serum proteins or both. This is in accord with earlier clinical observations that patients sensitive to horse dander may or may not develop allergic reactions when given equine antisera.

Other Mammalian Allergens. Epidermal antigens from virtually any mammal, including exotic species, may produce allergic symptoms. *Household pets* are an obvious source of sensitization, with hamsters and gerbils to be added to the list of more traditional dander sources in the home. Cow epidermal allergens also may be present in matting under rugs and carpets, though these have been largely supplanted by synthetic materials in newer homes. The *school* environment also may provide animal exposures, as it is not uncommon for rabbits, mice, guinea pigs, or hamsters to be kept in classrooms. Occupational exposures also may induce symptoms. Farm children may become sensitized to common domestic animals such as cattle, hogs, horses, sheep and goats. Laboratory exposures result in sensitivity to rabbits, rats, mice, guinea pigs, dogs, monkeys, or cats. Many garments are derived from animal epidermal sources, including various furs, cashmere, mohair, alpaca, vicuna, and camel's hair, but these processed materials are probably an infrequent cause of Type I hypersensitivity reactions.

Sheep's *wool* merits special comment since patients not infrequently report that the fuzz from wool aggravates their allergic respiratory symptoms or contact with wool flares their eczema. However, reactivity to wool may be due to irritation rather than to true allergy, because of the physical properties of wool. Indeed, in recent years there have been no serious attempts to demonstrate the existence of specific allergen(s) in processed wool. Many sources of used wool are likely to be contaminated with human dander and/or house dust allergen, and it has been observed that rabbit antisera to a purified house dust allergen may cross-react with wool extract.

Feathers. Many allergic patients, particularly those afflicted with perennial allergic rhinitis or perennial asthma, exhibit positive skin test reactions to feather extract. Previously, much emphasis was placed on feathers as an etiologic agent in these conditions. However, extracts of freshly plucked feathers often are inactive in patients who react strongly to extracts of aged feathers, suggesting the presence of house dust allergens in the latter. Indeed, based on skin testing with serial dilutions of house dust and feather extracts, Voorhorst, Spieksma and Varekamp (1969) found their activities to be indistinguishable. The presence of mites in both substances could explain such results. On the other hand, Berrens (1968) has reported that the active material in feather extracts differs chemically from purified house dust allergens.

Regardless of the nature of the active material, aged chicken, goose and duck feathers do in fact precipitate symptoms in some atopic individuals. The usual sources of exposure are pillows, comforters, quilts, jackets, sleeping bags, and beds. Rarely, feathers of canaries, parakeets, parrots, pigeons, turkeys, and sparrows have been reported to produce Type I hypersensitivity reactions (also see Chapter 47, regarding avian hypersensitivity pneumonitis). Since the feather allergen generally is a degradation product, most "feather"–sensitive patients can eat meat of the same fowl with impunity. For the same reason "feather"–sensitive patients do not experience allergic reactions from egg-containing vaccines unless they have a concomitant allergy to egg proteins. It is unfortunate that package directions with egg-containing vaccines often call for inquiry about "feather" allergy, as this creates unnecessary confusion and apprehension in the large group of allergic individuals who know they have positive skin test reactions to "feathers" but are not sensitive to egg proteins.

INSECT-DERIVED INHALANT ALLERGENS

In comparison with pollen and fungus allergy, the number of cases of well-documented inhalant respiratory allergy due to insect-derived material is relatively small, though these may well expand as further knowledge is accrued. The subject is complicated by the vast numbers of in-

TABLE 17–1 ARTHROPODS IMPLICATED AS POSSIBLE INHALANT ALLERGENS

Class	Order	Member
Arachnida		Spiders
		Mites, ticks
Crustacea		Sowbugs
		Daphnia (water flea)
		Shrimp (plankton)
Insecta	Orthoptera	Locusts
		Grasshoppers
		Cockroaches
		Crickets
	Isoptera	Termites
	Dermaptera	Earwings
	Ephemeroptera	May flies
	Hemiptera	Bedbugs
	Homoptera	Aphids
	Coleoptera	Beetles
		Bean weevil
	Neuroptera	Lancewing flies
	Trichoptera	Caddis flies
	Lepidoptera	Moths, butterflies
	Diptera	Houseflies
		Mushroom flies
		Sewer flies
		Midges
		Deer flies
		Black flies
	Siphonaptera	Rat fleas
	Hymenoptera	Honey bees

(Modified from Perlman, F.: Insects as inhalant allergens. J. Allergy 29:302, 1958.)

sect species. Table 17–1, modified from Perlman (1958), indicates types of arthropods that have been implicated as possible causes of Type I hypersensitivity.

Arthropods as Local or Indoor Allergen Sources. Some of the most convincing cases of inhalant insect allergy have involved occupational exposures; for example, entomologists and laboratory workers have become sensitized to beetles, cockroaches, grasshoppers, locusts, and moths, the latter also causing asthma in a patient who worked in a moth domicile raising moth larvae for fish bait (Stevenson and Mathews, 1967). Agricultural workers have experienced allergic respiratory symptoms from locally abundant concentrations of Mexican bean weevils, grain mites, and honey bees. The latter inhalant sensitivity is to be distinguished from allergic reactions to Hymenoptera stings (Chapter 53). Swarms of mushroom flies and box elder beetles (Murray, Brown and Bernton,

1970) have penetrated homes in sufficient numbers to produce sensitization.

Indoors there are relatively rare cases of documented inhalant allergy to bedbugs, houseflies, and water fleas (Daphnia); the latter are crustaceans which are used as fish food. *Mites* have been discussed before. The *cockroach* is receiving increasing attention as a potentially important inhalant allergen in homes. Almost half of economically disadvantaged patients in large urban areas in the United States have positive skin tests to cockroach extracts (Bernton, McMahon and Brown, 1972), and many of these reactions can be transferred by the P-K test. Bronchial provocation tests in skin-reactive patients in many instances show immediate or dual responses which can be inhibited by cromolyn sodium (Kang, 1976). Three active fractions have been purified from cockroach extracts, and antigen-induced histamine release from sensitized leukocytes has been demonstrated *in vitro* (Twarog et al., 1977). Cockroach feces and contaminated food also contain the allergen. On the other hand, inhalant *silk* allergy is disappearing with diminishing use of silk fabrics in North America, and the elimination of silk filters in processing vaccines for immunization. It continues to be of potential importance in the Orient. The allergen is contained in sericin, a gelatinous substance which binds silk fibers together.

Insect Materials as Disseminated Aeroallergens. This was first well documented by Parlato's description (1930) of *caddis fly* allergy. The larval form of these insects develops in lakes and rivers. When mature they rise to the surface, the adult flies emerge and fly to shore where mating takes place, and the female flies back over the water to deposit her eggs. Although numerous varieties of caddis flies are widely distributed, these insects swarm in sufficient numbers to produce allergic symptoms primarily in the area of Buffalo, New York. The season of exposure is June to late August, with the peak in mid-August. The allergenicity of these flies is very much related to the fact that they are covered with small hairs that break off and become wind-borne. Sensitized persons have positive skin tests to caddis fly extracts, the immunochemical composition of which has been studied by Shulman (1968).

At about the same time caddis fly allergy was discovered at the eastern end of Lake Erie, Figley (1929) described *May fly* allergy at the western end of the lake. Somewhat like the caddis fly, the May fly larvae develop in the water, and the adults emerge to swarm ashore in vast numbers in June and July. The adults live only a few hours, but during this time they shed a friable outer skin or pellicle. Debris from these pellicles and the vast numbers of dead insects accumulating near the lake shore produce sufficient airborne allergen to sensitize numbers of patients in lake shore communities near Toledo, Ohio. This disease is of diminishing importance, however, as the number of these flies has been decreasing, probably as a result of water pollution in western Lake Erie.

On the other hand, the *Douglas fir tussock moth* in the northwestern United States has become an increasing problem. A large part of the dermatitis and respiratory symptoms occurring in persons exposed to great numbers of these moths probably represents an irritant effect, but results of prick tests and passive sensitization of monkey lung for histamine release provide evidence for true Type I hypersensitivity in some cases (Perlman et al., 1976).

The possibility that many other types of insect debris might be the causes of much allergic disease has intrigued a number of investigators (Feinberg, Feinberg and Beniam-Pinto, 1956; Perlman, 1958). Some support for this possibility is found in the fact that skin testing large numbers of allergic patients with a battery of insect extracts results in positive reactions in one third to one half of the subjects! Furthermore, these reactions are observed most frequently in patients with seasonal allergic symptoms and least commonly in nonallergic individuals. A recent example is the finding that more than half of asthmatic patients in Japan have positive intracutaneous skin test reactions to moth or butterfly extracts (Kino and Oshima, 1978). In some cases RAST and bronchial provocation tests were positive. Interpretation of this kind of information, however, is more conjectural than conclusive. Correlations with the insect content of the "aerial plankton" in which we live are thwarted by the lack of technology for identifying the source of most airborne insect debris. Thus the degree to which hypersensitivity to various inhalant insect allergens is of clinical importance remains to be clarified. Immunochemical data regarding the known insect allergens have been reviewed by Shulman (1968), and relevant entomologic information has been compiled by Frazier (1969).

MISCELLANEOUS ALLERGENS OF PLANT ORIGIN

Kapok. Imported largely from Indonesia, kapok is the seedhair from kapok trees. It has been employed as stuffing for pillows, sleeping bags, mattresses, aquatic lifejackets and cushions for boats, the latter uses because of its marked buoyancy. Studies many years ago suggested some relationship between kapok and cottonseed allergens corresponding to their botanical relationship. However, the allergenicity of kapok articles is acquired largely with aging (Dhorranintra and Bunnag, 1977). Based on skin testing with serial dilutions of extracts, Voorhorst (1969) found old kapok, like feathers, to be indistinguishable from house dust allergen. On the other hand, there appear to be immunochemical differences (Berrens, 1966). In any case, kapok is a potentially potent allergen which should not be employed as a substitute for feather pillows or other allergenic stuffings.

Orris Root. The powdered rhizome from certain species of iris had physical properties and a fragrance that were almost ideal for use in face powder and certain other cosmetics. Although the root was widely used for these purposes about 40 to 50 years ago, so many patients developed respiratory allergic symptoms that its use has largely been abandoned in North America.

Pyrethrum. This widely used insecticide is prepared from pyrethrum flowers. These are members of the large Compositae family and thus are botanically related to ragweed. Accordingly, skin test reactivity and clinical difficulty from pyrethrum are particularly likely to occur in ragweed-sensitive patients. Aggravation of allergic respiratory symptoms from insect sprays and powders most often is on an irritant basis, but the additional possibility of specific sensitization needs to be considered when the offending material contains pyrethrum. Some patients have difficulty after the inside of an aircraft has been sprayed with pyrethrum.

Cottonseed. The water-soluble, proteinaceous material in cottonseed contains one of the most potent allergens for man. Occasionally it contaminates inexpensive cotton stuffing in upholstery, mattresses, and cushions. More substantial exposures to the allergen(s) arise from the use of cottonseed meal, which may be found in fertilizers and as a constituent of feed for cattle, hogs, poultry and dogs. Symptoms usually result from inhalation, but allergic reactions also can occur from ingesting cottonseed meal used in pan-greasing compounds and in foods such as some fried cakes, fig bars and cookies. The processing of cottonseed *oil* generally involves washing, bleaching, and distillation at over 400°C. It is extremely unlikely that any traces of allergen would retain their activity through these procedures, and this is fortunate in view of the extremely wide usage of cottonseed oil. Patients sensitized to the water-soluble allergen tend to have explosive, intermittent symptoms depending on their source of exposure. Because of the extreme sensitivity of some individuals, casual skin testing can lead to severe or fatal reactions. Prick testing is recommended in preference to or before injection of cottonseed extracts.

Flaxseed (Linseed). This also contains potent allergen(s). Although varying from time to time and place to place, some of the possible inhalant sources of flaxseed exposure are cattle and poultry feed, dog food, wave-setting preparations, shampoos and hair tonics, some brands of depilatories, patent leather, insulating materials, rugs, and some cloth containing flax. Ingestant sources include Roman meal, Malt-O-Meal, flaxseed tea, milk from cows fed flaxseed meal, cough remedies, laxatives, and muffins. The numerous sources of linseed oil are not of concern for the same reasons as mentioned regarding cottonseed oil.

The precautions described in skin testing with cottonseed should be observed in testing with flaxseed.

Castor Bean. After castor oil is expressed from the beans, there remains a residual castor pomace, which contains another very potent allergen(s). This may be incorporated in fertilizer; also used burlap sacks may be contaminated with this allergen. A colony of sensitized patients in the vicinity of a castor bean processing factory that contaminated the atmosphere with castor bean pomace has been reported. Castor beans also contain a toxin (ricin), and for skin testing it is important that detoxified material be used and that the aforementioned precautions for dealing with potent allergens be observed.

Other Inhalant Allergens from Bean Sources. In addition to its use in foods, *soy bean* meal has many commercial uses that may permit sensitization by inhalation: fertilizer, animal food, glue and adhesives, water-based paint, paper size, artificial wool, fire-fighting foam, water proofing, whipping powder, soothing bath preparations, and textile dressing (Fries, 1971). Recently we observed a laboratory worker who had an acute Type I hypersensitivity reaction from *Bandeiraea simplicifolia*, a bean source of anti-B lectin. Occupational allergy from *coffee bean* dust has been reported (Kaye and Freedman, 1961).

Vegetable Gums. Several vegetable gums have been added to a large variety of commercial products largely to improve their physical properties, but the pattern of gum usage has varied considerably at different times and in different places. For example, wave-setting lotions were the source of some of the best documented cases of vegetable gum allergy many years ago, but the hair sprays in common use today generally contain polyvinylpyrrolidone instead of vegetable gums. The gums most frequently reported to produce sensitization were Karaya or Indian gum, tragacanth, and acacia gum or gum arabic. Other gums are derived from quince seed, locust bean (carobseed), Irish moss (carrageenan), chickle, algin, agar, bassora, gelatin, ghatti, gum guar, mesquite, and pectin. Current information about inhalant sources is difficult to obtain, but vegetable gums still may be present in some brands of denture adhesive powders, tooth powders, wave-setting preparations, face powder, rouge, adhesives, and sizing materials and other substances used in printing and paper making. Vegetable gums also are used extensively in food products. Evaluation of possible gum allergy by skin testing requires employing several gums, since cross-reactions cannot be assumed. These allergens have not been assessed by modern immunochemical methods.

Miscellaneous Plant Inhalants. These include lycopodium (dusting powders), psyllium (laxative), and jute (burlap, rope, carpets).

OTHER INHALANT ALLERGENS

Fish odors can produce allergic respiratory symptoms in highly sensitive patients. Such persons also may be highly reactive to fish glue, such as LePage glue. Skin testing with these potent allergens can be dangerous; prick testing is recommended.

In Japan, asthma has been reported from *buckwheat* attached to buckwheat chaff in pillows. Inhaled *medications* also can sensi-

tize. Indeed this occurred so frequently with penicillin that its administration by inhalation has been largely abandoned. Intranasal insufflation of posterior pituitary preparations (Pituitrin) also caused considerable hypersensitivity. Inhalant allergy to pancreatic extract has been reported in parents of cystic fibrosis patients, caused by the parents' sprinkling the enzyme preparation on their small childrens' food (Dolan and Meyers, 1974).

OCCUPATIONAL EXPOSURES TO INHALANT ALLERGENS

Since problems with occupational allergy are seldom seen in pediatric practice, these will not be discussed here individually. However, since some adolescents entering

TABLE 17–2 SOME OCCUPATIONAL INHALANT ALLERGENS PRODUCING TYPE I HYPERSENSITIVITY REACTIONS*

Wood dusts
Western red cedar	Chan-Yueng et al., 1973
Abirnana	Booth, LeFoldt and Moffitt, 1976
Cocabolla	Eaton, 1973
Others	Sosman et al., 1969

Enzymes
Enzyme detergents	Zetterstrom, 1977
Trypsin	Colten et al., 1975
Pancreatin	Pepys and Davies, 1978
Papain	Dolovich et al., 1977

Wheat flour — Pepys and Davies, 1978

Other materials of plant origin
Coffee bean dust	Kaye and Freedman, 1961
Grain dust	Warren, Cherniack and Tse, 1974
Powdered tobacco and chicory	Jimenez-Diaz and Sanchez Cuenca, 1935

Simple chemical substances
Chloramine T	Feinberg and Watrous, 1945
Phthalic anhydride	Maccia et al., 1976
Meatwrappers' asthma	Andrasch et al., 1976
Trimellitic anhydride	Zeiss et al., 1977
Phenylglycine acid chloride	Kammermeyer and Mathews, 1973
Platinum salts	Freedman and Krupey, 1968
Toluene diisocyanate†	Butcher et al., 1976
Dimethyl ethanolamine	Vallieres et al., 1977
Amino ethyl ethanolamine	Pepys and Pickering, 1972
Persulfate salts	Pepys, Hutchcroft and Breslin, 1976
Amprolium hydrochloride	Greene and Freedman, 1976

*This list excludes pharmaceuticals.
†Immune mechanism questionable.

the work force may become sensitized through exposure at work, Table 17–2 lists some of the most common inhalant occupational allergens and references providing detailed information. This list pertains primarily to Type I hypersensitivity; hypersensitivity pneumonitis relating to occupational exposure is discussed in Chapter 47.

SUMMARY

Among the inhalant allergens other than pollen and fungi, "house dust" is of major importance, but identification of the allergenic substances in this heterogeneous material is difficult; mites appear to be important in some cases. Epidermal allergens from various mammalian species are common offenders which usually are easily recognized. Insects can produce allergic symptoms in localized areas, but their importance as widely disseminated aeroallergens remains to be defined. There are many other substances that occasionally act as inhalant allergens, and it is incumbent upon physicians caring for allergic patients to be familiar with these.

References

Aas, K.: Bronchial provocation tests in asthma. Arch. Dis. Child. 45:221, 1970.

Andrasch, R. H., Bardana, E. J., Jr., Hoster, F., and Pirofsky, B.: Clinical and bronchial provocation studies in patients with meatwrappers' asthma. J. Allergy Clin. Immunol. 58:291, 1976.

Bernton, H. S., McMahon, T. F., and Brown, H.: Cockroach asthma. Br. J. Dis Chest 66:61, 1972.

Berrens, L.: Kapok allergens. Int. Arch. Allergy 29:575, 1966.

Berrens, L.: On the composition of feather extracts used in allergy practice. Int. Arch. Allergy 34:81, 1968.

Berrens, L.: The allergens in house dust. Progr. Allergy 14:259, 1970.

Berrens, L., van Bronswijk, J. E. M. H., Young, E., and van Dijk, A. G.: A controlled study of allergen production in cultures of Dermatophagoides pteronyssinus. Acta Allergologica 30:390, 1975.

Booij-Nord, H., DeVries, H. J., Sluiter, H. J., and Orie, N. G. M.: Late bronchial obstructive reaction to experimental inhalation of house dust extract. Clin. Allergy 2:43, 1972.

Booth, B. H., LeFoldt, R. H., and Moffitt, E. M.: Wood dust hypersensitivity. J. Allergy Clin. Immunol. 57:352, 1976.

Bullock, J. D., and Frick, O. L.: Mite sensitivity in house dust–allergic children. Am. J. Dis. Child. 123:222, 1972.

Butcher, B. T., Salvaggio, J. E., Weil, H., and Ziskind, M. M.: Toluene diisocyanate (TDI) pulmonary disease: immunologic and inhalation challenge studies. J. Allergy Clin. Immunol. 58:89, 1976.

Chan-Yeung, M., Barton, G. M., MacLean, L., and Grzybowski, S.: Occupational asthma and rhinitis due to western red cedar (Thuja plicata). Am. Rev. Respir. Dis. 108:1094, 1973.

Cohen, M. B., Nelson, T., and Reinarz, B. H.: Observations on the nature of the house dust allergy. J. Allergy 6:517, 1935.

Colten, H. R., Polakoff, P. L., Weinstein, S. F., and Streider, D. J.: Immediate hypersensitivity to hog trypsin resulting from industrial exposure. N. Engl. J. Med. 292:1050, 1975.

Dekker, H.: Asthma and Milben. Munch. Med. Wochenschr. 75:515, 1928 (translated in J. Allergy Clin. Immunol. 48:251, 1971).

Dhorranintra, B., and Bunnag, C.: Cross reactions in skin tests between kapok and house dust allergenic extracts. Ann. Allergy 39:201, 1977.

Dolan, T. F., Jr., and Meyers, A.: Bronchial asthma and allergic rhinitis associated with the inhalation of pancreatic extracts. Am. Rev. Respir. Dis. 110:812, 1974.

Dolovich, J., Shaikh, W., Tarlo, S., Bell, B., and Hargreave, F. E.: Human exposure and sensitization to airborne papain. Ann. Allergy 38:382, 1977.

Eaton, K. K.: Respiratory allergy to exotic wood dust. Clin. Allergy 3:307, 1973.

Fagerberg, E., and Wide, L.: Diagnosis of hypersensitivity to dog epithelium in patients with asthma bronchiale. Int. Arch. Allergy 39:301, 1970.

Feinberg, S. M., and Watrous, R. M.: Atopy to simple chemical compounds–sulfone-chloramides. J. Allergy 16:209, 1945.

Feinberg, A. R., Feinberg, S. M., and Beniam-Pinto, C.: Asthma and rhinitis from insect allergens. I. Clinical importance. J. Allergy 27:437, 1956.

Figley, K. D.: Asthma due to May fly. Am. J. Med. Sci. 178:338, 1929.

Fontana, V. J., Wittig, H., and Holt, L. E., Jr.: Observations on the specificity of the skin test. The incidence of positive skin tests in allergic and nonallergic children. J. Allergy 34:348, 1963.

Frazier, C. A.: Insect Allergy. St. Louis, Warren H. Green, Inc., 1969.

Freedman, S. O., and Krupey, J.: Respiratory allergy caused by platinum salts. J. Allergy 42:233, 1968.

Fries, J. H.: Studies on the allergenicity of soy bean. Ann. Allergy 29:1, 1971.

Gerrais, P., Reinberg, A., Gerrais, C., Smolensky, M., and DeFrance, O.: Twenty-four-hour rhythm in the bronchial hypersensitivity to house dust in asthmatics. J. Allergy Clin. Immunol. 59:207, 1977.

Greene, S. A., and Freedman, S.: Asthma due to inhaled chemical agents — amprolium hydrochloride. Clin. Allergy 6:105, 1976.

Holford-Strevens, V., Wide, L., Milne, J. F., and Pepys, J.: Allergens and antigens of Dermatophagoides farinae. Clin. Exper. Immunol. 6:49, 1970.

Hooker, S. B.: Qualitative differences among canine danders. Ann. Allergy 2:281, 1944.

Ingham, P. E., and Ingham, D. M.: House dust mites and infant-use sheepskins. Med. J. Australia 1:302, 1976.

Jimenez-Diaz, L., and Sanchez Cuenca, B.: Asthma produced by susceptibility to unusual allergens: linseed, insects, tobacco and chicory. J. Allergy 6:397, 1935.

Kammermeyer, J. K., and Mathews, K. P.: Hypersensitivity to phenylglycine acid chloride. J. Allergy Clin. Immunol. 52:73, 1973.

Kang, B.: Study on cockroach antigen as a possible causative agent in bronchial asthma. J. Allergy Clin. Immunol. 58:357, 1976.

Kawai, T., Marsh, D. G., Lichtenstein, L. M., and Norman, P. S.: The allergens responsible for house dust allergy. I. Comparison of Dermatophagoides pteronyssinus and house dust extracts by assay of histamine release from allergic human leukocytes. J. Allergy Clin. Immunol. 50:117, 1972.

Kaye, M., and Freedman, S. O.: Allergy to raw coffee — an occupational disease. Canad. Med. Assoc. J. *84*:469, 1961.

Kino, T., and Oshima, S.: Allergy to insects in Japan. I. The reaginic sensitivity to moth and butterfly in patients with bronchial asthma. J. Allergy Clin. Immunol. *61*:10, 1978.

Leegaard, J., and Roth, A.: RAST in the diagnosis of hypersensitivity to horse allergens. A comparison with clinical history and *in vivo* tests. Clin. Allergy *7*:455, 1977.

Lindblad, J. H., and Farr, R. S.: The incidence of positive intradermal reactions and demonstration of skin sensitizing antibody to extracts of ragweed and dust in humans without history of rhinitis or asthma. J. Allergy *32*:393, 1961.

Maccia, C. A., Bernstein, I. L., Emmett, E. A., and Brooks, S. M.: *In vitro* demonstration of specific IgE in phthalic anhydride hypersensitivity. Am. Rev. Respir. Dis. *113*:701, 1976.

May, C. D., Lyman, M., Alberto, R., and Cheng, J.: Immunochemical evaluation of antigenicity of house dust extract. Specificity of dermal wheal reactions and responses to injections for immunotherapy. J. Allergy *46*:73, 1970.

McAllen, M. K., Assem, E. S. K., and Mannsell, K.: House-dust mite asthma. Results of challenge tests on five criteria with *Dermatophagoides pteronyssinus*. Br. Med. J. *2*:501, 1970.

Miyamoto, T., Oshima, S., Ishizaki, T., and Sato, S.: Allergenic identity between the common floor mite (*Dermatophagoides farinae* Hughes, 1961) and house dust as a causative antigen in bronchial asthma. J. Allergy *42*:14, 1968.

Miyamoto, T., Oshima, S., and Ishizaki, T.: Antigenic relation between house dust and dust mite (*Dermatophagoides farinae* Hughes, 1961) by a fractionation method. J. Allergy *44*:282, 1969.

Morita, Y., Miyamoto, T., Horiuchi, Y., Oshima, S., Katsuhata, A., and Kamal, J.: Further studies in allergic identity between house dust and the house dust mite, *Dermatophagoides farinae* Hughes, 1961. Ann. Allergy *35*:361, 1976.

Murray, F. J., Brown, H., and Bernton, H. S.: A case of asthma caused by box elder beetle. J. Allergy *45*:103, 1970.

Ohman, J. L., Jr., Lowell, F. C., and Bloch, K. J.: Allergens of mammalian origin. III. Properties of a major feline allergen. J. Immunol. *113*:1668, 1974.

Ohman, J. L., Kendall, S., and Lowell, F. C.: IgE antibody to cat allergens in an allergic population. J. Allergy Clin. Immunol. *60*:317, 1977.

Parlato, S. J.: The sand fly (caddis fly) as an exciting cause of allergic coryza and asthma. II. Its relative frequency. J. Allergy *1*:307, 1930.

Pepys, J., and Pickering, C. A. C.: Asthma due to inhaled chemical agents — amino ethyl ethanolamine in aluminum soldering flux. Clin. Allergy *2*:197, 1972.

Pepys, J., Hutchcroft, B. J., and Breslin, A. B. X.: Asthma due to inhaled chemical agents — persulfate salts and henna in hair-dressers. Clin. Allergy *6*:399, 1976.

Pepys, J., and Davies, R. J.: Occupational asthma. *In* Middleton, E., Jr., Reed, C. E., and Ellis, E. F. (eds.): *Allergy: Principles and Practice.* St. Louis, C. V. Mosby Co., 1978. pp. 819, 824.

Perlman, F.: Insects as inhalant allergens. Consideration of aerobiology, biochemistry, preparation of material, and clinical observations. J. Allergy *29*:302, 1958.

Perlman, F., Press, E., Googins, J. A., Malley, A., and Poarea, H.: Tussockosis: reactions to Douglas fir tussock moth. Ann. Allergy *36*:302, 1976.

Ponterius, G., Brandt, R., Hulten, E., and Yman, L.: Comparative studies on the allergens of horse dandruff and horse serum. Int. Arch. Allergy *44*:679, 1973.

Romagnani, S., Biliotti, G. Passaleva, A., and Ricci, M.: Mites and house dust allergy. III. *In vitro* lymphocyte transformation to house dust and mite (*Dermatophagoides pteronyssinus*) extract in atopic and nonatopic individuals. Clin. Allergy *3*:51, 1973.

Sarsfield, J. K.: Role of house-dust mites in childhood asthma. Arch. Dis. Child. *49*:711, 1974.

Shulman, S.: Insect allergy: biochemical and immunological analyses of the allergens. Prog. Allergy *12*:246, 1968.

Sosman, A. J., Schlueter, D. P., Fink, J. N., and Barboriak, J. J.: Hypersensitivity to wood dust. N. Engl. J. Med. *281*:977, 1969.

Spain, W. C., Gillson, R. E., and Strauss, M. D.: Comparative immunologic studies with salivary and epithelial extracts of the dog, cat and rabbit. J. Allergy *13*:563, 1942.

Stevenson, D. P., and Mathews, K. P.: Occupational asthma following inhalation of moth particles. J. Allergy *39*:274, 1967.

Twarog, F. J., Picone, F. J., Strunk, R. S., So, J., and Colten, H. R.: Immediate hypersensitivity to cockroach. Isolation and purification of the major antigens. J. Allergy Clin. Immunol. *59*:154, 1977.

Vallieres, M., Cockcroft, D. W., Taylor, D. M., Dolovich, J., and Hargreave, F. E.: Dimethyl ethanolamine–induced asthma. Am. Rev. Respir. Dis. *115*:867, 1977.

van Bronswijk, J. E. M. H., and Sinha, R. N.: Pyroglyphid mites (Acari) and house dust allergy. J. Allergy *47*:31, 1971.

Voorhorst, R., Spieksma, F. Th. M., Varekamp, H., Lenpen, M. J., and Lyklema, A. W.: The house-dust mite (*Dermatophagoides pteronyssinus*) and the allergens it produces. Identity with the house-dust allergen. J. Allergy *39*:325, 1967.

Voorhorst, R., Spieksma, F. Th. M., and Varekamp, H.: *House-dust Atopy and the House-dust Mite.* Leiden, Staflen's Scientific Publishing Co., 1969.

Voorhorst, R.: To what extent are house-dust mites (Dermatophagoides) responsible for complaints in asthma patients? Allergie u. Immunol. *18*:9, 1972.

Voorhorst, R.: The human dander atopy. II. Human dander, a complicating factor in the study of the relationship between house dust and dermatophagoides allergens. Ann. Allergy *39*:339, 1977.

Warren, P., Cherniack, R. M., and Tse, K. S.: Hypersensitivity reactions to grain dust. J. Allergy Clin. Immunol. *53*:139, 1974.

Zeiss, C. R., Patterson, R., Pruzansky, J. J, Miller, M., Rosenberg, M., and Levitz, D.: Trimellitic anhydride–induced airway syndromes: clinical and immunologic studies. J. Allergy Clin. Immunol. *60*:96, 1977.

Zetterstrom, O.: Challenge and exposure test reactions to enzyme detergents in subjects sensitized to subtilisin. Clin. Allergy *7*:355, 1977.

18

Manuel Lopez, M.D.
John E. Salvaggio, M.D.

Nonimmune Environmental Factors in Allergic Disease

This chapter considers the effects of climate, atmospheric pollution, and other nonimmune environmental factors on allergic disease. Because of the complex interrelationship between climate, meteorologic changes, air pollution, and home environment, it is often very difficult to define the effects and importance of each environmental factor on allergic disease. Environmental factors have been divided into domestic and urban for purposes of convenience, although it is recognized that their intimate relationship makes this classification somewhat arbitrary.

DOMESTIC ENVIRONMENT

The indoor home environment is of particular importance since children spend a substantial part of their life at home. Despite its importance, however, accurate data on the different indoor atmospheric components and their role in allergic disease are meager. The home environment is affected by such factors as air conditioning and heating systems, humidifiers, and family habits and hobbies. For example, heavy cigarette smoking in a home and frequent use of insecticides, aerosols, and other sprays are sources of significant indoor environmental insults. Cigarette smoke will be discussed as a prototype of domestic environmental factors important in allergic disease.

Many patients with rhinitis and bronchial asthma experience an increase in symptomatology when exposed to tobacco smoke, although the degree of intolerance varies considerably between individuals. Speer (1968) reported that eye irritation and nasal symptoms occurred in the vast majority of allergic nonsmokers when exposed to tobacco smoke; almost half also experienced cough, and over a fifth wheezed when in contact with smoke. Although the incidence of eye irritation was comparable in nonallergic nonsmoking individuals, nasal symptoms and cough occurred with half the frequency noted in allergic patients; wheezing occurred in fewer than 4 percent of nonallergic patients. The response even in allergic patients appeared to be irritative rather than allergic. The effect of passive or atmospheric cigarette smoke on production of respiratory symptoms in children in household environments is not known, but the overall percentage of respiratory symptoms has been reported to increase in proportion to degree of household smoking. An increased incidence of respiratory problems such as bronchitis and pneumonitis in infancy also has been associated with parental smoking, and several epidemiologic surveys have suggested an overall increase in the prevalence of respiratory disorders in children from homes in which parents smoke. Unfortunately, all such studies are fraught with difficulties in interpretation because of the many variables that may influence observations and that are extremely difficult to control. Moreover, an increase in respiratory problems has not been found in households of smokers by other investigators.

Allergy to tobacco smoke, defined by elicitation of wheal and flare skin reactions to tobacco leaf extracts and clinical improvement following immunotherapy, has been reported. Many clinical conditions have been associated with "allergic" manifestations to tobacco smoke, including various forms of dermatitis, rhinitis, asthma, cardiovascular disturbances, gastrointestinal symptoms, and headache. For the most part, studies on allergy to tobacco smoke have utilized tobacco leaf rather than smoke extracts and have been woefully deficient in experimental design. The issue of whether tobacco smoke sensitivity is due to allergic mechanisms or is entirely irritative has yet to be resolved (Rylander, 1974; Taylor, 1974). On the other hand, tobacco smoke has been reported to exert numerous effects on host defense mechanisms in man and experimental animals, such as decrease in mucociliary clearance of inhaled materials and increased bronchial irritability. Denudation of ciliated epithelium with squamous metaplasia of the epithelium and possible toxic effects of smoke on ciliary function *in vitro* and *in vivo* have also been reported. Tobacco smoke increases the number of alveolar macrophages, induces more cytoplasmic inclusions and lysosomal bodies, and depresses alveolar macrophage phagocytic and bactericidal activity. It also decreases mitogen-induced blastogenic responses of lymphocytes and promotes eosinophilia. Because of the irritant effects of cigarette smoke on the respiratory tract and the clinical sensitivity reported in many patients with allergic diseases, children with allergic disease and asthma in particular should avoid tobacco smoke. Thus, smoking should be eliminated as completely as possible from the allergic child's home.

Other common sources of irritants at home include fireplaces, room deodorizers, furniture and floor waxes, and cooking odors. Allergic patients, especially patients with asthma, are known to be affected by the inhalation of a wide variety of irritants. Possible reasons for this increased suscepti-

bility are discussed in Chapter 45. Nadel et al. (1965) have presented evidence that sensitization of vagal tracheobronchial irritant receptors is associated with an exaggerated bronchoconstrictor reflex and may be one cause of airway hyperreactivity in asthma. Connell (1963) has shown that repeated exposure to an allergen causes a decrease in the dose of the same or other allergens needed to induce nasal symptoms. This "priming" effect on the airways is likely to increase responsiveness to irritants such as smoke and air pollutants.

Children frequently have difficulty in identifying offending irritants in the environment and are less capable of avoiding them. For this reason, it is important that physicians and parents of an allergic child recognize and modify exposure to the many indoor irritants that can harm the child.

URBAN ENVIRONMENT

Air Pollution

Air pollution can be defined as the atmospheric accumulation of foreign airborne substances that are harmful to man, animals, or plants. In general, pollution is referred to as *smog,* a combination of fog and smoke. There are several types of smog (Table 18–1): Industrial smog is the dominant type in large industrialized areas such as New York, Chicago, and Tokyo and was the primary cause of the "London smog" of December 1952. It is produced by combustion of sulfur-containing fossil fuels, especially coal and crude oils. The second type, photochemical smog, accumulates in areas such as Los Angeles and Denver, which have a high density of automobiles, generally poor air drainage, and sufficient sunlight to induce photochemical reactions with nitrogen oxides and hydrocarbons. A third type of pollution is grouped in a miscellaneous category and arises from industrial sources such as mines, factories, and smelters. These vary with the individual locality and the industrial source. Several different types of pollution frequently coexist in a given locality.

Levels of air pollution are affected great-

TABLE 18–1 CLASSIFICATION AND COMPONENTS OF SMOG

Industrial Smog (London smog)
  Combustion of fossil fuels
    Oxides of sulfur
    Sulfuric acid
    Particulate matter

Photochemical Smog (Los Angeles smog)
  Automobile exhaust emission
    Ozone
    Nitrogen oxides
    Hydrocarbons

Miscellaneous
  Point sources

ly by weather conditions, but the most important meteorologic factors leading to the accumulation of pollutants are temperature inversions, which limit their vertical dispersion, and low wind velocity, which hinders their horizontal dispersion.

Data from epidemiologic studies, experimental human exposure, and animal studies leave little doubt that air pollution aggravates respiratory problems. Numerous studies have demonstrated an association between air pollution and acute respiratory illness in children residing in the more polluted areas. In most of the reported studies, children living in communities with pollution of the "London smog" type show diminished ventilatory function compared with children living in less polluted areas. The same difference has not been shown consistently with "Los Angeles smog," however. The role of air pollution in aggravating allergic symptoms and asthma is difficult to evaluate. Epidemiologic studies must take into consideration the multiplicity of pollutants and their mutual interactions and synergisms, in addition to the role of natural pollutants (e.g., pollen, mold spores) and meteorologic changes (temperature, humidity, wind velocity). On the other hand, information derived from short-term exposure to single agents under laboratory conditions cannot be equated with the realities of complex environmental conditions. With these limitations in mind, we will review some experimental and epidemiologic studies and selective acute air pollution episodes as they apply to patients with allergic diseases and asthma.

INDUSTRIAL SMOG

Sulfur Dioxide. Sulfur dioxide (SO_2), which is present in the atmosphere of urban areas as a result of combustion of fossil fuels, is a widely measured air pollutant, and its level has been used as the indicator of air pollution. For this reason, the effects of this type of pollution have been studied most frequently. Its atmospheric concentration averages from 0.1 to 0.4 PPM with occasional peaks of 1 to 1.5 PPM, as was reported at the height of the London smog episode of December 1952. At that time, concentrations averaged 1.34 PPM over a 48-hour period. In laboratory animals, very high concentrations of SO_2 (200–500 PPM) produced lesions similar to those noted in human chronic bronchitis. At lower concentrations, SO_2 produces bronchoconstriction and decreases mucociliary activity. Nadel et al. (1965) have shown that this type of bronchial constriction is due to vagal reflex mechanism involving irritant receptors. However, the changes described above occur with SO_2 concentrations that are highly irritant to the nasal mucosa (i.e., five to ten times the observed atmospheric levels of the most polluted areas). Long-term animal exposure to SO_2 in concentrations in the range of those encountered in urban areas have not been reported to cause adverse effects on pulmonary function or tissue damage (Alarie et al., 1972; Vaughan et al., 1969). Frank et al. (1962) demonstrated increased airways resistance in eleven nonatopic individuals exposed to SO_2 at a concentration of from 5 to 13 PPM for 5 to 30 minutes. One subject had bronchoconstriction with exposure to 5 PPM. Similar individual susceptibility to SO_2 has been shown by other investigators. Ayres and Buehler (1970) exposed subjects with and without pulmonary disease to high concentrations (50 PPM) of SO_2 and observed considerable variation in response. Patients with bronchitis and asthma had a significantly greater response. It appears that the variability in SO_2 effects among these different studies is due both to differing SO_2 concentrations and to biologic variability among healthy subjects. Approximately 10 percent of the population are "hyperreactors," showing increased airways resistance following SO_2 exposure. This may explain in part why only certain individuals from an exposed population will have adverse reactions to air pollution.

Patients with asthma appear to be particularly susceptible to short-term exposure to air pollution, and epidemiologic studies have implicated SO_2 as an etiologic factor (Carnow et al., 1969). Zeidberg and co-workers (1961) correlated increased wheezing on days with high ambient SO_2 over a 1-year period in adults and children with asthma. Similar results were obtained by Cohen et al. (1972) in a group of asthmatics in a small town located close to a coal-fired power plant, and by Girsh et al. (1967), who noted an increased asthma rate in children on days of high atmospheric pollution in Philadelphia. Other studies, however, have shown no correlation between SO_2 air levels and changes in symptoms in asthmatic patients (Derrick, 1970). It also is important to realized that in epidemiologic studies effects of SO_2 cannot be separated from those of other pollutants. Thus, correlations found between SO_2 levels and asthmatic symptoms do not necessarily imply a direct cause-and-effect relationship.

Sulfuric Acid. Accumulation of sulfuric acid in the atmosphere results from the oxidation of sulfur dioxide to sulfur trioxide; sulfur trioxide is hydrated to sulfuric acid when present in atmospheres with high water droplet content. Sulfuric acid is more irritating than SO_2 and induces severe cough and increased airways resistance (Sim and Pattle, 1957). The sulfuric acid content of industrial smog usually does not exceed 10 percent of the total sulfur content.

Carbon Monoxide. This compound (CO) is one of the more widely distributed air pollutants, resulting from heating, fuel combustion, industrial processes such as steel manufacturing, and refuse burning. Gasoline-powered vehicles are the largest source of ambient levels. Its concentration may vary widely in a given area. In urban areas, levels of 5 to 10 PPM are not uncommon. Peaks of 120 PPM have been reported in Los Angeles traffic and 40 PPM to 300 PPM have been reported on New York expressways. The effect of CO results primarily from its affinity for hemoglobin, displacing oxygen from red blood cells and resulting in impairment of tissue oxygenation. CO can impair human psychomotor performance at concentrations found in urban atmospheres, but it has little or no effect on respiratory function. No adverse effect of environmental CO has been reported in asthmatic patients.

Particulate Matter. Both liquid and solid particles are included in this group. They are identified according to size and physical stage as fog, mist, dust, smog, and soot. Chemical composition depends on the source of local emission, such as industrial and domestic furnaces, incinerators, exhaust emissions, and chemical industrial pollution (Vaughan, 1969). Particulate pollutants cause direct adverse effects on the bronchial tree, act as carriers of other pollutants, or act as catalysts potentiating the effect of other pollutants. For example, sodium chloride aerosols increase the irritant activity of SO_2.

It is virtually impossible to separate the effect of particles from that of other pollutants such as SO_2 originating from the same source and having related actions. In most studies, particulate matter and SO_2 are considered as a pollution mixture. In comparative studies, however, some investigators have implicated inert dust concentrations as a cause of higher morbidity rates in certain cities when concentrations of SO_2 were similar.

PHOTOCHEMICAL SMOG

Photochemical smog is formed in the atmosphere by chemical reactions between solar radiation, nitrogen oxide and hydrocarbons. Most hydrocarbons are emitted from motor vehicles, but other sources may include local industries and coal- and oil-fueled electric power plants. These photochemical reactions produce ozone, nitric oxide, and other oxidants. The oxidants act on organic substances present in the atmosphere, producing organic radicals that eventually degrade into carbon dioxide, carbon monoxide, water, and ozone. The net result of this reaction is so-called photochemical smog, which characterizes cities with warm, sunny weather and many automobiles. Adverse effects such as acute eye and respiratory tract irritation occur with the levels of photochemical smog present in many city environments. Schoettlin and Landau (1961) reported a significant increase in asthma attacks on days when the oxidant level was sufficiently high to irritate the eyes (0.25 PPM).

Ozone. Ozone (O_3) levels often serve as the index of photochemical smog since ozone constitutes the main component, contributing up to 90 percent of the total oxidant level. In an episode of heavy smog in the Los Angeles area in 1959, ozone reached a concentration of 0.99 PPM. Eye irritation is experienced with levels of 0.1 to 0.2 PPM, concentrations of 0.2 to 0.5 PPM reduce visual acuity, and levels of 0.3 to 1 PPM cause coughing and severe fatigue (Jaffe, 1967). Experimental exposure of normal subjects to 0.6 to 0.8 PPM of ozone for a period of 2 hours increases airways resistance and decreases vital capacity, forced respiratory volume and diffusion capacity (Young et al., 1964). As with other pollutants, there appears to be great variability in degree of individual susceptibility to the irritant effects. Bates et al. (1974) demonstrated increased airways resistance in normal subjects exposed to 0.75 PPM ozone for 2 hours. SO_2 added in concentration of 0.37 PPM, which ordinarily has no effect alone, enhanced the effect of ozone. DeLucia and Adams (1977) reported that inhalation of ozone during exercise can induce respiratory symptoms which are proportional to the intensity of exercise.

Nitrogen Dioxide. Nitrogen oxides are important constituents of automobile exhaust emissions and tobacco smoke. They are precursors of ozone under conditions favorable for photochemical reactions. Nitrogen dioxide (NO_2) usually is found in urban atmospheres in concentrations less than 1 PPM. The acute toxic effects of high concentrations of NO_2 are well demonstrated by the pulmonary insufficiency produced in farmers working in silos (silo filler's disease). Experimental exposure to NO_2 (1.6 to 2.5 PPM) increases airways resistance in healthy volunteers after 1 to 50 minutes of exposure. In the relatively low concentration found in urban areas, it is doubtful that NO_2 has a significant effect on airways resistance.

ACUTE AIR POLLUTION EPISODES

The clearest evidence for an association between air pollution and human health has been provided by the respiratory symptoms produced during acute air pollution episodes in which meteorologic conditions producing air stagnation resulted in a marked increase in atmospheric pollutants. The symptoms most frequently described during these episodes were those of irritation of the respiratory tract (lacrimation, rhinorrhea, cough, and increased mucus production) and, less frequently, gastrointestinal symptoms (nausea and vomiting). Although the general population was at risk, patients with chronic respiratory illness, including asthma, were more severely affected. Illustrative examples of selected episodes of acute air pollution are discussed below.

Meuse Valley, Belgium, 1930. During a period of 5 days, a thermal inversion with marked accumulation of atmospheric pollutants occurred in the heavily industrialized Meuse River Valley of Belgium. Thousands of individuals became ill with eye and nasal irritation, hoarseness, cough, and dyspnea. Sixty persons died. The greatest mortality occurred in older persons who had cardiac or pulmonary disease. Although pollutants were not measured, it has been estimated that sulfur dioxide concentrations ranged between 10 and 40 PPM during the episode.

London, 1952. From December 5 through December 8, 1952, the city of London was affected by an air inversion, and air pollutants reached the highest levels ever reported in that city. The smog was so severe that buses, automobiles and even trains were not allowed to run. Individuals developed nasal discharge, coughing, difficulty in breathing, nausea, and vomiting. Though the elderly were more severely affected, virtually everyone exposed developed symptoms. There were marked increases in emergency room visits and hospital admissions, and deaths from respiratory and circulatory illness were ten times greater than normal. Strong antipollution laws since put into effect, which include severe restrictions on the use of fireplaces and the burning of coal, have prevented a repetition of this disaster.

Donora, Pennsylvania, 1948. In 1948, Donora, an industrial town located on the Monongahela River had several industries, including a sulfuric acid plant, a steel mill, and a zinc-producing plant. In the last

TABLE 18–2   GUIDELINES FOR ASTHMATICS DURING PERIODS OF HIGH AIR POLLUTION

Avoid unnecessary physical activity.

Avoid smoking and smoke-filled rooms.

Avoid exposure to dusts and other irritants, such as hair sprays or other sprays, paint, exhaust fumes, smoke from any fire, or other fumes.

Avoid exposure to persons with colds or respiratory infections.

Try to stay indoors in a clean environment. Air conditioning may help, if available. Also charcoal filters and electrostatic precipitators may be helpful.

If it appears that the air pollution episode will persist or worsen, it may be desirable to leave the polluted area temporarily until the episode subsides.

The physician should consider formulation of specific instructions to be followed by the patient in case of an air pollution alert. The patient should know what medication to use, know when to call the physician, and know when to go to a hospital.

The physician's special guidelines should be written down and kept in a readily accessible place.

(From Weather and Air Pollution Committee, American Academy of Allergy.)

week of October 1948, the town experienced a 3-day thermal inversion, during which many residents became ill, and 17 died. The episode was the subject of a detailed epidemiologic study by the United States Public Health Service (Schrenck et al., 1948). Approximately 40 percent of the population was affected. The most frequent symptoms were respiratory. Elderly persons and patients with chronic respiratory problems were particularly affected, as were patients with a history of bronchitis and asthma. Eighty-six percent of people with a history of asthma had an attack during the inversion and over half had very severe symptoms. Unfortunately, in the report asthmatic patients were not separated from others with chronic obstructive lung disease other than by history. Preexisting cardiorespiratory disease appeared to be the most significant predisposing factor in patients who died.

Asthma and Severe Air Pollution. In summary, patients with asthma have increased symptoms when exposed to severe air pollution for a short time. The marked variability in responses of the asthmatic lung to a wide variety of stimuli such as meteorologic changes, nonspecific irritant gases, allergens, and viral infections renders the interpretation of air pollution studies and analysis of individual pollutants difficult. As a general rule, it is advisable for patients with asthma to take special precau-

tions during periods of increased atmospheric pollution. Table 18–2 lists guidelines for asthmatics during air pollution episodes, formulated by the Weather and Air Pollution Committee of the American Academy of Allergy.

Climate

Climate and atmospheric changes may affect allergic disease indirectly by promoting the growth of molds and pollen-producing plants, as well as facilitating the dispersion of these allergens. Spores from ascomycetes and lower basidiomycetes are discharged into the air during periods of high humidity, while pollen and spores from certain of the *Fungi Imperfecti* group are shed into dry wind. The atmospheric concentration and dispersion of aeroallergens and pollutants fluctuate with meteorologic conditions. Rain decreases the atmospheric concentration of pollen and most types of spores, although the concentration of other spores, such as ascospores, are increased. Concentrations of certain spores increase with rise in temperature, dew point, and relative humidity (Hirst, 1953). High wind velocity decreases local atmospheric concentration of mold spores and pollen but may increase their concentration in places distant from their source. In periods of thermal inversion, there may be increases in aeroallergens as well as marked increases in air pollutants. It is difficult to assess the effect of various climatic factors such as humidity, temperature, and barometric pressure on allergic patients because of the concomitant effect of these changes on allergens and other irritants that induce asthma.

Humidity

Patients with allergic disease frequently report exacerbations of symptoms associated with changes in humidity. In general, high humidity is considered detrimental in asthma and several studies have shown increased airways resistance in patients with pulmonary disease who are exposed to high humidity. On the other hand, heated air during the winter may dry respiratory mucosa and exacerbate respiratory symptoms. Exercise-induced asthma tends to be more pronounced in a dry, compared to a humid, environment (Oden et al., 1977), and epidemics of asthma in the city of New Orleans have been associated with periods of low rather than high relative humidity.

It is common practice to recommend home humidifiers for patients with respiratory symptoms, particularly during the winter months, but the benefit of home humidification has not been established. Rodriguez and co-workers (1975) showed that the use of mists to increase humidity can be harmful in many patients with asthma. Many humidifiers that produce cold water sprays may increase concentration of airborne salts that can act as respiratory irritants. Another complicating factor is the frequent contamination of home humidifiers with mold, thermophilic actinomycetes, free-living amoebae, and other sources of antigen that may exacerbate asthma or predispose to hypersensitivity pneumonitis.

In summary, there is anecdotal evidence that high humidity is detrimental for asthmatics, and there are some supporting data showing an increase in airway resistance associated with high humidity. However, this is not a consistent finding and an overall deleterious effect of high humidity on asthmatics has not been well documented. On the other hand, humidifiers have not been shown to be beneficial and are potentially harmful.

Ionization of the Atmosphere

Ionization of air occurs naturally during thunderstorms and from cosmic rays. Atmospheric ionization also can be induced by artificial methods such as high voltage, electric fields, and the use of radioactive materials. Air ionization occurs when electrons are removed (forming positive ions) or added (forming negative ions) to atoms in the air. The concentration of ions in the atmosphere is low and has been estimated at approximately 400 to 2000 ions per ml of air depending on such atmospheric conditions as humidity and concentration of dust particles. Normally the concentration of positive ions is slightly greater than that of negative ions. Negative ions usually are considered beneficial to health and positive ions detrimental, although there is little definitive evidence on this point. Krueger and Smith (1958) reported that positively charged CO_2 molecules inhibited ciliary activity, decreased mucus flow, increased ciliary vulnerability to trauma, and induced smooth muscle contraction under experimental conditions. Although considerable work has been published on air ionization and its biologic effects, inadequate controls, failure to eliminate other variables such as organic and inorganic particles, and unreliable ionization and monitoring equipment (in earlier studies) have made results difficult to interpret. Some recent studies indicate symptomatic improvement in patients with allergic disease following exposure to artificially increased negative atmospheric ions. In other studies, negative ions have had no beneficial effect (Blumstein et al., 1964; Jones et al., 1976; Davis, 1963).

Temperature and Barometric Pressure

Sudden decrease in temperature appears to be troublesome for certain asthmatics. Experimentally, a sudden fall in temperature can precipitate asthma attacks. The frequency of asthmatic attacks increases dramatically with influxes of cold air at the beginning of the winter season. Whether this is due to a direct effect of cold air on the bronchial mucosa, changes in atmospheric concentrations of environmental allergens and irritants, or to other factors has not been clarified. A review of studies from 1953 to 1956 in Western Europe (Tromp, 1968) indicated that strong atmospheric cooling was a major factor in the observed increase in asthma attack rates at the beginning of the winter months. Greenburg and co-workers (1966) also have reported an increase in the number of emergency clinic visits for asthma in New York City at the onset of cold weather. These investigators postulated that symptoms are due to an increase in dust, spores, and other particulate matter lying dormant and released by the use of heating systems rather than to a direct effect of cold air, although cold air may be playing an aggravating role. An association between asthma attack rates, certain climatic factors, and atmospheric spore and pollen concentrations also has been noted in studies in New Orleans (Salvaggio et al., 1971).

The effect of cold air on bronchial mucosa is not entirely clear. The upper airways are efficient in heating and humidifying inhaled air even under extreme conditions of cold. Nevertheless, some patients with chronic respiratory problems such as chronic bronchitis and asthma have increased symptoms when exposed to cold air, and increased airways obstruction has been documented in asthmatics under controlled experimental conditions (Ramsey, 1977; Strauss et al., 1977). The application of topical anesthetic to the nasal and pharyngeal mucosa has been reported to prevent cold-induced increases in airways resistance in asthmatic children (Rodriquez-Martinez et al., 1973), suggesting a reflex mechanism involving the upper respiratory tract for cold-induced bronchial constriction. Increasing humidity also significantly decreases postexercise asthma in patients breathing cold air, suggesting that temperature and humidity are significant interacting variables (Strauss et al., 1978). There appears to be marked variability between asthmatic patients in tolerance to cold air (Miller, 1965; Wells et al., 1960).

Although exposure to cold air can result in increased airway obstruction in asthma, it is likely that the observed increase in asthmatic symptoms during autumn is related to a combination of an increase in airborne pollen and/or molds, seasonal viral infec-

tions, and changes in weather conditions rather than to a sudden drop in temperature or change in humidity *per se*.

Asthma Epidemics

Asthma symptoms of an epidemic nature associated with a specific geographic area have been reported in the Tokyo-Yokohama area and in New Orleans. The occurrence of these so-called asthma epidemics gives further insight into the complex interrelationship between climatic variables, airborne allergens, and pollutants acting on a susceptible population.

Tokyo-Yokohama Asthma. The Tokyo and Yokohama area in Japan is the site of one of the largest industrial complexes in the world, and its topography offers an ideal trap for air pollutants. In 1954, Huber et al. reported an increased incidence of asthma among United States military personnel stationed in that area. Patients initially developed symptoms described as a "cold" during the fall and early winter; in subsequent years, patients experienced attacks of dyspnea and wheezing, occasionally refractory to treatment. Dramatic improvement usually occurred after patients left the area, although pulmonary abnormalities persisted in some patients. Individuals involved appeared to represent a heterogeneous group of people with symptoms of chronic bronchitis and asthma (Oshima et al., 1964; Spotnitz, 1965; Tremonti, 1970) that developed initially while living in the heavily polluted area of Tokyo and Yokohama. In asthmatic patients, symptoms probably were due to a combination of organic and inorganic pollutants present in the atmosphere at certain times of the year.

New Orleans Asthma. The city of New Orleans has been the site of periodic outbreaks of asthma occurring mainly during the months of September, October, and November. Patients involved are allergic asthmatics, as evidenced by strong personal and family history of atopic disease, wheal and flare skin reactivity to common allergens, and increased bronchial hyperreactivity to histamine and Mecholyl (Salvaggio and Klein, 1967). Although there was an initial suggestion that epidemics were associated with emissions of silica-containing particles from burning dumps or grain dusts from local grain elevators, further extensive air sampling has failed to demonstrate any consistent association. In a study comparing epidemic with nonepidemic days during September and October from 1963 to 1967, there was a significant association between increased hospital admission rates for asthma and low wind velocity, low relative humidity, and low temperature. Asthma outbreaks in 1967 and 1968 were correlated with high quantitative pollen and spores counts during those years (Salvaggio et al., 1971). High summer asthma visit rates were associated with high total mold spore counts, particularly counts of Basidiomycete and Deuteromycete spores. High asthma attack rates during September and early October were associated with high mean ragweed pollen concentrations. The largest and most consistent major epidemics in late October and November were associated with high total spore concentrations and apparent high concentrations of amorphous particles resembling decaying vegetable matter. These major "post–ragweed season" epidemics also were strongly correlated with conditions resembling those of thermal inversions, namely high barometric pressure and low wind velocity, temperature, and humidity. From these studies it appears that the asthma epidemics in New Orleans are due to an increase in atmospheric concentration of "natural" environmental allergens as a result of certain climatic conditions, which in turn act on a susceptible atopic asthmatic population.

Climate Therapy

Changing climate as treatment for severe asthma has been advocated since ancient times. In theory, an area with a dry climate with little pollen-producing vegetation, few industries, and a low density of automobiles should be advantageous for the allergic patient. On the other hand, changing climate may facilitate the development of sensitivity to new allergens in a susceptible individual. Unfortunately, there is a paucity of information on the effects of geographic changes on severity of symptoms and the development of new allergies. The multiplicity of environmental factors as well as the marked individual susceptibility to those factors make it almost impossible to prescribe a geographic location favorable for a given patient. For these reasons, recommendation for permanent climatic change for the allergic child seldom is justified. For the occasional instance in which this may be appropriate, it is wise to give the child a trial of several months in the new location before making a final decision about a permanent move.

References

Alarie, Y., Ulrich, C. C., Busey, W. M., Krumm, A. A., and MacFarland, H. N.: Long-term continuous exposure to sulfur dioxide in cynomolgus monkeys. Arch. Environ. Health 24:115, 1972.

Ayres, S. M., and Buehler, M. E.: The effects of urban air pollution on health. Clin. Pharmacol. Ther. 11:337, 1970.

Bar-Or, O., Neuman, I., and Dotan, R.: Effects of dry and humid climates on exercise-induced asthma in children and preadolescents. J. Allergy Clin. Immunol. 60:163, 1977.

Bates, T. V., Bell, G. N., Brunham, D. D., et al.: Short-term effects of ozone on the lung. J. Appl. Physiol. 32:176, 1972.

Bernstein, C., and Klutz, C. D.: Allergy survey in Florida in the light of present knowledge. J. Fla. Med. Assoc. 39:38, 1952.

Blumstein, G. I., Speigelman, J., and Kimbel, P.: Atmospheric ionization in allergic respiratory disease. Arch. Environ. Health 8:818, 1964.

Carnow, B. W., Lepper, M. H., Shekelle, R. B., and Stanler, J.: Chicago air pollution study: SO₂ levels and acute illness in patient with chronic bronchopulmonary disease. Arch. Environ. Health 18:768, 1969.

Cederlof, R., Friberg, L., and Jonsson, E.: Morbidity to uniovular twins in relation to smoking habits and residence. Primary Report. Nord. Hyg. Tidskr. 45:71, 1964.

Cohen, A. A., Bromberg, S., Beuchely, R. W., Heiderscheit, L. T., and Shy, C. M.: Asthma and air pollution from a coal fueled power plant. Am. J. Public Health 62:1181, 1972.

Connell, V. T.: Quantitative intranasal pollen challenges. III. The priming effect in allergic rhinitis. J. Allergy 43:33, 1963.

Davis, J. B.: Review of the scientific information on the effects of ionized air on human beings and animals. Aerospace Med. 34:35, 1963.

DeLucia, A. J., and Adams, W. C.: Effects of O₃ inhalation during exercise on pulmonary function and blood biochemistry. J. Appl. Physiol. 43:75, 1977.

Derrick, E. H.: A comparison between the density of smoke in the Brisbane air and the prevalence of asthma. Med. J. Aust. 2:670, 1970.

Frank, N. R., Amour, M. O., Worchester, J., and Whittenberg, J. L.: Effect of acute controlled exposure to SO_2 on respiratory mechanics in healthy male adults. J. Appl. Physiol. 17:252, 1962.

Fry, J., and Lond, M. D.: Effects of severe fog on a general practice. Lancet 1:235, 1953.

Girsh, L. S., Shubin, E., Dick, C., and Schulander, F. A.: A study on the epidemiology of asthma in children in Philadelphia: The relation of weather and air pollution to peak incidence of asthmatic attacks. J. Allergy 39:347, 1967.

Greenburg, L., Field, F., Reed, J., and Erhardt, C.: Asthma and temperature change: An epidemiological study of emergency clinic visits for asthma in three large New York hospitals. Arch. Environ. Health 12:561, 1966.

Hirst, J. M.: Changes in atmospheric spore content: Diurnal periodicity and the effects of weather. Trans. Br. Mycol. Soc. 36:375, 1953.

Huber, T. E., Joseph, S. W., Knoblock, E., Redfearn, P. L., and Karakawa, J. A.: New environmental respiratory disease (Yokohama asthma). A.M.A. Arch. Ind. Hyg. 10:399, 1954.

Jaffe, L. S.: The biological effects of photochemical air pollutants on man and animals. Am. J. Public Health 57:1269, 1967.

Jones, D. P., O'Connor, S. A., Collins, J. V., and Watson, B. W.: Effect of long term ionized air treatment on patients with bronchial asthma. Thorax 31:427, 1976.

Kornbleuh, I. H., Pierso, G. M., and Seicher, F. P.: Relief from pollinosis in negative ionized rooms. Am. J. Phys. Med. 37:18, 1958.

Krueger, A. P., and Smith, R. F.: The effects of air ions on the living mammalian trachea. J. Gen. Physiol. 42:69, 1958.

Miller, J. S.: Cold air and ventilatory function. Br. J. Dis. Chest 59:23, 1965.

Nadel, J. A., Salem, H., Tamplin, B., and Tokiwa, Y.: Mechanism of bronchoconstriction during inhalation of sulfur dioxide. J. Appl. Physiol. 20:164, 1965.

Oshima, Y., Ishizaki, T., Miyamoto, T., Kabe, J., and Makino, S.: A study of Tokyo-Yokohama asthma among Japanese. Am. Rev. Respir. Dis. 90:632, 1964.

Ramsey, J. M.: Time course of bronchoconstrictive response in asthmatic subjects to reduced temperature. Thorax 32:26, 1977.

Rodriguez, G., Branch, B. L., and Cotton, E. K.: The use of humidity in asthmatic children. J. Allergy and Clin. Immunol. 56:133, 1975.

Rodriquez-Martinez, F., Mascia, A. V., and Mellins, R. B.: The effect of environmental temperature on airway resistance in the asthmatic child. Pediatr. Res. 7:627, 1973.

Rylander, R.: Environmental tobacco smoke effects on the non-smoker. Report from a workshop. Scand. J. Respir. Dis. (Suppl.) 91:1, 1974.

Salvaggio, J., Hassleblad, V., Seabury, J., and Heiderscheit,

L. T.: New Orleans asthma: II. Relationship of climatologic and seasonal factors to outbreaks. J. Allergy 45:257, 1970.

Salvaggio, J. E., and Klein, R. C.: New Orleans asthma: I. Characterization of individuals involved in epidemics. J. Allergy 39:227, 1967.

Salvaggio, J., Seabury, J., and Schoenhardt, E. A.: New Orleans asthma V. Relationship between chairity hospital asthma admission rates, semi-quantitative pollen and fungal spores count, and total particulate aerometric sampling data. J. Allergy Clin. Immunol. 48:96, 1971.

Schoettlin, C. E., and Landau, E.: Air pollution and asthmatic attacks in the Los Angeles area. Public Health Reps. 76:545, 1961.

Schrenck, H. H., Heinmann, H., Clayton, C. D., Gafager, W. M., and Wexler, H.: Air Pollution in Donora, Pa.: Epidemiology of unusual smog episode of October, 1948. Public Health Bull. 306, Washington, D.C., 1948.

Schutzbank, F. B.: Climatotherapy in allergic disease. J.A.M.A. 139:1260, 1949.

Sim, V. M., and Pattle, R. E.: Effects of possible smog irritants on human subjects. J.A.M.A. 165:1908, 1957.

Slavin, R. G., et al.: Guidelines for asthmatic patients during air pollution episodes. J. Allergy Clin. Immunol. 55:222, 1976.

Smith, J. M.: The long term effect of moving on patients with asthma and hay fever. J. Allergy Clin. Immunol. 48:191, 1971.

Speer, F.: Tobacco and the non-smoker. Arch. Environ. Health 16:443, 1968.

Spotnitz, M.: The significance of Yokohama asthma. Am. Rev. Respir. Dis. 92:371, 1965.

Strauss, R. H., McFadden, E. R., Jr., Ingram, R. H., Jr., and Jaeger, J. J.: Enhancement of exercise-induced asthma by cold air breathing. N. Engl. J. Med. 297:743, 1977.

Strauss, R. H., McFadden, E. R., Jr., Ingram. R. H., Jr., Chandler, D. E., Jr., and Jaeger, J. J.: Influence of heat and humidity on the airway obstruction induced by exercise in asthma. J. Clin. Invest. 61:433, 1978.

Taylor, G.: Tobacco smoke allergy — Does it exist? Scand. J. Respir. Dis. 91(Suppl.):10, 1974.

Tremonti, L. P.: Tokyo-Yokohama asthma. Ann. Allergy 28:590, 1970.

Tromp, S. W.: Influence of weather and climate on asthma and bronchitis. Rev. Allergy 22:1027, 1968.

Vaughan, T. R., Jenelle, L. F., and Lewis, T. R.: Long-term exposure to low levels of air pollutants. Arch. Environ. Health 19:45, 1969.

Wells, R., et al.: Effects of cold air on respiratory airflow resistance in patients with respiratory tract disease. N. Engl. J. Med. 263:268, 1960.

Young, W. A., Shaw, D. B., and Bates, D. V.: Effect of low concentrations of ozone on pulmonary function in man. J. Appl. Physiol. 19:765, 1964.

Zeidberg, L. D., Prindle, R. A., and Landau, E.: The Nashville air pollution study: I. Sulphur dioxide and bronchial asthma. Am. Rev. Respir. Dis. 84:489, 1961.

19

J. W. Paisley, M.D.

Infection and Allergy

Contact with microorganisms represents a constant exposure to a large number of foreign antigens. Diseases due to hypersensitivity to microbial antigens and specific infections are dealt with in detail in subsequent chapters. In addition, infection with viruses, bacteria, or other agents causes tissue damage that can precipitate or aggravate allergic disease. This chapter describes the effects of infectious agents on tissue and considers selected aspects of the diagnosis and antimicrobial therapy of common pediatric infections.

TISSUE EFFECTS OF INFECTIOUS AGENTS

Knowledge of the interaction between microorganisms and living cells aids in the understanding of how these agents produce an altered immune state and of the effect of therapy on the associated symptoms.

Bacteria

The tissue-damaging potential of bacteria can be equated roughly with their extraordinary ability to proliferate if given adequate nutrition. The presence of large numbers of organisms, however, does not imply tissue destruction, as evidenced by carriage of billions of organisms in the normal pharynx. Similarly, multiplication within tissue is not a prerequisite for pathogenicity, as evidenced by *Bordetella pertus-*

sis or *Mycoplasma pneumoniae,* whose superficial sites of replication in the respiratory tract belie their destructive potential. The pathogenesis of bacterial disease is related in large part to a wide variety of substances elaborated by or present within pathogenic organisms.

Exotoxins. Exotoxins are polypeptides of varying size that either are elaborated directly into the medium, as with extracellular products of *Staphylococcus aureus,* or represent extensions of the cell wall which are extruded into the medium, as observed with *B. pertussis* (Olson, 1975). One or more exotoxins with varied biologic activities are produced by many bacterial species. Tissue damage by bacteria in many instances is ascribed to the exotoxins elaborated by the infecting organism, although the exact mode of exotoxin action often is unknown.

The enzymatic activities of some exotoxins, e.g., clostridial phospholipase, are well defined. Other exotoxins, however, have been characterized only phenomenologically, such as the lymphocytosis-promoting factor of *B. pertussis.* Some act intracellularly, such as diptheria toxin or *Pseudomonas aeruginosa* exotoxin A, which prevents protein synthesis by inhibition of elongation factor, an enzyme involved in the synthesis of the polypeptide chain (Iglewski and Kabat, 1975). Others act extracellularly, such as the hyaluronidase of group A streptococcus (Ginsburg, 1972).

Cell-damaging effects of toxins may be direct, resulting in rapid cell lysis, as with cell membrane dissolution by clostridial phospholipase, or in delayed cell death, as with interruption of protein synthesis by *Pseudomonas aeurginosa* exotoxin A. Other toxins, however, induce tissue effects indirectly. Examples include the histamine-sensitizing factor of *B. pertussis* and the erythrogenic toxins of group A streptococci, which potentiate the effects of endotoxin and streptolysin O (Ginsburg, 1972). The effect of some exotoxins depends partly on the immune response of the host. For example, the rash of scarlet fever may be produced only in individuals previously sensitized to erythrogenic toxin, a theory that would explain the low incidence of scarlet fever in infancy (Ginsburg, 1972; Kim and Watson, 1972).

The production of exotoxins and their participation in human disease can depend upon several factors, some not directly controlled by the bacteria themselves. Production of diphtheria toxin and *Escherichia coli* enterotoxin, for instance, is mediated through extrachromosomal (phage) DNA, a capacity that can be acquired or lost by individual bacterial strains. Thus, the presence or absence of phage as well as properties of individual bacterial strains dictate the likelihood of pathogenicity of bacteria present. The quantity of toxin production can be strain-dependent, and toxin production also can depend on a variety of environmental factors. A high phosphate concentration in the surrounding medium, for instance, inhibits the elaboration of staphylococcal phospholipase C, whereas high iron concentration inhibits diphtheria toxin production.

Although production and diffusion of exotoxin may be halted by antimicrobial therapy and humoral factors, cell destruction may proceed unaltered once toxin is fixed to tissue. Clinical symptoms may progress, therefore, despite "appropriate" therapy and organism eradication.

Endotoxin. In addition to diffusible toxins, gram-negative organisms contain biologically active substances associated with their outer cell walls. These substances, collectively termed endotoxins, are lipopolysaccharides consisting of an active core (lipid A) and a solubilizing carrier (polysaccharide) (Lüderitz et al., 1973). The pharmacologic effects of endotoxins,

too numerous to review in entirety, include the following: pyrogenicity; potentiation of vascular responses to catecholamine; induction of leukopenia followed by leukocytosis; activation of complement by the classic and alternative pathways; activation of Hageman factor; promotion of platelet aggregation; and action on the peripheral vascular supply resulting in tissue hypoxia, pooling of blood, and decreased intravascular volume (Kass and Wolff, 1973). Despite the numerous biologic effects of endotoxins, their role in human disease remains undefined (Kass et al., 1973).

Indirect Effects Due to Bacteria. As alluded to above, bacteria or their components also may damage tissue indirectly, often through immune mediators. Even in well-studied diseases such as rheumatic fever, the exact mechanism of tissue damage often is not clear. Potentially destructive immune reactions may be initiated either "nonspecifically" (complement activation by endotoxin) or through specific (antigen-antibody) interaction. Once complement is activated, cell destruction may occur directly via cell lysis, or indirectly through the action of lysosomal enzymes liberated by phagocytic cells attracted to the area by anaphylatoxins. Damage from participation of cell-mediated immune mechanisms also may result from lymphocyte cytotoxins. Immune response may intensify local damage caused by infection and, in fact, can be the predominant cause of tissue damage, as, for example, in children with measles who had been previously immunized with killed measles virus vaccine (Bellanti et al., 1969). Tissue damage distant from the site of infection may result from immune reactions to antigen released, as occurs in poststreptococcal glomerulonephritis. Autoimmune tissue destruction may result from antibodies to microbial antigens that cross-react with tissue antigens, although firm evidence for this mechanism in man is lacking (Read and Zabriskie, 1976).

Viruses

Whereas toxins elaborated by bacteria may play a major role in the pathogenesis of bacterial infection, direct cellular invasion is the prerequisite for viral disease.

TABLE 19–1 COMMON VIRAL AGENTS OF HUMAN DISEASE

Family	Species	Examples of Disease
DNA Viruses		
Herpes (>100 nm)	*H. simplex* (types 1,2)	Gingivostomatitis Herpes labialis Encephalitis
	H. zoster	Chickenpox Herpes zoster
	Epstein-Barr	Mononucleosis
	Cytomegalovirus	Mononucleosis-like syndrome Hepatitis Congenital infection
Adeno (50–100 nm)	Adenovirus (Types 1–31)	Respiratory infections Pharyngoconjunctival fever (types 3,7) Epidemic keratoconjunctivitis (type 8) Hemorrhagic cystitis (types 11,21)
Pox (>100 nm)	Variola Cowpox Vaccinia	Smallpox Cowpox Eczema vaccinatum Generalized vaccinia
Papova (<50 nm)	Papilloma	Common warts
Unclassified (<50 nm)	Hepatitis B	Serum hepatitis
RNA Viruses		
Orthomyxo (>100 nm)	Influenza (A,B,C)	Influenza
Paramyxo (>100 nm)	Parainfluenza (types 1–4)	Colds Croup Pneumonia
	Mumps	Parotitis Meningoencephalitis
	Measles	Rubeola
	Respiratory syncytial virus	Colds Bronchiolitis Pneumonia
Corona (50–100 nm)	Several types	Colds
Toga (50–100 nm)	Rubella Arbo (over 350 types)	German measles Equine encephalitis
Reo (50–100 nm)	Rotavirus	Infantile gastroenteritis
Picorna (<50 nm)	Polio (types 1–3)	Nonspecific febrile illness Paralytic polio
	ECHO (types 1–34)	Upper respiratory infection Aseptic meningitis
	Coxsackie (types A1–24, B1–6)	Hand-foot-mouth (type A-16, others) Herpangina (types A-2,4,5,6,8,10) Myocarditis
	Rhinovirus (over 113 types)	Colds
Unclassified (<50 nm)	Hepatitis A	"Infectious" hepatitis

Common viral agents and examples of human disease are listed in Table 19-1. As in the case of bacteria, viruses can damage tissue directly or indirectly.

The earliest event in viral infection is attachment to cell membranes, which in itself may result in lysis or fusion of cells. This is exemplified by the effect of paramyxoviruses on erythrocytes (Oldstone and Dixon, 1976). Inhibition of normal cell protein and messenger RNA synthesis also may be an early event. Preformed and newly synthesized viral proteins block polypeptide synthesis (Holland, 1967; Penman and Summers, 1965). With subsequent impairment of normal homeostasis and membrane stability, cell death may occur. Replication, assembly, and release of virions often correlate pathologically with cellular swelling, nuclear degeneration, and cell rupture. Cytopathic viruses also may cause leakage of cell lysosomal enzymes into the cytoplasm (Allison. 1967).

As a concomitant of cellular infection, viruses may produce alterations in cell membrane antigens, with the result that they are then viewed as "foreign" by the host. This leads to antibody production and sensitization of lymphocytes to these antigens and potential immunologically mediated tissue damage. Circulating antigen-antibody complexes have been found in various animal and human virus or virus-related infections, including hepatitis B and Epstein-Barr virus infections, and subacute sclerosing panencephalitis (Oldstone and Dixon, 1976). Their potential role in producing clinical symptoms such as arthritis and rash has been emphasized in hepatitis B infection (Alpert et al., 1971; Brzosko et al., 1974).

The importance of the participation of the complement system in some viral diseases is illustrated by the mouse model of lymphocytic choriomeningitis virus (LCM) infection. In contrast to normal mice challenged with LCM, mice rendered complement-deficient by cobra venom do not succumb to LCM challenge despite documented viral replication, specific antibody production, and the presence of sensitized immune cells (Oldstone and Dixon, 1971). In this same model, cell-mediated immunity also appears to play an important role in tissue damage. Irradiated or other-

wise immunosuppressed mice infected with LCM do not develop the severe disease seen in normal animals (Gilden et al., 1972). Both complement-dependent and independent chemotactic factors may be elaborated by virus-infected cells.

Viruses capable of latent infection may be associated with reactivation disease and persistent antigenic stimulation (Chang, 1971; NIH Workshop, 1976). Examples of latent viruses include members of the herpes family. Subacute sclerosing panencephalitis appears to represent reactivation of latent measles virus.

Other Microorganisms

Mechanisms of tissue damage similar to those described for bacteria and viruses are involved in infections due to many other agents, including fungi, parasites, and rickettsiae. Due in part to the slower propagation of some of these organisms, tissue destruction may be predominantly immune system–mediated. Two such syndromes, allergic bronchopulmonary aspergillosis and hypersensitivity pneumonitis related to fungal antigens, are discussed in Chapters 45 and 47.

CONSIDERATIONS IN DIAGNOSIS

Viral Infections

Due to the difficulty of routinely identifying viral pathogens, "viral infection" has been a wastebasket diagnosis for a variety of symptom complexes. An accurate etiologic diagnosis often can be made based on a particular clinical syndrome: the classic childhood exanthems or the typical distribution of vesicular lesions in Coxsackie hand-foot-mouth disease are examples. Immediate laboratory confirmation of viral infection occasionally can be obtained from cytologic studies, e.g., the presence of multinucleated giant cells in lesions due to herpes simplex. More often, however, a nonspecific clinical syndrome and the lack of simple diagnostic tests combine to preclude presumptive identification of the etiologic agent.

Culture of viruses in laboratory-adapted,

TABLE 19–2 SELECTED VIRUSES AND MYCOPLASMA ASSOCIATED WITH PEDIATRIC DISEASES

Disease	H. simplex	Parainfluenza	Influenza	RSV	Coronavirus	Adenovirus	Rhinovirus	Enterovirus	Rotavirus	M. pneumoniae	Comment
Febrile exanthem	±		±	±		++		+++		±	Erythema multiforme may be associated with M. pneumoniae.
Conjunctivitis	±					++		±			Nonspecific. mild conjunctivitis may be seen with a variety of respiratory infections.
Otitis media		±	±	+		±	±	±		±	Although often associated with upper respiratory infection, virus isolation from middle ear fluid is rare. M. pneumoniae usually causes bullous myringitis.
Pharyngitis	+	+				++	+	+		++	May also be caused by Epstein-Barr virus.
Vesicular exanthem	++							+++			
Cold		++	++	+	+	++	+++	++		+	
Laryngotracheobronchitis		+++	+	+		+	±	±		+	
Bronchiolitis		+	+	+++		+	+	±		+	
Pneumonia, viral		+++	+	+++		+	±	±		++	Common agents are viruses in infants, M. pneumoniae in older children.
Gastroenteritis, viral		±	±	±		±		+	+++	++	Nonspecific symptoms may be seen with a variety of respiratory viral infections, especially in infants.

*Symbols (± to +++) denote relative frequency of association of each agent with the disease entities.
References: Gardner, 1971; Glezen et al., 1967; Glezen et al., 1971; Goodwin et al., 1967; Shurin et al., 1978; Loda et al., 1968; Tilles et al., 1967; Zapikian et al., 1976.

living cell lines allows accurate diagnosis of many infections. The rapidity with which some viruses produce characteristic cytopathic effect in tissue culture (e.g., within 1 to 2 days for herpes simplex) makes viral culture a practical diagnostic tool for infections due to these agents. Growth of virus in tissue culture has potential therapeutic benefit as well, as antiviral drugs become available. Difficulties of routine viral culturing include the requirement for a specialized laboratory, the markedly greater expense compared to bacterial cultures, and the prolonged incubation time required for some agents (e.g., 4 weeks or longer may be necessary for the demonstration of cytomegalovirus). Recent new techniques, however, may play an important future role in the routine diagnosis of viral infections. These include direct visualization of virions in clinical specimens by electron microscopy and demonstration of viral antigens by fluorescent antibody staining of infected cells or by sensitive immunologic techniques such as the enzyme-linked immunosorbent assay (ELISA) (McIntosh et al., 1978; Hsiung, 1977).

The problems encountered in diagnosing mycoplasmal infections are similar to those of viral infections. The lack both of sensitivity and specificity of the cold agglutinin response in mycoplasmal infections in children has been emphasized (Clyde and Denny, 1967).

Bacterial Infections

The problem faced by the clinician dealing with bacterial infection is the opposite of that posed by viral disease. Instead of not being able to identify any pathogen, one often discovers too many. Bacteria play three roles in diseased tissue: *colonizer*, proliferating without producing damage; *secondary invader*, damaging previously abnormal tissue; and *primary invader*,

TABLE 19–3 NORMAL MICROBIAL FLORA FOUND IN VARIOUS BODY SITES

Skin*
- *Staphylococcus epidermidis*
- *S. aureus*
- *Propionibacterium acnes*
- *Lactobacillus* spp.
- *Corynebacterium* spp.
- Enterobacteriaceae
- *Candida* spp.

Conjunctiva
- *S. epidermidis*
- *S. aureus*
- *Streptococcus pneumoniae*
- *Viridans streptococci*
- *Lactobacillus* spp.
- *Corynebacterium* spp.
- *Neisseria* spp.
- *Hemophilus influenzae*

Middle ear
- None

Sinus
- None

Nasopharynx-throat
- *S. epidermidis*
- *S. aureus*
- *Viridans streptococci*
- *St. pneumoniae*
- *Lactobacillus* spp.
- *Corynebacterium* spp.
- *Neisseria* spp.
- *Hemophilus influenzae*
- Enterobacteriaceae

Anaerobes
- *Candida* spp.
- *Treponema* spp.
- *Herpes simplex*
- Adenoviruses

Lower respiratory tract
- None

Small intestine†
- *S. epidermidis*
- Group D streptococci (including enterococci)
- *Viridans streptococci*
- *Neisseria* spp.
- *Hemophilus* spp.
- Enterobacteriaceae
- Anaerobes
- *Candida* spp.

Large intestine
- *S. epidermidis*
- *S. aureus*
- Group D streptococci (enterococci, other)
- *Lactobacillus* spp.
- *Corynebacterium* spp.
- Enterobacteriaceae
- Anaerobes (including *Bacteroides, Clostridium* spp.)
- *Candida* spp.
- *Entamoeba coli*
- *Endolimax nana*
- *Trichomonas hominis*
- Adenoviruses
- Enteroviruses

*Compared to older children and adults, isolation frequency in infants is lower for *Corynebacterium* spp., higher for *S. aureus* and enterobacteriaceae.

†Progressing from duodenum to lower ileum, one obtains (1) fewer sterile cultures, (2) fewer oral flora, (3) more enterobacteriaceae, (4) higher organism concentrations.

References: Locatcher-Khorazo and Seegal, 1972; Skinner and Carr, 1974.

TABLE 19–4 COMMON BACTERIA, FUNGI, AND PARASITES ASSOCIATED WITH PEDIATRIC INFECTIONS

Infection	Streptococcus, group A	St. pneumoniae	S. aureus	S. epidermidis	N. gonorrhea	H. influenzae, non–type b	H. influenzae, type b	B. pertussis	Enterobacteriaceae	Anaerobes	M. pneumoniae	Chlamydia trachomatis	Candida spp.	Comments
Pyoderma	+++		+++											Bullous impetigo usually due to *S. aureus*.
Conjunctivitis Newborn[b]		+++	+		+				±			++		Inclusion body conjunctivitis caused by *Chlamydia*.
Infant and child	+'	++	+	+		++								
Otitis media[a] Newborn		+++	+	±		++			++					
Infant and child	+	+++	±			++	+		±	±				Chronic otitis media more often associated with staphylococci, anaerobes, and enterobacteriaceae.
Sinusitis[c]	±	+++	+			++			±	+				Anaerobes more common in chronic infections. Viral isolations include rhinovirus, influenza, parainfluenza.
Pharyngitis	+++										+		+	Thrush usually seen in infants or children on antibiotics.
Epiglottitis	+						+++							
Laryngotracheo-bronchitis	±		±				±							Vast majority of cases are viral.
Pneumonia, bacterial	+	+++	+				++	++			++	+		*C. trachomatis* and *B. pertussis* pneumonia primarily seen in young infants (<1 yr), *M. pneumoniae* in older children (>5 yr.).

[a] Diagnosed by tympanocentesis
[b] Newborn, <6 wks.; infant, 6 wks–2 yrs; child, >2 yrs
[c] Diagnosed by direct needle aspiration; data from older children, adults

TABLE 19–4. COMMON BACTERIA, FUNGI, AND PARASITES ASSOCIATED WITH PEDIATRIC INFECTIONS (Continued)

Infection	Streptococcus, group A	Streptococcus, group B	Streptococcus, group D[d]	St. pneumoniae	S. aureus	Listeria monocytogenes	N. gonorrhea	N. meningitidis	H. influenzae, type b	E. coli	Shigella	Salmonella	Yersinia enterocolitica	Enterobacteriaceae,[e] other	Campylobacter fetus	Giardia lamblia	Entamoeba histolytica	Comments
Meningitis Newborn	+	+++				+				++		+		+				Most common E. coli serotype is K1.
Infant and child				++	++			++	+++			±		±				Incidence of H. influenzae low after age 5 years.
Septic arthritis Newborn		+++			+		+			+		+		+				
Infant				±	+++			±	+++									N. gonorrhea primarily is sexually active age group.
Child	+			±	+++		++	±	+			±						
Osteomyelitis Newborn		+			+++		±			±		±		±				
Infant and child	+				+++				±			±						Chronic osteomyelitis usually S. aureus. Sickle cell anemia patients prone to Salmonella infections
Gastroenteritis, bacterial					±					+	+++	+++	+		+	+	+	Enterotoxins may be produced by E. coli, other organisms.
Cystitis, Pyelonephritis			+							+++		±		+				

[d]Includes enterococci
[e]Including Pseudomonas spp
[f]Excludes food poisoning
(From Axelsson and Bronson, 1973; Eichenwald and McCracken, 1978; Feingold et al, 1966; Shurin et al., 1978.)

damaging previously normal tissue. Intelligent therapeutic decisions necessitate differentiating between colonizing and invading organisms. Colonizing organisms usually need not be and often cannot be eradicated by antimicrobial therapy.

If the organism comes from a normally sterile site, such as the middle ear or blood, this distinction is rather easy to make. It is difficult or impossible, however, if the organism is cultured from a normally nonsterile site. The overlap between commensal and potentially pathogenic organisms is seen in Tables 19–2, 19–3 and 19–4. Identifying an organism as a pathogen, therefore, requires the fulfillment of at least one of several criteria:

1. Identification of an organism that is essentially never a commensal (e.g., *Corynebacterium diphtheriae* in the throat)

2. Isolation of an organism from a normally sterile site without contamination of the specimen

3. Histologic demonstration of tissue invasion by the organism

4. Demonstration of substances produced by an organism in sites distant from its site of replication (e.g., circulating botulinal toxin or *Hemophilus influenzae* type b antigenuria in a patient with pneumonia)

5. Demonstration of a specific serologic response to the organism

In clinical practice, identification of a pathogen usually is based on one of the first two criteria.

Proper specimen collecting is of paramount importance in the diagnosis of bacterial disease. Cultures of the respiratory tract are the best example of specimens invariably contaminated with normal flora. Examples include nasopharyngeal culture for the diagnosis of otitis media (Feingold et al., 1966), sinusitis (Axelsson and Bronson, 1973), or pneumonia (Mimica et al., 1971), and poorly collected sputum specimens for the diagnosis of pneumonia (Davidson et al., 1976). Organisms isolated from these specimens correlate poorly with organisms proven by more invasive sampling techniques to be responsible for local disease.

Interpretation of diagnostic bacterial cultures requires knowledge of the normal microbial flora. A partial list of "normal" indigenous organisms is presented in Table 19–3. Many potential pathogens, such as *H.*

influenzae type b, are not considered normal flora but may colonize healthy children transiently without causing disease (Michaels et al., 1976). Conversely, "normal" flora frequently is cultured in such common diseases as nonstreptococcal respiratory infections (Hable et al., 1971).

A variety of abnormal clinical states may alter indigenous flora without producing overt symptoms. Enterobacteria often colonize the skin and throat in hospitalized patients. Antibiotic therapy favors growth of yeast and resistant bacteria. Intestinal stasis and incompetence of the ileocecal valve may result in generalized bacterial overgrowth in the small bowel. Thus, a patient's clinical state must be taken into account when interpreting culture results.

It is apparent from the above considerations that one often cannot identify the exact etiologic agent of an infection associated with a normally nonsterile site or requiring a diagnostic procedure considered too invasive for routine use. Initial antimicrobial therapy, therefore, is directed against the most likely pathogens. Suggested drugs for selected pediatric infections are presented in Table 19–5. A comprehensive review of this subject has been recently published (Eichenwald and McCracken, 1978).

Use of antimicrobials as a "placebo" or for infections that are likely due to viruses — such as the common cold — is poor medical practice. Complications of antimicrobial therapy include idiosyncratic reactions, drug toxicity, drug allergy, disruption of protective normal flora, and induction of resistance in the microbial population. The emergence of ampicillin-resistant *H. influenzae* exemplifies the latter problem. In general, the more toxic or less studied the antimicrobial, the more specific are the indications for its use. In pediatrics a prime example is chloramphenicol, which is indicated for severe disease due to ampicillin-resistant *H. influenzae* type b but contraindicated for the routine treatment of otitis media.

Antimicrobial dosages in pediatrics vary with the severity of disease, the child's age and weight, and his ability to metabolize or excrete the drug. Recommended dosages of some common antimicrobials in children with normal renal and hepatic function are presented in Table 19–6.

TABLE 19–5 ANTIMICROBIAL TREATMENT OF COMMON PEDIATRIC INFECTIONS

| Infection | Classification | Antimicrobial[a] | |
		PRIMARY	ALTERNATIVE
Pyoderma	Impetigo	Penicillin	Erythromycin
	Bullous impetigo	Dicloxacillin	Cephalosporin
Otitis media[b]	Newborn	Ampicillin and aminoglycoside[c]	
	Child	Ampicillin	Penicillin (or erythromycin) and sulfonamide
Sinusitis		Ampicillin	Penicillin (or erythromycin) and sulfonamide
Pharyngitis		Penicillin	Erythromycin
Epiglottitis		Ampicillin[d]	Chloramphenicol
Pneumonia	Infant	Ampicillin[d]	Chloramphenicol
	Child		
	lobar	Penicillin	Cephalosporin
	diffuse	Erythromycin	Tetracycline
Meningitis	Neonate	Ampicillin and aminoglycoside	Chloramphenicol and aminoglycoside
	Child	Ampicillin and chloramphenicol	
Septic arthritis and osteomyelitis	Infant	Ampicillin[d] and oxacillin[e]	Chloramphenicol and oxacillin
	Child	Oxacillin	Cephalosporin
Gastroenteritis	*Shigella*	Trimethoprim-sulfamethoxazole	Ampicillin
	Salmonella[f]	Ampicillin	Chloramphenicol
Cystitis and Pyelonephritis		Sulfonamide	Ampicillin

[a]In all cases, therapy should be governed by results of gram stains of appropriate specimens, cultures, and susceptibility tests.

[b]Tympanocentesis indicated in newborns and in treatment failures.

[c]Gentamicin is currently the best-studied aminoglycoside for pediatric use, with the broadest range of activity in most areas of the country.

[d]In areas where ampicillin-resistant *H. influenzae* type b is prevalent, initial therapy of severe infections should include chloramphenicol.

[e]Nafcillin and methicillin are alternative agents.

[f]Treatment indicated only for neonates, severely ill children, or those infected with *S. typhi*. If ampicillin resistance is prevalent, chloramphenicol should be used.

TABLE 19-6 PEDIATRIC DOSAGES OF COMMON ANTIMICROBIALS

Antimicrobial	Route[a]	Dosage NEWBORN[b] (mg/kg/day)	Dosage CHILD (mg/kg/day)	(gm/day maximum)	Comment/Toxicity
Penicillin G, aqueous	P	65–150 q6–12[c] (200,000 units = 125 mg)	30–150 q4	12.0	
Penicillin G, procaine	P	30 q24	65–375 q12–24	1.5	
Penicillin, phenoxymethyl	O	–[d]	30–125 q6	4.0	
Ampicillin	O	–	50–100 q6–8	4.0	Rash, diarrhea
	P	100–200 q8–12	100–300 q4–6	14.0	
Amoxicillin	O	–	20–40 q6–8	8.0	Less diarrhea than ampicillin
Carbenicillin	P	225–400 q6–8	400–600 q2–4	36.0	Bleeding diathesis, hepatotoxicity
Methicillin	P	50–150 q8–12	100–300 q4–6	12.0	Nephrotoxicity, hemorrhagic cystitis, neutropenia
Oxacillin	P	50–150 q8–12	50–150 q4–6	6.0	Nephrotoxicity, hemorrhagic cystitis, neutropenia
Dicloxacillin	O	–	25–100 q6	4.0	
Cephalothin	P	40–60 q8–12	100–300 q4–6	12.0	
Cefazolin	P	–	25–100 q6	6.0	Longer half-life, less phlebitis than cephalothin
Cephalexin	O	–	40–100 q6	4.0	
Erythromycin	O	–	30–50 q6	4.0	Estolate may produce hepatotoxicity in older children
Tetracycline[e]	O	–	20–40 q6	2.0	Few indications in pediatrics Teeth staining, nephrotoxicity
	P	–	15–25 q12	0.3	
Clindamycin	O	–	10–25 q6–8	2.0	Primarily for severe infections due to penicillin-resistant *Bacteroides* spp. Pseudomembranous colitis
	P	–	15–40 q6	5.0	
Chloramphenicol	O	25–50 q12–24	50–100 q6	4.0	Reversible bone marrow suppression; aplastic anemia; cardiovascular collapse in neonates Blood levels must be monitored
	P	25–50 q12–24	50–100 q6	4.0	
Sulfonamide[f]	O	–	100–150 q6	6.0	Crystalluria, hematuria, rashes
Trimethoprim/ Sulfamethoxazole	O	–	5–20[g] q8–12	0.64	Neutropenia, thrombocytopenia (also, see sulfonamide)
Kanamycin	P	15–30 q8–12	15–30 q8	1.5	Nephrotoxicity, ototoxicity
Amikacin	P	15–22.5 q8–12	15–22.5 q8	1.5	Limited data on the use of tobramycin, amikacin in neonates
Gentamicin	P	5–7.5 q8–12	6–7.5 q6–8	0.4	Blood levels must be monitored for
Tobramycin	P	4–6 q8–12	5–7.5 q6–8	0.4	optimal therapy.

[a]P = parenteral, O = oral.

[b]Age less than 4 weeks. Lowest dose and longest interval are suggested for infants under 2000 gm birth weight and less than 7 days age. Higher values for larger, older neonates.

[c]Suggested frequency of administration. (Divide total daily dose listed into 2 to 6 doses, depending upon dosage frequency recommended).

[d](–) means drug not generally indicated and/or dosage not well established.

[e]Tetracycline, oxytetracycline, chlortetracycline.

[f]Sulfasoxazole, sulfadiazine, triple sulfa.

[g]Numbers refer to the dosage of trimethoprim in the fixed combination.

References

Allison, A.: Lysosomes in virus-infected cells. Perspect. Virol. *5*:29, 1967.

Alpert, E., Isselbacher, K.J., and Schur, P.H.: The pathogenesis of arthritis associated with viral hepatitis. N. Engl. J. Med. *285*:185, 1971.

Axelsson, A., and Bronson, J.E.: The correlation between bacteriological findings in the nose and maxillary sinus in acute maxillary sinusitis. Laryngoscope *82*:2003, 1973.

Bellanti, J.A., Sanga, R.L., Klutinis, B., Brandt, B., and Artenstein, M.S.: Antibody responses in serum and nasal secretions of children immunized with inactivated and attenuated measles-virus vaccines. N. Engl. J. Med. *280*:628, 1969.

Brzosko, W.J., Krawczynski, K., Nazarewicz, T., Morzycka, M., and Nowoslawski, A.: Glomerulonephritis associated with hepatitis-B surface antigen immune complexes in children. Lancet *2*:477, 1974.

Chang, Te-Wen: Recurrent viral infection. N. Engl. J. Med. *284*:765, 1971.

Clyde, W.A., and Denny, F.W.: Mycoplasma infections in childhood. Pediatrics *40*:669, 1967.

Davidson, M., Tempest, B., and Palmer, D.L.: Bacteriologic diagnosis of acute pneumonia. J.A.M.A. *235*:158, 1976.

Eichenwald, H.F., and McCracken, G.H.: Antimicrobial therapy in infants and children. J. Pediatr. *93*:337, 1978.

Feingold, M., Klein, J.O., Haslam, G.E., Tilles, J.G., Finland, M., and Gellis, S.S.: Acute otitis media in children. Am. J. Dis. Child. *111*:361, 1966.

Gardner, P.S.: Acute respiratory virus infections of childhood. *In* Banatvala, J.E. (ed.): *Current Problems in Clinical Virology*. Edinburgh, Churchill-Livingstone, 1971, pp. 1–32.

Gilden, D., Cole, G., Monjan, A., and Nathanson, N.: Immunopathogenesis of acute central nervous system disease produced by lymphocytic choriomeningitis. Parts I, II. J. Exp. Med. *135*:860, 874, 1972.

Ginsburg, I.: Mechanisms of cell and tissue injury induced by group A streptococci: Relation to post-streptococcal sequelae. J. Infect. Dis. *126*:294, 1972.

Glezen, W.P., Loda, F.A., Clyde, W.A., Senior, R.S., Sheaffer, C.I., Conley, W.G., and Denny, F.W.: Epidemiologic patterns of acute lower respiratory disease of children in a pediatric group practice. J. Pediatr. *78*:397, 1971.

Glezen, W.P., Clyde, W.A., Senior, R.J., Sheaffer, C.I., and Denny, F.W.: Group A streptococci, mycoplasmas and viruses associated with acute pharyngitis. J.A.M.A. *202*:119, 1967.

Goodwin, M.H., Love, G.J., Mackel, D.C., Berquist, K.R., and Ganelin, R.S.: Observations on the association of enteric viruses and bacteria with diarrhea. Am. J. Trop. Med. Hygiene *16*:178, 1967.

Hable, K.A., Washington, J.A., and Herrman, E.C.: Bacterial and viral throat flora. Clin. Pediatr. *10*:199, 1971.

Holland, J.: Inhibition of host-cell macromolecular synthesis by high multiplicities of poliovirus under conditions preventing virus synthesis. J. Mol. Biol. *8*:574, 1967.

Hsiung, G.D.: Laboratory diagnosis of viral infections: General principles and recent developments. Mount Sinai J. Med. *44*:1, 1977.

Iglewski, B.H., and Kabat, D.: NAD-dependent inhibition of protein synthesis by *Pseudomonas aeruginosa* toxin. Proc. Natl. Acad. Sci. USA *72*:2284, 1975.

Kass, E.H., and Wolff, S.M. (eds.): Bacterial lipopolysaccharides: Chemistry, biology and clinical significance of endotoxins. J. Infect. Dis. *128*(Suppl.):S1, 1973.

Kass, E.H., Porter, P.J., McGill, M.W., and Vivaldi, E.: Clinical and experimental observations on the significance of endotoxemia. J. Infect. Dis. *128*(Suppl.):S299, 1973.

Kim, Y.B., and Watson, D.W.: Streptococcal exotoxins: Biological and pathological properties. *In* Wannamaker, L.W., and Matsen, J.M. (eds.): *Streptococci and Streptococcal Diseases*. New York, Academic Press, 1972, pp. 34–49.

Locatcher-Khorazo, D., and Seegal, B.C.: *Microbiology of the Eye*. St. Louis, C.V. Mosby Co., 1972, pp. 13–23, 63–76.

Loda, F.A., Clyde, W.A., Glezen, W.P., and Senior, R.J.: Studies on the role of viruses, bacteria and *M. pneumoniae* as causes of lower respiratory tract infections in children. J. Pediatr. *72*:161, 1968.

Lüderitz, O., Galanos, C., Lehmann, V., Nurminen, M., Rietschel, E.T., Rosenfelder, G., Simon, M., and Westphal, O.: Lipid A: Chemical structure and biological activity. J. Infect. Dis. *128*(Suppl.):17, 1973.

McIntosh, K., Wilfert, C., Chernesky, M., Plotkin, S., and Mattheis, M.J.: Summary of a workshop on new and useful methods in viral diagnosis. J. Infect. Dis. *138*:414, 1978.

Michaels, R.H., Poziviak, C.S., Stonebreaker, F.E., and Norden, C.W.: Factors affecting pharyngeal *Haemophilus influenzae* type b colonization rates in children. J. Clin. Microbiol. *4*:413, 1976.

Mimica, J., Donoso, E., Howard, J.E., and Lederman, G.W.: Lung puncture in the etiological diagnosis of pneumonia. Am. J. Dis. Child. *122*:278, 1971.

National Institutes of Health Workshop: Current understanding of persistent viral infections and their implications in human disease — summary of a workshop. J. Infect. Dis. *133*:707, 1976.

Oldstone, M.B.A., and Dixon, F.J.: Acute viral infection: Tissue injury mediated by anti-viral antibody through a complement effector system. J. Immunol. *107*:1274, 1971.

Oldstone, M.B.A., and Dixon, F.J.: Immunopathology of viral infections. *In* Miescher, P.A., and Müller-Eberhard, H.J. (eds.): *Textbook of Immunopathology*. New York, Grune and Stratton, 1976, pp. 303–314.

Olson, L.C.: Pertussis. Medicine *54*:427, 1975.

Penman, S., and Summers, D.: Effects on host-cell metabolism following synchronous infection with polio virus. Virology *27*:614, 1965.

Read, S.E., and Zabriskie, J.B.: Immunological concepts in rheumatic fever pathogenesis. *In* Miescher, P.A., and Müller-Eberhard, H.J. (eds.) *Textbook of Immunopathology*. New York, Grune and Stratton, 1976, pp. 471–488.

Shurin, P.A., Howie, V.M., Pelton, S.I., Ploussard, J.H., and Klein, J.O.: Bacterial etiology of otitis media during the first six weeks of life. J. Pediatr. *92*:893, 1978.

Skinner, F.A., and Carr, J.G.: *The Normal Microbial Flora of Man*. London, Academic Press, 1974.

Tilles, J.G., Klein, J.O., Jao, R.L., Haslam, J.E., Feingold, M., Gellis, S.S., and Finland, M.: Acute otitis media in children. N. Engl. J. Med. *277*:613, 1967.

Zapikian, A.Z., Kim, H.W., Wyatt, R.G., Cline, W.L., Arrobio, J.O., Brandt, C.D., Rodriguez, W.J., Sack, D.A., Chanock, R.M., and Parrott, R.H.: Human reovirus-like agent as the major pathogen associated with "winter" gastroenteritis in hospitalized infants and young children. N. Engl. J. Med. *294*:965, 1976.

20

William A. Howard, M.D.

Medical Evaluation

The expanding concept of the diseases of hypersensitivity necessitates a more studied approach to patients with problems in this general area. Concern is not only with the problems of so-called Type I reactions of immediate hypersensitivity, usually IgE mediated, but with cytotoxic and cytolytic reactions, antigen-antibody complex disease, delayed hypersensitivity or cellular immune responses, and response to certain drugs and infectious agents. Sorting out these problems is the initial step in managing the patient with suspected allergy.

THE ALLERGY HISTORY

History-taking is probably one of the most sophisticated investigative techniques in medicine. To take an adequate history requires training, practice, skill, knowledge, understanding, empathy, and above all, patience. There is no substitute for a proper history, and it is no exaggeration to state that in the field of allergy it is the single most important tool available in establishing a diagnosis. There has been a tendency toward using forms, questionnaires, and computer printouts as aids to history taking; while such techniques may save time, there is no evidence that they produce a better history. Printed forms or outlines, many developed by pediatric allergists, will be useful in making certain that no part of the allergy history

is overlooked and will be invaluable in the clinic situation, where the quality of the history may vary widely, but only the physician can develop a historical pattern of illness in the patient that will be meaningful to him and helpful in management. The personal contact with the patient, the chance to observe the child's behavior, and to watch parent-child interactions, will be almost as important in the final summation as the medical information obtained.

As befits the most important part of the work-up, adequate time must be allowed for the full development of the history. The informant must never be made to feel hurried or under pressure, and must be encouraged to explore any parts of the history or respond to questions in a manner that will facilitate recognition and remembrance of the important parts of the story. The physician may wish to indicate the adequacy and reliability of the informant if this will have a bearing on the value of the information obtained.

The Chief Complaint

A chief complaint should be succinct, in as few words as possible, preferably using the informant's own expressions. Much can be learned from a parent's description of a child's presenting complaint, which may be more informative than a single term such as "asthma." If there is more than one presenting problem, they may be listed in the order of appearance, or perhaps in the order of severity, depending on the relationships between the complaints. Although there will be additional opportunities to explore temporal relationships, it is sometimes helpful to indicate the length of time the ailment has been present, or perhaps the year in which it was first noted.

The Present Illness

This is the portion of the history devoted to establishing the pattern of the patient's problems. The informant may not be able to give the information in just the sequence desired and may tend to ramble. Trying to keep the historian on target may be difficult, if not impossible, especially when the history is complicated or covers a long period of time. In such instances it is better to allow the patient free rein, only later filling in the gaps and creating coherence by careful questioning. Free association by the parent often brings out details that might have been omitted in a strict question and answer format.

Many histories will have definite beginnings, are relatively easy to follow, and make for a concise record. In others, the onset is indefinite and may date back to infancy or early childhood. In such instances it may be helpful to start the informant off with recollections of prenatal and perinatal problems, followed by a delineation of the infant's progress into his present complaint. This can be a useful procedure since one almost invariably learns much about the family and its background, creating a solid foundation on which to build a history.

Eventually it will be necessary to incorporate certain basic facts into the narrative. It is essential to know the details of the onset, and the circumstances surrounding the beginnings of the problem. These may include delineation of the patient's symptoms with respect to time of onset, both seasonal and time of day, location, special circumstances or exposures, the role of infection, frequency of occurrence, previous treatment and responses to medication, triggering factors, and any emotional impact on the child and his family. To complete the present illness it is necessary to summarize the child's immediate condition, and if possible, to indicate the family's reasons for seeking an allergy evaluation.

The Past History

Customarily, the past history is built around a review of systems, and enables the physician to uncover additional problems of medical significance, whether or not associated with the allergic complaints. However, it may be even more useful as a tool for filling in any gaps in the patient's story. One may elaborate on leads uncovered earlier so that the two elements, present illness and past history, together give a clear picture of the patient's medical problems.

The Family History

Here, interest not only centers on the immediate family but should also include the kindred known to the informant. The initial family history is often incomplete and unreliable, and in many instances the informant will volunteer additional information on a subsequent visit, after having had an opportunity to question other members of the family.

The principal queries will deal with the presence of allergies in other members of the family, since we consider allergy to be a heritable trait. Figures usually given suggest that if there is a unilateral family history of allergy, there is a 35 percent chance of allergy in the offspring; with a bilateral family history the chance increases to 65 percent. One should remember that the first indications of allergy, although commonly appearing at an early age, may be manifest at any time, and may not appear in the immediate family until after the proband presents with allergy.

A careful search should be made for other problems with an immune component, such as connective tissue diseases, autoimmune phenomena, and malignancy. Immunodeficiency states may be indicated by severe and unexplained illnesses or deaths in the family, especially those occurring in the first year of life. Cardiovascular-renal diseases in the family may be of importance, as may be the occurrence of recurrent or unusual infections.

The Environmental History

This is a unique and important element of history taking in the allergic individual, since many, perhaps all, of his allergens will be found somewhere in his surroundings, whether at home, school, work, or play. The significance of the environmental history may best be illustrated by the fact that it may be sufficient to establish the diagnosis; and elimination of the offending substance may be, in some instances, the only treatment required.

Environment includes the patient's room, the home, the neighborhood, the homes of friends and playmates, the school and its environs, the location of a part-time job, and even the family car. Materials used in the pursuit of hobbies or at work or play may prove to be significant sources of trouble. Table 20–1 lists a convenient environmental check list.

Environmental control measures will increase the likelihood of good results from specific immunotherapy with environmental allergens and should be an integral part of

TABLE 20–1 ENVIRONMENTAL HISTORY

Home
  Location: city, suburb, rural
  Renter or owner
  Outdoor factors: landscaping, flowering and pollinating plants in area
  Age of home; length of time in house (months, years)

Construction
  Type: frame, brick, other
  Basement: finished, unfinished, earth, none
  Crawl space: presence of vapor barrier

Heating and cooling
  Type: forced air, electric baseboard, space heater or wall furnace, radiator, fireplaces, other
  With *forced air:* type of filter (none, fiberglas, permanent, electrostatic) and frequency of filter change
  Cooling system: central, window, swamp

Mold and moisture
  Condensation or mildew: windows, walls, bath, basement, none
  Humidifiers: furnace, coldmist, steam (determine frequency of cleaning)
  Exhaust fans: kitchen, bathrooms

Clothes dryer
  Location: separate room, garage, kitchen, basement, porch, other
  Vent: outside, crawl space, none, other

Cleaning
  Vacuum: upright, canister
  Type of vacuum bag: permanent, disposable
  Other: broom, dry mop, wet mop

Patient's bedroom
  Location: basement, main floor, upper floor
  Number of children sharing room
  Flooring: Wood, tile or linoleum, area rug, wall to wall carpet
    Rug: Wool, cotton, synthetic, fiber, shag, pile
    Pad: felt, rubberized felt, rubber, synthetic, unknown, none
  Windows: curtains, drapes, shades, blinds, none
  Heating vent: near bed, opposite side room, none
  Beds (consider all beds in room):
    Mattress: innerspring, foam

  Springs: box or coil
  Beddings: synthetic, wool, cotton, other
  Pillow: feather, foam, synthetic, other
  Mattress pad: cotton, synthetic
  Spread: linty, nonlinty
  Furniture: dresser, desk, bookcase, chairs, nightstand, lamps, radio, TV, stereo, houseplants, books, toybox, shelves, washable toys, nonwashable toys
  Closet: clothing, shoes, toys and games, sports equipment, storage, other

Living room
  Flooring: wood, tile or linoleum, area rug, wall to wall carpet
    Rug: wool, cotton, synthetic, fiber, shag, pile, none
    Pad: felt, rubberized felt, rubber, synthetic, unknown, none
  Furniture: TV, upholstered chairs, upholstered sofa, toys or games, books, other
  Furniture content: innerspring, foam, down, synthetic, antique, fabric, other
  Throw pillows: kapok, cotton, synthetic, foam, none, other

Pets
  Type
  Where allowed in house: patient's bedroom, family (TV) room, outdoors only

Smoking
  By whom: none, mother, father, other

Plants
  Number
  Location

Other environmental factors (animals, smoke, other factors)
  Babysitter's home
  Other parent's or relatives' homes
  School or employment
  Vacation home or recreational vehicle, etc.

Hobbies (include those of patient and of family members)
  Indoor
  Outdoor

any treatment program. In some instances it may be appropriate to observe the effectiveness of such control measures before beginning injection therapy. This will emphasize the importance of the environment and may encourage parental cooperation.

Food History

Adverse reactions to foods quite commonly are blamed for many of the ailments of childhood, but it may be very difficult to establish a cause and effect relationship. In determining the role of foods it is important to differentiate between what the parents have observed personally with the ingestion of suspected foods and what they have been told to avoid, either on nonspecific grounds or because of positive skin tests to certain foods.

The food history may well be covered in the initial discussion, especially if foods are suspected as a cause of the patient's problems and adequate clues are available. Lacking this, it may be necessary to trace the food history back to the initial feedings, whether breast or bottle, the types of formulas, presence or absence of "colic," the time of addition of various solid foods, and the development of special likes or dislikes, all of which may be of significance.

The relationship of foods to gas, colic, vomiting, or diarrhea in the small child should be sought, as well as any connection to respiratory symptoms, including cough and wheeze, or eczema and hives. In some instances, foods may be noted in association with certain behavior difficulties such as the "tension-fatigue syndrome" (Chapter 59). Any shock organ may be involved.

Adverse reactions to foods may be both qualitative and quantitative, and it will be important to determine the frequency of feeding of a certain food, as well as the quantity eaten. One should note and describe any previous dietary manipulations which may shed light on the role of specific foods in etiology.

Social and Emotional History

As with any chronic or recurrent ailment that may interfere with daily activities, allergic diseases may have a considerable impact on the patient's emotional responses and his social adjustments. These may not be easy to elucidate, but may have much significance both in etiology and management of the underlying condition.

It will be important to ascertain something of the patient's daily routine, including school, sports, play, and hobbies. Does he get along well with others? What are his attitudes toward parents, siblings, playmates, schoolmates, and teachers and other adults? What is the child's self-image? How does he see himself in relation to others? Does he have sufficient self-esteem? How does he manage his illness? Does he accept certain limitations on his activities, and is he willing to assume some responsibility for taking medications and following treatment regimens as prescribed? The answers to these questions will be important in planning any treatment program. It is most important that the child understand and take part in long-term management. The child's participation encourages self-reliance and promotes acceptance of such constraints as may be placed on ordinary activities.

Conversations with the child will be helpful, especially if they can be conducted along light and friendly lines, at any time the opportunity presents itself. Most young patients need no encouragement to talk, and though this may be a bit confusing when taking a history, listening to the child may produce significant contributions to the general picture.

Previous Specific Therapy

Special considerations apply to the child who has had a previous allergy investigation and who is on specific immunotherapy, or whose parents have raised questions relating to injection therapy. One must get enough information to make a fair and critical evaluation of previous testing and response to treatment. If only symptomatic therapy has been employed, it is important to know what drugs were used, the dosage employed, and their efficiency. If immunotherapy has been utilized, it is essential to know the contents of the extract, the size and frequency of injections, the presence or absence of adverse reactions, and the results of therapy, including the parents' evaluation of the overall success of previous management.

The reasons a second opinion is being sought should be ascertained — whether it is the suggestion of the primary physician, the allergist, or the patient's family. The need for study should be carefully validated, and any recommendations to alter or discontinue current therapy should be made in consultation with the referring physician and the parents.

THE GENERAL EXAMINATION

Evaluation of the child with possible allergic problems requires a complete physical examination, emphasizing the need to consider the whole child. Satisfactory management can only be accomplished by a delineation of all problems, not just those related to allergy.

Height, weight, and age relationships are most important, and where possible, it is helpful to obtain prior values for comparison. These may help to indicate the long-term effects of disease states, allergic or otherwise, the results of steroid medication, and changes brought about by treatment.

Before the actual examination, careful observation will give much information concerning the severity of the illness, its impact on the child, whether he is upset or agitated, and how he reacts to those about him. Rate and depth of respirations, prolongation of expiration, and the presence or absence of cyanosis or pallor may be observed. Structural deformities may be noted, and one may look for clubbing of fingers and toes as evidence of chronic pulmonary disease.

Special emphasis must be placed on those systems of special interest to the allergist, each of which may have findings suggestive of allergic involvement.

Skin. Involvement of the skin is a characteristic of childhood allergy, and the manifestations are varied. Generalized eruptions such as atopic dermatitis and seborrhea may be visible, or may be indicated by history, in which case it will be essential to obtain an accurate description of the rash. Urticaria, angioedema, contact dermatitis, dry skin, and ichthyosis may be presenting complaints. Purpuric eruptions and telangiectasia

may accompany certain allergic and immunologic problems. The state of the child's nutrition often may be deduced from the general appearance of the skin, and dermatologic manifestations of systemic disease may be noted.

Eyes. Involvement of the eyes in seasonal allergies will be manifest by conjunctivitis, itching, stinging or burning, and excessive lacrimation. Conjunctival involvement may be bulbar, palpebral, or both. Chemosis with edema of the bulbar conjunctivae may occur. Puffiness of the eyelids is common in perennial allergic rhinitis, together with dark circles beneath the eyes, the so-called "allergic shiners." A deep transverse crease often is apparent in the lower eyelid lines.

Nose. The bridge of the nose may be broadened in the presence of chronic nasal allergy, and there may be a transverse crease above the tip of the nose, resulting from frequent nose-rubbing (the "allergic salute"). Nasal obstruction may be present, with pale or violaceous swelling of the turbinates, and may occasionally be complicated by a deviated septum or the presence of a pseudopolyp. True polyp formation in children is rare, and their presence should suggest a search for evidence of cystic fibrosis. Irritation about the external nares may be the result of a persistent nasal discharge, and dried or crusted mucus or blood in the anterior nares may be associated with recurrent epistaxis. Chronic or persistent mouth breathing may be accompanied by snoring or stertorous breathing and if prolonged may lead to the characteristic "adenoid" facies, with a deepened nasolabial fold, and some degree of malocclusion and overbite. A less appreciated finding which may result from persistent nasal obstruction is a characteristic appearance of the chest, with a mild funnel deformity in the area of the xiphoid, and some indentation of the rib cage at the level of the insertion of the diaphragm, with slight flaring of the costal margin.

Sinus involvement in allergic children is frequent, and the changes in the lining membranes tend to parallel the changes seen in the nasal mucosa. The ethmoid sinuses may become infected with any upper respiratory infection, resulting in chronic nasal discharge and postnasal drip. The hallmark of early maxillary sinus involvement (of allergic etiology) is flattening of the bony infraorbital ridge and the malar eminence, due to under-development of the sinus from failure of proper aeration. Secondary bacterial invasions of the allergic sinus may occur.

Ears. Simple inspection of the tympanic membranes may give some information about inflammation, but the use of pneumatic otoscopy will enable the observer to make a better assessment of middle ear disease and of the presence of fluid behind the drum. The drum that does not move, whether retracted or slightly full, will indicate significant middle ear pathology. More recently, tympanometry with impedance audiometry has come into use for the infant and small child, whose drums are difficult to examine, and who cannot cooperate in the usual hearing tests.

External otitis, with involvement of the ear canal, is somewhat more common in allergic children; and there is often some allergic involvement of the skin in the crease behind the ear, associated with other evidence of eczema or seborrhea. Infectious eczematoid dermatitis may be noted about the external ear in the presence of a pustular exudate from the middle ear, without an accompanying allergy.

Tonsils and Adenoids. The lymphoid tissue of Waldeyer's ring is an important part of the child's immune system and response to infection. It also participates regularly in allergic involvement of the nose and the nasal and oral phaynx. The tonsils will be found to be somewhat large during early childhood, in response to stimulation by infection and allergy, and after the age of 5 or 6 years will often regress spontaneously. Enlarged tonsils and adenoids may contribute to noisy breathing, and enlarged tonsils may cause enough obstruction to produce cor pulmonale. The tonsils may shrink considerably in size after an acute infection has subsided, and it is important to view the tonsils over a period of time in order to more accurately assess their role in the production of respiratory symptoms.

Chest. The chest deformity in asthma is generally quite mild, except in long-standing severe obstruction. One looks for a prominence in the upper chest with slight xiphoid depression and crowding of the lower rib cartilages. In severe instances it will be so marked as to produce the "pear-shaped" chest, with pigeon breast, and a more or less fixed chest wall. All of these changes are at least partially reversible with successful management of the underlying disease. Wheezing, with sonorous and sibilant rales and prolonged expirations, is typical of the child with asthma, but in the first year or two of life, mucus accumulation will produce a to-and-fro type of noisy breathing, with less evidence of the classic prolongation of expiration. The presence of increased secretions and the coarse and fine rales which are often heard may lead to a diagnosis of pneumonia, which may not necessarily be substantiated by x-ray studies. Consolidation in the child's chest may be a true pneumonia, but is often the result of a small area of atelectasis. Pulmonary findings will clear more quickly in the older child, while infants may keep a rattle for weeks.

Chest pain is often a subjective finding in the asthmatic, and although usually related to cough, it may be a sign of subcutaneous emphysema, pneumothorax, or mediastinal air.

Abdomen. Abdominal distention may accompany severe cough or wheeze, usually from swallowed air, and is more common in the younger age group. One may note that the small wheezing child is more comfortable in the supine position, since attempting to sit up causes the distended abdomen to push the diaphragm upward, further interfering with breathing.

LABORATORY EXAMINATIONS

The number and nature of the tests that may be performed to establish a diagnosis of allergy will vary with the specific complaint. Initial evaluation of the patient usually will include a complete hemogram (with differential cell count), nasal and stool smears for eosinophils when indicated, a tuberculin test (if not done in the preceding 6 months), a urinalysis, and an audiovisual assessment if possible. These tests may suggest a basic problem related to allergy, but a definitive diagnosis will depend upon more sophisticated tests. Most of these tests are discussed in other chapters, but it is appropriate to mention here that valuable information may be obtained from studies relating to resistance to infection, pulmonary function tests, and culture of appropriate fluids and secretions. X-ray studies will be required in some patients, especially the asthmatics, but every effort should be made to keep the exposure to x-rays at the minimum consistent with good patient care. The use of the skin test in diagnosis is discussed in detail in Chapter 21.

Herbert C. Mansmann, Jr., M.D.

21

Allergy Tests in Clinical Diagnosis

Atopic diseases are often exacerbated by specific allergic factors in a patient's environment and/or diet. The identification and elimination of these factors is an important step in treatment. Though a comprehensive history may suggest potential etiologic factors, allergy tests help to identify those of major importance. This chapter reviews allergy tests, their principles, uses, and limitations.

Allergy tests include skin tests, bronchial challenge tests and *in vitro* tests such as radioallergosorbent (RAST), leukocyte histamine release, lymphocyte transformation, or macrophage inhibitory factor (MIF) production. Other tests useful in diagnosis or follow-up of allergic children include hearing tests, tympanometry, lung function tests and exercise tolerance tests. Finally, there is a group of tests such as leukocytotoxic tests, end-point titration or provocative testing procedures that are "controversial," in that there is disagreement among physicians about their scientific basis and interpretation.

ALLERGY SKIN TESTS

Historical Background. In 1865, Blakely performed the first allergy skin test when he placed pollen from an anther of Italian rye grass on abraded skin and observed a wheal and flare reaction.

Though he published his "Experimental Researches on the Cause and Nature of Catarrhus Aestivus" in London in 1873, it attracted little attention. Not until 1907, when Von Pirquet described a scratch test for tuberculosis, did skin testing become a clinical procedure. In 1909 Smith and in 1917 Walker popularized the scratch test as a useful diagnostic technique in clinical allergy.

Mantoux in 1908 initiated intracutaneous testing for the diagnosis of tuberculosis. In 1912, Oscar Schloss in the United States adopted this procedure for diagnosing food allergy in children. The prick test, introduced by Lewis (1924) and Freeman (1930), is the preferred type of allergy skin test in England today.

The discovery by Prausnitz and Küstner in 1921 that allergic sensitivity could be transferred by serum to the skin of a non-allergic recipient led to the development of "passive transfer" skin testing and eventually to the discovery that nonhuman primates could serve as recipients for P-K tests. Wide developed an assay for specific IgE antibody (RAST) in 1967 that has replaced P-K testing in general.

Skin Response to Stimuli. The "triple response" of Lewis (1924) represents the primary skin response to mechanical stimulation. When skin is stroked lightly with a blunt instrument, pallor due to capillary constriction appears in 15 to 20 seconds. It increases in intensity for 30 to 60 seconds and then fades over 3 to 5 minutes.

With firmer pressure, a red rather than white line reflects capillary dilation, which occurs even if the circulation to the skin is obstructed or if nerves have degenerated. A stronger stimulus induces a flare outward from the red line, owing to arteriolar dilation mediated by a local axon reflex, which disappears only after nerves have been cut and have degenerated. With a still more intense stimulus, the local red reaction becomes paler and develops into a wheal, as histamine released from skin mast cells acts on endothelial cells to increase capillary permeability and permit escape of protein-rich plasma. Some individuals have unusually sensitive skin, in which distinct wheals may persist for half an hour or more (dermatographism).

This response may be modified by age, time of day, skin disease, and medication. Infants have an incomplete response, in which only the flare occurs. The wheal response develops slowly with increasing age. Circadian rhythms also affect skin responsiveness, which is lowest in the early morning and greatest in the evening. In skin diseases such as atopic dermatitis white dermatographism may predominate, i.e., only capillary constriction may occur (see Chapter 31). Endogenous or exogenous epinephrine, antihistamine drugs, and topical corticosteroids may also modify skin responsiveness.

Immunologically Induced Tissue Reactions. The skin may react in a variety of ways to antigen exposure, including immediate wheal and flare reactions, delayed "immediate" reactions, late cutaneous allergic responses, Arthus reactions, and delayed (tuberculin type) skin tests. A patient may react in more than one way to a single skin test, indicating that more than one type of response may occur.

The *immediate skin test* is a highly sensitive bioassay for detecting specific allergic antibodies to which the patient is immunologically sensitive. Like the triple response, it is dependent upon both humoral and neurogenic factors. When antigen placed onto or into the skin combines with mast cell–fixed antibody, histamine is released from mast cells. It induces a wheal by direct action on capillaries and a flare by arteriolar dilation acting through an axon reflex. The immediate reaction reaches its peak in 10 to 20 minutes and may fade rapidly or persist up to 1 hour. Skin window techniques also indicate a cellular response of both eosinophils and polymorphonuclear cells, possibly due to release of chemotactic factors in addition to histamine. The techniques of performing immediate skin tests and their interpretation are discussed later in this chapter.

Delayed Skin Reactions to "Immediate" Skin Tests. Infants and young children sometimes develop a "delayed-type" reaction of redness and induration at 12 to 48 hours after intradermal antigen injection, in the absence of an "immediate" skin test reaction. These reactions should be recorded, and the tests repeated in 3 to 6 months if the antigen appears to be clinically important, since such reactions may evolve into immediate-type reactions with time (Crawford and Roane, 1963). Delayed reactions appear to be immunologically specific and indicate prior allergen exposure. The immune mechanism underlying this unique type of skin reaction in small children is unclear.

The *late cutaneous allergic response (LCAR)* differs from the delayed type of "immediate" skin test in that it occurs after an "immediate" skin test reaction, peaking approximately 8 hours later (Umemoto et al., 1976). Moreover, LCAR occurs only after very large immediate skin tests. The LCAR often is the size of the flare of the initial immediate reaction. LCAR reactions (but not immediate reactions) are suppressed by corticosteroid therapy, but there has been no systematic study of this reaction in small children. There is evidence that the LCAR is mediated by IgE antibody, and it is presumed that the late reaction to antigen introduction into the skin has a clinical counterpart in natural exposure to the same antigen.

Arthus reactions are dependent upon precipitating antibody and can, like immediate hypersensitivity, be passively transferred with serum. Unlike immediate skin test reactions, which can be transferred only to man or subhuman primate, Arthus sensitivity can be transferred to guinea pigs and other laboratory animals. An Arthus reaction appears 3 to 6 hours after antigen administration, reaches a peak between 8 and 12 hours, and begins to resolve by 24 hours. Skin biopsies of the test show a diffuse cellular infiltrate in which eosinophils and lymphoid cells predominate. The Arthus reaction is inhibited by corticosteroids but not by antihistamines. A positive Arthus reaction is characteristic of allergic bronchopulmonary aspergillosis and of such illnesses as pigeon breeder's disease (Chapter 47).

Delayed (Tuberculin-Type) Skin Tests. The classic tuberculin reaction begins 12 hours after injection of antigen and becomes maximal at 48 to 72 hours, with a well defined area of induration surrounded by erythema. A very strong reaction may be characterized by edema, vesicles, or bullae and may result in residual pigmentation. Histologically, the perivascular lymphoid cell granulomata predominates. Positive patch tests in patients with contact dermatitis are another form of delayed-reaction skin tests (see Chapter 32). Typical tuberculin delayed-type hypersensitivity reactions to common antigen preparations (e.g., whole ragweed extract) also have been described in patients who demonstrate immediate wheal and erythema reactions as well. When tested with antigen E, a highly purified fraction of ragweed extract, only immediate reactions (without delayed reactions) have been observed (Green et al., 1967). It should be remembered, however, that patients are exposed naturally to the whole ragweed pollen granule, rather than to its antigen E component alone.

ALLERGY (IMMEDIATE) SKIN TESTS

General Considerations. Table 21–1 lists general rules to consider before initiating skin tests. Allergy skin tests are but one of the steps in diagnosing allergy. Although a positive test implies the presence of skin-sensitizing antibodies, its clinical relevance must be interpreted in the light of the patient's history and clinical course. It may indicate past, current, or developing allergic sensitivity. On occasion, a positive test may lack discernible clinical importance. *Skin tests cannot — nor are they intended to — replace a thorough history and physical examination, which must serve as the basis for their interpretation. A positive skin test is not proof that an allergic illness exists or that the allergen is clinically relevant.* Conversely, a negative test does not rule out the existence of an allergic problem or eliminate the clinical importance of a substance that may be inducing symptoms as an irritant rather than an allergen (e.g., tobacco smoke). Positive skin tests should be used as an aid in the development of logical environmental controls and as a guide to immunotherapy for those major allergens that cannot be avoided.

Skin testing must be performed by a valid technique with valid antigens before its results can be evaluated as must any laboratory test. A number of factors affect skin test results, including the specificity and potency of the testing antigen. While current methods of standardizing skin testing antigens are inadequate and antigens may vary from batch to batch, new immunochemical techniques

---

TABLE 21–1 GENERAL RULES FOR ALLERGY TESTS

1. Be sure that simpler, less expensive, and safer techniques have received an adequate trial.
2. Ask yourself: *Are the tests really necessary?*
3. Always *believe* the history. No matter how outlandish it may seem, accept it for a fact until cautious testing proves or disproves it. Consider the patient's safety above all else.
4. Avoid innumerable and casually selected allergens. Know *why* each test will help management.
5. Limit the number of tests done at any one time.
6. Test highly suspect allergens separately.
7. Record important allergic sensitivities in a highly visible, specific place in the patient's record.
8. Establish procedures to make certain that you or your office personnel do not inadvertently test the patient for factors to which he or she is anaphylactically sensitive.
9. Never perform any type of test without having emergency equipment immediately at hand.
10. Perform challenge tests only when the benefit makes the risk worthwhile. Document the decision to perform a test with written informed consent.

may overcome this major problem in the future. The physician interpreting skin tests must be aware that factors other than antigen specificity can also produce false positive or false negative reactions (Norman et al., 1976).

Antigen preparations which, in concentrations used for allergy testing, cause positive reactions to occur in a significant minority of the population (e.g., 10 percent of asymptomatic individuals) may be inducing these reactions on a nonimmune basis. Some preparations contain histamine, histamine liberators, or other vasoactive material and induce reactions in a large proportion of individuals on a pharmacologic basis (e.g., spinach) (May, 1976). Thus a positive skin test (especially a weakly positive one) is presumptive but *not definitive evidence for the presence of antibody.* False positive reactions may be induced also by preservatives or other materials in the antigen diluent, hence the necessity for always including a diluent control to rule out nonspecific reactivity.

"False positive" skin tests in patients suspected to be allergic to foods have been studied and reviewed recently by Bock et al. (1977; 1978). Their data suggests that the use of high concentrations of antigen (e.g., intradermal tests with food allergens) leads to overdiagnosis of food sensitivity. Although prick test results correlated better with clinical food sensitivity than did intradermal tests with the concentration of antigen employed, it is likely that intradermal tests would have correlated as well, had the concentration of antigen been reduced.

On the other hand, if the patient does not respond to injected histamine because, for instance, he or she has taken antihistamines before testing, a negative skin test may be invalid. *For this reason, a positive histamine control test should always be included in skin testing.* As noted previously, false negative reactions can occur also when there is not sufficient antigen in the testing solution to induce a response.

Allergy Testing Materials. Several hundred allergens have been identified that may have potential clinical relevance. Most are available for skin testing. Also available are allergens that have trivial or no perceivable relevance. To select appropriate allergens logically for testing from the many

available, the physician must know what environmental allergens are most prevalent in his or her area. Significant variations in the potency of antigens from different manufacturers as well as variations between lots from the same manufacturer pose further problems. Using antigens supplied by a single manufacturer will reduce this variation as much as possible; yet, clinically relevant but skin–test negative allergens might be positive with another manufacturer's solutions. Concentrated extracts for scratch or puncture testing usually are marketed in a glycerinated solution for preservation, though unglycerinated, aqueous extracts preserved with 0.4 percent phenol are also available. The physician should become familiar with the types of testing material available, their stability, and the techniques for handling them. The best source of this information is an established teaching medical center.

Indications for Testing. A detailed allergic evaluation is indicated for patients in whom empirical elimination of environmental or dietary factors fails to control allergic symptoms. In this category are infants and children who develop continuous, prolonged, or frequent intermittent respiratory illnesses and children of any age who develop persistent protracted respiratory symptoms of more than 4 weeks' duration or have recurrent seasonal illnesses and have objective evidence of allergy. Skin testing is an important means of identifying major allergic factors that are causing or exacerbating symptoms.

Selection of Factors for Testing. A detailed history of the seasonal occurrence of symptoms and of the patient's environment will identify the majority of allergenic factors to which the child is exposed. Most pediatric patients, especially the younger ones, require only a small number of tests. The physician must know what airborne allergens exist in the patient's geographical location (see Chapters 16 and 17) and must be willing to spend the necessary time in history taking to select the appropriate tests.

In general, it is best to restrict allergy testing to those factors that cannot be avoided. Housedust, for example, is one of the most frequent environmental allergens that affects children. Housedust — a ubiquitous allergen — is a complex substance derived from multiple constituents whose composition may vary with geographical location. It contains insect and fungal protein, various danders, and stable glycoprotein carrier molecules of plant and animal origin (Berrens, 1970; see also Chapter 17). A positive housedust test can help motivate the family to follow through with the housekeeping measures necessary to control housedust.

Mold allergy poses a special problem to many patients. Routine tests for common molds often are required. If the patient is not progressing satisfactorily or if there is mildew in the environment, mold plates can be exposed in several locations within the home, and the prevailing molds identified can be tested (see also Chapter 16).

Seasonal allergy problems occurring in the spring, summer, or fall are due largely to airborne pollens. Identification of the type of pollen responsible for symptoms requires not only knowledge of what pollens are generally prevalent in the area at different seasons but also specific botanical knowledge of the types of plants that are pollinating in the patient's area that particular year (see Chapter 16).

When an antigen is avoidable, such as dog or cat danders, the author feels that a skin test is unnecessary because atopic children ultimately become allergic to the animal, if they are not allergic to it already. The author believes the animal should be removed from the child's environment. On the other hand, many allergists feel that if a family is emotionally attached to a domestic animal, the evidence of a positive skin test is helpful in persuading the family either to eliminate the animal or to remove it from the child's immediate environment.

These same general points may be made about other environmental allergens such as feathers, kapok, and materials found in furniture and furnishings.

Allergy testing for food is controversial. Though allergy to foods precipitates respiratory allergy in children, its frequency, its importance in recurrent respiratory tract infections, and its effect on reactions to environmental factors is debatable (Hill, 1948). It is clear clinically that food allergy becomes progressively less important with increasing age (Foucard, 1973).

The judicious use of food skin tests often aids the physician and the parent in the evaluation of food allergy if a diet diary together with trial elimination of foods has not been successful (Dannaeus, 1977). The author tests for foods that the patient commonly eats and uses test results as a guide for elimination diets and for food challenges. For example, if a patient has a negative skin test to an important, frequently eaten food, the food should be withheld for a week and then an oral food challenge test should be conducted to establish the clinical importance. On the other hand, if the patient had a strongly positive test, that food would be eliminated and reintroduced for oral challenge after symptoms had cleared. The number of foods to be tested will depend upon age and symptoms. Skin testing for drug allergy, such as allergy to penicillin or insulin, is discussed in Chapter 54; skin testing for stinging insect allergy is described in Chapter 53.

Techniques of Testing

Table 21–2 lists precautions that must be observed before initiating skin tests. Two

TABLE 21–2 TESTING PRECAUTIONS

1. Skin test should *never* be performed unless a physician is available immediately to treat constitutional reactions.
2. Have emergency equipment at hand: rubber tourniquet, airways, laryngoscope, hand resuscitation bag, epinephrine, vasopresser agent, theophylline, injectable antihistamine, and oxygen must be available and an intravenous set with intravenous fluids should be checked routinely.
3. Do not test if the patient has moderate to severe symptoms; it is preferable not to test if *any* asthmatic symptoms are present.
4. Double-check known and suspected list by history.
5. Be certain that the test concentrations are known and are appropriate.
6. Determine and record medications patient is taking, and time of last dose.

basic techniques are employed in skin testing. In one, the antigen is placed onto abraded skin (scratch test) or on intact skin, which is then pricked by a sharp instrument (prick and puncture tests). In the second technique, the antigen is injected into the skin through a hypodermic needle. Scratch, puncture, and prick tests are less sensitive than intradermal tests, although they may give sufficient information to preclude the necessity for intradermal testing. Generalized reactions are also less likely to occur than with intradermal testing, *although anaphylactic reactions can occur in highly sensitive individuals even with scratch, prick, or puncture tests.*

The reader is referred to reviews concerning allergy skin testing (Rhyne, 1971; Zweiman, 1971; Aas, 1975, 1978; Slavin, 1974; Shapiro, 1977).

The skin over the test sites is cleaned with alcohol and marked with a felt tip or ballpoint pen. Both sides of the back midway to the spine or the volar surface of the forearms may be used for scratch, prick, or puncture tests. Intradermal tests should be done only on the forearms or lateral surfaces of the upper arm so that a constricting band can be used proximal to the test sites, should a systemic reaction occur. Test sites should be at least 3 cm apart. Both a positive and negative control test should be performed. Histamine phosphate is used for a positive control (1 percent solution for scratch, puncture, or prick tests and 0.01 percent solution for intradermal tests) and antigen diluting fluid for a negative control test.

Scratch Tests. The superficial layers of skin are abraded by a sharp instrument (e.g., 22 or 26 gauge needle or a scarifier) without drawing blood and a drop of antigen is applied over the scratch, taking care to avoid contaminating the extract remaining in the bottle with patient's serum. The site is observed for 20 minutes for the development of a wheal and flare response. The reaction is graded at its peak by comparing it with the histamine control, by recording the diameter of wheal versus erythema, or by other systems based on size of reaction.

The reaction is recorded conventionally as a negative to 4+ reaction. A positive (3+) test generally consists of a wheal at least 5 mm greater than the control, whereas in a 4+ test the wheal is asymmetrical, with "pseudopods" and a large surrounding flare.

Puncture Tests. The allergen extract is placed on the test site first; a sterile needle or similar sharp pointed instrument is passed through the extract into the superficial layers of skin. A new instrument should be used for each test. (Each instrument should be sterilized before being used for other patients.) Recently a plastic disposable device with eight heads, each with nine points, has been introduced for performing skin tests with glycerinated antigens, which may simplify puncture tests in children.

Prick Tests. This is a variation of the puncture test, in which the skin is lifted by the point of a needle from an oblique angle, after the needle is passed through the drop of allergen extract on the skin. Table 21–3 lists common errors in scratch, prick, and puncture testing.

Intradermal Tests. The allergen extract is injected intracutaneously from a 1 ml tuberculin syringe. Sufficient testing solution is injected to produce a 3 mm blob, estimated to be approximately 0.02 ml in volume. Before performing the test, it is important to express air from the syringe and

---

TABLE 21–3 COMMON ERRORS IN SCRATCH, PRICK OR PUNCTURE TESTING

1. Tests are too close together, so that overlapping reactions cannot be separated visually.
2. Technique is not identical for each site, i.e., different lengths of scratches or varying intensity of scratch or puncture.
3. Too much allergen solution, which causes spreading away from site.
4. Too many tests done at a time; suggest less than 20 in highly sensitive individuals.
5. Patient not checked for reaction frequently enough after testing. It is particularly important to check highly sensitive individuals early, and wipe away allergen if internal reaction develops rapidly. A mild reaction may be minimized in 20 minutes.

needle since the injection of a small amount of air may be interpreted mistakenly as a positive reaction. Tests should be read at 15 to 20 minutes and at 24 hours.

Intradermal testing is estimated to be approximately a hundredfold more sensitive in detecting specific skin-fixed antibody than is scratch testing. Intradermal testing also carries a greater risk of a systemic reaction because of a greater potential for systemic absorption of antigen. "False" positive reactions, that is, reactions caused by irritant factors in the antigen or those which do not appear to have clinical relevance, also occur more frequently with intradermal than with other types of skin tests. However, intradermal tests may identify important allergic factors which were missed by scratch or prick tests, especially in children under 3 years of age (Crawford, 1963; Reddy et al., 1978).

The following procedures will help to minimize adverse reactions to testing:

Eliminate tests or use more dilute antigen concentrations for allergens to which the patient is highly allergic by history.
Never use allergen concentrations stronger than 1:500 or 1:1000 weight by volume.
Limit the number of intradermal tests performed at one time.
In general, 15 or at most 20 tests should be the absolute maximum tested at one time.
Always do a pretest before using the full strength intradermal test antigen.

While many physicians perform a scratch test prior to an intradermal test (eliminating all antigens that produce a positive scratch test), others, including the author, prefer to test intradermally with serial dilutions of

TABLE 21–4 COMMON ERRORS IN INTRADERMAL TESTING

1. Test sites are too close together.
2. Too large a volume is injected.
3. Concentration is higher than necessary.
4. Person performing test neglects to prevent or observe "splash" resulting from air injection.
5. Antigen is injected subcutaneously instead of intradermally.
6. Intracutaneous bleeding site read as an adequate test.
7. Too many tests done at a time; suggest maximum of 10 per half hour in highly sensitive subjects.

the skin test antigen, beginning with one hundredth the concentration of the final antigen, followed by one tenth if the first test is negative and finally testing the full strength solution of 1:500 or 1:1000 w/v. By following these precautions, a large allergy center had no significant systemic reaction over a 20-year period (Van Arsdel, 1957). Common errors of intradermal testing are listed in Table 21–4.

Factors Affecting Skin Tests

Age. Skin test reactions may vary with age. Infants may react predominantly with only an erythematous flare, while older children develop both a wheal and a flare. The ability of most infants to respond by P-K reaction (Carey and Gay, 1934) and the fact that the skin of newborn infants and older infants responds to histamine and to codeine, a histamine releaser (Sulzberger and Baer, 1940), but to a lesser extent than adults, suggest that age in itself should not be a major deterrent for testing.

Circadian Rhythms. Skin test responses are elevated in the afternoon, peak in the late evening, and are at their lowest in the morning (Lee et al., 1977). One of many factors in the variation in skin test responses to the "same" antigen may be differences in time of day tested, but large differences (e.g., from markedly positive to negative) would not be expected on this basis.

Drugs. Since antihistamines are known to inhibit the effect of histamine on the skin, they have been traditionally withdrawn 12 hours before skin testing (Galant et al., 1972). However, antihistamines may suppress skin tests for a much longer period than is generally appreciated. Diphenhydramine may inhibit skin tests for 2 days and hydroxyzine for 4 days (Cook, 1973). Consequently, it would appear prudent to discontinue antihistamines for 2 and preferably 4 days before testing.

Parenteral epinephrine and isoproterenol have been reported to inhibit the immediate wheal and flare reaction (Kram et al., 1975). The effect of adrenergic agents on skin tests is relatively short-term (minutes to hours), however, and generally is mild.

Oral adrenergic agents probably should be withheld for 6 hours prior to testing; inhalant adrenergic drugs need not be withheld at all. Therapeutic doses of oral theophylline and terbutaline do not affect allergen or histamine skin tests significantly (Chipps et al., 1978).

Systemic corticosteroid drugs do not appear to interfere with antigen-induced histamine release. One week of daily methyl prednisolone therapy did not alter wheal and flare intradermal skin reactions to histamine nor did it affect reactions to the histamine releaser 48/80 (Slott and Zweiman, 1974), though it produced a significant eosinopenia and prevented local accumulation of eosinophils at the skin test site. Steroids need not be discontinued prior to skin testing.

Interpretations of Skin Tests. The validity of skin tests, like any other laboratory test, depends upon the interpretation and the use made of this information.

As a general rule, slight reactions tend to have minimal significance whereas strongly positive reactions, especially those associated with pseudopodial whealing, correlate highly with clinical sensitivity to the corresponding allergen. In general, the greater the reaction (i.e., the more antibody that is skin fixed), the more allergic the patient is to that antigen. A positive skin test indicates the presence of IgE antibody for that specific allergen, *but it does not necessarily indicate that the patient will develop symptoms when exposed to that substance.* Basically the physician uses the information obtained from allergy skin tests as a basis for immunotherapy, when indicated. Interpretation requires judgment, and the physician must correlate the test results with the history and with knowledge of the patient and the patient's family in formulating a rational plan of therapy.

Indications for Retesting. If symptoms progress or remain unchanged after 6 months of conscientious environmental or dietary control, it has been our practice to reevaluate the history and to retest those allergens that could be causing symptoms but which produced negative skin tests previously. Allergic patients who have just moved from another area may require retesting for local allergens if they are not doing well. On the other hand, if their symptoms are under control, it seems reasonable to continue previous therapy, if it meets acceptable standards. Such patients should be seen periodically, since symptoms may gradually recur as the patient becomes allergic to additional old or new environmental factors.

RADIOALLERGOSORBENT TESTS (RAST)

The RAST makes use of a "sandwich" technique, in which radiolabeled anti-IgE is used to quantitate the amount of specific IgE present in serum. Antigen is bound to an insoluble matrix such as Sephadex particles or a methylcellulose disc and is incubated with the patient's serum (Wide, 1967; Gleich, 1975).

If specific antibody is present, it will combine with the antigen on the insoluble matrix and will remain bound, whereas other proteins can be rinsed away. The matrix is next incubated with I^{125}-labeled anti-IgE, which in turn will bind to any IgE on the matrix. The bound anti-IgE remains while the unbound can be eliminated. The matrix is then "counted" in a gamma counter, and the results expressed quantitatively. The "count" is directly proportionate to the quantity of specific IgE bound to antigen.

In general, the RAST is less sensitive than the direct skin test and, like the skin test, its specificity is limited by the specificity of available antigen. Other major disadvantages are the limited number of available allergens, the significantly higher cost as compared to skin testing, and sometimes the length of time before test results are available.

Under certain circumstances, however, RAST testing may be a very useful clinical tool, e.g., in the presence of generalized atopic dermatitis or, infrequently, in uncontrollable asthma. The advantages of RAST include that it does not require intact skin for testing, it is reliable and safe, and it is not affected by medication.

As further research increases its sensitivity and more specific antigens become available, RAST should become more useful in diagnosing drug (especially penicillin) allergy and in situations such as hymenoptera sensitivity, in which direct skin testing may put the patient at special risk of anaphylaxis. However, like skin testing, *RAST is a laboratory test that does not make a diagnosis of allergy, and it must be interpreted on the basis of a thorough clinical evaluation.*

BRONCHIAL AND OTHER CHALLENGE TESTS

A variety of antigen challenge tests have been employed in the past, such as the direct instillation of dried pollen or other allergen or allergen extracts into the eye and nose in order to observe the reaction in 15 to 20 minutes. Such testing is tedious, potentially dangerous, and provides little more information than does skin testing.

On the other hand, bronchial challenge tests either with antigen, methacholine, or histamine may be of great value in research but may have limited clinical usefulness. Methacholine and histamine challenge tests make use of the fact that patients with asthma are 100 times more sensitive to these agents than are normals. Histamine and methacholine tests determine the dosage of these drugs which induces a 20 percent fall in the forced expiratory volume at one second ($FEV_{1.0}$). The tests are occasionally useful in diagnosing asthma (see Chapter 42). These procedures are safe if carried out by an experienced consultant, and bronchospasm is easily reversed by bronchodilator medication.

Bronchial challenge tests with antigen are of some value in identifying allergens that are responsible for exacerbating asthma. Unlike methacholine challenge, however, antigen challenge may be followed by a second response 5 to 8 hours later. The initial reaction can be reversed by adrenergic drugs, but the late reaction responds poorly to adrenergic agents though it does respond to corticosteroid medication.

Bronchial provocation testing with inhalant allergens is of some value in limited circumstances, in which identification of allergens responsible for provoking asthma is critical to patient care. Bronchoprovocation is a potentially dangerous procedure and is not necessary for the formulation of a ther-

apeutic regimen for most children. In those few for whom bronchoprovocation may be necessary, it should be performed in a hospital by physicians experienced in its use who are prepared to deal adequately with the possible complications of the test.

Oral challenges to food, a useful test in pinpointing foods that may be responsible for inducing potential life-threatening reactions, are discussed in Chapter 29.

EXERCISE TESTING

Exercise tolerance tests are important clinical tests in older children and adolescents in the diagnosis and management of asthma induced by exercise. Exercise testing can be carried out most simply by 6 minutes of free running up and down stairs or on a convenient sidewalk. Lung function can be monitored prior to exercise and for 20 minutes afterwards with a peak flow meter or simple spirometer. The diagnosis and management of exercise-induced asthma is discussed in detail in Chapter 46.

IN VITRO TESTS FOR CELLULAR RESPONSIVENESS

Various tests that measure cellular responses to antigen stimulation have been used in an attempt to identify antigens which may induce symptoms by any of a variety of immune mechanisms. Skin tests for delayed-type hypersensitivity have been reviewed in Chapters 1 and 6. Patch testing for contact hypersensitivity is reviewed in Chapter 32.

The presence of tissue eosinophilia is used as circumstantial evidence for the existence of an allergic reaction in or near the tissues involved. Although tissue or blood eosinophilia does occur frequently in IgE-mediated and perhaps in other immune tissue reactions, it may be present even though detectable immune mechanisms are absent, possibly reflecting release of "allergic" chemical mediators by nonimmune mechanisms. Also, the absence of eosinophilia does not rule out "allergy." In addition to examination of nasal, eye, bronchial and intestinal secretions and peripheral blood for eosinophils, tissue responses to antigen placed on abraded skin ("skin windows") have been used to implicate allergic responsiveness to suspected antigens. This procedure is too cumbersome to be useful in clinical practice.

In vitro tests for antigen-induced histamine release (e.g., from peripheral blood leukocytes) also have been used and are of value in examining mechanisms of antigen-induced histamine release. Neither these tests nor *in vitro* antigen-induced degranulation of human or animal basophils are of value in clinical practice. They are not more sensitive indicators of the presence of IgE antibody than are skin tests or RAST. Generally they add little to diagnosis and management of allergic disorders, though they may be useful in clinical research. Other tests such as *in vitro* antigen-induced proliferation of lymphoid cells, chemotactic assays, and macrophage inhibition factor (MIF) production are useful tools in research but add little to clinical management of allergy.

OTHER TESTS

A variety of tests useful in the diagnosis and for follow-up of allergic children are described elsewhere in this book. Among these are hearing tests and tympanometry (Chapter 37) and pulmonary function test (Chapter 42).

A number of techniques for diagnosis of food allergy based on empirical observation have become very controversial in medicine. These include *in vitro* leukocytotoxic food tests, end-point intracutaneous test titration, subcutaneous provocation testing, and sublingual provocation testing. These tests are discussed in Chapter 59.

References

Aas, K.: Diagnosis of immediate type respiratory allergy. Pediatr. Clin. North Am. *22*:33, 1975.

Aas, K.: The diagnosis of hypersensitivity to ingested foods. Clin. Allergy *8*:39, 1978.

Blakely, C. H.: Experimental Researches on the Cause and Nature of Catarrhus Aestivus (Hay Fever). London, 1873.

Berrens, L.: The allergens in house dust. Progr. Allergy *14*:259, 1970.

Bock, S. A., Buckley, J., Holst, A., and May, C. D.: Proper use of skin tests with food extracts in diagnosis of hypersensitivity to food in children. Clin. Allergy *7*:375, 1977.

Bock, S. A., Lee, W. Y., Remigio, L., Holst, A., and May, C.: Appraisal of skin tests with food extracts for diagnosis of food hypersensitivity. Clin. Allergy *8*:559, 1978.

Carey, T. N., and Gay, L. N.: Skin reactions in infants. Susceptibility of the skin of the newborn to passive atopic sensitization: Comparison with reactions to histamine. J. Allergy *5*:488, 1934.

Chipps, B. E., Talamo, R. C., Mellits, E. D., and Valentine, M. D.: Immediate (IgE-mediated) skin testing in the diagnosis of allergic disease. Ann. Allergy *41*:211, 1978.

Chipps, B. E., Teets, K. C., Saunders, J. P., Sobotka, A. K., and Lichtenstein, L. M.: The effects of oral theophylline on skin tests and histamine release. J. Allergy Clin. Immunol. *61*:171, 1978.

Cook, T. J., MacQueen, D. M., Wittig, H. J., Thornby, J. I., Lanton, R. L., and Virtue, C. M.: Degree and duration of skin test suppression and side effects with antihistamine. J. Allergy Clin. Immunol. *51*:71, 1973.

Crawford, L. V., and Roane, J. A.: Allergy skin testing in infancy. Southern Med. J. *56*:1250, 1963.

Dannaeus, A., Johansson, S. G. O., Foucard, T., and Ohman, S.: Clinical and immunological aspects of food allergy in childhood. I. Estimation of IgG, IgA and IgE antibodies to food antigens in children with food allergy and atopic dermatitis. Acta Paediatr. Scand. *66*:31, 1977.

Foucard, T.: A follow-up study of children with asthmatoid bronchitis. 1. Skin test reactions and IgE antibodies to common allergens. Acta Paediatr. Scand. *62*:633, 1973.

Galant, S., Zippin, C., Bullock, J., and Crisp, J.: Allergy skin test: I. Antihistamine inhibition. Ann. Allergy *30*:53, 1972.

Gleich, G. J., and Jones, R. T.: Measurement of IgE antibodies by the radioallergosorbent test. J. Allergy Clin. Immunol. *55*:334, 1975.

Gottlieb, P. M., Stupniker, S., and Askovitz, S. I.: The reproducibility of intradermal skin tests: A controlled study. Ann. Allergy *18*:949, 1960.

Green, G. R., Zweiman, B., Beerman, H., and Hildreth, E. A.: Delayed reactions to inhalant allergens. J. Allergy *40*:224, 1967.

Hill, L. W.: Food sensitivity in 100 asthmatic children. New Engl. J. Med. *238*:657, 1948.

Kram, J. A., Bourne, H. R., Maibach, H. I., and Melmon, K. L.: Cutaneous immediate hypersensitivity in man: Effect of systemically administered adrenergic drugs. J. Allergy Clin. Immunol. *56*:387, 1975.

Lee, R. E., Smolensky, M. H., Leach, C. S., and McGovern, J. P.: Circadian rhythms in the cutaneous reactivity to histamine and selected antigens, including phase relationships to urinary cortisol excretion. Ann. Allergy *38*:231, 1977.

Lewis, T., and Grant, R. T.: Vascular reactions of the skin to injury. Part II. Heart *11*:209, 1924.

May, C.: Lack of interference in skin tests by histamine in food extracts. Ann. Allergy *37*:8, 1976.

Norman, P. S., Marsh, D. G., and Tegnall, J.: Stability of allergen extracts diluted for testing. J. Allergy Clin. Immunol. *57*:231, 1976.

Prausnitz, C., and Küstner, H.: Studien über die ueberempfindlichkeit. Zbl. Bakt. I. Abt. Orig. *86*:160, 1921.

Reddy, P. M., Nagaya, H., Pascual, H. C., Lee, S. K., Gupta, S., Lauridsen, J. I., and Jerome, D. C.: Reappraisal of intracutaneous tests in the diagnosis of reaginic allergy. J. Allergy Clin. Immunol. *61*:36, 1978.

Rhyne, M. B.: Skin testing. Concepts and realities. Pediatr. Clin. North Am. *16*:227, 1971.

Schloss, O. M.: A case of allergy to common foods. Am. J. Dis. Child. *3*:341, 1912.

Shapiro, G. G., Bierman, C. W., Furukawa, C. T., and Pierson, W. P.: Allergy skin testing: Science or quackery? Pediatrics 59:495, 1977.

Smith, H. L.: Buckwheat poisoning. Arch. Int. Med. 3:350, 1909.

Slavin, R. G.: Skin tests in the diagnosis of allergies of the immediate type. Med. Clin. North Am. 58:65, 1974.

Slott, R. I., and Zweiman, B.: A controlled study of the effect of corticosteroids on immediate skin test reactivity. J. Allergy Clin. Immunol. 54:229, 1974.

Sulzberger, M. B., and Baer, R. L.: Whealing capacity of skin of newborn or young infant. Arch. Dermatol. Syph. 41:1029, 1940.

Umemoto, L., Poothullil, J., Dolovich, J., and Hargreave, F. E.: Factors which influence late cutaneous allergic responses. J. Allergy Clin. Immunol. 58:60, 1976.

Van Arsdel, P. P., Jr., and Sherman, W. B.: The risk of inducing constitutional reactions in allergic patients. J. Allergy 28:251, 1957.

Van Metre, T. E.: A simple method for keeping allergenic extracts at a temperature near 4° C during office use for skin testing and immunotherapy. J. Allergy Clin. Immunol. 59:341, 1977.

Walker, C.: Studies on the sensitization of patients with bronchial asthma to the different proteins found in the dandruff of the house and in the hair of the cat and the dog and to the sera of the animals. J. Med. Research 35:497, 1917.

Wide, L., Bennich, H., and Johansson, S. G. O.: Diagnosis of allergy by an in vitro test for allergen antibodies. Lancet 2:1105, 1967.

Zweiman, B.: Diagnostic procedures in atopic patients. In Montagna, W., and Billingham, R. E. (eds.): Advances in Biology of Skin. Vol. XI, Immunology and the Skin. New York, Appleton-Century-Crofts, 1971, pp. 123–140.

22

Jerome M. Buckley, M.D.
David S. Pearlman, M.D.

Controlling the Environment

The word environment comes from the old French "environner," meaning "to surround or encompass." The environment surrounding man can be divided into the *abiotic environment*, which consists of non-living factors (temperature, wind, humidity, the air and its nonliving contents, and radiation), and the *biotic environment*, which includes all living or recently living materials — plant and animal.

Moses Maimonides (1135–1204) recorded the following observation in his Treatise on Asthma (Muntner, 1963): "Your Highness (the King of Egypt) has already confided in me that the air in Alexandria is harmful to you and whenever you fear an attack of the illness (he was speaking of his asthma), you prefer to move to Cairo where the air is much drier and calmer, making the attack more tolerable for you." Maimonides later lists as one of his Six Obligatory Regulations For His Highness's Illness, "keeping clean the air which you breathe." Thus, as early as the twelfth century, a governmental body was made aware of the importance of clean air!

The number of substances found in man's environment that can induce allergic reactions is legion. In addition, numerous environmental substances precipitate or aggravate "allergic" symptoms by nonimmune mechanisms. For example, sneezing and burning or itching of the nose and eyes — symptoms characteristic of allergic reactions to pollens and animal danders — can be mimicked by contact with cigarette smoke, newsprint, petrochemical fumes, and other irritant factors. Such substances can also greatly aggravate allergic reactions in the eye and the respiratory tract. However, the mechanisms by which substances induce tissue damage are not considered in this chapter because the purpose of environmental control measures is to minimize the patient's contact with *any* factor that precipitates or aggravates symptoms of allergic disease.

Environmental control depends first on indentifying such factors. Except for the most striking associations, the patient or parents often will be unaware of many of the factors responsible for the problem, and a thorough history for possible offending environmental factors is the first step. *Where* (home, school, area of country, vacation cabin, friends' homes) and *when* (time of day, time of year) as well as other circumstances possibly related to the symptoms must be explored. Chapter 20 (Table 20–1) lists the many points to be covered in an environmental history. Allergy tests and, when appropriate, provocative challenges can help determine the causative agents. As implied above, environmental agents contributing to allergic disease do not always operate through allergic (i.e., IgE antibody-dependent) mechanisms, hence "allergy tests" may not be completely revealing.

With difficult problems, a visit to the home (Weiseman and Weiseman, 1964) or school can reveal unusual or unexpected environmental factors. The surrounding neighborhood, the nearby foliage and animals, the quality of housekeeping, the presence of animal hairs, filled ashtrays, or musty odors, or finding a child's bedroom cluttered with nicknacks and toys, for example, may provide the physician with specific information on which to base his advice on environmental control. (Of additional importance when the physician makes a home visit is the effect that such interest from the physician has on the willingness of the patient and parents to comply with instructions for environmental control.)

APPROACH TO ENVIRONMENTAL CONTROL

Environmental control must be rational, based on the known or suspected sensitivities of the child, and individualized according to the physical and financial resources of the patient's family. Controls must not be so rigid that siblings are neglected over concern for the patient. When expensive household alterations, equipment purchases, or total changes in life style are involved, the physician must be reasonably confident that these will benefit the patient. On the other hand, the physician will have to convince the family of the importance of carrying out the most crucial changes. Thus, the wise physician will take a middle road, recommending first those changes that are not harmful and that are easily accomplished and accepted by the family; recommendations for more extensive environmental manipulation may be in order if the initial changes are not sufficient.

In making recommendations for environmental control, it is important to consider the normal psychosocial growth of the child, in terms of the influence environmental manipulation may have on family life and on the child's life outside the home. For example, overprotecting the child from contact with domestic animals to which the child is minimally sensitive may result in severe limitation of the child's and family's normal activities and lead to family resentment toward the child. This can be just as detrimental to the child emotionally as failure to eliminate an animal, known to be a major allergen for the child, would be physically. Also, undue limitation of physical activity can discourage play and normal social interaction with other children at school. Here the goal should be full participation, even if it requires the use of medication.

As a general rule, it is wise to limit exposure to those common allergenic and irritating substances that can be inexpensively and conveniently removed. The more difficult it is to eliminate a factor because of psychologic reasons or for reasons of convenience or expense, the more evidence is needed implicating it as a cause of trouble before its elimination is recommended. Since "allergy" to various substances is a matter of degree, it may be sufficient to diminish contact with a substance, without eliminating it from the environment altogether. Mild sensitivity to the family dog, for instance, may be resolved satisfactorily by keeping the dog outside the house at all times or by confining the animal to the utility room when in the house.

Particular emphasis should be given to that part of the environment in which the child spends the greatest amount of time. The bedroom, therefore, in which the young child may spend half his life, and the older child, well over a third, is the focus of attention. Generally, extensive environmental control measures should be directed toward the bedroom, moderate measures toward the TV room, with less intense attention to other rooms of the house. However, for the child with severe allergic disease, extensive measures may be needed in the entire house, in relatives' homes, in the schoolroom, in a babysitter's home, and any other place the child frequents.

Worsening or precipitation of allergic disorders has been related to various atmospheric phenomena, such as storms, sudden changes in humidity or temperature, and air pollutants (Feinberg, 1974; Zweiman et al., 1972; Physicians' Guide to Air Pollution Episodes, 1972; also see Chapter 18). The mechanism by which these atmospheric or weather changes affect allergic diseases still is obscure, although some explanations have been proposed. Negative and positive ions in the air have been related to changes in respiratory function, mood changes, and aggravation of vascular headaches (Soyka and Edmonds, 1976; Krueger, 1973). Positive ions appear to inhibit broncho-ciliary clearance, thus increasing respiratory tract problems, whereas negative ions have a beneficial effect. Most of this information is testimonial, and there is little rationale at present for manipulating such factors in the home environment.

The literature is replete with information regarding the value of procedures for removing molds (Criep et al., 1958), methods of decreasing house dust and house dust mites (Sarsfield et al., 1974), the ability of dehumidifiers to decrease the humidity and the mold count within a household (Villaveces, 1971), the use of air conditioning to decrease pollen counts (Spiegelman and Friedman, 1968), and the removal of particulate matter such as dust and tobacco smoke via special filters, either electrostatic (Lefcoe and Inculet, 1971) or HEPA (High Efficiency Particulate Air) (King, 1973; Zwemer and Karibo, 1973). However, there is little data (Fontana and Rappaport, 1966) on the extent to which patients' symptoms are altered and, more particularly, on the extent to which the total course of the patient's disease is changed. Thus, physicians tend to rely on their own observations that individual patients improve on removal of certain factors from the environment and they extrapolate from their observations to what "makes sense" for other known or suspected inciting agents.

CONTROL OF TEMPERATURE, HUMIDITY, AND INDOOR AIR POLLUTANTS

Heating Systems. There are three basic types of controlled heating systems: (1) forced air systems, in which the air is heated and then forced (blown) throughout the house via a duct system, (2) electric heat, in which there are separate electric heating units in each room, and (3) hot water heat, in which water is heated and distributed to pipes in individual rooms, where heating occurs by radiation and convection. There also are radiant heating systems similar to hot water systems except that a metal conductor transfers heat from an energy source to the environment, and space heaters or floor furnaces with or without fans placed in a central location in the house. Various energy sources — natural gas, oil, coal, electricity — can be used for all of these. Hot water, electric, and other radiant heating systems are best for families of allergic individuals. Forced air systems, especially those without efficient filters or space heaters, are least desirable because air is blown through the house, carrying with it fine particles of dust. Moreover, forced hot air heat tends to be more drying than does heating by hot water. On the other hand, air which does not circulate cannot be filtered, humidified, or dehumidified effectively without the use of numerous room units. Taking this into account, one concludes that the least expensive all-purpose system to allow heating, humidification, and filtration is a forced air system.

Periodic cleaning (yearly) of the duct system is important, as is thorough cleaning of the system in a new house before it is first used since the duct system frequently is used for garbage and waste disposal during construction. Vents in the child's bedroom should be closed at night to minimize air turbulence, if adequate heating can still be maintained (keeping the bedroom door open may help).

For energy conservation, a heat pump can be considered. Special attention should be given to proper insulation — walls, doors, windows, and attic — not only to conserve energy but also to minimize air turbulence.

Cooling System. Cooling systems include everything from simple fans to sophisticated air-conditioning systems. Cooling systems also include attic exhaust-fan systems of two types: one which cools by pulling air from outside through the entire house, and another that simply cools hot attic air by circulating air through the attic. In the first type the system pulls outside materials, including pollens, molds, and dirt, through the house (no filters are involved). Such cooling systems that draw air through the house with no filtration are not advisable for allergic children. The second type of system is acceptable in that decreasing the temperature of attic air either can obviate the need for air conditioning or can lessen the amount needed to keep the house comfortable.

Evaporative coolers used in some areas

of the country as an alternative to refrigeration systems, because of water condensation, can be a source of mold growth if not cleaned properly. This generally is not a problem in the type of cold water cooling in which a fan is used to blow air over coils cooled by water completely enclosed in the system.

The most common type of air conditioning in use is the refrigeration type, in portable or central units. Portable air conditioners can, of course, handle only small areas of the house and may contain inadequate filters. With appropriate filters, however, such units can be especially effective for a bedroom if the bedroom door is kept closed. Using the unit's fan without refrigeration can bring in fresh, filtered air during the cooler time of night.

A central air conditioner is reasonably efficient in filtering larger allergens and irritant particles, but the system is often utilized in a way that does not help the allergic child. Because of the cost of operation, the system may be used for relatively

short periods — only in the hottest weather or only during the day. The windows are kept open at night for the cooler night air. For pollen- and mold-sensitive children, however, it is important to keep the bedroom windows closed during problem seasons to minimize allergen and irritant exposure (Seebohm, 1973). The least expensive means for temperature control is the most desirable. The child who lives in a climate in which for most of the year the bedroom is comfortable at night with the windows closed may do well with a portable air conditioning unit for the occasional hot nights during pollen season, without an investment in a central system being necessary.

Filtering Systems. Both central and portable systems are available. Frequently, a portable filtering system can be rented for a trial of at least a month (often the rental fee applies to purchase of the unit) to test its effectiveness and help determine whether purchase is worthwhile. The door and windows of the bedroom should be closed during such an evaluation.

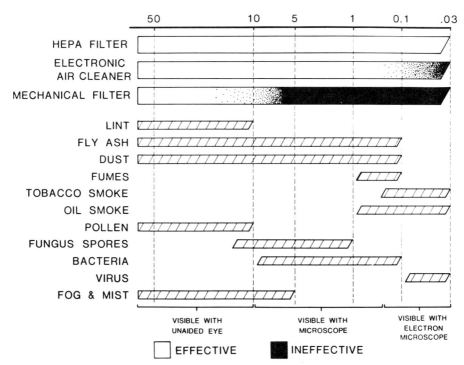

FIGURE 22–1. Effectiveness of various filtering systems in eliminating airborne particles that may precipitate or aggravate allergic diseases.

Mechanical Filters. The simplest type of filtering system is mechanical, employing filters of closely knit fibers that sift out particles of a given size, usually down to 10 microns (Fig. 22–1). These are adequate for most mold spores and pollens. However, house dust particles tend to be smaller. Moreover, cigarette smoke and various aerosols and animal danders are not adequately filtered. Mechanical filters should be changed monthly; more frequent changes are necessary in areas with high pollen and mold counts or with house dust problems.

Electrostatic Filters. These filters work by charging particles in an electric field and trapping them on an oppositely charged filter plate. Electrostatic filters have the potential of producing ozone, which is a respiratory irritant, and room electrostatic filters may intensify asthma in some patients because of ozone generation. Central units do not appear to cause as much of a problem as portable units, which generate ozone in closer proximity to the patient. Both self-cleaning and manually cleaned electrostatic filtration units are available. Self-cleaning is not generally satisfactory, however, and manually cleaned units with filtration cells that can be removed for cleaning are recommended, especially if the cells can be cleaned in a dishwasher. All electrostatic filters require a mechanical pre-filter and possibly a carbon filter of some nature to remove any gaseous particles.

High Efficiency Particulate Air Filter. HEPA filters are clearly the most effective filters available for removing particulate matter. They are not electrostatic and operate on a single filtration principle; ozone generation does not occur. Portable units are available, but at present there is no acceptable central HEPA filter system available for sizable living quarters because of the large blower capacity necessary to force air through a HEPA system. Extremely effective air filtration is possible for a few feet directly in front of the HEPA filter (Zwemer and Karibo, 1973), and generally, the flow of air is minimal, creating little feeling of blowing air and relatively little noise.

Unfortunately, while air filtration with these or any other filtration devices is theoretically helpful, it often fails to alter the patient's symptoms significantly. Of all the central filtration devices available today, the most desirable would seem to be a combination of a mechanical and an electrostatic filter, with added carbon filters as needed. HEPA filtration is recommended for portable units (King, 1973).

Humidification System. In some parts of the country, humidification of air in the home is desirable, whereas in other parts, dehumidification may be needed. For normal function of human mucous membranes, a humidity level between 25 and 40 percent is considered optimal. Household humidification should be held within this range to the extent practical. Where the regulatory device is located is important, since the humidity level is measured only at that point. Because humidification is necessarily somewhat uneven throughout the house, humidification may be adequate where the device is located — in the basement, for example — but inadequate in the bedroom, where the child spends a major portion of his time.

Advantages of proper humidification must be weighed against the potential hazard of increasing mold growth with excessively moist conditions. Molds grow best in a warm moist environment, especially in humidity greater than 50 percent and temperature above 37°C. Certain molds, however, survive in less favorable conditions. Humidifiers can act as sources of molds and bacteria, contributing to immediate type I hypersensitivity reactions and, in heavily exposed subjects, to hypersensitivity pneumonitis (Sweet et al., 1971; Tourville et al., 1972).

There are three types of humidifiers: reservoir, evaporator, and jet spray. The reservoir type is the most common. A wheel rotates in the reservoir of water, and air is blown over the wheel, picking up moisture as it passes. With evaporator and jet spray types of humidifiers, excess moisture is removed from the system by a drain. Without adequate drainage, pooling of moisture can encourage mold growth. The appropriate system for a particular house depends on the size, design, and heating system of the house, as well as meteorologic conditions in the area.

Portable humdifiers can be selected for

either hot or cold humidification. True humidifiers have a humidistat control that will shut the humidifier off when the relative humidity attains a certain level in the room. A vaporizer, on the other hand, adds moisture to the atmosphere without respect to the level of humidity. Without control of humidification, excessive moisture can readily encourage mold growth. (A good rule of thumb is that if rugs, beddings, windows or walls become damp, humidity is excessive.) Humidifiers and vaporizers must be cleaned regularly to control mold growth, which can become a major source of airborne mold spores.

Dehumidification. Dehumidification is necessary when a patient's symptoms are aggravated either by the excess humidity itself or by the mold growth that humidity facilitates (Villaveces, 1971). Most dehumidifiers are portable and use calcium chloride or refrigeration coils to remove moisture from air passed through them. Additives that come with humidifiers or dehumidifiers contain either sodium nitrite, a toxic chemical, or bleach. It is advisable, however, to use only water in operating the units and to periodically clean the units with chlorine bleach or a cleaner such as Lysol.

Information on cooling, heating, humidification and dehumidification load estimates (and a map giving climate correction factors) is available from the Association of Home Appliance Manufacturers (AHAM). Consumers Union of the United States,* a nonprofit organization which publishes an annual *Buying Guide* and the monthly *Consumer Reports* magazine, is an excellent source of information regarding specific equipment.

A patient's parents often ask about *tax deductions for the purchase of air filtration equipment or air conditioning.* Information is contained in Section 213, Code 2019 on Medical-Dental Expenses, subsection .015 of the U.S. Tax Code regarding capital expenditures. Although capital expenditures generally are not deductible, there can be a medical expense deduction to the extent that the amount of such expenditure

exceeds the amount of the increase in the value of the property. Since tax laws do change, the patient or parents should be advised to check with an accountant.

ENVIRONMENTAL CONTROL OF SPECIFIC ALLERGENS AND IRRITANTS

House Dust

House dust is a composite of various potentially allergenic materials, of which insect emanations and animal danders tend to be of particular importance (see Chapter 17). House dust is a universal irritant, and minimizing dust exposure is desirable for all children with allergic disorders. Although it is impossible to provide a "dust-free" environment, the aim is to achieve one that is "dust poor," particularly in the child's bedroom. All dust sources and dust catchers not essential to the bedroom or to other rooms in which the child spends considerable time should be eliminated. These include toys, models — essentially any object that collects dust. A minimal number of books should be allowed in the bedroom (bookcases should have closed shelves), and the bedroom closet should be used to store only the child's present seasonal clothes. To the extent possible, bedding should be of washable synthetic or synthetic blend materials and should be washed regularly.

Curtains should be of smooth material that can be washed and tumbled dry or tumbled on the "air-only" cycle to remove dirt and dust. Window shades are preferable to venetian blinds. If blinds are used, they can be cleaned conveniently by immersing them in a bathtub full of water. Short pile carpeting is easier to clean, traps less particulates, and sheds less than long pile or shag. The physician should let the family try all other bedroom control measures, including frequent vacuuming, before urging the replacement of bedroom carpeting. Linoleum and wood floors are easier to clean than carpeted floors, but some area rugs may be desirable, particularly in winter. Easily washed synthetic area rugs are advised. The bedroom should be cleaned thoroughly

---

*Consumers Union of the United States, 256 Washington Street, Mount Vernon, N.Y., 10050.

at least weekly, and lightly wet-dusted daily.

The child particularly sensitive to house dust should be encouraged to keep his or her room neat but should not help in dusting and vacuuming the room; rather, an alternative chore should be found. If it is necessary for the child to be involved in cleaning, protective disposable face masks, available in many drugstores, should be worn. Dust bags from the vacuum cleaner should be emptied outside the house. Forced air vents in the child's bedroom should be closed off to the extent compatible with keeping the room temperature comfortable (the vent may also be covered with three to five layers of cheesecloth). Windows should be closed, and fans should not be permitted. Pillows made of any material other than polyester and mattresses and box springs should be encased in impermeable plastic. A polyester mattress pad, or several sheets doubled over, should be used over the plastic. This is especially important for children with atopic dermatitis since sweating aggravates dermatitis. If possible, bunk beds should be separated since the child on the bottom bed receives increased dust exposure from the upper bunk. (Chapter 17 deals in detail with house dust.)

Fungi and Molds

Fungi and molds are ubiquitous, but their growth is especially encouraged in moist, warm conditions. It is the airborne spores from these organisms that constitute the major allergenic problem (see Chapter 16). Molds, rusts, and smuts are found on decaying vegetation, in soil, and on various plants (Wyse and Malloch, 1970); allergic symptoms associated with lawn mowing may in fact be related to sensitivity to molds which contaminate the lawn, rather than to grass pollen sensitivity. Limitation of such activities known or suspected to increase symptoms is of obvious importance.

Mold identification in the home is discussed in Chapter 16. Mold growth flourishes in damp areas of the home such as basements or crawl spaces, areas in which there have been leaks in the house,

in rubber carpet underpads soiled by leaks or by urine from animals, in bathrooms (especially shower stalls), window sills in moist climates, utility rooms (especially with washing machines), and humidifiers and vaporizers. Rubber and foam pillows and mattresses eventually may be contaminated by mold growth stimulated by body moisture and heat. Polyester pillows are recommended, and the mattress as well as the box spring should be enclosed in a plastic envelope and the zippers sealed with masking tape. For comfort, two (polyester) pads may be required. The number of houseplants should be minimized, or the soil-pot covered with aluminum foil to decrease dissemination of the mold spores by air currents.

Window frames, baths, showers, and other areas in which molds grow should be treated periodically with a Lysol or Clorox solution. The frequency is determined by the climate and household conditions, but such cleaning should be done at least every 3 months. These areas also should be rinsed with Zephiran Chloride, using a 12.5 percent solution or the 17 percent solution that can be purchased without prescription.

Particular attention should be directed to crawl spaces in moist areas of the country. The ground can be covered by black polyethylene sheets to decrease the moisture drawn into the house; standing water in the crawl space can be eliminated by installation of effective drains. In basements and crawl spaces, the use of trioxymethylene (crystalline paraformaldehyde) can be effective. The crystals are placed in an open 3 to 5 mm jar in different areas of the house, but the area must be closed as tightly as possible for 24 hours. (The number of jars depends on several factors: air circulation, humidity, amount of mold — details can be obtained from the manufacturer). The rooms must be well ventilated afterwards since formaldehyde is toxic and even small amounts of the vapor can be extremely irritating to respiratory membranes. Food should not be left exposed during the formaldehyde treatment. The frequency of this procedure also depends on climate and household conditions and can be determined by repeated mold cultures. The same treatment is good for summer or winter homes that are closed up for a portion of the year. (See Chapter 16 for other discussion on mold control.)

Animal Contacts

Animal Danders. For the most part, it is the dandruff, serum, and saliva from animals that are responsible for sensitivity rather than the animal hair. Individuals sensitive to a species of animal tend to be somewhat sensitive to all varieties of that species, although the degree of sensitivity may vary. Some varieties tend to be more sensitizing than others. It is a common belief that certain dogs (poodles, for instance) are "hypoallergenic" and rarely, if ever, cause sensitization. Unfortunately, this belief is incorrect, and severe sensitivity occurs to virtually all animals, including poodles and Chihuahuas (the animal associated with the myth of "taking one's asthma away").

As with allergy in general, the degree of animal sensitivity varies from patient to patient. For one patient, elimination of the animal from the environment may be required, whereas for another person, reduced contact may suffice. As a minimum control, animals should be kept out of the allergic child's bedroom at all times. In many cases, keeping the animal outdoors at all times is sufficient. If the animal is allowed even limited indoor contact (for instance, confinement to the utility room or basement), the dander can still be disseminated throughout the house by a forced air heating or cooling system. In cases of severe animal sensitivity, the animal should be eliminated altogether.

Animals should not be groomed in the house and certainly never by the person who is allergic to animal dander. Other animal contacts — at a babysitter's home or at school, for instance — may present a major problem and elimination of the animal from the classroom or changing babysitters may be necessary. A babysitter who has animals at home and comes to the child's home should be encouraged to wear clothes with which the animals have had little or no contact. Parents who have contact with animals to which the child is highly allergic should change clothes away from the house if feasible or, at least, upon entering the house.

Occasional animal contacts for the child who is not highly sensitive are permissible. For instance, the child who is only mildly sensitive to horse dander can be allowed to ride a horse occasionally if symptoms remain under control with simple medication. In order that a child who is allergic to animals may visit a home with animals — especially to stay there overnight — the animals should be removed temporarily, the rooms to be occupied should be cleaned thoroughly before the visit, and the bedding should be changed. Frequently, these measures together with pretreatment with antihistamines, bronchodilators and/or cromolyn will permit limited exposure to offending allergens, while allowing the child to participate in a normal activity, encouraging healthy psychosocial development. Similar principles apply to camping: if animals are a normal part of the camping experience, they should not sleep in the same cabin or tent with the allergic child nor travel in the same vehicle with the campers, and vehicles used for their transport should be thoroughly cleaned before use by campers.

A strong effort should be made to keep animals known to cause allergic problems out of the classroom. There is no justification for classroom animals if they make any child ill.

Animal Products. Fur coats and down pillows and sleeping bags should not be kept in the patient's closet or near the bedroom. Although it is usually permissible to wear a down jacket outdoors, it should not be stored in the child's bedroom. Rug pads, mattresses, and furniture stuffing made of various kinds of animal hair —including horse, cow, and hog — were common years ago and still are found in some homes. The extent to which hair in these products constitutes a significant allergenic source is unclear, since, as mentioned before, the hair shaft generally is not the culprit. Such organic material is a haven for mold growth, however, and probably should be eliminated from the home for children who are highly allergic to animals.

Individuals who are sensitive to fish and certain other animals may have problems with some glues. Certain glues used in model building, such as LePage's glue, are fish-derived; others, including Elmer's glue, are derived from other animal products.

Plant Contacts

Pollens. Airborne pollen and mold allergens float for considerable distances, hence foliage in the general area is of greater significance than the particular grass, trees, or shrubs in the patient's yard. A nearby tree or shrub with pollen to which the patient is allergic, however, may cause special problems, and if windows cannot be kept closed at all times during the pollen season (Seebohm, 1973), removal of such foliage may be important. In addition, if insect sensitivity is a problem, flowering plants that attract insects should be eliminated from the immediate environment.

The location of the bedroom in which the patient sleeps can be important. Selecting a room on the opposite side of prevailing wind direction, on the "cooler" side of the house in the summer to maximize the feasibility of keeping bedroom windows closed, can be helpful. Children highly sensitive to weed and other plant pollens should be discouraged from playing in fields in which these plants grow. Open fields near the house invite the growth of allergenic weeds; if possible, weeds should be cut short early during the weed pollen season to minimize pollination. In many areas, ordinances require landowners to control weed growth on open land, and a call to the local health department or other government agency may prod the property owner to cut the weeds or to use weed killer.

The child should be encouraged to bathe and change clothes after playing outside in grass or weeds; clothes worn by the child while playing outside should be kept outside the bedroom while waiting to be laundered. A family member in daily contact with allergens to which the child is highly allergic should be encouraged to change clothes and bathe upon entering the house if possible.

Flowers are insect pollinated and generally are not a significant problem for allergic children because of the heaviness of the pollen and the necessity for close contact with the plant for significant allergenic exposure. However, since pollen from flowers can be sensitizing and, with sufficiently close contact, can be a source of significant respiratory tract symptoms, large quantities of flowers in the house are discouraged. Some flowers can be more of a problem than others. It is wise to remember that ragweed is related to chrysanthemums, zinnias, marigolds, and dahlias, as they all are part of the sunflower (Composite) family. (See also Chapter 16 for additional discussion of pollen control.)

Plant Products

Pyrethrum. For individuals sensitive to ragweed, contact with pyrethrum, an insecticide derived from plants related to the ragweed family, should be avoided.

Kapok. Kapok is a plant fiber used in inexpensive pillows and mattresses and in some stuffed toys. It is also found in some old sleeping bags and in antique furniture as stuffing. Sensitivity to kapok can be severe, and the material should be eliminated from the immediate environment.

Cottonseed. Cottonseed is part of unrefined cotton and can be the source of extreme hypersensitivity. Refined cotton, as in cotton sheets, does not present a problem, but cottonseed associated with cotton linters used in innerspring mattresses and furniture may be a source of inhalant allergens. Cottonseed also is used in fertilizer and certain animal foods and baked goods. Because it is so highly refined, cottonseed oil rarely is a problem. However, cottonseed flour, the use of which as a protein supplement in foods is increasing, can induce acute allergic reaction in sensitive people.

Orris Root. Orris root was once a frequent component of cosmetics and is still found in some inexpensive cosmetics, some tooth powders, and bathing salts. It can cause severe allergic reactions.

Flaxseed. Sensitivity to flaxseed is uncommon, but can be severe. Flaxseed is found in chicken feeds and feeds for other animals, in hair setting lotions, shampoos, some insulating materials, rugs, and in some foods, such as Roman Meal Bread.

Vegetable Gums. Karaya, tragacanth, carobseed, acacia, chicle, and quinceseed gums are found in wave setting lotions (flakes off when dry), in medications as a filler, in sizing, in printing drying powders, and in hand lotions, chewing gums, chocolate substitutes, gelatin preparations, soft center candies, pie fillings, ice cream, gravies, cake icing, salad dressings, laxatives, toothpastes and powders, and mouthwashes. These may be allergens for some children.

Nonallergenic Materials

Although there are claims of allergic sensitivity to cigarette smoke, the significance of smoke as an allergen is unclear. On the other hand, smoke is a universal irritant and will exacerbate upper and lower respiratory tract problems (Lim, 1973). Contact with smoke should be minimized in all individuals with allergic diseases (Nadel and Comroe, 1961). Smoke exposure in the home must be eliminated. At a minimum, family members should refrain from smoking in the child's presence. Specifically this means no smoking in the same room or in the car with the patient. Preferably family members should avoid smoking in the house altogether, and smoking by visitors should be discouraged. Perfumes, cosmetics, various other odors (Horesh, 1966; Rosen, 1978; Engebretson, 1971), and hair sprays, also can exacerbate allergic respiratory disease either as allergens or irritants. Direct and indirect contact with these materials should be minimized in the home.

ENVIRONMENTAL CONTROLS AWAY FROM HOME

Traveling can pose a problem for the allergic patient. The patient should take along his or her own pillow; if the child is animal sensitive, a motel or hotel that does not permit animals should be chosen. The parents or patient needs to remember to take along medication and continue the regular medication schedule. A clinical summary and medication schedule from the patient's physician could be especially helpful.

In planning travel, the patient or parents should select a time of the year when problem airborne allergens in the area to be visited are at a minimum. Samter and Durham's book *Regional Allergy of the United States, Canada, Mexico, and Cuba* is a valuable information source. Written in 1955, it is out of print but may be obtained at medical libraries. A more recent publication by Alexander Roth (1978) dealing with the entire world also contains useful information.

RECOMMENDATIONS FOR CHANGES IN LOCATION

Only in rare circumstances, in those severe diseases in which rapid weather changes, cold, damp climates, or long, intense pollen seasons clearly are responsible for intractable symptoms, should a change in geographic location be considered. Even then, unless it is compatible with the psychosocial and financial well-being of the entire family, a change in location on medical grounds should not be encouraged. Although there is evidence that such a move may be helpful for a short period (Skoogh et al., 1976), more long-term studies are necessary. It is a common experience that an allergic disorder will remit or improve significantly after a move but then gradually recur — often to the same or even to a greater extent. This response is probably related to the acquisition of sensitivity to allergens in the new environment. On the other hand, moves away from certain kinds of environments, such as a ranch or farm or away from a factory producing air pollutants, can be critically important, if the patient is highly sensitive to the particular allergens in that environment.

References

Criep, L.H., Teufel, R.A., and Miller, C.S.: Fungicidal agents in the treatment of allergy to molds. J. Allergy 29:258, 1958.

Engebretson, G.R.: Allergies and odors arising from indoor environments. Am. J. Public Health 61:366, 1971.

Feinberg, S.M.: Environmental factors and host responses in asthma. Acta Allergol. *29*(Suppl. 11):7, 1974.

Fontana, V.J., and Rappaport, I.: Environmental control unit. N. Y. State J. Med. *66*:2913, 1966.

Horesh, A.J.: The role of odors and vapors in allergic disease. J. Asthma Res. *4*:125, 1966.

King, J.G.: Air for living — comparison of HEPA and electrostatic air filtration. Resp. Care *18*:160, 1973.

Krueger, A.P.: Are negative air ions good for you? The New Scientist, June 14, 1973, p. 668.

Lefcoe, N.M., and Inculet, I.L.: Particulates in domestic premises. I. Ambient levels and central air filtration. Arch. Environ. Health *22*:230, 1971.

Lim, T.P.K.: Airway obstruction among high school students. Am. Rev. Respir. Dis., *108*:985, 1973.

Maimonides, Moses: Treatise on asthma. *Medical Writings*. Vol. 1. Edited by S. Munter. Philadelphia, J.B. Lippincott, Co., 1963.

Nadel, J.A., and Comroe, J.H., Jr.: Acute effects of inhalation of cigarette smoke on airway conductants. J. Appl. Physiol. *16*:713, 1961.

Physicians' Guide to Air Pollution Episodes. J.A.M.A. *221*:19, 1972.

Rosen, H.: Hydrocarbons and Other Gasses as Related to the Field of Allergy. Clinical Allergy Based on Provocative Testing. Hicksville, New York, Exposition Press, 1978.

Roth, A. (ed.): *Allergy In The World – A Guide For Physicians And Travelers*. Honolulu, University Press of Hawaii, 1978.

Samter, M., and Durham, O.C.: *Regional Allergy Of The United States, Canada, Mexico, and Cuba*. Springfield, Illinois, Charles C Thomas, 1955.

Sarsfield, J.K., Gowland, D.G., Toy, R., and Norman, A.L.E.: Mite-sensitive asthma of childhood. Trial of avoidance measures. Arch. Dis. Child. *49*:716, 1974.

Seebohm, P.M.: Management of respiratory problems by nonallergists. 1. Allergic rhinitis. 2. Asthma. Postgrad. Med. *53*:52, 63, 1973.

Skoogh, B.E., Simonsson, B.G., Beiggren, A.G., et al.: Climate and environment change in patients with chronic airway obstruction. Arch. Environ. Health *31*:11, 1976.

Soyka, F., and Edmonds, A.: *The Ion Effect*. New York, E.P. Dutton & Co., Inc., 1977, pp. 58–80.

Spiegelman, J., and Friedman, H.: The effect of central air filtration and air conditioning on pollen and microbial contamination. J. Allergy, *42*:193, 1968.

Sweet, L.C., Anderson, J.A., Callies, Q.C., and Coates, E.O., Jr.: Hypersensitivity pneumonitis related to a home furnished humidifier. J. Allergy Clin. Immunol. *48*:171, 1971.

Tourville, D.R., Weiss, W.I., Wertlake, P.T., and Lendemann, G.M.: Hypersensitivity pneumonitis due to contamination of home humidifier. J. Allergy Clin. Immunol. *49*:245, 1972.

Villaveces, J.W.: The dehumidifier: Its indoor use in controlling molds and mold asthma — a personal case history. Ann. Allergy *29*:93, 1971.

Weiseman, R.D., and Weiseman, J.R.: Value of home visits in the treatment of the allergic patient. N.Y. State J. Med., *64*:1948, 1964.

Wyse, D.M., and Malloch, D.: Christmas tree allergy: mold and pollen studies. Can. Med. Assoc. J. *103*:1272, 1970.

Zweiman, B., Slavin, R.G., Feinberg, A.J., Falliers, C.J., and Aaron, T.H.: Effect of air pollution on asthma: A review. J. Allergy Clin. Immunol. *50*:305. 1972.

Zwemer, R.J., and Karibo, J.: Use of laminar flow device as an adjunct to standard environmental control measures in symptomatic asthmatic children. Ann. Allergy *31*:284, 1973.

Miles Weinberger, M.D.
Leslie Hendeles, Pharm. D.

23

Pharmacologic Management

PRINCIPLES OF MANAGEMENT

Asthma

A rational approach to the management of asthma requires a conceptual understanding of the disease and a definition of its particular clinical pattern in the patient to be treated (see Chapter 45). The treatment of asthma must be individualized according to frequency and chronicity of symptoms. Management of acute symptoms occurring on an infrequent, intermittent basis requires measures that relieve respiratory distress rapidly and effectively. Promptness of action, potency, and safety over the short run are the major considerations, without concern for long-term toxicity. Therefore, an inhaled sympathomimetic is the bronchodilator of first choice, whereas an orally administered drug like theophylline, which requires time to be absorbed and is slower in onset of action, is used as a secondary bronchodilator. The same reasoning justifies the short-term use of high-dose systemic corticosteroids when symptoms are not relieved by sympathomimetic agents and theophylline.

On the other hand, in management of the patient with chronic asthma, theophylline has been shown to be effective when administered continuously to prevent symptoms, without apparent "tolerance." Theo-

phylline, therefore, is recommended as the primary therapeutic agent in chronic asthma (Hambledon et al., 1977; Bierman et al., 1977). Cromolyn is an alternative to theophylline for the prevention of asthmatic symptoms. Although generally less effective than theophylline, dosage is standardized, and toxicity is virtually nonexistent. Oral or inhaled sympathomimetic drugs also are used to treat chronic asthma. Data related to control of symptoms with continuous use of these agents are limited, however, and the presence of decreasing effect over time gives reason for concern. Corticosteroids also may be needed when the continuous or frequently recurring symptoms of chronic asthma are unresponsive to bronchodilators (Ellul-Micallef and Fenech, 1975). Because of the potential long-term adverse effects of daily corticosteroid therapy, short-acting oral steroids are administered on alternate days or newer preparations such as beclomethasone dipropionate are administered by inhalation. As might be expected, the more severe the disease, the more medications are required for adequate control of asthma (Fig. 23–1).

Rhinitis

While environmental control is the most effective method of avoiding symptoms of allergic rhinitis, and injection therapy with

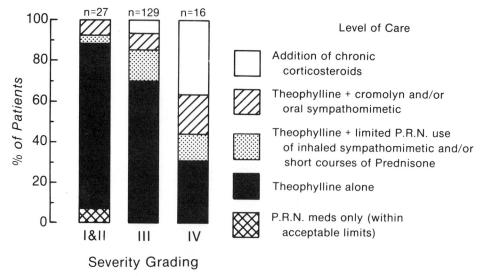

FIGURE 23–1. Relationship between asthma severity and a number of medications required for disease control in 172 patients with chronic asthma. Severity of disease increases from grades I through IV. (From Ekwo and Weinberger: Evaluation of a program for the pharmacologic management of children with asthma. J. Allergy Clin. Immunol. *61*:240, 1978.)

allergenic extracts may decrease sensitivity to inhalant allergens, pharmacologic management often is the most practical therapeutic approach. When chronic rhinitis occurs in the absence of identifiable allergens, there is no alternative to the use of drugs, and appropriate selection of medication usually can relieve symptoms. For several decades antihistamines have been the most commonly used drugs for allergic rhinitis. However, their effectiveness often is limited, and all too frequently there are annoying side effects including sedation, dry mouth, and irritability. Many patients therefore elect to tolerate symptoms rather than endure the side effects. The value of antihistamines is neither established nor disproved for symptoms of nonallergic chronic rhinitis.

Limitations in the effectiveness of antihistamines may relate as much to the method of drug administration as to the therapeutic index of the drug. Patients tend to take antihistamines after they develop symptoms, whereas if they took their medication *prior* to allergen exposure the antihistamine might be more effective since these drugs act as competitive antagonists to histamine. When used in this manner, antihistamines decrease symptoms of sneezing, rhi-

norrhea, nasal itching, and allergic conjunctivitis (Schaaf et al., 1979).

Other traditional pharmacologic measures for allergic rhinitis include orally active sympathomimetic agents such as ephedrine, pseudoephedrine, and phenylpropanolamine. These appear most effective for relief of nasal congestion.

Sodium cromolyn, an antiasthmatic drug that prevents mast cell degranulation and subsequent histamine release, also can reduce symptoms of allergenic rhinitis, particularly in patients with high levels of IgE (Handelman et al., 1977). However, it must be administered up to six times a day for maximal effectiveness.

Intranasal insufflation of topical corticosteroids such as beclomethasone dipropionate controls symptoms, particularly nasal congestion, more reliably than does cromolyn (Chatterjee et al., 1974). As a general rule, even topical corticosteroids should be reserved only for those patients who fail to respond to nonsteroid drugs.

In selected patients whose predominant symptom is rhinorrhea, particularly in those patients who suffer from "vasomotor" (chronic nonallergic and noninfectious) rhinitis, the use of an anticholinergic such as propantheline (Probanthine) may offer symptomatic relief.

Treatments to be avoided include (1) the use of repository injections of corticosteroids, because of marked suppressive effects on the hypothalamic-pituitary-adrenal axis, (2) the long-term use (longer than 2 weeks) of dexamethasone by nasal aerosol (Decadron Turbinaire) because of systemic absorption (Norman et al., 1967; Michels et al., 1967), and (3) prolonged use of topical nasal decongestants (greater than 5 days) because of rebound congestion and development of dependence *(rhinitis medicamentosa)*.

Anaphylaxis

Appropriate therapy for anaphylaxis warrants the prompt administration of a potent physiologic antagonist of the effects of histamine; the classic and most potent drug for this purpose is parenteral epinephrine. Antihistamines are appropriate therapy following the parenteral epinephrine since antigenic exposure may be continuing (as with an ingested food that is not yet completely absorbed). Antihistamines are *inappropriate* initial measures for treating the acute manifestations of anaphylactic reactions since they cannot reverse the rapid action of histamine already released. Antihistamines may *partially* prevent anaphylactic reactions, if administered prior to allergen exposure and release of histamine. Corticosteroids are of unproven value during acute anaphylaxis, unless the duration of the reaction is prolonged (see Chapter 52).

Chronic Urticaria

Urticaria responds promptly but briefly to injected epinephrine and oral epinephrine-like agents including ephedrine and pseudoephedrine which have been used for chronic urticaria with some effectiveness. The major pharmacologic treatment of chronic urticaria, however, has been the use of antihistamines, with hydroxyzine being perhaps the most popular (and probably one of the most effective). Cyprohep-

tadine has been reported to be specifically effective in some cases of cold urticaria (Wanderer and Ellis, 1971), but it also has some growth effects in children (increased appetite, increased linear growth, increased nitrogen retention) that have not been fully elucidated.

THERAPEUTIC AGENTS

Sympathomimetic Bronchodilators

Since 1906, when epinephrine was found to be a potent bronchodilator, adrenergic drugs have been studied extensively and a relationship identified between structure and function of sympathomimetic amines (Fig. 23–2). The therapeutic goal for the newer drugs has been greater selectivity for beta$_2$ (lung) adrenergic receptors (Table 23–1). Additionally, the newer agents are useful orally because of their resistance to degradation by intestinal enzymes. This resistance to enzymatic degradation also prolongs their duration of action. Synthetic sympathomimetic agents including metaproterenol, terbutaline, and albuterol (salbutamol), fenoterol and carbuterol are clinically available in many parts of the world. Currently only metaproterenol and terbutaline are available in the United States, though others are in clinical trials. Various formulations and dosages are given in Table 23–2.

Topical Aerosolized Sympathomimetic Drugs. Sympathomimetic drugs delivered by inhalation provide the most rapid and often the most effective means of relieving acute asthmatic symptoms. They probably are similar in potency to parenterally administered medications but have fewer side effects and are more suitable for self-administration (Hetzel and Clark, 1976). The metered dose inhaler is the most convenient method of administration; however, the desired response may be difficult to obtain in the severely dyspneic patient or younger child who is unable to inhale a sufficient quantity of the drug. For these patients, a solution of one of these agents, e.g., terbutaline (Bachus and Snider, 1977), can be given more successfully and distrib-

PHENYLETHYLAMINE

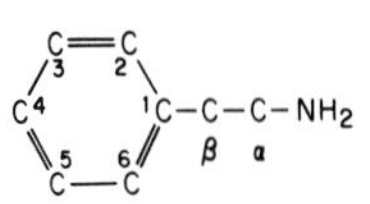

CATECHOLAMINE

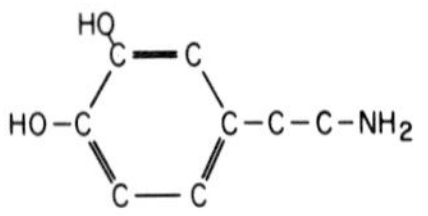

Drug Name	Structure	Major Receptor Activity	Oral Bioavailability In Conventional Doses	Approximate Duration Of Effect
NOREPINEPHRINE	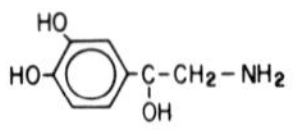	α	NO	<1 HOUR
PHENYLEPHRINE	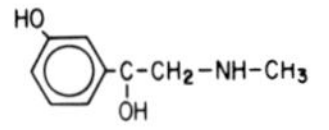	α	NO	<1 HOUR
EPINEPHRINE	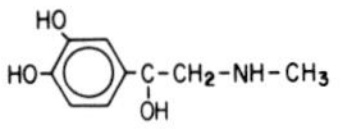	α, β_1, β_2	NO	<1 HOUR
EPHEDRINE	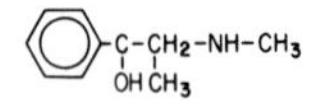	α, β_1, β_2 CNS	YES	4 HOURS
ISOPROTERENOL	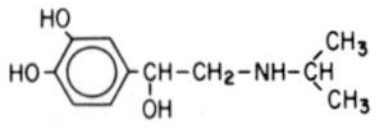	β_1, β_2	NO	<1 HOUR
ISOETHARINE	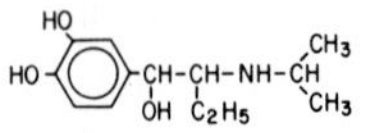	β_2	SOME	1 HOUR
METAPROTERENOL	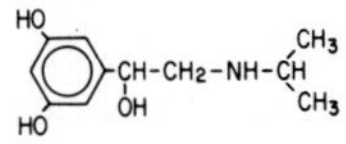	β_2	YES	4 HOURS
TERBUTALINE	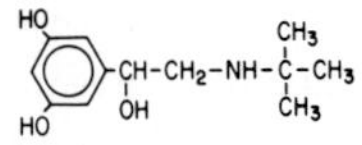	β_2	YES	6 HOURS
ALBUTEROL	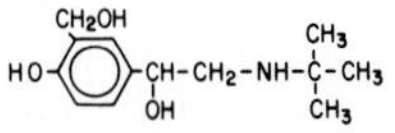	β_2	YES	6 HOURS

FIGURE 23–2. Structure and function of sympathomimetic amines. Adrenergic receptor activity is indicated by the conventional *α*, *β_1*, and *β_2*. Pharmacologic effects associated with the stimulation of these receptors are indicated in Table 23–1. (From Weinberger and Hendeles: Pharmacotherapy of asthma. Am. J. Hosp. Pharm. *33*:1071, 1976.)

TABLE 23–1. SELECTED PHARMACOLOGIC EFFECTS OF SYMPATHOMIMETICS

Clinical Effect	Receptor
Bronchodilation	$Beta_2$
Tremors	$Beta_2$
Tachycardia and arrhythmias	$Beta_1$
Hypertension	Alpha
Pallor	Alpha
Urinary retention	Alpha
Central nervous system stimulation	Not defined—dependent upon crossing blood-brain barrier

(Modified from Weinberger and Hendeles: Pharmacotherapy of asthma. Am. J. Hosp. Pharm. *33*:1071, 1976.)

TABLE 23–2 PREPARATIONS AND DOSAGE OF SYMPATHOMIMETIC DRUGS

Generic Name	Trademark Name(s)	Dose	Frequency	Preparations
PARENTERAL — SUBCUTANEOUS				
Epinephrine hydrochloride	Adrenalin		q 20 minutes × 3	Injection (solution) 1:1000 (1 mg/ml)
Terbutaline hydrochloride	Brethine Bricanyl	0.01 ml/kg up to 0.25 ml	q 30 minutes × 2	Injection (solution) 1:1000 (1 mg/ml)
PARENTERAL — INTRAVENOUS				
Isoproterenol hydrochloride	Isuprel	Begin with 0.1 μg/kg/min; increase by 0.1 μg/kg/min at 15 minute intervals until clinical response, heart rate greater than 180, or 0.8 μg/kg/min	Continuous infusion	Injection (solution) 1:5000 (0.2 mg/ml)
INHALATION				
Metaproterenol sulfate	Alupent Metaprel	2 inhalations (1.3 mg)	q 4 hours	Freon propelled metered dose inhaler, 0.65 mg/metered dose
Terbutaline	Brethine Bricanyl	0.5–1 mg diluted in 1.5 ml normal saline; delivered by air driven nebulizer	q 4 hours	Inhaler not available
ORAL				
Terbutaline	Brethine Bricanyl	1.25–5 mg	q 6–8 hours 3 times/day	Tablets, 2.5 mg and 5 mg
Metaproterenol	Alupent Metaprel	10–20 mg	q 4–6 hours 3 to 4 times/day	Tablets, 10 and 20 mg Syrup, 10 mg/5 ml

uted more evenly and completely throughout the airways if diluted in saline and administered over a few minutes by air driven nebulizer (e.g., Maximist, DeVilbiss) or manual air pump (e.g., standard 1¾-inch diameter or larger tire pump fitted with plastic tubing and an appropriate nebulizer). However, aerosolized sympathomimetics should not be administered by intermittent positive pressure breathing (IPPB) equipment because such equipment gives no additional benefit (Moore et al., 1972) but may increase the risk of pneumothorax (Karetzky, 1975).

When used in recommended dosage and under supervision, these agents are extremely safe. *The potential for abuse, however, with the subsequent possibility of paradoxical bronchoconstriction and toxicity from both the drug and/or freon propellant warrants care in prescribing this dosage form.* Specifically, when this form is prescribed it is wise to mark the prescription nonrefillable so that frequency of prescription need can be used to gauge frequency of drug use. These drugs should not be dispensed casually by emergency room or by other physicians *who are not taking full responsibility for the chronic ongoing care of the patients.* Misuse may be avoided if the drugs are used only as part of an overall program for asthma management, their use is under parental control if possible, and both patient and parents are warned thoroughly about drug misuse.

Isoproterenol, because of its rapid onset of action and potent intensity of effect, probably is the most useful diagnostic agent in testing bronchodilator response. Therapeutically, metaproterenol is the drug of choice among currently marketed preparations available in the United States (as of 1980) because of longer duration of action and apparent lesser degree of tolerance (Chervinsky and Belinkoff, 1969). As terbutaline, albuterol, carbuterol, or fenoterol become available, they may offer further therapeutic advantages since they have even longer durations of action.

Sympathomimetics with predominant vasoconstrictor activity are used as nasal decongestants. Phenylephrine (Neo-Synephrine) is most commonly used, but others such as oxymetazoline (Afrin) appear to have longer durations of action. All of these topical decongestants, however, should be used for only *short* periods (less than 5 days) to prevent rebound congestion and development of *rhinitis medicamentosa.* They should *not* be used in chronic rhinitis.

Parenteral Sympathomimetic Drugs. In acute asthma, epinephrine or terbutaline may be administered by subcutaneous injection as an alternative to inhaled sympathomimetic drugs; this is the route of choice in an asthmatic who is so dyspneic that aerosolized administration is ineffective. Epinephrine by injection is the drug of choice for anaphylaxis. Isoproterenol has been administered intravenously to avoid mechanical ventilation in children with respiratory failure (Parry et al., 1976) though it requires special precautions to avoid serious complications (see Chapter 45). Intravenous terbutaline or albuterol (salbutamol), when available, also may be effective with fewer associated cardiac effects (Johnson et al., 1978).

Oral Sympathomimetic Drugs. The original oral sympathomimetic, ephedrine, possesses a relatively weak bronchodilator effect and has been employed most commonly in combination with theophylline. When used in this manner, however, only a modest degree of additional bronchodilation results. Moreover, the addition of ephedrine to maximally therapeutic doses of theophylline results in synergistic toxicity. Newer agents such as metaproterenol and terbutaline do not appear to cross the blood-brain barrier as readily as ephedrine, and thus may exhibit proportionally less synergism with theophylline for central nervous system toxicity. The more potent beta$_2$ agonists, however, stimulate receptors on skeletal muscle, causing a relatively high incidence of dose-related tremor that can interfere with attainment of maximally effective bronchodilator dosage in many patients (Legge et al., 1971).

When compared with the inhaled route, the oral sympathomimetic bronchodilators have a slower onset of bronchodilation and are considerably less potent in blocking exercise-induced bronchospasm (Godfrey and Konig, 1975; Anderson et al., 1976). Moreover, they do not appear to be completely free of the acquired tolerance that is apparent for the inhaled sympathomimetics (Nelson et al., 1977). Since oral sympathomimetics also are frequently associated with uncomfortable systemic effects, their therapeutic role currently is not well defined. These agents are recommended as second-line bronchodilators that may be appropriate alone under some circumstances for mild acute symptoms, or for added oral bronchodilator therapy when optimal doses of theophylline do not provide adequate bronchodilation.

Oral sympathomimetics with alpha adrenergic activity appear to have some nasal decongestant effects and also may be of benefit in treating urticaria. Single doses of pseudoephedrine (Cantekin et al., 1977) or phenylpropanolamine (Dressler et al., 1977) decrease nasal airway resistance. The efficacy of these drugs in chronic therapy has not been well studied, however. Conventionally, ephedrine is used in doses up to 50 mg (depending on the size of the child and clinical response), pseudoephedrine in doses of 30 to 120 mg, or phenylpropanolamine in doses of 12.5 to 50 mg for nasal deconges-

tion, with administration intervals of 4 to 8 hours. Phenylephrine, also used orally as a nasal decongestant for some time, is not effective at recommended doses (Elis et al., 1967).

Monoamine oxidase inhibitors may potentiate the hypertensive effect of ephedrine by decreasing the metabolism of norepinephrine displaced from neuronal storage sites. This interaction has not been described for the newer agents, which have minimal alpha adrenergic properties.

Theophylline

Until recently, theophylline was used mainly as an acute bronchodilator. The elucidation of its pharmacokinetics and pharmacodynamics has enabled theophylline to be used more safely and with greater efficacy. Its bronchodilator effect increases progressively with serum concentration

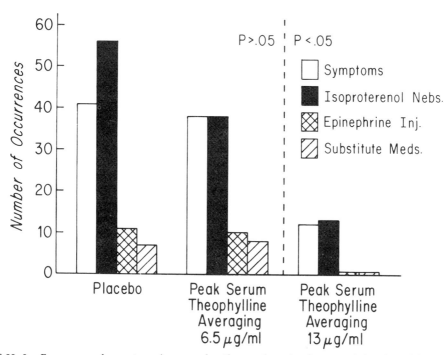

FIGURE 23–3. Frequency of symptoms (measured as the number of asthma attacks) and need for inhaled isoproterenol among 12 children with chronic asthma treated (double-blind) with placebo, an ephedrine-theophylline combination in conventional doses, and theophylline in doses that averaged twice the conventional recommendations. (From Weinberger and Bronsky: Evaluation of oral bronchodilator therapy in asthmatic children. J. Pediatr. 84:421, 1974.)

(Mitenko and Ogilvie, 1973) as does its ability to block exercise-induced bronchospasm (Pollock et al., 1977). Of particular importance has been the demonstration that theophylline can control the manifestations of chronic asthma when administered in doses that maintain serum concentrations between 10 and 20 µg per ml (Fig. 23–3). Tolerance, i.e., decreasing effect, does not appear to occur during chronic continuous use (Bierman et al., 1977).

Though theophylline may be more effective in some patients at serum concentrations over 20 µg per ml, the risk of toxicity increases progressively as serum concentrations exceed 20 µg per ml (Fig. 23–4). It should be noted that adverse drug effects also can occur in patients at low serum concentrations. While gastrointestinal effects, such as nausea, vomiting, occasional diarrhea, and central nervous system effects such as headache, irritability and nervousness commonly occur as serum concentrations exceed 20 µg per ml, seizures and deaths have been documented, generally at serum concentrations over 40 µg per ml, sometimes without a warning of the less serious adverse effects (Zwillich et al., 1975). Therefore, "pushing the dose to toxicity," especially without therapeutic monitoring, may be very hazardous.

Thus, for maximal therapeutic benefit with minimal risk, the "optimal" therapeutic range for theophylline in serum appears to be between 10 and 20 µg per ml (Weinberger, 1978). Dosage recommendations to attain these levels differ depending on whether the drug is used for treatment of symptoms or for continuous prophylactic therapy. The goal in relieving acute symptoms is to give the drug by a reliable and rapidly absorbed route of administration in a dose that reaches the therapeutic range as fast as possible, and then to maintain a dosage that keeps it there so long as it is needed. On the average, a "loading dose" of 7.5 mg per kg of ideal body weight will result in a serum concentration of about 15 µg per ml (Hendeles et al., 1978a). A conservative strategy is to administer 1 mg per kg for each 2 µg per ml of increase in serum concentration desired, initially aiming for the lower end of the therapeutic range to assure safety.

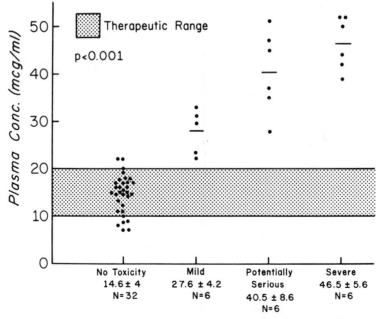

FIGURE 23–4. Relationship between serum theophylline concentration and adverse effects. Mild toxic symptoms: nausea or headache. Potentially serious symptoms: vomiting and/or tachycardia. Severe symptoms: arrhythmias and/or seizures (seizures occurred in two of these patients and one died). (From Hendeles et al., 1977a.)

Ratio of Concentration Achieved (µg/ml) to the Dose Administered (mg/k)
Peaks (r=.81)
Troughs (r=.83)
0
1
2
3
4
5
6
.2
.4
.6
.8
1.0
1.2
1.4
1.6
1.8
2.0
2.2
2.4
Clearance (ml/kg/min)

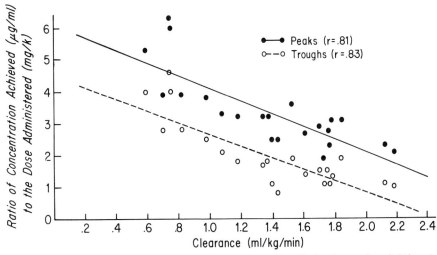

FIGURE 23–5. Relationship between theophylline clearance rate for elimination and peak (2 hour) and trough (6 hour) serum theophylline concentration when drug was administered continuously every 6 hours. (From Ginchansky and Weinberger: Relationship of theophylline clearance to oral dosage in children with chronic asthma. J. Pediatr. *91*:655, 1977.)

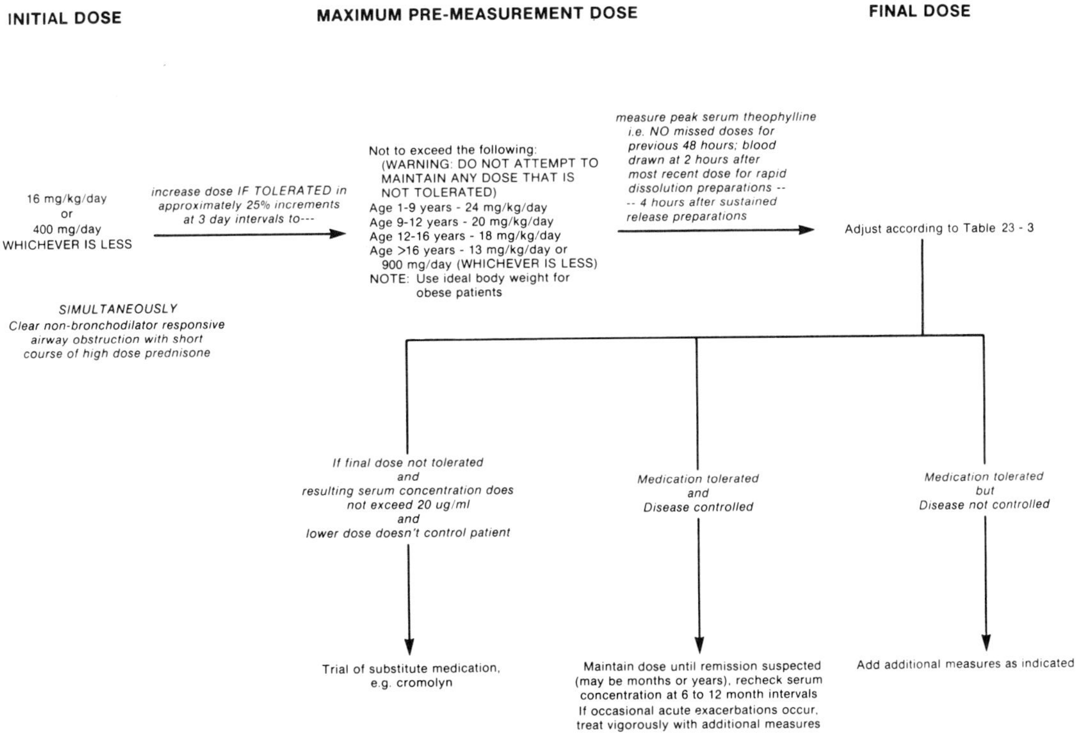

INITIAL DOSE
MAXIMUM PRE-MEASUREMENT DOSE
FINAL DOSE
16 mg/kg/day
or
400 mg/day
WHICHEVER IS LESS
increase dose IF TOLERATED in approximately 25% increments at 3 day intervals to---
Not to exceed the following:
(WARNING: DO NOT ATTEMPT TO MAINTAIN ANY DOSE THAT IS NOT TOLERATED)
Age 1-9 years - 24 mg/kg/day
Age 9-12 years - 20 mg/kg/day
Age 12-16 years - 18 mg/kg/day
Age >16 years - 13 mg/kg/day or 900 mg/day (WHICHEVER IS LESS)
NOTE: Use ideal body weight for obese patients
measure peak serum theophylline i.e. NO missed doses for previous 48 hours; blood drawn at 2 hours after most recent dose for rapid dissolution preparations -- -- 4 hours after sustained release preparations
Adjust according to Table 23 - 3
SIMULTANEOUSLY
Clear non-bronchodilator responsive airway obstruction with short course of high dose prednisone
If final dose not tolerated and resulting serum concentration does not exceed 20 ug/ml and lower dose doesn't control patient
Medication tolerated and Disease controlled
Medication tolerated but Disease not controlled
Trial of substitute medication, e.g. cromolyn
Maintain dose until remission suspected (may be months or years), recheck serum concentration at 6 to 12 month intervals
If occasional acute exacerbations occur, treat vigorously with additional measures
Add additional measures as indicated

FIGURE 23–6. Algorithm for determining optimal theophylline dosage for chronic therapy. Doses are expressed as 24-hour totals and should be divided to maintain serum theophylline concentrations as stable as possible on an around-the-clock basis. The dosing interval is guided by the individual patient's rate of theophylline elimination and the absorption characteristics of the product used. Products with rapid dissolution characteristics have rapid absorption and require administration at intervals of approximately 6 hours for most children and 8 hours for most nonsmoking adults. Reliably absorbed sustained-release preparations generally allow 8-hour dosing intervals for children; 12-hour intervals may be appropriate for adults with average or slower rates of elimination. (From Hendeles et al., 1978*b*.)

TABLE 23–3 FINAL DOSE ADJUSTMENT GUIDED BY MEASUREMENT OF SERUM THEOPHYLLINE CONCENTRATION* (See Figure 23–6)

Peak Theophylline Concentration (μg/ml)	Approximate Adjustment in Total Daily Dose	Comment
<5 5–7.5	100% increase 50% increase	If patient is asymptomatic, consider trial off drug; repeat measurement of serum concentration after dose adjustment.
8–10	20% increase	Even if patient is asymptomatic at this level, an increased serum concentration may prevent symptoms during a viral upper respiratory infection, heavy exposure to an inhalant allergen, or vigorous exertion.
11–13	Cautious 10% increase if clinically indicated	If patient is asymptomatic, no increase is necessary; if symptoms occur during upper respiratory infection or exercise, increase as indicated.
14–20	None	If "breakthrough" in asthmatic symptoms occurs at the end of dosing interval, change to sustained-release product and repeat serum theophylline measurements.
	Occasional intolerance requires a 10% decrease	If side effects occur, decrease total daily dose as indicated.
21–25	10% decrease	Even if side effects are absent.
26–30 31–35	25% decrease 33% decrease	Even if side effects are absent, omit next dose and decrease total daily dose as indicated; repeat measurement of serum theophylline concentration.
≥35	50% decrease	Omit next two doses, decrease as indicated, and repeat measurement of serum theophylline concentration.

NOTE—To avoid potential toxic reaction: (1) Assure that the sample represents a peak concentration obtained at steady state (e.g., no missed or extra doses—with close approximation of prescribed dosing intervals during previous 48 hours). (2) Use a reliable laboratory; if result appears questionable, repeat determination if not initially performed in duplicate. (3) The increase of 50% or 100% should be made in 25% increments at 2-day intervals to further assure safety and tolerance. The serum concentration may increase disproportionate to dosage increase as the therapeutic range is entered (Weinberger and Ginchansky: Dose-dependent kinetics of theophylline disposition in asthmatic children. J. Pediatr. *91*:820, 1977.)

*Modified from Hendeles, et al.: Guide to oral theophylline therapy for chronic asthma. Am. J. Dis. Child. *132*:876, 1978.

On initiating theophylline therapy for treatment of chronic asthma, it is best to begin with small doses administered around the clock and to increase the dose gradually until a serum concentration within the therapeutic range has been achieved. Too rapid increase in dosage may result in such side effects as nervousness, irritability, headache, and mild nausea even at serum concentrations below 10 μg per ml. These side effects that occur at subtoxic serum levels rapidly disappear in most patients as theophylline is continued, and the low initial dose with subsequent clinical titration generally avoids these caffeine-like effects altogether. A loading dose of theophylline should be reserved for those patients whose asthma symptoms are sufficiently severe to warrant these side effects. Chronic therapy is best initiated at low, well-tolerated doses (Hendeles et al., 1978b).

Final dosage requirements for continuous theophylline administration vary widely among individuals because of the remarkable interpatient variability in drug elimination (Fig. 23–5). The necessity to individualize dosage and to avoid adverse effects of theophylline has led to a scheme that both minimizes risk and simplifies the procedure so that multiple serum theophylline measurements usually are not necessary to determine dosage for chronic therapy (Fig. 23–6, Table 23–3). After selection of an initial dose with dosage increases as tolerated, serum theophylline measurement can be used to determine the final dose. A single serum theophylline measurement may suffice in many patients, whereas a second measurement may be required in some. When serum theophylline measurements are erratic and appear to correlate poorly with the prescribed dosage, problems in patient compliance, timing of the serum samples in relation to drug administration, or accuracy of the laboratory test should be questioned.

Theophylline clearance is relatively stable over time. Thus, once dosage is established and asthma is stable, younger children and adolescents probably require examination of serum theophylline only at 6- to 12-month intervals to readjust dosage for growth. Yearly levels are adequate for children during slower growth periods and for adults (Wyatt et al., 1978).

Clearance of theophylline, however, can be altered by specific physiologic and pharmacologic interactions, probably not all of which have been defined. Troleandomycin (TAO) profoundly affects theophylline clearance, increasing the serum theophylline concentration twofold (Weinberger et al., 1977). A related macrolide antibiotic, erythromycin, may have a similar though perhaps less potent effect on theophylline clearance (Kozak et al., 1977). These drug interactions, therefore, can result in theophylline toxicity by increasing serum theophylline levels. As mentioned previously, ephedrine, when administered with theophylline, results in increased toxicity *without* an increase in serum theophylline levels (Weinberger and Bronsky, 1975). Cigarette smoking increases theophylline elimination and thus increases dosage requirements if a stable serum theophylline concentration is to be maintained (Jenne et al., 1975). Conversely, patients who stop smoking may have a gradual (over months) return to a nonsmoking clearance rate and thus may develop potentially toxic serum concentrations (Powell et al., 1977). Liver disease (Piafsky et al., 1977a) and heart failure (Piafsky et al., 1977b) are examples of physiologic alterations that slow theophylline elimination and thus present a potential risk for toxicity if not recognized. Sustained fever associated with viral exanthem also appears to slow theophylline elimination and elevate serum levels (Chang et al., 1978).

Various theophylline formulations have been marketed over its 46 years of usage. In many cases, these have been based on misguided notions of the chemistry and absorption characteristics of the drug. The formulations identified as "salts" of theophylline, e.g., aminophylline, oxtriphylline, theophylline calcium salicylate, theophylline sodium glycinate, are little more than mixtures of a strong base with theophylline. At a physiologic pH, theophylline itself is a weak base and cannot form salts with a strong base. Only at very high pH does theophylline undergo tautomerism and become a weak acid capable of forming a salt with the ethylenediamine, choline, calcium salicylate, or sodium glycinate in these preparations. Theophylline also has been marketed in hydroalcoholic solutions in the belief that absorption will be improved. Recent studies show that theophylline is absorbed as effectively in aqueous solution, chewable tablets, or anhydrous tablets (Weinberger et al., 1978).

Other xanthine bronchodilators identified as theophylline derivatives include dihydroxypropyltheophylline (dyphylline or glyphylline), proxyphylline, and acephylline (the latter two are available in Europe). Dyphylline and proxyphylline are only one fifth to one tenth as active bronchodilators as theophylline. There is a serious question about the bioavailability of acephylline. Dyphylline (Lufyllin, Dilor), the only alternative xanthine bronchodilator on the American market, has a very short half life (2 hours in adults). Although a purported timed release preparation is available (Airets L.A.), bioavailability has not been established. Present data thus leave little indication for clinical use of xanthines other than theophylline (Hendeles and Weinberger, 1977).

In choosing a theophylline product, there is little reason to consider derivatives, salts, or hydroalcoholic solutions. Five categories of theophylline preparations warrant consideration (Table 23–4). When rapid absorption is desired, theophylline can be given parenterally using the intravenous solution (aminophylline). Alternatively, if a non-oral route is desired, the rectal solution (Somophyllin) generally appears to be absorbed rapidly. Rapid absorption (up to 85 percent in an hour) also occurs with oral liquid preparations and uncoated tablets which dissolve rapidly (Hendeles et al., 1977b).

For chronic therapy, especially in children, sustained-release formulations are preferable to overcome the usual short drug half-life and to improve compliance (Fig. 23–7). For children who cannot swallow capsules or tablets whole, the beads within a capsule can be sprinkled on a spoonful of soft food (e.g., applesauce) and washed down

TABLE 23–4   THEOPHYLLINE PREPARATIONS OF POTENTIAL USE IN PEDIATRICS*

Dosage Form	Trademark Name(s)	Anhydrous Theophylline Content
Tablet	Slo-Phyllin	100 mg scored
		200 mg scored
	Theophyl 225	225 mg scored
	Theophyl Chewable	100 mg double scored
	Theolair	125 mg scored
		250 mg scored
Oral liquid	Elixicon Suspension	20 mg/m
	Somphyllin Syrup	18 mg/ml
	Quibron Elixir†	10 mg/ml
	Slo-Phyllin GG Syrup‡	10 mg/ml
	Theophyl 225 Elixir	7.5 mg/ml (5% alcohol)
Sustained release	Slo-Phyllin Gyrocaps	60 mg capsules
		125 mg ”
		250 mg ”
	Theo-Dur Tablets	100 mg scored
		200 mg scored
		300 mg scored
	Theophyl S-R	125 mg
		250 mg
Rectal solution	Somophyllin	51 mg/ml
Intravenous solution	(Aminophylline U.S.P.)	21 mg/ml

*Modified from Weinberger: Theophylline for treatment of asthma. J. Pediatr. *92*:1, 1978.
†Guaifenesin, included in this product and in Slo-Phyllin GG, is not an active ingredient.
‡Warning: These brand names are used for two or more preparations containing different concentrations of theophylline; only the most useful is listed. Prescriptions for these products should specify the theophylline concentration.

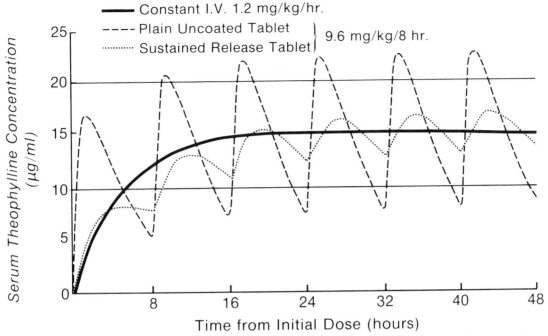

FIGURE 23–7. Expected serum theophylline concentration in an average child from a constant intravenous infusion, and during multiple oral dosing with a typical uncoated tablet and a bioavailable sustained-release tablet. The IV dose was selected to give a steady state concentration of 15 μg/ml when administered at a constant rate. This is contrasted with the same dose for 8 hours administered as the two oral dosage forms. (From Weinberger et al.: The relationship of product formulation to absorption of oral theophylline. New Engl. J. Med. 299:852, 1978.)

with a beverage; they will retain their sustained-release properties so long as the beads themselves are not chewed.

Cromolyn Sodium

This drug presented a new approach to asthma management. Cromolyn acts as a prophylactic agent, apparently by preventing or decreasing release of histamine and other chemical mediators; it has no bronchodilator, anti-inflammatory or antihistamine activity. As a result, *cromolyn sodium has no effect on acute symptoms of asthma.* Presumably activation or release of mediators by nonimmune as well as immune (allergic) mechanisms is affected since cromolyn has some efficacy in blocking exercise-induced bronchospasm and benefit from cromolyn is not reliably dependent on the presence of inhalant allergy. On the other hand, cromolyn is less effective than theophylline when used

optimally, in suppressing both exercise-induced bronchospasm (Pollock et al., 1977) and the symptoms of chronic asthma (Fig. 23–8). However, cromolyn is virtually nontoxic, even in overdose, and serious adverse effects have not been found except for a few reported allergic reactions. Cromolyn is administered in powder form by inhalation. The dosage generally is one (20 mg) capsule four times a day. Some patients will experience coughing or bronchospasm on inhaling cromolyn because it is irritating to their very reactive airways. In such patients the inhalation of isoproterenol before cromolyn may facilitate continuation of cromolyn. When cromolyn is prescribed, it should be used for 4 weeks' trial before it is assumed not to be effective, and the physician should observe the patient's method of using the Spinhaler. Some have suggested that larger doses occasionally may give more benefit, but this is not well established. Cromolyn is available in the United

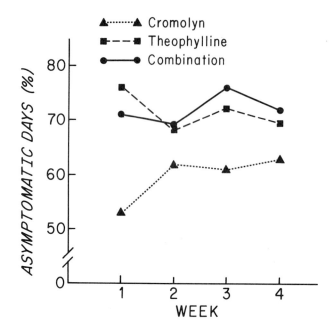

FIGURE 23–8. Weekly frequencies of asymptomatic days in 28 asthmatic children. While significant differences between cromolyn (cromoglycate) and theophylline were observed (p < 0.025), the differences between weeks were not significant for any of the three drug regimens (p > 0.1). (From Hambleton et al.: Comparison of cromoglycate (cromolyn) and theophylline in controlling symptoms of chronic asthma. Lancet 1:381, 1977.)

States exclusively in 20 mg capsules that are utilized with a turbo inhaler (Spinhaler) for delivery. Since cromolyn is dispensed in lactose, patients should rinse the mouth with water after inhaling a capsule, to forestall a possible increase in dental caries. It also is possible to deliver cromolyn to young children by dissolving the contents of a capsule in about 2 ml of water and administering the suspension by a Venturi-type nebulizer driven by compressed air.

Cromolyn has been used with moderate clinical efficacy as a solution for allergic rhinitis (Handelman et al., 1977) and conjunctivitis (Greenbaum et al., 1977). It must be administered up to six times a day in order to be effective clinically; this is inconvenient for most patients and has not been proven superior to antihistamines.

Corticosteroids

Corticosteroids are the only drugs that can reverse the airway obstruction in asthma that is unresponsive to bronchodilators (Fig. 23–9). However, their exact mechanism of action is unknown. They do not appear to affect spasm of bronchial smooth muscle, they do not affect the immediate response to antigen challenge (either by skin testing or inhalation), they do not prevent exercise-induced, methacholine-induced or histamine-induced asthma. However, they do facilitate bronchodilation by increasing the response of the airways to bronchodilators in one hour (Ellul-Micallef and Fenech, 1975), and increase PaO_2 in hypoxemic patients as early as 3 hours after administration (Pierson et al., 1974). Moreover, they can restore normal airway response to bronchodilators in patients who previously responded poorly if at all. Corticosteroids also diminish sputum production in the asthmatic and appear to decrease airway obstruction due to mucosal edema.

Corticosteroids are most potent when administered daily or several times daily. While there is virtually no toxicity when they are administered in high doses for short periods (days), prolonged daily therapy results in suppression of endogenous adrenal function, Cushingoid changes in appearance, growth suppression, posterior subcapsular cataracts, osteoporosis, and the other glucocorticoid metabolic effects. In an attempt to minimize the risks of long-term toxicity, prednisone or other *short-acting* corticosteroid (prednisolone, methylprednisolone) should be employed on an alternate-day basis when continuous prophylactic therapy is needed, using single early

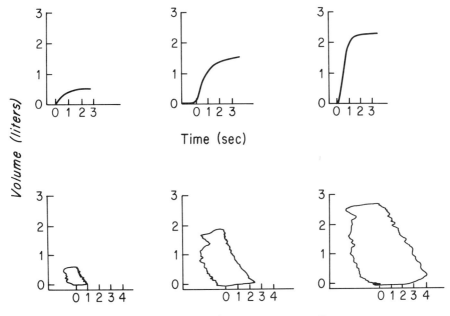

FIGURE 23–9. Time-volume (upper) and flow-volume (lower) spirometric tracings of a 12-year-old boy with chronic asthma. The first tracings were after maximum bronchodilator therapy (loading dose of theophylline, parenteral and inhaled sympathomimetics) at the time of his first visit. The second was performed after inhaled isoproterenol following 5 days of prednisone (40 mg twice daily), which relieved his asthmatic symptoms. Vital capacity, FEV_1, and flow rates all continued to improve to normal after 5 more days of prednisone (third tracing). (From Weinberger and Hendeles: Management of asthma. Postgrad. Med. J. *61*:85, 1977.)

morning doses (8 A.M. or before) every second day. Used on this basis, steroid therapy can lead to effective symptom suppression while minimizing the adverse effects (Harter and Novitch, 1966). More recently, the use of certain corticosteroid esters by inhalation, e.g., beclomethasone dipropionate and triamcinolone acetonide, has been demonstrated to suppress the symptoms of chronic asthma with little systemic corticosteroid effect when used in the recommended dose range. These newer inhalant steroid preparations have fewer systemic effects than dexamethasone.

Beclomethasone dipropionate was the first of the new generation of inhaled corticosteroids on the American market. Although initial reports suggested the absence of systemic effect when used in recommended doses, it now appears that some hypothalamic-pituitary-adrenal (HPA) dysfunction can occur when used in recommended doses, perhaps in the order of that seen with alternate-day prednisone therapy (Wyatt et al., 1978*b*). Thus, there appears to be little reason to choose inhaled beclomethasone dipropionate over alternate-day prednisone purely on the basis of pituitary adrenal function. However, for patients in whom the control of asthma is not adequate with alternate-day prednisone or in whom other adverse effects are apparent, beclomethasone dipropionate may offer therapeutic advantage.

Little or no growth suppression is associated with prednisone every other day in doses of up to 40 mg and possibly higher (Reimer et al. 1975). In fact, children with severe chronic asthma whose growth has been suppressed may experience growth acceleration with the use of a therapeutically effective alternate-day prednisone regimen. In our experience, when an alternate-day prednisone regimen is selected for therapy, children need at least 20 mg of prednisone per dose. Similarly, dosages of 400 μg per day or higher usually are generally needed when inhaled beclomethasone is used for chronic asthma. When one of the two chronic corticosteroid regimens is initiated, it generally is better to begin at the upper end of the recommended dose range, achieve control of systems, and diminish drug dosage to the lowest levels possible which control asthma. We generally recommend instituting alternate-day prednisone at a dosage for 40 mg for preadolescents and adolescents, at 30 mg for younger school age children down to the post toddler ages, at 20 mg every other day for toddlers and at 10 mg every other day for infants. Dosage reductions of 5 to 10 mg can be tried at 2-week intervals. Inhaled beclomethasone dipropionate probably is best administered at about 800 μg per day (four inhalations four times daily) with 50 to 100 μg per day dose reductions at 2-week intervals so long as symptoms are controlled.

In general, daily corticosteroid therapy to relieve acute symptoms requires 10 to 40 mg b.i.d. (depending on body size, e.g., 10 mg for infants, 40 mg for adolescents and adults); the use of this "clearing" dose prior to the onset of chronic therapy often will help insure the adequacy of the chronic therapeutic measures. Breakthrough symptoms during alternate-day prednisone or inhaled beclomethasone require the use of similar doses of daily prednisone when acute bronchodilator therapy is inadequate.

The most common adverse effect of inhaled beclomethasone dipropionate is oral thrush which generally responds readily to oral nystatin. It can be minimized by rinsing the mouth after medication. Pulmonary moniliasis is extraordinarily rare. Mild Cushingoid facies and some increase in appetite and accompanying weight gain occur commonly at higher doses of alternate-day prednisone although other adverse effects of long-term alternate-day oral steroid therapy are uncommon even at considerably higher doses.

While virtually any oral glucocorticosteroid can be used for acute symptoms, only prednisone, prednisolone, or methylprednisolone have sufficiently short duration of adrenal suppressive effect to allow the safety seen with alternate-day therapy. A single dose of longer acting corticosteroid such as dexamethasone appears to result in a prolonged systemic effect, and cannot be used to advantage on an alternate-day basis.

Product selection for inhaled corticosteroids in the United States is limited to beclomethasone dipropionate. For oral corticosteroid therapy, however, various alternative preparations are available (Table 23–5). Prednisone is the least expensive for chronic therapy; neither prednisolone nor methylprednisolone offers any advantage to justify the increased cost to the patient. The cost savings of alternate-day prednisone over inhaled beclomethasone dipropionate also is apparent.

Corticosteroids also are effective in the treatment of rhinitis. In general, systemic corticosteroids are warranted only occasionally, when allergic rhinitis and conjunctivitis are severe enough to be temporarily

TABLE 23–5   PREPARATIONS AND RELATIVE COSTS OF CORTICOSTEROIDS*

Dosage Form	Generic Name	Trademark Name(s)	1977 Costs for 20 mg of Prednisone or Equivalent ($)
Tablet	Prednisone	Deltasone	0.08
		Orasone	0.07
	Prednisolone	Delta-Cortef	0.19 (5 mg)
	Methylprednisolone	Medrol	0.63 (16 mg)
Injection	Methylprednisolone sodium succinate	Solu-Medrol	2.00 (16 mg)
Aerosol	Beclomethasone dipropionate	Vanceril, Beclovent	0.32 (400 μg)

*Modified from Weinberger and Hendeles: Antiasthmatic drugs. *In* Miller and Greenblatt (eds.): Handbook of Drug Therapy, Elsevier-North Holland, Inc., 1979.

disabling. The new generation of topical corticosteroids such as beclomethasone dipropionate appear particularly effective for allergic rhinitis when persistent nasal congestion unresponsive to oral decongestants is a dominant symptom. These are not yet commercially available in the United States; however, a baby nipple with the end cut open converts the intrabronchial inhaler to an intranasal form.

Antihistamines (H₁ Blockers)

The classic antihistamines competitively inhibit the physiologic effects of histamine (H_1 receptor activity) except for the stimulant effect on gastric acid secretion (H_2 receptor activity). In addition, they possess antiemetic, anticholinergic, sedative or CNS stimulating properties. These latter effects differ greatly among various antihistamines. There is little data demonstrating that differences in effects among the antihistamines relate to chemical structure; traditionally, however, antihistamines have been categorized into six groups according to chemical structure (Fig. 23–10). These categories, however, have little functional importance, since they do not predict relative efficacy or side effects. For example, diphenhydramine, which is strongly sedative, is in the ethanolamine group along with carbinoxamine, which rarely produces sedation.

Despite the plethora of antihistamines commercially available as single entities or in combination with other agents, few have been subjected to scientific study using double-blind placebo controlled techniques. Cook et al., (1973) did present evidence that hydroxyzine is more effective than diphenhydramine and other antihistamines in suppressing wheal size, both in extent and duration of action (see Fig. 23–10). Hydroxyzine also was shown to be more effective than diphenyhydramine and cyproheptadine in inhibiting histamine-induced pruritus (Rhoades et al., 1975). These studies strongly suggest a potential difference in clinical efficacy between hydroxyzine and other antihistamines.

Hydroxyzine, when administered on a constant daily basis can be particularly effective in preventive therapy for allergic rhinitis and conjunctivitis. Persistent side effects, particularly drowsiness and xerostomia, are uncommon in patients taking continuous hydroxyzine if therapy is initiated with a small dose at bedtime (25 mg) and increased progressively over a 10-day period, as tolerated, until an optimal dosage for adults of 150 mg per day is attained. In contrast to other symptoms of seasonal allergic rhinitis, nasal congestion does not appear to be suppressed by hydroxyzine (Schaaf et al., 1979). Orally administered alpha-adrenergic agonists (phenylpropanolamine or pseudoephedrine) on the other hand can be effective in relieving nasal congestion, justifying their use in combination with antihistamines for allergic rhinitis (Empey et al., 1976). In perennial nonallergic rhinitis, nasal congestion often is the dominant symptom and the role for antihistamines is less clear.

Drowsiness, dry mouth, irritability, or dizziness commonly may occur on initiating antihistamine therapy. These side effects, while annoying to some patients, rarely are serious. On the other hand, the patient should be warned that side effects may interfere with coordination or judgment and that driving a car or riding a bicycle in traffic should be avoided until the degree of adverse reaction is apparent. Urinary retention, anorexia, and constipation also can occur. In toxic doses, younger children may experience an excitation phase with hallucinations, incoordination, muscular twitching, fever, convulsions, and even cardiorespiratory collapse and death (Hestand and Teske, 1977). Chronic toxicity with any of the antihistamines is relatively rare. Cyproheptadine may stimulate the appetite and has been used for this purpose in patients with anorexia.

Previous warnings against the use of antihistamines in cases of coexisting allergic rhinitis and asthma probably have been exaggerated (Karlin, 1972). While the drying effect may present some hazard in the acute asthmatic attack, chlorpheniramine and hydroxyzine have a minor bronchodilating effect. This probably is not clinically significant and may relate to the anticholinergic effect of these two agents. There is little evidence that antihistamines alter the

HISTAMINE 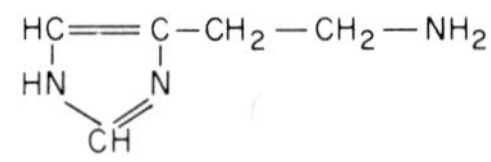

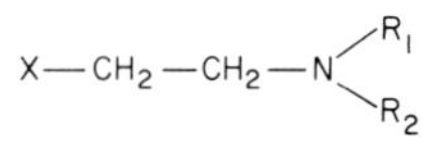

CHEMICAL GROUP	GENERIC NAME	BRAND NAME	H_1 BLOCKERS
Ethanolamine	Diphenhydramine	Benadryl	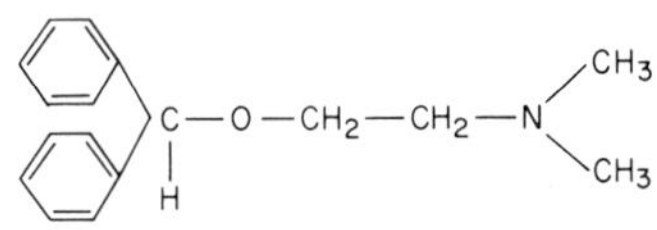
	Carbinoxamine	in Rondec	
	Clemastine	(Tavist)	
Ethylenediamine	Tripelenamine	Pyribenzamine	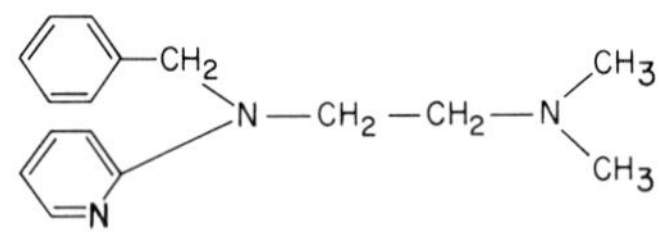
	Methapyriline	Histadyl	
Alkylamine	Chlorpheniramine	Chlortrimeton	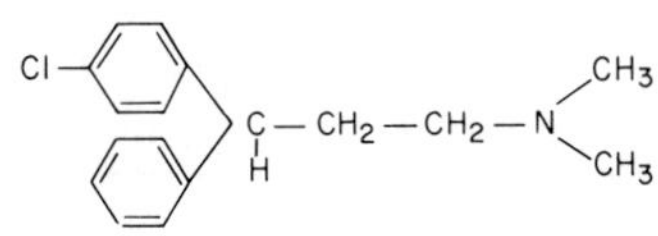
	Brompheniramine	Dimetane	
	Triprolidine	in Actifed	
Piprazine	Hydroxyzine	Atarax	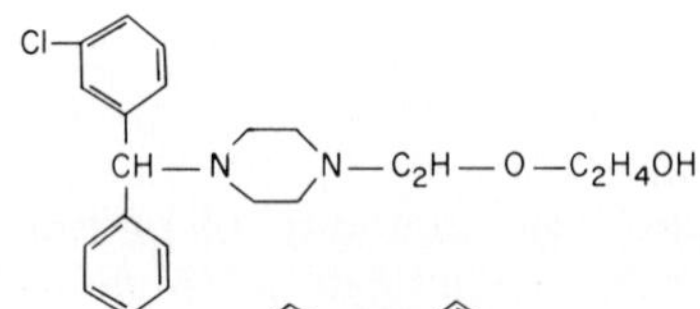
Piperidine	Cyproheptadine	Periactin	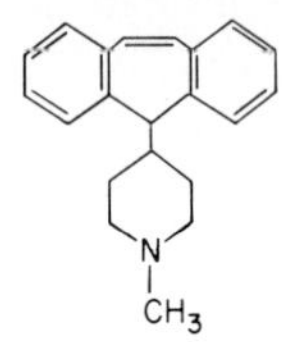
Phenothiazine	Promethazine	Phenergan	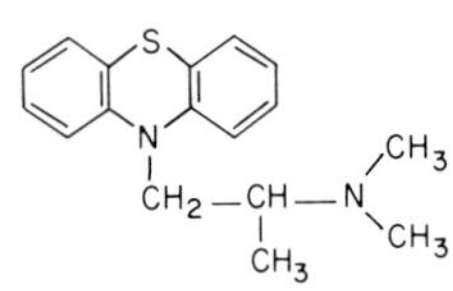
	Trimeprazine	Temaril	
	Methdilazine	Tacaryl	

FIGURE 23–10. *See legend on the opposite page.*

T½ (HRS)	WHEAL SUPPRESSION EXTENT (%)	DURATION (DAYS)	SIDE EFFECTS (RANK)	EEG EFFECT	COMMENT
3-4	31	1.9	3	Low energy-sedation	Therapeutic range (25-50 ng/m) Marked anticholinergic effect
14					Sedation infrequent
					Sedation infrequent
2-3	44	2.8	4	High energy-"overalertness"	
					In non-prescription sleep aids
12-15	34	2.4	5	High energy-"overalertness"	In many OTC products
36					
5					
3	63	4.3	2		
			1		Less effective than hydroxyzine in itch suppression. Uniquely effective in some cases of cold urticaria.
	51	2.8	2	Low energy-sedation	

FIGURE 23–10. Structure and pharmacologic properties of H₁ antihistamines. The extent and duration of wheal and flare suppression during a double-blind randomized study also are listed. Rank of 1 represents the highest frequency of side effects. (From Cook et al.: Degree and duration of skin test suppression and side effects with antihistamines. J. Allergy Clin. Immunol. *51*:71, 1973.)

frequency or severity of asthmatic symptoms.

The pharmacodynamics of antihistamines have not been studied in depth. Diphenhydramine has been examined more carefully than most. It appears to be effective at serum concentrations in the range of 25 to 30 nanograms per ml while toxicity commonly occurs when the serum concentration exceeds 50 μg per ml (Carruthers et al., 1978). A single 50 mg oral dose is poorly bioavailable, averaging 43 percent when compared to an intravenous dose. Since the half-life of diphenyhydramine (3 to 4 hours) is relatively constant among patients, increasing the dose beyond 50 mg is likely to increase side effects without substantially increasing beneficial effects. Despite the relatively short serum half-life, diphenhydramine exerts some suppressive effect on the wheal and flare response to allergenic extracts for an average of 1.8 days (Cook et al., 1973). Thus there appears to be little correlation between the elimination of the drug from the body and the duration of its antihistamine effect in the tissue, and commonly recommended prescribing practices for antihistamines (three to four times a day) may be inappropriate. Current dosage recommendations for antihistamines are generally not supported by appropriate clinical evaluation but instead are based largely on empirical custom.

Miscellaneous Therapeutic Agents

Anticholinergic Agents. Anticholinergic agents in the form of burning stramonium leaves and stramonium cigarettes have been used since the nineteenth century for the treatment of asthma and are still available for this purpose. Confirmation of the apparent bronchodilator effect of inhaling these drugs has more recently been supported in studies on atropine. The bronchodilator effect of even the newer anticholinergics, however, generally is weaker than that of theophylline or adrenergic bronchodilators. The use of inhalant anticholinergic drugs for asthma is experimental for the most part, and their role in asthma therapy has not been established.

Expectorants. Expectorants have been used traditionally in asthma but without documentation of effect on the viscosity of mucus. One study suggested benefit from iodides through some nonexpectorant mechanism of action, but benefit occurred in a small proportion of patients, and the frequency of toxicity was high (Falliers et al., 1966). The American Academy of Pediatrics Committee on Drugs recently has condemned the use of iodides, particularly in children and in women of childbearing age, because of the toxic and teratogenic potential and lack of substantial therapeutic benefit (American Academy of Pediatrics Committee on Drugs, 1976). Water also is used to encourage expectoration. While adequate hydration is part of supportive therapy for an acute exacerbation of asthma, overhydration is not advantageous and may complicate asthma therapy.

Antibiotics. Viral infection, rather than bacterial, has been associated with exacerbations of asthma (McIntosh et al., 1973; Minor et al., 1974). Adult asthmatics with "bronchitic" sputum do not have bacteria in the lower respiratory tract as determined by transtracheal aspirations (Berman et al., 1975), and antibiotics have little effect in treatment outcomes for childhood status asthmaticus (Shapiro et al., 1974). Thus, the indications for antibiotics in children with asthma or other allergic disorders are the same as in the child without allergic disease, namely, symptoms and signs of pyogenic infection.

Other Agents. Since asthma is a chronic disease with such a variable clinical course, a variety of unconventional methods of management become popular from time to time, ranging from arsenic as "Gay's Solution" to "megavitamin" treatment and acupuncture.

Newer agents should be introduced into regular patient care only as these agents offer clear therapeutic advantages over established drugs. With a disease that has as variable a clinical course as asthma, the physician must select appropriate drugs based on knowledge of their pharmacology that best suit the needs of the patient to assure effective control of asthma (Weinberger and Hendeles, 1977).

References

American Academy of Pediatrics Committee on Drugs. Adverse reactions to iodide therapy of asthma and other pulmonary diseases. Pediatrics 57:272, 1976.

American Thoracic Society. Committee on Diagnostic Standards for Non-Tuberculosis Respiratory Disease: Definition and classification of chronic bronchitis, asthma, and pulmonary emphysema. Am. Rev. Respir. Dis. 85:762, 1962.

Anderson, S.D., Seale, J.P., Rozea, S.P., et al.: Inhaled and oral salbutamol in exercise-induced asthma. Am. Rev. Respir. Dis. 114:493, 1976.

Bachus, B.F. and Snider, G.L.: The bronchodilator effect of aerosolized terbutaline. J.A.M.A. 238:2277, 1977.

Berman, S.Z., Mathison, D.A., Stevenson, D.D., et al.: Transtracheal aspiration studies in asthmatic patients in relapse with "infective" asthma and in subjects without respiratory disease. J. Allergy Clin. Immunol. 56:206, 1975.

Bierman, C.W., Shapiro, G.G., Pierson, W.E., et al.: Acute and chronic theophylline therapy in exercise-induced bronchospasm. Pediatrics 60:845, 1977.

Cantekin, E.I., Bluestone, C.D., Welch, R.M., et al.: Nasal decongestant activity of pseudoephedrine. Ann. Otol. Rhinol. Laryngol. 86:235, 1977.

Carruthers, S.G., Shoeman, D.W., Hignite, C.E., et al.: Correlation between plasma diphenhydramine level and sedative and antihistamine effects. Clin. Pharmacol. Ther. 23:375, 1978.

Chang, K.C., Bell, P.D., Lauer, B.A., et al.: Altered theophylline pharmacokinetics during acute respiratory viral illness. Lancet 1:1132, 1978.

Chatterjee, S.S., Nassar, W.Y., Wilson, O., et al.: Intra-nasal beclomethasone dipropionate and intra-nasal sodium cromoglycate: A comparative trial. Clin. Allergy 4:343, 1974.

Chervinsky, P., and Belinkoff, S.: Comparison of metaproterenol and isoproterenol aerosols: spirometric evaluation after two months therapy. Ann. Allergy 27:611, 1969.

Cook, T.J., MacQueen, D.M., Witting, H.J., et al.: Degree and duration of skin test suppression and side effects with antihistamines. J. Allergy Clin. Immunol. 51:71, 1973.

Dressler, W.E., Meyers, T., London, S.J., et al.: A system of rhinomanometry in the clinical evaluation of nasal decongestants. Ann. Otol. Rhinol. Laryngol. 86:310, 1977.

Ekwo, E., and Weinberger, M.: Evaluation of a program for the pharmacologic management of children with asthma. J. Allergy. Clin. Immunol. 61:240, 1978.

Elis, J., Laurence, D.R., Mattie, H., et al.: Modification by monoamine oxidase inhibitors of the effect of some sympathomimetics on blood pressure. Br. Med. J. 2:75, 1967.

Ellul-Micallef, R., and Fenech, F.F.: Effect of intravenous prednisolone in asthmatics with diminished adrenergic responsiveness. Lancet 2:1269, 1975.

Empey, D.W., Bye, C., Hodder, M., et al.: A double-blind crossover trial of pseudoephedrine and tripiolidine alone and in combination, for the treatment of allergic rhinitis. Ann. Allergy 34:41, 1976.

Falliers, C.J., McCann, W.P., Chai, H., et al.: Controlled study of iodotherapy for childhood asthma. J. Allergy 38:183, 1966.

Ginchansky, E., and Weinberger, M.: Relationship of theophylline clearance to oral dosage in children with chronic asthma. J. Pediatr. 91:655, 1977.

Godfrey, S., and Konig, P.: Suppression of exercise-induced asthma by salbutamol, theophylline, atropine, cromolyn, and placebo in a group of asthmatic children. Pediatrics 56 (Suppl):930, 1975.

Hambleton, G., Weinberger, M., Taylor, J., et al.: Comparison of cromoglycate (cromolyn) and theophylline in controlling symptoms of chronic asthma. Lancet 1:1381, 1977.

Handelman, N.I., Friday, G.A., Schwartz, H.J., et al.: Cromolyn sodium nasal solution in the prophylactic treatment of pollen-induced seasonal allergic rhinitis. J. Allergy Clin. Immunol. 59:237, 1977.

Harter, J.G., and Novitch, A.M.: Evaluation of steroid analogues in terms of suitability for alternate-day steroid therapy. J. Allergy 37:108, 1966.

Hendeles, L., Bighley, L., Richardson, R.H., et al.: Frequent toxicity from IV aminophylline infusions in critically ill patients. Drug. Intell. Clin. Pharm. 11:12, 1977a.

Hendeles, L., Weinberger, M., Bighley, L.: Absolute bioavailability of oral theophylline. Am. J. Hosp. Pharm. 34:525, 1977b.

Hendeles, L., and Weinberger, M.: Dyphylline, the "untheophylline" xanthine bronchodilator. Drug. Intell. Clin. Pharm. 11:424, 1977.

Hendeles, L., Weinberger, M., Bighley, L.: Disposition of theophylline following a single intravenous aminophylline infusion. Am. Rev. Respir. Dis. 118:97, 1978a.

Hendeles, L., Weinberger, M., Wyatt, R.: Guide to oral theophylline therapy for chronic asthma. Am. J. Dis. Child., 132:876, 1978b.

Hestand, H.E., and Teske, D.W.: Diphenhydramine hydrochloride intoxication. J. Pediatr. 90:1017, 1977.

Hetzel, M.R., and Clark, T.J.H.: Comparison of intravenous and aerosol salbutamol. Br. Med. J. 2:919, 1976.

Jenne, J., Nagasawa, H., McHugh, R., et al.: Decreased theophylline half-life in cigarette smokers. Life Sci., 17:195, 1975.

Johnson, A.J., Spiro, S.G., Pidgeon, J., et al.: Intravenous infusion of salbutamol in severe acute asthma. Br. Med. J., 1:1013, 1978.

Karetzky, M.S.: Asthma mortality associated with pneumothorax and intermittent positive-pressure breathing. Lancet 1:828, 1975.

Karlin, J.: The use of antihistamines in asthma. Ann. Allergy 30:342, 1972.

Kolotkin, B.M., Lee, C.K., Townley, R.G.: Duration of specificity of sodium cromolyn on allergen inhalation challenges in asthmatics. J. Allergy Clin. Immunol. 53:288, 1974.

Kozak, P.P., Cummins, L.H., Gillman, S.A.: Administration of erythromycin to patients on theophylline. J. Allergy Clin. Immunol. 60:149, 1977.

Legge, J.S., Gaddie, J., Palmer, K.N.: Comparison of two oral selective β_2-adrenergic stimulant drugs in bronchial asthma. Br. Med. J. 1:637, 1971.

McIntosh, K., Ellis, E.F., Hoffman, L.S., et al.: The association of viral and bacterial respiratory infections with exacerbations of wheezing in young asthmatic children. J. Pediatr. 82:478, 1973.

Minor, T.E., Dick, E.C., DeMeo, A.N., et al.: Viruses as precipitants of asthmatic attacks in children. J.A.M.A. 227:292, 1974.

Michels, M.I., Smith, R.E., Heimlich, E.M.: Adrenal suppression and intranasally applied steroids. Ann. Allergy 25:569, 1967.

Mitenko, P.A., and Ogilvie, R.I.: Rational intravenous doses of theophylline. New Engl. J. Med. 289:600, 1973.

Moore, R.M., Cotton, E.K., Pinney, M.A.: The effect of intermittent positive-pressure breathing on airway resistance in normal and asthmatic children. J. Allergy Clin. Immunol. 49:137, 1972.

Nelson, H.S., Raine, D., Doner, C., et al.: Subsensitivity to the bronchodilator action of albuterol produced by chronic administration. Am. Rev. Respir. Dis. 116:871, 1977.

Norman, P.S., Winkenwerder, W.L., Agbayani, B.F., et al.: Adrenal function during the use of dexamethasone aerosols in the treatment of ragweed hay fever. J. Allergy 40:57, 1967.

Parry, W.H., Martorano, F., Cotton, E.K.: Management of life-threatening asthma with intravenous isoproterenol infusions. Am. J. Dis. Child. 130:39, 1976.

Piafsky, K.M., Sitar, D.S., Rangno, R.E., et al.: Theophylline disposition in patients with hepatic cirrhosis. New Engl. J. Med. 296:1495, 1977.

Piafsky, K.M., Sitar, D.S., Rangno, R.E., et al.: Theophylline kinetics in acute pulmonary edema. Clin. Pharmacol. Ther. *21*:310, 1977.

Piersen, W.E., Bierman, C.W., Kelley, V.C.: A double-blind trial of corticosteroid therapy in status asthmaticus. Pediatrics *54*:782, 1974.

Pollock, J., Kiechel, F., Cooper, D., et al.: Relationship of serum theophylline concentration to inhibition of exercise-induced bronchospasm and comparison with cromolyn. Pediatrics *60*:840, 1977.

Powell, J.R., Thiercelin, J., Vozeh, S., et al.: The influence of cigarette smoking and sex on theophylline disposition. Am. Rev. Respir. Dis. *116*:17, 1977.

Rhoades, R.B., Leifer, K.N., Cohan, R., et al.: Suppression of histamine induced pruritus by three antihistaminic drugs. J. Allergy Clin. Immunol. *55*:180, 1975.

Reimer, L.G., Morris, H.G., Ellis, E.F.: Growth of asthmatic children during treatment with alternate-day steroids. J. Allergy Clin. Immunol. *55*:224, 1975.

Schaaf, L., Hendeles, L., Weinberger, M.: Hydroxyzine suppression of symptoms of seasonal allergic rhinitis. J. Allergy Clin. Immunol. *13*:129–133, 1979.

Shapiro, G.G., Eggleston, P.A., Pierson, W.E., et al.: Double-blind study of the effectiveness of a broad spectrum antibiotic in status asthmaticus. Pediatrics *53*:867, 1974.

Sly, R.M., Badiei, B., Faciane, J.: Comparison of subcutaneous terbutaline in the treatment of asthma in children. J. Allergy Clin. Immunol. *59*:128, 1977.

Vlagopoulos, T., Townley, R., Ghazanshahi, S., et al.: Comparison of the onset of action and bronchodilation effects of the anticholinergic agent SCH 1000 with isoproterenol. J. Allergy Clin. Immunol. *55*:99, 1975.

Wanderer, A.A., and Ellis, E.F.: Treatment of cold urticaria with cyproheptadine. J. Allergy Clin. Immunol. *48*:366, 1971.

Weinberger, M.: Theophylline for treatment of asthma. J. Pediatr. *92*:1, 1978.

Weinberger, M.M., and Bronsky, E.A.: Evaluation of oral bronchodilator therapy in asthmatic children. J. Pediatr. *84*:421, 1974.

Weinberger, M., Bronsky, E., Bensch, G.W., et al.: Interaction of ephedrine and theophylline. Clin. Pharmacol. Ther., *17*:585, 1975.

Weinberger, M., and Ginchansky, E.: Dose-department kinetics of theophylline disposition in asthmatic children. J. Pediatr. *91*:820, 1977.

Weinberger, M., and Hendeles, L.: Antiasthmatic drugs. *In* Miller, R.R., and Greenblatt, D.J. (eds.): *Handbook of Drug Therapy.* Elsevier-North Holland, Inc., 1979.

Weinberger, M., and Hendeles, L.: Management of asthma. Postgrad. Med. J. *61*:85, 1977.

Weinberger, M., and Hendeles, L.: Pharmacotherapy of asthma. Am. J. Hosp. Pharm. *33*:1071, 1976.

Weinberger, M., Hendeles, L., Bighley, L.: The relationship of product formulation to absorption of oral theophylline. New Engl. J. Med. *299*:852, 1978.

Weinberger, M., Hudgel, D., Spector, S. et al.: Inhibition of theophylline clearance by troleandomycin. J. Allergy Clin. Immunol. *59*:228, 1977.

Wyatt, R., Weinberger, M., Hendeles, L.: Oral theophylline dosage for the management of chronic asthma. J. Pediatr *92*:125, 1978*a*.

Wyatt, R., Waschek, J., Weinberger, M., Sherman, B.: Effects of inhaled beclomethasone dipropionate and oral alternate-day prednisone on pituitary-adrenal function in children with chronic asthma. New Engl. J. Med. *299*:1387–1392, 1978*b*.

Zwillich, C.W., Sutton, F.D., Neff, T.A., et al.: Theophylline induced seizures in adults; correlation with serum concentrations. Ann. Intern. Med. *82*:784, 1975.

Bernard A. Berman, M.D.
C. Warren Bierman, M.D.

24

Injection Therapy

IMMUNOTHERAPY (HYPOSENSITIZATION)

In 1903, Dunbar introduced the concept of injection treatment of allergic disease. He attempted to develop a passive "antitoxin," *pollantin,* which could be administered topically, by injecting "pollen toxin" into geese and horses; therapeutic results from this procedure were inconsistent. Subsequently, Noon and Freeman (1911) attempted to develop active "immunity" in patients with hay fever by injecting extracts of boiled grass pollen. These investigators reported beneficial results in the 20 grass pollen hay fever patients so treated, and this therapy soon was tried in America. In 1915 Cooke reported the first study in the United States on the (successful) treatment of hay fever by active immunization. Cooke believed, as had Noon and Freeman, that hay fever was caused by a toxin to which pollen injections induced an antitoxin that "desensitized" the patient to the pollen. By 1922, however, Cooke noted that in spite of clinical improvement, patients still had skin reactions to pollen injections. This reactivity he believed to be due to "unneutralized antibody," and he suggested the term "hyposensitization" in place of "desensitization."

By 1935, Cooke had discovered a substance in the blood of treated patients that could inhibit the Prausnitz-Küstner (PK) test. He called this factor "blocking antibody" and demonstrated that patients with ragweed hay fever would improve clinically if they were transfused with serum from treated patients. Loveless (1940) further characterized blocking antibody as a substance different from reaginic ("allergic") antibody, in its heat stability at 56° and its failure to bind to human skin. These observations led to a widespread belief that pollen injections ameliorated symptoms of hay fever by producing "nonallergic" antibody that neutralized pollen antigen.

The induction of circulating blocking antibody by allergy injection therapy has been documented extensively, but recent studies suggest that clinical improvement following injection therapy is not due simply to production of blocking antibody. Although the exact mechanism or mechanisms by which injection therapy works are not known, beneficial effects from therapy appear to be antigen-specific. In 1968, Norman and Lichtenstein suggested "immunotherapy" as a more appropriate term for the treatment of allergic disease by antigen injections. Immunotherapy has become the preferred term for the procedure, though it is used interchangeably with the older term, "hyposensitization," and with "allergy injection therapy."

ANTIGENS USED FOR IMMUNOTHERAPY

A wide variety of antigens have been employed for immunotherapy, ranging from housedust to foods. Many, but not all, have been subjected to controlled clinical trials, primarily in the past two decades. These

333

studies have helped to define the effectiveness of therapy with certain specific antigens and to provide insights into the possible mechanism(s) by which such therapy acts.

Housedust. Several controlled studies carried out both in America and in Europe have evaluated the efficacy of housedust immunotherapy. Over a 2 year period, 189 adult patients were studied in a controlled clinical trial (Braun, 1949). Seventy-eight percent of those treated with housedust injections improved, compared to 34 percent of patients who did not receive injections.

Aas (1971) performed a placebo-controlled study on children and carried out bronchial challenge tests before and after 3 years of therapy. Thirty-five of 51 patients treated with housedust injections had a 75 percent improvement on inhalation challenge with housedust antigen, as compared to 9 of 28 placebo-treated patients, a difference that was statistically significant. Warner (1978) reported a placebo-controlled trial on 51 perennially asthmatic children treated with a relatively dilute tryosine-absorbed *Dermatophagoides pteronyssinus* (mite) extract, an antigen that is believed to be the major allergen in housedust in Europe. Therapy was evaluated by following symptom and drug scores as well as by pre- and post-therapy bronchial provocation testing, studying both immediate and late (4 to 8 hours) responses to antigen inhalation. Symptom and drug scores were significantly better in the antigen-treated than in placebo-treated children. Although there was no difference between the two groups in the immediate response to bronchial inhalation challenge, 10 of 22 treated patients (compared to 1 of 15 untreated patients) lost their late bronchial reactions to antigen inhalation. Furthermore, the loss of late responses appeared to parallel clinical improvement.

Pollens. Ragweed has been the primary pollen studied in the United States. Johnstone (1957) in a placebo-controlled evaluation of immunotherapy for ragweed hay fever showed that patients with the highest tolerated dose of antigen had a significantly greater improvement in symptoms than patients who received low-dose therapy or placebo injections.

In another study, 18 children were given immunotherapy for ragweed hay fever and 17 served as controls (Sadan et al., 1969).

Symptom and medication scores were supplemented with measurements of antigen-induced histamine release *in vitro*. IgE levels, antigen-induced histamine release *in vitro*, and blocking antibody also were measured before and after treatment. Thirteen of the 18 treated children had fewer symptoms than any of the control children, and two became completely asymptomatic. The treated group showed a decrease in *in vitro* histamine release in most patients and an increase in blocking antibody, whereas there was little change in these measurements in most of the untreated patients. There were no group differences in changes in IgE levels. In a second study of 24 of these children, all were treated. Those patients who had received a placebo during the first year of therapy had a significant decrease in symptoms, while those previously treated maintained their protection (Levy et al., 1971).

A study carried out in both ragweed- and grass-allergic adults evaluated the specificity of pollen immunotherapy by treating only with ragweed antigen. Patients treated with ragweed antigen had decreased symptoms during the ragweed pollen season, but their symptoms did not differ from nontreated patients during grass pollen season. Grass pollen–induced histamine release from basophils remained the same before and after treatment, but ragweed-inducible histamine release diminished significantly in treated patients (Norman et al., 1978).

Animal Danders. In general, there is little indication for immunotherapy with animal danders. *Animals to which patients are allergic should be removed from their immediate environment.* Evidence for the efficacy of currently available animal extracts is meager. However, a study that employed a potent antigenic fraction of cat pelt was carried out in 10 patients, five treated and five serving as controls. In this study, active treatment resulted in decreased skin reactivity and a 10- to 100-fold fall in bronchial reactivity as compared to control patients (Taylor, 1978). Though this study showed that immunotherapy with potent cat antigen can *decrease* sensitivity to cat danders, a significant degree of sensitivity remained, with patients still reactive to sufficient animal exposure. Contamination with animal viruses is a potential hazard of immunotherapy to animal danders, and some cat dander extracts have been found to contain feline leukemia virus, which poses an unknown risk to the recipient.

Mold. Mold antigens are commonly used in the treatment of patients with rhinitis or asthma, when history and skin tests suggest that these agents play an etiologic role in the illness. Mold antigens appear to be effective in selected cases, but no well-controlled study on these antigens has been published to date.

Foods. Elimination of offending foods from the diet is the primary therapy of food allergy. Not only is there a lack of evidence for benefit from food immunotherapy, but also the posssibility of causing or exacerbating food allergy must be kept in mind. For example, in the past, egg-based vaccines that contained significant amounts of egg albumin have been implicated in inducing allergic reactions in egg-sensitive recipients. Similarly, patients who have been treated with milk injections to induce fever ("fever therapy") frequently have become allergic to milk and beef products.

Insects. Immunotherapy for hypersensitivity to stinging insects of the Hymenoptera group (bees, wasps, hornets, fire ants) is considered in Chapter 53. Although the whole body extract antigens used in years past were of dubious value, specific venom antigens are highly effective in protecting from anaphylaxis (Hunt, 1978). The effects of immunotherapy for large reactions to mosquito bites, studied many years ago, were unimpressive and such therapy is not utilized now for mosquito hypersensitivity. Immunotherapy for inhaled insect antigens such as Mayfly or Caddis fly has not been evaluated.

Drugs. Immunotherapy or desensitization may be useful in drug reactions that involve IgE antibody. Patients with penicillin allergy who require penicillin for effective therapy may be given the drug by "rush desensitization" techniques. Similarly, patients with insulin allergy may be "desensitized" to insulin. This is discussed more fully in Chapter 54.

Bacterial Vaccines. The use of bacterial vaccines to control "infectious" asthma has been the subject of controversy for years. Numerous clinical studies in children have shown that asthma results from viral rather than bacterial infections (Minor et al.,

1974). A double-blind study carried out in children showed no benefit for bacterial vaccine treatment (Fontana et al., 1965), as have numerous other studies. One pediatric study (Mueller et al., 1969) suggested that selected children might benefit from the procedure, although there was no overall difference between the treated and placebo groups. In 1978, the U.S. Food and Drug Administration withdrew most bacterial vaccines from the market. Those few that remain must be withdrawn by 1983 unless they can be proven safe and effective.

CONDITIONS THAT MAY RESPOND TO IMMUNOTHERAPY

Immunotherapy can be beneficial in the treatment of certain IgE-mediated disorders, such as *seasonal allergic rhinitis* (hay fever) (Frankland and Augustin, 1954; Johnstone, 1957; Sadan, 1969; Levy et al., 1971), *perennial allergic rhinitis* (Braun, 1949), and the *allergic component of asthma* (Johnstone, 1968; Aas, 1970; Aas, 1971; Warner et al., 1978; Taylor, 1978). Less clear is its usefulness in managing the complications of rhinitis such as *serous otitis media* or *sinusitis*. These complications occur in part because of obstruction of the eustachian tubes or sinus ostia by edematous nasal mucosa, and it is reasonable to expect that any therapy that decreases rhinitis may lead to improved middle ear and paranasal sinus functions.

There is little evidence that immunotherapy will benefit atopic dermatitis. However, it may benefit those patients who have coexisting respiratory allergy. Immunotherapy should be administered cautiously, since it may exacerbate the dermatitis if the antigen concentration is increased too rapidly, especially during pollen season.

Immunotherapy is of proven value in desensitization to certain drugs, such as penicillin and insulin, and in anaphylactic sensitivity to Hymenoptera stings. Immunotherapy has been administered for many other conditions including food allergy, migraine headache, vasomotor rhinitis, intrinsic (nonallergic) asthma, and chronic urticaria. There is no evidence, however, that it is beneficial in any of these conditions.

Immunotherapy decreases but rarely totally eliminates symptoms, and its beneficial effects vary widely from patient to patient. Some may show dramatic improvement, while others may have negligible or no improvement. Furthermore, even when immunotherapy controls the allergic component of hay fever or asthma, the underlying hyperreactivity of nasal mucosa and of the bronchi to various nonallergic stimuli may not change (Taylor, 1978).

MECHANISM(S) OF ACTION

Immunotherapy induces a number of immune changes in the host. The induction of "blocking antibody," described by Cooke (1935) and Loveless (1940), presumably results in interception of antigen before it has an opportunity to interact with cell-bound specific IgE, thereby diminishing the opportunity for antigen-induced IgE-mediated histamine release. The correlation between blocking antibody titers and symptom improvement is relatively poor, however, and recent investigations suggest that the effects of immunotherapy involve considerably more than the production of IgG antibodies.

Patients receiving immunotherapy for hay fever show an initial rise in specific IgE antibody levels for pollen antigen. As treatment progresses, specific IgE antibody levels gradually decline. Treated patients no longer demonstrate the seasonal increases in specific IgE antibody seen in untreated populations (Berg and Johannson, 1971; Yunginger and Gleich, 1973). Long-term treatment also produces a decrease in the sensitivity of mediator cells in many patients, with a resulting decrease in antigen-induced basophil histamine release; a stimulation of IgA and IgG blocking antibody in nasal secretions (Norman, 1978); a decrease in the proliferative response of T cells to antigen; and other changes such as decreased numbers of T lymphocytes with IgM antibody markers on their surfaces in some patients (Neiburger, 1978).

Of these changes, suppression of specific IgE antibody synthesis and the development of secretory "blocking" antibodies would appear to be of particular importance in reducing mucosal reactivity to aerosolized antigen. These blocking antibodies are capable of binding to ragweed antibody and presumably thereby of inhibiting IgE antibody-induced histamine release. Immunotherapy produced a fourfold increase in blocking antibody titers of both IgG and IgA class antibodies but did not alter the ratio of IgG to IgA blocking antibodies or to IgE antibodies in one study (Platts-Mills et al., 1976). Serum blocking antibody titers, in other words, do not accurately reflect local blocking antibody production. More studies are needed to determine the relationship between local blocking antibody production and clinical effects from immunotherapy.

STANDARDIZATION OF ANTIGENS USED FOR IMMUNOTHERAPY

The lack of highly specific potent antigens has been a limiting factor to effective immunotherapy. All commercially produced pollen extracts, for example, contain a number of protein antigens, but only a few are associated with the specific biologic activity of the extract. Some of the clinically unimportant material may produce adverse immune reactions that limit the amount of extract the patient can tolerate. The standardization of allergenic extracts has been a major problem since Noon first initiated pollen injections. Specific methods of standardization have varied from laboratory to laboratory, and the reactivity of a group of extracts may appear to differ by ten- to 100-fold in one test, but only two- or threefold in another test (Baer, 1978).

Initially, antigens were standardized on the basis of the amount of soluble protein that could be extracted from a given quantity of pollen. Noon defined his pollen unit as one-one millionth of the quantity of protein which could be extracted from 1 gram of pollen. This was superseded by a weight to volume system in which a given weight of dried extracted protein was diluted in a volume of solution. A further refinement converted the weight to volume system to a protein-nitrogen unit system in which the protein content of the solutions was determined and expressed in terms of units (1 P.N.U. - 0.00001 mg of N). Though all three systems are still in use, none determines the *specific allergen content*, so that different lots of antigen even from the same firm may vary widely in allergen potency. Accordingly, new methods of standardization are being developed, and in the United States federal standards are being set and gradually being made more stringent as techniques improve.

Ragweed was the first allergen to be fractionated, and four major antigenic components were identified. Antigen E was selected as the most important of these antigens. Many laboratories now standardize the antigen E content of ragweed extracts. More recently such techniques as radioallergosorbent tests (RAST) employing allergic human sera of known specific IgE antibody content, or isoelectric focusing have been utilized as a means of standardizing antigens for their specific allergen content. As further physicochemical characterization of major antigens in different pollens and molds and in housedust occurs, far more specific and effective treatment antigens can be expected.

PRINCIPLES OF IMMUNOTHERAPY

Immunotherapy is an adjunct to allergic management, not a substitute for it. The overall goal of allergic management is to minimize symptoms and reduce the need for drugs. The first priority is to identify major offending allergens and irritants and to eliminate them from home, school, or work environment. *Immunotherapy should be reserved for those allergic factors that cannot be eliminated and that appear to play a major role in the patient's allergic disease.* The patient and/or parent should be presented with the facts of what immunotherapy can and cannot do. They should understand that *immunotherapy can help control but not cure symptoms.* Furthermore, they should be offered a choice as to whether or not the benefits are worth the time, effort, and inconvenience. Immunotherapy appears to most benefit patients with the most severe symptoms and in whom skin and nasal sensitivity is the most pronounced (D'Souza et al., 1973).

Patient Selection. Severity and duration of the disease will have a strong bearing on recommending immunotherapy. Patients who have moderate or even severe respiratory symptoms during short, well defined pollen seasons of 1 to 3 weeks may well elect medication such as antihistamines, topical intranasal corticosteroid sprays, or even *short* courses of parenteral steroids, rather than immunotherapy.

Patients with multiple seasonal allergic symptoms may be candidates for immunotherapy, especially if the symptoms induce physical or emotional hardships that interfere with normal daily activities or reduce substantially the quality of life. For example, the patient may be unable to sleep or may cough so much at night that no one else in the house can sleep. Immunotherapy may relieve the symptoms sufficiently to allow the patient to function effectively at school or on the job. It also may lessen some of the complications of chronic allergic rhinitis, such as sinusitis, recurrent upper respiratory infections, and recurrent otitis media or effusion. Johnstone (1968) suggested that immunotherapy may lessen the development of allergic asthma, though this has yet to be confirmed.

Selection of Antigens. Any physician involved in the formulation of treatment programs for immunotherapy should be familiar with the principal allergen sources in the geographic area. Extracts of local varieties of grass and ragweed should be included in the injections if the clinical and laboratory results indicate sensitivities to these substances. Allergen sources with a minor role in the patient's clinical picture, such as trees that pollinate only 2 or 3 weeks each year, may be omitted in favor of symptomatic treatment during the critical period. In cases in which different members of the same plant family are known to strongly cross-react, the physician can select the most prevalent members of the group for inclusion in the treatment program and discard the others. While several antigens may be combined safely in the same mixture, the use of an excessive number of antigens should be avoided, especially those of minor importance. Attempts to include extracts of every possible allergen may diminish the overall effectiveness of immunotherapy. Patients receive suboptimal doses of the clinically significant allergens and get little benefit from the others. In treating young children, a special effort should be made to combine extracts into one vial to minimize the number of injections per visit.

To be condemned is the practice by some firms that market allergens of making up a

TABLE 24–1 SAMPLE INSTRUCTION SHEET FOR IMMUNOTHERAPY

Dr._____ **Patient**_____**Date**_____

Schedule of dosages for treatment with Allergens Solution.

Please read special direction sheet before giving any injections.

The treatments are to be given regularly once each week until the maximum tolerated dose listed is reached, then they are to be given at intervals of _____ weeks.

Please continue injections at the maximum tolerated dose until the patient is reevaluated in this office.

Each solution is five or ten times the strength of the preceding solution. Unfavorable reaction may prevent advancing the dosage as rapidly as indicated in the following schedule. *It may be necessary to go back to a well-tolerated dose and increase by smaller increments than indicated in this schedule, if the reaction is an inch (2.5 cm) or greater. Do not increase dose if the interval between injections is more than 2 weeks.*

In the event that treatments are inadvertently missed and the patient's injections are spaced more than four weeks apart, then the dose must be reduced to avoid the possibility of a systemic reaction.

Start with Solution _____

	Sol. 1	Sol. 2	Sol. 3	Sol. 4
All the doses in any one vertical column must be completed before the next column is started.	0.10 cc	0.10 cc	0.05 cc	0.05 cc
	0.15 cc	0.15 cc	0.10 cc	0.07 cc
	0.25 cc	0.25 cc	0.15 cc	0.10 cc
	0.35 cc	0.35 cc	0.25 cc	0.15 cc
	0.50 cc	0.50 cc	0.35 cc	0.20 cc
			0.50 cc	0.25 cc
				0.30 cc
				0.40 cc
				0.50 cc

Maintenance dosage: _____ cc Solution _____ Administer every _____ weeks

Please, at each visit, under *Remarks,* make a brief note as to how the patient has been as *regards the allergic condition* since the previous visit. Without this cooperation, maximum benefit cannot be obtained from the consultation. *The patient should bring this record along on follow-up consultation.*

Date	Solution	Amount given	Any local reaction	Any general reaction	Remarks

treatment mixture arbitrarily on the basis of a skin test sheet submitted by a physician, without regard to history, symptoms, or the patient's clinical course.

PRINCIPLES OF TECHNIQUE

Preparation of Solutions. Treatment antigens should be prescribed individually for each patient by the physician supervising therapy, and a copy of the prescription retained by the consultant physician, preferably on the patient's chart. The antigen set and its container should be labeled clearly with the patient's name, specific contents, antigen concentrations, and the expiration date of the solutions. Color coding labels according to concentration further safeguards against a mistake in dosage. Clearly written instructions for administration should accompany the antigen set (Table

TABLE 24–2 GENERAL INFORMATION AND PRECAUTIONS FOR INJECTIONS OF ALLERGEN SOLUTIONS

1. Treatments should be administered under the direct supervision of a licensed physician.

2. Keep all solutions in the dark, in the refrigerator.

3. Never give an injection unless you have on hand a syringe containing epinephrine hydrochlorine (Adrenalin) 1:1000 for use in case of a reaction.

4. Cleanse the skin with 70 percent alcohol before injection. Use a 0.5 or 1.0 cc tuberculin syringe and administer in the arm subcutaneously. **Always pull back the piston of the syringe before an injection of allergen solution.** If blood appears in the syringe, always change the position of the needle point to make sure that the solution is not injected into a blood vessel.

5. Always keep the patient under observation for 20 to 30 minutes after an injection.

6. Reduce the dosage 50% during the pollen season if the patient is having moderate to severe symptoms.

7. If a systemic reaction occurs (usual manifestations: hives, acute hay fever, paroxysmal coughing, asthma, cyanosis, flushing, perspiration, nausea, vomiting, dizziness, fainting or collapse), place a tourniquet around the patient's arm above the site of the injection and inject 0.25 cc of epinephrine into the site of the allergy injection and 0.25 cc in the opposite arm. Repeat the epinephrine at 15-minute intervals for three doses as necessary, and release the tourniquet occasionally so that you do not embarrass the circulation. Administer oxygen by mask. Give 200 mg of hydrocortisone by injection as soon as possible after the onset of a severe reaction. An antihistamine (e.g., chlorpheniramine 10 mg) also may be injected intramuscularly.

   If the patient continues to have respiratory distress, begin an intravenous infusion with 5% glucose in normal saline, insert oral airway, and transfer to nearest hospital.

   Subsequent doses of allergen must be reduced.

8. If the patient experiences trouble because of injections, such as sore arms or more general forms of reactions, it may not be possible to proceed as rapidly as indicated in the schedule. Under such circumstances, it is better practice to go back to a well-tolerated dose and to increase, if possible, by smaller increments than those originally suggested. Conversely, some patients may be able to tolerate more rapid increases than those indicated on the schedule. This depends upon the judgment of the attending physician.

9. In our experience, the perennial method of treatment is the most effective regimen for the patient. With this technique, injections are continued all year. The frequency is determined by the patient's clinical response. Usually, if the patient is doing well after the initial program of immunization is completed, the frequency can be reduced to every 2 weeks, then every 3 weeks, and finally to once a month.

10. **In the event that treatments are inadvertently missed and the patient's injections are spaced more than 4 weeks apart, the dose must be reduced to avoid the possibility of a systemic reaction.** For each week beyond 4 weeks, the dose is decreased by 50%. For example: if the patient had last received 0.50 cc and the interval between injections was eight weeks, then the patient's dosage should be reduced one full bottle.

11. The presence of mild allergic symptoms (mild wheezing or hay fever) is not a contraindication for administering the injection.

24–1) and should include a schedule that lists the dosage and frequency of injections during the period of increasing antigen concentration, the projected maintenance dosage, the frequency of maintenance injections, and the specific emergency procedures to be followed in case of adverse reactions (Table 24–2).

Perennial and Preseasonal Immunotherapy. The selection of an appropriate treatment schedule involves a choice between two forms of therapy, *perennial* and *preseasonal*. Both approaches involve weekly or biweekly injections of allergen in increasing doses until a maximum tolerated dose is reached.

In preseasonal therapy, injections are begun 3 to 4 months before the anticipated onset of the pollen season. The goal is to reach the maximum tolerated dosage by the beginning of the season, at which point the treatment is discontinued until the following year.

With perennial immunotherapy, the patient is placed on a year-round maintenance schedule when the highest tolerated dose has been reached. Clinical and immunologic evidence suggests perennial treatment allows the patient to tolerate a higher cumulative dose of antigen, which results in better clinical protection than preseasonal therapy allows. Once maintenance dosage has been reached, the frequency of maintenance injections depends on the patient's symptoms. In general, the goal is to reach a monthly maintenance schedule, though some allergists prefer to increase the injections to every 2 weeks immediately before the pollen season.

Though perennial treatment for pollen allergies may be started during the pollen season, if the initial dose is small, it probably is wiser to wait until the end of the season, especially if the patient has extreme sensitivity or if the symptoms are severe. Pollen-sensitive patients who have reached a maintenance level before the season begins should receive a slightly reduced dose during the season. This minimizes the chance of a sudden systemic reaction due to the combination of injected and inhaled pollens.

A third treatment technique, developed originally in the 1930s, may be used for certain specific substances such as penicillin, insulin, or anaphylactic sensitivity to stinging insects. This procedure, called "rush desensitization," usually requires that the patient be hospitalized, with an intravenous infusion running and appropriate emergency equipment immediately at hand. Injections of allergen extract are administered every 15 to 30 minutes for up to 2 days. The rationale behind this approach is to gradually bind circulating IgE antibodies and to achieve a state of "antigen excess." Patients subjected to rush desensitization must be monitored very carefully for the appearance of severe local and systemic reactions. In general, only life-threatening clinical conditions justify the risk associated with this procedure (Chapter 54).

Initial Dose. The initial dose of allergen extract must be adjusted carefully to the sensitivity of the patient. Severity of clinical symptoms, intensity of skin test reactions, prior history of systemic reactions, and the patient's age should be considered. Young children usually tolerate a more concentrated dose than do adolescents or adults. For patients with moderate sensitivity, the customary starting dose is in the range of 1:10,000 to 1:100,000 weight-by-volume of the anticipated final dose. Some allergists prefer to determine the starting point by performing serial skin tests beginning at 1:1,000,000 and increasing the skin test concentrations tenfold with each test, selecting as the beginning dosage a solution which is 5 to 10 times as dilute as that producing a positive test. If the patient tolerates the first injection of dilute extract without a significant local reaction, therapy can proceed at weekly or biweekly intervals with increments of 0.05 to 0.10 ml, depending on the individual treatment schedule. When the dose reaches 0.50 ml, the entire process should begin again, with 0.05 to 0.10 injection of an extract which is 5 to 10 times stronger than the original. Any local reaction larger than 2 cm, or a systemic reaction, requires an adjustment in the dosage schedule.

Maintenance levels usually are reached in 3 to 6 months, depending on the sensitivity of the patient. At that time, the interval between injections may be increased gradually, depending on the patient's symptoms. For many patients the maintenance dose is 0.50 ml of a 1:50 or 1:100 w/v extract. In many cases, however, this dose and/or concentration cannot be reached without severe reaction, necessitating a lower dosage for maintenance.

Who Should Administer Allergy Injections? Allergy injections should be administered only by trained personnel *under the direct supervision of a physician, with the physician immediately available.* Appropriate emergency equipment and a syringe of aqueous 1:1000 epinephrine must be within reach. Once the consulting physician has established a diagnosis and a suitable treatment program, the administration of immunotherapy may be turned over to the patient's primary physician. Because of the risk of anaphylaxis, *parents never should be permitted to administer injections at home.* It is important that the patient return once or twice a year to the consultant for follow-up examination. At these visits the consultant reviews the patient's progress, performs a physical examination, orders laboratory tests if appropriate, adjusts the antigen dosage schedule if necessary, determines if there are any side effects, and provides the referring doctor with a detailed report.

Pre-Injection Precautions. Vials containing allergenic extracts should be stored in a refrigerator but not in the freezing compartment. Color-coding labels and dosage sheets provide a further safeguard against mistakes. Serious reactions can occur if the wrong concentration is administered; always cross-check the vial against the treatment card and ask the patient to repeat his or her name and address, and perhaps birth date.

Administration. The injection of antigen should be given in the upper, outer aspect of the arm, midway between the shoulder and elbow, staying away from the elbow and shoulder joints. This permits sufficient space for a tourniquet in the event of a systemic reaction. To minimize the pain of injection, the extract should be administered with a 25 gauge ⅝-inch needle. The injection should be given deep subcutaneously, and great care should be taken *not* to inject antigen directly into the bloodstream.

Long-term storage of allergy extracts diminishes their potency; thus special precautions are necessary when changing vials. The maintenance dose should be reduced 1 full dilution (e.g., from 1:100 to 1:1000) on changing from an old to a newly prepared

antigen. If the treatment schedule is disrupted by a patient's vacation or illness, the dose should be adjusted based on the time elapsed. If 2 to 4 weeks have passed, the previous dose should be repeated. Beyond 4 weeks, the dose should be dropped 50 per cent for every week missed.

Reactions. Following the injection, the patient should be instructed to wait at least 20 minutes before leaving the physician's office. The patient should be examined by the physician or by the office assistant before being permitted to leave.

If the patient does experience a systemic reaction — rhinorrhea, nasal itching, hoarseness, tight chest, generalized hives, extreme weakness — 0.1 to 0.25 ml of 1:1000 aqueous epinephrine should be administered subcutaneously into the injection site and an equal amount into the opposite arm. A tourniquet should be applied proximal to the site to slow the absorption of the antigen. If necessary, additional epinephrine and injectable antihistamines may be used (see Chapter 52).

Many patients develop small wheals at the injection site, resembling mosquito bites. These do not require any attention in the treatment schedule. On the other hand, the dose should be repeated rather than increased (if not on maintenance dosage) if the wheal is 1 to 2 cm in diameter. If the wheal is larger than 2 cm, the next injection should be reduced by 0.10 to 0.30 ml. Continued local reaction should be discussed with the allergist. If reactions occur after 3 or 4 months of therapy, the patient may have reached his or her maximal tolerated dose.

Large local reactions indicate that the patient has a significant potential for developing a systemic reaction, and the dose must be reduced accordingly. *Systemic reactions can occur even in the absence of prior local reactions,* however.

Delayed reactions generally appear between 12 and 24 hours after the injection and may be either local or systemic. Delayed local reactions resemble large soft bruises and can be treated with an oral antihistamine, aspirin, or the local application of an ice pack. If a delayed local reaction occurs, the dosage should be adjusted by the consultant.

Delayed systemic reactions are the most difficult to recognize. They usually appear as a slight or moderate flare-up of the patient's symptoms, with increased rhinorrhea or sneezing, for example. This type of reaction is not serious, but it indicates that the patient has received too large a dose of antigen and that the allergist should be consulted. Continued mild overdoses are responsible for dramatic "cures" following cessation of immunotherapy.

Duration of Therapy. The first year of immunotherapy generally is considered a trial period. If the patient responds favorably, the maintenance injections are continued until the patient has been relatively free of symptoms for a year or more. The entire treatment program may last from 1 to 5 years, with an average duration of 3 years. Patients with asthma often require a longer course. Some patients relapse when injections are stopped and must resume therapy for continued relief.

Not all patients benefit from immunotherapy, and some patients may not improve until the second year of treatment. Treatment failures may be due to inadequate dosage, inactive extracts, or an incorrect diagnosis. Patients who improve initially and then experience an increase in symptoms in a later season may have acquired additional allergies or developed another condition. For example, vasomotor rhinitis and intrinsic asthma will not respond to immunotherapy.

Treatment failures often are due to neglect of environmental controls. The patient or parent may believe that immunotherapy negates the need to eliminate allergenic factors from the environment. If this is the case, the physician must educate the patient and family again about the goals of allergic management and limitations of immunotherapy.

TYPES OF ANTIGEN PREPARATIONS AVAILABLE

Aqueous Extracts. The original antigen administered by Noon and Freeman was protein extracted from grass pollen by boiling. Because boiling inactivated some proteins, room temperature extraction was substituted in buffered saline solution. Such buffered aqueous antigens have had the most widespread use, and their clinical and immune effects have been studied in greatest depth.

There have been no well-documented adverse effects other than the occurrence of local or systemic reactions to injections. Although these cannot be avoided entirely when high dose therapy is used, these reactions can be handled easily if appropriate emergency equipment is immediately available. Aqueous immunotherapy has been studied in pregnancy, and no adverse maternal or fetal effects have appeared (Metzger et al., 1978). (Nevertheless, it is wise to be conservative with regard to *instituting* immunotherapy during pregnancy). Aqueous extracts have a major disadvantage in that therapeutic effectiveness requires multiple injections over a prolonged period of time. Local and systemic reactions also limit the total amount of antigen which can be administered. With ragweed, for example, 50 to 100 μg antigen E is the maximal amount that can be administered in a year of therapy (Norman and Lichtenstein, 1978).

Alum-Precipitated, Pyridine-Extracted Antigens. In an effort to increase the antigenic stimulus while decreasing the number of local and systemic reactions, a pyridine-extracted alum-precipitated antigen was introduced (Allpyral). This antigen became the center of great controversy in the late 1960's when a study of ragweed immunotherapy showed it to be without potency for ragweed antigen (Lichtenstein et al., 1968). At the same time, other authors showed inhibition of histamine release and development of blocking antibody to grass pollen antigens (Weinstock and Starr, 1970). The differences in immunogenicity appeared to be related to a step in the extraction process that denatured the ragweed antigen but not grass antigen. A subsequent study of alum pyridine grass antigen confirmed that it was equivalent clinically and immunologically to aqueous grass antigen (Bierman, 1972). Studies of other alum-pyridine antigens have not been performed.

Alum-Precipitated, Aqueous-Extracted Antigens. Though alum-precipitated pollen antigens were first introduced almost four decades ago (Stull et al., 1940), in depth studies were not carried out until the 1970's. Therapy with alum-precipitated ragweed antigens showed them to be effective in stimulating blocking antibodies. Amelioration of symptoms was similar to that attained with aqueous extracts, with fewer injections and fewer local and systemic reactions (Norman and Lichtenstein, 1978). Similar results were obtained using alum-precipitated grass antigens (Bierman et al., 1972). The effectiveness of other alum-precipitated antigens has yet to be determined.

CONTROVERSIAL ANTIGENS AND TECHNIQUES

In allergy treatment, a number of techniques have evolved, enjoyed a period of popularity and been discarded ultimately, when they were proved to be ineffective, naively conceived in the light of new knowledge, or potentially harmful.

Histamine "Desensitization." With the identification of histamine as a mediator of the allergic reaction, histamine injections were introduced to treat a variety of "allergic" disorders between 1930 and 1950. Histamine was either administered intravenously or by serial injections for such disorders as vascular headache, known as "histamine cephalgia" (Hanes, 1969; Horton, 1941). This form of therapy is no longer employed.

Antigen Emulsification in Oil. Antigens were emulsified in mineral oil to slow absorption and permit the administration of a large total dosage in a single injection. This procedure was popularized as a "one-shot" treatment for hay fever. In addition to significant systemic reactions, local reactions consisting of sterile abscesses or mineral oil tumors are associated with such therapy. Evidence that mineral oil injections can induce myelomas in mice led to abandonment of this procedure (Potter, 1962).

Oral Desensitization to Foods. Another technique popularized for treatment of food allergy was oral desensitization, that is, the administration of progressively increasing dosages of the food to which the child is allergic. Though this is still practiced by some physicians, there is no immunologic evidence of effectiveness.

Controversial Techniques. Techniques such as antigen titration and sublingual drops for allergy are centers of current controversy. These are discussed in Chapter 59.

PROSPECTS FOR THE FUTURE

Current research on therapeutic antigens involves their chemical modification by such substances as formalin (allergoids), ultraviolet light, urea, and polymerization; the isolation of purified specific antigens; and therapeutic techniques such as topical (intranasal) immunotherapy.

Allergoids. Benefits from chemical modification of allergens have been documented primarily in the use of allergoids, which are allergen extracts that have been treated with formaldehyde to reduce their allergenic properties but not their ability to stimulate presumably protective antibodies. Early studies with both grass and ragweed pollen extracts have shown that allergoids are well tolerated by patients and that they can induce IgG antibodies that block histamine release to pollen extracts (Marsh et al., 1972). In a double-blind controlled study of allergoids involving 50 ragweed-allergic individuals followed over four pollen seasons, half of the group received conventional pollen ragweed extract and the other half received allergoids. After the first season, patients treated with allergoids had higher titers of IgG antibodies to ragweed antigens than did the group treated with conventional aqueous antigen. They also experienced somewhat fewer clinical symptoms. By the third season, patients treated with aqueous extracts had achieved the same average IgG levels as the first group, when all patients appeared to have reached an immunologic plateau. The advantage of allergoids appears to be that they stimulate blocking antibodies earlier in therapy and induce fewer local and systemic reactions than aqueous extracts.

Urea Denatured Antigens. Another technique, involving urea denatured antigen E, has been less successful. Antigen E of ragweed consists of two polypeptide chains held together by noncovalent forces. Urea causes these chains to dissociate, producing a mixture that is 10,000 times less allergenic than native allergen. Ishizaka (1975) showed that the mixture of dissociated chains was capable of partially suppressing ongoing IgE antibody responses to antigen E in mice, presumably by the stimulation of suppressor T cells. In limited clinical trials, the urea denatured material was well tolerated but had only minimal clinical and immune effectiveness.

Polymerized Antigens. These represent yet another approach to antigen modification to increase safety and effectiveness of immunotherapy. Studies of polymerized whole ragweed and of polymerized ragweed antigen E (Metzger et al., 1976; Patterson et al., 1978; Bacal et al., 1978) showed that such antigens can induce chemical and immune protection equivalent to that obtained with aqueous antigens with fewer associated local or systemic reactions.

Ultraviolet Irradiated Antigens. These have been studied primarily in Europe (Henocq et al., 1973). Housedust antigens irradiated with ultraviolet light lose their ability to induce positive skin tests or induce bronchial reactions. When used for immunotherapy they appeared to protect as well as standard antigens. No American studies have been carried out.

Isolation of Purified Specific Antigens. This technique has already improved the effectiveness of immunotherapy for Hymenoptera anaphylaxis (Hunt et al., 1978);

and the identification of the specific allergen of ragweed pollen has improved the quality of ragweed antigens. The progress in identification and purification of other specific antigens (Chakrabarty, 1979) should improve the specificity and effectiveness of immunotherapy in general.

Topical (Intranasal) Immunotherapy. Intranasal immunotherapy is an example of the search for new therapeutic techniques. The success of intranasal immunization for certain viral diseases (e.g., influenza) stimulated trials of this technique for hay fever. Though initial studies showed some induction of local blocking antibodies, results in general have been inconsistent (McLean et al., 1979; Nickelson et al., 1979). Further studies will make use of more potent topical antigens.

References

Aas, K.: Bronchial provocation tests in asthma. Arch. Dis. Child. 45:221, 1970.

Aas, K.: Hyposensitization in house dust asthma. Acta Paediat. Scandinav. 60:264, 1971.

Bacal, E., Zeiss, C. R., Suszko, I., et al.: Polymerized whole ragweed: An improved method of immunotherapy. J. Allergy. Clin. Immunol. 62:289, 1978.

Baer, H.: Standardization of antigens. J. Allergy Clin. Immunol. 6:206, 1978.

Berg, T., and Johansson, S. G. O.: In vitro diagnosis of atopic allergy IV: Seasonal variations of IgE antibodies in children allergic to pollens. Int. Arch. Allergy 41:452, 1971.

Bierman, C. W., Pierson, W. E., and Van Arsdel, P. P., Jr.: The effect of long-term pollen immunotherapy in children on leukocyte histamine release. J. Allergy Clin. Immunol. 59:111, 1972.

Bruun, E.: Control examination of the specificity of specific desensitization in asthma. Acta Allergy 2:122, 1949.

Chakrabarty, S., Ekramoddoullah, A. K. M., Kisil, F. T., and Sehon, A. H.: Isolation of a highly purified allergen from Kentucky blue grass pollen. J. Allergy Clin. Immunol. 63:192, 1979.

Cooke, R. A.: The treatment of hay fever by active immunization. Laryngoscope 25:108, 1915.

Cooke, R. A.: Studies in specific hypersensitiveness IX. On the phenomenon of hyposensitization. J. Immunol. 7:219, 1922.

Cooke, R. A., Barnard, J. H., Hebard, S., et al.: Serologic evidence of immunity with co-existing sensitization in a type of human allergy (hay fever). J. Exper. Med. 62:733, 1935.

D'Souza, M. F., Pepys, J., Wells, I. D., et al.: Hyposensitization with Dermatophagoides pheronopsinus in house dust allergy: A controlled study of clinical and immunological effects. Clin. Allergy 3:177, 1973.

Dunbar, W. P.: Zur Urache und specifischen Heilung des Heufiebers. Munich, Roldenbourg, 1903.

Frankland, A. W., and Augustin, R.: Prophylaxis of summer hay fever and asthma. Lancet I:1055, 1954.

Freeman, J.: Further observations on treatment of hay fever by hypodermic innoculation of pollen vaccine. Lancet II:814, 1911.

Fontana, V. J., Salanitro, A., Wolfe, H., et al.: Bacterial vaccine and infectious asthma. J.A.M.A. 193:895, 1965.

Hanes, W. J.: Histamine cephalgia resembling tic douloureux. Headache 8:162, 1969.

Henocq, E., Garcelon, M., and Berrens, L.: Photo-inactivated allergens. Clin. Allergy 3:461, 1973.

Horton, B. T.: The use of histamine in the treatment of specific types of headaches. J.A.M.A. 116:377, 1941.

Hunt, K. J., Valentine, M. D., Sobotka, A. K., et al.: A controlled trial of immune therapy in insect hypersensitivity. New Engl. J. Med. 299:157, 1978.

Ishizaka, K., Okudaira, H., and King, T. P.: Immunogenic properties of modified antigen E. II. Ability of urea-denatured antigen and α-polypeptide chain to prime T cells specific for antigen E. J. Immunol. 114:110, 1975.

Johnstone, D. E.: Study of the role of antigen dosage in the treatment of pollenosis and pollen asthma. Am. J. Dis. Child. 94:1, 1957.

Johnstone, D. E., and Dutton, A.: The value of hyposensitization therapy for bronchial asthma in children — a 14 year study. Pediatrics 42:793, 1968.

Levy, D. A., Lichtenstein, L., Goldstein, E. O., et al.: Immunologic and cellular changes accompanying the therapy of pollen allergy. J. Clin. Invest. 50:360, 1971.

Lichtenstein, L. M., Norman, P. S., and Winkenwerder, W. L.: Antibody response following immunotherapy in ragweed hay fever: Allosyral vs whole ragweed extract. J. Allergy 41:49, 1968.

Loveless, M. H.: Immunologic studies in pollenosis. I. The presence of two antibodies related to the same pollen antigen in the serum of treated hay fever patients. J. Immunol. 38:25, 1940.

Marsh, D. G., Lichtenstein, L. M., Norman, P. S., et al.: Induction of IgE-mediated immediate hypersensitivity to group I rye grass pollen allergen and allergoids in non-allergic man. Immunology 22:1013, 1972.

McLean, J. A., Mathews, K. P., Bayne, N. K., et al.: A controlled study of intranasal immunotherapy with short ragweed extract. J. Allergy Clin. Immunol. 63:166, 1979.

Metzger, W. T., Patterson, R., Zeiss, C. R., et al.: Comparison of polymerized and unpolymerized antigen E in immunotherapy of ragweed allergy. New Engl. J. Med. 295:1160, 1976.

Metzger, W. J., Turner, E., and Patterson, R.: The safety of immunotherapy during pregnancy. J. Allergy Clin. Immunol. 61:268, 1978.

Minor, T. E., Baler, J., Dick, E., et al.: Greater frequency of viral respiratory infections in asthmatic children as compared with their nonasthmatic siblings. J. Pediat. 85:472, 1974.

Mueller, H. L., and Lang, M.: Hyposensitization with bacterial vaccine in infectious asthma. J.A.M.A. *208*:1379, 1969.

Neiburger, R. G., Neiburger, J. B., and Dockhorn, R. J.: Distribution of peripheral blood T and B lymphocyte markers in atopic children and changes during immunotherapy. J. Allergy Clin. Immunol. *61*:88, 1978.

Nickelson, J. A., Wypuch, J. I., and Arbesman, C. E.: Clinical and immunological response to local nasal immunotherapy. J. Allergy Clin. Immunol. *63*:166, 1979.

Noon, L.: Prophylactic inoculation against hay fever. Lancet *1*:1952, 1911.

Norman, P., Winkenwerder, W., and Lichtenstein, L.: Immunotherapy of hay fever with ragweed antigen E. J. Allergy *42*:93, 1968.

Norman, P. S.: Bronchial reactivity and immunotherapy. J. Allergy Clin. Immunol. *61*:281, 1978.

Norman, P. S., Lichtenstein, L. M., and Tignall, J.: The clinical and immunologic specificity of immunotherapy. J. Allergy Clin. Immunol. *61*:370, 1978.

Norman, P. S., and Lichtenstein, L. M.: Comparison of alum-precipitated and unprecipitated aqueous ragweed pollen extracts in the treatment of hay fever. J. Allergy Clin. Immunol. *61*:384, 1978.

Patterson, R., Suszko, I. M., Zeiss, C. R., et al.: Comparison of immune reactivity to polyvalent monomeric and polymeric ragweed antigens. J. Allergy Clin. Immunol. *61*:28, 1978.

Platts-Mills, T.A.E., von Maur, R. G., Ishizaka, K., et al.: IgA and IgG antiragweed antibodies in nasal secretions. J. Clin. Invest. *57*:1041, 1976.

Potter, M., and Boyce, C. R.: Induction of plasma cell neoplasm in strain BALB/C mice with mineral oil and mineral oil adjuvants. Nature *193*:1086, 1962.

Sadan, N., Rhyne, M. B., Mellits, E. D., et al.: Immunotherapy of pollenosis in children: New Engl. J. Med. *280*:623, 1969.

Stull, A., Cooke, R. A., Sherman, W. B., et al.: Experimental and clinical study of fresh and modified pollen extracts. J. Allergy *11*:439, 1940.

Taylor, W. V., Ohman, J. L., and Lowell, F. C. Immunotherapy in cat-induced asthma. J. Allergy Clin. Immunol. *61*:283, 1978.

Warner, J. O., Price, J. F., Soothill, J. F., et al.: Controlled trial of hyposensitization to *Dermatophagoides pteronyssinus* in children with asthma. Lancet *II*:912, 1978.

Weinstock, M., and Starr, M. S.: Studies in pollen allergy: II. Comparison of leucocyte sensitivity and levels of blocking antibody in hay fever subjects administered allpyral or pollaccine. Int. Arch. Allergy *37*:385, 1970.

Yunginger, J. W., and Gleich, G. J.: Seasonal changes in serum and nasal IgE concentrations. J. Allergy *51*:174, 1973.

25

D.E. Johnstone
J.F. Soothill

Prevention of Allergic Disease

A number of allergic diseases, such as eczema, asthma, and rhinitis, are strongly associated with the state of atopy — a familial, antigen-nonspecific predisposition to produce and react with skin-sensitizing (mainly IgE) antibodies to common environmental antigens, particularly inhalants and foods. The state is antigen-nonspecific, in the sense that most individuals react in this way to numerous antigenically different substances.

Though atopy is strongly familial (Van Arsdel and Motulsky, 1959), it is clear from studies in identical twins (in whom concordance is not 100 percent) that the state of atopy is not based solely on genetic factors but that environmental factors contribute as well. Because atopic disease often develops early in life and for other reasons, it is likely that the antigenic experience of the neonate may be important in producing damaging sensitization upon which subsequent atopic disease is largely based. This suggests the possibility of preventing atopic disease by eliminating, reducing, or altering exposure to allergens commonly involved in atopic disease, particularly in the early months of life. Atopic disease also may be prevented or ameliorated even after sensitization has occurred by avoidance of or hyposensitization to certain antigens (Chaps. 22 and 24). Since vulnerability of atopic individuals to sensitization is antigen-nonspecific and includes a wide variety of allergens, such individuals can be protected against further sensitization by avoiding highly sensitizing environments later in life. This chapter will cover factors predisposing to childhood atopy, prevention of atopic disease, and practical measures for protecting the child at risk.

FACTORS PREDISPOSING TO CHILDHOOD ATOPY

Inheritance

The genetic background to atopic disease is both strong and complex. About half the offspring of an atopic parent are atopic (even more if both parents are atopic) (Van Arsdel and Motulsky, 1959), but the particular atopic syndrome differs not only between families but also among individuals in the same family. This suggests polygenic inheritance (Chap. 3); some of the genetic and environmental factors that affect the expression of atopic disease are recognized or suspected (vida infra).

Atopy and Immunodeficiency

The observation that children who are known to be immunodeficient often develop allergic (including atopic) diseases led to the suggestion that there may be far more extensive immunopathologic manifestations from relatively minor immunodeficiency than generally appreciated (Soothill, 1976); specifically, a persistent pathologic hyper-response of one ordinarily protective mechanism may occur as a result of failure of effective antigen handling by another. For example IgA, the principal secretory immunoglobulin, performs a major protective role at mucosal surfaces. Buckley and Dees (1969) showed that in IgA-deficient subjects there is an increased frequency of precipitins to food antigens. Kaufman and Hobbs (1970) found that there was a significantly increased proportion of abnormally low serum immunoglobulins in atopic subjects (greater than 2 S.D. below the normal mean), especially for serum IgA. However, since many subjects in the atopic group had high values, the means of the atopic group did not differ from those of the controls. Transient immunodeficiency, especially in infancy, is recognized as a cause of frequent infection. A prospective study of newborn offspring of atopic parents showed that before symptoms had developed, those who later became atopic (most developed eczema) had lower IgA levels than those who did not develop symptoms, though the difference between the two subgroups had disappeared by one year (Taylor et al., 1973). This greatly strengthens the probability in the authors' opinion that IgA deficiency led to the development of atopic disease since it was present prior to manifest disease. It also strengthens our view that neonatal antigen experience in an immunodeficient host is important for allergic sensitization.

Other immunodeficiencies also may contribute to the development or aggravation of atopic disease, particularly deficiencies in the antibody–complement–phagocyte pathway. Two common defects have been associated with atopy: a defect in yeast opsonization (a defect of an undefined component of the alternative pathway of complement which is defective in 5 percent of the general population but about 27 percent of atopic individuals), and a defect in the second component of complement (low levels are found in about 1.5 percent of the general population but about 22 percent of atopic individuals) (Turner et al., 1978). Support for the fact that these defects are primary, that is, they are not secondary to atopic disease, comes from the finding that they are mutually exclusive;

if in an atopic child one is defective, the other is normal. Many children with a rarer deficiency in neutrophil mobility are atopic (Hill et al., 1974). Also, there is a high incidence of atopy in subjects homozygotic or heterozygotic for cystic fibrosis (Warner et al., 1976). The association of atopy with this range of defects of functions strongly suggests that defective antigen handling is a general basis of atopy.

An alternative theory relating immunodeficiency to atopy is based on the role of T helper and T suppressor cells in experimental induction of IgE antibody (Tada, 1975). According to this concept, the propensity for increased IgE antibody formation results from defective T cell suppression in atopic individuals. This concept is derived from experimental animals, and there is no evidence that it applies in atopic humans.

Atopy and Tissue Type

Some immunopathologic diseases are linked to specific tissue types (Chap. 3), and some studies have shown an association with atopy. Marsh et al. (1973) reported weak linkages between certain tissue types and the IgE antibody response to specific pollen-derived antigens. Although the antibody response was associated with tissue types, atopic disease, e.g., hay fever, was not. Such association might not be expected since the atopic state is antigen-nonspecific. On the other hand, Thorsby (1978) reported that atopic disease was linked to HLA types A1 and B8, but Krain and Teresaki (1973) reported linkage to A3 and B7. This apparent disagreement was clarified by studying tissue types of patients presenting with different syndromes; Soothill et al. (1976) found that whereas HLA A1 and B8 were more frequent in individuals with eczema, A3 and B7 were more frequent in those with hay fever. Limited data suggest that these relationships hold, regardless of which immunodeficiency may underlie the development of atopy. Thus, consistent with evidence of polygenic inheritance, we have an explanation of the varied syndromes in atopy: Any one of several mechanisms of immunodeficiency may cause an increased IgE antibody response, but the atopic disease or syndrome is independently controlled by other factors that can be related to tissue type.

Atopy and Place of Birth

Atopy is less common in "developing" than "developed" countries (Godfrey, 1975). Morrison Smith's (1973) study of immigrants to Britain confirmed the lower incidence of asthma in children of African origin born outside Britain, but offspring of parents of African origin who were born in Britain had at least as frequent an incidence as indigenous non-African children. This suggests that the difference in incidence of asthma among the African children was environmental rather than genetic. Thus, there appears to be a damaging environmental factor for infants in "developed" countries that is lacking in "underdeveloped" ones. There are at least three possible mechanisms for this: the effect of worm infections, more common in Africa than in Britain; possible death from infection of the relatively immunodeficient in Africa; and difference in infant feeding. Only the latter can be applied usefully for allergy prevention (vida infra).

Atopy and Season of Birth

Reports that in Europe asthma occurs more frequently in children born in late autumn (Soothill et al., 1976) also suggest that seasonal differences in neonatal antigen contact are important for the development of atopy. Possible relevant environmental antigens are not known; possibilities include the high activity of *Dermatophagoides pteronyssinus* in this season and the high prevalence of respiratory virus infections that occur in the winter months during the time of the "physiologic deficiency" of IgG in infancy. Reports that viral infections contribute to the development of or precipitation of atopic disease need reappraisal following the recognition of the role of immunodeficiency in allergy. It is possible that atopic disease and manifest respiratory virus infection may be related to the same immunodeficiency. Other nonseasonal neonatal events may well also play a role in the development of atopic disease, as is suggested by the association of asthma with obstetric compli-

cations and with neonatal surgery (Salk et al., 1974; Johnstone et al., 1975).

Infant Feeding

Ingestion of antigens (food and bacterial) that gain entry to the circulation is important in turning on the immune response in the neonate. A variety of immune responses occur that include local and systemic antibody formation (especially IgA), partial tolerance (Chase, 1946), and specific reduction of antigen entry through the intestinal mucosa by development of a capacity for partial antigen exclusion (Walker et al., 1972). Though these responses occur simultaneously to the same antigen stimulus, variations in responses are inherited independently (Swarbrick et al., 1978, and unpublished data). It is clear that imbalance of these complex responses could lead to allergy to food. This has led to a hypothesis that for the infant, foods regarded as especially allergenic may play a part in the general development of allergy. Following the report of Grulee and Sanford (1936) that eczema occurred more frequently in artificially fed babies, Glaser and Johnstone (1953) reported that avoidance of cow milk and certain other feedings (see later for details) did prevent atopic allergy in genetically susceptible children. However, these children were fed on soy preparation, which is now recognized as allergenic.

Another hypothesis for the observed effects of diet on allergic sensitization may be offered. Artificially fed babies have a somewhat different intestinal flora than do breast-fed babies, with a predominance of *E. coli* (Bullen et al., 1977); the effect of immunodeficiency on this is not yet known, but it may exaggerate the burden of *E. coli* in the intestinal tract. An effective way of producing IgE antibodies in an experimental animal is to administer very small doses of antigen (it can be by mouth) at the same time as a strong adjuvant (Jarrett et al., 1977). *E. coli* endotoxin is a powerful adjuvant. It is speculated that the artificially fed, slightly immunodeficient child may fail to control the *E. coli* flora sufficiently so that excessive entry of *E. coli* endotoxin acts as a potent adjuvant, resulting in IgE antibody formation to environmental allergens, food, and other normally swallowed substances. By this mechanism, the propensity to sensitization to ingested nonfood allergens also could be enhanced.

A prospective study showing that a regimen that included exclusive breast feeding prevented eczema (Matthew et al., 1977) may be interpreted according to either hypothesis (see next section for details). The observation that the minority of breast-fed babies who received some supplementary feeds have as high an incidence of eczema as did bottle-fed babies is suggestive of the latter mechanism, since it is known that the flora of the breast-fed babies who receive supplements is more like that of a bottle-fed baby than that of babies who are exclusively breast-fed (Bullen et al., 1977). Probable mechanisms for the differences in intestinal flora secondary to feedings with other than human milk are saturating protective lactoferrin with iron and buffering the acidity of the normal (breast-fed) gut (Bullen, 1976).

PREVENTION OF ATOPIC ALLERGY

Antenatal Prevention

If the association between atopic disease (particularly asthma) with a particular birth season (late autumn in Britain) is confirmed as a general phenomenon, counseling of highly atopic families aimed at avoidance of birth in these months through appropriate contraceptive measures may well reduce disease prevalence. Similarly, in view of the apparent association of obstetric complications and neonatal surgery with an increased incidence of atopic disease, reduction of antenatal and perinatal complications by good prenatal care may be beneficial. Also, Kuroime et al. (1976) suggested that maternal avoidance of certain foods (generally the more sensitizing) to reduce fetal contact may prevent sensitization. Prospective studies examining the effects of these measures have not yet been performed.

Neonatal Infant Feeding

Glaser and Johnstone (1953) conducted a retrospective study to test a hypothesis that the genetically vulnerable child might be less likely to develop manifestations of atopic disease if certain sensitizing antigens were excluded from the diet early in life. Withholding certain sensitizing foods from the mother during pregnancy and excluding wheat, egg, fowl, and dairy products from the child's diet for the first nine months of life (the diet was soy-based) resulted in a significant lowering of the incidence of atopic dermatitis. Of the infants on the diet who did develop eczema, only 15 percent developed subsequent respiratory allergy compared to 60 percent of their eczematous siblings who were permitted a nonrestricted diet from birth.

In a subsequent prospective study, Johnstone and Dutton (1966) compared a similar soy-based diet with *ad libitum* feeding of a diet of cow milk, human milk, or both in 235 infants. Of 115 infants on the restricted diet, 9 developed asthma and 8 allergic rhinitis, whereas of 120 infants on the control diet, 28 developed asthma and 40 developed allergic rhinitis.

In a prospective controlled study of an antigen avoidance regimen, Matthew et al. (1977) showed the value of breast feeding in the prevention of eczema. A history of allergies in both parents was taken antenatally. If one or both had atopic disease, mothers were asked to participate by avoiding pets and antigenic bedding, utilizing measures to reduce house dust, and by breast feeding exclusively for three months or more. Nineteen mothers chose not to participate, and their offspring acted as controls. Significantly fewer children (2 of 23) on the regimen developed eczema in the first 6 months than did children in the control group (9 of 19). Also, at six months serum IgE levels were significantly lower in the "regimen" group than in the control group. Evidence that the neonatal period is especially important for sensitization leading to disease came from the follow-up to one year, during which time feeding was conventional; though the serum IgE of the group on the regimen rose to that of the control, only one more subject developed eczema. A few infants on the regimen received supplementary feeds and so were excluded from the regimen group; the relative incidence of eczema in this group was as high as in the bottle-fed group. This, and the fact that the preventive effect is not 100 percent, may explain why some retrospective studies of the effect of infant feeding on the development of atopic disease have not shown effects; it also suggests that the effects observed were attributable mainly to the dietary differences, rather than to the other environmental manipulations that were part of the protocol.

These data need to be confirmed by a larger study. It is too early to determine whether other atopic disease such as asthma is prevented by this kind of dietary and environmental manipulation. Since human milk may contain some foreign food antigens (Kaplan and Solli, 1977), allergen avoidance by lactating mothers also may be an important consideration in allergy prevention.

In contrast to these three positive studies, Halpern et al. (1973), in a multicenter study, did not detect benefit from avoiding cow milk either by breast feeding or by substitution of soy formula. The low frequency of allergy in all groups in that study, however, is surprising and unexplained. More work is needed to identify the optimal period for dietary manipulation, but exclusive breast feeding for three to four months (using only dextrose water supplements to satisfy additional water requirements) is compatible with current feeding practice and is readily achievable by most mothers.

Avoidance of Allergenic Substances

Atopic individuals with a propensity to develop IgE antibodies to common inhalant antigens are more vulnerable than others to develop respiratory disease when exposed to highly sensitizing industrial environments, such as those found in the enzyme detergent and platinum industries. Excluding such atopic individuals from this type of employment has led to the successful reduction in the incidence of disease among platinum workers (Juniper et al., 1977).

This extremely important approach has yet to be established formally in childhood, but we already recommend elimination of pets, institution of dust control, and other similar measures in the homes of infants with atopic dermatitis to minimize further sensitization (Sarsfield et al., 1974). It is clear that sensitization can occur at any stage in life in a genetically susceptible individual, and almost everyone can be sensitized under appropriate circumstances if the exposure is sufficiently intense.

PREVENTION OF SYMPTOMS AFTER SENSITIZATION

Avoidance of provoking antigens is discussed in detail in Chapter 22, although explanation of the principle belongs here. With acute single antigen allergies, such as urticaria due to tomatoes or asthma due to cats, the effect of antigen avoidance is often obvious, complete, and profoundly satisfying. With multiple-antigen allergies associated with less clear-cut symptoms, confirmation of cause and effect may require three withdrawals and reintroductions, preferably blind (Goldman et al., 1963). Some patients with allergy, especially postinfectious cow milk allergy (Harrison et al., 1976), may recover before the cycles are complete, which neither disproves the diagnosis of allergy nor the usefulness of the treatment. Some allergy may be so severe that challenge tests with foods may be dangerous. Nonetheless, avoidance of substances to which the child is allergic should be as complete as possible, especially in infancy. Such foods should be reintroduced periodically to see if the sensitization persists. (For example, some infants highly allergic to milk may be able to tolerate at least small quantities of milk in later childhood.)

Avoidance of inhalant allergens is often more difficult, but trial evidence has shown that house dust control is effective in relieving childhood asthma (primarily due to Dermatophagoides in Britain), and pet and mold avoidance also may be effective (Sarsfield et al., 1974).

Hyposensitization is discussed in detail in Chapter 24. The predominance of Dermatophagoides allergy in European childhood asthma has led to its use in hyposensitization. Studies employing aqueous extracts (Aas, 1971; Taylor et al., 1974) have been followed by a study of tyrosine-associated extract (Warner et al., 1978). This latter study showed that the main effect of the treatment was on the late bronchial reaction in children with asthma (Chap. 45). With the loss of the late reaction, the children's asthmatic symptoms were controlled without drug therapy even though IgE or immediate allergic reactions (e.g., immediate response on skin test or immediate bronchial challenge) were not altered by treatment.

PRACTICAL MEASURES FOR PROTECTING AN AT-RISK CHILD

This background knowledge, incomplete though it is, justifies the following measures. The effects rarely will be complete, but we believe that they will prevent disease in some and reduce disease even in very vulnerable infants.

Feeding

Exclusive breast feeding is recommended for a minimal period of three months. Mothers should avoid feeding neonatal supplements other than glucose and water if possible. Failing that, soy formulas may be preferable to modified cow milk formulas. There is suggestive evidence that during lactation, mothers should be on a diet free of egg, wheat, and milk and perhaps nuts and chocolate; it is important to check the nutritional adequacy of the diet. Alternatively, the Glaser-Johnstone program for dietary prophylaxis may be tried. This program consists of discussing the diet with the parents before the baby is born. In the newborn nursery, care is taken to see that the baby is not fed cow milk formulas. If the mother cannot nurse her baby, a soybean formula is fed in place of cow milk. During the infant's first nine or ten months, the following foods are *avoided entirely*: cow milk, beef, veal, cheese, ice cream, egg (yolk and white), and wheat. Care must be taken to give the baby adequate nutrition. It is essential that the diet be sufficiently flexible so that it contains appropriate vitamins and other nutrients to avoid potential dietary deficiencies.

Environment

While very few young parents have the economic resources to provide the ideal environment for their new infant, certain environmental measures can be carried out even by those on a very restricted budget. Ideally, the home should be new with radiant or hot water heating, should be appropriately insulated, and should have centrally controlled humidity. As minimal measures, the parents should avoid houses that are excessively moist or have circulating hot air heating that cannot be filtered. Clothes dryers must be vented outside to avoid excessive mold growth and lint. While controlled humidity of 35 to 40 percent is desirable to avoid excessive dryness of skin and mucous membranes, care must be taken to avoid a substantial growth of mold spores in the humidifier.

Environmental measures are particularly important in the bedroom to reduce the child's exposure to house dust and Dermatophagoides. Impervious smooth floors that are easily cleaned, total plastic encasings of pillows and mattresses, sealing zippers on plastic mattress covers with masking tape, and avoidance of nonwashable stuffed toys, heavy drapes, house plants, and other difficult to clean items should be encouraged.

Pets, such as dogs, cats, birds, gerbils, and other small rodents, should be excluded from the home and should *never* be permitted in the child's bedroom.

Smoking should not be permitted in the home, and parents should not expose their children to smoke in other confined spaces, such as the family car. Not only is tobacco smoke an irritant, but an increasing body of evidence also indicates that it predisposes to an increased susceptibility and prolonged course of respiratory viral infections, especially in infants and young children.

Hobbies and Careers

At-risk children should be encouraged to adopt hobbies that do not subject them to highly sensitizing substances. In career planning, the potential adverse effects of prolonged exposure to highly sensitizing industrial environments or prolonged contact with animals or animal products, pollens, and other allergenic vegetable materials must be considered along with the child's talents and interests to guide him or her into a field most compatible with his or her medical condition.

References

Aas, K.: Hyposensitization in house dust allergy in asthma. Acta Pediat. Scand. *60*:264, 1971.

Atherton, D. J., Sewell, M., Soothill, J. F., Wells, R. S., and Chilvers, C. E. D.: A double blind controlled crossover trial of an antigen avoidance diet in atopic eczema. Lancet *1*:402, 1978.

Buckley, R. H., and Dees, S. C.: Correlation of milk precipitins with IgA deficiency. N. Engl. J. Med. *281*:465, 1969.

Bullen, C. L., Tearle, P. V., and Stewart, M. G.: The effect of "humanized" milks and supplemented breast feeding on the fecal flora of infants. J. Med. Microbiol. *10*:404, 1977.

Bullen, J. J.: Iron-binding proteins and other factors in milk responsible for resistance to Escherichia coli. *In* Ciba Symposium *42*: Acute diarrhea in childhood, Elsevier, Oxford, 1976.

Chase, M. S.: Inhibition of experimental drug allergy by prior feeding of the sensitizing agent. Proc. Soc. Exp. Biol. Med. *61*:257, 1946.

Glaser, J., and Johnstone, D. E.: Prophylaxis of allergic disease in newborns. J.A.M.A. *153*:620, 1953.

Godfrey, R. C.: Asthma and IgE levels in rural and urban communities of The Gambia. Clin. Allergy *5*:201, 1975.

Goldman, A. S., Anderson, D. W., Sellars, W. A., Saperstein, S., Kniker, W. T., Halpern, S. R., et al.: Milk allergy. 1) Oral challenge with milk and isolated milk proteins in allergic children. Pediatrics *32*:425, 1963.

Grulee, C., and Sanford, H.: The influence of breast feeding and artificial feeding in infantile eczema. J. Pediatr. *9*:223, 1936.

Halpern, S. R., Sellars, W. A., Johnson, R. B., Anderson, D. W., Saperstein, S., and Reisch, J. S.: Development of childhood allergy in infants fed breast milk, soy or cow milk. J. Allergy Clin. Immunol. *51*:139, 1973.

Harrison, M., Kilby A., Walker-Smith, J. A., France, N. E., and Wood, C. B. S.: Cow's milk protein intolerance; possible association with gastroenteritis, lactose intolerance and IgA deficiency. Br. Med. J. *1*:1501, 1976.

Hill, H. R., and Quie, P. G.: Raised serum IgE level and defective neutrophil chemotaxis in three children with eczema and recurrent bacterial infections. Lancet *1*:183, 1974.

Jarrett, E. E.: Activation of IgE regulatory mechanisms by transmucosal absorption of antigen. Lancet *2*:223, 1977.

Johnstone, D. E., and Dutton, A.: Dietary prophylaxis of allergic disease in children. N. Engl. J. Med. *274*:715, 1966.

Johnstone, D. E., Roghmann, K. L., and Pless, I. B.: Factors associated with the development of asthma and hayfever in children. Pediatrics *56*:398, 1975.

Juniper, C. P., Howe, M. J., Goodwin, B. F., et al.: Bacillus subtilis enzymes: A seven year clinical, epidemiological and immunological study of an industrial allergen. J. Soc. Occup. Med. *27*:3, 1977.

Kaufman, H., and Hobbs, J. R.: Immunoglobulin deficiencies in an atopic population. Lancet *2*:1061, 1970.

Krain, L. S., and Teresaki, P. I.: HLA antigens in atopic dermatitis. Lancet *1*:1059, 1973.

Kuroime, T., Oguei, M., Matsumura, T., Iwasaki, I., Kanbe,

V., Kawahe, S., and Negishi, K.: Milk sensitivity and soya sensitivity in the production of eczematous manifestations in breast fed infants with practical reference to intrauterine sensitization. Ann. Allergy *37*:41, 1976.

Kaplan, M. S., and Solli, N. J.: Immunoglobulin E in breast-fed atopic children. J. Allergy Clin. Immunol. *64*:122, 1979.

Marsh, D. G., Bias, W. B., and Hsu, S. H.: Association of the HL-A7 cross reacting group with a specific reaginic antibody response in allergic man. Science *179*:691, 1973.

Matthew, D. J., Taylor, B., Norman, A. P., Turner, M. W., and Soothill, J. F.: Prevention of eczema. Lancet *1*:321, 1977.

Morrison Smith, J.: Skin tests and atopic allergy in children. Clin. Allergy *3*:269, 1973.

Salk, L., Grellong, B. A., Straus, W., and Dietrich, J.: Perinatal complications in the history of asthmatic children. Am. J. Dis. Child. *127*:30, 1974.

Sarsfield, J. K., Gowland, G., Toy, R., and Norman, A. L. E.: Mite sensitive asthma of childhood. Trial of avoidance measures. Arch. Dis. Child. *49*:716, 1974.

Soothill, J. F.: Some intrinsic and extrinsic factors predisposing to allergy. Proc. R. Soc. Med. *69*:439, 1976.

Soothill, J. F., Stokes, C. R., Turner, M. W., Norman, A. P., and Taylor, B.: Predisposing factors and the development of reaginic allergy in infancy. Clin. Allergy *6*:305, 1976

Swarbrick, E. T., Stokes, C. R., and Soothill, J. F.: The absorption of antigens after oral immunization and the simultaneous induction of specific systemic tolerance. GUT *20*:121, 1978.

Tada, T.: Regulation of reaginic antibody formation in animals. Prog. Allergy *19*:122, 1975.

Taylor, B., Norman, A. P., Orgel, H. A., Stokes, C. R., Turner, M. W., and Soothill, J. F.: Tansient IgA deficiency and pathogenesis of infantile atopy. Lancet *2*:111, 1973.

Taylor, B., Sanders, S. E., and Norman, A. P.: A double blind control trial of house mite fortified dust vaccine in childhood asthma. Clin. Allergy *4*:34, 1974.

Thorsby, E.: HLA-type bestemmelser i sykdomsdiagnostikk. Tidsskr. Nor. Laegeforen. *98*(19–21):961–962, 1978.

Turner, M. W., Mowbray, J. F., Harvey, B. A. M., Brostoff, J., Wells, R. S., and Soothill, J. F.: Defective yeast opsonization and C2 deficiency in atopic patients. Clin. Exp. Immunol. *34*:253, 1978.

Van Arsdel, P. P., and Motulsky, A. G.: Frequency and hereditability of asthma and allergic rhinitis in college students. Acta Genet. *9*:101, 1959.

Walker, W. A., Isselbacher, K. J., and Bloch, K. J.: Intestinal uptake of macromolecules; effect of oral immunization. Science *177*:608, 1972.

Warner, J. O., Norman, A. P., and Soothill, J. F.: Cystic fibrosis heterozygosity in the pathogenesis of allergy. Lancet *1*:990, 1976.

Warner, J. O., Price, J. F., Soothill, J. F., and Hey, E. N.: Controlled trial of hyposensitization to dermatophagoides pteronyssinus in children with asthma. Lancet *11*:912, 1978.

Clifton T. Furukawa, M.D.
Thomas A. Roesler, M.D.

26

Psychologic Aspects of Allergic Disease

One of the factors affecting allergic diseases is the child's "emotional climate." Equally important is the somatopsychic effect that the illness itself has on that climate. Emotions alone do not cause allergic disease. A child must first have the biologic substrate that allows allergic symptoms to occur. However, emotional factors can trigger allergic symptoms in biologically sensitive individuals, and allergic symptoms can cause serious emotional stress for the individual and for his or her family.

The cause of allergic symptoms is complex. To understand allergic diseases, one must be able to look at all aspects of the illness. It is important for the clinician to be able to focus in both directions — to appreciate the effect of the emotional environment on symptoms and also to recognize the effect of symptoms on the emotional environment.

Allergic symptoms play an integral part in an illness made up of many factors. These factors interrelate in such a way that if one factor is changed, the others all are affected. Thus, if a child's symptoms change for the better or worse, that change will have direct effects on the child's overall environment. Conversely, a change in the child's environment will directly affect symptoms (Mattsson, 1975; Knapp et al., 1976; and Minuchin et al., 1975, 1978).

We propose to use this perspective of both psychosomatic and somatopsychic effects to provide a general overview of the evaluation, diagnosis, and treatment of the psychologic aspects of allergic diseases.

HISTORICAL NOTES

For a long time, the prevailing view of asthma as a psychophysiologic illness was based on the writing of French and Alexander (1939, 1941), who primarily studied adult asthmatics. They postulated that emotions affected organ systems through the sympathetic nervous system, and correlated physiologic responses with emotional states. Thus, they likened the asthmatic's wheeze to a "stifled cry," which resulted because the patient could not express his feelings openly. In their psychoanalytically oriented view, asthma was a disease with symptoms triggered by the unconscious fear of losing the mother.

Others have viewed asthma as a conditioned response in the true Pavlovian sense. In 1886, many years before the development of the behaviorist school, MacKenzie described an asthmatic patient who wheezed at the sight of a paper rose in a bell jar. Although conditioned responses may play a role in asthma in some patients, behavioral therapy has not been as effective as drugs such as theophylline and steroids in treating severe asthma.

Another area of considerable interest has been the discussion of personality traits and how they relate to various psychosomatic conditions. For example, Wolff (1953) postulated that asthmatics tend to be persons who get themselves in situations where they feel "left out in the cold" and therefore experience the physiologic response of red, wet, and swollen respiratory membranes. Several large scale studies have been conducted to determine if distinct personality traits in asthmatics could be identified by psychologic testing. No clear picture has emerged (Fitzelle, 1959).

Currently, the general systems theory seems to explain psychophysiologic phenomena more thoroughly. Much of the interest in the psychologic aspects of asthma centers on the role it plays in the family. There are two principal sources for this interest. The first was based on observations of severely ill asthmatics sent to residential treatment centers (Purcell, 1969). The second was derived from the treatment of severely asthmatic patients with family therapy. Purcell and co-workers identified from among children sent to a residential center a subgroup who improved rapidly when taken from their families. These same children quickly worsened upon returning home. The crucial factor was determined to be the presence of the other members of the family.

In other studies, Liebman et al. (1974) took a group of similar youngsters and treated them in their families. By changing the relationships between family members, the researchers were able to change significantly the course of the children's illnesses. All seven children in the original study were steroid-dependent before treatment and steroid-free afterwards. Only one of the seven continued to require emergency room visits after the treatment. Follow-up showed continued good results.

These studies involved more severely affected asthmatics than are usually seen by a primary care physician. There are only a few studies of patients with mildly to moderately severe asthma, but they support the idea that emotional stress is related to the severity of asthma (Williams and McNicol, 1975).

SOMATOPSYCHIC ASPECTS OF ALLERGIC DISEASES

In spite of medical progress, allergic diseases often are chronic illnesses with emotional components that may have an impact on both the child and the family. Further, many patients have more than one allergic problem. A general overview follows of the somatopsychic aspects of various allergic diseases.

Allergic Rhinitis

Allergic rhinitis is not an attractive illness. Because of a continuous nasal discharge, children often wipe their noses with the whole hand, beginning with the tip of the fingers and proceeding to the base of the palm ("allergic salute"), and may develop a line across the bridge of the nose ("allergic pleat"). They often mouth breathe, which leads to "adenoidal facies." Their constant rhinorrhea, snorting, coughing, throat clearing, and opened-mouth chewing may alienate peers and adults, who try to avoid them. The children themselves are unaware of their disease and feel rejected without knowing why.

Children with allergic rhinitis may develop school problems because they often suffer from lack of sleep. The resulting chronic fatigue leads to decreased attention span and to learning disorders, which can be intensified by serous otitis. The fluctuating hearing loss sometimes caused by serous otitis may be mistakenly interpreted as deliberate "inattention," by parents, teachers, and even physicians. Furthermore, the frequent "colds" of children with allergic rhinitis cause them to miss more school than their peers, which further compounds peer maladjustment and accentuates learning difficulties.

Another complication of children with nasal allergy can be a diminished sense of smell. This can lead to poor eating habits and to failure to gain weight or even to weight loss. Since mealtime is an important intrafamily social activity, constant nagging about eating adds to the child's insecurity and heightens intrafamily tension.

Food Allergy

Children with food allergy also can pose difficult intrafamily mealtime problems. The allergy may require the entire family to alter its diet, or it may exclude the child from the family's diet, thus adding to intrafamily tensions. The parents may resent having to fix two meals, while the siblings may feel "left out" because of the attention accorded their brother or sister. Equally great is the social impact of not being able to eat regular food at school, at restaurants, and at friends' homes.

Atopic Dermatitis

Children with eczema itch constantly. Their rash, complicated by frequent skin infection, discourages normal social interaction with peers. Children may be embarrassed, particularly in physical education classes, when required to undress. Also, unsympathetic teachers may compound the problem by inferring that the rash is caused by uncleanliness or psychologic problems. The child is apt to develop a poor self-image, which may be intensified by the symptoms of respiratory and gastrointestinal allergy that are frequently associated with atopic dermatitis. Scratching at night interferes with adequate sleep. Scratching in the day distracts from other activities and learning.

Asthma

Symptoms from asthma may be as mild as intermittent cough or as severe as imminent respiratory failure. Asthma may or may not be perceived as a handicap, depending on the prior experience of the child. Some children with severe pulmonary obstruction may not be aware of their condition until they experience normal health. On a more subtle level, those with exercise-induced asthma may consider it normal to cough or wheeze with exertion. Also, mechanisms of coping with asthma vary considerably among families, spanning the entire spectrum from overreaction to denial.

The emotional impact of asthma generally correlates with the severity of the disease. When a severe attack occurs, the child becomes very anxious and may even worry about dying. When the child must focus all energies upon the work of breathing, everyone feels that *something* must be done. All family plans and activities are disrupted. If severe asthma occurs frequently, social development stops because

school attendance and active play with other children becomes difficult.

If the family cannot cope with the stress, family resources may become exhausted, and the parents may even separate. Anger, blame, and guilt are common in dealing with asthma. The asthma attack disrupts normal life, and some children discover it to be a powerful tool to manipulate life events. The physician may even unwittingly reinforce this manipulation.

PSYCHOSOMATIC PROBLEMS OF ALLERGIC CHILDREN AND PSYCHOSOMATIC FAMILIES

Distinguishing psychosomatic problems from somatopsychic ones allows these problems to be viewed from a distinctive reference point. Somatopsychic problems are emotional problems that follow physical symptoms. Psychosomatic problems represent physical symptoms that follow emotional situations.

The study of emotional situations that precede psychosomatic problems (symptoms) has yielded important information about the nature of psychosomatic diseases. Minuchin and co-workers (1978) have postulated the existence of certain types of family behavior that elicit psychosomatic symptoms in children. In Minuchin's work, these families are referred to as "psychosomatic families." It has been shown that an asthmatic child living in this type of family often will not respond to proper medical treatment. It is postulated that the asthma serves a special function in the family and has, in fact, become a usual and necessary part of family life.

Standardized videotaped interviews of families of children with severe asthma suggest that they have certain traits in common that are quite similar to those of families of children with anorexia nervosa or brittle diabetes. These characteristics include overprotection, rigidity, enmeshment (a quality of overinvolvement in the affairs of other family members), and an inability to resolve conflict. In addition, the ill child participates in unresolved marital discord. Within the model put forth by this group, the care of the sick child becomes a substitute for resolving conflict in family life.

These families are good at protective responses, but lack the communication skills necessary to resolve family problems.

Coping

In chronic disease, "coping" can be equated to "cure." Coping ability is dependent upon the severity of the disease and upon the available medical, economic, social, and emotional resources. These variables are never constant, but if resources are constantly taxed by severe disease, even those with excellent coping abilities can be overwhelmed. Alternately, those with few resources can be overwhelmed by relatively minor problems. It is, therefore, important that the physician evaluate the impact of the disease on the family. For example, the simple recommendation "take medication X every 6 hours" may be difficult because the dosing schedule interferes with work or sleep schedules or because the cost of medication is a financial problem.

The normal family has several important functions: one is to protect its members and a second is to prepare children to live and grow as individuals. When a family member becomes ill, the other members become concerned and increase their protective functions. This family response promotes the healing process by protecting the vulnerable person from as much stress as possible. Though an acute illness stretches the fabric of family life, the family makes the necessary accommodation in the way most in keeping with its usual equilibrium. When the illness is over, the sick person gets well and the family returns to its regular pattern.

With a chronic illness, a different solution is necessary, because the protective stance so necessary in response to acute illness may, in the long run, inhibit emotional development in the chronically ill child and may interfere with the second important function of the family — providing the child the chance to be an individual, within a secure environment.

In a family dealing with chronic disease, some of the features of the acute response become incorporated into daily routine. A new equilibrium is established, taking into account the changed circumstances of family life. All relationships are affected. The person (often the mother) who takes over the nursing, nurturing, and protection of the sick child will have less time for other things, including her spouse and other children in the family. All of these changes can be considered part of a normal family response to the stress of chronic illness.

Rees (1963) randomly selected from a normal sample a group of asthmatics and their families. He found that in 44 percent of the families, the parental attitudes were described as satisfactory. In 44.5 percent of the families, overprotection was a factor; in 4.5 percent, rejecting attitudes were a problem. Most families meet the challenge well and continue to provide for the basic needs of their members.

In considering normal coping behavior, it is necessary to make some comments about the greater community as well. Normally, school personnel, peers, and even the patient's physician find a middle ground between overconcern and denial in their treatment of the ill child and his family. However, a teacher or physician who is oversympathetic can retard the ill child's movement toward increasing self-reliance, while a nonconcerned attitude can endanger the child's health.

Table 26–1 provides a schematic view of normal developmental issues taken from the perspective of the individual, the family, and the peer group. The table is designed to give the clinician a quick tool to identify major developmental themes. These developmental issues will help the clinician assess the normality of the child's and family's coping patterns.

Behavior Problems of Allergic Children

The child who discovers that allergic symptoms can be used to manipulate life situations is the rule rather than the exception. It is the role of other people in the child's life to insure that this tool is not used too often or to the child's detriment.

Allergic symptoms are more than just part of a pattern of illness. They are also events in the life of the child, family, school, and community. As such, they have the power to shape the responses of

TABLE 26–1   NORMAL ISSUES AND CONCERNS OF CHILDREN
WITH CHRONIC ALLERGIC DISEASES

Age (years)	Individual Issue	Family Issue	Peer Group Issue
0–2	Child must develop trust that basic needs will be met.	Parents need extra support. Siblings need attention.	
3–5	Tendency for a child to feel guilty for being ill and that illness is punishment for bad behavior.	Care must be taken to allow the separation of parent and child to proceed as normally as possible. Siblings need attention.	Child needs to be exposed to peers in as normal a setting as possible.
6–11	Child needs education about the illness and needs to build competency as an individual.	Locus of control of treatment is shifting from parents to child. Siblings need attention.	Parents need to encourage peer group interaction, including exercise to full extent tolerated by child.
12–18	Child is concerned about the stigma of being chronically ill.	Normal adolescent issues of gaining distance from the family become entangled with parental concern about child's health. Siblings need attention.	Adolescent may have difficulty integrating into the peer group because of being different.

other people. Looked at from this perspective, wheezing can be equivalent to fighting, crying, lying, or flattering. It can be used to achieve the same ends. When these ends are not healthy long-term goals for the child in question, the child has a behavior problem.

Difficulty arises when parents are afraid of the symptom. If they are afraid to send their child to school because he or she is wheezing, for example, the child will understand that wheezing is a powerful tool and an effective means of avoiding school.

A common behavior problem of allergic children is failure to comply with prescribed medical regimens. Often, noncompliance serves the same function for the child as his allergic symptoms. It can become a tool with which to manipulate the environment. However, not all noncompliance can be considered "acting out" on the part of the child. Other factors (e.g., communication problems between physi-

cian and family, economic constraints) that can cause noncompliance are discussed in the next section.

EVALUATION AND DIAGNOSIS

A thorough evaluation of a child with psychosocial problems associated with allergic disease should include a structured psychosocial interview, a complete physical exam, and an evaluation of the rest of the family. Table 26–2 outlines the approach given here. This approach has been helpful in our office practice.

The physician should obtain a detailed history of the family experience with allergic illness. The history should include — in addition to the age of onset and the severity of current symptoms — the reaction of the patient and of the family members who do not have allergic diseases. What trauma has the illness induced? How much

TABLE 26–2 DIAGNOSIS OF SIGNIFICANT PSYCHOSOCIAL PROBLEMS

I. Historical data

    A. Patient and family asthma experience
        1. Age of onset, frequency of attacks, severity
        2. Disruption of life, e.g., school, trips
        3. Economic impact — work loss, medical costs

    B. Effect of environmental changes
        1. Variation with vacations, trips, weekends, holidays
        2. Variation between one home versus another

II. Medical findings

    A. Physical
        1. Physical stigmata, e.g., allergic facies, barrel chest, etc.
        2. Development appropriate to age, e.g., size, social interactions, sexual maturity?
        3. Mental status — appropriate for age and circumstance?
    B. Laboratory
        1. Pulmonary function — correlation with history and physical
        2. Allergy factors — skin test data
    C. Medications — schedule, side effects, misuse, compliance

III. Personal and family factors
    A. Physician-patient interaction
    B. Psychosocial assets
    C. Family
        1. Relationships between patient, siblings, parents, extended family
        2. Family resources for dealing with disease
        3. "Locus of control"
        4. Family style of interaction

school has the patient missed? How frequently has the child had to visit the doctor or go to the hospital emergency room? How much disruption has there been of the family's trips and vacations, day and night schedules, ownership of pets and farm animals, and choice of home or job? The economic impact of the disease on the family should also be explored. It is especially important to note if the severity of asthma varies as the child moves from one household to another (such as in a broken marriage), or as he travels away from home.

Since some patients may have significant psychiatric disease that is unrelated to their allergies, it is important to perform a mental status examination in questionable instances.

During the physical examination, allergic facies, barrel chest, or other stigmata that may affect the child's body image should be noted. The appropriateness of the youngster's behavior in the clinical setting and in his relationship to friends and adults should be ascertained. Whether or not the youngster is large or small for age or un-

derdeveloped sexually can also have a significant impact.

Laboratory tests should focus upon whether or not physical findings correlate with the apparent severity of the disease. For instance, if one finds excellent pulmonary function in a person who appears to have severe asthma, significant psychosocial problems may be present. Skin test results and other laboratory tests may be important in assessing the cause-effect relationship of various external factors. These can then be weighed against possible psychologic factors. Positive skin tests, the presence of nasal eosinophils and high IgE titers suggest the presence of environmental allergy but do not rule out the possibility of a psychosomatic component to the child's disease.

Evaluating the Role of Medication

As part of the evaluation, the role of medications in the child's life should be investigated. Medications may induce a variety of problems:

1. Side effects, such as somnolence or agitation (antihistamine, theophylline, decongestants, adrenergics), obesity and acne (steroids), gastric distress (theophylline, antibiotics), and even psychosis (steroids);

2. Unpleasant interactions between parent and child because of medication taste, schedule, or mode of administration (inhaled powders, sprays, suppositories or rectal solutions);

3. Misuse because of misunderstanding or manipulation by the child.

When evaluating a patient's response to medication, the physician must be aware of individual patient characteristics, as well as his or her own response to the patient. It is recognized that some patients exaggerate and others minimize the difficulties encountered with their diseases. Asthmatics with high or low extremes of "panic-fear" traits request medications inappropriately (Dahlem et al., 1977). The response of the physician to these patients varies. "Sensitive" physicians tend to prescribe on less objective data, and their prescribing tends to be in relation to the amount of panic or fear shown by their patients (Kinsman et al., 1977). Thus the physician must not only recognize patient traits but also be aware of his or her own response to them.

Other aspects of physician-patient interactions can affect the therapeutic outcome. These include time spent with the patient and family, educational endeavors in the office and community, social and racial bias, interactions of the physician with the child versus the parent, and manipulative attempts between child, parents, and physician.

Compliance with the prescribed medical regimen is one of the most important factors to be evaluated. At present, laboratory tests to measure compliance have been developed for only a few medications. Urine tests for cortisol can determine whether or not steroid preparations are used as directed; urinary excretion of beta adrenergic drugs and cromolyn can be measured; and serum theophylline levels are readily available. Once proper theophylline dosage has been established by serum levels, any spot check of serum or salivary theophylline level can document whether or not the pa-

tient is compliant (Eney and Goldstein, 1976). Failure of patient compliance can result from any one or more of the following:

1. Lack of understanding of the disease, its cause and course
2. Lack of understanding of how medications and other prescribed measures work
3. Problems from medication side effects
4. A difficult medication schedule
5. A negative attitude about medications
6. Inability to handle the responsibility of medications
7. Rebellion against family or physician
8. Secondary gain from being sick

If compliance is the problem, the reason for noncompliance can be treated by education, counseling, or a change in regimen.

Evaluating the Role of the Family

Part of the clinician's evaluation should include a review of the child's functioning in social areas: Is the child making a satisfactory adjustment to school and peer group? Is he or she having behavioral problems at home or in the community? Does the patient have a satisfactory self-image? Most clinicians have a natural feel for the limits of normal office behavior of children in various age groups. This can be an excellent guide when asking about how the child functions in other situations.

It is important not to focus all one's attention on the index patient. Once some idea of the patient's psychosocial adjustment has been obtained, the physician should assess the family situation by asking some of the following questions. Are there any problems with the siblings? Do they feel neglected? Does either parent feel he or she is spending too much or too little time with the ill child? Are there sources of emotional support other than the immediate family? Do the spouses have enough time for themselves and for each other? Have they been able to get away by themselves lately? Often a physician needs only give a family "permission" to satisfy neglected needs to produce a healthy effect on the entire family.

Some families will have difficulty meeting the demands of the medical care system. Their past experiences need to be evaluated to determine how families can best function to meet the child's needs. Those patients with many psychosocial assets tend to be better able to follow medical regimens than those with few, so it is important to determine the extent and adequacy of patient and family support systems (deAraujo et al., 1972). It would, for instance, be unreasonable to ask an unemployed family to purchase expensive equipment or furnishings for better environmental control.

Another area that needs to be explored is the "locus of control." The physician needs to determine who in the family is responsible for control of the disease. When the child is very young, parents will be in total control of the treatment process. As the child grows older, more and more of the responsibility for the illness should be assumed by the child and relinquished by the parents. The physician will want to evaluate the appropriateness of the agreement between parents and children about who assumes responsibility for various aspects of treatment. Some parents will want to shift too much responsibility onto the child, whereas some will find it difficult to let go of their control. The physician must be aware of his or her own role. Some parents will not give the physician enough responsibility, and some will expect too much of him or her.

The presence or absence of the following family characteristics should be noted carefully.

1. *Rigidity:* Is the family flexible and able to try new solutions to problems?

2. *Overprotectiveness:* Do parents and child protect each other to an unreasonable degree? Is the sick child given as much freedom and "space" as his symptoms will permit?

3. *Enmeshment:* Are members of the family overinvolved with each other's business? Do family members complete each other's sentences and speak for one another?

4. *Lack of generational boundaries:* Are children inappropriately involved in parents' conflicts and decisions?

5. *Lack of conflict resolution:* Are families able to resolve conflicts, rather than ignoring them or letting them drag on unnecessarily?

These five family characteristics are often present in families with serious emotional problems, which can affect the course of the child's illness and lead to further complications.

In summary, most patients who have allergic disease improve when the cause is determined and eliminated, and appropriate drugs are prescribed. Some patients, however, may not improve or may actually get worse. If more intense therapy is not successful, suspect noncompliance. When a complying patient worsens, the diagnosis needs to be re-evaluated. For instance, in a patient with a chronic cough the real problem may be sinusitis, gastroesophageal reflux, a foreign body in the bronchus, bronchopulmonary aspergillosis, or psychologic problems that require intervention.

TREATMENT

There is a great deal the primary care physician can do to treat the emotional aspects of allergic diseases. He or she needs to be aware of the types of problems that can arise, should practice good medicine, treat the compliance problems, educate the patient and the family, aid the family in increasing coping skills, screen for serious pathology, and refer to a consultant when the problem involves too much time or is unusually complicated.

Good Medical Practice

Good medical practice, especially the conscientious use of proper medications, is the first step toward effective psychological treatment of allergic children. When medication is properly prescribed and regulated, the potentially serious side effects of commonly used drugs can be minimized. More importantly, many somatopsychic symptoms can be prevented before they have a chance to develop into a psychological illness.

Compliance Problems

The benefits of even the best medical practice can be negated by poor patient cooperation. Failure of a child or the family to comply with treatment can be a frustrating experience for the physician. Nevertheless, it is a fundamental part of the physician's responsibility to deal with the problem and try to determine its cause. Is the problem the child's (doesn't like taste) or the parent's (afraid to give medicine, so doesn't insist)? If so, the physician may be able to prescribe a better-tasting or more easily administered alternate drug. He can educate the parents about the drug, its benefit to risk ratio, side effects, and signs of toxicity. He can demonstrate the best technique for administering the medication. He can also teach the parents to reinforce acceptance of the medication with social and material rewards.

A common problem is that of the noncompliant teenager. With this problem, it is essential to *document* noncompliance *before* confronting the patient and family. Theophylline blood levels provide such documentation, and confrontation can lead to education, which should include suggesting methods to guarantee proper dosing.

Education

Education is a major factor in treatment. The amount of time a physician is willing to spend on education will have a significant effect on the patient and his family. This can take place in the traditional form of the office consultation in which aspects of the illness are discussed between doctor and patient. The physician may want to use his office staff or other specially educated individuals to talk about allergic diseases with his patients either singly or in groups. Several types of texts with programmed instruction have been prepared for children and parents (Parcel, 1975). Children can be referred to special summer camps where there is an emphasis on learning to live with their illness. State Lung Associations are developing community based programs for children and parents (Smith, 1976). The focus of the educational efforts in each of these settings is on the anatomy, physiology, and treatment of asthma.

A theme running throughout the treatment of psychologic factors in allergy is the attempt to increase the coping skills of the

family. A physician may want to do this by expanding the network of social support available to the family. A referral to a social agency may be necessary.

Most counseling efforts in the office aim at increasing coping skills. A very important function the physician can play is to help the family set norms of appropriate behavior for children and parents. The physician can watch family interaction and suggest when a child can take more responsibility for the illness, or conversely, advise parents to treat the illness more seriously.

Referral for Psychiatric Consultation

Beyond counseling, one function of the primary care physician is to recognize signs of serious psychopathology in their developing patients. Table 26–3 is a schematic presentation of signs of failure of normal psychologic development. To correspond with Table 26–1, it is divided into three perspectives: the individual focus, the family focus, and the peer group focus. It should provide the reader with a guide to help screen for significant pathology. The presence of any of the "symptoms" appearing on Table 26–3 in a chronically ill child can be a signal that development is not proceeding normally. These patients should be evaluated carefully, with consideration of further treatment or referral.

Referral of the allergic child for psychiatric consultation or treatment will depend on the child's symptoms and the primary physician's knowledge and attitude. The most obvious reasons for referral are psychiatric problems independent of allergic disease, such as psychosis, encopresis or fire setting or other severe behavior problems.

Table 26–3 lists conditions that require psychiatric help. Whether the physician refers or tries to manage these conditions depends on his knowledge, his comfort with psychologic issues, and his available time. Regressive behaviors, poor self-image, social immaturity, and overprotective parenting, for example, will often respond to education and counseling in the office. It is up to the individual clinician to recognize his or her own limits. As allergic diseases are chronic in nature, problems which are not resolved can be expected to recur at a later

TABLE 26–3   SIGNS OF FAILURE OF NORMAL PSYCHOLOGIC
DEVELOPMENT IN ALLERGIC CHILDREN

Age (years)	Individual Focus	Family Focus	Peer Group Focus
0–2	Failure to thrive	Parental exhaustion Potential for separation or divorce Symptoms in siblings	
3–5	Regressive behavior, e.g., soiling, sleep disturbance	Parent-child symbiosis	Pseudomature child who talks well with adults but cannot mix with peers
6–11	Inadequate self-image Withdrawal and anxiety symptoms	Overprotective parent-child relation- ship, resulting in immature child and overworked parent	Social inadequacy—child who cannot do age appropriate things, e.g., ride a bicycle, build a treehouse, and partici- pate in Brownies or Cub Scouts
12–18	Depression Inability to move toward identity definition	Acting out "Adolescent rebellion" Compliance issues	Social ostracism or inclusion in peer group as the "sick kid"

age. For example, a mother who cannot allow her 4 year old out of her sight for a minute may well have problems when the child is expected to go to school at age 6. Her problems may recur at the age of puberty and again in the late teens, when it is time for the child to leave the family.

When the clinician decides to refer, he should try to select a therapist whose skills meet his patient's needs. It is imperative that the therapist chosen has been appropriately educated about the allergic disease for which the patient is referred. Since therapists may have diverse training, skills, and philosophical orientations, the referring physician should be familiar with the consultant's personality and therapeutic techniques. Three general types of psychiatric treatment are currently in use: insight therapy, behavior modification, and family therapy. Insight therapy appears appropriate for treatment of intrapsychic issues such as feelings of self-worth, depression, and identity development. Behaviorists concentrate on measurable behavior and reinforcement patterns. Family therapists focus on how people interrelate in the home environment of the patient.

A referral for behavioral therapy is indi-

cated when the child's primary problem is refusal to take medications or other unhealthy behaviors that have become reinforced by his illness. Treatment consists of a carefully planned program of positive rewards for acceptable behaviors (Micklich, 1977). A referral for family therapy is indicated when the child is functioning better outside of the family than in it, and the characteristics of "psychosomatic families" are clearly present.

Treatment for "psychosomatic" families consists of disengaging the patient's symptoms from the family conflicts, encouraging the family to function independently, and helping the family members to resolve conflict. Final stages in the therapy include working with the parents to resolve marital issues and helping the patient join his or her peer group.

Other treatment approaches for specific problems include hypnosis, systematic desensitization, and biofeedback. Hypnosis has been used in adults with asthma to decrease anxiety levels, with a resulting decrease in the frequency of attacks (Maher-Laughman, 1976). The results of systematic desensitization, with or without biofeedback techniques, have been equivocal; but the technique may be helpful in certain panic-prone children. The technique embodies elements of relaxation training that might have a place in the treatment of asthma (Davis et al., 1973). Relaxation exercises are easy to teach to patients and are useful techniques for the clinician to learn.

Occasionally, children with very severe asthma may need referral to a residential treatment center, either as a way of obtaining better control of the physical environment or of the psychological environment. Such separation from the family is a reasonable method of treatment if family structure is concurrently altered. Otherwise, the gains made in the treatment center in increased autonomy and self-esteem will be lost when the child returns home.

There is no easy answer to the question of when to refer a patient for psychologic therapy. The determining factors involve the patient, family, community, and especially the physician. Referral is often not for the asthma or allergies *per se*. Rather, it is because of the child's or family's psychologic response to the illness. The object of referral is to help the patient cope and to improve the quality of interpersonal relationships. Interdisciplinary collaboration between primary care physician and consultants is essential to ensure optimal physical and mental health for allergic children and adolescents.

References

Dahlem, N. W., Kinsman, R. A., and Horton, D. J.: Panic-fear in asthma: Requests for as-needed medications in relation to pulmonary measurements. J. Allergy Clin. Immunol. *60*:295, 1977.

Davis, M. H., Saunders, D. R., Creer, T. L., and Chai, H: Relaxation training facilitated by biofeedback as a supplemental treatment in bronchial asthma. J. Psychosom. Research *17*:121, 1973.

deAraujo, G., Dudley, D. L., and Van Arsdel, P. P. Jr.: Psychosocial assets and severity of chronic asthma. J. Allergy Clin. Immunol. *50*:257, 1972.

Eney, R. D., and Goldstein, E. O.: Compliance of chronic asthmaticus with oral administration of theophylline as measured by serum and salivary levels. Pediatrics *57*:513, 1976.

Falliers, C. J.: Treatment of asthma in a residential center. Ann. Allergy *28*:513, 1970.

Fitzelle, G. T.: Personality factors and certain attributes toward child rearing among parents of asthmatic children. Psychosomatic Med. *21*:209, 1959.

French, T. M., and Alexander, F.: Psychogenic factors in asthma. Am. J. Psychiat. *96*:87, 1939.

French, T. M., and Alexander, F.: Psychogenic factors in bronchial asthma. Psychosom. Med. Monograph 4, No 1, 1941.

Kinsman, R. A., Dahlem, N. W., Spector, S., and Staudenmayer, H.: Observations on subjective symptomatology, coping behavior, and medical decisions in asthma. Psychosom. Med. *39*:102, 1977.

Knapp, P. H., Mathe, A. A., and Vorhon, L.: Psychosomatic aspects of bronchial asthma. *In* Weiss, E. B., and Segal, M. S. (eds.): *Bronchial Asthma — Mechanisms and Therapeutics*. Boston, Little, Brown and Co., 1976.

Liebman, R., Minuchin, S., and Baker, L: The use of structural family therapy in the treatment of intractable asthma. Am J Psychiat. *131*:535, 1974.

MacKenzie, J. N.: The production of "rose asthma" by an artificial rose. Am. J. Med. Sci. *91*:45, 1886.

Maher-Laughman, G. P.: Hypnosis in bronchial asthma. *In* Weiss, E. B., and Segal, M. S. (eds.): *Bronchial Asthma: Mechanisms* and *Therapeutics*. Boston, Little, Brown and Co., 1976.

Mattsson, A: Psychologic aspects of childhood asthma. Ped. Clin. North Am. Vol 22 (No. 1), Feb. 1975.

Miklich, D. R., Renne, C. M., Creer, T. L., et al.: The clinical utility of behavior therapy as an adjunctive treatment of asthma, J. Allergy Clin. Immunol. *60*:285, 1977.

Minuchin, S., Rosman, B., and Baker, L.: *Psychosomatic Families; Anorexia Nervosa in Context,* Boston, Harvard University Press, 1978.

Minuchin, S., Baker, L., Rosman, B., et al.: Psychosomatic illness in children: A new conceptual model. Arch. Gen. Psychiatry, *32*:1021, 1975.

Parcel, G. S.: *Teaching My Parents About Asthma*. Medical Illustration Service, Galveston, Tex. 77550. University of Texas Medical Branch.

Purcell, K., et al.: The effect on asthma in children of experimental separation from the family. Psychosom. Med. *31*:144, 1969.

Rees, L: The significance of parental attitudes in childhood asthma. J. Psychosom. Res. *7*:181, 1963.

Smith, S: The family asthma program: A pioneer program. Am. Lung Assoc. Bull., June 1976.

Williams, H. E., and McNicol, K. N.: The spectrum of asthma in children. Ped. Clin. North Am. *22*:43, 1975.

Wolff. H. G.: *Stress and Disease*. Springfield, Ill., Charles C Thomas, 1953.

27

Dennis L. Christie, M.D.

Diagnosis and Treatment of Gastrointestinal Tract Diseases

The discussion of the gastrointestinal tract will be divided into two sections since disorders of each section can result in quite different clinical syndromes due to or aggravating allergy. Disorders of the esophagus and stomach may be manifested by pulmonary symptoms such as aspiration of gastric contents with recurrent pneumonia or asthma. Disorders of the small and large bowel are manifested by nutritional disorders, diarrhea, or both, ranging from malabsorption syndromes with failure to thrive to a number of different diarrheal diseases.

THE ESOPHAGUS AND STOMACH

Abnormalities in esophageal function have been associated with aspiration pneumonia for several decades (Urschel, 1967). However, the spectrum of pulmonary diseases caused by esophageal dysfunction has not been evaluated critically in a pediatric population. Many of the symptoms of patients with abnormal esophageal function can be confused with allergic respiratory disease and must be differentiated from other diseases associated with similar symptoms.

Physiology

The esophagus is a hollow muscular organ that extends from the pharynx at the

sixth cervical vertebra to the stomach at the gastroesophageal junction. The length of the esophagus varies from 7 to 14 cm in the infant to approximately 35 cm in the adult. It is lined by stratified squamous epithelium and has two muscle layers, an inner circular and an outer longitudinal. In the upper one-third of the esophagus, the muscle layers are composed of striated voluntary fibers, while the remaining esophagus contains only smooth muscle.

Two sphincters are present in the esophagus. The upper esophageal sphincter consists of the muscle of the cricopharyngeus. This muscle arises from the cricoid cartilage of the larynx and forms a band of muscle that acts as a sphincter. This sphincter is approximately 3 cm long and has a resting pressure of up to 140 mm Hg. The upper esophageal sphincter relaxes with swallowing, which occurs in a sequence after pharyngeal contraction but before esophageal peristalsis (Fig. 27–1). The upper esophageal sphincter acts as a barrier to reflux of gastric contents into the hypopharynx.

The lower esophageal sphincter is a physiologic zone of high pressure separating the body of the esophagus from the fundus of the stomach. No anatomic sphincter has been demonstrated at the gastroesophageal junction, but intraluminal esophageal manometrics have shown that this area has a resting pressure of approximately 15 to 30 mm Hg (Fig. 27–2). Lower esopha-

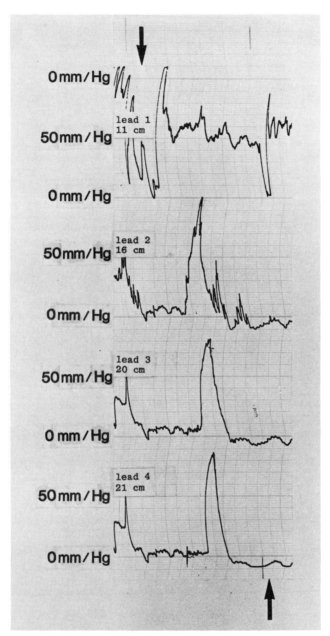

FIGURE 27–1. Esophageal manometer tracing of a normal swallow, showing relaxation of the upper esophageal sphincter in Lead 1 followed by a peristaltic wave in the body of the esophagus in Leads 2–4.

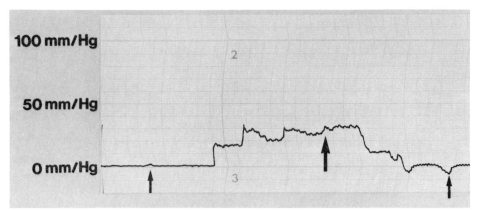

FIGURE 27–2.   A high pressure zone (large arrow) of approximately 26 mm Hg separating the stomach (positive deflection on left) from the esophagus (negative deflection on right).

geal sphincter pressure will drop to 0 within 2.5 seconds after swallowing is initiated. The pressure will then return to its normal elevated state approximately 10 seconds after deglutition when the esophageal peristaltic wave passes the lower esophagus. The lower esophageal sphincter is believed to be the most important barrier to prevent reflux of gastroduodenal contents into the esophageal lumen.

Symptoms and Signs of Esophageal Dysfunction

Since the major function of the esophagus is the transportation of food from mouth to stomach and prevention of reflux of gastric material back into its lumen, most symptoms of esophageal disease in infants and young children are related to feeding.

Regurgitation and vomiting are the most common symptoms of gastroesophageal disease in infants. Regurgitation refers to the effortless expulsion of gastric contents during or after feeding. Regurgitation can occur whether the infant is upright, supine, or prone and can range in amount from a few milliliters to several ounces. The vomiting occurring with esophageal dysfunction is secondary to an incompetent lower esophageal sphincter. The vomitus is forceful and projectile and usually occurs during or within 1 hour after feeding. No clinical dis-

tinction can be made from the vomiting secondary to gastroesophageal reflux, pyloric stenosis, peptic ulcer disease, duodenal web, or food allergy.

"Colic" is a symptom so vague and difficult to characterize that many different etiologies have been incriminated, including gastroesophageal reflux and food allergy. Infants with significant regurgitation or vomiting may fail to thrive or may gain weight abnormally slowly in the first several months of life because they fail to retain sufficient calories.

Dysphagia is a symptom unique to the esophagus, but it is not commonly recognized in pediatric patients. Dysphagia is defined as a difficulty in swallowing and is seen characteristically when solid material is swallowed. Older children will describe the feeling of food catching in their throats, and they may be able to point to a location in the substernal area.

Heartburn is the sensation of burning beneath the substernal area, with radiation to the neck. It occurs primarily when the patient is lying supine or when the patient increases intra-abdominal pressure by positional changes or exercise. Older pediatric patients may associate "throw up burps" with heartburn.

Aspiration of swallowed food particles and liquid secondary to reflux of gastric contents may induce respiratory symptoms in infants and children. Aspiration occurs because of abnormalities in function of the pharyngeal and laryngeal swallowing mechanisms or because of esophageal obstruction, gastroesophageal reflux, or esophageal motor disorders. Severe lung damage may occur when gastric fluid with a pH of 2.5 or less is aspirated. Aspiration pneumonia and an ''asthma-like'' syndrome with dyspnea, cyanosis, wheezing, rales, rhonchi, and occasional gross pulmonary edema were recognized with aspiration of gastric contents following general anesthesia (Mendelsohn, 1946). Aspiration of smaller quantities of gastric contents may induce significant bronchospasm (Wynne and Modell, 1977). Children with esophageal reflux and aspiration may have nocturnal episodes of coughing, shortness of breath, tachypnea, and vomiting (Carre, 1960). Their recurrent attacks of wheezing and coughing may be associated with radiographic evidence of pneumonitis over a period of months to years, though they may be free of symptoms between attacks. Though many infants and children with recurrent pulmonary disease due to gastroesophageal reflux have such esophageal symptoms as vomiting, regurgitation, dysphagia, or heartburn (Christie et al., 1978), some may not (Danus et al., 1976).

Patients with repeated episodes of aspiration are commonly diagnosed as having ''asthmatic bronchitis,'' bronchitis, or asthma. Clinical differentiation between these patients and those with extrinsic asthma may be difficult.

Differential Diagnosis

Pharyngeal and laryngeal disorders are common causes of aspiration. Anomalies such as cleft lip and palate, choanal atresia, Pierre Robin syndrome, or laryngeal cleft are associated with oropharyngeal dysphagia and can be associated with aspiration. Patients with such neurologic abnormalities as cerebral palsy, familial dysautonomia, or Werdnig-Hoffmann disease, which are associated with incoordinated laryngeal or pharyngeal swallowing, may aspirate during feeding (Fig. 27–3).

Esophageal obstruction occurs in patients with achalasia, esophageal stricture, or an upper esophageal foreign body. Up to 10 percent of patients with achalasia develop aspiration pneumonia with symptoms of wheezing or chronic bronchitis with recurrent pneumonia (Anderson, 1953) (Fig. 27–4). A chest x-ray film may show aspiration pneumonitis. Complications include lung abscesses, bronchiectasis, asthma, emphysema, and pulmonary fibrosis.

Esophageal stricture, a complication of

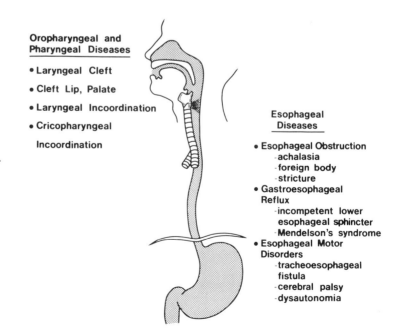

Oropharyngeal and Pharyngeal Diseases

- Laryngeal Cleft
- Cleft Lip, Palate
- Laryngeal Incoordination
- Cricopharyngeal Incoordination

Esophageal Diseases

- Esophageal Obstruction
  - achalasia
  - foreign body
  - stricture
- Gastroesophageal Reflux
  - incompetent lower esophageal sphincter
  - Mendelson's syndrome
- Esophageal Motor Disorders
  - tracheoesophageal fistula
  - cerebral palsy
  - dysautonomia

FIGURE 27–3. Causes of aspiration pneumonia.

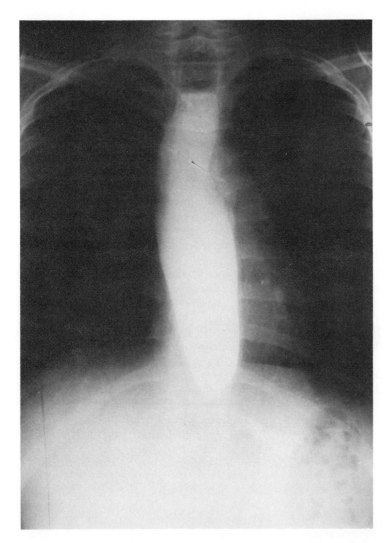

FIGURE 27–4. Barium esophagram demonstrates dilated esophagus in a child with recurrent pneumonia from achalasia with aspiration.

gastroesophageal reflux, can cause aspiration if the esophagus above the stricture becomes grossly dilated. Such patients may awaken at night coughing and choking because of "overflow of food" and secretions from the esophagus into the posterior oropharynx during sleep (Fig. 27–5).

Abnormal esophageal motility may result in aspiration pneumonia if food and acid are not cleared from the esophagus during deglutition. These patients are also at risk for severe esophagitis with subsequent stricture and esophageal ulcer because the esophageal mucosa is exposed to acid for prolonged periods of time. In infants and children this occurs with tracheoesophageal fistula or mental retardation (Parker et al., 1979).

Gastroesophageal reflux may result in aspiration because an incompetent lower esophageal sphincter will not prevent reflux of gastric contents when patients are in a recumbent position. Two clinical syndromes appear to be present in infants and children with aspiration secondary to gastroesophageal reflux. The "recurrent pneumonia" patients present with episodes of cough, fever, and tachypnea, usually worse at night. These patients will have interstitial pneumonia or lobar consolidation on chest x-rays. They will be completely well between periods of aspiration. The "asthmatic bronchitis syndrome" patients have recurrent episodes of bronchitis and coughing with significant wheezing. Both groups of patients generally have symptoms of eso-

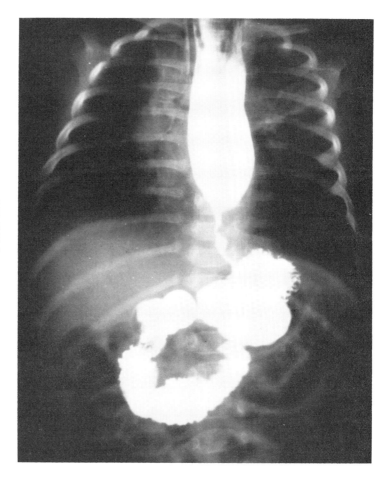

FIGURE 27–5. Narrow esophageal stricture at gastroesophageal junction is identified by barium esophagram. Fifteen-month-old child had dysphagia and recurrent pneumonia.

phageal disease along with respiratory symptoms.

Asthma and Gastroesophageal Reflux. The question of whether extrinsic asthma may be worsened or precipitated by gastroesophageal reflux and aspiration remains to be determined. Before one can attribute significant asthmatic symptoms to reflux, all other causes of respiratory pulmonary disease must be excluded. Some authors have demonstrated gastroesophageal reflux in children with severe asthma (Byrne, 1978; Shapiro, 1979). However, it is not clear that their gastroesophageal reflux is responsible for the severity of their asthma.

Tests for Esophageal Dysfunction

Barium esophagography and cineesophagography are the basic screening tests for evaluation of esophageal function.

All patients with suspected aspiration should have a careful study of posterior oropharyngeal function and peristalsis in the body of the esophagus. The radiologist should be able to diagnose gastroesophageal reflux in the majority of patients under the age of 2 years. The barium swallow should also exclude abnormalities in cricopharyngeal function or abnormalities in the oropharynx that may lead to aspiration. There is a definite correlation between severity of gastroesophageal reflux by barium esophagram and protracted pulmonary disease (Darling et al., 1978).

Gastroesophageal scintiscan: If a barium esophagram does not show evidence of reflux, the gastroesophageal scintiscan may be useful to demonstrate episodes of reflux into the esophagus in pediatric patients (Christie et al., 1978) (Fig. 27–6). This test consists of instilling water with a small amount of ^{99m}technetium sulfur colloid into the stomach. Reflux of material into

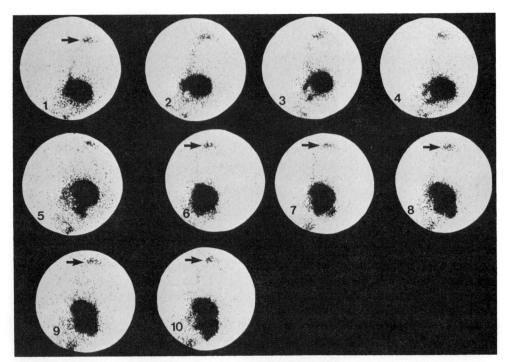

FIGURE 27–6.   Gastroesophageal scintiscan demonstrates reflux into oropharynx (arrows).

the esophagus is measured with a gamma camera. Patients can be scanned for at least 30 minutes after ingestion of the technetium sulfur colloid for esophageal reflux. A modification of this test, the gastropulmonary scan, may prove to be the definitive test to diagnose aspiration secondary to esophageal reflux (Reich et al., 1978). In this test, technetium sulfur colloid is placed in the stomach with a regular meal and the patient's lungs are scanned several hours after ingestion of the radioactive material. Radioactivity in the lung parenchyma is diagnostic of aspiration. Recent studies have demonstrated that 24 hour pH monitoring may also be useful in some patients with recurrent aspiration secondary to esophageal disease (Jolley et al., 1978) (Fig. 27–7).

The acid reflux test is the most sensitive means to diagnose gastroesophageal reflux and consists of instilling a 0.1 N HCl in the stomach and of placing a pH probe 5 cm above the lower esophageal sphincter (Christie and Mack, 1978). Pressure is applied to the abdomen or the patient performs certain maneuvers to increase ab-dominal pressure. A drop in pH to less than 4 in the body of the esophagus is diagnostic of gastroesophageal reflux. Esophageal manometrics with open-tipped tubes with side orifices measure esophageal peristalsis accurately. Motility data can easily be obtained of normal swallowing, relaxation of the upper and lower esophageal sphincters, and quantitation of lower esophageal sphincter pressure and peristaltic wave amplitude and duration.

Treatment

Treatment of pulmonary disease associated with esophageal dysfunction is medical. Surgery should not be considered unless the episodes of pneumonia or bronchospasm are life-threatening or when medical therapy has failed. Infants should be placed upright at night, should have thickened feedings and should receive antacids every 4 hours while awake. Older children should sleep with the head of their bed on 8 inch blocks. They should eat their evening meal at least four hours prior to bedtime. Antacids

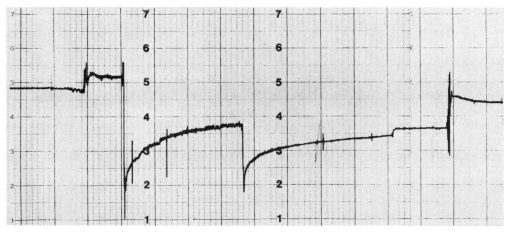

FIGURE 27–7. Twenty-four hour pH monitoring demonstrates reflux in an infant with a drop in pH to 3. (Each large square equals two minutes.)

may be useful in decreasing severity of esophagitis and in increasing gastric pH. Pharmacologic therapy has not been evaluated completely. Theophylline may increase symptoms by relaxing the esophageal sphincter and permitting further reflux. Atropine-like drugs induce similar adverse effects. The action of the H2 antihistamines has not yet been studied in children.

THE GASTROINTESTINAL TRACT

Physiology

Normal absorption and digestion of fats, carbohydrates, and proteins from the diet depend upon three stages of digestion: the intraluminal stage, the intestinal stage, and the removal stage. The intraluminal stage is characterized by secretion of pancreatic enzymes and bile salts into the lumen of the small intestine. Long-chain triglycerides are hydrolyzed by pancreatic enzymes and formed into water-soluble micelles. During the intestinal stage, disaccharides are digested at the surface of the small bowel mucosa. Subsequently, the byproducts of carbohydrate, fat, and protein are transported across the small bowel and removed to capillaries or lymphatics.

Normally, approximately 60 to 100 gm of fat are ingested daily in the adult diet, the majority being long-chain triglycerides. These long-chain triglycerides are insoluble in water and must be acted upon by pancreatic lipase to form free fatty acids, 2-monoglycerides, and free glycerol. The by-products of lipase action on triglycerides are formed into water-soluble micelles by the action of bile salts. Absorption of these lipolytic products from the micelles takes place in the duodenum and jejunum (Gray, 1978).

The main carbohydrate constituents in the diet in the adult are starch, sucrose, and lactose. Approximately 400 mg of carbohydrate is ingested daily, usually in the form of starch and sucrose. However, in infants the majority of carbohydrate may be from lactose. A quart of cow milk contains about 50 gm lactose. Starch is composed of two polysaccharides, amylose and amylopectin. Amylase from the pancreas will break the 1,4 bonds of amylose, yielding maltose and maltotriose. Hydrolysis of amylopectin yields alpha limit dextrins, maltose, and maltotriose. The alpha limit dextrins are further hydrolyzed by the action of isomaltase, an enzyme found at the brush border of the small bowel. Sucrose is digested by the action of sucrase to glucose and fructose. Finally, lactose is digested by lactase, yielding galactose and glucose. Deficiency in isomaltase, sucrase, or lactase in young infants can result in watery, acid diarrhea with dehydration and failure to thrive (Gray, 1975).

Protein digestion starts in the stomach by the activity of pepsin upon the peptide bonds of the aromatic L-amino acids. Pancreatic proteases are secreted into the duodenum in an inactivated form. Trypsinogen is activated into trypsin by enterokinase, an enzyme found in the brush border of the duodenal mucosa. Trypsin then stimulates inactive peptidases from the pancreas. These endopeptidases are capable of breaking peptide bonds to form free amino acids and peptides. The peptides and free amino acids are then transported across the intestinal mucosa.

The majority of absorption and digestion of food occurs in the upper part of the small intestine, which is approximately 280 cm long and 5 cm in diameter in an adult man. The small intestine is composed of serosa, muscularis, submucosa, and mucosa. The mucosal surface of the small bowel is lined with columnar epithelium. The surface of the absorptive cells is covered by a microvillous membrane, which comes into contact with luminal contents. This membrane facilitates absorption of nutrients and contains disaccharidases and peptidases for digestion of disaccharides and peptides. Outpouchings of mucosal epithelium, called villi, are present to increase the absorptive and digestive surfaces that are exposed to the intraluminal nutrients.

In the premature and term infant, digestive processes can be much different than later in life. Firstly, efficiency of fat absorption does not reach normal adult standards until over 6 months of age. Several factors seem to be involved. Lipase activity is low in the neonate, and bile acid concentrations present in the lumen of the small intestine are below the critical micellar concentration necessary for normal fat absorption. Carbohydrate digestion and absorption may also not be normal, as compared to the adult. Lactase activity does not fully develop until the end of gestation, so that lactose intolerance can occur in the first few days of life. Also, amylase activity is below normal in the full-term infant, and remains low during the first several months of life. Protein absorption is also unique, because the neonate can absorb whole protein through the small bowel mucosa. This function may be an important route of antigen absorption. The significance of macromolecular absorption in early infancy, as it relates to disease states, has yet to be determined.

Maldigestion is defined as a failure to absorb a dietary constituent because of abnormal or inadequate digestion. Malabsorption is defined as a failure to transport food by-products across the small bowel mucosa into the lymphatics or portal vein branches. Normal daily stool weight averages approximately 200 gm per day of which 80 percent is water. An increase in the weight of the stool can be defined as diarrhea. This increased stool weight can be secondary to increased water content as well as fat, electrolytes, or carbohydrates.

Diarrhea. There are four types of diarrhea: (1) osmotic diarrhea, (2) secretory diarrhea, (3) diarrhea secondary to abnormal intestinal motility, and (4) diarrhea caused by the absence of a normal active ion absorption process. Osmotic diarrhea is due to an accumulation of poorly absorbable products in the lumen of the small intestine. Usually osmotic diarrhea is caused by failure to transport a carbohydrate such as lactose. The osmotic pressure of the luminal contents within the small bowel results in a pressure gradient that causes water to be secreted into the lumen of the duodenum and jejunum. Osmotic diarrhea can be distinguished clinically because fasting stops the diarrhea. The osmolality of the diarrheal stool is generally greater than twice the concentration of the sodium and potassium found in the diarrheal stool (mEq Na + mEq K × 2). Reducing substances in osmotic diarrhea can be identified by placing a Clinitest tablet into an equal volume of liquid stool and water.

Secretory diarrhea is generally caused by small bowel disease. This diarrhea results from increased hydrostatic and tissue pressure resulting in passive secretion into the small intestine or from active secretion by small bowel mucosal cells. Secretory diarrheal stools are extremely large and will continue even after the patient has fasted. The osmolality of the stool in a secretory diarrhea is generally equal to twice the concentration of the sodium and potassium in the stool.

Diarrhea secondary to an abnormality in intestinal motility is predominantly seen in patients who have either an extremely rapid transit time or in patients who have stasis syndrome with bacterial overgrowth and secondary steatorrhea.

Also, diarrhea may result from failure to absorb ions normally because electrolytes are not transported actively across the small bowel mucosa (Phillips, 1972; Krejs and Fordtran, 1978).

Diagnostic Principles

History and physical examination are important in the diagnosis of chronic diarrhea caused by gastrointestinal allergy, as noted in Table 27–1. It is important to note when specific proteins have been introduced into the diet. Profuse diarrhea and vomiting can immediately follow cow or soy milk ingestion. It is useful to determine whether the diarrhea is made worse by certain carbohydrates, such as lactose or sucrose. The infant with cow milk protein sensitivity can have eczema or asthma. A sibling may have had similar symptoms in early infancy.

TABLE 27–1 APPROACH TO DIAGNOSIS OF GASTROINTESTINAL DISEASE ASSOCIATED WITH ALLERGY

Step 1: Obtain data base
"Allergic" symptoms
Compatible gastrointestinal symptoms
Exposure to milk protein, soy, gluten
Family history of allergy
Evidence of allergic disease — eosinophilia, elevated IgE, nasal eosinophils, bronchospasm
Step 2: Document abnormal gastrointestinal function
Serum D-xylose
Lactose tolerance
Serum carotene
Stool-reducing substances
Fecal leukocytes
72-hour stool fat
Serum albumin
Step 3: Confirm diagnosis
Observe response to allergen-free diet
Rechallenge when gastrointestinal tests are normal and observe:
Symptoms
Effects on GI functions
Effects on biopsy
Step 4: Treatment
Avoid protein in diet (soy and milk, until age 2; gluten, for life)
Systemic steroids for eosinophilic gastroenteritis if necessary

Physical examination in infants with significant chronic diarrhea will show decreased weight as compared to height and head circumference, which may be normal. The abdomen can be distended and tympanitic. Muscle wasting and pretibial edema are sometimes present.

After a thorough physical examination and history, the physician must try to answer two questions: (1) *What part of the gastrointestinal tract is responsible for the diarrhea?* (2) *What is the disease process?* Large-volume diarrhea without evidence of blood or fecal leukocytes usually means small bowel involvement. Frequent small bloody stools accompanied by tenesmus indicate large bowel disease. Whether the diarrhea is secretory or osmotic should be determined. The stools must then be evaluated for qualitative fat, fecal leukocytes, blood, reducing substances, and parasites. If evidence for upper gastrointestinal disease is present because of abnormal qualitative stool fat or positive reducing substances, specific tests to evaluate function of the small bowel, function of the pancreas, and liver must be done. These would include a one-hour serum xylose and tests for carotene, sweat chloride, alkaline phosphatase, bilirubin, and hepatocellular enzymes. A low carotene means fat malabsorption is present but does not locate the site. An abnormal xylose test is an indication for small bowel biopsy. The majority of infants and children with small bowel mucosal disease, whether caused by celiac sprue, cow milk protein, or soy protein, will have abnormal screening tests. The definitive diagnosis depends upon abnormal findings on mucosal biopsy, either of the small or large bowel, and response to withdrawal of the offending protein.

Specific Tests

Table 27–2 lists the laboratory tests useful in evaluation of allergic gastrointestinal disease.

Xylose Tolerance Tests. Several tolerance tests have been devised to assess small bowel mucosal function. The one-hour serum D-xylose test was originally conceived to evaluate small bowel mucosal

TABLE 27–2 LABORATORY TESTS USEFUL IN EVALUATION OF ALLERGIC
GASTROINTESTINAL DISEASE

	Normal	Meaning of Test
TOLERANCE TESTS		
Serum D-xylose (5 gm orally)	> 20 mg/dl at 1 hour	Abnormal in severe small bowel mucosal disease
Lactose tolerance test (2 gm/kg)	No diarrhea, abdominal distention, cramps following challenge; rise in blood glucose of > 20 mg/dl	Abnormal response in patients with deficiency of lactase enzyme in small bowel mucosa
Sucrose tolerance test (2 gm/kg)	Same as lactose tolerance test. Rise in blood glucose of > 40 mg/dl	Abnormal response in patients with deficiency of sucrase-isomaltase enzyme in small bowel mucosa
SERUM TESTS		
Carotene (must be on carotene diet, green, yellow vegetables)	> 100 µg/dl	Low in any disease where fat malabsorption is present, especially in small bowel mucosal disease
Albumin	> 3.2 gm	Low in diseases causing protein loss in gastrointestinal tract
Red blood cell folate	< 60 ng/ml	Decrease in small bowel mucosal disease
STOOL TESTS		
Fecal leukocytes	No leukocytes by methylene blue stain	Increased in inflammatory diseases of intestine, primarily colon
Reducing substances	0 to trace reducing substance in stool	Indicates malabsorption of carbohydrate
72-hour fecal fat	> 3.5 gm fat/day (coefficient fat absorption: > 95% over 6 months; > 90% 0 to 6 months)	Quantitates fat malabsorption
24-hour stool weight	< 200 gm	Formed stool > 400 gm usually means steatorrhea. Stool < 100 gm — steatorrhea unlikely

disease in infants and children with celiac sprue. Xylose is a five-carbon monosaccharide that is absorbed across the small bowel mucosa. The xylose absorption test is used to differentiate small bowel mucosal disease from intraluminal causes of steatorrhea. Abnormal renal function and ascites invalidate the urinary test. Vomiting and delayed gastric emptying of xylose also can cause abnormally low blood and urinary concentrations. The one-hour serum xylose test is performed by giving infants and children who weigh less than 30 kg, 5 gm of D-xylose after an overnight fast. The xylose levels are obtained prior to the xylose challenge and one hour later. Serum xylose levels of less than 20 mg/dl are abnormal. The one-hour serum xylose level will be less than 20 mg/dl in the majority of patients with severe small bowel mucosal disease, whether it is caused by celiac sprue, cow milk protein, or soy protein sensitivity. However, it may be normal in patients with mild to moderate villous abnormalities of the small bowel mucosa (Christie, 1978).

Lactose Tolerance Test. The lactose tolerance test is a screening test for lactase deficiency in the small intestine. The infant is fasted overnight and given 2 gm/kg of lactose in a 10 percent solution. Blood glucose levels are measured every 15 minutes for an hour. All stools passed within 24 hours after the lactose challenge are analyzed for the presence of reducing substances. Reducing substances are evaluated by obtaining 10 drops of liquid stool. To this is added 20 drops of water and a Clinitest tablet. Any more than a trace of reducing substance is abnormal. Blood levels should rise to greater than 20 mg/dl over fasting levels. Patients with small bowel mucosal disease can have secondary disaccharidase deficiency and, therefore, an abnormal lactose tolerance test. The test will also be abnormal in patients with primary lactase deficiency. It is important to make sure that a patient with suspected cow milk protein sensitivity has a normal lactose tolerance test prior to challenge with a cow milk protein formula that contains lactose.

Sucrose Tolerance Test. The sucrose tolerance test is performed by giving the infant or child 2 gm/kg of sucrose in a 10 percent solution after an overnight fast. Serum levels of glucose are obtained at 15-minute intervals for one hour. A rise greater than 40 mg/dl in the serum is considered normal for the sucrose tolerance test. Liquid stools are again collected for analysis of sucrose. However, if sucrase deficiency is suspected, the stool must first be hydrolyzed with dilute hydrochloric acid before the Clinitest tablet is added. Patients with the rare sucrase-isomaltase deficiency will have an abnormal sucrose tolerance test, and some patients with small bowel mucosal disease from other causes may also have an abnormal result.

A sucrose or lactose tolerance test is not considered to have an abnormal result unless the patient has clinical symptoms after the challenge. Most infants with disaccharidase enzyme deficiency will have diarrhea, cramping, abdominal pain, and abdominal distention immediately following the challenge. Some patients receiving lactose will not show normal rises in blood glucose levels after the oral dose is given (Paige et al., 1978). However, unless clinical symptoms are present, these patients should not be considered as being lactase deficient.

Fat Absorption Test. Only two fat absorption tests are used widely in pediatric practice in the United States. Serum carotene is used as a screening test for fat malabsorption in patients who are eating a diet containing adequate amounts of vegetables.

Carotene is a precursor of vitamin A and its absorption depends upon normal fat transport across the small bowel mucosa. Normal plasma carotene levels are greater than 100 μg/dl. Levels between 50 to 100 μg/dl are borderline; levels less than 50 μg/dl are considered to be unequivocally abnormal. Serum carotene will be low in pancreatic insufficiency, in small bowel mucosal disease, and when impaired intraluminal micelle formation is present. A 72-hour quantitative fecal fat measurement is useful to document the presence of steatorrhea. Infants and children must have an adequate fat-containing diet before the test is contemplated. Normally, there is less than 3.5 gm of stool fat per 24 hours.

Stool Fecal Leukocyte Test. Obtaining a stool smear for fecal leukocytes is useful in patients with inflammatory bowel disease involving the colon predominantly. In infants with a diagnosis of cow or soy milk protein colitis, a methylene blue stain for fecal leukocytes should be obtained prior to proctosigmoidoscopic examination or rectal biopsy. Fecal leukocytes are not seen in patients with small bowel mucosal disease unless acute inflammation is present, as can be seen in a small percentage of infants with acute viral enteritis.

When blood and fecal leukocytes are present in the stools, proctosigmoidoscopic examination is performed to evaluate the possibility of colitis. The absence of ramifying blood vessels and the presence of friability are indications of inflammation.

Biopsy. Small bowel biopsy is performed by passing a multipurpose biopsy capsule to the ligament of Trietz. Two specimens are obtained for analysis. For proper interpretation, the biopsy must be oriented and mounted properly. Only the central core of the specimen should be evaluated (Perera et al., 1975). If done properly, a small bowel biopsy can give specific diagnosis such as lymphangiectasia, eosinophilic gastroenteritis, giardia, or immunodeficiency. A flat small bowel biopsy usually indicates sprue or, less commonly, severe cow or soy milk protein sensitivity.

The use of small bowel biopsy is indicated in any infant with significant diarrhea and failure to thrive, even when screening tests are equivocal. This is especially true in patients found to have an isolated deficiency of a specific nutrient such as folate, vitamin B$_{12}$, calcium, or iron.

Rectal biopsy should be performed to look for granulomas, crypt abscesses, and ganglion cells.

X-Ray Examination. Upper gastrointestinal and small bowel follow-through radiographs are less useful in evaluation of chronic diarrhea in young infants than in older children. Small bowel mucosal detail is difficult to interpret. However, the findings of thickened folds in the duodenum, jejunum, or ileum are an indication for small bowel biopsy. When the possibility of a structural abnormality, such as malrotation with volvulus, exists, radiographs are indicated.

A barium enema should be done only when there is no evidence of acute inflammation in the colon and at least one week after rectal biopsy. The barium enema is less useful in allergic gastrointestinal disease, except in the rare patient with soy or milk protein colitis or in the ileocolitis seen in patients with eosinophilic gastroenteritis.

Food Challenges. Food challenges are useful in identifying foods to which the patient is specifically allergic. However, since anaphylaxis can occur in some patients, such food challenge should not be performed unless emergency equipment is on hand (see Chapter 52 on anaphylaxis). Food challenge is best avoided if there is a likelihood of anaphylaxis. Biopsies of the organ suspected to be involved (stomach, small bowel, colon) should be done before and after challenge.

Other Tests of Intestinal Function. Other tests that can be useful in selected patients with allergic disease of the gastrointestinal tract are a prothrombin time, a serum albumin, and a serum folate. Prothrombin time is prolonged in patients with vitamin K malabsorption, which can be secondary to small bowel mucosal disease or abnormal micelle formation in the small bowel mucosa. The serum folate level may be abnormal when the upper small intestine is damaged. It will be normal in pancreatic insufficiency or when micelle formation is abnormal. After performing screening tests of gastrointestinal function, challenge with the offending protein is required for definitive diagnosis.

Principles of Care

After the specific diagnosis of a gastrointestinal disease has been made, appropriate therapy should be initiated. An infant with definite cow or soy milk protein sensitivity should avoid this protein until approximately 2 years of age. All labels on any food must be read before allowing the infant to eat it. Any foods containing casein, lactalbumin, whey, or cow milk protein must be avoided. Soy protein is commonly found in baby junior foods and cereals, and all labels again must be scrutinized (see Tables 27-3 and 27-4). The child diagnosed as having celiac sprue must be on a gluten-free diet for life.

A patient found to have eosinophilic gastroenteritis can first be treated by diet elimination if there is a reasonable history of a specific food precipitating gastrointestinal symptoms. As a general rule, elimination diets are not consistently useful in stopping symptoms in patients with eosinophilic gastroenteritis. The standard therapy for eosinophilic gastroenteritis is a trial of low-dose corticosteroids. Generally, 1 mg per kg of body weight per day, or not more than 20 mg per day, is indicated. Sometimes patients who can be managed on alternate-

TABLE 27-3 COW MILK PROTEIN–FREE DIET

Allowed	Avoid
Soy milk formulas	Cow milk formulas
Isomil	Fresh milk
Soyalac, i-Soyalac	Cream
ProSobee	Canned milk
Neo-Mull-Soy	Cheese
	Casein
Special formulas	Lactalbumin
Pregestimil	Cured whey
Portagen	Malted milk
Nutramigen	Butter
Meat base	Margarine
Vivonex	Milk-based pudding
	Flour mixtures
	Lunch meats
	Commerical meat patties
	Hamburgers
	Sweets
	Creamed foods
	Gravies

TABLE 27–4 SOY BEAN PROTEIN–DIET

Allowed	Avoid
Cow milk protein formulas	Soy milk formulas
Enfamil	Soy flour
SMA	Textured vegetable protein
Similac	Soy sauce
Low Birth Weight Similac	Coffee substitutes
Advance	Soya ice cream products
	Meat extenders
Special formulas	Worcestershire sauce
Pregestimil	Hollywood bread
Portagen	
Nutramigen	
Vivonex	
Meat base	

day low-dose therapy will become asymptomatic in a period of weeks to months.

Patients found to have specific nutrient deficiencies, such as folate, vitamin B_{12}, or iron, should be treated with appropriate doses of these substances. As a rule, once the nutritional deficiency has been reversed, further therapy on a long-term basis will not be indicated.

On rare occasions, an infant may be intolerant to both cow and soy milk protein as well as special hydrolyzed protein formulas. In this case, long-term breast milk therapy or an elemental diet, such as Vivonex, is indicated. The elemental diet contains

TABLE 27–5 GASTROINTESTINAL DISEASES ASSOCIATED WITH ALLERGY

Cow Milk Protein Sensitivity
  Eosinophilic gastroenteritis of infancy
  Nonspecific small bowel mucosal disease
    Acute onset
    Delayed onset
  Intractable diarrhea syndrome of early infancy
  Nonspecific colitis
  Iron deficiency anemia associated with gastrointestinal blood loss
  Enterocolitis in low-birth-weight infants
Soy Protein Sensitivity
  Nonspecific small bowel mucosal disease
  Nonspecific colitis
Eosinophilic Gastroenteritis
  Stomach and small bowel
    Allergic
    Nonallergic
  Colon
  Esophagus
Celiac Sprue

only free amino acids and glucose polymers and contains a small amount of linoleic acid to eliminate the possibility of essential fatty acid deficiency. Elemental diets should be reserved for the patient who has definitely demonstrated intolerance to other standard and specialized formulas and where human breast milk cannot be supplied on a long-term basis.

Oral sodium cromoglycate has been advocated as a form of therapy for patients who have adverse reactions to specific foods (Vaz et al., 1978). No data are available as to long-term use of this drug for food sensitivity. Controlled double-blind studies comparing cromoglycate with placebo are necessary before routine use can be advocated.

GASTROINTESTINAL DISEASE SYNDROMES ASSOCIATED WITH (OR CONFUSED WITH) ALLERGY

Cow Milk Protein Sensitivity

Allergy to cow milk protein continues to cause debate among physicians as to its existence, diagnosis, and treatment. Every conceivable gastrointestinal symptom including diarrhea, vomiting, colic, constipation, bloody stools, flatus, abdominal pain, and regurgitation has been attributed to cow milk allergy. Other symptoms such as wheezing, rhinorrhea, and eczema also are commonly associated (Buissert, 1978). Estimates as to frequency in pediatric patients vary from 0.3 to 7.5 percent (Collins-Williams, 1962).

Several specific allergic syndromes caused by cow milk protein sensitivity have been described (see Table 27–5).

The most common type of cow milk protein sensitivity presents in the first 6 to 8 months of life. Symptoms include chronic diarrhea, failure to thrive, recurrent vomiting, and an increased incidence of atopic dermatitis, rhinitis and "asthma-like" symptoms. Anaphylaxis has been reported. Two types of clinical presentations are evident. The acute onset disease is seen in the first weeks of life and is characterized by frequent watery stools, systemic symptoms of fever, and abdominal distention. Differentiation from acute viral enteritis is difficult. Profound metabolic acidosis and shock secondary to massive fluid loss may occur.

The delayed onset disease takes several weeks to months before symptoms are apparent. These infants have failure to thrive, wasted buttocks, abdominal distention, and large, bulky stools. The disease can be confused easily with celiac sprue if gluten already has been introduced into the diet. Small bowel biopsy in the two types of cow milk protein sensitivity shows mild to severe mucosal damage. The lesion is nonspecific; plasma cells and lymphocytes are present in the lamina propria, and the villi are generally moderately abnormal, showing blunting and increased branching. A flat small bowel biopsy cannot be differentiated from the nonspecific flat lesion seen in celiac sprue. Clinical response to a gluten-containing, cow milk–protein-free diet would be necessary when the small bowel biopsy is completely flat in order to differentiate between the two diseases.

Intractable diarrhea of early infancy is a term used to describe a condition characterized by chronic diarrhea for longer than 2 weeks, resulting in significant weight loss. These infants often have diarrhea even when not eating, and some are unable to tolerate even simple monosaccharides. Biopsies of the small intestine generally show severe mucosal damage. The differential diagnosis includes infectious, metabolic, and anatomic causes (Branski, 1978). Evidence exists that intractable diarrhea of early infancy can be caused by cow milk protein sensitivity. It is likely that the acute onset cow milk protein sensitivity described above is the one that can lead to intractable diarrhea if not recognized early in the patient's clinical course.

Cow milk protein sensitivity colitis has been described (Gryboski et al., 1966). Affected infants have bloody diarrhea beginning in early infancy, usually before 5 months of age. Fecal leukocytes are present, and proctosigmoidoscopic examination shows induced and spontaneous friability. Rectal biopsies show acute inflammation in the lamina propria, crypt abscesses, and mucus depletion. Differential diagnosis for this entity includes Hirschsprung's disease with enterocolitis and infectious etiologies such as the shigella and salmonella diarrheas.

In 1964 Wilson, Heiner, and Lahey identified three infants with iron deficiency anemia and gastrointestinal *blood loss secondary to whole cow milk protein ingestion* (Wilson et al., 1964). Since their original description, they have reported another 17 infants with similar findings (Wilson et al., 1974). These patients have occult gastrointestinal blood loss while on whole cow milk. Anemia persists in spite of iron therapy. A significant percentage also demonstrate low total serum protein, presumably from gastrointestinal loss. Diagnosis depends upon the demonstration of gastrointestinal bleeding while on whole cow milk protein, cessation of blood loss with whole cow milk protein removal, and return of bleeding with reintroduction.

Enterocolitis in low-birth-weight infants secondary to cow milk protein and soy protein has been reported (Powell, 1976). The two infants had severe abdominal distention, bloody diarrhea, vomiting, and a "sepsis-like" picture following ingestion of cow milk and soy protein. Radiographs demonstrated intramural gas in the intestine. Both infants had a recurrence of symptoms at ages 7 and 8 months.

The diagnosis of cow milk protein sensitivity as it affects the gastrointestinal tract is controversial because of a lack of standardized criteria. Goldman set forth the following as necessary before the diagnosis of cow milk sensitivity could be made: (1) symptoms subside after milk withdrawal; (2) symptoms recur in 48 hours following milk introduction; (3) three challenges should be positive and should be similar as to onset, duration, and clinical features; and (4) symptoms disappear after each challenge is discontinued (Goldman et al., 1963). Recent investigators, however, have demonstrated abnormal small bowel mucosal biopsies within 24 hours of cow milk protein challenge in asymptomatic infants (Iyngkaran et al., 1978); and others have described symptoms occurring several days to weeks after introduction of cow milk (Kuitunen et al., 1975). Until further studies resolve the questions as to diagnosis and etiology, small and/or large bowel biopsy in infants suspected to have cow milk protein sensitivity is warranted. Diagnosis should be based upon (1) changes in postchallenge small bowel or colonic biopsy compared to prechallenge biopsy and (2) clinical symptoms when cow milk protein is introduced. Infants found to have abnormal biopsies after cow milk protein challenge but who are asymptomatic should continue on cow milk formula and be followed to see if symptoms occur.

Soy Protein Sensitivity

Soy protein also has the potential for causing gastrointestinal disease. Severe reactions to soy protein have been documented, and both small bowel and colonic involvement can occur (Ament and Rubin, 1972; Halpin et al., 1977). Some infants react to cow milk protein as well.

Clinical symptoms are similar to those of the acute and delayed-onset cow milk protein sensitivity diseases. Diagnosis depends upon (1) clinical symptoms following soy protein challenge and (2) small or large bowel biopsy after soy protein challenge.

Eosinophilic Gastroenteritis

Eosinophilic gastroenteritis is a disease characterized by infiltration of eosinophils into the mucosa and muscle layers of the stomach and duodenum. Clinical characteristics depend upon the layer of intestine involved. Klein and colleagues proposed that the disease be divided into three categories: (1) primary mucosal disease with malabsorption and protein loss; (2) primary muscle layer disease with recurrent obstructive symptoms, usually gastric outlet obstructions; and (3) primary serosal disease with eosinophilic ascites (Klein et al., 1970).

The mucosal form of the disease seems to be caused by food allergy. As mentioned previously, cow milk protein has been incriminated in this syndrome. Waldman et al. (1967) described a group of infants and children with edema, growth retardation, hypoalbuminemia, hypogammaglobulinemia, peripheral eosinophilia, and anemia. The majority also had other manifestations of allergy such as asthma, eczema, and allergic rhinitis. Small bowel biopsies demonstrated eosinophilic infiltration.

Caldwell et al. (1975) demonstrated gastrointestinal symptoms of epigastric pain, cramps, and diarrhea following ingestion of raw egg white in a patient with eosinophilic gastroenteritis. A rapid rise in serum IgE levels also was documented. Katz and colleagues (1977) described six children with systemic allergic symptoms of asthma, rhinitis, or urticaria. Four had growth retardation; only two had chronic diarrhea. Clinically, all children had peripheral eosinophilia, iron deficiency anemia, gastrointestinal blood loss, hypoalbuminemia, hypogammaglobulinemia, and elevated serum IgE levels. Gastric biopsies in all six children showed eosinophilic infiltration, necrosis, and regeneration of surface and glandular epithelium. Small bowel biopsies also were abnormal. Finally, Caldwell and colleagues (1978a) have further defined the allergic basis for the mucosal type of eosinophilic gastroenteritis. They demonstrated a marked rise in serum IgE in a child following wheat ingestion, with an abnormal number of jejunal IgE-producing plasma cells. This child also demonstrated allergy to fish, egg, and peanuts and had suffered from growth retardation, iron deficiency, and protein-losing enteropathy. Though the evidence supports an allergic basis for the mucosal form of eosinophilic gastroenteritis in most patients, not all patients improve on avoidance of the allergen and, in some, no allergic factors are evident.

Diagnosis of the mucosal eosinophilic gastroenteritis can be made by biopsy of gastric or small bowel mucosa. The mucosal abnormality in the small bowel can be patchy and variable so that multiple biopsies may be necessary. Katz et al. (1977) advocate using gastric biopsies for diagnosis. The mucosal form of eosinophilic gastroenteritis should be suspected when an atopic child shows marked growth retardation or diarrhea. Laboratory findings in this disease include low serum albumin and gammaglobulins, as well as iron deficiency anemia. Protein loss in the gastrointestinal tract can be demonstrated by chromium-labeled albumin studies.

When eosinophilic gastroenteritis involves primarily the muscle layers of the stomach or small intestine, recurrent obstruction is common. These patients show epigastric pain, postprandial vomiting, and weight loss. Upper gastrointestinal radiographs show gastric outlet or small bowel obstruction. Surgical specimens demonstrate infiltration of submucosal and muscle layers with eosinophils. Both serosal and mucosal involvement can be present. Patients with primarily muscle layer involvement do not have allergic manifestations. Recent investigators have demonstrated normal serum immunoglobulin, serum complement, and serum IgE in seven patients with eosinophilic gastroenteritis and obstruction (Caldwell et al., 1978*b*). None had clinical allergy or food hypersensitivity.

The serosal form of eosinophilic gastroenteritis is most rare. Patients present with ascites, as well as symptoms related to mucosal or muscle layer involvement. Ascitic fluid from these patients contains many eosinophils.

Two recent variants of eosinophilic gastroenteritis syndrome have been reported. Haberkorn et al. (1978) described a patient with ileocolitis found to have eosinophilic gastroenteritis. The original diagnosis had been ileocolonic Crohn's disease, but subsequent biopsies and radiographs demonstrated involvement in proximal small bowel and stomach.

Dobbins and colleagues (1977) described a patient with dysphagia, heartburn, and pain with swallowing who had a life-long history of asthma and allergic rhinitis. He was found to have eosinophilic infiltration in the squamous epithelium of the esophagus as well as his small intestine. Landres et al. (1978) reported another case of dysphagia secondary to eosinophilic gastroenteritis. Biopsies in this patient showed predominant infiltration into muscle layers of the esophagus.

Eosinophilic esophagitis must be suspected in patients with allergic respiratory disease who have associated dysphagia. Esophageal motility studies can demonstrate abnormal motor function. Systemic steroid therapy may be useful in ameliorating symptoms.

Celiac Sprue

Celiac sprue usually presents between 12 and 24 months of age. However, because of the early introduction of gluten-containing cereals in the first weeks of life, the disease is now being diagnosed in early infancy. Infants with celiac sprue are underweight for age and have a history of chronic diarrhea, anorexia, and vomiting. The stools are large, bulky, and malodorous. Physical examination reveals an infant with abdominal distention and marked wasting of musculature.

A variety of abnormalities occur which are related to malabsorption of vitamins and protein and include hypoalbuminemia, hypocalcemia, a prolonged prothrombin time, hypo-

magnesemia, and low serum carotene. Steatorrhea is documented by a 72-hour collection for fecal fat.

The diagnosis of celiac sprue is made by (1) small bowel biopsy revealing a nonspecific flat lesion and (2) response to a gluten-free diet. Because treatment consists of a life-long gluten-free diet, a small bowel biopsy is essential to the diagnosis.

The differential diagnosis for celiac sprue consists of any disease causing malabsorption with failure to thrive in early infancy. These include giardiasis, lymphangiectasia, cystic fibrosis, and cow milk protein and soy protein sensitivity. Infants found to have a flat small bowel biopsy when cow milk protein sensitivity is considered will need rechallenge with gluten and another small bowel biopsy at a later date to exclude celiac sprue.

OTHER GASTROINTESTINAL PROBLEMS

Nonspecific Diarrhea Syndrome (Irritable Colon Syndrome)

A common gastrointestinal problem in pediatrics is the infant or young child who has intermittent diarrhea lasting for several weeks to months but who continues to grow normally in spite of the diarrhea. The diarrhea is usually episodic in nature but can be continuous for prolonged periods of time (Davidson and Wasserman, 1966). These infants pass three to ten semisolid to water stools daily. The first stool in the morning tends to be of normal consistency. Subsequent stools usually are liquid and contain mucus; undigested vegetable fibers such as carrots or peas may be passed in the stools. The patients grow normally, without a fall-off in height and weight, even though the diarrhea may last for several months. They have no clinical evidence of malabsorption syndrome (Burke and Anderson, 1975).

Family history can be useful because adult family members give a history of functional bowel disease, generally constipation, diarrhea, or abdominal pain, with some frequency (Jorup, 1952). The infant may have had colic or constipation in the first several months of life.

Diagnosis of nonspecific diarrhea of early

infancy must take into account the fact that certain gastrointestinal illnesses can cause a similar clinical picture, such as post-gastroenteritis syndrome and *Giardia lamblia* infection. Post-gastroenteritis syndrome occurs after a nonspecific illness, usually viral. Recent evidence supports the concept that human rotavirus (HRV) is a common cause of gastroenteritis under 5 years of age. This virus always invades the small intestinal mucosa, causing a small intestinal lesion with secondary disaccharidase deficiency (Schreiber et al., 1977). Infants who have continued diarrhea after viral infection have a combination of malabsorption and maldigestion secondary to damage to the small bowel mucosa. For some reason, the damage caused by the viral illness is slow to resolve, and secondary disaccharidase deficiency may persist for several weeks. In *Giardia lamblia* infection, patients can have abdominal pain, lactose intolerance, intermittent diarrhea, and increased flatus — all secondary to the infestation. These patients do not always show frank malabsorption, although they can demonstrate a picture compatible with celiac sprue (Raizman, 1976).

In some infants thought to have nonspecific diarrhea syndrome, protein sensitivity may be the cause of the intermittent diarrhea. Certainly, infants with cow milk protein or soy protein sensitivity may present a similar clinical picture; these infants will generally, however, demonstrate abnormalities by tolerance tests such as xylose, lactose, and sucrose oral carbohydrate challenges. Fall-off in weight also is commonly seen in these latter entities; there also may be a history of atopic disease in the patient, and peripheral eosinophilia may be present.

Thus, the diagnosis of a nonspecific diarrhea syndrome is made by exclusion of specific disease entities. Several stool specimens should be obtained and tested for reducing substances and fecal leukocytes. If stool cultures are negative for bacterial pathogens and no reducing substances or fecal leukocytes are present in the stools, one has evidence against small bowel and large bowel disease. However, with suspicion that a secondary disaccharidase intolerance may be present, both lactose and sucrose tolerance tests must be done to exclude these possibilities. The integrity of the small bowel mucosa can be evaluated by a one-hour serum xylose examination. A normal serum carotene level is evidence against significant fat malabsorption. If all screening tests are normal and the patient demonstrates an ability to gain weight over a period of weeks, then the physician can be confident that significant bowel disease does not exist. An associated positive family history or early infancy constipation or colic are also helpful clues to the diagnosis of nonspecific diarrhea syndrome. In selected cases, however, small bowel and rectal biopsies may be necessary to completely exclude any abnormality in the intestine.

The etiology of chronic nonspecific diarrhea is not known. Some authors believe that it is a variant of irritable bowel syndrome seen in adults. These children may develop recurrent episodes of abdominal pain associated with diarrhea later in childhood. The attacks of abdominal pain and loose stools may coincide with illness or stressful environmental situations (Almy, 1978). Almy believes that colic in the neonate may be the first clinical manifestation in infants and children who will develop chronic, nonspecific diarrhea. Colic in these children is secondary to excessive air swallowing with abnormal peristalsis in the rectum. Constipation in early infancy is the next clinical syndrome, perhaps associated with nonspecific diarrhea in later life. Passage of small, hard, dry, pellet-like stools for several months is common, regardless of change in formula or diet. Almy identifies the older patient after age 4 who develops abdominal pain at times associated with intermittent diarrhea. No unifying hypothesis is available to explain the variations seen in the syndrome, and it may be that, with increased diagnostic techniques, fewer cases will be classified as this "nonspecific diarrhea."

Treatment of nonspecific diarrhea syndrome is difficult because of failure to understand the underlying physiology. Certainly, dietary treatment is unnecessary and has been demonstrated not to be useful. Patients thus should be maintained on a normal diet appropriate for their age. Antispasmodics have not been consistently useful in this entity, and certainly drugs such as Lomotil or Imodium are not indicated. Some authors advocate bulk-forming agents such as psyllium seed (Metamucil or Konsyl) or bismuth-containing agents (Pepto-Bismol). However, there are no controlled studies to substantiate the efficacy of these agents. Other investigators have advocated the use of broad-spectrum antibiotics, though they are not often effective (Davidson and Wasserman, 1966).

Chronic Recurrent Abdominal Pain of Childhood

Chronic recurrent abdominal pain of childhood is a common entity occurring during the school years, particularly during the ages 5 to 10. It must be differentiated from specific gastrointestinal diseases that cause a similar pattern. In approximately two-thirds of the cases the child will complain of pain located in the periumbilical area of the abdomen. Less often, it will be localized to the epigastric area. The pain may recur intermittently from weeks to months, only to disappear completely. The pain can be either cramping in nature, a dull ache, or can be sharp and specifically localized. The severity of the pain is difficult to assess because, at times, it will interfere with school and play, but in other situations will be hardly noticeable. The attacks of pain occur at any time during the day or prior to bedtime; only rarely will it awaken the child from sleep. There does not seem to be any association with ingestion of specific foods or activities. There often are accompanying symptoms such as dizziness, headaches, numbness, and leg aches (Liebman and Thaler, 1978). There are no other associated gastrointestinal symptoms, however.

In evaluating the patient with chronic recurrent abdominal pain, organic causes must be excluded first. Pain that is associated with objective gastrointestinal signs is not functional. Specifically, patients with recurrent vomiting, hematemesis, melena, weight loss, or bloody diarrhea should not be considered as having functional abdominal pain. If the pain is located in the upper quadrants of the abdomen or lateralizes to the flank areas, further diagnostic studies are need to exclude organic disease. Other associated symptoms that will point to organic disease are "heartburn," regurgitation, a history of jaundice, dysuria, urgency, frequency, hematuria, seizure disorder, or chronic diarrhea.

The physical examination in recurrent abdominal pain of childhood will be within normal limits. There is no evidence of allergic disease by physical examination. Rectal examination is generally unremarkable, although some investigators have described hard, small stools in the rectal ampulla (Stone, 1970). If the pain pattern is typical of recurrent abdominal pain of childhood and the physical examination is completely normal, only a few screening tests will be necessary to exclude other diseases. A complete blood count, sedimentation rate, urinalysis, and stool examination for occult blood and fecal leukocytes are the most useful screening tests in the majority of patients. However, if other associated symptoms and signs are present, then liver function tests, urine amylase, and radiographic studies of the gastrointestinal tract are indicated. If radiographic studies are needed, a small bowel series should be included in the evaluation of the upper gastrointestinal tract so that patients with inflammatory bowel disease in the distal ileum may be diagnosed early. Intravenous pyelogram usually is not necessary except when there is evidence of an abnormality in urinalysis or where the pain is lateralized. Proctoscopic examination can be useful and must be employed if there is evidence of blood or fecal leukocytes on serial stool examination. Recurrent vomiting, hematemesis, or evidence of tenderness or guarding in the epigastric area are indications for upper gastrointestinal radiograph and, in selected patients, fiberoptic endoscopy (Ament, 1977).

The most frequent causes of recurrent organic abdominal pain are diseases involving the urinary tract and include hydronephrosis and urinary tract infection. Diseases involving the upper gastrointestinal system, including peptic ulcer, are the second most common disease entities involved. The majority of patients with peptic ulcer, however, will have a history of recurrent vomiting or will have some localizations of the pain to the upper abdomen. Often there will be a family history of peptic ulcer disease.

The etiology of recurrent abdominal pain in childhood is not understood. Causes have been attributed to food allergy, constipation, abdominal migraine, irritable colon, and neurological factors. However, no unifying hypothesis is available to explain all possible entities. Family history is generally negative for definitive gastrointestinal diseases although some investigators have described gastrointestinal symptoms and headaches as being present in a significant percentage of parents (Apley, 1975).

Treatment consists of excluding other diseases and reassuring the parents and child that significant illness is not present. Counseling can be useful in selected situations. Long-term use of analgesics should be avoided. A regular diet is prescribed, since there is no evidence that diet restriction is helpful. Neither antispasmodics nor antacids are effective.

References

GASTROINTESTINAL DISEASES ASSOCIATED WITH ALLERGY

Almy, T. P.: Irritable bowel syndrome. *In* Sleisenger, M. H., and Fordtran, J. S. (eds.): *Gastrointestinal Disease: Pathophysiology, Diagnosis, Management.* Philadelphia, W. B. Saunders, 1978, p. 1587.

Ament, M. E., and Rubin, C. E.: Soy protein — another cause of the flat intestinal lesion. Gastroenterology *62*:227, 1972.

Ament, M. E., and Christie, D. L.: Upper gastrointestinal fiberoptic endoscopy in pediatric patients. Gastroenterology *72*:1244, 1977.

Anderson, H. A., Holman, C. B., and Olsen, A. M.: Pulmonary complications of cardiospasm. JAMA *151*:608, 1953.

Apley, J.: *The Child with Abdominal Pain,* Blackwell Scientific Publications, Oxford, 1975.

Branski, D.: Intractable diarrhea of infancy. *In* Lebenthal, E. (ed.): *Digestive Diseases in Children.* Grune & Stratton, New York, 1978, p. 351.

Buisseret, P. D.: Common manifestations of cow's milk allergy in children. Lancet *1*:304, 1978.

Burke, V., and Anderson, C. M.: The irritable colon syndrome. From "Other Disorders of the Large Intestine," *Paediatric Gastroenterology.* Oxford, Blackwell Scientific Publications, 1975, p. 469.

Byrne, W. J., Euler, A. R. and Strobel, C. T.: Recurrent pulmonary disease in children: A complication of gastroesophageal reflux. Gastroenterology *74*:1016A, 1978.

Caldwell, J. H., Tennebaum, J. I., and Bronstein, H. A.: Serum IgE in eosinophilic gastroenteritis. Response to intestinal challenge in two cases. New Engl. J. Med. *292*:1388, 1975.

Caldwell, J. H., Sharma, H. M., and Hurtubise, P. E.: Eosinophilic gastroenteritis and extreme allergy: Immunopathological comparison with nonallergic gastrointestinal disease. Gastroenterology *74*:1016, 1978*a.*

Caldwell, J. H., Mekhjian, H. S., Hurtubise, P. E., et al.: Eosinophilic gastroenteritis with obstruction: Immunological studies of seven patients. Gastroenterology *74*:825, 1978*b.*

Carre, I. J.: Pulmonary infections in children with a partial thoracic stomach ("hiatus hernia"). Arch. Dis. Child. *35*:481, 1960.

Christie, D. L.: Use of the one-hour blood xylose test as an indicator of small bowel mucosal disease. J. Pediatr. *92*:725, 1978.

Christie, D. L. and Mack, D. V.: Evaluation of the pH probe test for gastroesophageal reflux in pediatric patients. Clinical Research *26*(2):173A, 1978.

Christie, D. L., and Rudd, I. G.: Radionuclide test for gastroesophageal reflux (GER) in children. Pediatr. Research *12*(409A):432, 1978.

Christie, D. L., O'Grady, L. R., and Mack, D. V.: Incompetent lower esophageal sphincter and gastroesophageal reflux in recurrent acute pulmonary disease of infancy and childhood. J. Pediatr. *93*:23, 1978.

Collins-Williams, C.: Cow's milk allergy in infants and children. Int. Arch. Allergy *20*:38, 1962.

Danus, O., Casar, C., Lanain, A., et al.: Esophageal reflux — an unrecognized cause of recurrent obstructive bronchitis in children. J. Pediatr. *89*:220, 1976.

Darling, D. B., McCauley, R. G. K., and Leonidas, J. C.: Gastroesophageal reflux in infants and children: Correlation of radiological severity and pulmonary pathology. Radiology *12*(7):735, 1978.

Davidson, M., and Wasserman, R.: The irritable colon of childhood: Chronic nonspecific diarrhea syndrome. J. Pediatr. *69*:1027, 1966.

Dobbins, J. W., Sheahan, D. J., and Behar, J.: Eosinophilic gastroenteritis with esophageal involvement. Gastroenterology *72*:1312, 1977.

Goldman, A. S., Anderson, D. W., Jr., Sellers, W. A., et al.: Milk allergy. I. Oral challenge with milk and isolated milk protein in allergic children. Pediatrics *32*:425, 1963.

Gray, G. M.: Mechanisms of digestion and absorption of food from gastrointestinal disease. *In* Sleisenger, M. H., and Fordtran, J. S. (eds.): *Gastrointestinal Disease: Pathophysiology, Diagnosis, Management.* Philadelphia, W. B. Saunders, 1978, pp. 241–250.

Gray, G. M.: Carbohydrate digestion and absorption: Role of the small intestine. N. Engl. J. Med. *292*:1225, 1975.

Gryboski, J. D., Burkle, F., and Hillman, R.: Milk-induced colitis in the infant. Pediatrics *38*:299, 1966.

Haberkern, C. M., Christie, D. L., and Haas, J. E.: Eosinophilic gastroenteritis presenting as ileocolitis. Gastroenterology *74*:896, 1978.

Halpin, T. C., Byrne, W. J., and Ament, M. E.: Colitis, persistent diarrhea, and soy protein intolerance. J. Pediatr. *91*:404, 1977.

Iyngkaran, N., Robinson, M. J., Sumithran, E., et al.: Cows' milk protein-sensitive enteropathy. Arch. Dis. Child. *53*:150, 1978.

Jolley, S. G., Johnson, D. G., Herbst, J. J., et al.: An assessment of gastroesophageal reflux in children by extended pH monitoring of the distal esophagus. Surgery *84*:16, 1978.

Jorup, S.: Colonic hyperperistalsis in neuro-labile infants. Acta Paediatr. Stockh. *41*:596, Suppl 85, 1952.

Katz, A. J., Goldman, H., and Grand, R. J.: Gastric mucosal biopsy in eosinophilic (allergic) gastroenteritis. Gastroenterology *73*:705, 1977.

Klein, N. C., Hargrove, R. L., Sleisenger, M. H., et al.: Eosinophilic gastroenteritis. Medicine *49*:299, 1970.

Krejs, G. J., and Fordtran, J. S.: Diarrhea. *In* Sleisenger, M. H., and Fordtran, J. S. (eds.): *Gastrointestinal Disease: Pathophysiology, Diagnosis, Management.* Philadelphia, W. B. Saunders, 1978, pp. 313–335.

Kuitunen, P., Visakorpi, J. K., Savilahti, E., et al.: Malabsorption syndrome with cow's milk intolerance. Arch. Dis. Child. *50*:351, 1975.

Landres, R. T., Kuster, G. G. R., and Strum, W. B.: Eosinophilic esophagitis in a patient with vigorous achalasia. Gastroenterology *74*:1298, 1978.

Liebman, W., and Thaler, M. M.: Pediatric consideration of abdominal pain and the acute abdomen. *In* Sleisenger M. H., and Fordtran, J. S. (eds.): *Gastrointestinal Disease: Pathophysiology, Diagnosis, Management.* Philadelphia, W. B. Saunders, 1978.

Mendelson, C. L.: The aspiration of stomach contents into the lungs during obstetric anesthesia. Am. J. Obstet. Gynecol. *50*:191, 1946.

Paige, D. M., Mellitis, E. D., and Chiu, F.: Blood glucose rise after lactose tolerance testing in infants. Am. J. Clin. Nutr. *31*:222, 1978.

Parker, F., Christie, D. L., and Cahill, J.: Incidence and significance of gastroesophageal reflux in tracheoesophageal fistula. J. Pediatr. Surg. *14*(1):5, 1979.

Perera, D. R., Weinstein, W. M., and Rubin, C. E.: Small intestinal biopsy. Human Pathol. *6*:157, 1975.

Phillips, S. F.: Diarrhea: A current view of the pathophysiology. Gastroenterology *63*:495, 1972.

Powell, G. K.: Enterocolitis in low-birth-weight infants associated with milk and soy protein intolerance. J. Pediatr. *88*:840, 1976.

Raizman, R. E.: Giardiasis: An overview for the clinician. Digestive Diseases *21*:1070, 1976.

Reich, S. B., Earley, W. C., Ravin, T. H., et al.: Evaluation of gastro-pulmonary aspiration by a radioactive technique: Concise communication. J. Nuc. Med. *18*:1079, 1977.

Schreiber, D. S., Trier, J. S., and Blaclow, N.: Recent advances in viral gastroenteritis. Gastroenterology *73*:174, 1977.

Shapiro, G. G., and Christie, D. L.: Gastroesophageal reflux in steroid dependent asthmatic youths. Pediatrics *63*(2):207, 1979.

Stone, R. T., and Barbero, G. J.: Recurrent abdominal pain in childhood. Pediatrics *45*:732, 1970.

Urschel, H. C. Jr., and Paulson, D. L.: Gastroesophageal reflux and hiatal hernia. J. Thoracic Cardiovasc. Surg. *53*:20, 1967.

Vaz, G. A., Tan, L. K-T., and Gerrard, J. W.: Oral cromoglycate in treatment of adverse reactions to foods. Lancet *1*:1066, 1978.

Waldman, T. A., Wochner, R. D., Laster, L., et al.: Allergic gastroenteropathy. New Engl. J. Med. *276*:761, 1967.

Wilson, J. F., Heiner, D. C., and Lahey, M. E.: Studies on iron metabolism. IV. Milk-induced gastrointestinal bleeding in infants with hypochromic microcytic anemia. JAMA *189*:568, 1964.

Wilson, J. F., Lahey, M. E., and Heiner, D. C.: Studies on iron metabolism. V. Further observations on cow's milk-induced gastrointestinal bleeding in infants with iron deficiency anemia. J. Pediatr. *84*:335, 1974.

Wynne, J. W. and Modell, J. H.: Respiratory aspiration of stomach contents. Ann. Int. Med. *87*:466, 1977.

H. Peter Chase, M.D.
Jacqueline Dupont, Ph.D.

28

General Nutritional Considerations

Eighty percent of people in industrialized countries eat an adequate diet and have little or no need for nutritional supplements. In fact, obesity is generally a greater problem than undernutrition. However, the 20 percent with inadequate nutrition include infants with low iron intake; preschoolers with excessive dislikes for various vegetables, meats or milk who may develop specific nutrient deficiencies; teenagers who are constantly "on the go" or on a "diet" and eat only a small variety of foods; teenagers who are pregnant; the elderly; and, perhaps most of all, children with other diseases who develop chronic undernutrition. It is important for the physician to have adequate skills in nutritional history taking and physical examination to detect dietary deficiencies.

BASIC PRINCIPLES

The first principle of nutrition is: *Eat a varied diet.* Most individuals, except those with malabsorption, will thus obtain adequate quantities of all the known (and unknown) nutrients.

A second principle of nutrition has particular relevance to the allergist, who might be eliminating various foods from a child's diet in search for a food allergy. It is: *Whenever a food is omitted from a diet, it must be replaced with another food of equivalent nutritional value.* Figure 28–1

illustrates a case of a child in which this rule was ignored. The infant pictured was admitted to the hospital at age 13 months, after having been placed on a fruit, vegetable, and cereal diet at age 8 months following an episode of diarrhea. The diarrhea had been exacerbated when milk was reintroduced; the physician made a diagnosis of "food allergy" and prescribed a completely milk-free diet. This child's serum protein on admission was 4.3 grams per dl with an albumin of 2.1 grams per dl. She had generalized edema, puffy cheeks ("chipmunk facies"), skin striae, discolored coarse hair that fell out easily, a protuberant abdomen, and classic protein-calorie malnutrition (kwashiorkor). "Iatrogenic" kwashiorkor, resulting from dietary restrictions — including restrictions for "food allergy" — is now the most common manifestation of this disease in the United States. It can be avoided entirely if the second principle listed above is followed.

A third general principle for children is: *A plotting of height and weight on a growth grid is the best screening tool for undernutrition.* Children with nutritional deficiencies generally do not grow normally. In fact, in any child with inadequate growth, nutritional deficiency should be considered. It may then be important to consider the next principle.

Know what a child is eating. The most useful tool in doing this is the 3-day diet record, which usually requires the assis-

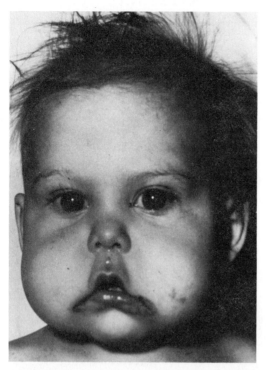

FIGURE 28–1. An 8-month-old girl who presented with kwashiorkor after having been on a milk-free diet for 4 months prescribed for "milk allergy." She had puffy cheeks, coarse strawlike hair that fell out easily, bilateral angular stomatitis of the mouth, a large liver, skin striae, and edema.

tance of a dietitian or nutritionist. The parent (or child if old enough) records as accurately as possible the kind and amount of food consumed by the patient over the 3-day period. The total calorie intake and the percentages of recommended daily allowances (RDAs) for the many nutrients (see Table 28–1) can then be calculated and appropriate modifications can be suggested. A computer program is now available in many hospitals to help with these calculations. A 24-hour diet history also can be used, but it is less accurate owing to limitations of memory as well as possible day-to-day variations. Once the dietary analysis data are available, foods can be added or substituted (using foods of equivalent nutritional value) as needed.

ESSENTIAL NUTRIENTS

Calories

Inadequate calorie intake is the most common cause of failure to thrive in the infant without obvious cardiovascular, endocrine, genitourinary, or other major congenital malformations. Failure to thrive is defined as "not growing as well as expect-

TABLE 28–1 RECOMMENDED DAILY DIETARY ALLOWANCES (RDA)*

		Infants	Children	Adolescents	Adults
Vitamin A	(IU)	1,500	2,500	5,000	5,000
Vitamin D	(IU)	400	400	400	400
Vitamin E	(IU)	5	10	25	30
Vitamin K	(mg)	Not established, but probably 0.03 to 1.5 μg/kg/day			
Vitamin C	(mg)	35	40	55	60
Vitamin B_1	(mg)	0.3	1.2	1.4	1.4
Vitamin B_2	(mg)	0.4	1.2	1.4	1.4
Vitamin B_6	(mg)	0.6	0.9	1.8	2.0
Niacin	(mg)	5	12	18	18
Folic Acid	(μg)	50	200	400	400
Vitamin B_{12}	(μg)	0.3	1.5	5	5
Calcium	(g)	0.4	0.8	1.2	0.8
Phosphorus	(g)	0.2	0.8	1.2	0.8
Iodine	(μg)	25	80	140	125
Iron	(mg)	6	10	18	10–18
Magnesium	(mg)	40	200	350	350
Zinc	(mg)	5	10	15	15

*As set by the Food and Nutrition Board, National Academy of Sciences – National Research Council for oral intake. Values are approximations, as they may vary slightly by age and sex.

ed by standard measurements." Inadequate calorie intake often is caused by improper formula dilutions or inadequate feedings. A general rule for adequate daily caloric intake in childhood after the first year is 1000 calories plus 100 calories for each year of age. In undernutrition, weight generally is affected more than height, which, in turn, is affected more than head circumference. Head circumference reflects brain growth, which can be impaired only with severe prolonged undernutrition in infancy (Chase and Martin, 1970). Severe failure to thrive, or "marasmus" (Fig. 28–2), is defined as "a state in which the child weighs less than 60 percent of the expected mean weight for age and in which there is no edema." If inadequate caloric intake is suspected, the treatment of choice is a "trial of feeding" which involves observing the infant in a medical center where food intake can be closely followed to determine if weight gain occurs when the infant receives an adequate calorie intake. If the child does not gain weight in 1 to 2 weeks while receiving an adequate intake, a more extensive medical workup should be considered.

An excess of calorie intake over calories expended results in obesity. As with most disorders, obesity is better prevented than treated. If it does occur, treatment at the earliest age possible is important. Obesity in infancy is associated with a greater likelihood of obesity in later life (Knittle, 1972). Two factors associated with childhood obesity are the early introduction of solids in infancy (prior to four months) and the obesity of parents. Treatment of obesity should be initiated as early as possible and should include: (a) modification of food intake, using regular analyses of diet records; (b) nutrition education; (c) group or individual psychiatric help; and (d) increasing physical activity. Family behavior modification techniques may be helpful in changing any of these factors.

Vitamins

Vitamins are essential organic compounds not made in adequate quantities in the body. Vitamins A, D, E and K are the "fat soluble" vitamins; the other vitamins are classified as "water soluble." Deficiencies of fat soluble vitamins occur more frequently in industrialized countries than do deficiencies of water soluble vitamins since the latter are usually supplemented in flour and bread products. Supplementation of water soluble vitamins is allowed because any excessive intake is easily excreted in the urine whereas excessive intake of fat soluble vitamins is poorly excreted, and may lead to acute and/or chronic toxicity syndromes. Signs of deficiency of water soluble vitamins can be seen temporarily when large quantities are withdrawn suddenly; for example, when a person has been on megavitamin therapy or has been taking large doses of vitamin C. Recommended daily allowances of the various vi-

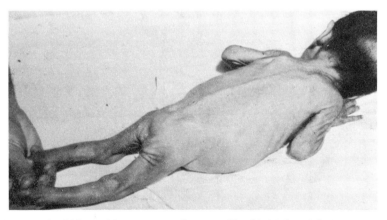

FIGURE 28–2. A 5-month-old boy with marasmus who was still at his birth weight (2900 grams), owing to neglect. Note the lack of subcutaneous fat, the lack of gluteal muscles, the protuberant abdomen, and the hair loss from spending so much time lying on his back in bed. He doubled his weight in 1 month but has remained permanently impaired in head growth and intellectual function.

TABLE 28–2 VITAMINS

Vitamin	Major Physiologic Importance	Laboratory Tests	Signs of Deficiency	Signs of Excess	Treatment of Deficiency
A	Growth, night vision, maintenance of epithelium	Serum vitamin A level (normal ≥ 20 μg/dl)	Follicular hyperkeratosis, corneal changes; changes in tongue papillae; night blindness	Scaly skin (fingers and hands), irritable, bone pain, gum hypertrophy, pseudotumor cerebri	15,000 IU's p.o. × 10 days (can give 1 shot IM)
D	Growth, bone and muscle metabolism, calcium and phosphorus homeostasis	Serum calcium, phosphorus and alkaline phosphatase; bone radiographs show cupping and fraying at bone ends	Convulsions or tetany (infant); cranial bossing; rib beading; wide wrists; leg bowing	Nausea, polyuria, diarrhea, weight loss, renal or tissue calcification	2500 IU's daily × 2–4 wks, plus calcium and phosphorus
E	Potent antioxidant, fertility, muscle metabolism, regulate prostaglandin synthesis	Peroxide hemolysis of RBCs; serum vitamin E level	In premature infant, anemia; reticulocytosis; thrombocytosis; edema	Possible gastrointestinal upset, muscle weakness, disturbed muscle function	200 IU's daily (25–50 IU's daily in an infant)
K	Blood clotting	Prolonged prothrombin time; low levels of factors II, VII, IX and X	Bleeding	Hemolytic anemia, increased bilirubin	1 to 5 mg of K, given IV; may need twice weekly
C	Growth, wound healing, collagen and "ground substance" formation	Plasma level < 0.2 mg/ml; bone radiographs	Bleeding gums (especially with severe form, scurvy); pains; subperiosteal hemorrhage; rib beading	—	100 to 500 mg/day, P.O. IM or IV
B_1 (thiamin)	Nerve function, energy and protein metabolism, cardiovascular function	Low urinary level (< 50 μg/dl); reduced RBC–transketolase	Anorexia; neurologic changes (particularly with severe form, beriberi) such as polyneuritis, fatigue, cardiac changes	—	20 to 50 mg/day, P.O. IM or IV in divided doses for 2 wks
B_2 (riboflavin)	Energy metabolism, maintenance of epithelium	Low urinary level (< 50 μg/dl)	Fissures at both corners of mouth and/or in nasolabial folds; cheilosis; tongue changes	—	40 to 50 mg/day, P.O., IM or IV until symptoms gone
B_6 (pyridoxine)	Neurologic function, coenzyme in amino acid and other metabolism	Tryptophan loading test	Anemia; convulsions (infant); gastrointestinal upset	—	10 to 50 mg/day–IV or IM
Niacin (nicotinic acid)	Growth, neurologic function, maintenance of epithelium, energy metabolism	Low urinary nicotinamide (< 0.5 mg/g creatinine)	With pellagra, skin rash (brown and scaly) in exposed areas; tongue changes; diarrhea	—	50 to 500 mg/day, P.O. IV or IM with other B vitamins
Folic Acid and B_{12}	Synthesis of red blood cells (both); peripheral nerve function (B_{12}); normal fetal development (folic acid)	Serum folate (normal > 3 ng/ml) or B_{12} level (normal = > 120 pg/dl), macrocytic anemia	Macrocytic anemia (both); peripheral nerve changes and glossitis (B_{12})	—	5 mg folic acid orally, twice daily. B_{12} = 15–25 μg/d orally (more for pernicious anemia)

tamins are given in Table 28–1; some specific functions and signs of deficiency and toxicity are shown in Table 28–2.

Amino Acids

Amino acids are essential for protein synthesis. The eight amino acids essential for the human are: leucine, isoleucine, lysine, methionine, phenylalanine, threonine, tryptophan, and valine. In addition, histidine is essential for infants. Eighty percent of protein intake in industrialized countries is from animal protein and generally is adequate in amino acid balance, whereas 80 percent of protein intake in Third World countries is from vegetable protein, which tends to have a poor balance of amino acids. Proteins of the two major grains, wheat and rice, are low in lysine and threonine. Corn (or maize) is low in tryptophan, which is a precursor for niacin synthesis. Soy beans are low in methionine. It is possible to get a balanced complement of amino acids by a judicious mixture of grains and legumes, but not from any one vegetable or grain source alone. The amino acids from such a mixture also may not be absorbed as efficiently as from animal protein. It is difficult for infants and children to consume sufficient amounts of vegetables and grains to obtain adequate amino acids for growth. Full-blown protein malnutrition is called "kwashiorkor," a term applied to children who are between 60 and 80 percent of the expected weight for age and who have edema. Children who have edema and weigh less than 60 percent of the expected weight for age are said to have "marasmic kwashiorkor." An infant with kwashiorkor may have any of the signs described in the previous section on basic principles. The diagnosis is confirmed by a low serum albumin and/or total protein. The total protein may be falsely elevated because of an increase in gamma globulin secondary to the frequent infections that occur in children with malnutrition. Treatment should consist of feeding a formula with the simplest nutrients available. Complex sugars and proteins may not be digested because intestinal disaccharidase and dipeptide hydrolase enzyme levels are low in malnutrition. An excessive osmotic load must be avoided, and intravenous alimentation may be necessary if diarrhea is severe. Since fat may have accumulated in the heart, liver, and other tissues, rapid intravenous infusions of blood or other products are hazardous in early therapy owing to poor myocardial function and too rapid shifts in body fluids.

Fatty Acids

Linoleic acid is an essential fatty acid in the human, although it may be replaced by one of its metabolites, arachidonic acid. Both of these polyunsaturated fatty acids are precursors for prostaglandin synthesis. Infants fed formulas deficient in linoleic acid may show poor growth, a scaly skin rash, diarrhea, and frequent infections (Hansen et al., 1963). Total intravenous feeding not accompanied by fat emulsions is a major cause of fatty acid deficiency. Children with malabsorption such as those with cystic fibrosis, sprue, celiac syndrome, or intestinal resections may develop both fatty acid and fat soluble vitamin deficiencies. (Chase and Dupont, 1978). In general, 3 percent of calorie intake should be from linoleic acid. Breast milk contains 5 percent of calories as linoleic acid, commercial formulas 3 to 4 percent, and cow milk 1 percent. Intralipid usually is given as a 10 percent emulsion that contains 50 percent of calories as linoleic acid. A 2 kg infant requiring 300 calories per day would need 3 percent of calories as linoleic acid (9 calories); fat contains 9 calories per gram, therefore 1 gram of linoleic acid would be required. This is found in 20 cc of Intralipid 10% Fat Emulsion.

Polyunsaturated fatty acids (primarily linoleic acid) also are important in reducing serum cholesterol levels. Children from families with a history of early heart attacks, or who have a parent with known hyperlipoproteinemia, should be screened routinely for increased serum cholesterol and triglyceride levels (Chase et al., 1974). When increased cholesterol levels are found, dietary changes should include increasing polyunsaturated fats and decreasing saturated fats and cholesterol intake. A reduction in simple sugar intake and increase in exercise also may help to lower triglyceride levels.

Minerals

Trace Elements. The trace elements make up less than 0.01 percent of body weight and include iron, copper, zinc, manganese, and iodine. Iron and iodine have long been known to be essential. Recently, specific syndromes associated with deficiencies of copper and zinc have been recognized in humans. *Trace elements are not included in formulated foods, fortified cereals, most vitamin pills or in soft drinks, and may be inadequate in a teenager's "fast-food" diet.* Fruits and vegetables and whole grain cereals are particularly valuable as sources of these nutrients.

Iron. Iron deficiency remains the greatest single nutritional deficiency in the U.S. The National Preschool Nutritional Survey of 1974 found 30 percent of preschoolers in the lowest socioeconomic group and approximately 15 percent of preschoolers in other socioeconomic groups to have hemoglobins less than 11 g at 1.5 years, which is the peak age of deficiency. Prematures and small-for-gestational age infants are particularly susceptible owing to their lack of iron stores and their rapid postnatal growth. In 1976, the American Academy of Pediatrics recommended supplementation from one or more sources (e.g., cereal, milk) for all infants (Committee on Nutrition, 1976). They recommended that supplementation start no later than 4 months of age in term infants or 2 months in preterm infants and continue through the remainder of the first year of life at least. Most infants need about 7 mg of elemental iron per day. The amount in milk varies from 12 mg/L (Similac) to lower levels found in some of the soy products (e.g., Mulsoy = 4 mg/L), cow milk (1 mg/L) and human milk (1.5 mg/L). Although breast milk is deficient in iron, the iron that is present may be absorbed more efficiently than iron in cow milk.

The anemia of iron deficiency characteristically is hypochromic and microcytic; laboratory diagnosis should start with examination of the blood smear. Treatment consists of giving 6 mg per kg body weight per day of the ferrous form, usually divided into two or three doses. Treatment should continue for 1 or 2 months after the hemoglobin is normalized, to rebuild iron stores.

Copper. Copper deficiency occurs most frequently in infants receiving total intravenous nutrition without copper supplements, but also is found in infants with malabsorption and in small premature infants (Heller et al. 1978). Leukopenia and neutropenia, bone changes (including osteoporosis, metaphysial spur formation, and soft tissue calcification), poor growth, and anemia may all be seen. Low serum copper levels are diagnostic and blood ceruloplasmin levels also may be low. The RDA is 6 ppm (0.6 mg/L), a level now present in most commercial milks. Cow milk has only 0.15 mg/L, whereas human milk has approximately 0.45 mg/L. Additions of 20 to 30 mg per kg body weight per day of elemental copper (as copper sulfate) to intravenous solutions will prevent the development of copper deficiency in total parenteral alimentation.

Zinc. Zinc deficiency was first associated with severe growth deficiency and delayed sexual maturation in Egypt and Iran. More recently zinc supplements have been shown to increase growth in apparently normal North American infants (particularly males). Some infants with failure to thrive, poor appetite, and poor taste acuity (hypogeusia) will respond to zinc therapy (Hambidge, 1977). Acrodermatitis enteropathica is an inborn error of zinc metabolism, and some infants receiving total intravenous nutrition without zinc supplementation will develop a rash similar to that of acrodermatitis. Zinc also is important as a metalloenzyme (e.g., for alkaline phosphatase) and as a coenzyme in the release of vitamin A from the liver. Thus, low serum zinc levels should be considered when vitamin A levels are low. Zinc is better absorbed from breast milk than from cow milk, and is now routinely added to many commercial formulas. Administration of 1 mg Zn (e.g., as zinc sulfate) per kg body weight per day is adequate to treat zinc deficiency. The RDA for zinc for older children is 10 mg per day.

UNDERNUTRITION AND THE IMMUNE RESPONSE

Malnutrition is known to increase the susceptibility to infection, and entire books have been written on this subject (Scrimshaw et al., 1968). In malnourished children, both antibody production and phagocytic activity may be defective. Iron deficiency alone can diminish the antibody response.

Cell mediated immunity also is diminished (Nutrition Reviews, 1976) by generalized undernutrition. Thymus-dependent (T) lymphocyte number may be diminished and function may be affected. Cutaneous anergy may be found in undernourished children, and a negative TB skin test may be present with active tuberculosis.

BREAST MILK

No chapter on nutrition would be complete without reiteration of the knowledge that human milk is made for human infants. Table 28–3 gives the composition of human and cow milk for some of the nutrients that differ in the two milks. Both milks have low levels of fat soluble vitamins, particularly of vitamin D. Cow milk is especially low in vitamin E, whereas human milk is especially low in vitamin K and pyridoxine. In addition to the many other advantages of breast milk, there are suggestions that avoidance of cow milk, using breast milk, may have prophylactic value for "high risk" infants of parents with histories of allergic disorder (see Chapter 25).

FAD DIETS

As emphasized in the Basic Principles section, *any diet that does not provide all*

TABLE 28–3 COMPOSITION OF MILKS

		Human Milk	Cow Milk
Protein	(g/dl)	1.5	3.3
Fat	(g/dl)	3.5	3.7
Carbohydrate	(g/dl)	6.0	4.5
Sodium	(mEq/L)	7	25
Potassium	(mEq/L)	14	36
Calcium	(mEq/L)	17	61
Phosphorus	(mEq/L)	9	53
Vitamin A	(μg/dl)	53	34
Vitamin D	(IU/dl)	0.4	0.3–1.0
Vitamin E	(mg/dl)	0.35	0.1
Vitamin K	(μg/dl)	1.5	6
Pyridoxine	(μg/dl)	11	48

of the essential nutrients is dangerous if followed for a long enough time. We have seen infants with kwashiorkor resulting from inadequate protein feeding, under the guise of the dangerous Zen-macrobiotic diet (in which the infant may end up receiving only cereal) and from an improperly balanced vegetarian diet. Reducing diets of every sort imaginable have been suggested, tried, and shown successful. However, they teach the person or family nothing about the good eating habits necessary when the "diet of the month" is abandoned. In addition, there are other hazards with such diets (e.g., deaths associated with the liquid protein diet, hypercholesterolemia associated with the low carbohydrate diet).

Another fad in recent years has been the use of large doses of vitamins in "therapeutic" ("megadoses") rather than "physiologic" doses. The use of vitamin C to prevent the common cold has been shown in numerous studies to have, at best, only a slight effect on the severity and duration of symptoms, and no effect on the incidence of colds (Committee on Nutrition, 1977). Similarly, *megavitamin therapy,* sometimes called the "orthomolecular approach," has been used in the treatment of nonspecific mental retardation, psychoses, autism and hyperactivity. These terms all refer to the use of dosages several times the physiologic need for one or more nutrients. *There have been no proper scientific clinical trials showing their benefit.*

It also should be realized that *"natural forms" of vitamins or foods are chemically identical to synthesized counterparts, with cost being the only differential.* The lack both of nutritional knowledge and of assertiveness on the part of physicians has, unfortunately, aided in the spreading of nutritional fads.

HELPFUL HINTS IN DIETARY ALTERATIONS

The first suggestion is to understand the basic nutritional considerations, as outlined above. Second, make sure that all the nutrients desired are present in the correct quantities in the food or supplement being consumed. For example, in one case families of children with cystic fibrosis were told that consumption of trace minerals with the child's vitamin supplement would be worthwhile. It was hoped that zinc would be among the trace minerals, but on investigation zinc was found to be present in adequate quantities in only one of the several preparations selected by the families. (It happened to be one of the least expensive preparations.) Reference to Table 28–1, which lists the RDA for various nutrients, will help ensure nutritional adequacy in any dietary manipulations undertaken.

Brief comments and "helpful hints" about various dietary considerations are given below:

Caffeine. Is tasteless and occurs in coffee (90 mg/cup), tea 75 mg/cup), cola drinks (30 mg/cup), and chocolate bars (20 mg/oz). It may keep children awake at night.

Calcium. High in cow milk ($\simeq$ 300 mg/cup), cheese ($\simeq$ 200 mg/oz), fish ($\simeq$ 50 mg/oz) egg ($\simeq$ 27 mg/egg), tortillas, and green leafy vegetables. Supplements are generally required if a milk-free diet is to be continued for longer than 2 weeks (also give vitamin D).

Calcium Supplement: Calcium gluconate (9% calcium): Infants = 3–6 gram/day; children = 6–10 grams/day; adults = 8 grams 3 times daily.

Cholesterol. See text under Fatty Acids. If serum level high, intake should be restricted to less than 300 mg per day. High in eggs and liver. Increasing polyunsaturated fat intake and restricting saturated fats can be more effective in lowering serum cholesterol than cholesterol restriction.

Copper. See section on minerals. Low in milk. Present in water and most fruits and vegetables. Can give 100 to 500 mEq of elemental copper per day as 1 percent copper sulfate (usually a total dose of copper sulfate of 1 to 3 mg/day) to treat deficiency in an infant.

Dextrose. A synonym for glucose. The United States food industry used nearly one billion pounds in 1972 in sweetening our food. It is formed by breaking down other disaccharides. High intake is related to dental caries and high serum triglyceride levels.

Fiber. Chemically defined as the portion of plant food resistant initially to hydrolysis by acid, and subsequently resistant to alkali. Most grains contain some cellulose fiber. Fruit may contain pectin. Inhabitants of industrialized countries who eat refined starches receive $\simeq$ 2 to 10 grams of crude fiber per day, compared to the 10 to 15 grams per day eaten by persons in Third World countries. Intake may be important in lowering serum cholesterol levels and in prevention of diverticulosis of the colon by enhancing fecal flow. Possible beneficial effects in other conditions are still unproven.

Gluten. See Chapter 29, on special diets. A protein — found in wheat, rye, oats, and barley — that must be restricted in gluten-induced enteropathy.

Goat Milk. Deficient in folic acid; has a high leucine content.

Iodine. Necessary for thyroxin formation. Present in soil and water in some geographic areas, and generally supplemented in iodized salt. Generally need 80–140 μg per day.

Iron. See section on Minerals. Infants need about seven mg of elemental iron (ferrous form) per day; treatment of deficiency consists of giving 6 mg per kg per day, usually in two or three doses.

Lactose. A disaccharide of galactose and glucose. The enzyme lactase is present in lowest quantity of the three disaccharidases in the gastrointestinal mucosa, and is thus most apt to be deficient with acute or chronic diarrhea or malnutrition. Adults of some pigmented races frequently lack the adult isoenzyme of lactase. It is the main sugar of milk. A lactose-free diet should exclude milk and most milk products.

Leucine. An essential amino acid that can stimulate insulin production and induce hypoglycemia. Cow milk has twice and goat milk three times as much as human milk.

Phosphorus. High in cow milk ($\simeq$ 300 mg/cup). Phosphorus can be given as a mixture of K and Na acid phosphate, giving 0.1 to 1.0 gram per day of elemental phosphorus. (The elemental phosphorus varies with the preparation used.)

Potassium. High in milk and orange juice ($\simeq$ 10 mEq/cup). Some fruits (e.g., apricot, cantaloupe) and vegetables (e.g., beans, cabbage, carrots) have 15 mEq/cup (1 mEq = 40 mg). May need to restrict in renal disease or supplement in diarrhea. Can give KCl in milk or juice in a level up to 60–80 mEq/L although it may cause gastrointestinal upset.

Purines. May wish to restrict when lowering uric acid. High in liver, kidney, sweetbread, organ meats, anchovies and sardines, with most other meats in the "intermediate-high" group, along with peas, spinach, lentils, beans, seafood, poultry and oatmeal.

Sodium. The average adult in the U. S. takes 100–300 mEq (3–7 grams) per day, compared to the usual daily requirement of about 40 mEq (1.5 gram). A "mild" restriction is 4 grams per day, a "moderate" restriction is 2 grams per day and a "strict" restriction is 500 mg per day. Most sodium is consumed as table salt. Milk has about 125 mg (5.4 mEq) per cup. Restriction may be necessary with renal disease or hypertension. Children with CF may need salt tablets (0.5 to 1.0 gram) in the hot summer, but salt tablets are not needed by most persons.

Sucrose. A disaccharide containing 1 mol of dextrose (glucose) and 1 mol of fructose per mol of sucrose. About 22 billion pounds were consumed in the U.S. in 1972. See dextrose.

Zinc. See section on Minerals. Present in meats and fish, and to a lesser extent nuts and unrefined cereal or bread. Zinc acetate (or sulfate — which sometimes causes GI irritation) in a dose of 1 mg elemental zinc per kg body weight for 3 to 6 months is adequate to treat zinc deficiency.

References

Chase, H. P., and Dupont, J.: Abnormal levels of prostaglandins and fatty acids in blood of children with cystic fibrosis. Lancet *ii*:236, 1978.

Chase, H. P., and Martin, H. P.: Undernutrition and child development. New Engl. J. Med. *282*:933, 1970.

Chase, H. P., O'Quin, R. J., and O'Brien, D.: Screening for hyperlipidemia in childhood. J.A.M.A., *230*:1535, 1974.

Committee on Nutrition, American Academy of Pediatrics: Iron supplementation for infants. Pediatrics *58*:765, 1976.

Committee on Nutrition, American Academy of Pediatrics: Health foods, and fad diets. Pediatrics. *59*:460, 1977.

Hambidge, K. M.: The role of zinc and other trace metals in pediatric nutrition and health. Pediatr. Clin. North Am. *24*:95, 1977.

Hansen, A. E., Wiess, H. F., Boelsche, A. N., Haggard, M. E., Adam, D. J. D., and Davis, H.: Role of linoleic acid in infant nutrition: Clinical and chemical study of 428 infants fed on milk mixtures varying in kind and amount of fat. Pediatrics *31*:171, 1963.

Heller, R. M., Kirchner, S. G., O'Neill, J. A., Hough, A. J., Howard, L., Kramer, S. S., and Green, H. L.: Skeletal changes of copper deficiency in infants receiving prolonged total parenteral nutrition. J. Pediatr. *92*:947, 1978.

Knittle, J. L.: Obesity in childhood. A problem in adipose tissue cellular development. J. Pediatr. *81*:1048, 1972.

Lymphocyte number and function in protein malnutrition. Nutrition Reviews. *34*:208, 1976.

Scrimshaw, N. S., Taylor, C. E., and Gordon, J. E.: *Interactions of Nutrition and Infection.* WHO, Geneva, 1968.

GENERAL NUTRITION TEXTBOOKS

Goodhart, R. S., and Shils, M. D.: *Modern Nutrition in Health and Disease,* 5th edition. Lea & Febiger, Philadelphia, 1976.

Pike, R. L., and M. L. Brown: *Nutrition, An Integrated Approach,* 2nd edition. John Wiley and Sons, New York, 1975.

29

Lloyd V. Crawford, M.D.

Allergy Diets

Trial elimination diets, diet diaries, and food challenges can be helpful diagnostic and therapeutic procedures in the management of allergic disorders in children. Though *in vivo* and *in vitro* laboratory tests may be of some value, the clinical history, trial elimination diets, diet diaries, and food challenges are the most important techniques in identifying food allergens responsible for symptoms. A major weakness of diagnostic elimination diets and food challenges, however, is that they may not differentiate food allergy fron nonallergic food intolerance. In food challenges, double-blind technique is more reliable than open visible testing but may be impractical.

Food hypersensitivity tends to be more prevalent in the first few months of life, and its incidence declines in later childhood. It can be important, however, at any age, throughout childhood or adult life. Food allergy is more frequently suspected and proved in the first few months of life, when only limited numbers and types of foods have been ingested. Specific conditions in which trial diets may be helpful include atopic dermatitis, urticaria, gastrointestinal allergy, perennial allergic rhinitis, and, occasionally, asthma. There is no substantiated value for the routine use of elimination diets in the treatment of chronic perennial asthma.

The simplest type of elimination diet is a short period of elimination of those foods suspected of playing a role in the patient's disorder. If improvement results in 1 or 2 weeks, the suspect food is then returned to the diet in an attempt to provoke clinical manifestations. If elimination of the suspect foods fails to improve symptoms, elimination trials based on probability may be tried next. If no improvement results from this diet and suspicion of food sensitivity still remains, a more extensive restrictive elimination diet may be used as a diagnostic tool, but only for a short time. *Only specific food allergens should be eliminated for long periods.*

If diagnostic trial diets identify a specific food allergen, treatment consists of eliminating the offending food or foods, *always keeping in mind the necessity for nutritional adequacy of the diet* (see Chapter 28). Young children often develop clinical tolerance to food allergens as they grow older. A food allergen may be eliminated for 6 to 12 months, and the allergenic food reincorporated into the diet to determine whether tolerance has developed. Children are less likely to develop tolerance to fish and nut allergens than to milk, eggs, wheat, vegetables, and fruit. There is no justification for restricting multiple foods from the diet for long periods of time solely on the basis of a positive skin test.

SINGLE FOOD ELIMINATION

Many parents of infants and children with food allergy will be suspicious that a single food is causing the allergy. Sensitivity to a single food such as milk, egg, or wheat is common in the first 6 months, but the child often develops concurrent sensitivity to one or more foods or inhalant allergens.

Cow milk allergy is relatively common in America. The incidence of milk allergy varies greatly in different studies, from 0.3 per cent (Collins-Williams, 1956) to 7 per cent (Clein, 1954) in the general pediatric population, to 14 per cent (Goldman et al., 1963) up to 30 per cent (Bachman and Dees, 1957) in the allergic pediatric population. A single elimination diet for possible milk allergy consists of complete elimination of milk and milk products for 7 to 10 days. An excellent choice for a milk substitute is a casein hydrolysate with added corn oil, sugar, starch, vitamins, and minerals, such as Nutramigen or Pregestimil. The older infant or child should be instructed to avoid other dairy products also, including cheese, yogurt, butter, and ice cream. The parents should be supplied with a list of other sources of milk. Detailed instructions regarding diets and recipes for food without milk may be obtained from the American Dietetic Association; the Professional Services Department of the Chicago Dietetic Supply House (1750 W. Van Buren Street, Chicago, Illinois); or the Ralston-Purina Company (Checkerboard Square, St. Louis, Mo.). A second choice

for a substitute for cow milk is a soybean formula. (The physician should be aware, however, that soybean is a member of the legume family and can itself cause allergic reactions). Table 29–1 lists infant's formulas available as cow milk substitutes. The various soybean preparations usually provide an excellent milk substitute and are adequate nutritionally. Reintroduction of milk, using a heat-denatured formula, may be attempted in 3 to 6 months if the milk allergy has been mild; in cases of moderate allergy, 6 to 12 months; in severe cases, 1 to 2 years.

A single food can be hidden easily in the processing of other foods, and the patient or parent will need additional guidance in order to totally eliminate the food. Common foods, such as egg and corn, are frequently found in such food mixtures as mayonnaise, salad dressings, and margarine. A problem occasionally encountered in food allergy and elimination diets is cross-sensitization among members of the various food groups. For example, a child may have an obvious clinical reaction to peanut butter but have a more obscure reaction to the other legumes, i.e., peas, navy beans, string beans, or soy. When allergy to a food does exist, careful observation for any possible symptoms produced by ingestion of a related food is also important. The biologic classification of foods

TABLE 29–1 FORMULA SUBSTITUTES FOR MILK ALLERGY

Product	Manufacturer	Protein Source	Carbohydrate Source	Fat Source
Nutramigen	Mead Johnson	Enzymatic hydrolysate of casein	Sucrose, tapioca	Corn
Pregestimil	Mead Johnson	Enzymatically hydrolyzed milk protein	Glucose, tapioca	Coconut, corn
Isomil	Ross	Soy protein isolate	Corn sugar, sucrose, corn starch	Corn, coconut, soy
Mull-soy	Syntex	Soy flour	Sucrose, invert sucrose	Soy oil
Neo-Mull-Soy	Syntex	Soy protein isolate	Sucrose	Soy oil
Nursoy	Wyeth	Soy protein isolate	Corn syrup, sucrose	Oleo, coconut, safflower, soy
Prosobee	Mead Johnson	Soy protein isolate	Corn sugar, sucrose	Soy

(see Chapter 15) is helpful in identifying cross-sensitivities that might exist.

"PROBABILITY" MULTIPLE-ELIMINATION DIET

When a careful allergic history fails to identify a single food, but food allergy still is suspected, it often is prudent to institute a diet that eliminates two or three foods that are considered to have a "high" index of probability for sensitization. This type of trial diet should be carried out for a minimum of 2 to 3 weeks. In children over the age of 2 years, milk, chocolate, and cola are suggested food allergens to be eliminated first. This type of probability diet is more reliable if the patient keeps a symptom score for 2 weeks before the trial diet to compare with the symptom score obtained during the 2-week trial. Interpretation of the trial diet results is based on comparison of the symptom scores before and after the diet. Equivocal differences in patient symptom scores are considered a negative trial; a positive trial is one during which symptom scores are 50 per cent or less of the pre-trial scores. If improvement has been considered indefinite on the trial diet, the trial period should be continued an additional 2 weeks. If the probability multiple-elimination diet results in a positive trial, single specific foods should then be reinstituted by an open visible or double-blind oral provocation challenge to demonstrate specificities. If there is no improvement during the trial period, then the combination of foods to be considered for elimination, based on "probability," is corn and wheat. The elimination of corn and wheat is particularly difficult, and patients must be educated to read (and interpret) labels on foods. If the trial elimination of corn and wheat results in no improvement of symptom scores, the next candidates for an elimination trial are eggs and legumes. A comprehensive list of dietary sources of cow milk, corn, egg, and wheat are available from the American Dietetic Association; the Professional Services Department of the Chicago Dietetic Supply House; and National Dietary Foods Association, Cincinnati, Ohio 45724.

EXTENSIVE ELIMINATION DIETS

If elimination of a single suspect food or use of a probability multiple-elimination diet has failed to implicate a specific food allergy, more extensive elimination diets may be tried. Extensive elimination diets should be used as a diagnostic tool only for a short period of time. The following are suggested extensive elimination diets for infants: under 3 months of age, milk substitute alone; 3 to 6 months, milk substitute and rice cereal; 6 months to 2 years, milk substitute with vitamin supplement, rice cereal, applesauce and pears, carrots and squash, and lamb. In 7 to 10 days, if there has been no change in symptomatology, the diet is abandoned. However, if the allergic syndrome disappears or markedly improves, foods can be added to the diet one at a time by family groups at intervals of 4 or 5 days. If any food exacerbates the allergy, that food should be eliminated from the diet for 6 months before another trial.

The use of more standard extensive elimination diets are indicated in the older child and the adolescent. Rowe (1931) initially developed and popularized these types of diets. The basic Rowe standard elimination diets are available through most hospital dietetic departments. They also have been modified and reproduced in many textbooks (Golbert, 1972; Grogan, 1977). Allergy Diet 1 (Table 29–2) is suggested for older children and adolescents, although it is similar to the extensive elimination diet of infancy. These types of extensive elimination diets are used primarily for those children who have daily symptoms; they are not recommended for those who have intermittent allergic symptoms. The Allergy Diet 2 (Table 29–3) is a basic cereal, milk, and egg-free diet and is a useful diet for the older child and adolescent. Allergy Diet 2 is somewhat less restricted than Allergy Diet 1. Standard extensive elimination diets are adequate diagnostic procedures for the majority of children with suspected food allergy. On rare occasions, there may be an indication for a 3- to 4-day fasting diet with intravenous supplement. Flexical (Mead-Johnson) is a nutritionally balanced elemental formula that supplies protein in a predigested elemental form, with carbohydrate and fat in a single readily digestible form.

TABLE 29–2 ALLERGY DIET 1

All fruits and vegetables, except lettuce, must be cooked.

Foods and Beverages Allowed:

Lamb	Water
Poi	Pineapple
Rice	Apricot
Rice cereals	Cherries
Rice wafers	Blueberry
Lettuce	Salt
Artichokes	Sugar (cane or beet)
Beets	Synthetic vanilla extract
Spinach	Tapioca
Celery	
Sweet potatoes	

Any vegetable oil, such as olive oil, Crisco, or Spry, *except* oleomargarine.*

Avoid:

Milk
Tea
Coffee
Cola
Soft drinks
Chewing gum
All medications except those prescribed by the doctor
All foods not listed under *Foods and Beverages Allowed*

Instructions:

Stay on basic diet for_____days.   **Result**

Then, on_____, add_____, alone, first thing in A.M. _____

Next, on_____, add_____, alone, first thing in A.M. _____

Next, on_____, add_____, alone, first thing in A.M. _____

Next, on_____, add_____, alone, first thing in A.M. _____

Next, on_____, add_____, alone, first thing in A.M. _____

Next, on_____, add_____, alone, first thing in A.M. _____

Next, on_____, add_____, alone, first thing in A.M. _____

Keep a diet diary as instructed.

*Kosher pareve oleomargarines and Mazola Margarine contain no milk.

(From Golbert, T. M.: Food allergy and immunologic diseases of the gastrointestinal tract. *In* Patterson, R. (ed.): *Allergic Diseases, Diagnosis and Management.* Philadelphia, J. B. Lippincott Co., 1972, p. 362.)

TABLE 29–3 ALLERGY DIET 2 (Cereal, Milk, Egg-Free Diet)
MODIFIED FROM ROWE'S CEREAL-FREE 1-2-3 DIET

All fruits and vegetables, except lettuce, must be cooked.

Foods and Beverages Allowed:

Lamb	Arrowroot
Chicken, turkey	Potatoes, potato chips
Beef, all beef wieners	Rice
Ham (boiled), bacon	Yams or sweet potatoes
	Tapioca*
Lettuce	
Artichokes	Lentils
Beets	Navy beans
Spinach	Kidney beans
Celery	Asparagus
Soy beans	Water
Soy milk	Ginger ale
Soy bean sprouts	White soda

Pineapple ⎫
Apricot   ⎪
Cherry   ⎬ and their juices
Blueberry ⎪
Plum   ⎪
Prune   ⎭

Poi
Olive oil
White vinegar
Vanilla extract

Any vegetable shortening or oleomargarine that contains no milk solids†
Salt
Cane or beet sugar
Maple syrup or maple flavored cane syrup

Avoid:
Tea
Coffee
Cola
Soft drinks
Chewing gum
All medications except those prescribed by the doctor
All foods not listed under *Foods and Beverages Allowed*

Instructions:

Stay on basic diet for_____days.   **Result**

Then, on_____, add_____, alone, first thing in A.M. _____

Next, on_____, add_____, alone, first thing in A.M. _____

Next, on_____, add_____, alone, first thing in A.M. _____

Next, on_____, add_____, alone, first thing in A.M. _____

Next, on_____, add_____, alone, first thing in A.M. _____

Next, on_____, add_____, alone, first thing in A.M. _____

Next, on_____, and_____, alone, first thing in A.M. _____

Keep a diet diary as instructed

*Minute Tapioca may contain citric acid. Use whole or pearl tapioca.
†Kosher pareve oleomargarines, Mazola Margarine, Crisco and Spry contain no milk.
(From Golbert, T. M.: Food allergy and immunologic diseases of the gastrointestinal tract. *In* Patterson, R. (ed.): *Allergic Diseases, Diagnosis and Management.* Philadelphia, J. B. Lippincott Co., 1972, p. 363.)

FOOD DIARY AND ORAL FOOD TESTING

While elimination diets are suitable for children with suspected food allergy that recurs frequently, a food diary often is more valuable in suspected cases of food allergy in which symptoms occur at infrequent intervals. A food diary consists of a detailed record of all types of foods ingested and a record of when ingestion occurred in relation to the occurrence of allergic symptoms. The diet is unrestricted when a diet diary is used as a diagnostic tool. All food, drugs, and beverages taken 24 hours before each flare-up are recorded in chronologic order. After three recurrences, an attempt is made to identify a food that has been ingested in common as to time and symptoms produced in all three episodes. When interpreting the food diary, it is mandatory that the physician have a knowledge of food families. If a food allergen is suspected from a diet diary, that food family is withheld for a period of time depending on the frequency with which symptoms have occurred. If improvement results, a food challenge is undertaken. If this results in an apparent clinical reaction, the food is eliminated from the diet for a longer period.

An open oral provocative trial is best undertaken while the patient is under the direct observation of a physician. However, this is not always possible, and many times parents may supervise the testing. The technique of open provocative testing that this author uses is as follows: a challenge test to an eliminated food is done when allergic symptoms are minimal, using only one test food on a single day. On an empty stomach (in the morning) the patient is given the test food in double its usual amount, in an attempt to provoke symptoms. After the challenge, the child is observed for a period of 24 hours for development of symptoms. *It is too risky – and usually unnecessary – to attempt to use food challenges for foods that have caused anaphylaxis.*

Blind oral food challenges are more reliable and may eliminate the misleading interpretations that occur with open testing (May, 1978). They also are more time-consuming, however, and often are impractical. In older children, the suspect food is fed blind and encapsulated in opaque, colored capsules. In young children, the suspect food is mixed with other food materials. An unequivocal single positive reaction to a double-blind challenge is considered sufficient for diagnosis. If a patient fails to have an immediate type reaction to 8 grams of the dried food, the food probably does not constitute a significant food allergen, responsible at least for IgE-mediated food sensitivity. If the double-blind food challenge has been equivocal, a repeat challenge with double the dose may be performed in 2 weeks.

DYE FREE DIETS

The frequency of adverse reactions to color dye additives in food and drugs is controversial. The following FD&C dyes are the five most commonly used: FD&C Blue No. 1, Brilliant Blue FCF; FD&C Red No. 2, Amaranth; FD&C Red No. 4, Ponceau SX; FD&C Yellow No. 5, Tartrazine; FD&C Yellow No. 6, Sunset Yellow. When adverse reactions to food colors are demonstrated, they often cannot be proved to be mediated by an immune mechanism. Aspirin is a common cause of urticaria, and aspirin-sensitive children also may react to tartrazine and other azo dyes and benzoic acid compounds that are added to drugs and foods. Approximately 25 percent of children who have urticaria with aspirin develop urticaria when they ingest tartrazine dye. Parents of these children should have a list, as up-to-date as possible, of tartrazine-containing foods and drugs. A large number of drugs contain tartrazine dye, and it is almost impossible to obtain a complete list because drugs are put on or taken off the market so frequently. Reference texts provide information regarding drugs that contain tartrazine (Harnett et al., 1978). Table 29–4 lists common sources of azo and benzoic acid dyes in foods.

NONALLERGIC CONDITIONS AFFECTED BY DIET MANIPULATION

Ingestion of food and additives may cause adverse reactions that mimic hypersensitivity reactions via nonimmune mech-

TABLE 29–4 FOODS OFTEN CONTAINING AZO DYES OR BENZOIC ACIDS

Azo Dyes
Candy, caramels, Lifesavers, fruit drops, filled chocolates
Soft drinks, fruit drinks, ades
Jellies, jams, marmalade, fruit yogurts, ice cream, pie fillings, puddings (vanilla, butterscotch, chocolate), caramel custard, whips, dessert sauces, powdered cream
Crackers, cheese puffs, chips, cake and cookie mixes, waffle and pancake mixes, some brands of macaroni and spaghetti, bakery goods except for plain rolls
Mayonnaise, salad dressing, catsup (certain brands), mustard, remoulade, bearnaise and hollandaise sauces, other sauces
Mashed rutabagas, purees, packaged soups and some canned soups
Canned anchovies, herring, sardines, fish balls, caviar, cleaned shellfish
Colored toothpastes

Benzoic Acid Compounds
Soft drinks, ciders, fruit drinks, ades
Jellies, jams, marmalade, fruit gelatins, stewed fruit sauces
Cheese, low calorie margarines, salad dressings, remoulade, hollandaise, bearnaise and mustard sauces
Refrigerated preserves of herring, sardines, anchovies, shellfish, and fish

(From Sly, R. M.: *Pediatric Allergy—Medical Outline Series.* Flushing, N. Y., Medical Examination Publishing Co., Inc., 1977, p. 201.)

anisms. Dietary manipulation may adversely affect or may ameliorate numerous conditions in children. Diet, for instance, may improve or worsen disaccharidase deficiency, gluten-sensitive enteropathy, and cystic fibrosis related to food intolerance.

The physician should, therefore, be aware that when major food manipulation is undertaken, aggravation or improvement of the condition does not necessarily identify the mechanism by which that particular foodstuff affects the condition.

References

Bachman, K. D., and Dees, S. C.: Milk allergy II. Observations on incidence and symptoms of allergy to milk in allergic infants. Pediatrics 20:400, 1957.

Clein, N. W.: Cow's milk allergy in infants. Pediatr. Clin. North Am. 1:949, 1954.

Collins-Williams, C.: The incidence of milk allergy in pediatric practice. J. Pediatr. 48:39, 1956.

Golbert, T. M.: Food allergy and immunologic diseases of the gastrointestinal tract. In Patterson, R. (ed.): *Allergic Diseases—Diagnosis and Management.* Philadelphia, J. B. Lippincott Co., 1972.

Goldman, A. S., Anderson, D. W., Sellars, W. A., Saperstein, S., Kniker, W. T., Halpern, S. R., et al.: Milk allergy 1. Oral challenge with milk and isolated milk proteins in allergic children. Pediatrics. 32:425, 1963.

Grogan, F. T.: Elimination procedures in the diagnosis of pediatric allergic problems. In Crawford, L. (ed.): *Pediatric Allergic Diseases—Focus on Clinical Diagnosis.* Flushing, N. Y., Medical Examination Publishing Co., Inc., 1977, p. 175.

Harnett, J. C., Spector, S. L., and Farr, R. S.: Aspirin idiosyncrasy. In Middleton, E., Jr., Reed, C. E., and Ellis, E. (eds.): *Allergy Principles and Practice.* St. Louis, C. V. Mosby Co., 1978, p. 1002.

May, C. D., and Bock, S. A.: Adverse reactions to food due to hypersensitivity. In Middleton, E., Jr., Reed, C. E., and Ellis, E. (eds.): *Allergy Principles and Practice.* St. Louis, C. V. Mosby Co., 1978, p. 1159.

Rowe, A. H.: *Food Allergy, Its Manifestations, Diagnosis and Treatment.* Philadelphia, Lea & Febiger, 1931.

Guinter Kahn, M.D. **30**

Principles of Diagnosis and Treatment of Skin Disorders

The skin is composed of three distinct structural compartments: the epidermis, dermis, and subcutaneous tissue.

Epidermis. The outermost portion of the epidermis is composed of a horny compaction of dead, keratinized cells called the stratum corneum. It varies greatly in thickness (15 to 700 μ), forms the major barrier that resists penetration of the skin, and provides for internal homeostasis. The thicker the stratum corneum, the better the protection. Teleologically, a thick stratum corneum allows for frequent contact with foreign material by the palms and soles, minimizing possible trauma and irritation from such contact.

Epidermal cells originate as a single band of columnar cells called the stratum basale, which rests primarily on the basement membrane (Fig. 30–1). This basal layer acts to rejuvenate the epidermis and produce the cells above it, called prickle cells, which move upward and accumulate large granules to form a thin granular layer. The granules gradually disappear, and the cells flatten to become the compact layer of keratin called the stratum corneum. About 14 days are required for the migration of a cell from the basal layer to the stratum corneum; approximately 14 more days are needed for the cell to traverse upward through the stratum corneum to be shed. The combination of the bottom, forming layer (stratum basale) and the upper, shielding layer (stratum corneum) provides

the dermis with a self-regenerating protective cover. Skin diseases usually disrupt this cover, often altering the rate of epidermal regeneration and percutaneous absorption (persorption).

Persorption of chemicals through the epidermis occurs to an extreme degree in premature infants, and less in infants, children, and adults. Most compounds placed on the skin of prematures can be found in the urine and saliva only minutes later. Compounds are absorbed faster through the skin when the stratum corneum (the prime barrier) is made more permeable by trauma, heat, or hydration. The use of occlusion to facilitate topical penetration of inflamed skin takes advantage of all three conditions.

Melanocytes are also found in the epidermis, interspersed among the basal columnar cells. They are derived from neural tissue and function to synthesize melanin, which pigments the skin. About one of every six cells in the basal layer is a melanocyte.

The basal layer has the pluripotential to replenish the epidermis and to produce appendageal structures such as sweat glands. An eccrine sweat gland consists of a coiled base that leads into a duct that traverses the dermis and epidermis. Eccrine sweating is stimulated by warmth, exertion, nausea, fever, and drugs such as alcohol, pilocarpine, and acetylcholine. It is reduced by cold, dehydration, diminished metabolism, and anticholinergic drugs. Apocrine sweating is stimulated by emotional factors and

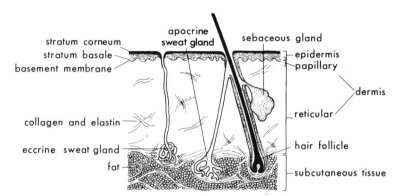

FIGURE 30–1. Diagram of the structure of the skin. (Modified from Kahn, G. (ed. and trans.): *Rassner's Atlas of Dermatology*. Baltimore, Urban and Schwarzenberg, 1978, p. 130.)

adrenergic drugs but not by heat. Apocrine sweat glands enter the pilosebaceous unit as illustrated in Figure 30–1.

The basement membrane divides the epidermis from the dermis and holds the two layers together. It is this area in which local tissue edema can force the skin to separate and form bullae, a phenomena that occurs easily in infants and children but less readily with increasing age.

Dermis. The dermis is a tough heterogeneous mixture of collagen, elastin, reticulin, and mucopolysaccharides. Cellular components include fibroblasts, mast cells, and histiocytes. While the epidermis acts as a barrier to the outside world, the tough tissue of the dermis acts to support it and serves as a conduit to guide nerves and blood and lymphatic vessels to their end position in the uppermost (papillary) layer of the dermis, under the basement membrane. The dermis also serves to support the pilosebaceous unit, consisting of an arrectores pilorum muscle, a hair, and its attendant sebaceous apparatus. Nerves of the skin are distributed in a random fashion except for direct innervation of hair follicles or sweat glands. Nerves do not innervate sebaceous glands or the epidermis in general. Special end organs in the upper dermis allow exquisite tactile sensory perception. These cutaneous nerve endings, high in the dermis, receive elementary impulses indirectly via the epidermis and allow perception of heat, cold, touch, pain, pressure, and location.

Subcutaneous Tissue. Beneath the dermis, a layer of subcutaneous fat padding gives form to the exterior of the body and serves as a protective insulating buffer for the internal structures. The subcutaneous tissue consists of fat cells, fibrous tissue, nerves, blood vessels, occasional reticuloendothelial cells and transient white blood cells (Solomon et al., 1978).

DEVELOPMENTAL ASPECTS OF SKIN PHYSIOLOGY

Our knowledge about the changes that occur in the skin through infancy, childhood, and into adult life is appallingly sparse. A summary is given in Table 30–1 (Montagna, 1965). Various hormones have profound effects on individual components of the skin, those associated with sexual maturation having perhaps the most widely recognized effects. "Adolescent" hormonal effects begin at about the age of 8 years. The sebaceous unit enlarges and produces increased amounts of triglycerides. The apocrine apparatus grows and secretes glandular material, which is degraded by bacteria to form odiferous end products. These changes frequently precede by years the appearance of secondary sexual characteristics. Sebum production and glandular size are diminished by estrogens and increased by androgens.

Cell proliferation and differentiation appear to be regulated by intracellular levels of cyclic nucleotides, which are controlled in part by the actions of adrenergic agents and other chemical mediators normally accessible to the skin. Although all the structures with which they are associated have not been delineated, four specific kinds of receptors have been associated with nucleotide activation in the epidermis: beta-adrenergic receptors predominate in the epidermis, whereas both alpha and beta receptors occur in the dermis. Alpha receptors are found only in dermal blood vessels. All of the cells involved with the mediation of immune responses, including mast cells, basophils, lymphocytes, and polymorphonuclear leukocytes, can be found scattered in the dermis in varying numbers and proportions, depending upon the pathologic process involving the skin. Proliferation, antibody and mediator formation, and other functions associated with these cells also presumably are under the regulatory influence of cyclic nucleotides. A more detailed discussion of these cells, mediators, and their interrelationship is found throughout the text.

TABLE 30–1 SUMMARY OF AGE-RELATED SKIN CHANGES

Skin pH	About 6.5 for first 2 days of life; about 5 for the next 4 days; thereafter about 4.5 (Solomon and Esterly, 1973).
Percutaneous absorption (persorption)	Prematures have substantially greater persorption than infants, children, and adults. No proven differences between infant and adult skin (Leyden et al., 1977). However, consideration must be given to the greater skin surface in proportion to weight in infants, as compared to adults.
Contact irritancy	No proven differences between infant and adult skin (Leyden et al., 1977) (excluding premature infants).
Blister formation	Occurs more easily on the skin of infants and children. The younger the child, the more readily blisters form.
Melanocytes	Evenly distributed, not functioning until birth (light complexioned black newborn). Soon after birth, regional variation in distribution of melanocytes begins, e.g., pigment in nipples, face, and genitalia increases. Progressive loss of melanocytes occurs at a rate of about 11 percent per decade.
Hair	Hairs of newborn are fine (vellus type) and lightly pigmented. After birth they are replaced by coarser, pigmented (terminal type) hair. Grouped follicles (three or more) per pilosebaceous unit do not occur until age 20 years. The number of hairs decreases progressively from birth to senescence; hair loss is not noted until 25 percent of the hair is missing.
Contact allergy	The incidence of contact sensitization gradually increases until the eighth year of life, when adult reactivity is reached.
Sebaceous glands	They are well developed at birth due to maternal androgens. They involute during childhood, enlarge and become functional at 8 to 10 years, and continue to develop through adolescence. Increase in surface free fatty acids, triglycerides, and wax esters parallels increased glandular activity (Strauss et al., 1976).
Apocrine glands	Enlarge during childhood, become functional at age 8 to 10. Axillary sweating begins a few years before puberty.
Eccrine glands	Nonfunctional at birth. Perspiration begins at 2 to 5 days; complete activity not achieved until age 2 to 3 years. Density of glands per cm^2 is greater in children than adults.
Nerve endings	There is a continuous reduction in the number of touch corpuscles (specialized Meissner's and Pacini's nerve endings) from birth to old age, whereas free nerve endings undergo no changes.
Collagen	Becomes increasingly mature (stable) with maximal changes between birth to age 2 years. Mucopolysaccharide concentration decreases with age, especially hyaluronic acid.

DIAGNOSTIC PRINCIPLES

History and Physical Examination

A nondermatologist will feel more comfortable describing skin disorders by noting their size, shape, color, texture, tenderness, location, number, and odor. Definitions of commonly used dermatologic descriptive terms can be found in Table 30–2. Dermatologic history-taking is an underestimated art that can be extraordinarily helpful in dermatologic diagnosis. The history should begin with variations of the following core questions:

1. What is the patient's complaint?
2. When did it begin, and on what part of the body?
3. How has it changed?
4. What makes it better or worse?
5. What was the effect of any medication tried?
6. Who has recently treated it? (This question may tell you more about the patient and the patient's relationship to his or her disease than most personality screening tests).

From this core information most patients will give peripheral details and are grateful for the invitation to talk freely of their affliction. At this point, look at the skin. The remainder of the history is composed of questions secondary to the revelations of the initial history and of the physical findings. It is here that core knowledge in dermatology, allergy, and pediatrics bears fruit. Family history may be important in atopy, acne, psoriasis, ichthyoses, bullous diseases, and many genodermatoses. Environmental history may reveal irritant eruption, the causes of which may vary from bubble gum to bubble baths, and which may be secondary to hobbies or habits. Keep in mind that dermatitis from irritant contactants is far more common than dermatitis from allergens in children and adolescents. Remember that shoe allergy or contact dermatitis is more common than fungal infection on the feet of children. Prevalence of a disease is extremely

TABLE 30–2 COMMON DERMATOLOGIC LESIONS

Macule	A change in color that is level with the skin; i.e., it is visible but not palpable and is less than 1 cm in diameter
Patch	A macule larger than 1 cm in diameter
Papule	Solid elevation less than 1 cm in diameter
Nodule	Solid elevation more than 1 cm in diameter
Wheal	Transitory (minutes to hours) solid elevation of the skin, synonymous with hive and urtica
Vesicle	Clear fluid-filled elevation less than 1 cm in diameter, while blister refers to similar lesions of any size
Bulla	Clear fluid-filled elevation more than 1 cm in diameter, synonymous with bleb
Pustule	A purulent vesicle which can become larger and form a *furuncle, abscess* or *carbuncle; boil* is the general term
Cyst	Sac of liquid or semi-solid material
Excoriation	Artefact produced by scratching or picking
Fissure	Linear cleavage
Scale	Exfoliation of dead epidermis
Crust and scab	Coagulated, dried serum or blood on the skin
Erosion	Superficial denudation
Ulcer	Deep denudation or loss of tissue
Scar	Fibrous replacement of skin

important in dermatologic evaluation; e.g., it is common for pityriasis rosea to occur in small endemic clusters. Know which diseases itch and when they itch the most (e.g., scabies itch more at night) and which do not itch (e.g., pityriasis rosea generally, psoriasis, and secondary syphilis), and which are transmissable (e.g., warts, molluscum contagiosum, scabies, and venereal diseases).

When taking the history and doing the physical examination, remember that infants and children differ from adults in that their skin is more reactive. Children more frequently have superficial bacterial infections; mucosal infections of herpes simplex and candidiasis (thrush); bullous reactions (e.g., congenital syphilis, mastocytosis); irritant reactions (contact *allergy* is uncommon); nevus development (pigmented, vascular); genodermatoses often characterized by masses, bullae, or dystrophic skin and adnexa; and eczematoid eruptions, which vary from seborrheic to candidal, to atopic, to irritant dermatitis.

Cross-associations may be of key importance in history-taking. For example, is there a background of diabetes in the child who has recurrent candidiasis? If the candidiasis is chronic and mucocutaneous, is there an associated endocrinopathy or immunologic deficiency? Is the skin infection recurrent? Is it accompanied by recurrent infections of other systems? Should one consider an immune deficiency or a deficiency in other host factors? Is there a family history of similar problems? After extracting all possible information from the history and physical examination, use the laboratory as necessary to complete the diagnostic evaluation.

LABORATORY METHODS

Potassium Hydroxide Preparations for the Demonstration of Fungi, Parasites, and Ova. Scrape the lesion with a dull-edged scalpel blade. Place the material on a glass slide. Add a drop of 20 percent KOH. Apply a cover slip. To diagnose fungal diseases, heat gently over a flame until a bubble appears. The specimen is then ready for microscopic examination. If a fungus is suspected, similar scrapings should be placed onto Dermatophyte Test Media (C.A. Baker Labs, Inc.) or Sabaraud's media for culture.

Bacterial Cultures. These should be done in a similar manner, except that the skin must be thoroughly cleaned with 70 percent alcohol 2 minutes prior to removing cells or tissues. After resident organisms are removed by alcohol swabbing, it is best to apply a sterile compress to the area for a few minutes before debriding or lifting off crust, scale, or blister coverings to expose the underlying exudative material for culture. For fluctuant lesions, the exudate is collected directly through a needle or on a sterile cotton swab. Gram stain and culture provide a direct method to determine if lesions contain pathogenic bacteria. Antibiotic sensitivity studies provide therapeutic guidelines for diseases that produce crusts, scales, blisters, or abscesses (e.g., impetigo, ecthyma, furunculosis, folliculitis). For deep infections (e.g., erysipelas, *Hemophilus influenzae* cellulitus), 0.5 cc of preservative-free sterile saline injected into the site of origin (if known), then aspirated back into the syringe and onto the culture plate, may reveal the causative agent. Blood cultures and determination of serum factors that may reflect infection (e.g., DNase B for streptococcal infection) may be more helpful in many cases. Request sheep blood agar media if beta-hemolytic streptococci are suspected, chocolate agar if gonorrhea is suspected.

Cytodiagnosis of Certain Viral Infections. The use of electron microscopy or animal testing is rarely required by practicing physicians. However, cytodiagnosis (Tzanck smear) is a valuable tool that quickly identifies herpes simplex, herpes zoster, and varicella. It is performed by scraping the base of a fresh vesicle and staining the material with Giesma stain. A diagnosis can be available in a few minutes using this simple technique: Pinch an early vesicle between the forefinger and thumb to prevent bleeding. Remove the blister top with a scalpel and scrape the floor of the blister. Spread the scrapings on a clear glass slide. Allow it to air dry, then stain with Giemsa material. Using a low-power microscope, look for the giant cells of herpes simplex, herpes zoster, or varicella (Fig. 30–2).

Wood's Light Examination. Long wave ultraviolet light induces greenish fluores-

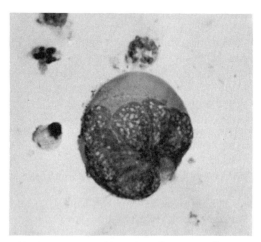

FIGURE 30-2. Multi-nucleated giant cell gently scraped from base of herpes simplex vesicle (magnified 480×). Note the adjacent white blood cells for size comparison.

cence in *hairs* infected by *Microsporum* fungi. Physicians tend to overuse the Wood's light for fungal examination. *The Wood's light reveals only one species of fungus in the hair, so that lack of fluorescence does not rule out tinea capitis.* The Wood's light does *not* reveal the presence of common dermatophytes on the skin, but does produce golden fluorescence outlining the area of tinea versicolor infection. This is the only fungal infection of glabrous skin for which the Wood's light is useful; this infection is not common in children. Bacterial infections caused by *Corynebacterium* organisms may fluoresce orange-pink. *Pseudomonas* metabolites fluoresce light green. Wood's light is useful in detecting white fluorescence of vitiligo or pigment loss; also, the darkness of hypermelanotic lesions is intensified.

Tests for Dermographism. Neither pressure tests nor injections of cholinergic agents in the skin are sensitive (see Chapter 40). The application of an ice cube for 5 to 10 minutes on a patient suspected of having cold urticaria is a valuable diagnostic aid (see Chapter 34).

Patch Test. At the appropriate concentration, suspected substances are applied under occlusion to the normal skin of the back for about 48 hours. The patch test and the scratch and intradermal tests are discussed in Chapters 32 and 21, respectively.

Darkfield Examination. This examination and related blood studies for venereal disease are beyond the scope of this text. However, these diseases should be kept in mind in the differential diagnosis of diagnostically perplexing dermatologic problems.

Skin Biopsy. This may give only limited information when the histologic picture is merely suggestive, but it does aid in limiting the diagnostic possibilities. Biopsy results are not diagnostic of infectious and papulosquamous processes and are nonspecific for most subacute and chronic dermatoses. *A specific diagnosis can be obtained from the skin biopsy for most tumors and for some forms of ichthyosis and bullous diseases.* Clinical correlation helps to confirm the histologic result and is of particular value in limiting the differential diagnosis. The clinician can receive maximal return on his biopsy investment by supplying detailed information about the history, physical findings, and differential diagnostic possibilities to the dermatopathologist.

Direct and Indirect Immunofluorescent Tests. These tests are useful to detect immunoglobulins and complement in biopsy specimens and serum, and they can be helpful in lupus erythematosus and chronic bullous diseases of childhood.

THERAPEUTIC PRINCIPLES

The following discussion of therapy for skin diseases is intended as a general therapeutic guideline. It omits the use of pastes, powders, and oils which are without proven value, compounds which can do more harm than good, such as gentian violet and iodochlorhydroxyquin, and topical preparations for which there are superior therapeutic alternatives. Sunscreens, shampoos, and acne therapeutics are considered in other chapters in relation to specific skin disorders.

1. Learn the normal course of the disease. For instance, many diseases of the newborn are transient. A few days' delay in treating nondescript papular erythematous lesions in the first weeks of life may reflect the therapeutic wisdom of the practitioner (Solomon and Esterly, 1973).

2. The more severe and acute the dermatitis, the more delicate and gentle should be the therapy (Weinberg et al., 1975).

3. If the condition is not widespread, treat locally. Learn only a few topical remedies; know how to use them well.

4. Soaks and compresses using water alone are as beneficial for erosive, weeping, or acute dermatitis as those with any chemical added to the water. Using water alone offers fewer side effects, less expense, and less inconvenience to the patient.

5. Common towels make excellent dressings. To improve patient compliance, always consider accessibility and cost in treatment.

6. The following agents are of no proven value in the treatment of diseases of the skin and are *contraindicated* because of adverse effects frequently associated with their use: topical anesthetics, topical antihistamines, topical proteolytic enzymes, topical vitamins, cornstarch, boric acid, and hexachlorophene.

7. Soaps are useful cleansers, but irritate. The least harsh include Keri, Basis, Neutrogena, Oilatum, and Dove. (The harshest include Ivory, Lowila, Zest, and Irish Spring.) Whereas dryness and irritation from soaps are common, allergic sensitization to the perfumes, antiseptics, and chemicals in soaps is rare.

8. Of the topical antiseptic agents, chlorhexidine gluconate in 4 percent alcohol (Hibiclens) is recommended. Its bactericidal spectrum is broad, and its ability to remain active on the skin for prolonged periods is substantial. It also is virtually free of side effects, does not stain, and produces little discomfort on open wounds. It is not approved for routine use on the newborn at this time because of insufficient test data (Peterson et al., 1978).

9. Learn to use two types of salves in dermatology: a dry salve (cream) for oily, moist, and intertriginous surfaces, and an oily salve (grease) for dry surfaces. Eucerin is an inexpensive cream which is half aquaphor and half water. Others include Unibase, Plastibase, Polysorb, Hydrosorb, Keri, and Lubriderm. These creams can be made drier (less greasy) by adding water until they become a lotion. (Lotions are more drying than creams and are valuable for treating hairy surfaces.)

10. Petrolatum is an inexpensive ointment. Others include Aquaphor, lard, Crisco, and Albolene. They can be made less greasy by adding Eucerin or other creams. Petrolatum is the standard ointment of dermatologic therapy. It is composed of long chain hydrocarbons from petroleum. It never causes contact allergy and provides a continuous (occlusive) cover. To moisturize skin, soak it for several minutes in water, then cover the water-laden wet skin with petrolatum. A large variety of chemicals can be dispersed evenly in petrolatum for effective presentation to the skin.

For drying moist or intertriginous surfaces after application of a cream, air blown from any source is valuable. Creams are made from fatty solids by adding emollients that allow water to mix into the material, converting it into an opaque substance (cream). The amount of water in the fat determines how drying it will be. Creams are absorbed into the skin, making them cosmetically acceptable, because they do not feel tacky or sticky. Their surface layer is discontinuous, i.e., they are not occlusive. Creams can become rancid unless preservatives are added. The more chemicals found in creams (emollients, preservatives), the greater is the possibility for creams to be allergenic or irritant. In general, medications in creams are not as effective as medications in ointments. Nevertheless, medicated creams (steroids, for example) outsell medicated ointments in the United States in the ratio of about 20 to 1. (The reverse is true in England, where ointments seem to be better tolerated.) In certain disorders such as atopic dermatitis, ointments may be too occlusive, so creams are applied over moisturized skin.

11. Rubbing alcohol is an inexpensive antiseptic, but it stings on open wounds. Its drying effect can be altered by the addition of glycerin, 5 percent to 25 percent. Adding more than 10 percent glycerin to rubbing alcohol converts it into a moisturizing solution, because of the hygroscopic properties of glycerin compared to the evaporation-induced dryness of alcohol. Other liquid bases (lotions) include Calamine, Aveeno and Cetaphil.

12. The following are examples of medications that can be added to the vehicles petrolatum, Eucerin, or alcohol with glycerin:

1 percent hydrocortisone to relieve inflammation

1 percent phenol to relieve itching

2–6 percent salicylic acid to decrease scaling eruptions and acne

Hydrocortisone and its derivatives are found in commercial preparations in many strengths, and, therefore, have varying benefits and dangers. Phenol in concentrated solutions can cause kidney disease. In the usual 0.5 percent to 2 percent concentrations, it rarely causes sensitization or side effects; but when used on open surfaces, it may cause dizziness. Camphor may be used in its place. Salicylic acid can sensitize (rare) and cause salicylism. If stronger concentrations are required, use them only on small areas.

13. Twice daily application of topical corticosteroid preparations appears optimal. More frequent application probably wastes the medicine. Hydrocortisone salves may be strengthened by increasing hydrocortisone concentration, occluding the area with plastic wrap, or using stronger corticosteroid congeners. Application under plastic wrap makes cortisone about ten times more effective. Applying the medication under a warm, wet towel compress–especially covered with plastic wrap — also enhances the penetration of topical preparations. (Hydrating and heating the stratum corneum reduces its barrier capability). Therefore, medication is best applied after a bath, while the skin is warm and moist. Occlusion using plastic wrap is not tolerated by all children. Plastic wrap is potentially dangerous for use with infants because it can cause suffocation. A small proportion of patients with atopic dermatitis will not tolerate occlusion because of pruritus and infection. The plastic wrap should not be left on more than 8 hours, since infection may be generated after a longer period.

Corticosteroid salves and lotions are now available in so many forms and strengths that there is a detailed science of their optimal use (Stoughton, 1975). The inexperienced can safely manage various diseases with 1 per cent hydrocortisone. More potent steroids, such as betamethasone or triamcinolone (0.1 per cent), may be tried for as long as 1 month. Formulations now available, however, have become sufficiently potent to produce systemic side effects. These agents include Diprosone, Florone,

Halog, Lidex, Topicort, Topsyn, Aristocort (0.5 percent) and Kenalog (0.5 percent). A physician inexperienced with these strong agents should never use them for generalized diseases, nor should he use them in intertriginous areas. They should be employed only for short periods of time in other local areas. In general, the more potent topical steroid preparations should be reserved for the armamentarium of those physicians with broad experience in the use of corticosteroids.

Local side effects of topical corticosteroids (Hill and Rostenberg, 1978) include the following:

Sebaceous effects. Perioral dermatitis, rosacea-like dermatitis, steroid acne, aggravation of preexisting folliculitis, and granuloma gluteale infantum (large red nodules in the diaper area).

Atrophic effects. Cigarette-paper–like wrinkling, delayed wound healing, and exacerbation of existing ulceration. Favorite sites of atrophy include: perianal, characterized by erythematous, smooth, shiny, telangiectatic areas that are often pruritic and tender; digital, causing pencil-sharpened–like atrophy of the distal digits; intertriginous, causing striae at anatomical sites of occlusion and also causing purpura, ecchymosis, and telangiectasia.

Immunologic effects. Altered local response to dermatophyte infections, causing tinea incognito; conversion of ordinary scabies into the "Norwegian" type. (See Chapter 35.)

Cosmetic effects. Hypertrichosis of the face; hypopigmentation.

Endocrinologic effects. The incidence of iatrogenic Cushing's syndrome from topical corticosteroids has risen dramatically for the past 5 years. Even experienced physicians need to be reminded that 1 per cent hydrocortisone under occlusion has the potential to induce the same side effects as the strongest known topical steroids applied with or without occlusion (Baden, 1978).

14. Hydroxyzine (Atarax, Vistaril) is the best overall antihistamine preparation for relief of itching and inflammation. Recommended dosage is about 5 to 10 mg per year of age, per day, divided into two to four doses. Dosage is adjusted on an individual basis according to its effectiveness and according to the sedation it produces.

15. If an antibiotic is indicated for a skin infection, it should be used systemically.

References

Baden, H.: Hydrocortisone vs. high-potency corticosteroid ointments. Arch. Dermatol. *114*:798, 1978.

Hajime, I., Adachi., Halprin, K. M., et al.: Cyclic AMP accumulation in psoriatic skin: differential responses to histamine, AMP, and epinephrine by the uninvolved and involved epidermis. J. Invest. Derm. *70*:250, 1978.

Hill, C. J. H., and Rostenberg, A.: Adverse effects from topical steroids. Cutis *21*:624, 1978.

Leyden, J. J., Katz, S., Stewart, R., and Kligman, A. M.: Urinary ammonia and ammonia-producing microorganisms in infants with and without diaper dermatitis. Arch. Dermatol. *113*:1678, 1977.

Montagna, W (ed.): *Advances in Biology of the Skin.* Vol. 6. New York, Pergamon Press, 1965, pp. 1–273.

Peterson, A. F., Rosenberg, A., and Alatary, S. D.: Comparative evaluations of surgical preparations. Surg. Gyn. Ob., *146*:63, 1978.

Solomon, L. S., and Esterly, N. B.: *Neonatal Dermatology.* Philadelphia, W. B. Saunders Co., 1973, pp. 11–42.

Solomon, L. S., Esterly, N. B., and Loeffel, E. D.: *Adolescent Dermatology.* Philadelphia, W. B. Saunders Co., 1978, pp. 1–27.

Stoughton, R. B.: Perspectives in topical glucocorticosteroid therapy. Prog. Dermatol. *9*:7, 1975.

Strauss, J., Pochi, P. E., and Downing, D. T.: The sebaceous glands. Twenty five years of progress. J. Invest. Dermatol. *67*:90, 1976.

Weinberg, S., Leider, M., and Shapiro, L.: *Color Atlas of Pediatric Dermatology.* New York, McGraw-Hill Co., 1975, pp. xvii–xxx.

31

Gary S. Rachelefsky, M.D.
Alvin H. Jacobs, M.D.

Atopic Dermatitis

Atopic dermatitis (AD) is principally a disorder of infancy and early childhood. It is characterized by extreme pruritus and persistent — often frantic — scratching, which induces papulation, excoriations, bleeding, oozing and crusting, secondary infection, and, ultimately, thickening or lichenification. Although the dermatitis can occur on any area of the body, there are typical locations of involvement that vary according to age (*vida infra*). The designation "atopic" dermatitis arises because it frequently occurs in individuals with a personal or family history of atopic respiratory disorders.

Diagnostic criteria for AD (Hanifin and Lobitz, 1977) are presented in Table 31–1. Virtually all patients with atopic dermatitis manifest findings thought to be related to a "skin susceptibility" to development of the dermatitis: increased sweating; decreased cutaneous oil production; abnormal vascular responses such as white dermatographism; and a decreased itch threshold, with increased itching from heat, abrasion, psychologic tension and infection. Scratching appears to be an essential ingredient in the pathogenesis of the dermatitis. Itching, which induces scratching, seems to be the common factor through which allergic, irritant, and other factors contribute to the development of the disorder (Furukawa, 1979). Atopic dermatitis, in other words, behaves as "an itch that rashes."

INCIDENCE

Halpern et al. (1973) in the United States noted a 4.3 percent incidence of AD in 1753 children from birth through 7 years of age; similar studies in Great Britain have revealed an incidence of approximately 3 percent in infants and an incidence of about 1 percent in school children, with a slight predilection for females over males. No racial predilection exists. It is more prevalent in city dwellers and more common in industrialized areas. Sixty percent of children with atopic dermatitis develop the disorder by 1 year of age; an additional 30 percent develop it before 5 years of age. The remainder develop their dermatitis in later childhood or early adult life.

PATHOGENESIS

The pathogenetic basis of atopic dermatitis is unclear, but speculation in recent years has centered on three areas: abnormal skin physiology and biochemistry, β adrenergic blockade, and specific immune abnormalities.

Physiologic Aberrations

Sweat Production. AD patients have an increased tendency toward sweating, and

TABLE 31-1 DIAGNOSTIC CRITERIA FOR ATOPIC DERMATITIS

Absolute Features

Must have each of the following:
1. Pruritus
2. Typical morphology and distribution:
   a. Flexural lichenification in adults
   b. Facial and extensor involvement in infancy
3. Tendency toward chronic or chronically-relapsing dermatitis

plus

Two or more of the following features:
1. Personal or family history of atopic disease (asthma, allergic rhinitis, atopic dermatitis)
2. Immediate skin test reactivity
3. White dermographism and/or delayed blanch to cholinergic agents
4. Anterior subcapsular cataracts

or

Four or more of the following features:
1. Xerosis/ichthyosis/hyperlinear palms
2. Pityriasis Alba
3. Keratosis pilaris
4. Facial pallor/infraorbital darkening
5. Dennie-Morgan infraorbital fold
6. Elevated serum-IgE
7. Keratoconus
8. Tendency toward nonspecific hand dermatitis
9. Tendency toward repeated cutaneous infections

From Hanifin, J. M., and Lobitz, W. C.: Newer concepts of atopic dermatitis. Arch. Dermatol. *113*:663, 1977.

they develop increased itching with sweating. With any stimulus to sweating (hot weather, exercise, emotional tension), the patient with AD has increased pruritus, increased scratching, and increased dermatitis.

Sebum Production. Decreased numbers of dermal glands lead to diminished sebum formation, increased water loss, and xerosis, especially in winter months. Also, increased cholesterol with decreased unsaturated fatty acids and wax esters of skin surface lipids in patients with AD may contribute further to excessive dryness.

Vascular Responses. Children with AD characteristically demonstrate paradoxical vascular reactions to mechanical and pharmacologic stimuli. Pressure with a blunt instrument (Lobitz, 1976) on the normal skin as well as on involved skin results in a white line without urticaria (white dermatographism) rather than in the normal erythema and wheal formation (triple response of Lewis). Skin temperature, especially of the

extremities, of patients with AD tends to be abnormally low; temperature adaptation of the extremities to external temperature changes is abnormal, with slower warming and faster cooling than normal.

Topical application of nicotinic acid esters produces blanching rather than erythema. Acetylcholine or methacholine injected intradermally into normal skin induces erythema, sweating, and pilomotion — actions that are not blocked by atropine. When administered to AD skin, these agents induce gradual blanching, sometimes preceded by erythema. This "delayed blanch" reaction is inhibited by atropine and is thought to be secondary to capillary dilation and increased permeability, which results in local edema of surrounding tissue.

Chemical Mediators. Elevated acetylcholine concentrations in blood and skin parallel disease severity. Norepinephrine stores in the skin, and blood levels of kininogens also are increased in AD (Michaelsson, 1969). Intracutaneous administration of serotonin, kallikrein, and histamine will induce blanching or only slight erythema, compared to the marked erythema that occurs in normal skin. Prostaglandin E administration induces a delayed vasodilatory response (Juhlin and Michaelsson, 1969), though there is a normal response to intradermally injected saline and epinephrine.

Some patients with AD have increased levels of histamine in both uninvolved and involved skin. Numbers of mast cells may be normal or increased in involved skin (Mihm et al., 1976). Intramuscular injection of histamine produces a greater than normal increase in skin temperature, whereas an intracutaneous injection produces less edema than normal. Abnormal histamine levels and altered responsiveness to histamine may be of particular relevance to the increased pruritus in AD, since the sensation of itching appears to be mediated by certain pain fibers, and there is evidence that histamine is a chemical mediator of cutaneous pain (Rosenthal, 1977).

The Relationship of Atopic Dermatitis to Beta Adrenergic Blockade

Szentivanyi (1968) proposed that partial blockade of the beta adrenergic receptor system is the constitutional basis for asthma and possibly other atopic disease (see Chapter 14). Various observations are consistent with this hypothesis. Increased sensitivity of the sweat glands to cholinergic stimulation and the heightened responses to alpha adrenergic stimulation reported in AD could reflect decreased beta adrenergic activity. Patients with AD pretreated with propranolol, a beta receptor blocking agent, do not have the expected increased sweat response to locally injected acetylcholine, suggesting that they already have maximal beta adrenergic blockade (Hemels, 1970). Since the level of intracellular cyclic AMP (cAMP) in certain neurons appears to control their excitability, increased itching could result also from decreased intracellular cAMP due to reduced beta receptor activity in local neurons (McAfee and Greengard, 1972).

Possible beta adrenergic blockade is suggested by differences between AD and normal skin in tissue culture. Catecholamines suppress the DNA synthesis of normal skin, but not that of AD skin; this has been interpreted as reflecting preexisting beta adrenergic blockade (Reed et al., 1976). Epidermal mitosis also is influenced by beta adrenergic factors: beta adrenergic stimulation decreases mitosis in normal skin but not in AD skin. This could explain the lichenification in AD (as a reflection of abnormal proliferation of epithelial cells) (Reed et al., 1976). *In vitro* leukocyte studies also have shown decreased responsiveness to beta adrenergic stimulants. Also, lymphocyte and granulocyte responses to beta adrenergic agents are decreased in patients with AD and asthma (Busse and Lee, 1976), whereas responses to prostaglandin E are normal, suggesting that the site of impairment is at the level of the beta receptor. Whether beta adrenergic blockade accounts for the decreased blood flow (blanching) following local injection of acetylcholine or histamine or whether this response is due to increased alpha adrenergic activity is not clear.

On the other hand, evidence against beta adrenergic blockade in the pathogenesis of AD includes normal activity of adenyl cyclase, phosphodiesterase, and cyclic adenosine monophosphate–dependent protein kinase in skin of patients with AD; a normal increase in cAMP after isoproterenol stimulation; and normal enzyme kinetics for glucose metabolism in isolated sweat glands from AD skin (Cotton and Van Rossum, 1973).

Immune Derangements in Atopic Dermatitis

Abnormalities in the Humoral Immune System. Serum levels of IgG, IgM, and IgA generally are normal or elevated in atopic dermatitis; serum IgD levels are decreased in some adults with AD. Elevations in IgG and IgM levels, when they occur, are thought to be secondary to chronic skin infection. Individuals with AD may have many positive immediate wheal and erythema skin test reactions to common environmental antigens, and the number of positive skin tests may correlate with disease severity (Rajka, 1961). Total serum IgE is elevated in approximately 80 percent of patients, and generally the severity of skin involvement is proportional to the IgE level. Those with highest levels tend also to have respiratory allergy. Patients with increased IgE also have specific IgE antibody to a variety of inhalant and food antigens. However, specific IgE antibody detected by skin testing does not correlate as well .with specific IgE determined by RAST in patients with atopic dermatitis (55 percent correlation) as it does in respiratory allergic disorders (Hoffman et al., 1975).

The role of IgE antibody in the pathogenesis of AD is unclear. Approximately 20 percent of individuals with AD have normal or low serum IgE levels; serum IgE levels may remain elevated even with resolution of the skin rash; elevated serum IgE has been observed in a significant proportion (25 to 50 percent) of patients with various nonatopic skin diseases (e.g., dyshidrosis, acne, bullous pemphigoid, neurodermatitis, contact dermatitis, psoriasis, and pityriasis rubra pilaris); and "eczema" has been observed in patients with X-linked agammaglobulinemia who have low to absent IgE levels. In addition, there has been generally poor correlation between the presence and level of IgE antibodies, and exacerbation of dermatitis on challenge with corresponding allergens.

Low serum IgA levels also occur in atopic dermatitis (Kaufman and Hobbs, 1970). Taylor et al. (1973) observed transient IgA deficiency at age 3 months, which preceded the development of atopic dermatitis in infants of allergic parents. They suggested that low gut IgA facilitated allergic sensitization by easier influx of allergens through the intestinal mucosa.

The number of B lymphocytes in blood may be normal or elevated in atopic dermatitis, depending upon the technique of measurement and the cell marker used (Luckasen et al., 1974; Hovmark, 1977; Rachelefsky et al., 1976; and Thestrup-Pedersen et al., 1977). The number of circulating cells that bear IgE surface markers also may be elevated in some patients with AD (Carapeto et al., 1976).

Abnormalities in Cell-Mediated Immunity (CMI). Cell-mediated immunity may be abnormal in AD. Clinically, patients with AD have an increased susceptibility to viral infections (vaccinia, herpes simplex, warts, and molluscum contagiosum) and to

fungi (*Trichophyton rubrum*). Patients with AD are less readily sensitized (contact dermatitis) to dinitrochlorobenzene and Rhus extract than normal persons and may have diminished delayed-type skin test reactions to tricophyton and candida organisms and streptokinase-streptodornase. However, this could be secondary to the disease process or to therapy with topical steroids: Uehara (1977) observed transient suppression of established tuberculin reactivity during active dermatitis, suggesting that the presence of dermatitis may play a role in the diminished *in vivo* CMI in AD.

In general, decreased numbers and diminished function of T cells in patients with AD parallels disease activity: the more severe the AD, the greater the T cell abnormalities observed (McGeady and Buckley, 1975; Rachelefsky et al., 1976; and Thestrup-Pedersen et al., 1977).

Some patients with high serum IgE titers appear to have a serum factor that inhibits T cell rosette formation (Hanifin and Gottlieb, 1974), and peripheral blood lymphocytes from some of these patients respond abnormally when cultured *in vitro* with T cell mitogens PHA (phytohemagglutinin) and Con A (concanavalin A) or B cell mitogen PWM (pokeweed mitogen) (Anderson and Hjorth, 1975; Grove et al., 1975; Hovmark, 1977; Rachelefsky et al., 1976). *In vitro* reactivity to tuberculin, lipopolysaccharides, and tetanus toxoid is normal, whereas there are suppressed reactions to candida organisms (McGeady and Buckley, 1975) and herpes simplex antigen (Hovmark, 1977).

Abnormalities in Leukocyte Movement. *In vitro* monocyte chemotactic responsiveness is depressed in some patients with AD (Synderman et al., 1977) and appears to be related to age; i.e., those over 11 years have a greater defect than those between 6 and 10 years (Fischer et al., 1977). The depressed monocyte response does not correlate with total serum IgE levels, eosinophil counts, and symptom scores, but it may be associated with a plasma inhibitor (Hanifin et al., 1977). Defective monocyte chemotaxis present in immunodeficiency with thrombocytopenia and eczema (Wiskott-Aldrich syndrome) also appears to be due to increased levels of circulating lymphocyte-derived chemotactic factor.

Depressed neutrophil chemotaxis observed in some adults with AD may be due to a serum inhibitor present in some persons only during active disease (Rogge and Hanifin, 1976). Neutrophil chemotaxis appears to be normal in children with AD.

Atopic Dermatitis and Immunodeficiency States. The eczema of the Wiskott-Aldrich syndrome is indistinguishable clinically from that of AD. Increased serum IgE and depressed CMI have been noted. Patients with hyper-IgE with undue susceptibility to infection (Buckley's syndrome) have recurrent staphylococcal skin infections, recurrent candidiasis, and, in many instances, a skin rash that may be confused with AD, even though it actually has a different appearance (Buckley, 1978). Some patients with ataxia-telangiectasia or X-linked agammaglobulinemia also have a dermatitis that can be mistaken for atopic dermatitis.

IgE and T Cell Function. The exact relationship between AD and IgE is not clear. Current evidence suggests that the primary abnormality in patients with AD could be abnormal T cell regulation, which, in turn, may lead to increased IgE antibody production. Suppressor T cells control the rate of IgE (and other) antibody production in animals. Removal of T cells augments antibody response to protein and polysaccharide antigens; reconstitution with thymocytes suppresses this enhanced response. T cells also appear important in regulating IgE production in man, and decreased numbers of T cells or depressed suppressor T cell function can result in excessive production of IgE antibody, as seen in human neoplastic and immunodeficiency disease.

Atopic dermatitis thus may be a multifactorial disease, in which a spectrum of physiologic, adrenergic, and immune abnormalities coexist. The relative importance of the factors may vary with differences in genetic influences on them and with age, environmental factors, infection, and therapy.

HISTOLOGIC FEATURES OF ATOPIC DERMATITIS

Two basic skin lesions occur in atopic dermatitis and are classified as vesicular or lichenified on the basis of their gross appearance (Mihm et al., 1976). *Vesicular lesions* are confined mostly to the epidermis and consist histologically of intercellular edema (spongiosis) with vesicle formation, epidermal hyperplasia, and an inflammatory cell infiltration with lymphocytes and macrophages. Only an occasional neutrophil, eosinophil, or basophil is seen. Mast cells are not increased in number, though they appear to be hypogranulated. The superficial venous plexus (SVP) is altered, with hypertrophy of endothelial cells and reduplication and thickening of vascular basement membranes. The stratum corneum is markedly thickened, with retention of cellular debris.

Histologic examination of *lichenified lesions* reveals irregular hyperplasia of epidermis with minimal intercellular edema, and marked thickening of the papillary dermis with increased numbers of lymphocytes and monocytes or macrophages. Mast cells are increased in number but do not appear to be degranulated. Changes in the SVP are similar to those of vesicular lesions but are more prominent and also involve the venules in the reticular dermis. Dermal nerves are abnormal, exhibiting demyelinization, fibrosis, and occasional vacuolated areas (lipids). Similar but less marked abnormalities of the SVP and venules occur in clinically normal skin of AD patients, but epidermal hyperplasia, intercellular edema, and cellular infiltrates are minimal.

CLINICAL FEATURES AND COURSE

Figure 31–1 illustrates the typical distribution of AD at various ages. We divide our discussion here into infantile stage (up to 2 years), the childhood stage (2 to 12 years), and the adolescent and adult stage (12 years and after.)

Infantile Stage (Figs. 31–2 and 31–3). Atopic dermatitis rarely begins earlier than 8 weeks of age, though seborrheic dermatitis may precede and coexist with it (Figs. 31–4, 31–5, and 31–6). Lesions generally first appear on the cheek, characterized by erythema that is dry and chapped in appearance. The lesions may progressively in-

Text continued on page 418.

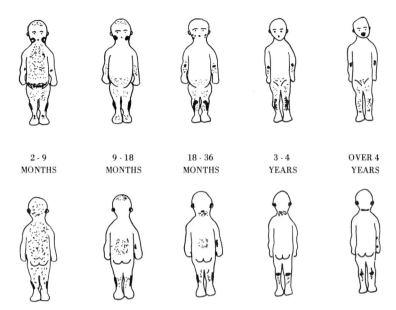

FIGURE 31–1.   Distribution of atopic dermatitis in relationship to age. (Adapted from: Sedlis, E.: Natural history of infantile eczema: its incidence and course. *In* Holt, E. L. (ed.): Conference on infantile eczema. J. Pediatr. *66* (part 2):153, 1965.)

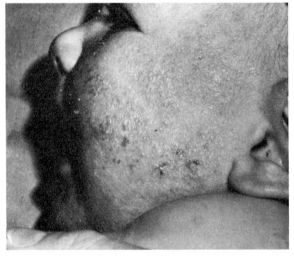

FIGURE 31–2.   Eight-month-old infant with atopic dermatitis; note excoriations.

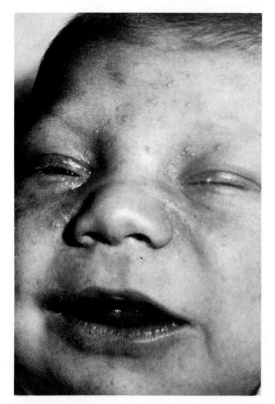

FIGURE 31–3. Nine-month-old infant with impetiginized atopic dermatitis.

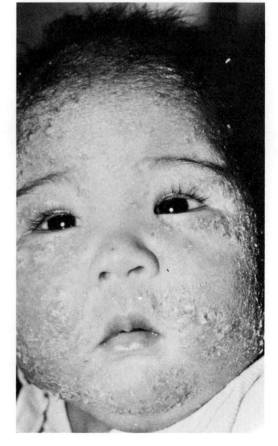

FIGURE 31–4. This infant has seborrheic dermatitis. There is erythema and scaling but no evidence of excoriation. The scale is yellow and greasy.

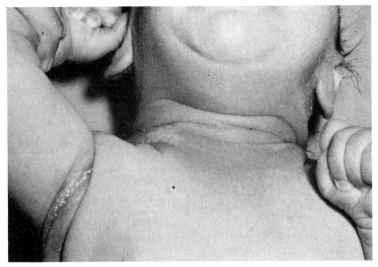

FIGURE 31–5. The typical intertrigo of seborrheic dermatitis in infancy. It is non-pruritic.

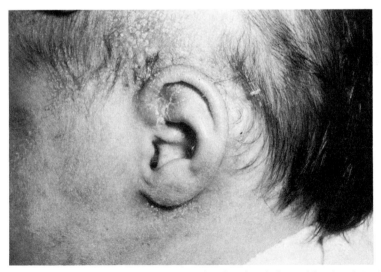

FIGURE 31–6. Greasy scale in the external ear and scalp of an infant with seborrheic dermatitis.

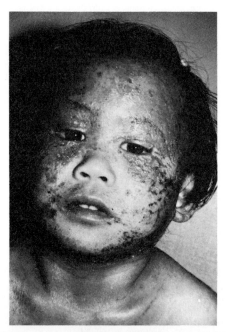

FIGURE 31-7. Three-year-old with severe atopic dermatitis. The extensive deep excoriations are evidence of this child's misery.

volve the forehead and scalp, extremities, trunk, ears, and anorectal area. Initially, involvement of the extremities is on extensor surfaces. Fingersucking leads to finger involvement. Papules and vesicles predominate; scratching induces oozing and crusting and sometimes secondary infection. Itching usually is intense, causing the infant to be irritable and interfering with sleep. By 18 months of age, the dermatitis may involve extremities completely. Frequently, it is most prominent in flexor creases.

Childhood Stage (Figs. 31-7, 31-8, and 31-9). This stage is frequently a continuation of the infantile stage, though a period of apparent "cure" may intervene. The child often is anxious, irritable, and hyperactive. Dry skin (xerosis) is a constant feature and is particularly prominent on the hands; fissures at the corner of the mouth are not unusual. Flexural involvement (antecubital and popliteal fossae, flanks, and back of neck) becomes more marked (see Fig. 31-9); the face is less involved, except for the ear lobes and skin behind the ears.

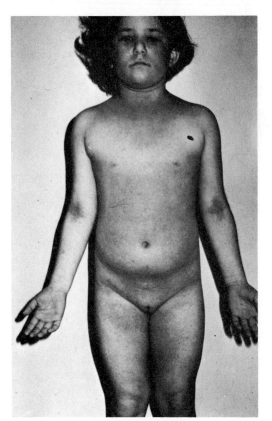

FIGURE 31-8. This 9-year-old girl shows generalized erythema with the typical flexural involvement of atopic dermatitis.

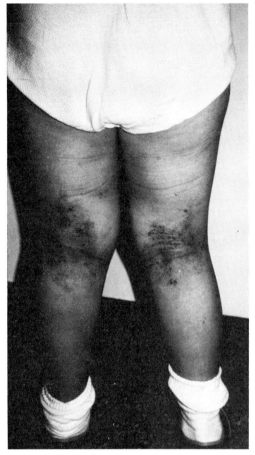

FIGURE 31–9.   Excoriated, eczematized popliteal fossae in a typical atopic child.

Lesions are less eczematous (acute) and appear drier. They are characterized by small papules, 0.5 to 1.5 mm in diameter, discrete, dome-shaped, and often vesicular. Scratching causes the papules to enlarge and crust, and results in large areas of lichenification, with peripheral discrete papules.

Adolescent and Adult Stage (Figs. 31–10 through 31–13).   By adolescence, the patient has developed dermatitis that consists of large plaques of lichenification surrounded by crusted papules, most prominent in antecubital and popliteal fossae, face, neck, eyelids, wrists, hands and feet (see Figs. 31–10 and 31–11). Dry skin continues to be a persistent problem, especially in winter. Secondary infection, due primarily to group A beta hemolytic streptococci or to staphylococci, is manifested by serous exudation and crusting.

COMPLICATIONS

It is a common misconception that most children will outgrow their dermatitis by 2 or 3 years of age. *For many patients, this is a life-long disease;* approximately 20 percent of children with dermatitis at age 2 years will have dermatitis into adulthood. It also is a harbinger of respiratory atopic disease in as much as 75 percent of cases.

Skin Infection.   Bacterial and viral skin infections (impetigo, folliculitis, abscesses, vaccinia, molluscum contagiosum, and herpes virus infection) are common in atopic dermatitis (Figs. 31–14 and 31–15). *Staphylococcus aureus* colonizes the dermatitis of almost all patients. Group A beta hemolytic streptococci or staphylococci (especially phage type III) or both frequently play important roles in the exacerbation of AD. Staphylococcal pustules accompany severe

Text continued on page 423.

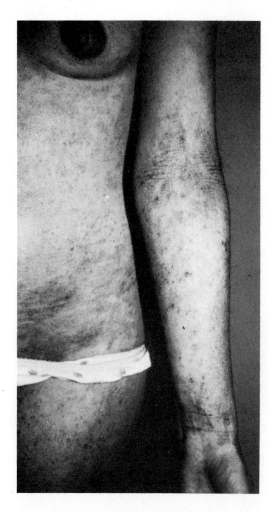

FIGURE 31–10. Adolescent girl with chronic atopic dermatitis, showing excoriation and lichenification.

FIGURE 31–11. This adolescent girl with chronic atopic dermatitis shows excoriation and lichenification of the neck. Also note the apparent follicular prominence ("goose bumps") which is characteristic of the atopic skin.

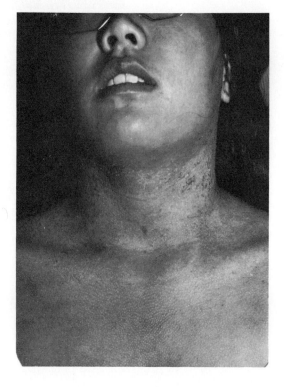

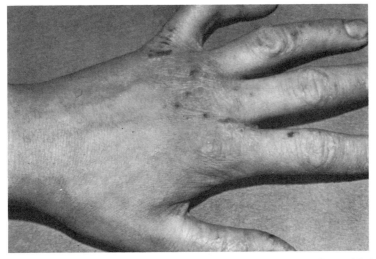

FIGURE 31–12.   Involvement of the hands is very common in atopics beyond infancy.

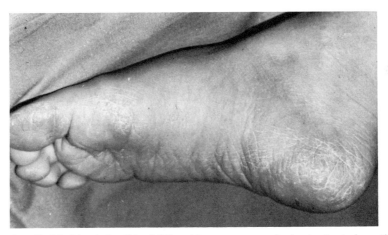

FIGURE 31–13.   So-called "athlete's foot" in childhood is more commonly due to atopic dermatitis than to tinea pedis.

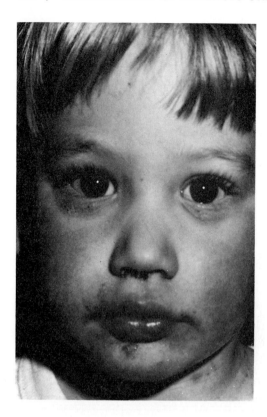

FIGURE 31–14.   This child demonstrates two common features of atopic dermatitis. First, because of allergic conjunctivitis he rubs his eyes and has developed lichenification of his lower lids. Second, as a complication of his allergic rhinitis, he has developed impetigo in the nostril which is already spreading to other areas of this susceptible skin.

FIGURE 31–15.   This young man with chronic atopic dermatitis has developed eczema herpeticum after contact with a friend's "cold sore."

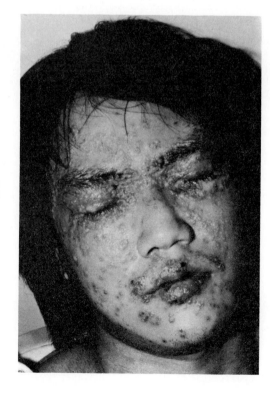

exacerbations of atopic dermatitis (Hanifin and Rogge, 1977). A combination of local factors (abnormal stratum corneum) and systematic factors (abnormal chemotaxis and defective phagocytosis) contributes to bacterial colonization and skin infection.

Patients with atopic dermatitis are highly susceptible to infection with cowpox virus (vaccinia) and are at risk with even accidental contact with a recently vaccinated person. Eczema vaccinatum has been estimated to occur once in 8.7 to 50 million vaccinia inoculations, largely in children under 5 years of age. It was the leading cause of death in the New York City mass vaccination program in 1946. It has become a rare complication since smallpox vaccination has been discontinued. Herpes simplex infection (see Fig. 31–15) resembles eczema vaccinatum and can vary from mild to fatal disease. Clinical manifestations of eczema vaccinatum are indistinguishable from eczema herpeticum (also known as Kaposi's varicelliform eruption). Both are characterized by groups of umbilicated vesicles and pustules, predominantly involving sites of both active and quiescent dermatitis, that is, areas of skin not involved with dermatitis. Hyperimmune vaccinia gamma globulin is of value in treating eczema vaccinatum;

herpes simplex immune globulin is not effective in eczema herpeticum.

Eye Complications. An increased incidence of keratoconus occurs in AD. Bilateral anterior or posterior subscapular cataracts have been reported in 1 to 16 percent of patients with AD, depending on the author, and appear to be independent of severity of dermatitis or its therapy. However, systemic steroid usage also can induce posterior subscapular cataracts in susceptible individuals.

Nephritis. Acute glomerulonephritis due to skin infections with nephritogenic strains of group A beta hemolytic streptococcus is not uncommon (see Chapter 67). Urine examination is particularly important in children with skin infections caused by this organism.

DIFFERENTIAL DIAGNOSIS

Seborrheic dermatitis occurs primarily in early infancy; it has certain features which resemble atopic dermatitis (Table 31–2) and may coexist with AD. An adult form begins in the pre- and early adolescent period and is related to androgenic stimulation of sebaceous glands. The infantile form of sebor-

TABLE 31–2 FEATURES DISTINGUISHING SEBORRHEIC AND ATOPIC DERMATITIS IN INFANCY

	Seborrheic Dermatitis	Atopic Dermatitis
Family history	Usually none	History of atopic disorders
Age of onset	Usually under 2 months	Usually over 2 months
Distribution	Scalp; any flexures, especially genitoanal; in older child, eyebrows, eyelids	Cheeks, forehead, extensor surfaces of limbs (Flexural involvement in older patients)
Lesions	Erythema with greasy, yellowish scales. Sharply demarcated flexural lesions	Erythema, papules, vesicles No scales (may be *crusted*) Tapering
Pruritus	Minimal	Severe (a hallmark of the disease)
Laboratory findings	Eosinophilia absent; negative skin tests	Eosinophilia; positive skin tests (especially for egg white) frequent
Prognosis	Usually clear in 3–4 weeks, up to 2 months. No associated defects	Prolonged course. High incidence of associated allergic rhinitis and asthma

rheic dermatitis (see Figs. 31–4, 31–5, and 31–6) starts between the second and tenth week of life, with a peak onset between the third and fourth week. It frequently clears spontaneously within 3 or 4 weeks. The essential features are erythema and scaling. Pruritus and papulovesicles characteristic of AD are absent. Sharply defined, round or oval patches extend peripherally and may coalesce. The patches are covered by adherent scales, which are yellowish-brown and greasy on the scalp and smaller and white in flexural areas. The eruption commonly begins on, and may be confined to, the scalp, but classically also involves the flexures symmetrically. It can become secondarily infected, especially with *Candida albicans*.

Leiner's disease (erythroderma desquamativum) is an exfoliative dermatitis of early infancy and is thought to be an extreme form of seborrheic dermatitis. It frequently is associated with marked enlargement of regional lymph nodes and with protracted diarrhea. Improvement has occurred with a variety of therapeutic regimens; antiseborrheic medications are the treatment of choice. A rare fatal familial form of this disease, in which there is dysfunction of the fifth component of complement (C5), is associated with failure to thrive, diarrhea, and recurrent sepsis due to staphylococci and gram-negative bacilli. The abnormal C5 is associated with a specific defect in the phagocytosis of baker's yeast particles, which can be corrected *in vitro* by normal serum or the addition of purified human C5. Infusion of fresh plasma or blood is an effective form of therapy. Other members of the family also exhibit defective opsonizing activity. Prognosis and course of this variant of Leiner's disease is unknown.

Cutaneous candidiasis commonly seen in infants and young children should never be confused with AD. The lesions most commonly occur in the warm, moist, intertriginous areas. The lesions are erythematous with sharply demarcated scalloped borders, usually with overhanging scales with satellite vesicopustules. Pruritus may be intense. Therapy is discussed in Chapter 35.

A variety of metabolic, immunodeficiency, and congenital skin disorders have associated skin rashes that resemble atopic dermatitis. These include *phenylketonuria, ahistidinemia, Hartnup syndrome, Hurler's syndrome, Wiskott-Aldrich syndrome, ataxia-telangiectasia, severe combined immunodeficiency, X-linked agammaglobulinemia, congenital eczematoid dysplasia, hereditary acrokeratosis,* and *acrodermatitis enteropathica.*

Other cutaneous diseases that may be confused with AD include *lichen simplex chronicus, contact dermatitis, drug reactions, nummular dermatitis,* and *chronic exfoliative dermatitis. Psoriasis* may begin in early childhood and also can be confused with AD. *Fungal infections,* especially those with secondary contact dermatitis due to topical treatment, may resemble acute AD.

Chronic dermatitis of the hands or feet may occur with active AD on other parts of the body but frequently is seen as a separate entity (see Figs. 31–12 and 31–13). One may see a noninflammatory vesicular eruption of the hands that comes and goes without a specific pattern. *Dyshidrotic eczema* is characterized by inflammatory lesions of the digits, palms, or soles. It begins as an annular vesiculopustular eruption that is pruritic. It is recurrent and eventually results in inflamed, exfoliating skin. *Contact dermatitis* of the hands and feet may be caused by multiple substances, including metal, rubber, and topical medications (see Chapter 32).

CLINICAL EVALUATION OF THE CHILD WITH ATOPIC DERMATITIS

History and Physical Examination

The diagnosis of AD can be made with reasonable certainty from history and physical examination.

History. The history should establish the way in which the dermatitis developed, when and where it first began, how it progressed, when it became most severe, its current distribution, and symptomatology. Details of treatment also are important: what topical medication, skin care, and systemic therapy have been prescribed? Did these medications help or make the dermatitis worse? Parents should be encouraged to bring in all medications so that their content can be determined. Not infrequently the dermatitis may have been worsened by treatment with topical medication containing such substances as organic iodides, antibiotics, antihistamines, or anesthetics.

A possible relationship to dietary or environmental factors may provide important information. For example, in the infant, the relationship of the onset or exacerbation of dermatitis to the type of milk or solid foods in the diet may suggest allergy to some food, while specifics of diet alterations or restrictions may provide clues to possible iatrogenic dietary deficiencies. In the older child the onset or exacerbation of dermatitis coincident with a move to a different house, installation of new carpet, or acquisition of a new pet will suggest environmental factors.

The history should explore other problems that may occur in association with atopic dermatitis, such as recurrent skin infections, gastrointestinal problems (chronic or recurrent diarrhea and/or failure to thrive), upper respiratory problems (recurrent "colds" and/or otitis), and/or lower respiratory problems (recurrent bronchitis, "bronchiolitis," or asthma).

A family history of atopic dermatitis, allergic rhinitis, and asthma is common in the patient with atopic dermatitis. There is an impression that the families of such patients have a greater than normal incidence of other dermatoses, particularly a tendency to xerosis, or dry skin. It is important to identify not only possible allergic factors in the environment but also factors such as wool carpeting or use of "bubble bath" which may irritate the skin and intensify itching.

Physical Examination. Performing a physical examination on a small child with a generalized dermatitis often is a trial for the physician. Frequently, the child is unhappy, irritable, resists examination, cries incessantly, and scratches paroxysmally when his or her clothing is removed. Height and weight measurements are important, since children may show growth retardation as a result of the disease or from therapy or dietary restrictions. The distribution of the dermatitis may provide clues to causative factors; open weeping areas or pustules may be signs of skin infection. A diagram of involved areas is useful. The degree of dryness present in the skin that is not actually inflamed should be noted. The response of the skin to pressure with a blunt instrument, such as a tongue blade, also can be determined during the examination. Since atopic dermatitis frequently coexists with respiratory allergy, the ears should be examined by pneumatic otoscopy, the membranes of the nose for signs of nasal allergy, and the lungs for rales or wheezes. If spleen or liver is palpable it should be noted, as should the temperature of extremities relative to the environmental temperature. Note also the length of the nails. Lymphoid tissue should be assessed: lymphadenopathy local to the area of dermatitis is not unusual, but rarely it may point to a lymphomatous condition of which the dermatitis may be a part. Sparse tonsillar and other lymphoid tissue may be a clue to immune deficiency.

LABORATORY STUDIES

There are no laboratory tests that establish a diagnosis of AD. Increased levels of circulating eosinophils frequently are present, though the degree of eosinophilia does not appear to correlate with either severity of dermatitis or presence of other atopic manifestations. On the other hand, certain tests are indicated to identify complications of the disease or of therapy.

A hematocrit is important to rule out iron deficiency anemia secondary to dietary restrictions; a blood smear also should be examined to verify adequate platelets. A nasal smear may suggest associated allergic rhinitis. Skin infections should be cultured in order to identify the proper antibiotic for therapy. Skin responses to various pharmacologic agents and tests for immune abnormalities are detailed elsewhere, but such tests rarely are of practical use in diagnosis or treatment. Histologic examination of the skin rarely is necessary for diagnosis.

While the validity of allergic skin tests in implicating causative factors in atopic dermatitis is controversial, they may provide useful information in some patients. In children who have been placed on severely restricted and sometimes nutritionally inadequate diets, negative food skin tests are useful in persuading anxious parents to liberalize the child's diet. In children sensitive to environmental factors, skin tests to factors in the environment, e.g., dog or cat dander, may identify specific factors that will induce itching. In children with coexistent respiratory allergy, skin testing is useful in identifying factors that are important in allergic rhinitis or asthma, even though these tests may not have direct relevance to the eczema. Testing for specific serum IgE may be helpful in the young child or the one with extensive skin involvement who can not be adequately skin-tested.

TREATMENT

Treatment is discussed in two sections. The first concerns the care of the skin; the second outlines general measures in the overall management of the patient.

Care of the Skin

Acute Phase. When AD is first seen in the acute phase, with inflammation, oozing, and crusting, it is important to recognize that secondary infection usually is present and systemic antibiotic therapy must be instituted promptly. Reduction of inflamma-

tion and removal of crusts and exudate are best done with intermittent cool, wet dressings applied open over the inflamed skin; this reduces inflammation, decreases pruritus, and aids in the removal of crusts and exudate. Two or three layers of gauze, Kerlix, or linen are thoroughly moistened with Burow's solution and loosely applied to the involved areas for 15 to 30 minutes four times daily. The dressings are dipped in the solution every 10 to 15 minutes during application to prevent drying and sticking. Burow's solution (aluminium acetate solution 1:40) is prepared by dissolving one tablet or packet of Domeboro in a quart of cool tap water. Therapy with wet compresses should not be used for more than 3 days.

Subacute and Chronic Phase. Several approaches to therapy of the subacute and chronic phase are in use, based on the recognition that the dry skin of atopic dermatitis is due to a lack of sufficient water in the stratum corneum. The drier the skin, the greater the itching. Washing with water removes the water-soluble substances that retain the water in the horny layer, resulting in increased dryness and itching after bathing. One approach to therapy completely avoids bathing with water. Another technique involves the liberal use of emollients along with steroid preparations applied to the active dermatitis, utilizing bathing.

MODIFIED SCHOLTZ REGIMEN

1. **No bathing with either soap or water should be done.** The only exception to this no-bathing rule is the use of a moist washcloth to clean the groin and axillary area.

2. **Clean entire skin surface at least twice daily with a nonlipid cleansing lotion.** Cetaphil lotion, consisting primarily of water, acetyl alcohol, sodium laurel sulfate, and propylene glycol, is used. Apply lotion liberally and rub it in until it foams. Then gently wipe off, leaving a film of lotion on the skin to aid in retention of water in the horny layer of the skin. No oily or greasy lubricants or topical ointment preparations are allowed. They are occlusive and increase sweat retention, thus intensifying pruritus. Avoid tar preparations; they can be irritating and may cause folliculitis and promote infection.

3. **Topical steroid treatment.** Inflamed or pruritic areas of the dermatitis are treated by topical application of fluorinated corticosteroids. Either a solution or cream formulation should be used, not an ointment base (see Table 31–3). All acutely inflamed areas should clear promptly with the topical steroid preparation. If they fail to clear, suspect infection or noncompliance. In most instances, if the entire program is followed, inflammation clears in 2 to 3 weeks.

4. **Continuing treatment.** After acutely inflamed areas have responded, improvement can be maintained by adhering to the no-bath routine and Cetaphil cleansing. Topical steroids are then needed only occasionally, with flare-ups of the dermatitis. The weakest topical preparation clinically effective should be used. When the skin has remained clear of eruption for several months, a brief cool bath is allowed once or twice monthly, always followed by a liberal application of the lipid-free lotion. Most patients can tolerate a brief, lukewarm bath as often as once weekly after their skin has remained clear for several more months. Cetaphil lotion must be continued daily for cleansing and lubrication.

EMOLLIENT REGIMEN

1. **Emollients are used liberally to treat the patient's excessively dry skin.** Emollients range from oil-in-water preparations (hydrophilic ointment) to more occlusive water-in-oil preparations (aquaphor). The patient or parent should be given several emollients and encouraged to determine which one works best and should apply it at least four times daily.

2. **Topical steroid treatment.** A long-acting fluorinated topical steroid is sparingly applied to inflamed areas two or three times daily, either in cream or ointment form — whichever appears to be most effective.

3. **Special baths are used to add water to the skin.** During a particularly dry or inflamed stage, bathing two or three times a day may be encouraged. The recommended procedure is for the patient to soak in water alone for a few minutes to hydrate skin, then add bath oil and remain in the bath for another couple of minutes. The skin is partly dried; then the cream is applied. Limited bathing is otherwise permitted, using a commercial bath oil in the water, such as Lubath or Alph-Keri Oil, and using a superfatted or modified soap, such as Basis or Neutrogena. Children who have extensive excoriation or oozing complain of considerable pain and burning from baths in plain water. These symptoms can be minimized by adding sufficient sodium chloride to provide an isotonic bath (2-1/2 tablespoonfuls of table or rock salt to 1 gallon of water).

4. **Local or systemic side effects may result from halogenated steroid preparations.** Local side effects are most likely when preparations are used for long periods under a plastic wrap (occlusive wraps). Local side effects include atrophy of the skin with erythema and telangiectasis, which produces thinning of the skin, related to the breakdown of collagen. Rosacea and perioral dermatitis along with striae may occur, especially after occlusive treatment. Other side effects reported have been ecchymoses, hypopigmentation, and hypertrichosis. Of importance in young children is the rebound phenomenon that may occur when fluorinated steroids are applied to the face. A frequent complaint is burning and stinging. Adrenosuppression, hypertension, and cushingoid appearance have been described in a few patients treated chronically with halogenated corticosteroids, especially when preparations have been applied with occlusive wraps to a large portion of skin. Hydrocortisone cream is safer for facial and intertriginous areas. Lesions near the eye should be treated with ophthalmic hydrocortisone.

TABLE 31–3 ORDER OF POTENCY* OF TOPICAL CORTICOSTEROIDS

I. Diprosone ointment 0.05%
   Halog cream 0.01%
   Lidex cream 0.05%
   Lidex ointment 0.05%
   Topicort ointment 0.25%
   Topsyn gel 0.05%
II. Aristocort cream 0.5%
   Diprosone cream 0.05%
   Flurobate gel (Benisone gel) 0.025%
   Topicort cream 0.25%
   Valisone lotion 0.1%
   Valisone ointment 0.1%
III. Aristocort ointment 0.1%
   Cordran ointment 0.05%
   Kenalog ointment 0.1%
   Synalar cream (HP) 0.2%
   Synalar ointment 0.025%
IV. Cordran cream 0.05%
   Kenalog cream 0.1%
   Kenalog lotion 0.025%
   Synalar cream 0.025%
   Valisone cream 0.1%
V. Desonide cream 0.05% (Tridesilon Creme)
   Locorten cream 0.03%
VI. Topicals with hydrocortisone,
   dexamethasone, flumethasone,
   prednisolone, and methyl prednisolone

*Group I is the most potent, and potency decreases with each group to the least potent — Group VI. There is no significant difference among agents within any given group.

From Stoughton, R. B.: A perspective of topical corticosteroid therapy. *In* Farber, E. M., and Cox, A. J. (eds.): *Psoriasis: Proceedings of the Second International Symposium.* New York, York Medical Books, 1977, p. 224.

Both approaches are presented, since patients who fail to respond to one may respond to the other.

GENERAL MEASURES

Control of Infection. Inflammation, oozing, and crusting usually are associated with bacterial infection. If skin cultures are positive, treatment consists of a 7- to 10-day course of oral penicillin or erythromycin, since the offending organisms most commonly are Group A beta hemolytic streptococcus and *Staphylococcus aureus*. The role of penicillin-resistant staphylococci has not been evaluated, though in the authors' experience such organisms are rarely seen. Topical antibiotic preparations are best avoided since they are potentially sensitizing and less effective than systemic medication.

Antihistamines. The antipruritic action of antihistamines may be beneficial in therapy, and their long-term use may be necessary in severe atopic dermatitis. Their clinical effectiveness appears to be related in large part to sedation. This may limit antihistamine use during the day. The choice of antihistamine depends on the physician's experience and on the side effects in individual patients. Hydroxyzine (Atarax, Vistaril) appears to be the most effective. Begin with 10 mg every 6 hours, increasing the dose 5 mg every 3 to 5 days until itching is minimized or intolerable side effects (e.g., sleepiness, lethargy) occur. Children tolerate this drug better than adults. Another frequently used antihistamine is diphenhydramine (Benadryl), which appears to have a greater sedative effect than hydroxyzine. It is important to emphasize that antihistamines must be prescribed on a regular basis to help prevent or control pruritus. thus interrupting the itch-scratch cycle. Nighttime use only may not be sufficient to control the scratching. Antihistamines never should be applied topically because of the risk of sensitization and secondary contact dermatitis.

Dietary Management. The role of dietary restriction in the therapy of atopic dermatitis is controversial. Many pediatricians and pediatric allergists are convinced that the dermatitis in some patients is exacerbated by foods. Many dermatologists are equally convinced that dietary manipulation is futile in managing atopic dermatitis. It is possible that pediatricians and dermatologists see different subpopulations of AD. Perhaps patients in whom food allergy is an important factor are managed by their primary physician or are referred to allergists and not referred to dermatologists for the most part. Unfortunately, no well-controlled studies have been performed. A conceptual model suggests that eczema may result from skin susceptibility with or without allergic responsiveness; importance of food allergy in "allergic" patients with

AD is thought to depend upon the degree of allergic sensitivity, the allergenicity of the food, and the quantity absorbed and not neutralized (Furukawa, 1979). Radioallergosorbent tests of serum from children with atopic dermatitis show that much IgE is specific for food or inhalant allergens (Church et al., 1976).

On the basis of current knowledge, it would appear prudent to try an elimination diet for a defined period (see Chapter 29), as an adjunct to appropriate skin care and other general measures, keeping in mind the child's nutritional needs for growth and development. At the end of a 4- or 6-week trial, a normal diet should be resumed unless there is substantial evidence that specific foods are important exacerbating factors.

Many studies have examined diet as a way of avoiding atopic dermatitis (Glaser and Johnstone, 1953; Johnstone and Dutton, 1966; Halpen, 1973; Mathew, 1977). These are discussed in Chapter 25.

In general, breast feeding, food avoidance, and elimination diets may be useful in the management of AD. Controlled studies examining the effects of these procedures on AD, however, are needed to clarify their role in therapy.

Environmental Control. Specific irritants and allergens should be eliminated from the home. The child allergic to house dust or animal danders can develop an exacerbation of dermatitis from direct contact with these factors. Details of environmental control are discussed in Chapter 22. Irritating and rough clothing, especially woolens, should be avoided, as should occlusive synthetic-fabric clothing, which may induce sweating and increased itching. Cold weather, hot, humid weather, or rapid temperature changes also may increase itching. Ointments with lanolin, perfume, or preservatives (e.g., parabens) are potential sensitizers and should be avoided. New clothing and sheets should be washed prior to use to remove sizing and other chemicals with which they may have been treated. Harsh enzymatic detergents should be avoided, and clothes rinsed thoroughly to eliminate residual detergent.

Often the patient scratches at night during sleep, and it may be necessary to apply cotton socks or gloves to reduce skin damage from scratching. Sleeping directly on plastic should be avoided and fingernails should be kept short.

A daily symptom-activity diary may be useful in identifying additional environmental factors that may have been overlooked in the initial evaluation. The reasons for these recommendations should be explained to parents and patients old enough to understand, and they should be encouraged to ask questions about them.

Psychologic Factors. Psychologic factors may play a role in certain patients with AD. No specific psychic disturbance or predisposition in a particular personality has been observed. Latent hostility, emotional lability, and maternal overprotection often exists. The constant pruritus, its disturbance of sleep of both patient and parent, and cosmetic impact all may induce somatopsychic symptoms. Further, emotional tension may increase pruritus. It is important for the physician to give friendly, sympathetic support to the parents and patient, with assurance that with appropriate care the dermatitis will not result in permanent disfigurement (see Chapter 26).

Allergy Injection Therapy. There is little evidence that allergy injection therapy (immunotherapy; hyposensitization) is helpful in controlling atopic dermatitis, although it may benefit those patients who have coexisting respiratory allergy. When used for this purpose in patients with AD, it should be administered cautiously since it may exacerbate the dermatitis if the antigen concentration is increased too rapidly, especially during the problematic pollen season.

Systemic Corticosteroids. Oral or intramuscular corticosteroids should be avoided in the treatment of children with atopic dermatitis. Whether they are *ever* justified is controversial. The authors of this chapter differ in opinion; Jacobs recommends against the use of corticosteroids in atopic dermatitis under any circumstance. Rachelefsky agrees with those physicians who feel that systemic corticosteroids are useful for a few specific indications, such as initial therapy of an acute exacerbation, clearing the skin sufficiently to perform skin testing, and controlling severe disease in order to begin effective topical therapy. The physician must be aware that the dermatitis frequently flares when systemic steroids are discontinued.

References

Anderson, E., and Hjorth, N.: B lymphocytes. T lymphocytes and phytohemagglutinin responsiveness in atopic dermatitis. Acta Derm. Venereol. 55:345, 1975.

Buckley, R. H.: Immunologic deficiency and allergic disease. In Middleton, E., Reed, C. E., Ellis, E. F. (eds.): Allergy — Principles and Practice. St. Louis, C. V. Mosby Co., 1978.

Busse, W. W., and Lee, T. P.: Decreased adrenergic responses in lymphocytes and granulocytes in atopic eczema. J. Allergy Clin. Immunol. 58:586, 1976.

Carapeto, F. J., Winkelmann, R. K., Jordon, R.: T and B lymphocytes in contact and atopic dermatitis. Arch. Dermatol. 112:1095, 1976.

Church, J. A., Kleban, D. G., and Bellanti, J. A.: Serum immunoglobulin E concentrations and radioallergosorbent tests in children. Pediatr. Res. 10(2):97, 1976.

Cotton, D. W. K., and Van Rossum, E.: Hexokinase, glucose-6-phosphate dehydrogenase and malate hydrogenase in the isolated sweat glands of normal and atopic subjects. Br. J. Dermatol. 89:459, 1973.

Fischer, T. J., Rachelefsky, G. S., Gard, W. E., and Stiehm, E. R.: Defective monocyte chemotaxis in atopic dermatitis. Ann. Allergy 38:308, 1977.

Furukawa, C. T.: Recent immunologic findings relating food allergy to atopic dermatitis. Ann. Allergy 42:207, 1979.

Glaser, J., and Johnstone, D. E.: Prophylaxis of allergic disease in newborn. JAMA 153:620, 1953.

Grove, D. I., Reid, J. G., and Forbes, I. J.: Humoral and cellular immunity in atopic eczema. Br. J. Dermatol. 92:611, 1975.

Halpern, S. R., Sellars, W. A., Johnson, R. B., Anderson, D. W., Saperstein, S., and Reisch, J. S.: Development of childhood allergy in infants fed breast, soy or cow milk. J. Allergy Clin. Immunol. 51:139, 1973.

Hanifin, J. M., and Gottlieb, B. R.: IgE inhibits T-cell rosette formation. Clin. Res. 22:328A, 1974.

Hanifin, J. M., and Lobitz, W. C.: Newer concepts of atopic dermatitis. Arch. Dermatol. 113:663, 1977.

Hanifin, J. M., and Rogge, J. L.: Staphylococcal infections in patients with atopic dermatitis. Arch. Dermatol. 113:1383, 1977.

Hanifin, J. M., Bauman, R., and Rogge, J. L.: Chemotaxis inhibition by plasma from patients with atopic dermatitis. Clin. Res. 27:198A, 1977.

Hemels, H. G. W. M.: The effect of propanolol on the acetylcholine-induced sweat response in atopic and non-atopic subjects. Br. J. Dermatol. 83:313, 1970.

Hoffman, D. R., Yamamoto, F. Y., Geller, B., Haddad, Z.: Specific IgE antibodies in atopic eczema. J. Allergy Clin. Immunol. 55:256, 1975.

Hovmark, A.: An in vitro study of depressed cell-mediated immunity and of T and B lymphocytes in atopic dermatitis. Acta Derm. Venereol. 57:237–242, 1977.

Johnstone, D. E., and Dutton, A. M.: Dietary prophylaxis of allergic disease in children. New Engl. J. Med. 274:715, 1966.

Juhlin, L., and Michaelsson, G.: Cutaneous vascular reactions to prostaglandins in healthy subjects and in patients with urticaria and atopic dermatitis. Acta Derm. Venereol. 49:251–262, 1969.

Kaufman, H. S., and Hobbs, J. R.: Immunoglobulin deficiencies in an atopic population. Lancet ii:1061, 1970.

Lobitz, W. C.: Atopic dermatitis. J. Dermatol. 3:39, 1976.

Luckasen, J. R., Sabad, A., Goltz, R. W., and Kersey, J. H.: T and B lymphocytes in atopic eczema. Arch. Derm. 110:375, 1974.

Mathew, D. J., Norman, A. P., Taylor, B., Turner, M. W., and Soothill, J. F.: Prevention of eczema. Lancet 1:321, 1977.

McAfee, D. A., and Greengard, P.: Andenosine 3'-5' monophosphate: Electrophysiological evidence for a role in synaptic transmission. Science 178:310, 1972.

McGeady, S. J., and Buckley, R. H.: Depression of cell-mediated immunity in atopic dermatitis. J. Allergy Clin. Immunol. 56:393, 1975.

Michaelsson, G.: Cutaneous reactions to kallikrein and prostaglandins in healthy and diseased skin. Thesis. Uppsala: Soderstrom and Finn, 1969.

Mihm, M. C., Soten, N. A., Dvorak, H. F., Austen, F. K.: The structure of normal skin and the morphology of atopic eczema. J. Invest. Dermatol. 67:305, 1976.

Rachelefsky, G. S., Opelz, G., Mickey, M. R., Kiuchi, M., Terasaki, P. F., Siegel, S. C., and Stiehm, E. R.: Defective T cell function in atopic dermatitis. J. Allergy Clin. Immunol. 57:569, 1976.

Rajka, G.: Prurigo Besnier (atopic dermatitis) with special reference to the role of allergic factors: II. The evaluation of the results of skin reactions. Acta Derm. Venereol. 41:1, 1961.

Reed, C. E., Busse, W. W., and Lee, T. P.: Adrenergic mechanisms and the adenyl cyclase system in atopic dermatitis. J. Invest. Dermatol. 67:333, 1976.

Rogge, J. L., and Hanifin, J. M.: Immunodeficiencies in severe atopic dermatitis. Arch. Dermatol. 112:1391, 1976.

Rosenthal, S. R.: Histamine as the chemical mediator for cutaneous pain. J. Invest. Dermatol. 69:47, 1977.

Synderman, R., Rogers, E., and Buckley, R. H.: Abnormalities of leukotaxis in atopic dermatitis. J. Allergy Clin. Immunol. 60:121, 1977.

Szentivanyi, A.: The beta-adrenergic theory of the atopic abnormality in bronchial asthma. J. Allergy 42:203, 1968.

Taylor, B., Norman, A. P., Orgel, H. A., Stokes, C. R., Turner, M. W., and Soothill, J. F.: Transient IgA deficiency and pathogenesis of infantile atopy. Lancet II:111, 1973.

Thestrup-Pedersen, K., Ellegaard, J., Thulin, H., and Zachariae, H.: PPD and mitogen responsiveness of lymphocytes from patients with atopic dermatitis. Clin. Exp. Immunol. 27:118, 1977.

Uehara, M.: Atopic dermatitis and tuberculin reactivity. Arch. Dermatol. 113:1226, 1977.

Frank Parker, M.D. # 32

Contact Dermatitis

PATHOGENESIS

Contact dermatitis is an inflammatory reaction of the skin which exhibits a characteristic histology. Its causes are numerous. When an external agent causes contact dermatitis, reactions occur as a result of one of two processes. If the external agent damages skin cells directly (e.g., damage from strong alkali and acids) an *irritant contact dermatitis* results. In contrast, the second process, *allergic contact dermatitis,* is an acquired immune reaction that results from contact with allergens (sensitizers), which are abundant in the environment. The immune reaction is cell-mediated (delayed-type hypersensitivity), in which contact chemicals act as haptens, combine with epidermal proteins, and form a complete antigen that induces sensitization. Upon repeat contact with the sensitizer, sensitized lymphocytes move into the

area of contact and induce an inflammatory reaction.

CLINICAL FEATURES AND PATHOLOGY

Though allergic sensitization can occur as soon as 7 to 10 days after first contact with the allergen, frequently it does not develop for many years. Once allergy develops and as long as it persists, subsequent encounters with the sensitizer produce dermatitis within 24 to 72 hours at any place on the skin where contact occurs.

It is difficult to differentiate allergic contact dermatitis from irritant dermatitis clinically and pathologically (Rosenberg, 1957). However, several features may help to distinguish between irritant and allergic contact reactions, as outlined in Table 32–1. Everyone exposed to an irritating sub-

TABLE 32–1 FACTORS HELPING TO DISTINGUISH BETWEEN IRRITANT AND ALLERGIC CONTACT DERMATITIS

	Irritant	Allergic
NUMBER OF PATIENTS AFFECTED	Many who come in contact	Few who come in contact
EXTENT OF DERMATITIS	Localized closely to areas of contact	Spread of dermatitis beyond exact areas of contact
TIME OF REACTION AFTER CONTACT	Within few hours of exposure	24–72 hours after exposure
SKIN REACTION	Red, scaling — if very acute, bullous Often painful	Often red and vesicular Itching common

stance in sufficient concentration will develop an irritant dermatitis, whereas only a small percentage of individuals exposed to the antigen will develop an allergic dermatitis.

Irritant reactions are localized in the precise area of contact. Moreover, an erythematous or bullous eruption occurs within a few hours of contact with the irritant, while the allergic contact reaction characteristically occurs 24 to 72 hours after exposure.

The acute phase of contact dermatitis, whether allergic or irritant, is characterized by redness, swelling, and the formation of papules due to vascular dilatation, perivascular infiltration of lymphocytes, and edema of the dermis. As the inflammatory reaction proceeds, intraepidermal edema (spongiosis) occurs, leading to vesicle formation. With disruption of vesicles, the skin weeps, oozes, and crusts (Fig. 32–1). Pruritus is an invariable and intolerable associated symptom, particularly of allergic

contact reactions. As the dermatitis becomes chronic, the skin becomes lichenified (leathery thickening with accentuation of skin lines), fissured, and scaly (Fig. 32–2).

Initially, allergic contact dermatitis is confined to the site of allergen contact, and indeed its unique distribution pattern often suggests the diagnosis of a contact reaction. Thus, reactions on ears, particularly the helix, may be due to shampoos or hair sprays. Otitis externa may be caused by sensitizing medications applied to the ear canals, particularly neomycin (Jensen, Allen, Mordecai, 1966) (see Fig. 32–1). Often, the piercing of earlobes is a precipitating factor in nickel sensitivity. The penis and scrotum may react to sensitizers conveyed to these areas by the hands. The vulvar and perivulvar areas may be sites of reaction to sensitizers in bubble baths. Reactions on the feet may be mediated by sensitivity to rubber substances, dyes, or

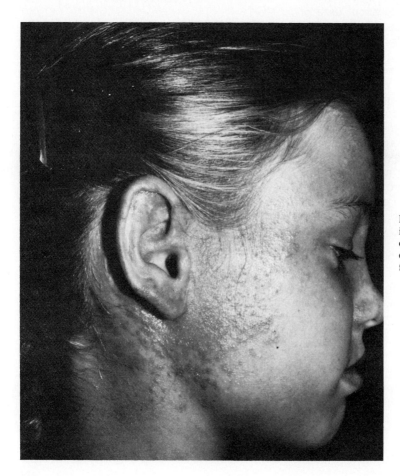

FIGURE 32–1. An acute, weeping dermatitis caused by allergic contact dermatitis to applications of a cream containing neomycin for otitis externa.

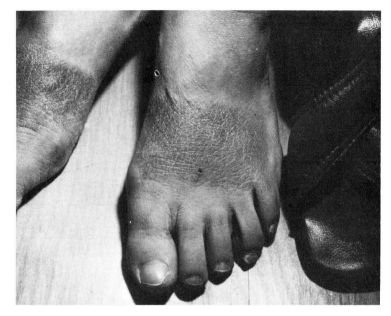

FIGURE 32–2. Chronic eczema, with lichenification of the skin. Note the sharp borders to the skin reaction, outlining the areas where sandal straps came in contact with the skin. This is an allergic contact dermatitis to paraphenylenediamine used in the leather.

metals used in the manufacture of shoes (see Fig. 32–2). In severe cases, the dermatitis initially localized to areas of allergen contact will disseminate over wide areas of the body (so-called "auto-eczematization"), so that the dermatitis may not conform precisely to areas of initial allergen contact (Parish, Rook, and Champion, 1963).

Occasionally, contact dermatitis may have a clinical appearance different from that just described (Fregert, 1974). Certain

TABLE 32–2 THE SIX MOST COMMON SENSITIZERS

1. Rhus: poison ivy, oak or sumac

2. Paraphenylenediamine: a chemical used in hair and fur dyes, leather processing, rubber vulcanizing and printing inks which cross-reacts with azo and aniline dyes, "caine" preparations and sulfonamides

3. Nickel compounds

4. Rubber compounds

5. Ethylenediamine: commonly used as a preservative in various cream medications such as Mycolog cream (but not Mycolog ointment), antihistaminic creams and ophthalmic solutions

6. Dichromates used in textile inks, paints and leather processing (Fisher, 1973)

rubber chemicals can cause a purpura-like dermatitis. Zirconium and beryllium can cause a granulomatous dermatitis. Certain contactants, particularly neomycin and nickel, have been reported to produce a "dermal" contact reaction in which the eczematous element is absent, but an edematous, urticaria-like inflammation occurs.

The six most common sensitizers causing allergic contact dermatitis are noted in Table 32–2. Certain topical medications that produce sensitization in adults, such as mercury, benzocaine, and antihistaminics, also produce dermatitis in children. Often, concentrations of medications that are not sensitizing in adults produce dermatitis in children.

Many household substances, including polishes, waxes, solvents, detergents, disinfectants, and insecticides, are potent irritants. Highly perfumed oils, toilet soaps, and powders also can cause a dermatitis, especially in body folds where these preparations may accumulate. For this reason, the use of nonperfumed oils, powders, and soaps free of antiseptics is recommended for infants. Further, when the infant begins to crawl, dermatitis of the legs, knees, and elbows can develop as a result of exposure to floor wax or polish, rough rug fabrics, and dust. Coveralls prevent these reactions.

TYPES OF CONTACT DERMATITIS

Diaper Dermatitis

Diaper dermatitis, the most common form of dermatitis in infancy, presents as erythema or, in severe cases, papulovesicular areas or even eroded bullae over the external genitalia and buttocks that become secondarily infected, often sparing the creases. The eruption can spread to include the lower half of the abdomen and thighs. In male infants, the reaction may occur as a urethral meatal ulcer, causing painful urination.

Diaper dermatitis is produced by prolonged contact with urine or feces or by residual antiseptics, soaps, or detergents in the diapers. Many authorities have implicated ammonia produced by bacteria in the urine and stool as the irritative substance, but this mechanism of diaper rash has probably been overemphasized (Jacobs, 1978).

The management of diaper dermatitis includes frequent changes of diapers, with careful cleaning of the skin with mild soap and water to rid the skin of urine and feces. Occlusive plastic clothing materials over diapers should be avoided. The new types of diapers with inner linings of synthetic hydrophobic fibers that allow passage of urine to the outer cotton layers keep the skin relatively dry and free of urine. When the diaper area is severely inflamed, the skin can be cleaned with mineral or olive oil rather than soap and water. Topical steroids, such as 1 percent hydrocortisone cream several times a day, and frequent use of a thick protective paste such as zinc oxide ointment will decrease the inflammatory response and protect the inflamed skin from direct contact with urine and feces. Occasionally, if 1 percent hydrocortisone cream does not cause improvement in the dermatitis, stronger fluorinated topical steroid preparations can be used two to three times a day for short periods of time (5 to 7 days), but longer use may cause severe dermal atrophy and stria formation and possibly may cause systemic effects by steroid absorption through the inflamed skin.

Other causes of diaper dermatitis include moniliasis, seborrheic dermatitis, impetigo, atopic dermatitis, and psoriasis. In general, when the eruption involves sites of the most intimate contact with the diaper such as the convexities of the buttocks, medial thighs and perineum, with sparing of the folds, contact dermatitis is the likely cause. In infancy, irritant dermatitis is most common, whereas contact allergy becomes more likely after infancy. Sharply demarcated rashes in the folds suggest intertrigo due to sweat retention, heat and moisture, often with secondary bacterial infection. Seborrheic dermatitis often manifests in this way and can be diagnosed if "cradle cap" is found, together with an erythematous rash in the axillae, neck folds, and the retroauricular areas. If satellite, erythematous-based pustules are seen studding the borders of the lesions in the folds, candida infection is likely. A band of erythema at the margins of the diapers, so-called "tide mark" dermatitis, is characteristic of an irritant reaction to recurring wetting and drying at the borders of the diapers. Large vesicles and bullae in the diaper area often are due to bullous impetigo.

Foot Dermatitis

Dermatitis of the feet may be due to allergic sensitization to ingredients in the shoes, particularly rubber (monobenzyl ether of hydroquinone, an antioxidant; tetramethylthiuram, an accelerator), leather (potassium dichromate and formaldehyde, tanning agents, or paraphenylenediamine used in dyeing leather), or metals used in the box toes of shoes (nickel sulfate). Most frequently, shoe dermatitis begins on the dorsal aspect of the big toe with eventual extension to other toes and then onto the feet, with sparing of the interdigital webs (see Fig. 32–2).

In children, eczematous reactions on the feet often are not allergic contact reactions but are related to friction of tight-fitting shoes or to excessive perspiration, in which case the eruption often is seen on the toes and interweb areas, owing to maceration from unabsorbed sweat (Fisher, 1973; Gibson, 1963).

Another common eczematous foot reaction seen in children is chronic scaling and fissuring over the soles of the feet and toes, related to atopic dermatitis. Although tinea pedis can mimic eczematous reactions, fungal infections of the feet are unusual in young, prepubertal children.

Contact dermatitis of the feet must be diagnosed by appropriate patch tests. If identified, the allergens may be avoided by wearing cotton liners, surgitube or Kellenex inside shoes or square toe socks.* If this mechanical protection does not help, special shoes made to order, free of the specific allergens, can be purchased.†

Allergic contact dermatitis of the feet will respond to topical fluorinated steroid ointments several times a day, with occlusive plastic wrapping at night. This increases the humidity under the wraps, accelerating the penetration of topical steroids. Frequent use of emollients between the steroid applications prevents dryness and fissuring.

Clothing Dermatitis

Contact dermatitis in children can be caused by woolen clothing or rough cuffs and collars, which, when wet, readily irritate the skin. Residues of soap and detergents in laundered clothes also can cause an irritant dermatitis. Children's flame resistant night clothing and wash and wear clothes that contain formaldehyde resins may produce dermatitis in areas of increased sweating, particularly in the axillae, sides of the neck, antecubital fossae, and inguinal areas.

Often, formaldehyde resin patch tests are nonreactive in sensitized children. Patch testing with small pieces of the suspected fabric may be more accurate.

Once it is determined that clothing dermatitis is produced by specific wearing apparel, these clothes should be avoided. New clothing made of 100 percent polyester, acrylic, or cotton usually is well tolerated. The additional use of topical steroids

and emollients will bring the dermatitis readily under control.

Soap and Detergent Dermatitis

Subacute primary irritant dermatitis usually is brought about by prolonged bubble baths, too frequent bathing, use of excessive amounts of bubble bath concentrations, or a combination of these factors. Children with atopic dermatitis who normally tend to have xerotic skin often are severely affected. They should use soaps containing added oils, and use emollients liberally to treat this form of dermatitis.

Cosmetic and Medication Dermatitis

Infants and children may acquire cosmetic dermatitis by contact with cosmetics worn by the mother and other attendants or applied in play; adolescent girls may experiment with a broad range of cosmetics. Perfumes, lipstick, nail polish, and hair dyes all can cause allergic reactions, which can be identified with patch tests to the various suspected substances. The physician should alert the patient with a suspected contact allergy to cosmetics of allergenic substances that may be found in cosmetics. Patch tests to prove these suspicions should be done, and the patient should then avoid cosmetics with the specific substances in them. Many times these are listed on the cosmetics; the trend is toward manufacturers being required to list the various materials used in each cosmetic. If ingredients are not listed, it may be necessary to write specific manufacturers to determine if an offending substance is used in their cosmetic line. Aside from paraphenylenediamine hair dyes, preparations containing formaldehyde or its resins, and cosmetics containing parabens or photosensitizers, the bulk of cosmetics in general use are "hypoallergic," since the products have been carefully screened before being marketed.

The application of various over-the-counter and prescription topical medications to cuts, scratches, bites, or sunburn can induce allergic contact dermatitis. Common offending substances in these topical preparations include various "caine" substances (benzocaine, surfacaine, metycaine), antihistamines (Antistine, Benadryl,

*Tru Last, purchased from J. W. Landenberger and Co., 3800 Caster Avenue, Philadelphia, Pennsylvania 19124.

†Foot-So-Port Shoe Company, Oconomowoc, Wisconsin 53066 or Julius Alfschul, Inc., 117–125 Graltan Street, Brooklyn, New York 11237.

and Pyribenzamine), antibiotics (especially penicillin, streptomycin, and neomycin), and medications containing ethylenediamine.

Local anesthetics, especially benzocaine, found in a variety of anti-itch, anti-sunburn and anti–poison oak preparations are particularly potent sensitizers and readily cross-react with paraphenylenediamine (dye), sulfonamides, and azo dyes, as well as with para-aminobenzoic acid (PABA), found in such preparations as sunscreening agents. Xylocaine (lidocaine) and Carbocaine (mepivacaine) are not related to the other "caines" and do not commonly cause contact dermatitis.

Topical antihistamines also cause allergic dermatitis, whereas oral antihistaminics seldom cause sensitization. However, if the patient was previously sensitized topically, oral antihistaminics may cause a generalized skin reaction. The common use of calamine lotion with Benadryl added (Caladryl) is to be condemned, as this frequently causes contact allergic reactions. The antihistamines Antistine, Phenergan, and Pyribenzamine are ethylenediamine derivatives and are particularly active topical sensitizers.

Ethylenediamine is one of the most common skin sensitizers in the United States. It is found in Mycolog Cream, a medication that should be avoided, but is not found in Mycolog Ointment (Fisher, 1973). It also is present in many ophthalmic solutions and may be a common cause of contact dermatitis of the eyelids. Ethylenediamine cross-reacts with aminophylline (a combination of theophylline and ethylenediamine). The administration of aminophylline to patients previously topically sensitized to ethylenediamine causes generalized dermatitis, though these persons tolerate theophylline without reaction.

Topical antibiotics, particularly penicillin, neomycin, and streptomycin, are potent sensitizers (Rees, 1964). Penicillin and streptomycin never should be used topically. Neomycin is present in a host of creams, ointments, and other topical medications as well as in some cosmetics and soaps (Epstein, 1958). Once a person is topically sensitized to neomycin, systemic administration of streptomycin or kanamycin — both of which cross-react with

neomycin — may cause a generalized dermatitis (Epstein and Wenzel, 1962). Neomycin commonly induces sensitization when applied for otitis externa (Fig. 32–1). Erythromycin rarely induces topical sensitization and can be used safely on the skin.

The parabens, which are substances commonly added to topical creams for their bacteriostatic and antioxidant preservative action, also frequently cause allergic contact dermatitis. These substances are found in some topical steroid creams and lotions (but not ointments), emollients, and antimicrobial creams. At times, sensitization to parabens in steroid creams may result in an exacerbation of the dermatitis. As a result, the patient or the physician may apply increasing amounts of the steroid cream, setting up a vicious cycle and inducing an intense dermatitis. The physician should always inquire as to what the patient or the patient's parents have been applying to any dermatitis!

Plant Dermatitis

Poison ivy, sumac, and oak are common causes of allergic contact dermatitis in children. Poison ivy (Rhus) dermatitis is a summer disease caused by contact with the oleoresin of the plant. Frequently pets, particularly long-haired dogs, contact the plant and transmit the oleoresin to the child. Ingestion of poison oak oleoresin or marked cutaneous involvement may induce acute nephritis. Often, the streaks of dermatitis where the plant has rubbed against the skin suggest the diagnosis (Fig. 32–3).

Vicks Vaporub contains several plant substances (oil of turpentine, oil of eucalyptus, and oil of cedar) that may irritate or sensitize a child's skin.

Topical steroids usually will control plant dermatitis, but in severe and extensive cases a short course of oral steroids may be necessary.

Perioral Dermatitis

In children, the lips and adjacent skin are commonly irritated. Often this is caused by a habit of licking. Saliva trapped between the thumb and mouth of a thumb-sucking

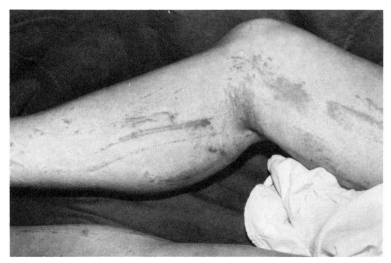

FIGURE 32–3. An acute contact dermatitis on the legs. Note the "lines" of erythema and vesicles where the leaves of the poison ivy plant brushed along the legs of this sensitive individual.

child may produce a dermatitis of the lips and cheeks. Likewise, children who are salivating because of tooth formation or eruption may suffer with a facial dermatitis. Children whose eating habits permit foods such as spinach, carrots, and citrus fruits to remain on the cheeks may suffer from a perioral dermatitis due to the irritation by food juices. This dermatitis may closely resemble atopic eczema. Rubber-sensitive children may acquire a perioral dermatitis from chewing rubber pencil erasers or rubber bands.

Topical 1 percent hydrocortisone cream and adherent pastes such as zinc oxide will clear the dermatitis and serve as a protective barrier to saliva or irritating fluids.

Atopic Dermatitis and Contact Dermatitis

Rarely, atopic infants who are allergic to eggs or fish acquire marked edema, urticaria, and flare of the atopic eczema of the skin or oral mucosa from contact with the foods to which they are allergic. Although children with atopic dermatitis are no more likely to develop contact dermatitis to potential sensitizers than other children (indeed, there is some evidence that such children are less readily sensitized to topical substances), they often develop contact allergic reactions because they are exposed

so frequently to topical medications during their long course of therapy. It is important that the physician caring for these patients not use potential sensitizers and that the patients and their parents be warned about the use of proprietary medications containing substances that carry a high risk of sensitization. They especially should avoid the use of topical antibiotics (neomycin, particularly Mycolog Cream), antihistaminics, ethylenediamine, and paraben-containing medications.

DIAGNOSIS AND TREATMENT

Patch Testing

The patch test is indispensable in proving the cause of allergic contact dermatitis. However, it should not be performed when the dermatitis is acute, or when there is extensive skin involvement, since under these circumstances the patch test may cause a general exacerbation of the dermatitis. Systemic corticosteroid therapy, even in doses sufficient to suppress the dermatitis, will not completely suppress a strongly positive patch test, so that patients can be patch-tested reliably while receiving oral steroids (O'Quinn and Isbell, 1969). Similarly, oral antihistaminics do not significantly influence the patch-test reaction. However, topical corticosteroids can be suppressive

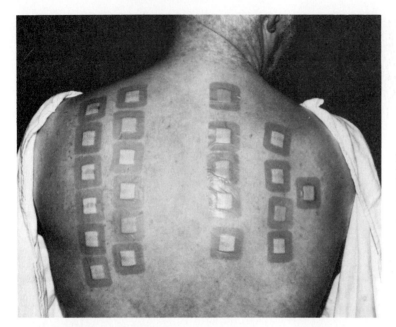

FIGURE 32–4. A series of patch tests in place over the upper back.

and should be avoided in the area of patch testing for several days before testing.

Patch testing is performed by applying standard and suspected antigens on gauze and adhesive strips such as Band-Aids to the back, where they should be kept in place for 48 hours (Fig. 32–4). Tests are read 20 minutes after removing the patches. As a rule, the site of a positive reaction itches and appears as vesicles on an edematous red base, exactly outlining the area covered by the allergen (Fig. 32–

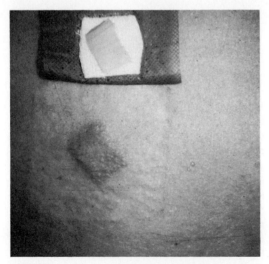

FIGURE 32–5. A 3+ positive patch test reaction showing erythema, papules, and vesicles of the skin, precisely mimicking the eczematous reaction.

5). When there is a questionable reaction, such as mild erythema, it is worthwhile reexamining the site 72 to 96 hours later (Fisher, 1973). Redness that persists or increases probably signifies an allergic reaction. Erythema that fades in 24 hours is most likely not due to an allergic reaction. The following grading system is conventional:

No erythema	0
Erythema	1+
Erythema and papules	2+
Erythema, papules and vesicles	3+
Marked edema and vesicles	4+

Positive patch tests may be due to irritants, but in general, irritants burn rather than itch, and they induce a skin reaction sooner than do sensitizers. Strong irritants can cause a reaction in a few hours. A primary irritant reaction tends to remain confined to the site of application and fades rapidly after the site has been uncovered, while allergic reactions tend to spread beyond the site, persist and even become more intense for several days after the patch is removed.

Treatment of Contact Dermatitis

After the diagnosis of an acute contact dermatitis is made by patch testing, the offending antigen(s) and any substances that cross-react with the antigen should be removed from the patient's environment.

The dermatitis is treated to control the inflammation and itching. Topical steroids and, in cases of severe widespread reactions, oral steroids are begun immediately. In addition, application of cool wet compresses (with water or Burow's solution, 1:20 dilution) for 25 minutes three times a day in the acute, vesicular, oozing, and weeping stages of the dermatitis rapidly dries up the vesicles and oozing, relieves itching, and debrides and cleans the skin surface. In the chronic phases, when the dermatitis is dry, thickened and fissured, topical steroid ointments and emollients used between steroid applications will resolve the inflammation and alleviate the dryness.

Oral antipruritic medications such as hydroxyzine, cyproheptadine, or diphenhydramine hydrochloride all are useful in helping to control the intolerable itching associated with the dermatitis. Secondary infection (impetiginization) of the dermatitis is a common finding; if present, it should be treated with appropriate systemic antibiotics.

References

Epstein, S.: Dermal contact dermatitis from neomycin. Ann. Allergy 16:268, 1958.

Epstein, S., and Wenzel, F. J.: Cross sensitivity to various "mycins." Arch. Derm. 86:183, 1962.

Fisher, A. A.: Contact Dermatitis, 2nd ed. Lea & Febiger, Philadelphia, 1973.

Fisher, A. A., et al.: Contact dermatitis due to ingredients of vehicles. Arch. Derm. 104:286, 1971.

Fregert, S.: Manual of contact dermatitis. Munksgaard, Copenhagen, 1974.

Gibson, W. B.: Sweaty sock dermatitis. Clin. Pediatr. 2:175, 1963.

Jacobs, A. H.: Eruptions in the diaper area. Pediatr. Clin. of North Am. 25:209, 1978.

Jensen, C. O., Allen, H. J., and Mordecai, L. R.: Neomycin contact dermatitis superimposed on otitis externa. J.A.M.A., 195:1975, 1966.

O'Quinn, S. E., and Isbell, K. H.: Influence of oral prednisone on eczematous patch test reactions. Arch. Derm. 99:380, 1969.

Parish, W. E., Rook, A. J., and Champion, R. H.: A study of auto-immune allergy in generalized eczema. Br. J. Dermatol. 77:479, 1963.

Rees, B. R.: Cutaneous reactions to antibiotics. J.A.M.A., 189:685, 1964.

Rosenberg, A., Jr.: Primary irritant and allergic eczematous reactions. Arch. Derm. 75:547, 1957.

33

Gail G. Shapiro, M.D.

Urticaria and Angioedema

Urticaria ("hives") is a pruritic eruption characterized by erythematous, edematous wheals of various sizes which blanch when pressed. The eruption is migratory. An individual wheal lasts from minutes to no more than 48 hours. However, urticarial lesions may recur in crops for an indefinite period of time (in some cases, years). Physiologically, the urticarial eruption mimics the triple response described by Sir Thomas Lewis: initial vasodilatation results in erythema, which is followed by increased vascular permeability and edema (or "wheal") formation and further erythema (or "flare") due to axon reflex vasodilatation. Though various mediators have been implicated in urticaria, histamine is the only mediator that has been shown to induce a pruritic erythematous wheal and is the only mediator universally accepted as a causative agent. Histologically urticaria is characterized by dilatation of small blood vessels and by edema which results in flattened rete pegs, widened dermal papillae, and separation of collagen bundles and fibers in the superficial dermis. There is minimal perivascular cellular infiltration. Angioedema is a similar reaction but confined to the deeper dermis and subcutaneous tissue. Since both urticaria and angioedema are concomitants of the same physiologic reaction, they are discussed together.

The incidence of urticaria and angioedema is extremely high. Over 20 percent of the population has had hives at some time (Mathews, 1974). Acute urticaria may occur in any age group and is the type most often seen in children. Chronic urticaria (urticaria that persists for 3 months or more) is more common in young adults than in children and adolescents.

Acute urticaria usually can be controlled symptomatically with antihistamine drugs and elimination of inciting factors (based on history). Often it is self-limited, and no underlying cause can be identified. The probability of identifying an underlying cause of chronic urticaria is much less than for acute urticaria. In the experience of most allergists, an underlying cause for chronic urticaria can be identified in fewer than half the cases.

The physician can deal with urticaria most successfully by having an appreciation of the basic mechanisms that can induce it and by employing a diagnostic approach that is thorough without being unnecessarily costly.

MECHANISMS

Histamine is a major mediator of urticaria, but whether it is the only mediator capable of inducing full-blown urticaria is not clear. Histamine is released from mast cells through a variety of immune and non-immune mechanisms. An important immune mechanism is Type I hypersensitivity, mediated by IgE and possibly some IgG_4 antibodies bound to mast cells which may interact with antigens causing histamine release. Urticaria resulting from Type I reactions is the easiest to investigate, since the reaction occurs shortly (frequently within minutes) after allergen contact,

440

and a good history often will identify the offending substance.

Activation of either the classic or alternative complement pathways may cause urticaria through the production of anaphylatoxins. The classic pathway is activated by antigen-antibody reactions involving IgM or IgG antibody. The alternative pathway can be activated by polysaccharides, by lipopolysaccharides (e.g., bacterial endotoxins), and possibly by dyes, drugs, and antigen-IgA complexes. Urticaria related to immune complex disease and to infectious diseases probably results at least in part from complement activation.

Some drugs induce the release of histamine by acting directly on the mast cell or indirectly through nonimmune pathways. Aspirin, indomethacin, and related drugs are thought to block prostaglandin synthetase, which decreases intracellular prostaglandin levels in mastocytes, thus altering mastocyte stability and facilitating histamine release (Szczeklik et al., 1977). Physical agents such as heat, light, and pressure may cause urticaria in some individuals by a variety of mechanisms (Chapter 34). Bradykinin, a product of blood coagulation, and other kinins are potent vasodilators capable of increasing vascular permeability. Though, unlike histamine, kinins do not cause pruritus, they may contribute to urticaria by increasing vascular permeability. The importance of kinin system activation, either alone or in conjunction with histamine release, remains undefined. Defective protease inhibitor levels have been found in some individuals with chronic urticaria, suggesting that this absence may encourage the generation of anaphylatoxins and kinins that cause or modulate urticaria (Doeglas and Bleumink, 1975). SRS-A (slow reacting substance of anaphylaxis), liberated by IgE-dependent mechanisms, also may contribute to the production of urticaria.

It should be clear that urticaria is a final common pathway for a variety of immune and nonimmune reactions. Although the mechanism of mediator release and production of urticaria can be identified in some cases, often both the causative agent and underlying pathogenesis of urticaria are unknown. Urticaria is not limited to atopic individuals; rather, it occurs frequently in nonallergic individuals.

CAUSES OF URTICARIA

Major etiologic factors producing urticaria can be categorized as follows:

Foods
Drugs
Inhalant allergens
Physical agents
Insect bites
Infectious disease
Noninfectious systemic disease
Hereditary conditions
Psychic factors

Foods. Various foods, most commonly eggs, peanuts, berries, fish, and shellfish, induce hives by IgE-mediated mechanisms. Frequently, the offending food is easily identified by history, since the reaction generally occurs immediately or a short time after the food is ingested. Food dyes such as tartrazine and benzoate derivatives also may induce hives through nonimmune mechanisms. With tartrazine, this reaction may be related to effects on prostaglandin synthetase as noted for aspirin-related drugs.

Drugs. Drugs that most commonly cause urticaria are penicillin, sulfonamides, aspirin, insulin, vaccines, and allergenic extracts. Allergic reactions may be immediate, within minutes to an hour of exposure, or may occur hours or days or weeks after exposure, depending on the mechanism involved. Aspirin and related compounds such as tartrazine (used to color medications and foods), indomethacin, and most of the anti-inflammatory drugs used in rheumatic diseases (Szczeklik et al., 1977) can produce or aggravate urticaria, possibly through inhibition of prostaglandin synthetase, as described before. Other drugs that release histamine by direct action on mast cells include morphine, meperidine (Demerol), codeine, polymyxin, tubocurarine, and stilbamidine. Drugs and antisera prepared from animals can induce a serum-sickness syndrome that includes urticaria.

Inhalants. Inhalant allergens infrequently cause urticaria. Occasionally an atopic individual may develop hives by walking in tall grass, or being licked by a dog, owing to direct skin contact with substances to which he or she is allergic. There usually is an obvious history for this type of exposure, and allergic respiratory symptoms frequently accompany urticaria. Urticaria can be a component of inhalant-induced anaphylaxis.

Physical Agents. Cold, light, and heat are capable of inducing hives in certain individuals. Urticaria induced by heat, emotional stress, and physical exertion is known as "cholinergic urticaria." These physical agents may cause urticaria in a variety of ways. Urticaria due to physical agents is discussed in detail in Chapter 34.

Pest Bites. Of special importance in childhood is the hive-like reaction to biting insects such as fleas or to bites by mites (chiggers or jiggers) or the larvae of a duck and snail parasite (swimmer's itch). This reaction — characterized by papules, vesicles, and hives — is known as papular urticaria and must be differentiated from true urticaria. The eruption typically is located on uncovered skin surfaces such as the extremities, and the lesions remain localized rather than migrating as in true urticaria. The eruption is an allergic (? type IV) reaction to the proteins of the pest's oral secretion or of the pest itself, and it resolves only after the offending organisms are eliminated.

Infectious Disease. Viral infections are common causes of acute urticaria in children and adolescents. Viruses may activate the classic or alternative complement cascade directly to produce anaphylatoxins, or indirectly when cleared by the host's antiviral antibodies. Several viral infections are known to be associated with urticaria, including infectious hepatitis, infectious mononucleosis, certain Coxsackie virus infections (Mathews, 1974), and infections by some strains of mycoplasma.

Parasites known to elicit urticaria are ascarids, ancylostomes, strongyles, filariae, echinococci, schistosomes, trichinae, *Toxocara* species, and *Fasciola* species (Warin and Champion, 1974).

Scattered case reports associate urticaria with candidal and tinea infections and with bacterial "foci of infection" (dental abscess and sinusitis). However, there is no proof that these associations are more than coincidental (Mathews, 1978). Systemic staphylococcal infection appears capable of inducing urticaria. There also is suggestive data relating beta hemolytic streptococcal infection to acute but not to chronic urticaria.

Noninfectious Systemic Disorders. Many systemic illnesses may be accompanied by urticaria. Rheumatic disorders, particularly systemic lupus erythematosus, and necrotizing vasculitis are accompanied by urticaria-like lesions. However, these lesions histologically have more marked perivascular infiltration as well as damage to the vessel wall and are a form of vasculitis. The rash associated with juvenile rheumatoid arthritis may be misinterpreted as urticarial and may be present for several weeks before other signs or symptoms of the disease are noted. Urticaria may accompany lymphoreticular malignancy. In adults, urticaria may occur with carcinoma of the colon, rectum, or lung. However, urticaria is rarely, if ever, the presenting complaint in an individual who does not show signs of the primary disease.

Urticaria occurring with hyperthyroidism and urticarial exacerbations with menses suggest a relationship between endocrine imbalance and urticaria.

Urticaria pigmentosa, or mast cell infiltration of the skin, may be so widespread as to cause a total marbelized coloration of the body by brownish pigmented mast cells that occur in large masses. Mast cell infiltration may be apparent as an isolated lesion only. Typically, trauma to the collections of mast cells causes redness and urticaria, as the mast cells release histamine upon pressure. Both the generalized form of mast cell infiltration known as systemic mastocytosis (in which various organs besides skin are involved, especially GI tract and bone marrow) and the widespread cutaneous form (urticaria pigmentosa) are recognized in early childhood. Patients with isolated mast cell infiltrations may grow into adulthood without having a physician recognize the unusual nature of their "birthmark."

Chronic urticaria may accompany selective IgA deficiency in pediatric patients (Buckley and Dees, 1967). Since secretory IgA acts to prevent penetration of foreign antigen, its deficiency may permit urticariogenic antigens to enter the circulation more readily than normal (Bonifazi et al., 1977). Other immunoglobulin deficiencies have been noted in patients with urticaria and recurrent infection (Buckley and Dees, 1967).

Hereditary Disorders. Several rare inherited disorders that are associated with urticaria include familial forms of cold and heat urticaria and vibratory angioedema.

Alpha-1-antitrypsin deficiency and decreased antichymotrypsin activity have been reported in some cases of cold urticaria and idiopathic angioedema (Doeglas and Bleumink, 1975). Urticaria may be associated with a syndrome of amyloidosis, severe deafness, and limb pain. Hereditary angioedema, while rare, is the most common of the inherited conditions. While it is usually discussed in the context of urticaria and angioedema, it is a disease unrelated to histamine release. Since its mechanism and characteristics are unique, it will be discussed in a separate section.

Psychologic Factors. Though frequently implicated in the etiology of and often associated with chronic urticaria, tension and anxiety are not clearly the cause and may be the result of the disease. Many authors have related waxing and waning of urticaria to emotional states. Psychologic factors certainly contribute to recalcitrant hives, whether or not they caused them.

DIAGNOSTIC EVALUATION

The physician must remember to prescribe appropriate medication to control hives while investigating possible causes and ways of eliminating the condition. At the onset, the physician should reassure the patients that urticaria is rarely if ever the sole presenting sign of a serious, life-threatening problem. Acute urticaria that is not associated with angioedema or respiratory compromise is self-limited and generally does not require extensive evaluation. History and physical examination usually identify obvious problems. The diagnostic approach is noted in Table 33–1.

History

A detailed history is of paramount importance. New drug and food ingestion must be sought carefully; the physician must remember to ask about commonly overlooked products such as aspirin, vitamins, cold remedies, laxatives, gums, toothpastes, food colorings, and additives such as tartrazine or benzoates. Recent immuniza-

TABLE 33–1 DIAGNOSIS OF CHRONIC URTICARIA

General

Detailed history and food diary
Physical examination
Laboratory studies
    Complete blood count and differential sedimentation rate
    C_3, C_4, CH_{50}
    ANA
    IgG, A, M
    SGOT, SGPT
    T_4
    Monospot test
    Urinalysis
Challenge with physical agents

Add, in Specific Situations

Food elimination and challenge
Allergy skin tests
Examination of stool for ova and parasites
Roentgenograms of foci of infection suggested by physical examination
Skin biopsy
Culture for ova and parasites, bacteria or fungi as appropriate

tions or injections of any kind should be looked for, and the patient should be questioned about recent acquisitions including plants, animals, and stuffed furniture. Possible relationships of the hives to physical agents, insects, systemic disease, and hereditary conditions should be investigated. While taking the history, the physician can gain some insight into the patient's emotional state and explore the possible psychologic components of the disease.

A 2 to 4 week food-symptom diary can be a helpful diagnostic tool. IgE-mediated urticaria usually occurs within minutes or hours after contact with an inciting allergen. By keeping a record of the relationship of ingested foods and other contactants to hive outbreaks, offending factors may be identified.

Physical Examination

The physician should look for any possible association of urticaria with other disease states, such as infection, rheumatic disease, or neoplasm, and for signs of allergic disease such as hay fever, eczema, or asthma. The character of the hives may give important diagnostic clues. For instance, yellow hives may occur with viral hepatitis; persistent lower extremity vesicles and papules occur with papular (insect-related) urticaria; minute intensely pruritic wheals with large areas of surrounding erythema are characteristic of cholinergic urticaria; pigmented skin that urticates on pressure is indicative of urticaria pigmentosa; and the edema of hereditary angioedema characteristically is nonpruritic (Mathews, 1974).

Elimination and Challenge

Occasionally the patient and physician become concerned about the relevance of foods or additives in the pathogenesis of urticaria and are unable to clearly establish a cause and effect relationship by history or by means of the food diary. The only way either to prove or to dispel concern over a possible association is with a strict elimination diet, during which the patient is allowed to eat one freshly prepared meat, grain, fruit, and vegetable for an entire week. If hives continue to appear, an alternate choice from each family of food can be selected. If hives still continue, it is unlikely that foods or additives are important. On the other hand, if the hives cease, new foods can be added one at a time at 2 to 3 day intervals until the hives reappear.

The final proof is a challenge with the supposed offending substance in a quantity that would ordinarily be consumed. If a food diary suggests an offending food or drug, direct challenge can be tried during a quiescent interval in the course of the urticaria and should provoke an exacerbation if there is a cause-effect relationship.

Laboratory Tests

If the history and physical examination fail to uncover the cause of chronic urticaria and angioedema, laboratory studies should be performed to rule out systemic diseases that may be associated with hives. These tests usually are negative, but they will reassure both physician and patient that the hives are not caused by serious disease.

Allergy skin testing is of dubious value as a general test in urticaria. When urticaria is caused by allergy, the history usually will identify the offending food or drug. When factors such as pollens cause urticaria, there should be a history of direct exposure and, generally, associated respiratory symptoms. Skin testing may be helpful in ruling out penicillin allergy or extreme sensitivity to a food prior to an oral challenge.

A complete blood count, differential white blood cell count, and erythrocyte sedimentation rate are useful in evaluating the patient for infection, noninfectious rheumatic systemic disease, and leukemic processes. If the history suggests parasitic infestation or if the patient has significant eosinophilia, stool specimens should be examined for ova and parasites. A urinalysis should be performed to rule out infectious and inflammatory disease states. Complement assays for C3, C4, and total hemolytic complement should be performed to rule out rheumatic disease with immune complex formation, and an antinuclear antibody test performed to rule out systemic lupus erythematosus. A monospot test will help identify or rule out infectious mononucleosis; the SGOT and SGPT, anicteric hepatitis; and T4, hyperthroidism. Since a variety of immunoglobulin abnormalities such as selective IgA deficiency have been found in adults and children with urticaria, quantitative immunoglobulin levels should be performed.

If the history or the physical examination suggests an infectious etiology of the urticaria, certain cultures or diagnostic radiology may be indicated. A throat culture or streptozyme test can be used to determine whether there is a beta hemolytic streptococcal infection, for example. It should be noted that cases of dental abscesses and sinus infections associated with urticaria are anecdotal reports.

Challenges with physical agents such as cold are simple measures that may provide a great deal of information (see Chapter 34). Skin biopsies may occasionally be helpful in diagnosing unusual forms of vasculitis that present as chronic urticaria. In adults, a skin biopsy diagnosed a subgroup of patients with urticarial-like lesions due to necrotizing vasculitis (Soter, 1977). Many of these patients had arthritis and arthralgia, abnormal sedimentation rate, and abnormal complement levels. There is no known pediatric counterpart of the syndrome.

TREATMENT

Initial therapy with appropriate drugs provides symptomatic relief while the cause is investigated. In acute severe urticaria, an injection of subcutaneous epinephrine (1:1000 epinephrine hydrochloride, 0.01 ml/kg [ml per kg of body weight] up to 0.3 ml total volume) usually provides immediate temporary relief. This should be followed with oral antihistamines administered around the clock, either by frequent dosing or with timed release preparations. Hydroxyzine (Atarax, Vistaril), diphenhydramine (Benadryl), cyproheptadine (Periactin), and azatadine maleate (Optimine) are among the more effective antihistamines for hives. Diphenhydramine (Benadryl) is recommended in a dosage of 1.25 mg/kg q 6 hr. Hydroxyzine, 10 to 25 mg every 6 hours, is particularly effective for cholinergic urticaria. Cyproheptadine, 2 to 4 mg orally four times daily, and azatadine maleate (Optimine), 1 to 2 mg every 6 to 8 hrs, tend to be effective for cold urticaria. Optimal dosage depends on the individual patient's tolerance and the beneficial effects produced. Initial dosages should be increased gradually until hives are controlled or until such side effects as drowsiness become intolerable. Unfortunately, since little is known about the clinical pharmacology of antihistamines in children, specific dosage recommendations are somewhat arbitrary.

Sympathomimetic drugs that have vasoconstrictive properties, such as ephedrine, may be useful adjuncts to antihistamine therapy. Terbutaline has been reported to be helpful in controlling chronic urticaria but required one week of administration before an effect was evident, (Kennes et al., 1977). The histamine H_2-receptor antagonist cimetidine may occasionally benefit patients with chronic urticaria, but its use for this purpose is experimental at present. A recent report documents synergism of H_1- and H_2-receptor antagonists in the treatment of urticaria pigmentosa (Gerrard and Ko, 1979), lending weight to the possible value of the combination in other forms of urticaria. Cromolyn

has recently been shown to be effective in blocking clinical manifestations of systemic mastocytosis, suggesting that mast cell physiology may be pharmacologically modified by this drug if taken orally (Sofer et al., 1979).

Although steroids are effective in some patients in controlling urticaria, they rarely are indicated. Administration should be reserved for such threatening events as laryngeal edema, since the risks of chronic steroid therapy outweigh the benefits. When steroid treatment is necessary, the drug should be tapered to single alternate-day doses, using the smallest dosage possible to control symptoms. One should administer antihistamine and sympathomimetic agents concurrently to minimize steroid requirements, and should warn the patient of the potential adverse effects of steroids.

COURSE

On long term follow-up, chronic urticaria persisted an average of 6 months; angioedema, 1 year; and urticaria with angioedema approximately 5 years (Champion, 1969). Unless it is a manifestation of systemic disease, urticaria is a self-limited disease without sequelae if managed appropriately.

HEREDITARY ANGIOEDEMA

Hereditary angioedema (HAE) is an inherited disorder of the complement system that is due to lack of the biologically active C_1 esterase inhibitor (C1INH). In 85 percent of patients C1INH is totally absent, and in the remainder it is present but biologically nonfunctional. The disease is transmitted as an autosomal dominant trait with incomplete penetrance. The disorder is characterized clinically by circumscribed areas of nonpitting, *nonpruritic* edema of skin and mucous membranes that are often but not always related to trauma. Involvement of the gastrointestinal tract results in cramping or diarrhea. Swelling usually develops over hours; it may be so severe as to be disfiguring, but usually resolves within 72 hours. Since laryngeal edema is the commonest cause of death, the physician must be prepared to treat with intubation or tracheostomy in crises.

Diagnosis rests on determination of C4 level. If C1INH is absent, the classic pathway from C1 to C4 to C2 is continually activated and C4 will be depressed even when the patient is asymptomatic. Since C2 is present in greater quantities than C4, it may exist at normal levels in an affected individual who is asymptomatic, and it will decline only during an acute episode of swelling. The nonpruritic character of the edema produced seems to be due to activation of a specific peptide. HAE results from fibrinolysis of this peptide, which enhances permeability of postcapillary venules.

Therapy with antifibrinolytic agents such as epsilon-aminocaproic acid and tranexamic acid has been useful. These agents prevent fibrinolysis and inhibit the activation of C1 by plasmin and immune complexes, apparently stabilizing C1 regardless of the initiating stimulus (Kaplan, 1977). Oxymetho-lone and danazol are two relatively nonvirilizing androgens that induce synthesis of C1INH, and are useful in treatment and prevention of angioedema. It appears that patients with HAE possess the gene for the C1 inhibitor, but its expression is suppressed. Androgenic steroid hormones overcome this suppression, possibly by changing messenger RNA synthesis, which results in production of functional C1INH (Gelfand et al., 1976). Antifibrinolytic agents are the drugs of choice in prophylaxis and treatment of spontaneous attacks of hereditary angioedema in children, since steroid androgenic agents have virilizing side effects on the developing child. Every effort should be made to avoid trauma, because trauma is the major initiating factor in the swelling of HAE.

References

Bonifazi, E., Meneghini, C.L., and Cece, A.: Pathogenic factors in urticaria in children. Dermatologica *154*:65, 1977.

Buckley, R.H., and Dees, S.C.: Serum immunoglobulins. III. Abnormalities associated with chronic urticaria in children. J. Allergy. Clin. Immunol. *40*:294, 1967.

Champion, R.H., Roberts, S.D.B., Carpenter, R.G., et al.: Urticaria and angioedema. A review of 554 patients. Brit. J. Derm. *81*:588, 1969.

Doeglas, H.M.G., and Bleumink, T.: Protease inhibitors in plasma of patients with chronic urticaria. Arch. Dermatol. III:979, 1975.

Gelfand, J.A., Sherins, R.J., Alling, D.W., and Frank, M.M.: Treatment of hereditary angioedema with danazol. New Engl. J. Med. *295*:1444, 1976.

Gerrard, J.W., and Ko, C.: Urticaria pigmentosa: Treatment with cimetidine and chlorpheniramine. J. Pediatr. *94*:843, 1979.

Kaplan, A.P.: Mediators of urticaria and angioedema. J. Allergy Clin. Immunol. *60*:324, 1977.

Kaplan, A.P.: Urticaria and angioedema. *In* Middleton, E., Reed, C.E., and Ellis, E.F. (eds.): *Allergy: Principles and Practices.* St. Louis, C. V. Mosby Co., pp. 1080–1099, 1978.

Kennes, B., DeMauberge, J., and Delespess, G.: Treatment of chronic urticaria with beta$_2$-adrenergic stimulant. Clin. Allergy *7*:35, 1977.

Mathews, K.P.: A current view of urticaria. Med. Clin. N. Am., pp. 185–205, 1974.

Mathews, K.P.: Chronic urticaria revisited. J. Allergy Clin. Immunol. *61*:347, 1978.

Rosen, F.S., and Austen, K.F.: Androgen therapy in hereditary angioneurotic edema. New Engl. J. Med. *292*:1476–1477, 1976.

Sheldon, J.M., Mathews, K.P., and Lovell, R.G.: The vexing urticaria problem: Present concepts of etiology and management. J. Allergy *25*:525, 1954.

Soter, N.A.: Chronic urticaria as a manifestation of necrotizing vasculitis. New Engl. J. Med. *296*:1440, 1977.

Soter, N.A., Austen, K.F., Wasserman, S.I.: Oral disodium cromoglycate in the treatment of systemic mastocytosis. N. Engl. J. Med. *301*:465, 1979.

Szczeklik, A., Gryglewski, R.J., and Czerniawsda-Mysik, G.: Clinical patterns of hypersensitivity to non-steroidal anti-inflammatory drugs and their pathogenesis. J. Allergy Clin. immunol. *60*:276, 1977.

Warin, R.P., and Champion, R.H.: Urticaria. London, W. B. Saunders Co., Ltd., 1974.

Alan Wanderer, M.D.

34

Physical Allergy

Hypersensitive responses to various physical stimuli, such as heat, cold, pressure and light, may result in urticaria or other dermatologic reactions. As a group these have been referred to as "physical allergies," which may be a misnomer since immune mechanisms have been established for only a few disorders (Kaplan, 1977). The primary care physician should become acquainted with these disorders since they may be important factors in 15 to 20 percent of patients with chronic urticaria. Some of these disorders, such as cold urticaria and deep pressure urticaria, are associated with significant morbidity, and evaluation by a dermatology or allergy consultant may be indicated.

MECHANICAL FACTORS

Dermographism ("write-on skin") is an increased propensity to induce a wheal and flare reaction after mechanical stroking of the skin. Wheals may occur from scratching or secondary to pressure from constraining clothing. Dermographism may develop early in life; this constitutional type can be lifelong. An idiopathic acquired form may develop at any age and often improves spontaneously 1 to 2 years after onset. A rarer form, delayed dermographism, has been described, in which symptoms occur 4 to 6 hours after skin stroking. Dermographism can develop secondary to generalized mastocytosis or as a result of other conditions (Table 34–1). In particular, dermographism

may occur in association with chronic urticaria, which can create diagnostic confusion.

The gradual onset of deep, painful swelling 4 to 6 hours after pressure application to the skin is referred to as deep pressure urticaria. The diagnosis often is missed because of difficulty in correlating pressure to delayed swelling. Another entity, hereditary vibratory angioedema, induces pruritus and swelling within minutes after vibratory stimulation.

The dermographic reaction occasionally can be transferred by injecting the serum of symptomatic patients into skin of normal individuals (passive transfer). The serum factor is associated with immunoglobulin E (Newcomb and Nelson, 1973), implying that an immune mechanism is operative. The responsible antigen in this reaction has not been identified.

The diagnosis of dermographism can be made by stroking the skin with a blunt object. The whealing response develops within 10 minutes after stroke pressure has been applied, as opposed to delayed pressure urticaria and delayed dermographism in which responses develop 4 to 6 hours after mechanical stimulation of the skin. A differential diagnosis of dermographism is listed in Table 34–1. Occasionally the diagnostic evaluation requires a skin biopsy to rule out chronic mastocytosis or other disorders, such as scabies.

The drug of choice for treatment of dermographism is hydroxyzine hydrochloride (Atarax). Recommended doses are 10 to 25

447

mg orally, three to four times a day in children 6 years and older, and 10 mg orally, three times daily for those under age 6 years. Tolerance to skin pressure reportedly develops in some patients after chronic skin exposure to sunlight. Deep pressure urticaria is not responsive to antihistamines and can best be controlled with systemic steroids.

TABLE 34–1 CLASSIFICATION OF HYPERSENSITIVITY TO PHYSICAL FACTORS

I. Mechanical
  A. Dermographism
    1. Primary
      a. Constitutional
      b. Idiopathic acquired
    2. Secondary
      a. Systemic mastocytosis
      b. Chronic urticaria
      c. Drug reaction (e.g., penicillin)
      d. Hyperthyroidism
      e. Insect stings
      f. Scabies infestation
  B. Delayed dermographism
  C. Delayed pressure urticaria
  D. Vibratory hereditary angioedema

II. Photosensitivity disorders
  A. Solar urticaria
    1. Six types, classified according to wavelength of light
    2. Erythropoietic protoporphyria (Type VI)
  B. Photosensitizing agents
    1. Phototoxic
    2. Photoallergic
  C. Miscellaneous
    1. Polymorphic light eruption
    2. Lupus erythematosus

III. Thermal
  A. Heat sensitivity
    1. Cholinergic urticaria
    2. Localized heat urticaria

IV. Cold urticaria
  A. Familial
  B. Acquired
    1. Primary
    2. Secondary
      a. Cryoglobulinemia
        (1) Essential
        (2) Viral
        (3) Neoplastic
          (a) Multiple myeloma
          (b) Chronic lymphatic leukemia
      b. Cryofibrinogenemia
      c. Paroxysmal cold hemoglobinuria
      d. Cold agglutinin
  C. Delayed

PHOTOSENSITIVITY DISORDERS

Urticaria that develops after brief sunlight exposure is termed solar urticaria. Wheals occur within minutes after exposure to light and fade after 30 minutes. Generalized sun exposure occasionally can result in systemic symptoms such as bronchospasm and hypotension. Symptoms typically develop during the third or fourth decade and persist for a variable time. There are six types of solar urticaria, classified according to the wavelengths of light that precipitate the whealing response. An immune mechanism may be operative in Type I or IV since solar sensitivity can be transferred by injecting serum from affected individuals into skin of normal individuals. In one patient, the serum factor responsible for passive transfer capability has been identified as IgE (Sams, 1970). Type VI, or erythropoietic protoporphyria (EPP), is caused by an inherited metabolic disorder characterized by increased protoporphyrin production in erythrocytes, plasma, and feces.

Diagnosis of solar urticaria is based on history that exposure to sunlight will induce wheals of short duration. It may be established by testing with a source of light of variable wavelengths such as a monochromator. EPP or Type VI should be considered in all cases of photosensitivity of a lifetime duration, especially if there is a family history of a similar disorder. Type VI photosensitivity may begin as urticaria but often develops into a chronic dermatitis of the face, including the nose, pinnae, and infraorbital skin. This diagnosis can be confirmed by microscopic demonstration of erythrocyte fluorescence.

Photodermatitis may develop from an interaction of drugs or chemical agents with light energy (Baer and Harber, 1965). There are two types of photosensitivity reactions, phototoxic and photoallergic. Phototoxic responses are nonimmune and occur on first contact with the offending agent after exposure to sunlight. Clinically the reaction resembles a sunburn and develops a few hours

TABLE 34-2 PHOTOSENSITIZING DRUGS AND AGENTS

Class of Agent	Example	Mechanism	Route of Exposure
Antibiotics	Demethylchlortetracycline (Declomycin)	PT*	Oral
Antifungal agents	Griseofulvin	PA†	Oral
Antihistamines	Promethazine HCl (Phenergan)	PA	Topical Oral
Antiseptics	Hexachlorophene	PA	Topical
Artificial sweeteners	Cyclamate	PA	Oral
Coal tar derivatives	Hair dyes	PT	Topical
Diuretics	Thiazides	PA	Oral
Furocoumarins	Perfumes	PT	Topical
Oral contraceptives	Estrogens	PA	Oral
Oral hypoglycemics	Tolbutamide	PA	Oral
Sunscreens	Para-aminobenzoic acid	PA	Topical
Tranquilizers	Chlorpromazine (Thorazine)	PT PA	Oral

*Phototoxic
†Photoallergic

after light exposure. Photoallergic reactions exhibit features of an immune response in that they require prior exposure to the agent and occur only in a small number of patients. The typical photoallergic rash is eczematoid, but it may exhibit pleomorphic features such as urticaria or papulovesiculation. Table 34-2 lists many common drugs and agents that can elicit photodermatitis.

Polymorphic light eruption (PLE) and discoid or systemic lupus erythematosus should be considered in the differential diagnosis of photosensitivity, since they can induce chronic pleomorphic skin eruptions after sunlight exposure. A skin biopsy and appropriate serologic tests (see Chapters 64 and 65) may be required to rule out collagen vascular disorders. PLE presents as a chronic inflammatory dermatosis in reaction to sunlight and is most common in North American Indians.

The mainstay of therapy for solar urticaria involves sun avoidance, which includes the use of sunscreens (para-aminobenzoic acid in ethanol; titanium oxide). Ordinary window glass serves as an effective sunscreen for solar urticaria that is sensitive to short wavelengths in the ultraviolet range. In addition, gradual repeated exposure to sunlight may induce a state of tolerance. Symptoms of EPP and PLE may be controlled by treatment with beta-carotene (Solatene). Possible photosensitizing agents or drugs also must be eliminated.

HEAT SENSITIVITY

Induction of small wheals 2 to 3 mm in diameter after exercise or emotional stress is referred to as cholinergic urticaria. The wheals are exceptionally pruritic and may be associated with more generalized symptoms of cholinergic stimulation, such as lacrimation, salivation, diarrhea, and bronchospasm (Moore-Robinson and Warren, 1968). This condition often develops in adolescence and can improve after several years. There is apparent hypersensitivity to cholinergic mediators, and typical lesions can be reproduced by intradermal injections of 0.05 ml of 0.02 percent methacholine (Mecholyl). Another type of heat sensitivity, referred to as localized heat urticaria, can be induced by direct contact of skin with a heat stimulus (Delorme, 1969). Systemic symptoms, such as loss of consciousness, may develop if large areas of skin are stimulated by heat. Potential danger may develop if systemic symptoms develop while bathing in warm water.

The treatment of choice for cholinergic urticaria is hydroxyzine hydrochloride (Atarax). The dosage schedule is identical to that recommended for dermographism. In addition, a single dose of 10 to 25 mg 2 or 3 hours before a planned activity may prevent symptoms. Localized heat urticaria can be effectively controlled with cyproheptadine hydrochloride (Periactin), using 2 to 4 mg orally, one to three doses daily.

COLD SENSITIVITY

Cold urticaria is a disorder characterized by induction of wheals and/or angioedema after exposure to cold stimulation. Symptoms usually are confined to areas exposed to cold temperatures, such as the hands and face. Extremely sensitive individuals may develop generalized urticaria, angioedema, hypotension, and bronchospasm during activities such as swimming in cold water. Deaths from drowning have occurred, and patients with this disorder should be forwarned of the dangers of swimming. The diagnosis of cold urticaria can be confirmed by application of an ice bag to the forearm for 5 to 10 minutes. A wheal will develop after the skin has been allowed to rewarm.

Primary acquired cold urticaria is the most common type of cold urticaria and can occur at any age. It appears to be immunologically mediated in many patients, since serum immunoglobulin factors (IgE, IgM) have been shown to transfer cold sensitivity into the skin of normal recipients (Houser et al.,

TABLE 34–3 LABORATORY TESTS TO BE CONSIDERED IN THE DIAGNOSTIC EVALUATION OF COLD URTICARIA

Complete blood count
Erythrocyte sedimentation rate
Mono spot test
Antinuclear antibody
Australian antigen
Serum cryoglobulin
Serum cryofibrinogen
Cold agglutination
VDRL
Bone marrow, skeletal series, skin biopsy (if indicated by history or physical examination)

1970; Wanderer et al., 1971). The natural course of primary cold urticaria is gradual improvement over 2 to 5 years, although patients may remain symptomatic for life. Acquired cold urticaria may develop secondary to several disorders (see Table 34–1). Table 34–3 lists various laboratory procedures appropriate for evaluation of acquired cold urticaria.

A familial form of cold urticaria has been described that develops in infancy and is transmitted as an autosomal dominant disorder. Following cold exposure, its characteristic features include rash (urticaria, but more commonly an erythematous papular eruption), fever, arthralgia, and leukocytosis. There is no known mechanism to explain this variant of cold sensitivity.

Cyproheptadine hydrochloride (Periactin) is the treatment of choice for suppressing primary cold urticaria (Wanderer et al., 1977). Average therapeutic doses are 2 to 4 mg orally four times a day, although doses as low as 2 mg orally twice a day may be effective. Tolerance to cold can be achieved by gradual cold exposure (Bentley-Phillips et al., 1976), although this technique is not successful in all cases and generally should be avoided because of possible induction of anaphylactoid reactions.

References

Baer, R.L., and Harber, L.C.: Photosensitivity induced by drugs. J.A.M.A. *192*:147, 1965.

Bentley-Phillips, C.B., Black, A.K., and Greaves, M.W.: Induced tolerance in cold urticaria caused by cold-evoked histamine release. Lancet 63–66, July 10, 1976.

Delorme, P.: Localized heat urticaria. J. Allergy *43*:284, 1969.

Houser, D.D., Arbesman, C.E., Ito, K., and Wicher, K.: Cold urticaria. Immunologic studies. Am. J. Med. *49*:23, 1970.

Kaplan, A.P.: Mediators of urticaria and angioedema. J. Allergy Clin. Immunol. *60*:324, 1977.

Moore-Robinson, M., and Warin, R.P.: Some clinical aspects of cholinergic urticaria. Br. J. Derm. *80*:794, 1968.

Newcomb, R.W., and Nelson, H.: Dermographia mediated by immunoglobulin E. Am. J. Med. *54*:174, 1973.

Sams, W.M.: Solar urticaria. J. Allergy *45*:295, 1970.

Wanderer, A.A., St. Pierre, J.P., and Ellis, E.F.: Primary acquired cold urticaria. Double-blind comparative study of treatment with cyproheptadine, chlorpheniramine and placebo. Arch. Dermatol. *113*:1375, 1977.

Wanderer, A.A., Maselli, R., Ellis, E.F., and Ishizaka, K.: Immunologic characterization of serum factors responsible for cold urticaria. J. Allergy *48*:13, 1971.

RECOMMENDED GENERAL REFERENCES

Fitzpatrick, T.B.: Dermatology in General Medicine. New York, McGraw-Hill Book Co., 1971.

Mathews, K.P.: A current view of urticaria. Med. Clin. North Am., *58*:185–205, 1974.

Warin, R.P., and Champion, R.H.: Urticaria. London, W. B. Saunders, Ltd., 1974.

35

Mickey J. Mandel, M.D.
William Lee Weston, M.D.

Other Skin Disorders

In this chapter, the more common congenital and hereditary disorders of the skin, infectious dermatoses, and other skin disorders with features that sometimes raise the question of "allergy" or immunodeficiency are considered. In some instances, immune mechanisms have been implicated in the pathogenesis of the disorder. The reader also is directed to the general references of dermatology listed at the end of the chapter for more comprehensive review of these disorders.

HAIR LOSS

Although alopecia (hair loss) of any type is rare in childhood, its occurrence usually produces considerable anxiety in the patient, parent, and doctor. Sixty percent of hair loss must occur in a single area before it can be detected clinically. The three most common types of alopecia in children are alopecia areata, trichotillomania, and tinea capitis. Tinea capitis is considered in this chapter in the section on fungal diseases.

Hair loss may occur secondary to otherwise unrelated scalp pathology, and the scalp should be inspected closely for variation of color and the presence or absence of infiltrative changes. With scalp nodules or tumors, nevus sebaceous or epidermal nevus should be considered. Scalp thickening is a feature of linear scleroderma or a posttraumatic lesion such as a burn. Atrophy of the scalp has been associated with lupus erythematosus and lichen planus.

Alopecia Areata. Alopecia areata is characterized by complete loss of hairs in circular, localized patches, which may be singular or multiple. The hairless patches are most prominent on the scalp but may occur in the eyebrows, eyelashes, or body hair. Regrowth of hair will occur within a year in almost all cases, but alopecia will recur in 40 percent of affected children within 5 years, with repeated cycles of hair regrowth and alopecia of increasing severity. When hair loss starts in the occiput and proceeds along the lateral margins to the frontal scalp, prognosis of recovery is poor. This pattern (ophiasis) frequently leads to alopecia totalis, loss of the entire scalp hair. Alopecia areata is identified by the presence of "exclamation point hairs," that is, hairs which appear thin proximally, with thick and broken distal ends. Cell-mediated immune mechanisms are thought to be important in alopecia (Ipp and Gelfand, 1976; Kern et al; 1973). Dense lymphocytic perifollicular infiltrates can be seen preceding hair loss. Direct lymphocyte injury of hair follicles has not been demonstrated, however. Alopecia areata has been associated with thyroid disease, pernicious anemia, adrenal insufficiency, and vitiligo. Treatment is supportive. Intralesional glucocorticosteroid injections have resulted in hair regrowth in some children, but there have been a few reported cases of blindness after injections of steroids in the frontal scalp area. In alopecia totalis, a cosmetic hair piece may be helpful.

Trichotillomania. Compulsive hair pulling may be observed in children and occasionally in infants, who seem to obtain satisfaction from this action. The vertex, other parts of the scalp, eyebrows, and eyelashes are involved with diminishing frequency. The hair shafts may be broken at different lengths and perifollicular petechiae may be seen. Trichotillomania should not be confused with the persistent traction in girls who wear ponytails, or use hair curlers or tight braiding techniques, producing traction alopecia. Treatment is psychologically oriented and supportive with the objective of reducing anxiety. Some dermatologists also recommend applying an oil to the hair so the child cannot pull it.

ECTODERMAL DISORDERS

Congenital Ectodermal Defect. Anhidrotic ectodermal dysplasia is associated with the triad of hypotrichosis, anodontia, and anhidrosis. The hair itself is thin, sparse and dry, but alopecia is never complete. The facies suggest congenital syphilis. Late erupting cone-shaped teeth are seen. Because of an inability to sweat, elevation of body temperature upon physical exertion is common. In warm weather, increase in body temperature may be sufficiently marked to progress to heat stroke. The absence of mucus glands in the upper and lower respiratory tract predisposes to frequent symptoms of respiratory tract infection. An increased incidence of allergic rhinitis and asthma with elevated IgE has been reported

in this disorder. Mental deficiency is uncommon. This disorder has features of both autosomal dominant and X-linked recessive inheritance.

Another form of congenital ectodermal defect, hidrotic ectodermal dysplasia, is associated with sparse scalp hair, poor dentition, and hypoplastic nails, but the eccrine sweat glands are active. Children with this autosomal dominant disorder have normal facial features.

Ichthyosis. Increased keratinization with with excessive scaling is the hallmark of ichthyosis. A widely accepted classification of ichthyotic disorders, listed in Table 35–1, is based upon normal or increased epidermal cell turnover. Control of excessive keratinization can be accomplished with alpha-hydroxy acids, such as 5 percent pyruvic, citric, lactic, or salicylic acid in petrolatum (Van Scott and Yu, 1974). Techniques of increasing skin hydration by frequent application of lubricants to wet skin is an essential part of therapy. Patients with ichthyosis frequently are more comfortable in humid climates.

Keratosis Pilaris. Keratosis pilaris is a familial hyperkeratosis of follicular orifices, with plugging of the infundibulum of the hair follicle. It is thought to be inherited as an autosomal dominant disorder. It commonly appears in early childhood and persists through adolescence. The characteristic "goose flesh" appearance is seen predominantly on the extensor surfaces of the arms and thighs, although it can appear on the face

TABLE 35–1 FOUR MAJOR TYPES OF ICHTHYOSIS

Name	Age at Onset	Clinical Features	Histology	Inheritance
Ichthyosis with normal epidermal turnover				
Ichthyosis vulgaris	Childhood	Fine scales, deep palmar and plantar markings	Decreased to absent granular layer; hyperkeratosis	Autosomal dominant
X-linked ichthyosis	Birth	Palms and soles spared; thick scales that darken with age; corneal opacities in patients and carrier mothers	Hyperkeratosis	X-linked
Ichthyosis with increased epidermal turnover				
Epidermolytic hyperkeratosis	Birth	Verrucous, yellow scales in flexural areas and on palms and soles	Hyperkeratosis, vacuolated reticular spaces in epidermis	Autosomal dominant
Lamellar ichthyosis	Birth; collodion baby	Erythroderma, ectropion, large coarse scales, thickened palms and soles	Hyperkeratosis, many mitotic figures	Autosomal recessive

and eyebrows. Individual lesions are red papules with a dry, central scale. Treatment consists of avoiding tight clothes, using topical keratolytic agents such as retinoic acids, alpha-hydroxy acids, or salicylic acid, and skin hydration by standard dermatologic hydration and lubrication techniques.

BULLOUS DISEASE

Epidermolysis Bullosa. Epidermolysis bullosa is characterized by hemorrhagic blisters that occur with slight trauma. Epidermolysis bullosa is a spectrum of disorders ranging from nonscarring to scarring forms. Whether scarring occurs is related to the cellular layer of the epidermis or dermis at which separation occurs. Table 35–2 classifies these disorders. Treatment consists of using systemic antibiotics for infection and replacing fluid, electrolyte, and protein losses. Protective dressings such as zinc oxide or petrolatum can be used. Skin cooling improves resistance to blister formation. Skin friction on palms and soles can frequently be reduced by 5 percent glutaraldehyde applied every 2 to 3 days. Minimal handling also is an important aspect of therapy, since even minimal trauma may lead to hemorrhagic blisters (Jarrett, 1976).

DISORDERS OF PIGMENTATION

Vitiligo. Vitiligo is an acquired idiopathic depigmentation, with borders sharply circumscribed by normal or hyperpigmented skin. The most frequently affected sites are the face, neck, sternal area, arms, and dorsal surface of the hands; but the condition may be generalized. It is thought to be due to an autoimmune mechanism. Antibodies to melanin-producing cells have been detected (Hertz et al., 1977).

There is some association between vitiligo and hyperthyroidism, adrenocortical insufficiency, pernicious anemia, and diabetes. There also is a reportedly increased frequency of vitiligo associated with IgA deficiency syndromes, as well as an increased association with combined occurrence of antithyroid antibodies and the HL-A I3 haplotype. Histologically, there is a complete absence of dopa-positive melanocytes. Pruritus may occur after sunburn of vitiliginous areas but also can occur without sun exposure. Treatment is mainly supportive, but intralesional steroids, oral psoralens, artificial keratin staining, and tattooing all have been used with varying success (Retornax et al., 1976).

Leukoderma. The acquired hypopigmentation of skin that is produced by specific substances or occurs secondarily to der-

TABLE 35–2 TYPES OF EPIDERMOLYSIS BULLOSA

Name	Age at Onset	Clinical Features	Histology	Inheritance
Nonscarring types				
Epidermolysis bullosa simplex	Birth	Hemorrhagic blisters over the lower legs; cooling prevents blisters	Disintegration of basal cells	Autosomal dominant
Recurrent bullous eruption of the hands and feet (Weber-Cockayne syndrome)	First few years of life	Blisters brought out by walking	Cytolysis of suprabasal cells; dyskeratotic	Autosomal dominant
Junctional bullous epidermatosis (Herlitz disease)	Birth	Erosions on legs, oral mucosa; severe perioral involvement	Separation between plasma membrane of basal cells and PAS-positive basal lamina	Autosomal recessive
Scarring types				
Epidermolysis bullosa dystrophica, dominant	Infancy	Numerous blisters on hands and feet	Separation of PAS-positive basal lamina; anchoring fibrils lost	Autosomal dominant
Epidermolysis bullosa dystrophica, recessive	Birth	Repeated episodes of blistering, secondary infection and scarring— "mitten hands and feet"	Separation below PAS-positive basal lamina; anchoring fibrils lost	Autosomal recessive

matitis is known as leukoderma. This has been shown in association with occupational dermatitis (e.g., from rubber garments as well as phenolic detergent germicides). These forms are rarely seen in children, however. The postinflammatory form of leukoderma is seen with a variety of inflammatory skin diseases, including pityriasis rosea, herpes zoster, psoriasis, atopic dermatitis, secondary syphilis, and morphea. Treatment consists of removing the offending substance and treatment of the underlying dermatosis. Leukoderma usually is reversible.

Pityriasis Alba. Pityriasis alba presents in children and adolescents as hypopigmented, scaly, oval patches, usually on the face, upper arms, neck, and shoulders. Histologically a mild dermatitis is seen. Pruritus, when it occurs, usually is mild. Treatment consists of hydration and lubrication techniques or application of topical low-potency steroids.

Incontinentia Pigmenti. This uncommon dermatosis usually affects female infants. When it does affect males, it tends to be lethal. There are three characteristic stages of the disorder: vesiculobullous, verrucous or papillomatous, and hyperpigmented. The lesions tend to be arranged in a linear or grouped fashion, mainly on the flexor surfaces of the extremities and the lateral trunk. Eosinophil counts are elevated in most cases. Other ectodermal defects include skin, hair, and dental; neurologic and ocular defects are found in 30 percent of patients with this disorder. Abnormalities in skin pigmentation tend to disappear by adulthood. There is no known treatment. Genetic counseling is important in families with this disorder (Carney, 1976).

SKIN INFECTIONS

Bacterial Infections (Pyodermas)

Coagulase positive *Staphylococcus aureus* and Group A beta-hemolytic streptococci are the major bacterial organisms that cause skin infections, although a variety of other bacteria can infect the skin. Skin infection should be treated with systemic rather than topical antibiotic therapy (see Chapter 19). Antibiotics should be selected by culturing the invad-

ing organism and determining antibiotic sensitivity if appropriate.

Superficial bacterial infection of the upper epidermis results in *impetigo*. Impetigo due to beta-hemolytic streptococci presents as a thick, stuck-on, honey-colored crust that can extend without central clearing. In addition to local spread, infection can lead to streptococcal-induced acute glomerulonephritis. The staphylococcal infections usually present with bullous lesions that rupture and crust in several days with central healing. The lesions also can appear circinate and can occur at any site of injury.

Ecthyma is a deeper infection than impetigo, with penetration to the superficial dermis. It is characterized by a firm, dry crust surrounded by erythema and a purulent exudate. In addition to systemic antibiotics, the use of topical tap water compresses to soften crusts and frequent cleansing with soap and water are important (Ferrieri, et al., 1972).

Bacterial invasion into the lower dermis, with obstruction of local lymphatics, results in *cellulitis*. Cellulitis presents clinically as ill-defined erythematous "plaques" that are hot and tender. It may be associated with painful regional lymphadenopathy, and septicemia may occur. The organisms usually responsible for cellulitis include beta-hemolytic streptococci and staphylococci. *Erysipelas* is a superficial, slowly progressive form of streptococcal cellulitis, occurring most frequently on the face. Cellulitis caused by *Haemophilus influenzae* may present with bluish discoloration of the affected areas. Treatment of cellulitis includes systemic antibiotic therapy and immobilization of the affected area. The patient should be hospitalized for treatment if constitutional symptoms are present.

Folliculitis (infection of hair follicles) presents with pustulation of the opening of multiple follicles. The staphylococcus is the most common causative agent. Treatment involves removal of the follicular obstruction by the use of cold, wet compresses or keratolytics, and antibiotics. Skin abscesses (*furuncles* and *carbuncles*) present as acute erythematous, firm, tender nodules with ill-defined borders. Abscesses may originate at the base of hair follicles or apocrine glands or occur unassociated with any specific skin element. The causative organism usually is *Staphylococcus aureus*. Treatment includes incision and drainage, in addition to appropriate antibiotic therapy (Fritch, 1971).

The *scalded skin syndrome* presents as a sudden onset of red, painful macular lesions that occur periorally and periorbitally, in flexural areas of the neck, in the axillae, and in popliteal, antecubital, and groin areas. Frequently, slight skin pressure results in pain and in separation of the epidermis, hence an appearance similar to scalded skin. The condition is secondary to a circulating staphylococcal toxin, elaborated by organisms on the skin or elsewhere (e.g., nasopharynx, abscesses). Staphylococci of phage group II, types 71, 55, 3A, 3B, and 3C are responsible. This syndrome occurs in various forms: Ritter's disease of the newborn, toxic epidermal necrolysis, staphylococcal scarlet fever, and bullous impetigo. Because the disease usually is induced by penicillin-resistant organisms, penicillinase-resistant synthetic penicillins generally are recommended for therapy. When penicillin is contraindicated, erythromycin or cephalosporins should be used. Steroids are contraindicated, and topical therapy is not efficacious (Elias et al., 1977).

Scarlet fever, usually due to beta-hemolytic streptococci, group A, is considered with exanthematous diseases, in Table 35–3. Systemic penicillin is the treatment of choice.

Superficial Fungus Infection

Fungi proliferate in the superficial layers of the epidermis, nails, and hair; they generally do not invade the lower epidermis. Fungus infections can be difficult to diagnose and frequently are confused with contact dermatitis, seborrheic dermatitis, psoriasis, miliaria, folliculitis, rosacea, as well as other forms of cutaneous infection. Location as well as appearance of the lesions are important clues to diagnosis.

Diagnostic tests for fungus infection include the microscopic examination of scales dissolved in potassium hydroxide; Wood's light examination for fluorescent hairs; and fungal culture. Fine, thin scales (two to three cell layers thick) are scraped from the border of the suspected fungal lesion, placed on a clean microscopic slide and covered with one to two drops of 10 percent potassium hydroxide (KOH). A cover slip is applied, and using the 10× objective with reduced illumination, the preparation is examined for long branching hyphae. Fungi are readily cultured at room temperature with Sabouraud's agar for morphologic identification. In suspected tinea capitis, broken hairs or fluorescent hairs should be extracted with a forceps and examined. Wood's light examination is not useful for tinea corporis, cruris, or pedis but is valuable in detecting white or yellow fluorescence of broken hairs in tinea capitis.

Tinea versicolor consists of scaly, polycyclic macules that may be hyper- or hypopigmented. It usually is easy to diagnose, and it attracts little other than cosmetic concern. It is caused by a saprophytic yeast, *Pityrosporum orbiculare* and its mycelial form, *Malassezia furfur*. It is more commonly seen in a hot, humid climate. Examination of the affected areas with the Wood's light shows an orange fluorescence. Microscopic examination using KOH preparations will frequently show a "spaghetti and meatball" pattern of short, curved hyphae and small spores. Cultures will show a yeast-like growth. This condition is best treated with topical sulfur preparations such as selenium sulfide (Selsun), applied for 24 hours on two consecutive nights. This should be repeated in 2 weeks. Repigmentation may take 3 to 6 months. Recurrence of tinea versicolor is common.

Infection with *Candida albicans* assumes many forms. It occurs as a diaper area dermatitis, a vaginitis or vulvovaginitis, in the oral mucosa as "thrush," in the angles of the mouth as perleche, and on the fingers involving the cuticles or nails. It involves the skin most commonly as a simple intertrigo, a pruritic eruption characterized by a sharply demarcated red rash at the site of skin apposition and friction. Candidal intertrigo has an increased incidence in patients with diabetes, hypo- or hyperparathyroidism, or hypocalcemia. Chronic mucocutaneous candidiasis frequently is associated with abnormalities of the immune system (see Chapter 8). Pharyngeal candidiasis also can be a complication of beclomethasone therapy for asthma. Candidal vulvovaginitis occurs most frequently in diabetes, pregnancy, or secondary to the use of broad-spectrum antibiotics. Treatment consists of using nystatin (Mycostatin), clotrimazole (Lotrimin), haloprogin (Halotex) or miconazole (Micatin) (Carter and Olansky, 1974). In diaper dermatitis the most important therapeutic consideration is keeping the area dry by frequent diaper changes. Substances such as cornstarch should not be used as they can promote candidiasis. With paronychial infections, topical anticandidal medications used under occlusive dressings may be required. The use of 3 percent thymol in chloroform frequently is helpful in drying the paronychial area.

The treatment of fungal infections has improved greatly with the advent of griseofulvin, which should be used if there is involvement of the hair or nails (Blank, 1965). Griseofulvin is a fat soluble chemical and should be taken after a fatty meal. The dose is usually 10 to 20 mg per kg of body weight per day. Children with tinea capitis should be treated for a minimum of 6 weeks, and for 3 months if there is nail involvement. Topical antifungals, including tolnaftate (Tinactin), haloprogin (Halotex), miconazole (Micatin), and clotrimazole (Lotrimin), are useful for fungal infections of the body and are of equal efficacy. These should be applied three times a day and continued for 1 to 2 weeks after the skin is clear. A kerion (a boggy fluctuant lesion with pustule formation) infection should be treated with griseofulvin, as well as systemic steroids to suppress the inflammatory response. It should be remembered that the treatment can clear the existing infection but does not change the individual's susceptibility to reinfection.

Tinea capitis, or *ringworm of the scalp,* presents with erythema and scaling. The infection produces a circumscribed area of hair loss with short, thickened hairs. *Microsporum canis* and *Trichophyton tonsurans* account for the majority of tinea capitis infections. Infections with organisms derived from domestic animals tend to be particularly inflammatory, and kerion formation is common. Kerion is thought to represent a delayed hypersensitivity response to the invading fungus. A yellow-green fluorescence of the hair seen using Wood's light is helpful diagnostically. Griseofulvin is effective therapy, along with hygienic measures, including regular cleaning of combs and daily shampoos.

Tinea corporis occurs on the trunk and extremities as sharply demarcated annular lesions of erythematous papules with scaling, often with encircling chains of small, confluent vesicles. Lesions may coalesce to form a confluent dermatitis. *Trichophyton mentogrophytes* and *Microsporum canis* are usually responsible for tinea corporis in children.

Tinea cruris occurs in the inguinal area or upper inner surface of the thighs, as symmetric, sharply marginated erythematous areas with central clearing. The borders of the lesions frequently are raised. It may be associated with a fungus infection of the feet and toenails. *Trichophyton rubrum, Trichophyton mentagrophytes,* and *Epidermophyton floccosum* are the most frequently causative organisms. Oral griseofulvin at 10 to 20 mg per kg of body weight per day for 4 weeks or tolnaftate applied topically twice daily are the drugs of choice.

Tinea pedis or *"athlete's foot"* most often is seen in postpubertal males as pruritic blisters on the instep of the foot. It also may present with fissuring between the toes; most commonly it is brought to the parents' attention by the associated intense itching. Toenail involvement also occurs. "Athlete's foot" usually affects one foot but occasionally both may be involved. Atopic dermatitis of the feet, which mimics tinea pedis, is more common in prepubertal children than is tinea pedis and tends to be symmetrical. Tinea pedis also must be differentiated from contact dermatitis. Application of topical antifungal agents such as tolnaftate twice a day is recommended. Griseofulvin occasionally is required.

Tinea unguium (onychomycosis) is a chronic infection of the nails of the feet and hands. It presents as whitish to yellow discoloration of the nails, which occurs with loosening of the nail plate from the nail bed. There eventually is thickening of the distal nail plate and crumbling. Toenails are affected much more often than fingernails. Most frequently, one or two nails are involved; it is rare for tinea unguium to involve all nails or even show equal involvement of the nails affected. (If all nails are involved, psoriasis or lichen planus should be considered.) The organisms most commonly responsible are *Trichophyton rubrum* and *Trichophyton mentagrophytes*. Griseofulvin is the drug of choice.

VIRAL INFECTIONS

Herpes Virus Group. The DNA virus–herpes virus group includes the common cutaneous pathogens, herpes simplex virus and the varicella-zoster virus. Infection with herpes simplex virus characteristically is manifest in the form of grouped vesicles or grouped erosions. Two types of viruses have been identified: Type I, usually involving the head and nongenital areas, and Type II, involving primarily the genital area (Spruance et al., 1977). Each type can occur in any location, however.

Primary inoculation herpes simplex usually presents as severe ulcerations associated with high fever, lymphadenopathy, vesiculation, desquamation, and ulcerations. The ulcerations most often are found in the mouth (gingivostomatitis) and vaginal area (vulvovaginitis). This clinical syndrome lasts for 2 to 3 weeks and involves children between 1 and 5 years of age. Recurrent herpes is commonly seen in children and adults. Infection recurs despite demonstrable levels of serum herpes virus antibodies. The virus is thought to remain latent in nerve ganglia. Triggering factors such as sun exposure, trauma, irritation, and premenstrual and emotional factors somehow activate the virus, which presumably travels through the nerve to the skin or mucosa, where it replicates and produces clinical infection. Disseminated herpes simplex can be seen in infants from birth to 3 years of age. Viremia results in liver, lung, and central nervous system involvement. Death usually occurs from herpes encephalitis.

Kaposi's varicelliform eruption (or eczema herpeticum) is a disseminated cutaneous herpes simplex infection seen particularly in individuals with atopic dermatitis. Vesiculation may originate in areas of inflamed skin, but the infection can become generalized and is fatal in a small proportion of cases. This same type of reaction also can be seen with cowpox virus (eczema vaccinatum), but with the current lack of widespread immunization to smallpox, generalized infection due to vaccinia virus may be of historical interest.

Diagnosis of infection by herpes simplex virus can be made by examining scrapings of the blister base for multinucleated giant cells. Virus cultures and antibody studies will confirm the diagnosis. Treatment is symptomatic and deals mainly with drying the lesions. This can be accomplished by frequent application of isopropyl alcohol or flexible collodion that contains ether.

Herpes zoster is characterized by several areas of grouped vesicles that occur within several adjacent dermatomes. It can occur at any age group but is more common in adults. In children, it generally is not painful and has a mild course of approximately 10 to 14 days. Treatment is supportive and consists of cool baths and the use of drying agents.

Varicella (Chickenpox). Varicella occurs in children between 2 and 8 years of age, although adults can be affected. The incubation period lasts 15 to 20 days. Symptoms of a low-grade fever and malaise have their onset up to 2 days before the rash. The fever lasts 5 to 6 days. The basic lesions are vesicles, but may appear in all stages (macules, papulovesicles, vesicles, and crusts) and occur in three- to five-group crops. They are more profuse on the trunk than on the extremities and can occur on mucous membranes. The duration is usually 8 to 9 days, and the seasonal occurrence is late fall, winter, and spring.

Molluscum Contagiosum. Molluscum contagiosum, produced by a pox virus that affects only humans, presents clinically as umbilicated and usually grouped papules. Most commonly, the abdomen, inner thighs, perianal region, or eyelids are affected. The papules have a central umbilicated comedo, which on expression extrudes a rather firm, whitish body. Lesions may be localized or generalized and usually persist. The natural course is unknown. Treatment consists of minor destructive measures such as curettage or the use of local vesical-producing chemicals such as cantharidin (Cantharone).

Warts. Warts are epithelial tumors, caused by the human papova virus. They appear as skin-colored papules with irregular, scaly surfaces. Warts are observed in varying sizes, shapes, and locations, and have been designated as digitate, flat, palmar, plantar, subungual, and genital. The natural course of warts is variable, but fre-

TABLE 35–3 DIFFERENTIAL DIAGNOSIS OF EXANTHEMATOUS DISEASE

Disease	Incubation Period	Prodrome	Exanthem	Enanthem	Other Diagnostic Features
Measles	9–14 days	3 days Cough, coryza, conjuctivitis	Red, maculopapular, confluent, face to feet, lasts 7–10 days, may desquamate	Koplik's spots	Cough prominent
Rubella	10–18 days	Usually none	Pink, maculopapular, discrete, spreads rapidly, lasts 3–5 days	None or faint	Lymphadenopathy may be prominent
Roseola infection	10–14 days	3 days Fever; "well child"	Rose, macular, discrete, fleeting	None	Child remains well Occasional febrile convulsion with first rise in temperature
Fifth disease (erythema infectiosum)	About 7–14 days	None	"Slapped cheek," lace-like rash on extremities, may reappear, lasts 7–14 days	Variable	Rash characteristic May appear when extremity is warmed (bathing, clothing, etc.)
Scarlet fever	2–5 days	1–2 days Fever, vomiting, sore throat	Red, punctate, sandpaper feel, confluent blush, lasts 7 days, desquamation	Red pharynx, tonsillitis, palatal petechiae, strawberry tongue	Circumoral pallor, increased rash in skin folds, "toxic" child
Enterovirus infection	Variable (usually short)	Variable	May resemble any of above ECHO—petechial Coxsackie—vesicular	Variable	Concurrent familial illness, gastroenteritis, epidemic locally

quently lesions will disappear within 3 to 8 months. There are many successful therapeutic approaches, each designed to destroy the wart-infected epidermis. These include surgical excision and the use of liquid nitrogen, tretinoin (Retin-A), 40 percent salicylic acid plaster, 25 percent podophyllin in alcohol, and cantharidin (Cantharone) (Binney et al., 1976). Spontaneous involution is never followed by scarring; aggressive destructive therapy can be, however.

Coxsackie Virus. Hand, foot, and mouth disease caused by Coxsackie virus infection (A-16, most commonly, but also A-5 and A-10) affects children more often than adults and frequently occurs in epidemics. After a 3- to 5-day incubation period, 2 to 4 mm erythematous papules and vesicles appear on the oral mucosa, hands, and feet and spread rapidly. Spontaneous resolution usually occurs in 7 to 10 days. Treatment is supportive.

Herpangina presents as painful blisters on an erythematous base, located on both sides of the oral cavity and near the uvula. These may rupture and form small, superficial, grayish-white ulcerations. There can be prodromal symptoms of nausea, malaise, fever, intestinal disorders, and occasional meningeal irritation. Herpangina is highly contagious, most commonly affecting children between 1 and 7 years of age. Coxsackie viruses A-2, A-4, A-6, A-8, and A-10 have been implicated as causative agents. Other Coxsackie group A virus infections may be associated with morbilliform or petechial eruptions with fever.

ECHO Virus Infections. Infection with ECHO viruses can lead to syndromes with various types of skin eruptions. ECHO type 9 virus produces a macular to maculopapular eruption, occasionally with petechiae. It occurs mainly in young children and affects the face, trunk, and extremities, including the palms and soles. Lesions resembling Koplik's spots may occur on the buccal mucosa. The "Boston exanthem" is associated with a macular erythematous eruption in children, sometimes with accompanying vesicle formation on the extremities. Other ECHO virus infections are associated infrequently with erythematous macular eruptions.

The common childhood exanthematous diseases are summarized in Table 35–3.

INFESTATIONS BY INSECTS

Scabies. During the current worldwide pandemic, scabies has become a relatively common cause of pruritic dermatitis. Scabies in babies and children often poses a difficult diagnostic problem, however. Linear burrows appear on the wrists, ankles, fingerwebs, nipples, anterior axillary folds, genitalia, and on the face in infants. Frequently, a generalized papular, pruritic dermatitis without obvious burrows is present that is confused with atopic dermatitis or contact dermatitis. Lesions may be secondarily infected or lichenified from frequent scratching. Topical therapy prior to establishment of the diagnosis may complicate the diagnosis. Microscopic examination of skin scrapings will identify the female mite, eggs, or feces. Scrapings are best obtained directly from the lesions, especially from unscratched burrows or vesicles. Mites are most often found in the fingerwebs and genitalia. Gamma benzene hexachloride is an effective topical scabicide, but it must be used cautiously, as neurotoxicity has been reported (Solomon et al., 1977). Application to the body from the neck down for 4 hours is recommended. It is then washed off with a bath. Other scabicides such as Eurax or a 6 to 8 percent sulfur in petrolatum base may be substituted. All members of the family should be treated.

Norwegian Scabies. In retarded children or in immunodeficiency states, scabies will present with thickened scales in a generalized distribution that mimics ichthyosis. Mites are identified easily on microscopic examination of skin scrapings.

Pediculosis. Pediculosis, or louse infestation, frequently presents with pruritus that is most intense at night. Excoriated papules or pustules or both are observed. There may be gelatinous nits(eggs) attached to the scalp or other body hair. Similar symptoms may be present in other members of the family. Treatment includes use of gamma benzene hexachloride and mechanical removal of nits. The use of dilute vinegar compresses followed by a shampoo and combing will facilitate removal of nits.

Papular Urticaria. Papular urticaria presents as pruritic grouped erythematous papules, with a central red papule and surrounding wheal. It frequently occurs on the extremities but occasionally may be generalized in distribution. The papules usually last for a few days but can last for weeks or months. Papular urticaria generally results from bites of insects such as fleas, mites, and bedbugs. Treatment consists of removing offending insects, if identified, and symptomatic therapy with antihistamines and topical glucocorticosteroids. Secondary infections should be treated with antibiotics. Households or other areas that may be the source of causative insects should be disinfected (Massie, 1974).

SUN SENSITIVITIES

Sun sensitivities in children may be manifested as sunburn, polymorphous light eruption, erythropoietic protoporphyria, lupus erythematosus, or photodermatitis (see also Chapter 34). Sunburn results from wavelengths of ultraviolet light between 290 and 320 nm (UVB). Pain and erythema in sunburn are produced by prostaglandin release. Treatment is mainly prophylactic, using sunblocks such as 5 percent PABA in alcohol, zinc oxide, or titanium dioxide — sunscreens designed to block UVB. Aspirin taken orally and indomethacin employed topically help prevent burning. Wet dressings and low-potency topical glucocorticosteroids help ameliorate symptoms and signs following sunburn. Photodermatitis also can occur from psoralen-containing plants such as figs, citrus fruits, buckwheat, ragweed, and celery. Frequently drugs such as thiazide diuretics, ethanolamine antihistamines, phenothiazine tranquilizers, tetracyclines, and sulfonamides may produce cutaneous symptoms associated with sun exposure (Frain-Bell, 1973).

Polymorphous light eruption presents as vesicular, eczematous, or urticarial lesions in sun-exposed areas, occurring 24 to 36 hours after sun exposure. The eruption tends to be worse during the early spring, with some clearing during middle and late summer as more tanning occurs in the skin. The disorder occurs commonly in North American Indians, in whom it appears to be transmitted as an autosomal dominant trait. Biopsy of affected areas shows dense lymphocytic infiltrates in the dermis. This histologic picture together with the delay in appearance of the eruption after sun exposure has suggested

the involvement of cell-mediated immune mechanisms in this disorder. Polymorphous light eruption can be induced by both short and long wavelengths of ultraviolet light. Consequently, sunscreens with the most extensive blocking activity, such as RVP and SunGuard, should be used when sun exposure cannot be avoided. Topical glucocorticosteroid treatment is helpful in ameliorating the eruption, but spontaneous resolution frequently will occur 2 to 4 days after the appearance of the rash.

Erythropoietic protoporphyria presents with burning and itching after a few minutes of sun exposure and can be confused with "allergic" photosensitivity. Despite severe symptoms, few skin changes are seen. There may be small papules over the dorsum of the hand and erythema and edema of the face, or frank angioedema. It is autosomal dominant and often presents by 2 to 3 years of age. Diagnosis is established by demonstration of a high concentration of protoporphyrin in red cells, by fluorescence microscopy. Oral beta-carotene (Solatene) in doses of 15 to 100 mg per day has been shown to be effective in the majority of patients with erythropoietic protoporphyria (Mathews-Roth et al., 1977). A complete blocking sunscreen such as RVP should be used, and susceptible individuals should be covered by protective clothing when exposed to direct sunlight.

NONALLERGIC URTICARIAL ERUPTIONS

Urticaria Pigmentosa (Mast Cell Disease). Urticaria pigmentosa, intradermal collections of mast cells, occurs in three forms. In the most common form, cutaneous lesions arise in infancy or early childhood but improve at puberty. Systemic lesions, if present, are few in number. A second form arises in adolescence or adult life. Spontaneous regression in this form does not occur. There are multisystem lesions, and the clinical course is static. A third form is systemic mast cell disease with progressive involvement of the liver, spleen, intestinal tract, meninges, bones, and bone marrow. This may progress to mast cell leukemia and occurs most often in adults.

Cutaneous lesions appear as multiple brownish maculopapules which urticate on stroking (from liberation of histamine). Itching and erythema also occur consequent to histamine liberation. Large collections of mast cells may appear as brownish nodules and plaques. Solitary large cutaneous nodules may appear. A diffuse erythrodermic type occurs in early infancy and presents with a generalized brownish-red, soft infiltration of the skin. Children develop urticarial lesions and multiple blisters both spontaneously and with traumatic stroking. Skin biopsy will establish the diagnosis.

Avoidance of histamine-releasing drugs, such as codeine, is important. Anesthetics and cytotoxic drugs should be given with caution. Even the topical use of salicylic acid esters in sunscreens or the penetrant vehicle dimethylsulfoxide can provoke histamine release. Hot baths, strenuous exercise, alcohol, spicy foods, as well as trauma, can evoke generalized itching and urticaria (Sahihi and Esterly, 1972).

REACTIVE ERYTHEMAS

Erythema Multiforme. The reactive erythemas in children consist of erythema multiforme and erythema nodosum. The target or iris lesion is the pathognomic eruption of erythema multiforme. It also can present with erythematous half-circles, polycyclic erythema, urticaria, bullae, and erosions. Lesions occur characteristically on the extensor and distal surfaces of the extremity, occasionally with involvement of the palms and soles. The trunk rarely is involved. When mucous membranes are involved, the syndrome is known as the Stevens-Johnson syndrome. There are no characteristic laboratory findings of the syndromes. Interference with eating, drinking, and other normal functions can occur with mucous membrane involvement, and eye involvement can lead to blindness. Lesions observed represent vasodilatation, edema, and leakage of red blood cells into the skin.

The pathogenesis of erythema multiforme is unknown, but the syndrome can be precipitated by infection with various agents (herpes simplex and *Mycoplasma* organisms in particular) and by various chemotherapeutic agents, long-acting sulfonamides, and other pharmacologic agents. It is presumed that hypersensitivity mechanisms are in-

volved, but evidence for an allergic basis of this syndrome is meager. Ordinarily, spontaneous healing occurs in 10 to 14 days, although the Stevens-Johnson syndrome may last for 6 to 8 weeks. Treatment includes removal of possible offending drugs, symptomatic treatment with oral antihistamines, and cold compresses and wet dressings. Treatment with systemic steroids has been claimed to be beneficial in some cases; although there is no firm evidence for their effectiveness, they should be considered in severe cases (Kauppinen, 1972; Rasmussen, 1976).

Erythema Nodosum. Erythema nodosum presents as painful erythematous nodules, commonly on the anterior surface of the legs. Its onset parallels the appearance of a cell-mediated immune response to specific infectious agents, which appear etiologic in this condition. Circulating immune complexes have been implicated in erythema nodosum as well. The beta-hemolytic streptococcus is the most common infectious agent involved, although erythema nodosum may be associated with other infections such as coccidioidomycosis, histoplasmosis, and tuberculosis. Sensitivity to sulfonamides or to birth control pills also has been associated with erythema nodosum. Treatment consists of removal of offending drugs and treatment of infection. Prednisone, 1 to 2 mg per kg of body weight per day for 2 to 3 weeks may be employed if severe pain occurs, and intralesional injections of steroids may be beneficial (Blomgren, 1972; Fine, 1969).

VASCULITIS

Henoch-Schönlein purpura, the principal vasculitis seen in children, is associated with bleeding into the skin. Lesions may originate with an urticarial component, with development of central petechiae and ecchymoses that can progress to form hemorrhagic vesicles, bullae, and ulcers. Palpable purpura is the major cutaneous lesion in vasculitis. Fever and malaise, arthralgia (Schönlein's purpura), and abdominal pain with melena (Henoch's purpura) may develop. In a third of the cases, gross hematuria associated with either focal or diffuse glomerulonephritis is found. Renal involvement accounts for the 3 percent mortality rate of this disease. Urinalysis should be done routinely to rule out the renal complications. The symptoms last approximately 1 month, but recurrence develops in about 40 percent of the cases. There is no effective treatment of the primary disease. Circulating immune complexes are thought to be responsible for this necrotizing vasculitis.

OTHER COMMON SKIN DISORDERS

Acne. Acne is a disorder of sebaceous follicles. Excessive scale production in the follicular wall results in plugging of the sebaceous follicle with cells that have a propensity to stick together. This results in an accumulation of keratin under the skin surface, which appears as a "whitehead." With distention of the follicular pore, admixture of keratin and pigmented follicular cells results in a "blackhead." Although whiteheads and blackheads are noninflammatory in themselves, overgrowth of follicular bacteria may result in formation of an inflammatory papule or pustule. Thus, acne can present as white or black comedones, erythematous papules, malodorous cysts, abscesses, or draining sinuses and can result in permanent scarring. The most common areas of involvement include the face, scalp, chest, and trunk, where sebaceous glands are most numerous. Acne associated with drug eruptions (for example, secondary to the use of iodides) frequently shows a uniform stage of lesions, commonly over the lower back, arms, and legs.

Treatment is directed at decreasing the process of pilosebaceous plugging, and decreasing inflammation. Topical benzoyl peroxide 5 and 10 percent gels (a bacteriostatic agent) and retinoic acid (tretinoin or vitamin A acid) 0.05 to 0.1 percent cream and 0.025 percent gels are beneficial. (These decrease the stickiness of follicular cells and thus discourage plug formation.) Oral tetracycline and erythromycin are concentrated in sebaceous follicles, and are remarkably effective therapeutically by reducing the number of follicular bacteria (Kaminester, 1978). They can be used on a long-term basis, in doses of 250 mg to 1.5 grams per day. Cysts may be incised, drained, and packed if necessary. Small cysts respond well to intralesional injection of triamcinolone acetonide at 5 to 6

mg per cc, but atrophy can result from this procedure. The ingestion of chocolate, cola drinks, and other foodstuffs has not been shown to aggrevate acne in general, but may possibly do so in certain individuals. There is no evidence that food allergy is involved in acne. Trauma to the skin by manipulation of acne lesions predisposes to rupture of sebaceous follicles and increases inflammatory changes associated with acne. Patients should be made aware of the importance of leaving their skin alone, employing only acceptable techniques of skin hygiene. Many cosmetic creams are comedogenic, and their use should be discouraged. Sun exposure may appear to be helpful at first, but sunburn or prolonged sun exposure frequently worsens acne.

Miliaria. Miliaria develops when sweat is trapped in eccrine sweat ducts. Two types are recognized, related to the level in the epidermis at which sweat gland obstruction occurs. In miliaria crystallina, the obstruction is within the stratum corneum and the lesions appear as 1 to 2 mm superficially grouped vesicles without erythema. This is more common in the intertriginous areas, particularly in newborns. In miliaria rubra, the obstruction occurs in the deep epidermis, and the eruption appears as erythematous grouped papules which may progress to pustules. Heat and high humidity aggravate the condition. Cooling the skin is most helpful in preventing or alleviating the condition. Keratolytic agents frequently are helpful, such as 3 percent salicylic acid in a cream or alcohol base.

Nummular Eczema. Nummular eczema appears as coin-shaped, vesicular or papulovesicular erythematous patches, and often is associated with dry skin. It does not appear to be related to atopic dermatitis. It occurs mainly in adults but can be seen in children and preferentially affects the relatively dry extensor surfaces of the legs and arms. It commonly is seen in the winter and fades in the summer. It should be differentiated from tinea corporis, atopic dermatitis, pyoderma, drug eruptions, and contact dermatitis. Treatment consists of skin hydration and the use of topical tars and topical glucocorticosteroids.

Dyshidrotic Eczema. Dyshidrotic eczema occurs most frequently in adolescents and presents with vesicles along the lateral margins of fingers and toes. It also can occur on the plantar and palmar surfaces. The vesicles may rupture and progress to an erythematous or nonerythematous scaly dermatosis. Pruritus can occur, but it is not universal. Skin irritation from soaps and detergents and other factors such as emotional stress can aggravate the condition. Treatment involves the use of drying agents such as tannic acid, skin hydration, and avoidance of irritating substances. Topical steroids and keratolytic agents also can be beneficial.

Pityriasis Rosea. Pityriasis rosea begins with an erythematous scaly, large oval plaque with central clearing ("Herald Patch"), which precedes a generalized rash on the trunk by 1 week to 1 month. The generalized rash consists of multiple erythematous papules 3 to 6 mm long on the trunk. These oval plaques frequently run parallel in their long axes and follow Langer's lines of skin cleavage. Itching may occur and sometimes can be extremely bothersome. The condition lasts 6 to 8 weeks and seldom recurs. An "inverse" form of pityriasis rosea occurs primarily in the groin, thigh, and axillary areas. Differential diagnosis includes secondary syphilis, tinea corporis, and drug eruptions. Treatment consists of reassurance to the patient and the use of oral antihistamines to control itching. Some dermatologists employ ultraviolet light therapy (Plemmons, 1975). The presumed etiology is a viral infection, since it may occur in epidemics.

Psoriasis. Psoriasis occurs as erythematous papules covered by thick, white scales. The guttate (rain drop) type develops 2 to 3 weeks after a streptococcal infection; it is commonly seen on the trunk and occurs more frequently in children than adults (Nyfors, 1975). The chronic form of psoriasis presents thick, large (5 to 10 cm) scaly plaques. These are seen on the knees, elbows, and scalp. In all forms of psoriasis the thickened epidermis is actively proliferating, with a cell turnover four to five times faster than normal. Treatment is aimed at diminishing epidermal turnover time, with the use of coal tar, sun exposure, topical steroids, and keratolytic agents. Psoriasis is controllable, but not curable. Mild forms may be controlled with the use of topical glucocorticosteroids applied twice daily for 4 to 8 weeks. More severe forms are treated with topical coal tar preparations such as 1 percent crude coal tar ointment or a tar gel preparation (Estar, Psorigel) applied twice daily for 4 to 6 weeks. Daily sun exposure in addition to application of coal tar preparations is advised. Photochemotherapy of psoriasis ("PUVA treatment") is experimental and is not advised for children.

References

Binney, M. L., et al.: Warts. Br. J. Dermatol. 94:667, 1976.

Blank, H.: Antifungal and other effects of griseofulvin. Am. J. Med. 39:831, 1965.

Blomgren, S. E.: Conditions associated with erythema nodosum. NY J. Med. 72:2302, 1972.

Carney, R. G., Jr.: Incontinentia pigmenti. Arch. Dermatol. 112:535, 1976.

Carter, V. H., and Olansky, S.: Haloprogin and Mycostatin therapy for cutaneous candidas. Arch. Dermatol. 110:81, 1974.

Elias, P. M., Fritsch, P., and Epstein, E. H., Jr.: Staphylococcal skin syndromes. Arch. Dermatol. 113:207, 1977.

Ferrieri, P., et al.: The natural history of impetigo. J. Clin. Invest. 51:2851, 1972.

Fine, R. M.: Chronic erythema nodosum. Arch. Dermatol. 100:33, 1969.

Frain-Bell, W.: The photosensitive child. Trans. St. Johns Hospital Dermatologic Society. 59:159, 1973.

Fritch, W. C.: Therapy of impetigo and furunculosis. JAMA 214:1862, 1971.

Hertz, K. C., Kirkpatrick, C. H., and Katz, S. I.: Autoimmune vitiligo: Detection of antibodies to melanin-producing cells. N. Engl. J. Med. 297:634, 1977.

Ipp, M., and Gelfand, E. W.: Antibody deficiency and alopecia. J. Pediatr. 89:728, 1976.

Jarrett, M.: Diagnosis and treatment of epidermolysis bullosa. South. Med. J. 69:113, 1976.

Kaminester, L. H.: Acne. JAMA 239(20):2171–2172, 1978.

Kauppinen, K.: Cutaneous reaction to drugs. Acta Dermatol. Venerol. 52:supp. 68, 1972.

Kern, F., et al.: Alopecia areata: Immunologic studies and treatment with prednisone. Arch. Dermatol. 107:407, 1973.

Massie, F. S.: Papular urticaria: Etiology, diagnosis and management. Cutis. 13:980, 1974.

Mathews-Roth, M. M., Pathak, M. A., Fitzpatrick, T. B., et al.: Beta carotene therapy for erythropoietic protoporphyria and other photosensitivity diseases. Arch. Dermatol. 113:1229, 1977.

Nyfors, A., and Lemhold, K.: Psoriasis in children. Br. J. Dermatol. 92:437, 1975.

Plemmons, J. A.: Pityriasis rosea, an old therapy revisited. Cutis 16:120, 1975.

Price, V. H.: Office diagnosis of hair shaft defects. Cutis 15:231, 1975.

Rasmussen, J. E.: Erythema multiforme in children. Br. J. Dermatol. 95:181–186, 1976.

Retornax, G., Betuel, H., Ortonne, J. P., and Thivolet, J.: HL-A antigens and vitiligo. Br. J. Dermatol. 95:173, 1976.

Sahihi, T., and Esterly, N. B.: Atypical diffuse cutaneous mastocytosis. Am. J. Dis. Child. 124:133, 1972.

Solomon, L. M., et al.: Gamma benzene hexachloride toxicity: A review. Arch. Dermatol. 113:353, 1977.

Spruance, S. L., et al.: The natural history of recurrent herpes labialis. N. Engl. J. Med. 297:69, 1977.

Van Scott, E. T., and Yu, R. J.: Control of keratinization with alpha-hydroxy acids and related compounds. Arch. Dermatol. *110*:586, 1974.

GENERAL REFERENCES

Braverman, I. M.: *Skin Signs of Systemic Disease.* Philadelphia, W. B. Saunders Co., 1970.

Korting, G. W.: *Diseases of the Skin in Children and Adolescents. A Color Atlas.* Philadelphia, W. B. Saunders Co., 1970.

Odland, G. F.: *The Skin.* Seattle, University of Washington Press, 1971.

Shelley, W. B.: *Consultations in Dermatology with Walter B. Shelley.* Philadelphia, W. B. Saunders Co., 1972.

Shelley, W. B.: *Consultations in Dermatology II with Walter B. Shelley.* Philadelphia, W. B. Saunders Co., 1974.

Solomon, L. S., and Esterly, N. B.: *Neonatal Dermatology.* Philadelphia, W. B. Saunders Co., 1973.

Solomon, L. S., Esterly, N. B., and Loeffel, D.: *Adolescent Dermatology.* Philadelphia, W. B. Saunders Co., 1978.

Weinberg, S., Leider, M., and Shapiro, L.: *Color Atlas of Pediatric Dermatology.* New York, McGraw-Hill Book Co., 1975.

36

Kenneth M. Grundfast, M.D.
Charles D. Bluestone, M.D.

Principles of Diagnosis and Treatment of Upper Respiratory Tract Disease

The Nose and Paranasal Sinuses

Kenneth M. Grundfast, M.D.

NOSE

Anatomy and Physiology

In the simplest terms, the nose can be thought of as a mucous membrane–lined conduit for air. The nose humidifies and alters the temperature of inspired air, provides resistance to airflow necessary for normal lung function, interacts with the lungs via neural reflexes, and contains specialized nerve endings that provide the sense of smell.

Nasal Skeleton

Though the nose is relatively small, it is compact and efficient. Anatomically it is composed of four parts: the bony pyramid (nasal processes of frontal bone, frontal processes of maxilla and nasal bones); the upper lateral cartilages; the lower lateral cartilages; and the septum (Fig. 36A–1). Superiorly (cephalad), the upper lateral cartilages extend beneath the nasal bones, but laterally and caudally, they become thin and delicate, forming a pliable area called the

nasal valve. In the nasal valve region, a portion of the upper lateral cartilages moves with respiration toward and from the septum. The cartilage in this area does not collapse completely with inspiration because the upper lateral cartilages curl away from the septum.

The nostrils and tip of the nose are shaped by the lower lateral or alar cartilages. Each of these cartilages is a thin, flexible plate bent upon itself in such a manner as to form both the medial and lateral walls of the nostril of one side of the nose. The columella that separates the two nostrils is formed by the lower margin of the septal cartilage, the medial portions of the two alar cartilages, and the bony anterior nasal spine together with a covering of skin. Thus, the external nose is a pyramidal structure enclosing a space where ambient air can be inhaled and modified and where eddy currents can be created that will bring vaporized molecules in contact with olfactory receptors.

Internal Nose

The walls and floor of the nose are rigid. The roof is arched from anterior to posterior,

466

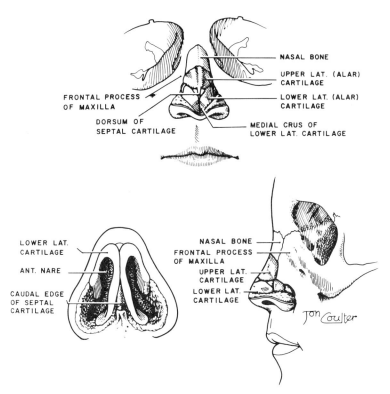

FIGURE 36A–1. Structural framework of the nose.

but the floor is level. Internally, the nose opens posteriorly into the pharynx through the two oval choanae. The transverse diameter of the nasal cavity is narrow above and wider below. The shape and location of structures within the nose serve to direct the airflow. The septum divides the nose into right and left nasal air passages. The skeletal portion of the septum is composed of the quadrangular septal cartilage anteriorly, the perpendicular plate of the ethmoid superiorly, the vomer and rostrum of the sphenoid posteriorly, and the crests of the maxillary and palatine bones inferiorly. Spurs and various deformities can involve any portion of the cartilaginous or bony septum, resulting in abnormal airflow through the nose and sometimes obstruction. Erectile tissue within the mucous membrane on both sides of the septum can adjust septal thickness and control airflow under varying atmospheric conditions.

The three turbinates protrude from the lateral wall of the nose. The inferior turbinate or concha is largest, most prominent, and most easily seen on intranasal examination.

The inferior turbinate is a separate bone, while the middle and superior turbinates are portions of the ethmoid bone (Fig. 36A–2). It is important to realize that the ostia that connect the paranasal sinuses with the nose lie hidden in the meatus between the turbinates. The middle meatus, underneath the middle turbinate, contains the ostia that connect with the maxillary sinus, the middle and anterior ethmoid air cells, and the frontal sinus. The posterior ethmoid air cells connect with the superior meatus, underneath the superior turbinate. The sphenoid sinus has an ostium lying in the sphenoethmoidal recess located superiorly and posteriorly in the nose. The nasolacrimal duct opens into the inferior meatus beneath the junction of the anterior and middle third of the inferior turbinate.

The lateral wall of the middle meatus contains the most intricate anatomy. The hiatus semilunaris is the deep gutter lying between the bulging ethmoid bulla and the hook-shaped uncinate process of the ethmoid bone. The anterior funnel-shaped end of the hiatus is called the infundibulum. The frontal sinus discharges its secretions into a region of the middle meatus known as the frontal recess, located above and anterior to the infundibulum. Within the hiatus semilunaris, the three or more distinct openings anteriorly are the ostia of the anterior ethmoid cells, while the larger opening lying more posteriorly is the ostium of the maxillary sinus. Secretions from the frontal sinus may reach the hiatus semilunaris by flowing posteriorly from the adjacent frontal recess.

The bones and cartilages that form the framework of the nose are covered by periosteum or perichondrium. Inside the nose, the covering is a thick, richly vascular mucous membrane. This highly specialized mucous membrane of the nose is continuous with a similar mucous membrane lining the paranasal sinuses, eustachian tube, middle ear, mastoid air cells, and the tracheobronchial tree.

Mucous Membrane

The respiratory epithelium is composed mostly of pseudostratified columnar cells surmounted by cilia. It is not uniform in structure at all levels of the respiratory tract. In fact, its microstructure seems to be adapted for the type of airstreams flowing over it. In the anterior third of the nose, especially on the rounded ends of the turbinates where the air is likely to be cold, dry, and unfiltered, the respiratory epithelium has no cilia, and the surface cells resemble squamous cells rather than columnar cells. The epithelium covering the medial aspect of the turbinates and adjacent septum is composed of long columnar cells with short, irregular surface cilia. Within the middle and inferior meatus where airflow is gentle, the epithelium is composed of short columnar cells with lengthy cilia. The sinuses, which usually

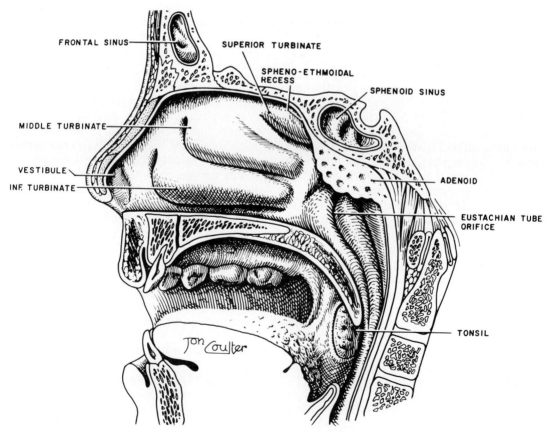

FIGURE 36A–2. The lateral wall of the nose.

receive only minute quantities of expired air, are lined by a thin epithelium.

The dense vascularity and plethora of glands within the stroma of the submucosa of the nose warm and moisten inspired air. The glands are of the racemose type and contain both serous and mucous cells. In addition, varying numbers of goblet cells lying between the surface columnar cells contribute to the secretion. The number of goblet cells is not constant but may vary with conditions that alter airflow patterns and possibly with inflammation or infection.

The cilia seem to function almost automatically. In fact, the contraction of the cilium can be observed even after most of the underlying cell has been removed. A single cilium will continue to stroke as long as a small amount of cytoplasm remains attached to it. The movements of the cilia in any given area of epithelium appear to be synchronous and purposeful, stroking in unison without bumping or distorting each other. Each stroke has a powerful rapid phase in one direction, with the cilium straight and stiff, followed by a slower phase of recovery during which the cilium bends. In this way, secreted mucus is moved in one direction.

Ciliary motion can be influenced by the following factors (Ballantyne and Groves, 1971).

Drying. Adequate moisture is necessary for normal ciliary function. Prolonged breathing of excessively dry air, inadequate secretion by mucosal glands, or both can lead to drying and impairment of ciliary activity. Conditions such as deviation of the nasal septum, which deflects the inspired air stream, produce excessive local evaporation, increased viscosity of the nasal mucus, stasis of the mucous blanket, and impaired ciliary activity.

Temperature. Ciliary activity is depressed by both low and high temperatures. Ciliary activity ceases at about 7 to 10°C and is depressed by temperatures above 35°C.

Acid-base Balance. Ciliary activity is decreased by low pH and stops completely at pH 6.4. It is increased by modest increases in pH.

Topical Medications. Epinephrine hydrochloride (1:10,000) applied to the ciliated cells for 20 minutes causes reversible inhibition of ciliary activity; with a 1:1000 solution this occurs in a much shorter time. However, ephedrine sulfate (0.5 percent solution) does not affect ciliary action.

Mucous Blanket

The so-called "mucous blanket" is a thin, sticky, continuous, highly viscid secretion that extends into all spaces within the nose, sinuses, eustachian tube, middle ear, mastoid, pharynx, and bronchial tree. The cilia propel it continuously along with particles that have been trapped by it. The pH remains at a relatively constant 7.0. The mucus in the sinuses moves through the ostia into the nose. The mucous blanket in the nose moves posteriorly through the choanae into the pharynx, where mucus is swallowed. Gastric secretions destroy bacteria and other minute particles that have been trapped by the mucus.

Blood, Nerve Supply, and Lymphatic Drainage

The sphenopalatine branch of the internal maxillary artery provides arterial supply to the turbinates, meatus, and septum. The anterior and posterior ethmoid branches of the ophthalmic artery supply the ethmoid and frontal sinuses and the roof of the nose. A branch of the superior labial artery and infraorbital and alveolar branches of the internal maxillary artery supply the maxillary sinus, while the pharyngeal branch of the internal maxillary artery is distributed to the sphenoid sinus.

The arterioles of the nasal respiratory mucosa are distinctive because they lack an internal elastic membrane, and the vascular endothelial basement membrane is continuous with the basement membrane of smooth muscle cells in the wall of the arteriole. In addition, the endothelial basement membrane is exceptionally porous. As a result, the subendothelial musculature of these vessels may be influenced more readily than other blood vessels by agents such as histamine and systemically administered vasoconstrictors (Nygind, 1978).

Within the lamina propria of the nasal mucosa are small, regular capillaries. Below the surface epithelium, the capillaries are larger and have fenestrations. The fenestrae are small areas in the endothelial lining where the endothelial cell consists only of a thin single membrane. This membrane and the porous basement membrane, reinforced by pericytes, constitute the only barrier between blood plasma and tissue fluid and provide for rapid passage of fluid through the vascular wall.

Veins within the nose form a cavernous plexus underneath the mucous membrane. The plexus is especially well developed over the middle and inferior turbinates and the lower portion of the septum where it forms erectile tissue. Venous drainage is principally through the ophthalmic, anterior facial, and sphenopalatine veins. The venous system of the nose, paranasal sinuses, and orbit communicate freely through valveless veins. Venous stasis related to nasal congestion can cause dark circles or discoloration beneath the eyes known as "allergic shiners."

In some areas of the nose, cavernous sinusoids are interposed between the capillaries and venules, predominantly in the basal part of the lamina propria of the turbinates. These cavernous sinusoids can be regarded as specialized capillaries that provide the nasal mucosa with an ability to adapt and respond to the varying demands of the nasal airway.

Lymphatic drainage of the nose is divided into an anterior and posterior network. The anterior network drains along the facial vessels toward nodes in the submaxillary glands. Most of the anterior nose, the vestibule, and the preturbinal area are drained by this system. The posterior network drains the major portion of the nose, and it forms three channels. The superior group, from the middle and superior turbinates and adjacent septum, form channels passing above the eustachian tube to drain into retropharyngeal nodes. The middle group, passing below the eustachian tube, serves the inferior turbinate, inferior meatus, and a portion of the floor and drains into the external jugular chain of lymph nodes. The inferior group, from the septum and part of the floor, drain through lymph nodes along the internal jugular vein.

The nerve supply to the nose is complex. The olfactory mucosa, located high in the nose, is characterized by the presence of "special sense" receptor nerve cells whose central processes unite to form small nerve fiber bundles that pass through the cribriform plate to enter the brain. These nerves constitute the neuronal pathway for the sense of smell. The anterior and posterior ethmoid nerves, branches of the ophthalmic division of the trigeminal nerve, supply pain, temperature, and touch sensations to the mucous membrane in the lateral wall anterior to the turbinates and meatus and the corresponding area of the septum. Nasal branches of the sphenopalatine ganglion containing fibers of the maxillary division of the trigeminal nerve supply pain, temperature, and touch sensations to much of the rest of the nasal mucosa. Parasympathetic supply originates in the facial nerve, where preganglionic fibers course to the sphenopalatine ganglion. The postsynaptic parasympathetic fibers enter all branches of the sphenopalatine ganglion and are distributed to the glandular epithelium within the nose. It is stimulation of these fibers that results in secretion from the glands in the nasal mucosa. The sympathetic fibers are derived from the white *rami communicantes* of spinal nerves T_1 through T_3. The sympathetic fibers course through the spenopalatine ganglion without synapsing, then are distributed to the nasal mucosa. Stimulation of the sympathetic fibers causes vasoconstriction of the vessels supplying the nasal mucosa, whereas stimulation of the parasympathetic system *dilates* blood vessels. The subepithelial cavernous sinusoids are kept partially constricted by continuous sympathetic stimulation. As the sinusoids account for a large part of nasal blood volume in the turbinates, changes in the autonomic innervation can cause considerable changes rapidly in the thickness of the nasal mucosa and, in turn, can affect the degree of nasal patency (Nygind, 1978).

Both the secretory and contractile myoepithelial elements of the human nasal glands are under parasympathetic control in contrast to the salivary glands, which possess a dual autonomic nerve supply. However, since the secretion of glands depends upon their blood supply, secretion of the nasal glands is indirectly affected by sympathetic nerve fibers through the innervation of blood vessels.

Glands

The glands of the lamina propria of the nasal mucosa consist of anterior serous glands and scattered seromucous glands. The openings of the serous glands are comparatively large, and the serous ducts often have an ampullated area near the area where the duct bends toward the surface. The seromucous glands are smaller and more numerous than the serous glands. Specialized cells in the seromucous glands contribute to the formation of secretions. Proteinaceous secretion is released from the glandular cells of the secretory tubules, then as the secretion passes through the mucous secretory tubules, large amounts of mucus are added. This combined primary secretion is collected in a collecting duct that is able to modify and control the ion and water concentration of the final glandular secretion. In the ciliated duct, goblet and ciliated cells form the mucociliary transport apparatus that assists in the expulsion of secretion from the gland opening.

Secretion

Nasal fluid is a mixture of mucus secreted by goblet cells and seromucous glands, serous fluid from the anterior serous glands and seromucous glands, a transudate from plasma, condensed water from the expired air, tears, cells and microorganisms. The major components of the fluid are water (95 to 97 percent), mucin (2.5 to 3 percent), electrolytes (1 to 2 percent), and proteins that are partly derived from plasma and partly synthesized locally in the mucosa (Nygind, 1978). The mucin forms long threads or fibrils, giving nasal secretion its viscoelastic properties. Electrolyte concentrations are similar to those in serum, with the exception of potassium, which is about three times higher in nasal secretions. With nasal hypersecretion resulting from respiratory infections, there is a decrease in sodium, chloride, calcium, and protein concentration in the secretion. However, in the nasal secretion that results from allergen challenge, potassium concentration decreases and protein concentration increases, possibly owing to increased transudation from plasma induced by allergic mediators.

Immunity

Secretory IgA (dimer + secretory component) is the principal immunoglobulin found in nasal secretion. It is transferred to the secretion by an active process. The dimer IgA is found in plasma cells surrounding the exocrine glands in the lamina propria of the nasal and sinus mucosa. The secretory component that is produced in the glandular cells binds to the IgA to form secretory IgA. Secretory IgA covers the mucosal surface of the mucous membrane and acts to protect against invasion of microorganisms. It inhibits the adherence of microorganisms to the surface and neutralizes viruses.

Although IgG is an immunoglobulin found mostly in the blood, it does pass from blood to tissue fluid and, to a lesser degree, from tissue fluid to secretion. Inflammation increases the permeability of blood vessels and epithelium, allowing larger amounts of IgG antibodies to reach the surface of the mucous membrane. Although there are normally relatively few IgG-producing plasma cells in nasal mucosa, their number increases with chronic nasal infection.

IgE is of great importance in allergic nasal disease. Unlike IgA, IgE is not linked with a secretory component but is transported actively through the epithelium.

Functions of the Nose

The major functions of the nose are olfaction, filtration, and humidification and warming of air for respiration. With ordinary tidal breathing airflow is low in the nose and odors are not usually perceived unless they are strong. In order to sense an odor, air must be brought higher into the nose where the olfactory receptors are situated. This is accomplished by sniffing, that is, fixing the rib cage and abruptly moving the diaphragm down. Nasal polyps or any mechanical obstruction within the nose that alters airflow patterns can impair the sense of smell.

Air conditioning is probably the most important function of the nose. The three nasal valves that serve to regulate and direct nasal airflow are termed the liminal, turbinal, and septal valves. The turbinates serve to further direct the flow of air and create controlled air turbulence within which the nose facilitates filtration, warming, and humidification of inspired air. The air is warmed by rapid heat transfer from blood in the capillary networks and venous sinuses.

The ability of the nose to cleanse air of particulate matter depends upon the nature of the particles. Allergenic particles, such as pollen, dust, and dander are partially filtered from inspired air in the nose. Size, shape, and density of the particles are important. In general, the larger and heavier the particles, the sooner they will be filtered from inspired air and deposited within the nose. Some particles form aggregations, and some hygroscopic dusts take on water, becoming larger until they reach an equilibrium determined by vapor saturation at the ambient body temperature (Hinchcliff and Harrison, 1976). Bacteria, although small, may form agglomerates or may be included in droplets. Viruses can also be enclosed in droplets. All of these then behave as larger particles and are trapped by the nasal mucous blanket. Factors such as particle inertia, density, and surface area, as well as velocity and turbulence of airflow, affect air filtration in the nose.

A large portion of foreign material in inspired air is deposited in the anterior third of the nose. After passing through the anterior nares, the flow rate of inspired air decreases as it is filtered through the hairs in the vestibule. The flow rate increases at the nasal valve region, then decreases in the preturbinal area as it strikes the anterior blunt ends of the inferior and middle turbinates. The shape of the turbinates induces turbulence and directs airflow backward instead of up. As the air flows posteriorly toward the choanae, it deposits particles. Additional deposition occurs even after air passes through the choanae into the pharynx. Noxious gases contained in inspired air diffuse into the mucous blanket.

The Nose and Pulmonary Function

It is important to realize that the nose is one integral unit functioning in concert with other portions of the respiratory system. Normal aeration of pulmonary alveoli depends upon the maintenance of an adequate resistance to the flow of air within the tracheobronchial tree. The nose furnishes from 50 to 70 percent of the total respiratory resistance. Nasopulmonary and nasobronchial reflexes increase bronchial tone in cases of nasal obstruction and also increase pulmonary resistance while decreasing compliance. Thus, nasal obstruction can increase pulmonary resistance while decreasing compliance.

Nasal Cycle

The term "nasal cycle" refers to the alternating changes in patency of the right and left nasal cavitites. Congestion, then decongestion of the erectile tissues of the nasal mucosa of the lateral wall and septum occur in rhythmic sequence in most individuals. As one nasal chamber opens and mucosal glands secrete, the erectile tissues of the opposite chamber fill with blood, and secretions of the mucosal glands diminish. The cycle is controlled by peripheral autonomic centers in the sphenopalatine and stellate ganglia. The cycle seems to be most active during adolescence when hormonal factors may act on nasal erectile tissue. Head position and body posture can influence hydrostatic pressure of blood in the head and, in turn, influence the nasal cycle. Vasoconstrictor nose drops can interrupt this cycle temporarily.

Protective Mechanisms

The sneeze is a simple yet important nasal reflex. Irritation of the nasal mucosa causes sneezing and associated cardiorespiratory responses. Such irritation may be due to allergic, autonomic, and psychologic factors. Ciliary propulsion of mucus is a protective mechanism in that it aids in the expulsion of foreign matter. Noxious stimuli increase nasal secretions. Immunoglobulins in nasal secretions (primarily IgA) can inactivate viruses. Lysozymes present in nasal secretions may aid in bacterial defense. When the mucociliary defenses fail and organisms invade the tunica propria or stroma of the mucosa, phagocytosis becomes important. Fibroblasts, ameboid wandering cells, undifferentiated mesenchymal cells, mast cells, and histiocytes also play a role in the removal of debris, pollen, bacteria, or other foreign material. Polymorphonuclear leukocytes are the active phagocytes in acute infection; histiocytes are active in subacute and chronic inflammation.

Examination of the Nose

Before examining the inside of the nose, the external nose should be inspected. The shape of the upper bony portion and lower cartilaginous portion should be noted. Palpation of the bony nasal dorsum can reveal deformities not apparent on inspection. Abnormal contour of the nasal alae, displacement of the septum, or a retracted columella may contribute to nasal obstruction. A transverse crease across the lower third of the nose at the junction of the bulbous soft portion and the more rigid bony dorsum suggests chronic nasal rubbing associated with allergic rhinitis. Persistent nasal obstruction with intranasal edema can cause broadening of the bony dorsum of the nose.

The internal nose is best examined with the aid of a nasal speculum to spread the nares and with bright illumination reflected from a headlight or head mirror into the nose. A knowledge of normal anatomic landmarks is essential. Edematous, pale bluish turbinates often are seen in children with allergic rhinitis. Purulent discharge in the middle meatus is indicative of sinusitis (Fig. 36A–3). Nasal polyps in children are more likely to be associated with cystic fibrosis than an allergic diathesis. Since masses such as a meningocele or an encephalocele can be mistaken for benign polyps, biopsy should not be performed without thorough investigation. Small, superficial, unexplained, nonhealing lesions in the nasal mucosa warrant biopsy. However, when the total extent and origin of an intranasal mass cannot be adequately judged on intranasal examination, it is wise to obtain radiographic studies of facial bones and paranasal sinuses before proceeding to biopsy.

When there is significant swelling of the nasal mucosa, examination is not complete until a topical vasoconstrictor such as phenylephrine hydrochloride or ephedrine sulfate has been applied to shrink the mucous membrane and allow better visualization of the entire nasal chamber.

A flexible fiberoptic or a rod lens telescopic nasopharyngoscope is useful in close examination of the posterior nose and nasopharynx. Prior to insertion of these instruments and prior to nasal biopsy, it is advisable to use 5 percent lidocaine hydrochloride (Xylocaine) as a topical anesthetic. The small nasopharyngeal mirror inserted posterior to the soft palate gives a view of the

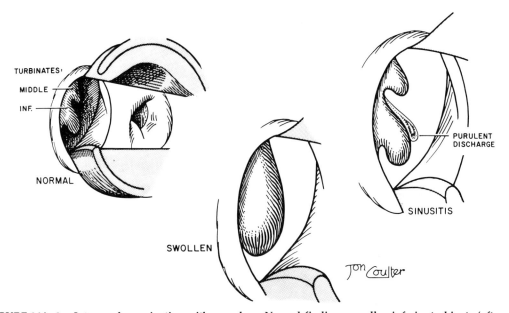

FIGURE 36A–3. Intranasal examination with speculum. Normal findings; swollen inferior turbinate (often associated with allergic rhinitis); findings in sinusitis.

choanae and eustachian tube orifices, but use of the mirror requires considerable skill and practice.

Nasal Smear Cytology

Since intranasal inspection may not always lead to a definitive diagnosis, it is sometimes helpful to obtain a specimen from the inside of the nose for cytologic study. A method for nasal cytologic examination is described in detail by Bryan and Bryan (1974). This is accomplished by gently passing a wire applicator thinly wrapped with cotton along the floor of the nose and up under the inferior turbinate three times in each side of the nose. The motion should be one of wiping rather than dabbing or blotting. After each wiping, the contents on the probe are gently rolled, not smeared, onto a glass slide. Next, the slide is fixed by placing it in a solution of 95 percent alcohol and ether (reagent quality) for five minutes. Alternatively, a commercial spray fixative can be used. Wright-Geimsa stain is applied for approximately 30 seconds, then immediately flooded for 30 more seconds with a buffer of pH 6.4 to 6.8. The slide is then washed with distilled water. Deliberate understaining is advisable so that the stained epithelial cells do not obscure the mast cells.

Evaluation of the Nasal Cytogram

Cytologic examination of a nasal smear for accumulations of eosinophils is helpful in differentiating allergic disorders from conditions such as viral or bacterial infections or tumor (Chap. 39).

The nasal cytogram can be helpful in differentiating nasal allergy from nasal infection. Intracellular structural changes can be seen when wipe smears from nasal secretions are stained with Papanicolaou's stain. Ciliated cells undergo distinctive destructive changes in the presence of viruses that cause the common cold. The mass degeneration and destruction of ciliated cells is termed "ciliocytophoria." A unique feature of the cytopathic effect is the separation of the nucleus-containing basal portion from the ciliated apical portion. Prior to separation of the cell, there is margination of pyknotic chromatin masses attached to inclusion material within the nucleus. There is increased granulation of the cytoplasm, and a halo can be seen around the nucleus before the ciliated cell constricts and finally breaks into two parts (Fig. 36A–4). Examination of nasal smears for ciliocytophoria can be helpful in identifying response to viral infection either with or in contrast to allergic and bacterial inflammation.

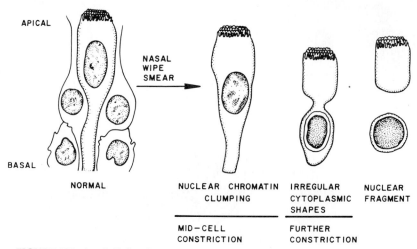

RESPONSE OF NASAL EPITHELIAL CELLS TO VIRAL INFECTION

FIGURE 36A–4. Cellular changes occurring in response to nasal viral infection.

Cytochemistry

Several cytochemical stains have been adapted for use on nasal smears in order to delineate specific chemical features of normal and altered columnar epithelial cells. Himes and Moriber stain makes it possible to identify deoxyribonucleic acid, proteins, and polysaccharides; periodic acid–Schiff (PAS) reagents can be used to demonstrate aldehyde reactions. Naphthol yellow S is a dye that combines with amino acids and thereby demonstrates protein components. The Feulgen stain localizes DNA, while the methyl green-pyronin stain shows areas of RNA within the columnar epithelial cell. Thus, by using several staining techniques, DNA, RNA, protein, and polysaccharides can be identified and localized.

Observing properly stained cellular components obtained from a wiped nasal smear can give clues to the factors that are causing cellular alterations within the nasal mucosa. Table 36–1 summarizes ways in which the cellular response to allergic inflammation differs from the cellular changes that occur in response to viral inflammation (common cold).

Rhinomanometry

Rhinomanometry is the measurement of nasal respiratory function. Several devices have been designed that are capable of measuring pressure, resistance, and volume of nasal airflow. Measurements can be made quickly and easily, and children usually tolerate the test procedures without becoming frightened. Analysis of rhinomanometric data has revealed that a fundamental function of the nose is to act as a servomechanism for matching the impedance of the upper respiratory tract to that of the lower. The nose also is involved in matching the impedance of the entire respiratory tract to alveolar ventilation, balancing a demand for oxygen with energy expended, and modulating the mechanical efficiency of respiration (Williams, 1970). Although rhinomanometry was once considered purely a research tool, it now is useful in clinical situations. Rhinomanometry can be helpful in determining whether an obstruction is caused primarily by engorgement of nasal mucosa or by adenoid hypertropy. Also, rhinomanometry can be utilized as a means for monitoring the effectiveness of medical or surgical measures in the treatment of chronic nasal obstruction.

PARANASAL SINUSES

General Considerations

The paranasal sinuses are a series of mucosa-lined pneumatic cavities that sur-

TABLE 36–1 CELLULAR RESPONSE TO ALLERGIC VS. VIRAL INFLAMMATION

Cellular Component	Allergic	Viral
Polysaccharide	Increase in cytoplasm	No appreciable amount seen in cytoplasm unless patient is also allergic — PAS negative
DNA	No visible disturbance of chromatin DNA	Consistent structural patterns of disturbed chromatin DNA
Protein	Less intense protein staining in goblet cells as compared to cells seen on smear from normal mucosa	More intense protein staining seen in cells that are degenerating
Cilia	Loss of cilia with remnants of cilia frequently seen; fragile cell membranes	Cilia remain intact and motile; as cells degenerate, apical ciliated end breaks away from basal nucleus–containing end
Other	Negative Sudan black B and oil red 0 stain for fats; small amounts of fatty acids	Inclusion material, apparently RNA (RNA positive, Feulgen negative) seen in nucleus and cytoplasm

Modified from Bryan, M. P., and Bryan, W. T. K.: Cytologic diagnosis in allergic disorders. Otolaryngol. Clin. North Am. 7(3):637, 1974.

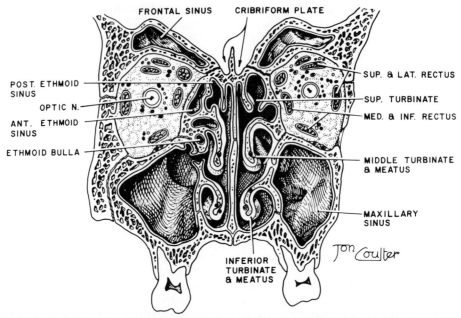

FRONTAL SINUS   CRIBRIFORM PLATE

POST. ETHMOID SINUS

OPTIC N.

ANT. ETHMOID SINUS

ETHMOID BULLA

SUP. & LAT. RECTUS

SUP. TURBINATE

MED. & INF. RECTUS

MIDDLE TURBINATE & MEATUS

MAXILLARY SINUS

INFERIOR TURBINATE & MEATUS

FIGURE 36A–5. Sagittal section through the nose showing the relationship of the sinuses to nasal landmarks (see text).

round the nose and lie adjacent to the orbit (Fig. 36A–5). Some of the sinuses begin to develop during fetal life, others during early childhood. Pneumatic expansion continues throughout the childhood years until early adulthood. The mucoperiosteum lining of the sinuses contains cilia and mucous glands, though they are sparser than in the nasal mucosa. The sinus mucosa is covered with a layer of mucus that is propelled by the cilia toward the ostia. The mucosa is able to regenerate if portions are damaged by infection, injury, chemicals, or surgery. However, regenerated mucosa appears to be more susceptible to infection because it has fewer cilia and goblet cells than normal mucosa and may be scarred.

Functions

The function of the paranasal sinuses is not clear. They may have an olfactory function since inspired air is evenly distributed within them, a resonating function in voice production, and a protective function in producing mucus to moisten the nasal chambers. In addition, they lessen the weight of the skull.

Maxillary Sinus

The maxillary sinus is the first of the cavities to develop. A small ridge develops superior to the inferior turbinate and projects medially into the middle meatus at approximately ten weeks of gestation. This is the rudimentary uncinate ridge. Just posterior and superior to this ridge, a mucosal evagination slowly extends laterally into the maxilla and expands. The maxillary sinus cavity, measuring approximately 7x4x4 mm, is present at birth. As the facial structures grow anteroinferiorly away from the skull after birth, the maxillary sinus also expands in the same direction at the rate of 2 mm vertically and 3 mm anteroposteriorly each year. By the age of twelve years, the floor of the sinus lies on a horizontal level with the floor of the nasal chamber. Anatomically, the floor of the maxillary sinus is closely related to the maxillary teeth. As a tooth erupts, the space vacated by it becomes pneumatized by the expanding sinus lumen. Expansion is complete after the permanent teeth erupt, with a final volume of 14 to 15 ml.

Since the lumen of the sinus grows progressively from above downward, the younger the patient, the more likely it is that the floor of the sinus lies above the level of the floor of the nasal chamber. In young children, the needle must be directed superiorly in order to enter the maxillary sinus to irrigate it or to obtain secretions for culture.

The ostium of the maxillary sinus is round or oval, approximately 4 mm in diameter, and lies in the middle meatus. Within the sinus, the ostium is located immediately below the orbital floor, at the highest point of the maxillary antrum. Therefore, in the upright position, secretion must completely fill the antrum or ciliary action must move secretion cephalad to the ostium to discharge into the nose.

Ethmoid Sinuses

The ethmoid sinuses consist of a group of three to fifteen air cells within the ethmoid bone on each side of the nose. These sinuses begin to develop during the fifth month of intrauterine life as numerous evaginations from the fetal nasal chamber. At first these evaginations are mere slits, but they develop rapidly, assuming a round or globular shape as they expand within the ethmoid bone. The air cells eventually abut each other, with thin, bony walls between the mucosa-lined air cells. The expansion of the ethmoid group of cells usually continues until late puberty. The ethmoid cell block, sometimes termed the ethmoid labyrinth, is pyramidal in shape, being wider posteriorly (where it abuts the sphenoid bone) than anteriorly (where it meets the lacrimal bone). Even though growth of the air cells results in air sinuses that are of different size and shape, the ostium of each ethmoid sinus is at the site of the cell's initial evagination from the fetal nasal chamber.

The ostia of the ethmoidal sinuses are the smallest of all the paranasal sinuses, measuring only 1 to 2 mm in diameter. Perhaps it is the small luminal diameter that makes these ostia so susceptible to occlusion by mucosal edema or growth of polyploid granulation tissue. Usually the ostia of the anterior ethmoidal cells are even smaller than those of the posterior ones.

The lamina papyracea is the thin bony plate that separates the ethmoid sinus air cells from the orbit. Occasionally, natural dehiscences occur in this bone so that there is communication between the ethmoid sinus and the orbit.

Orbital cellulitis usually occurs between the ages of six and nine years and is the most common complication of acute sinusitis in children (usually acute ethmoiditis). The infection spreads from the ethmoid mucosa through a natural dehiscence, via the vascular foramina or by a thrombophlebitis of veins communicating between the sinus and the orbit.

Frontal Sinus

The nasofrontal region is an evagination of the anterosuperior part of the middle meatus. At three to four months of fetal life, furrows develop in this region; then during subsequent development there is gradual deepening of the furrows and the formation of a single large pit or several small pits. These pits can be recognized at birth; as they continue to expand, their growth pushes one or two of them upward into the frontal bone. By six years, the sinus has grown sufficiently large to be radiographically visible in the frontal bone. The upward expansion continues, with the cell at first lying closer to the posterior table than to the anterior one before it finally becomes situated in the cancellous bone midway between the two tables. On rare occasions, the frontal sinus develops as an extramural expansion of one of the ethmoid air cells. Sometimes the frontal sinus fails to develop altogether, and usually the right and left chambers are of unequal size.

When the sinus develops directly as an extension of the whole frontal recess, the ostium of the sinus drains directly into the anterior upper part of the middle meatus. When the frontal sinus originates from a frontal recess furrow or from one of the cells of the ethmoidal infundibulum, drainage is into the nose via a nasofrontal duct.

The proximity of the sinus to the bone marrow of the frontal bone permits spread of infection from the sinuses into the marrow and bloodstream. Consequently, abscesses in the frontal bone can complicate frontal sinusitis.

Sphenoid Sinus

The sphenoid sinus begins to develop in the fourth month of fetal life as a posterior evagination from the nasal capsule into the sphenoid bone. Usually, the sinus is round; however, it sometimes expands by diverticula off the main lumen into the various parts of the sphenoid bone. Hence, the greater wing of the sphenoid bone often contains a pneumatic extension, and the lesser wing sometimes also contains an extension.

The sinus is classified as nonpneumatic, presellar, or sellar, depending upon the degree of pneumatization relative to the location of the pituitary fossa. Large sellar sinuses will sometimes expand so widely that the internal carotid artery and nerves adjacent to the sinus lumen appear as ridges on the bony wall of the sinus. The optic, ophthalmic, and mandibular divisions of the trigeminal or vidian nerve may lie separated from the sinus mucosa by only a thin layer of bone.

The ostium of the sphenoid sinus usually is round and located one half to one third of the way up the face of the sphenoid sinus. It usually lies 2 to 5 mm from the dura and the same distance from the midline. It is hidden from view by the superior turbinate during anterior rhinoscopy.

Methods of Examination

The sinuses are examined primarily by palpation and transillumination. Transillumination is done with a high intensity narrow beam light source applied to the hard palate or front of the maxilla (maxillary sinuses), or to the inferior aspect of the supraorbital rim (frontal sinuses). Results of transillumination testing are often equivocal and of questionable clinical importance.

Tenderness on palpation of a sinus is a sign of acute sinusitis. Although it has been customary for an examiner to tap on the patient's forehead or malar eminence to elicit tenderness, children are sometimes frightened by the sudden pain that results from percussion of the wall of an inflamed sinus. Rather, it is better to exert increasing pressure gently at the sites depicted in Figure 36A–6. It is helpful to ask the child to let you know if the pressure causes pain and, if so,

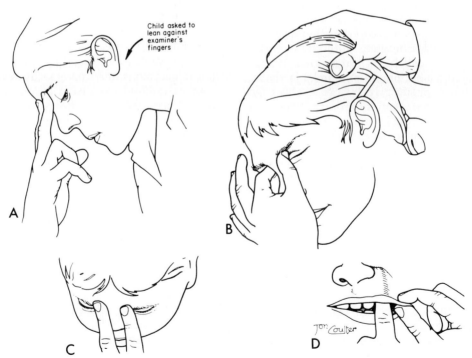

FIGURE 36A–6. Method of palpating paranasal sinuses. *A* and *B*–frontal sinuses; *C*–ethmoid sinuses; *D*–maxillary sinus.

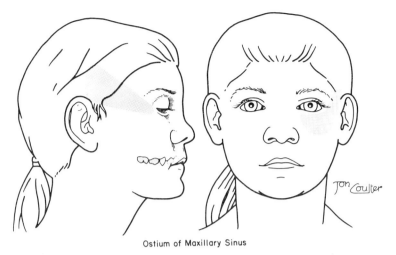

Ostium of Maxillary Sinus

FIGURE 36A–7. Referred pain from ostium of maxillary sinus.

whether the pain is greater on the left or right side.

Pain from sinus disease can be referred to areas adjacent to the involved sinus. Pain from inflammation and irritation of a maxillary sinus ostium can be referred to the infraorbital and temporal areas or to the maxillary premolar teeth (Fig. 36A–7). Pain from the frontal sinus can be perceived as coming from within the eye or in the area of the temporomandibular joint (Fig. 36A–8). Irritation of the frontonasal duct can cause pain in the premolar teeth. Pain from the sphenoid sinus can cause occipital pain, vertex pain, or a deep-seated headache (Fig. 36A–8).

Radiography

In adults with sinus disease, sinus radiographs may show changes ranging from mucosal thickening, changes in air–fluid levels, to partial or complete opacification of one or all sinuses. However, since radiographic findings must be correlated with clinical signs and symptoms, there is a wide varia-

FIGURE 36A–8. Patterns of referred pain.

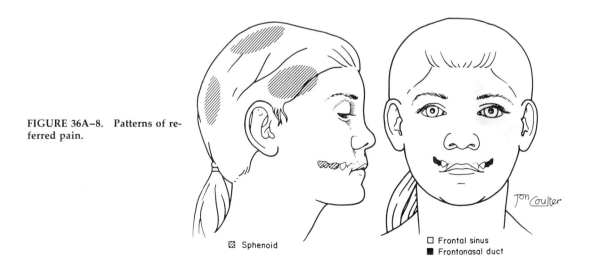

▨ Sphenoid

□ Frontal sinus
■ Frontonasal duct

tion in the radiographic appearance of normal sinuses, and many findings may be subtle. For example, it is difficult to decide when mucosal thickening is within normal limits and when it indicates response to infection or allergy.

In children, the interpretation of sinus radiographs becomes even more complicated since there is a variation between individuals in the rate at which sinuses develop. It can be difficult to differentiate pathologic opacification from poorly developed or late-to-develop sinuses. Further, the interpretation of abnormal sinus radiographs has become controversial. For instance, Caffey (1967) believed that opacified sinuses on radiographs could result from redundant sinus mucosa or from fluid from tears. Shopfner and Rossi (1973) studied sinus radiographs from 329 children to define criteria for interpreting sinus films. In this series only half of the children who were diagnosed as having sinusitis on clinical grounds had radiographic evidence of sinusitis. Fifty-seven percent of children without clinical evidence of sinusitis had radiographic findings that were considered abnormal according to their criteria. Abnormal paranasal sinus films were present most commonly in children with upper respiratory infections without clinical evidence of sinusitis. Unfortunately their study has been interpreted widely by pediatricians as demonstrating that sinus radiographs in children are of no value rather than that the significance of radiographic findings depends upon correlation with history and physical findings.

Another widespread misconception is that the paranasal sinuses cannot be visualized in very young children. Ethmoid sinuses can be visualized by radiography in children as young as 10 months. The three radiographic views that are most useful in evaluating paranasal sinus pathology in children are the posteroanterior (Caldwell) view, the occipitomental (Waters) view, and the lateral view. The posteroanterior view demonstrates the frontal sinuses and the superior ethmoid cells. The occipitomental view best demonstrates developmental or pathologic changes in the maxillary sinus. The lateral view provides considerable information about all the paranasal sinuses. It demonstrates the thickness of the anterior wall and the anteroposterior depth of the frontal sinus and the anteroposterior depth of the sphenoid sinuses. Although the right and left maxillary sinuses are superimposed in a lateral view, the thickness of the walls of the maxillary sinuses and the relationship of the antral floor to the teeth is demonstrated. The nasopharynx, adenoids, tonsils (if enlarged), and palate are well-visualized in the lateral views.

Radiographic findings that tend to substantiate a clinical diagnosis of allergic rhinosinusitis are thickening of paranasal sinus mucosa and sometimes polyps visible within the sinus. Representative sinus radiographs are shown in Chapter 40.

References

Adams, L., Boies, L., and Paparella, M.: Boies' Fundamentals of Otolaryngology, 5th ed. Philadelphia, W. B. Saunders Co., 1978.

Ballantyne, J., and Groves, J.: Scott-Brown's Diseases of the Ear, Nose and Throat, 3rd ed. London, Butterworth and Co., 1971.

Bernstein, L. (ed.): Surgery of the nasal sinuses. *Otolaryngol. Clin. North Am.*, W. B. Saunders Co., Philadelphia, 1971.

Bryan, M.P., and Bryan, W.T.K.: Cytologic diagnosis in allergic disorders. *Otolaryngol. Clin. North Am.*, 7(3):637, 1974.

Caffey, J.: Pediatric X-Ray Diagnosis, 5th ed. Chicago, Year Book Publishers, Inc., 1967.

Clemis, J. (ed.): Allergy in otorhinolaryngology, *Otol. Clin. North Am.*, 7(3): October, 1974.

Dodd, G.D., and Jing, B.: Radiology of the Nose, Paranasal Sinuses and Nasopharynx. Baltimore, Williams and Wilkins Co., 1977.

Hajek, M.: Pathology and Treatment of the Inflammatory Diseases of the Nasal Accessory Sinuses. St. Louis, C.V. Mosby Co., 1926.

Hinchcliff, R., and Harrison, D. (eds.): Scientific Foundations of Otolaryngology. Chicago, Yearbook Medical Publishers, 1976.

Nygind, N.: Nasal Allergy. Oxford, Scientific Publications, 1978.

Ritter, F.N.: The Paranasal Sinuses — Anatomy and Surgical Technique, 2nd ed. St. Louis, The C.V. Mosby Co., 1978.

Shopfner, C., and Rossi, J.: Roentgen evaluation of the paranasal sinuses in children. J. Radiol. *118*:176, 1973.

Williams, H.L.: Report of Committee on Standardization of Definitions, Terms, Symbols in Rhinomanometry of the American Academy of Ophthalmology and Otolaryngology (A.A.O.O.), Rochester, Minn., A.A.O.O., 1970.

The Ear

Charles D. Bluestone, M.D.
Kenneth M. Grundfast, M.D.

Allergic disorders can involve any of the mucous membrane–lined air-containing spaces of the middle ear, mastoid, and nose as well as the paranasal sinuses. Knowledge of the anatomy and physiology of the ear provides the basis for an understanding of the pathophysiology of its involvement in allergic disorders of the upper respiratory tract.

Anatomically, the ear may be divided into five portions: the auricle (pinna), external canal, eardrum, tympanum (middle ear space), and the inner ear.

AURICLE

The auricle (or pinna) consists of a thin piece of yellow fibrocartilage covered with skin and connected with surrounding parts by ligaments and muscles. The skin is firmly adherent on the anterior surface and looser on the posterior surface. The lymphatic drainage of the posterior surface drains to nodes at the mastoid tip, from the tragus and upper part of the anterior surface to parotid lymph nodes, and from the inferior part to nodes immediately caudal to the lobule.

Contact dermatitis of the auricle frequently is due to cosmetics, hair sprays, hair dyes, and jewelry. Seborrheic dermatitis both in early infancy and in adolescence may involve the auricle as well as the scalp. In young children, ear discomfort associated with inadequate middle ear ventilation may induce scratching and excoriation of the auricles.

THE EXTERNAL AUDITORY CANAL

The external auditory canal is about 2.5 cm in length in adults and usually less than 2 cm in length in young children. It is S-shaped in that its general direction is upwards and backwards in the outer cartilaginous part, then slightly downward and forward more medially in the bony part that meets the eardrum. In newborn or young infants, the bony canal has not yet formed, and the eardrum lies in an almost horizontal position. As a result, the external canal is more or less collapsed upon the surface of the eardrum. Since the infant's ear canal is almost entirely composed of cartilage, it is relatively distensible. For this reason, in infants movement of the ear canal on tympanometry may appear to indicate good eardrum movement even when a middle ear effusion is present.

The external auditory canal is the only cul-de-sac in the human body lined by skin. The skin of the outer one third is closely adherent to the cartilage and contains tiny hairs, sebaceous glands, and ceruminous glands. Almost all the sebaceous glands open into the lumina of the hair follicles. The ceruminous glands are simple coiled tubular structures with cuboidal secretory cells surrounded by an outer myoepithelium. Contraction of the myoepithelium compresses the lumen of the tubule and expels the contents. The ceruminous glands lie in the deeper portion of the dermis, and the ducts from the glands reach the epidermis, emptying either into the lumen of a hair follicle or on the free epidermal surface.

Earwax (cerumen) is the product of both sebaceous and ceruminous glands and can be "wet" or "dry." The type of earwax that a person has is genetically inherited, the wet type being dominant. Though it has no antibacterial, antifungal, or insect repellent properties, cerumen provides protection for the eardrum by acting as a vehicle for the collection and removal of epithelial debris and contaminants. It also provides lubrication and prevents desiccation of the epidermis. The skin of the ear canal and caudal

481

portion of the auricle may become macerated and edematous from chronic ear drainage. Since the cartilage of the auricle is continuous with the cartilaginous portion of the external ear canal, movement of the auricle or tragus results in severe pain in diffuse external otitis but usually not in otitis media. However, even in the child with severe external otitis, middle ear disease should be considered as an etiologic factor. The eardrum must be visualized and inspected for perforations despite an edematous, macerated, or excoriated ear canal.

THE TYMPANIC MEMBRANE

The tympanic membrane (eardrum) is an elliptical disc composed of three layers: an outer layer of epidermis, a middle fibrous layer, and an inner mucous membrane layer. The eardrum is nearly conical in shape with its concave surface toward the external ear canal. The lateral (short) process of the malleus protrudes from the surface of the eardrum toward the ear canal. The smaller portion of the eardrum above the short process is called Shrapnell's membrane, or the pars flaccida. The larger portion below the short process is the pars tensa. The eardrum forms the lateral wall of the middle ear space and is frequently involved in middle ear disease.

THE EUSTACHIAN TUBE

The eustachian tube connects the middle ear and mastoid air cells directly to the nasopharynx and indirectly to the nasal cavities and palate (Fig. 36B–1). In the adult, the anterior two thirds of the eustachian tube is cartilaginous and the posterior third bony, but in the infant, the bony portion is relatively longer. The lumen of the eustachian tube is shaped like two cones with the apex of each directed toward the middle. The aural orifice of the tube is oval in shape, measuring 5 mm high and 2 mm wide in the adult. The nasopharyngeal orifice in the adult is 8 to 9 mm in diameter, appearing as a vertical slit at right angles to the base of the skull, but in the infant this opening is 4 to 5 mm and oblique owing to the more horizontal position of the cartilage. The mucosal lining of the cartilaginous portion is similar to that of the nasopharynx and contains mucous glands. The mucosa in the protympanic portion of the eustachian tube is similar to that of the middle ear and contains both mucus-producing elements and cilia.

Usually the eustachian tube is closed, but it opens during swallowing, yawning, and sneezing, permitting the air pressure in the middle ear to equalize with atmospheric pressure. The tensor veli palatini is the only muscle related to active tubal opening (Cantekin et al., 1979A; Honjo et al., 1979). No constrictor muscle of the tube has ever been demonstrated, and closure has been attributed to the relaxation of the tensor muscle with passive return of the tubal walls to a condition of approximation. The eustachian tube has at least three physiologic functions with respect to the middle ear (Fig. 36B–2): *ventilation* of the middle ear to equilibrate air pressure in the middle ear with atmospheric pressure and to replenish oxygen that has

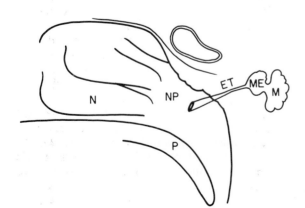

FIGURE 36B–1. Eustachian tube system. *N*, nasal cavity; *NP*, nasopharynx; *P*, palate; *ET*, Eustachian tube; *ME*, middle ear; *M*, mastoid.

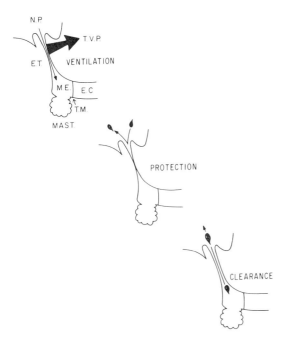

FIGURE 36B–2. Three physiologic functions of the eustachian tube in relation to the middle ear. *NP*, nasopharynx; *ET*, Eustachian tube; *TVP*, tensor veli palatini muscle; *ME*, middle ear; *Mast*, mastoid; *TM*, tympanic membrane; *EC*, external canal.

been absorbed, *protection* from nasopharyngeal sound pressure and secretions, and *clearance* of secretions produced within the middle ear into the nasopharynx. Assessment of these functions has been helpful in understanding the physiology and pathophysiology of the eustachian tube, as well as in the diagnosis and management of patients with middle ear disease.

Physiology of the Eustachian Tube

The normal eustachian tube is functionally obstructed or collapsed at rest (Fig. 36B–3A). Intermittent active opening of the tube maintains near-ambient pressures in the middle ear (Fig. 36B–3B) (Bluestone and Beery, 1976). When active opening of the eustachian tube is inefficient, functional collapse of the tube may persist (Fig. 36B–3C) until a pressure gradient develops between the middle ear cavity and the nasopharynx sufficient to assist tubal function passively (Fig. 36B–3D). The negative middle ear gradient is caused by the absorption of middle ear gas

and appears to be common in children who may have moderate to high negative middle ear pressures on tympanometry but normal eustachian tube function otherwise (Beery et al., 1975).

Eustachian tube function also may vary according to season (Beery et al., 1979*B*). Serial studies on children with tympanostomy tubes revealed better eustachian tube function in the summer and fall than in the winter and spring. Considerably more research is needed to elicit in-depth knowledge of eustachian tube–middle ear physiology.

Causes of Eustachian Tube Dysfunction

The eustachian tube can be obstructed by intrinsic or extrinsic factors. Congenital, traumatic, neoplastic, degenerative, metabolic, inflammatory, and idiopathic conditions can lead to eustachian tubal abnormalities.

Craniofacial anomalies, such as Down's, Crouzon's, Apert's, and Turner's syndromes, as well as cleft palate, are associated with middle ear disease, probably because of abnormal tensor veli palatini muscle function.

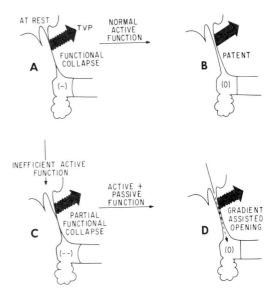

FIGURE 36B–3. Diagrammatic representation of physiologic ventilation of the middle ear during active opening of the eustachian tube by the tensor veli palatini muscle. An alternative mechanism for ventilation is gradient-assisted opening of the eustachian tube (see text).

Some children and adults with middle ear disease appear to have a congenital defect that results in patency or functional obstruction of the tube, possibly owing to an abnormal relation between the eustachian tube and the tensor veli palatini muscle. This may account for racial differences in the prevalence and incidence of otitis media. Native Americans (Eskimos and American Indians) have a higher incidence of otitis media than Caucasians, while Negroes have an incidence of otitis media that is half that of Caucasians. There is also some evidence that otitis media is more prevalent in certain families (Doyle, 1979).

Dentofacial abnormalities may be associated with abnormal eustachian tube function as well as with a deviated nasal septum. In these conditions eustachian tube function may improve with correction of the defect. The role of allergy is discussed in Chapter 38.

Relationship of Eustachian Tube Dysfunction to Middle Ear Disease

Otitis media may result from eustachian tube obstruction, abnormal patency, or both (Bluestone et al., 1979). Either functional or mechanical factors may lead to eustachian tube obstruction. The eustachian tube may collapse functionally because of increased tubal compliance, an abnormal active opening mechanism, or both. Functional eustachian tube obstruction is common in infants and younger children because of insufficient cartilaginous support of the eustachian tube and because age-related anatomic features prior to puberty in the craniofacial base predispose to inefficient function of the tensor veli palatini muscle. Children with cleft palates have effusions because of functional obstruction (Bluestone, 1971; Doyle et al., 1979). Intrinsic or extrinsic factors may obstruct the eustachian tube mechanically. Intrinsic obstruction results most commonly from acute or chronic inflammation of the mucosal lining (due to infection or possibly allergy) but may also be associated with polyps or a cholesteatoma (Bluestone et al., 1977, 1978). Extrinsic obstruction could result from increased extramural pressure, which occurs in the supine position or from peritubal compression from a tumor or possibly an adenoid mass (Bluestone et al., 1972b, 1975). Swallowing when the nose is obstructed induces positive nasopharyngeal pres-

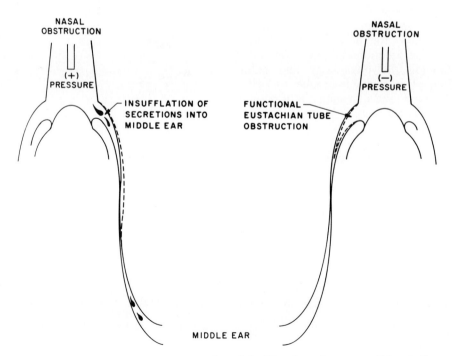

FIGURE 36B–4.   Diagrammatic representation of the "Toynbee phenomenon" (see text).

sure, which might insufflate infected secretions into the ear followed by a negative phase, which could lead to further obstruction ("Toynbee phenomenon," Fig. 36B–4) (Bluestone et al., 1974, 1975).

In the extreme form of abnormal patency, the eustachian tube is open even at rest. A patulous tube allows air as well as nasopharyngeal secretions to flow from the nasopharynx into the middle ear readily and results in "reflux otitis media." A semipatulous eustachian tube may be obstructed functionally as a result of increased tubal compliance, and the middle ear may have negative pressure, an effusion, or both. Nasopharyngeal secretions may be insufflated into the middle ear as a result of nose-blowing, sneezing, crying, or closed-nose swallowing. Increased patency of the tube may be due to abnormal tube anatomy or to a decrease in the extramural pressure such as that which occurs with weight loss.

PHYSICAL EXAMINATION OF THE EARS

The position of the patient for otoscopy depends upon age and cooperation, the clinical setting, and the preference of the examiner. Otoscopic evaluation of the neonate and young infant is best performed on an examining table. The parent or an assistant is necessary to restrain the baby since movement interferes with an adequate evaluation. However, infants and young children can be evaluated while sitting on the parent's lap. When necessary, the child may be restrained by the parent, who uses one hand to hold both wrists against the child's abdomen, the other to hold the child's head firmly against the parent's chest, and the legs can be held between the thighs, if necessary. Cooperative children can be evaluated while sitting in a chair or on the edge of an examination table.

All obstructing cerumen must be removed from the canal so that the external canal and tympanic membrane can be adequately visualized. This usually can be accomplished with the aid of an otoscope with a surgical head and wire loop or a blunt cerumen curette or by gently irrigating the ear canal with warm water employing a dental irrigator (Waterpic). Impacted cerumen can be softened by the instillation of a combination of glycerine and peroxide otic drops (equal parts mixture) and then irrigated at a later date. However, if an immediate diagnosis is required, the cerumen should be skillfully cleaned under direct vision (otoscope or otomicroscope) without traumatizing the canal walls, since any bleeding will obscure the tympanic membrane. After thorough cleaning, the external canal should be inspected for signs of inflammation.

Proper assessment of the tympanic membrane and its mobility are accomplished by the use of the pneumatic otoscope in which the diagnostic head has an adequate seal. Precise otoscopy is limited currently by certain deficiencies in the design of commercially available otoscopes. In many models, an airtight seal is difficult to obtain because of leaks within the otoscope head or between the stiff ear speculum and the external auditory canal. A small section of rubber tubing placed over the tip of the ear speculum aids in obtaining a seal with the ear canal. Many otolaryngologists prefer to use a Bruenings or Siegle otoscope with the magnifying lens, both of which are excellent to assess drum mobility since they have an almost airtight seal.

Inspection of the tympanic membrane should include the following: position, color, degree of translucency, and mobility. The assessment of the light reflex is of limited value in the evaluation of tympanic membrane–middle ear pathology. The normal eardrum should be in the neutral position, the short process of the malleus being visible but not prominent. Mild retraction of the tympanic membrane usually indicates the presence of middle ear negative pressure, in which case the short process of the malleus and posterior mallear fold are prominent and the manubrium of the malleus appears foreshortened. Severe retraction (atelectasis) of the tympanic membrane is characterized by a prominent posterior mallear fold and a short process of the malleus with a severely foreshortened manubrium. In such an ear, a horizontal line may be visible below the umbo of the malleus, which is the tympanic membrane resting on the promontory of the cochlea. However, the tympanic membrane may be severely retracted without the presence of high negative middle ear pressure when assessed by pneumatic otoscopy or tympanometry. This retraction presumably is due to previous high negative middle ear pressure with subsequent fixation of the ossicles and ligaments of the middle ear. Fullness of the tympanic membrane is apparent initially in the posterosuperior portion of the pars tensa and the pars flaccida since these two areas are the most highly compliant parts of the tympanic membrane (Khanna and Tonndorf, 1972). The short process of the malleus usually is obscured. The fullness may be due to increased air pressure, effusion, or both within the middle ear. In the most extreme condition, a bulging tympanic membrane involves the entire eardrum, in which instance the malleus usually is obscured.

The normal tympanic membrane has a ground-glass appearance; a blue or yellow color usually indicates a middle ear effusion visualized through a translucent tympanic membrane. A red tympanic membrane alone may not be indicative of a pathologic condition since the blood vessels of the drum may be engorged as the result of crying, sneezing, or blowing the nose. It is important to distinguish between translucency and opacity. The normal tympanic membrane should be translucent. The observer should be able to see through the drum to visualize the middle ear landmarks, i.e., the incudostapedial joint, promontory, round window niche, and the chorda tympani nerve. If a middle ear effusion is present medial to a translucent drum, an air–fluid level or bubbles of air may be visible, which can be differentiated from scarring of the tympanic membrane by altering the position of the head or by visualizing movement of the fluid during pneumatic otoscopy. If sufficient negative pressure can be applied with the pneumatic otoscope, the line frequently seen when a severely retracted membrane touches the cochlear promontory will disappear; i.e., the drum will pull away from the promontory. Inability to visualize the middle ear structures indicates opacification of the drum, which usually is the result of thickening of the tympanic membrane, and/or effusion. Battery-operated otoscopes should have the batteries replaced frequently to provide the maximum intensity of light to enable the examiner to "look through" the tympanic membrane.

Abnormalities of the tympanic membrane–middle ear are reflected in the pattern of tympanic membrane mobility when first positive and then negative pressure is applied to the external auditory canal with the pneumatic otoscope, a technique described by Siegel in 1864. This is achieved by first applying slight pressure on the rubber bulb (positive pressure) and then, after momentarily breaking the seal, releasing the bulb (negative pressure). At ambient middle ear pressure, the normal tympanic membrane moves inward with slight positive pressure in the ear canal and outward toward the examiner with slight negative pressure. The motion observed is proportional to the applied pressure and is best visualized in the posterosuperior portion of the tympanic membrane. A middle ear effusion and/or high negative pressure dampens the movement of the eardrum. If a monomeric membrane or atrophic scar — secondary to an old perforation — is present, mobility of the tympanic membrane can be more readily assessed by observing the movement of the flaccid area.

Figure 36B–5 shows the relationship between the assessment of mobility of the tympanic membrane with the pneumatic otoscope and the middle ear contents and pressure. As compared with the normal tympanic membrane when the middle ear contains only air at ambient pressure (Frame 1), a hypermobile eardrum (Frame 2) is seen most frequently in children whose membranes are atrophic or flaccid. The mobility of the tympanic membrane is greater than normal when even slight positive and negative external canal pressure are applied. Hypermobile tympanic membranes have been associated with subsequent loss of drum stiffness due to abnormal function of the eustachian tube (Elner et al., 1971), which probably is related to wide fluctuations in middle ear pressures. A middle ear effusion occurs rarely with hypermobile drums even when there is high negative middle ear pressure. Tympanic membrane mobility to both positive and negative pressure is decreased with ambient middle ear pressures if the drum is thickened as a result of tympanic membrane inflammation or scarring or if a partial middle ear effusion is present (Frame 3).

When the eardrum is maximally retracted because of negative middle ear pressure (Frames 4 to 6), it cannot be deflected further with positive ear canal pressure. However, applied negative pressure equivalent to that of the middle ear will permit the eardrum to return toward the neutral position (Frame 4). When the middle ear pressure is even lower, there may be only slight outward mobility of the tympanic membrane (Frame 5) because of the limited negative pressure that can be exerted through the otoscope. One must be careful not to assume that the return of the tympanic membrane to the resting retracted position is a normal response to positive pressure. If the eardrum is severely retracted with extremely high negative middle ear pressure or if there is middle ear effusion, or both, the examiner is not able to produce significant outward movement (Frame 6).

The tympanic membrane that exhibits fullness (Frame 7) will move to applied positive pressure but not to applied negative pressure if some air is present (Frame 7). This occurs commonly in the initial stage of acute otitis media with effusion. A full tympanic membrane with positive middle ear pressure without an effusion is seen frequently in neonates and in younger infants who are crying during the otoscopic examination and in older in-

	TYMPANIC MEMBRANE POSITION*		EXTERNAL CANAL PRESSURE+				MIDDLE EAR	
			POSITIVE		NEGATIVE		CONTENT	PRESSURE
			LOW	HIGH	LOW	HIGH		
1.	NEUTRAL	EXT. CANAL / MIDDLE EAR	1+	2+	1+	2+	AIR	AMBIENT
2.	NEUTRAL		2+	3+	2+	3+	AIR	AMBIENT
3.	NEUTRAL		0	1+	0	1+	AIR OR AIR AND EFFUSION	AMBIENT
4.	RETRACTED		0	0	1+	2+	AIR OR AIR AND EFFUSION	LOW NEGATIVE
5.	RETRACTED		0	0	0	1+	AIR OR EFFUSION AND AIR	HIGH NEGATIVE
6.	RETRACTED		0	0	0	0	AIR OR EFFUSION OR BOTH	VERY HIGH NEGATIVE OR INDETERMINATE
7.	FULL		0	1+	0	0	AIR AND EFFUSION	POSITIVE OR INDETERMINATE
8.	BULGING		0	0	0	0	EFFUSION	POSITIVE OR INDETERMINATE

*POSITION AT REST (SOLID LINE) AND WITH APPLIED PRESSURE (DOTTED LINE)

+DEGREE OF TYMPANIC MEMBRANE MOVEMENT AS VISUALIZED THROUGH THE OTOSCOPE; 0 = NONE, 1+ = SLIGHT, 2+ = MODERATE, 3+ = EXCESSIVE

FIGURE 36B–5. Pneumatic otoscopic findings related to middle ear contents and pressure (see text).

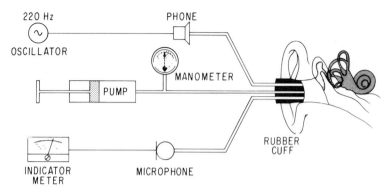

FIGURE 36B–6. Schematic design of electroacoustic impedance bridge.

fants and children after sneezing, nose blowing, or swallowing when the nose is obstructed. When the middle ear–mastoid air cell system is filled with an effusion and little or no air is present, the mobility of the bulging tympanic membrane (Frame 8) is severely decreased or absent to both applied positive and negative pressure.

Otomicroscopy. Many otolaryngologists employ the otomicroscope to improve the accuracy of diagnosis of otitis media and related conditions, since the microscope provides binocular vision and, therefore, depth perception, a better light source, and greater magnification. For most conditions, microscopic examination is impractical and generally not necessary. However, when diagnosis by pneumatic otoscopy is in doubt, then the otomicroscope is an invaluable diagnostic aid.

LABORATORY TESTS

Impedance Testing

The electroacoustic impedance bridge (Fig. 36B–6), which measures three basic middle ear functions — tympanometry, middle ear muscle reflex, and static compliance — has provided an invaluable tool in identifying middle ear disease.

The electroacoustic impedance bridge provides an objective assessment of the mobility of the tympanic membrane and the dynamics of the ossicular chain, intra-aural muscles with their attachments, and the middle ear cushion. Its design permits the introduction of a signal through one of three small openings in the probe tip, which is sealed in the external auditory canal. A portion of the signal is transmitted into and through the tympanic membrane and middle ear, and a portion is reflected into the ear canal and recorded by the microphone circuit of the ear probe. The reflected signal is related to the mechanical properties of the tympanic membrane. Air pressure within the ear canal is varied through the third aperture of the probe either manually or automatically. With this arrangement, impedance can be monitored at varying air pressures. The measurement of impedance changes at the tympanic membrane with a dynamic air pressure load is termed tympanometry, and when there is a static pressure load, static compliance can be measured. Details of tympanometry and of the interpretation of tympanograms are discussed in Chapter 37.

Tests of Ventilatory Function

The ventilatory function of the eustachian tube can be assessed by manometry, sonometry, and tympanometry. Sonometry is only available for investigation in the laboratory, but the other two tests can be used in the clinical setting. The principles of these tests are discussed, although detailed description of techniques is beyond the scope of this text. In general, one set of tests is designed to examine eustachian tube function when the tympanic membrane contains a ventilating tube or perforation, while the other measures eustachian tube function when the membrane is intact.

Manometry. The simplest manometric technique consists of connecting the ear canal to a pressure monitoring device using a catheter with an airtight seal. The middle ear pressure can be measured directly if the drum contains ventilating tubes or a perforation (intratympanic manometry). Air pressure can be increased or decreased in the ear canal with a syringe or air pump connected to the catheter with a valve. Different levels of positive or negative middle ear pressures can be created, and the ability of the eustachian tube to equilibrate to ambient pressures can be tested directly as the subject swallows. A variation of this method, the "force-response test" (Cantekin et al., 1979b), is able to distinguish between inefficient active opening and structural abnormalities of the eustachian tube.

When the tympanic membrane is intact, middle ear pressure must be inferred from pressure changes in the ear canal (extratympanic manometry). These recordings are of little value for assessing tubal function because the small volumes displaced by changes in middle ear pressure are more than offset by changes in temperature and atmospheric pressure.

Inflation-Deflation Test. The inflation-deflation test measures the ventilatory function of the eustachian tube through a perforation of the drum or tympanostomy tube using a pump-manometer portion of an impedance bridge (Bluestone et al., 1972a) or a controlled syringe pump and manometer (Bluestone et al., 1977). The test consists of the application of enough positive pressure to the middle ear to force open the eustachian tube. The pressure remaining in the middle ear after passive opening and closing is termed the closing pressure. Further equilibration of pressure is by swallowing, which induces the tensor veli palatini muscle to contract (Rich, 1920; Cantekin et al., 1979a; Honjo et al., 1979) and permits air to flow down the tube. The pressures can be monitored on a strip chart recorder; the pressure remaining in the middle ear after passive and active function is termed the residual positive pressure. In the deflation tests, low negative pressure is applied to the middle ear and is equilibrated by active tubal opening. The pressure remaining in the middle ear after swallowing is termed the residual negative pressure. In certain instances, the ability of the tube to open actively in response to applied low positive pressure also is assessed.

Failure to equilibrate the applied negative pressure during the test indicates locking of the eustachian tube during the test. This type of tube is considered to have increased compliance or is "floppy" in comparison to the tube with normal function.

Forced Response Test. A new technique has recently been developed to test eustachian tube function in subjects with *non-intact* tympanic membranes (Cantekin et al., 1979b). During this test, the middle ear is inflated at a constant flow rate, forcing the eustachian tube open. Following the forced opening of the tube, the pump will continue to deliver a constant airflow rate, maintaining a steady stream of air through the tube. Then the subject is instructed to swallow in order to assess the active dilation of the tube. This test enables the investigator to study the passive response of the eustachian tube as well as the active response due to the contractions of the tensor veli palatini muscle, which displaces the lateral walls from the cartilage-supported medial wall of the tube. Thus, the clinician can determine if tubal dysfunction is due to the material properties of the tube or to a defective active opening mechanism.

Microflow Displacement Tests. Determinations of eustachian tube function in individuals with intact tympanic membranes may be made by volume displacement measurements using microflow techniques. When the drum is moving, airflow is produced in the external ear canal. This flow is recorded by a flowmeter and then integrated to give quantitative measurements of volume displacement. Displacements as small as one microliter have been recorded with up to 95 percent accuracy.

Indirect Methods Using Tympanometry

Eustachian tube function can be evaluated clinically in subjects with intact tympanic membranes using tympanometry to measure resulting middle ear pressures.

Resting middle ear function can be determined reliably. A single measurement of normal resting middle ear pressure does not necessarily indicate normal eustachian tube function, but a measurement of negative middle ear pressure is presumptive evidence of eustachian tube dysfunction.

Toynbee and Valsalva Tests. These procedures give a semiquantitative indication of the ability of the eustachian tube to equilibrate to positive and negative pressures in the middle ear (Bluestone, 1975). After a tympanogram, the subject is asked to perform a Toynbee maneuver, which should produce negative middle ear pressure. If it doesn't, the subject probably has tubal dysfunction. If it does, the subject is asked to swallow in an attempt to equilibrate the negative pressure. If with a single swallow equilibration is not complete, repeated swallows are performed, and the pressure remaining in the middle ear is termed the residual negative pressure. A similar test measures the ability of the eustachian tube to allow equilibration to positive middle ear pressure. One problem with these tests is the inability to control the degree of positive and negative pressure generated in each individual.

Holmquist's test involves using a device to create a negative pressure in the nasopharynx and to induce a pressure of (negative) 400 mm H_2O in the middle ear (Holmquist, 1969, 1972). Otherwise it is similar to the Toynbee test. However, it frequently results in false positive results (Siedentop et al., 1978).

The inflation-deflation test assesses the ability of the subject to equilibrate up to 200 mm negative or positive air pressure in the ear canal (Bluestone, 1975). After an initial tympanogram, a pressure of + 200 mm H_2O is placed in the ear canal, which causes an inward deflection of the tympanic membrane and an increase in middle ear pressure (inflation). If the eustachian tube is normal, middle ear pressure should equilibrate with that in the nasopharynx. The deflation test is similar but uses negative middle ear pressure.

The patulous eustachian tube test compares the tympanogram when the patient is breathing normally with that while the patient holds his or her breath. A fluctuation in the tympanometric line that coincides with breathing indicates a patulous tube. These changes can be exaggerated by forced inspiration and expiration through one nostril or by Toynbee's test.

Indications for Testing Eustachian Tube Function

The most direct method to test eustachian tube function available to the clinician today is the inflation-deflation method through a perforation of the tympanic membrane or a tympanostomy tube. Since most patients have either functional obstruction or an abnormally patent tube, no other test procedures may be needed. However, if the tube appears to be totally blocked anatomically, then further testing must be performed. Retrograde-prograde radiographic contrast studies of the eustachian tube should be performed to determine the site and cause of the obstruction. Most cases of mechanical obstruction are due to inflammation at the bony end of the eustachian tube, which usually will resolve with medical or surgical management. However, if no cause of pathologic conditions in the middle ear is obvious, roentgenographic studies should be performed to rule out the possibility of neoplasm of the nasopharynx.

Since resting middle ear pressure may provide an indirect measurement of eustachian tube function, serial tympanograms may be helpful in patients with symptoms such as fullness, snapping, or popping in the ear, fluctuating hearing loss, tinnitus, or vertigo.

Any patient with recurrent acute or chronic otitis media with effusion should have eustachian tube function studies as part of the otolaryngologic and audiologic workup, since the type of medical and/or surgical treatment may depend on the test results.

References

Beery, Q. C., Bluestone, C. D., and Cantekin, E. I.: Otologic history, audiometry and tympanometry as a case finding procedure for school screening. Laryngoscope 85:1976, 1975.

Beery, Q. C., Doyle, W. J., Cantekin, E. I., and Bluestone, C. D.: Longitudinal assessment of ventilatory function of the eustachian tube in children. Laryngoscope, 89:1446, 1979.

Bluestone, C. D.: Eustachian tube obstruction in the infant with cleft palate. Ann. Otol, Rhinol. Laryngol. 80(Suppl. 2), 1, 1971.

Bluestone, C. D., Paradise, J. L., and Beery, Q. C.: Physiology of the eustachian tube in the pathogenesis and management of middle ear effusions. Laryngoscope 82:1654, 1972a.

Bluestone, C. D., Wittel, R., Paradise, J. L., and Felder, H.: Eustachian tube function as related to adenoidectomy for otitis media. Trans. A.A.O.O. 76:1325, 1972b.

Bluestone, C. D., Beery, Q. C., and Andrus, W.: Mechanics of the eustachian tube as it influences susceptibility to and persistence of middle ear effusions in children. Ann. Otol, Rhinol. Laryngol. *83*:(Suppl. 11):27, 1974.

Bluestone, C. D.: Assessment of eustachian tube function. Handbook of Clinical Impedance Audiometry, New York, American Electromedics Corp., 1975.

Bluestone, C. D., Cantekin, E. I., and Beery, Q. C.: Certain effects of adenoidectomy on eustachian tube ventilatory function. Laryngoscope, *85*:113, 1975.

Bluestone, C. D., and Beery, Q. C.: Concepts on the pathogenesis of middle ear effusions. Ann. Otol. Rhinol. Laryngol. *85*(Suppl. 25):182, 1976.

Bluestone, C. D., Cantekin, E. I., and Beery, Q. C.: Effect of inflammation on the ventilatory function of the eustachian tube. Laryngoscope *87*:493, 1977.

Bluestone, C. D., Cantekin, E. I., Beery, Q. C., and Stool, S. E.: Function of the eustachian tube related to surgical management of acquired aural cholesteatoma in children. Laryngoscope *87*:1155, 1978.

Bluestone, C. D., Cantekin, E. I.: Design factors in the characterization and identification of otitis media and certain related conditions. Ann. Otol. Rhinol. Laryngol. *88*(Suppl. 60):13, 1979.

Cantekin, E. I., Bluestone, C. D., Saez, C., Doyle, W. J., and Phillips, D.: Normal and abnormal middle ear ventilation. Ann. Otol. Rhinol. Laryngol. *86* (Suppl. 41):1, 1977.

Cantekin, E. I., Doyle, W. J., Reichert, T. J., Phillips, D. C., and Bluestone, C. D.: Dilation of the eustachian tube by electrical stimulation of the mandibular nerve. Ann. Otol. Rhinol. Laryngol. *88*:40, 1979*a*.

Cantekin, E. I., Saez, C. A., Bluestone, C. D., and Bern, S. A.: Airflow through the eustachian tube. Ann. Otol. Rhinol. Laryngol. *88*:603, 1979*b*.

Clemis, J. D.: Identification of allergic factors in middle ear effusions. Ann. Otol. Rhinol Laryngol. *85* (Suppl. 25):234, 1976.

Doyle, W. J., Cantekin, E. I., Beery, Q. C., and Bluestone, C. D.: Eustachian tube function in cleft palate children. Ann. Otol. Rhinol. Laryngol. in press, 1980.

Draper, W. L.: Secretory otitis media. Laryngoscope *78*:636, 1967.

Elner, A., Ingelstedt, S., and Ivarsson, A.: The elastic properties of the tympanic membrane system. Acta. Otolaryngol. *72*:397, 1971.

Holmquist, J.: Eustachian tube function assessed with tympanometry. Acta Otolaryngol. *68*:501, 1969.

Holmquist, J.: Tympanometry in testing auditory tubal function. Audiology *11*:209, 1972.

Honjo, I., Okazaki, N., and Kumazawam, T.: Experimental study of the eustachian tube function with regard to its related muscles. Acta Otolaryngol. *87*:84, 1979.

Khanna, S. M., and Tonndorf, J.: Tympanic membrane vibrations in cats studied by time-averaged holography. J. Acoust. Soc. Am. *51*:1904, 1972.

Lim, D. J., Liu, Y. S., Schram, J., and Birck, H. G.: Immunoglobulin E in chronic middle ear effusions. Ann. Otol. Rhinol. Laryngol. *85* (Supp. 25):119, 1976.

McGovern, J. P., Haywood, T. J., and Fernandes, A.: Allergy and secretory otitis media. J.A.M.A. *200*:134, 1967.

Mogi, G.: Secretory IgA and antibody activities in middle ear effusions. Ann. Otol. Rhinol. Laryngol. *85* (Suppl. 25):97, 1976.

Siedentop, K. H., Loewy, A., Corrigan, R. A., and Osenar, S. B.: Eustachian tube function assessed with tympanometry. Ann. Otol. Rhinol. Laryngol. *87*:163, 1978.

37

Jerry L. Northern, Ph.D.

Diagnostic Tests in Ear Disease

The testing of hearing is not always a simple task. The precipitating causes of auditory disorders may be intermittent or permanent, and the resultant hearing loss may be progressive, transient, or variable. The evaluation of hearing involves expensive electronic equipment, careful selection of tests and appropriate sites for testing. Equipment must be calibrated regularly and personnel must be trained appropriately. Early identification of children with hearing loss is exceedingly important to their intellectual and social development.

Although we speak of the measurement of hearing, we are actually measuring behavior. All variables that influence day-to-day behavior will also influence performance during a hearing test. The total person must be considered during testing; his or her response may be influenced by illness, lethargy, other competing stimuli, inattentiveness, boredom with the task, emotional problems, mental retardation, neurologic disease, or simple unwillingness to cooperate. The environmental ambient noise level may also provide distraction. Thus, hearing testing should be done in a relatively quiet room — away from flushing water pipes, open windows, or noisy hallways or waiting rooms.

THE NATURE OF HEARING LOSS

Hearing loss can be generally categorized as conductive or sensorineural impairment.

When a combination of both types of hearing loss occurs, we speak of a mixed auditory disorder.

Conductive impairment occurs when a problem exists in the external ear canal, tympanic membrane, or middle ear cavity that interferes with the transmission of sound along the normal physiologic air conduction pathway. Most conductive hearing losses can be ameliorated through treatment. Although conductive hearing losses may often resolve spontaneously, frequently some residual of the pathologic condition will persist and may be cumulative, intensifying the hearing loss in the next episode. The conductive hearing loss is characterized by a hearing loss for air conduction sounds, while sounds conducted to the inner ear directly by the bone conduction mechanism are heard normally. Causes of conductive hearing loss include foreign objects or debris in the external auditory canal, problems associated with tympanic membrane movement, otitis media, and congenital abnormalities. Early identification of conductive hearing impairment allows resolution of the disease process during its elementary stages. A conductive hearing loss is considered significant when it interferes with general communication processes.

Sensorineural hearing loss occurs when damage has been sustained by the sensory cells of the organ of Corti within the cochlea or by the fibers of the auditory nerve. Sensorineural hearing losses are commonly

492

overlooked because the external auditory canal and the tympanic membrane will appear normal in a physical examination. Such hearing loss is nearly always irreversible. Treatment consists of auditory training in the use of hearing aids, and special education training such as lip reading to develop speech and language. Young children with severe sensorineural hearing loss will have difficulty in the development of normal speech and language. Common causes of sensorineural hearing loss include viral and bacterial infections, drug ototoxicity, excessive noise exposure, congenital abnormality, and head trauma. The sensorineural audiogram is characterized by equivalent air conduction and bone conduction threshold values. Early identification of sensorineural hearing loss is extremely important for the total development of the child. Undetected hearing loss in children may lead to speech and language problems and can be responsible for school learning or behavior problems.

Hearing loss must be identified as unilateral or bilateral. The child with a totally deaf ear and a normal hearing ear may function quite well in most situations but may fail the hearing screening test. Further, the examiner must quantitate the degree of hearing loss in each ear, e.g., whether mild, moderate, severe or profound.

TUNING FORK TESTS

The basic implement for the hearing examination is the tuning fork. Tuning fork tests were introduced in the early 1800's and were named for the physicians who first described the techniques. The tuning fork should be struck just loudly enough for the patient to hear the tones.

The *Weber test* is a bone conduction test performed by placing a vibrating tuning fork on the forehead or skull midline. If a unilateral hearing loss is reported by the patient, and the tuning fork tone lateralizes to (is heard loudest by) the ear with a loss, a conductive hearing loss is indicated. When the tone lateralizes to the better ear, the poorer ear has a sensorineural hearing loss or has the worse sensorineural loss of the two ears. When the patient has a symmetrical hearing loss of any type or has bilateral normal hearing, the tone in the Weber test is heard in the middle of the head.

The *Rinne test* compares the patient's hearing by air conduction with the hearing by bone conduction. The vibrating tuning fork is placed alternately against the mastoid bone and beside the external ear canal. The patient is asked to indicate in which position the tone is heard loudest. The normal hearing patient and the patient with sensorineural hearing loss will hear the tone louder when the tuning fork is in front of the pinna, i.e., better by air conduction than bone conduction (AC>BC). This finding is known as a *positive* Rinne test. The conductive hearing loss patient, with an air-bone difference of 25 to 30 dB or more, will hear the tone better when the stem of the tuning fork is pressed against the mastoid bone behind the pinna. This finding is recorded as BC>AC, or a *negative* Rinne test. In the Rinne test, each ear is evaluated separately.

There are several drawbacks to the use of tuning forks in the assessment of hearing. Children younger than 6 years of age, and even some adults, find it difficult to report correctly how they hear the tuning fork tones; it is often difficult to isolate one ear for tuning fork test purposes without masking the opposite ear with a Barany noisemaker; the technique of tuning fork test procedures is poorly standardized; recording of results varies from clinic to clinic; overtones are easily created by striking the tuning fork too hard; and it is nearly impossible to quantify the intensity of the tuning forks to estimate the patient's hearing level accurately. The value of understanding the principles of the tuning fork tests is that they mimic the technique of modern audiology.

AUDIOMETRY

Hearing Screening

Audiometric screening should be provided for all preschool age children old enough to cooperate and school age children as part of every well child checkup. Even the slightest hearing loss can cause speech disorders and learning problems. Children with hearing loss often develop behavior problems because their inability to hear shortens their attention span and interferes with their ability to understand instructions and with social communication. Children with even mild hearing loss from otitis media may develop retardation in reading and arithmetic skills, which will necessitate special remedial teaching.

Approximately 5 percent of all school children have hearing losses sufficient to warrant additional evaluation. Ninety percent of these losses are correctable medically if detected early. If a special effort is not made to identify them, however, they may go unnoticed and may result in significant speech and hearing problems.

Hearing screening should be administered to all preschool children, kindergarteners, and primary school children. The importance of screening in the early grades is evident from reports indicating that 63 percent of all ultimate hearing losses will be identified by screening in kindergarten and 85 percent by screening at the third grade level.

The basic instrument needed for hearing screening is the portable screening audiometer. This instrument provides a means for conducting screening tests. Portable audiometers are manufactured by numerous special instrument companies and are relatively inexpensive. They should be recalibrated at regular intervals.

The most generally accepted frequencies for screening are 1000, 2000, 4000, and 6000 or 8000 Hz. This selection has been found to be a satisfactory compromise in the usually high ambient noise level that causes too many false positive tests at 250 and 500 Hz. The screening level recommended by the American Speech and Hearing Association is 20 dB at 1000, 2000 and 4000 Hz. If 20 dB is not heard at 4000 Hz, a 25 dB screening tone can be used.

Hearing tests should be conducted by an individual who has had appropriate training and should be done in a quiet room away from street noises, foot traffic, visual distractions, and other disturbances, which may result in an inaccurate or unreliable hearing test.

The child should be comfortably seated to one side and slightly behind the audiometer, with the chair at a 45° angle to it in a position that the tester can see his or her face during the test. The child should not be able to see the other children or the operation of the audiometer dials.

The audiometer headset must be placed carefully and snugly over the ears, with the red receiver on the right ear and the blue receiver on the left ear. The receiver openings should be lined up directly with the canal openings of the ears. The child's hair must be pushed back so it is not interposed between the ear and the receiver. Glasses should be removed.

The child is told to listen for faint sounds or "beeps" and is instructed to indicate when he or she hears the tone by raising his or her hand when the tone is present and dropping it when the tone ceases. Younger children can be taught to respond to the tone by dropping a colored stick into a box or by similar techniques that convert the test into a "game." Missed tones should be retested several times to rule out false negative results.

Threshold Audiometry

Children who have a hearing loss detected by screening audiometry should have a full pure tone audiogram. Many factors must be taken into consideration to obtain a reliable audiometric test result. The location of the testing room is important, since ambient noise may obscure auditory thresholds. The audiometer must be in perfect operating condition and must be calibrated at least every six months. The audiologist must know when and how to use masking and how to instruct the patient about the test procedures. Positioning of the headset, earphones, and bone oscillator is important, since poor placement can produce incorrect threshold measurements. The patient must feel comfortable during the test since such factors as the test chair, the temperature, the time of day, the patient's interactions with the tester, and patient motivation will affect the reliability of the test. Other important factors include age, intelligence, reaction time, and previous experience with hearing tests. The techniques of manipulating the audiometer are very simple; the techniques of evaluating the hearing in frightened or sick children can be difficult.

Air Conduction. Basic audiometry generally includes pure tone air conduction and speech tests, as well as pure tone bone conduction tests. Air conduction refers to the measurement of audiometric thresholds to signals heard by the patient through earphones mounted on a headset. The patient's ear with the best hearing is always tested first.

Several psychophysical procedures can be used to arrive at the threshold measurement. The best technique is an ascending method in which the threshold is measured by increasing the intensity of the stimulus progressively from inaudibility to audibility. The stimulus is increased in 10 dB steps until the patient hears the tone; the stimulus is then decreased in 5 dB steps until the patient no longer perceives it. The threshold is "bracketed" until a level is determined at which the tone is heard 50 percent of the time.

With a typical patient who understands instructions easily, the air conduction test begins with a sample pure tone stimulus of 40 or 50 dB (or even louder if necessary), which the patient can hear easily. Once the patient has been oriented to the tone and the testing procedure, the signal is reduced to a very low level (0 dB), and the ascending approach is begun. The first frequency to test is 1000 Hz, because it is the easiest of the test tones to hear. Following 1000 Hz, most audiologists test 2000, 4000, 8000, 500, and 250 Hz in sequence for each ear. Any time the tester wishes to check on the patient's reliability, the threshold at 1000 Hz can be reestablished quickly.

Bone Conduction. Thresholds in this test are established in the same fashion. With the use of the standard headband, the bone vibrator from the audiometer is placed on the mastoid behind the test ear, without touching the pinna and with the ears unoccluded by earphones. Thresholds for pure tones are determined with the same frequency sequence and ascending technique described for air conduction measurements. Bone conduction test frequencies range from 250 to 4000 Hz, and the intensity output is limited to 60 or 70 dB.

Bone conduction measurements are somewhat more difficult than air conduction measurements because vibrations are transmitted to the entire skull, including both cochleas, and, therefore, it is not always clear which ear is hearing the sound. The audiologist must keep in mind that in certain situations the test signals presented to one ear are actually perceived in the nontest ear. Unless he or she is constantly on the lookout for these situations, it is easy for erroneous findings to be measured and recorded. The audiologist controls which ear is being tested by bone conduction by masking the opposite ear via an air conduction earphone.

Masking. Masking is a technique in which a sound is presented to the nontest ear to remove it from the test procedure. The preferred masking sound is white noise, a random noise source with equal energy at all frequencies. Masking is probably the most difficult portion of the basic audiometry technique to master. In air conduction measurements, masking must always be considered when the threshold of the test ear is 40 to 50 dB different from the possible cochlear (bone conduction) response of the opposite ear. The primary mode for lateralization, or cross-hearing, of the test tone is through bone conduction. Therefore, during air conduction measurement, if there is a difference of 40 dB or more between the unmasked air conduction thresholds of the ears, the better ear must be masked when testing the poorer ear.

During bone conduction testing, the masking situation is critical. Since it is difficult to know which cochlea is being stimulated by the bone-conducted test signal, many audiologists always mask as a matter of course. The masking earphone is placed over the nontest ear, and the other earphone is placed on the patient's temple. The test ear is never occluded during bone conduction testing.

Several techniques are available for determining how much masking should be used. The reader should examine any introductory audiology textbook for additional information. Use of the correct masking level is important since too little masking or too much masking may result in erroneous audiometric results.

TYMPANOMETRY

The most common cause of ear disease in children is medically treatable middle ear pathology. All too often, traditional hearing tests fail to identify these impairments accurately.

Serous otitis media is the most widespread cause of hearing disorders in 5 and 6 year old children. During their first year in school, 20 percent of children have otitis media at least once. The average hearing loss in cases of serous otitis media is only 14dB; comparison of audiometric testing and otoscopic examination revealed that less than 50 percent of cases of middle ear pathology were identified by audiometry alone.

A technique for the *objective* assessment of the functional status of the middle ear mechanism is currently available. This method is known as tympanometry. Tympanometry has been shown to be very sensitive to the slightest presence of mild disease of the tympanic membrane or middle ear. The tympanometry technique is easily mastered by clinicians and technicians. Meaningful and valid information concerning the status of the auditory mechanism is readily obtained from nearly every patient. The procedure is quick, efficient, and tolerated well by children.

By definition, tympanometry is the objective measurement of tympanic membrane compliance (mobility) as a function of air pressure change in the external auditory canal. A tympanogram is a graphic representation of membrane compliance at specified values of air pressure between plus and minus 200 mm H_2O. Tympanic membrane compliance is a function of the air pressure on either side of the tympanic membrane. Maximum compliance of the tympanic membrane occurs when air pressure in the middle ear cavity is equal to air pressure in the external auditory canal. Thus, the measurement of maximum compliance provides the exact value of the existing middle ear pressure. Middle ear pressure is controlled by the function of the eustachian tube.

The knowledge of middle ear pressure is important clinical information. When the process of aeration in the middle ear is halted, as in partial or complete obstruction of the eustachian tube, the now static air in the middle ear space is absorbed by the blood vessels in the mucosal lining. This situation produces negative air pressure in the middle ear space, causing transudation of fluid and retraction of the tympanic membrane. If the aeration process of the middle ear cavity is blocked for an extended period of time, fluid may totally fill the middle ear space. Thus, the early identification of negative middle ear pressure may permit the physician to practice preventive medicine and avoid otitis media.

There have been numerous studies reporting normative data on the uses of tympanometry and middle ear pressure measurements, and confirming their value as a clinical tool with children and adults. Tympanometry resolves many of the disadvantages of conventional audiology and otologic assessment. It requires little cooperation from children, since no overt response is required. Total visualization of the tympanic membrane is not necessary to determine accurate tympanometric measurements, thereby eliminating the need to remove cerumen from every patient's ear. However, if the tympanogram is flat, it is essential that the cerumen be removed, since a plug of ear wax or a foreign body can produce a tympanogram which resembles an effusion.

Technique

The electroacoustic impedance meter is attached to the patient's head by a traditional audiometry-type earphone headset. An air-tight seal is obtained with a small metal probe inside a soft, rubber cuff and inserted into the patient's ear canal. The probe has three small holes. From one hole a low-frequency probe tone is emitted; the second hole is an outlet for an air pressure system creating positive, negative or atmospheric air pressure between the hermetically sealed probe tip and the tympanic membrane; the third hole leads to a pick-up microphone which measures the reflected level of the probe tone in the ear canal.

At the start of the tympanometry test, the eardrum is put into a position of poor compliance with a positive air pressure in the external ear canal. When the eardrum is not free to vibrate easily, sound is reflected from the tympanic membrane back into the ear canal and the instrument records a relatively high intensity level for the 200 Hz probe tone. As the air pressure against the eardrum is reduced, the normal eardrum begins to vibrate, passing the entrapped 200 Hz sound intensity through to the middle ear and cochlea. The vibration of the eardrum causes a reduction in the intensity of the 220 Hz tone as measured by the probe in the external ear canal. The compliance change of the tympanic membrane is recorded by the instrument as a relative change of the sound in the closed external ear canal cavity.

As air pressure variation approaches the point of maximum compliance of the eardrum, the mobility of the eardrum increases and the sound intensity of the probe tone decreases. At maximum compliance, most of the probe tone intensity is transmitted by the eardrum into the middle ear, thus creating a relatively low sound pressure level in the external ear canal. As air pressure is further reduced, lower than the point of maximum compliance, the eardrum again loses its ability to vibrate because of unequal air pressure in the canal and middle ear, thereby reflecting more sound back into the ear canal and creating an increase in the sound pressure level of the probe tone (Fig. 37–1).

Thus, the sound pressure level of the 220 Hz probe tone in the closed external ear canal is directly determined by the compliance of the eardrum. A high amount of reflected sound energy is measured when the tympanic membrane is stiff and immobile, as in such pathologic conditions as otitis media, ossicular fixation, or cholesteatoma. In contrast, normal eardrum mobility creates relative changes in sound pressure level by reflecting and absorbing probe tone energy as a function of the air pressure in the external auditory canal.

Clinical Uses of Tympanometry

The clinical uses of tympanometry are numerous. In addition to the evaluation of tympanic membrane mobility, tympanometry may be used to measure middle ear pressure, to identify perforations of the tympanic membrane, to follow onset and resolution of otitis media, and to confirm patency of ventilation tubes placed in the

tympanic membrane for treatment of otitis media. With experience and familiarity with the equipment and procedures, the clinician becomes adept at interpretation of tympanograms and makes significant diagnostic judgments.

Three basic patterns of tympanograms likely to be observed that can be related to specific middle ear conditions are discussed below and shown in Figure 37–2:

Normal Middle Ear Function: Figure 37–2A illustrates configurations typical of normal middle ear function. A normal tympanogram shows the point of maximum compliance at or near normal atmospheric pressure (0 mm H_2O air pressure), ranging between ±50 mm H_2O relative compliance.

Poorly Mobile Tympanic Membrane: Figure 37–2B shows tympanograms characterized by low relative compliance, in which definite peak points of maximum compliance may not be observed. These patterns are referred to as "flat" tympanograms. This type of curve is found in stiff middle ear conditions and may be indicative of presence of fluid or a perforation of the tympanic membrane. Patent ventilation tubes also result in "flat" tympanograms. In the cases of tympanic membrane perforation or patent ventilation tubes, the air forced in by tympanometry fills the entire middle ear cavity and the external ear canal. No compliance change occurs with reduction in air pressure, thus the appearance of a flat tympanogram. Excessive cerumen build-up in the external auditory canal will also demonstrate a flat tympanogram, but only, however, when the ear canal is totally occluded.

Retracted Tympanic Membrane: Figure 37–2C illustrates tympanogram patterns characteristic of retracted tympanic membrane. These curves exhibit relatively normal compliance; however, the point of maximum compliance occurs at a negative air pressure value. Negative air pressure values in the middle ear may be related to fluid in the middle ear, and persistence of this pattern indicates poor eustachian tube function.

Utilizing these patterns and descriptions of basic configurations of tympanograms, tympanometry is particularly valuable in audiologic and otologic assessment of school-age and younger children. As an objective method to follow the progression of middle ear pathology, tympanometry is of notable value to physicians and nurses. Blank tympanograms (flowsheet type) may be placed in the patient's chart, and these

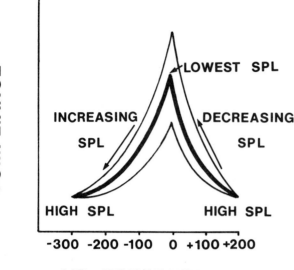

FIGURE 37–1. The tympanogram is a graphic record of change in sound pressure level (SPL) in the external ear canal as pressure is varied.

measurements recorded each time the patient is seen for treatment of otitis media. Prior to otologic disease and assuming the ear to be otherwise healthy, a normal tympanogram is displayed. Onset of the disease coincides with the obstruction of the eustachian tube, thereby creating a negative pressure value in the middle ear. This early stage of pathology yields a retracted tympanic membrane tympanogram. Progression of the disease results in a build-up of fluid in the middle ear cavity. Compliance of the tympanic membrane is reduced in this condition, and a flat tympanogram is demonstrated. As the disease is treated and the fluid condition begins to disappear, again a retracted tympanic membrane pattern will occur. Observation of this progression can prove useful in evaluating the effectiveness of prescribed medication for treatment. With the return of the middle ear to its normal status upon resolution of the diseased state, a normal tympanogram will once again be exhibited. The ear with otitis media may go through the entire disease process with less than a 10 dB change in hearing levels.

Tympanometry and Allergy

The role of allergy in recurrent middle ear effusions continues to be a controversial topic. Allergy affects the ear by obstructing the eustachian tube and by increasing the secretion of mucoid material from the middle ear mucosa. Usually diagnosis is made on history and seasonal symptoms, and therapy is directed at elimination of the cause or attainment of hyposensitization. Identification and management of allergic factors requires special skills and a great commitment of time, as well as complete audiometric and otologic evaluation.

Two studies have evaluated the middle ear problems in allergic children. Fernandez et al. (1977) compared results of pneumatic otoscopy and tympanometry in 102 children with allergic rhinitis or asthma. These authors concluded that tympanometry is an important adjunct to the evaluation of allergic children, supplying objective evidence of middle ear disease when none is evident by physical examination.

Bierman and Furukawa (1978) compared audiometric-otologic-tympanometric workups on newly diagnosed allergic children seen in 1975 with data gathered on similar patients seen from 1966 to 1969, when tympanometry was not available. The yield of abnormal ear findings was 51 percent in 488 patients seen in 1975, a significant increase over the 23 percent with abnormal ear findings during the 1966 to 1969 period. Of pa-

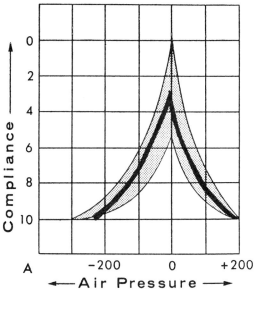

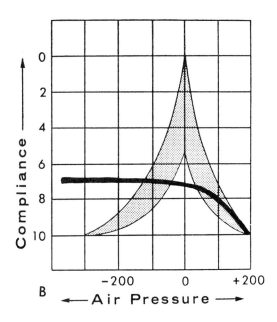

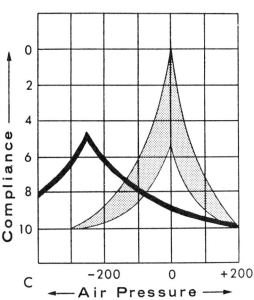

FIGURE 37–2. *A*, Normal tympanograms. A normal tympanogram shows the point of maximum compliance at or near normal atmospheric pressure (0 mm H$_2$O air pressure) ranging between ±50 mm H$_2$O relative compliance. *B*, Poorly mobile tympanic membrane tympanograms. Poorly mobile tympanic membrane tympanograms are characterized by low relative compliance where definite peak points of maximum compliance may not be observed. *C*, Retracted tympanic membrane as indicated by tympanograms. Retracted membrane tympanograms exhibit relatively normal compliance; however, the point of maximum compliance occurs at a negative air pressure value 150 mm H$_2$O.

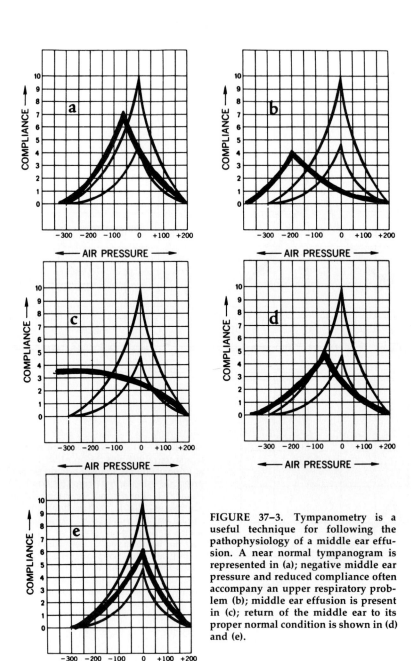

FIGURE 37–3. Tympanometry is a useful technique for following the pathophysiology of a middle ear effusion. A near normal tympanogram is represented in (a); negative middle ear pressure and reduced compliance often accompany an upper respiratory problem (b); middle ear effusion is present in (c); return of the middle ear to its proper normal condition is shown in (d) and (e).

tients seen in 1975 with abnormal tympanometry as the pathologic ear indication, 50 percent developed audiometric or otoscopic abnormalities in the subsequent 3 to 6 months; only 13 percent of those with no initial abnormal ear findings ultimately developed audiometric or otoscopic pathology. These investigators reported tympanometry to be a practical, useful addition to pediatric allergy practice, and recommended its routine use in every child referred for respiratory allergy, recurrent otitis, or delayed speech development.

There is no question that under proper circumstances and when adequate time exists, the most thorough evaluation of auditory problems is accomplished through the use of otoscopic examination, auditory threshold testing, and tympanometry. However, when less than optimal conditions prevail, we advocate the use of tympanometry as the most efficient and sensitive indicator of middle ear pathology.

References

Bierman, C. W., and Furukawa, C. T.: *Medical management of serous otitis in children*. Pediatrics *61*:768, 1978.

English, G. (ed.): *Otolaryngology: A Textbook*. Hagerstrom, Md., Harper Row Publishers, 1976.

Fernandez, D., Gupta, S., Sly, M., and Frazer, M. Tympanometry in allergic children. Ann. Allergy, *36*:105, 1977.

Jerger, J. (ed.): *Handbook of Clinical Impedance*. New York, American Electromedics Copr., 1975.

Martin, F.: *Introduction to Audiology*. Englewood Cliffs, N.J., Prentice-Hall, Inc., 1975.

Northern, J. (ed.): *Hearing Disorders*. Boston, Little, Brown and Co., 1976.

Northern, J., and Downs, M.: *Hearing In Children*. Baltimore, Md., Williams and Wilkins Co., 1974.

38

William E. Pierson, M.D.
James A. Donaldson, M.D.

Diseases of the Ear

Diseases of the middle ear may result from direct or indirect obstruction or malfunction of the eustachian tube or from pathologic processes of the middle ear itself. The final result is the accumulation of fluid in the middle ear and hearing loss (Bluestone et al., 1972; Lim et al., 1972; Sade, 1966). When the process is acute and self-limited, the long-term effects may be minimal. When the process is chronic, it can result in severe and sometimes persistent adverse effects on speech development and/or cognition, especially in the young child (Brannon and Murray, 1966; Lloyd et al., 1967; Holm and Kunze, 1969).

Middle ear fluid most commonly is purulent, serous, or mucoid (Lupovich and Harkins, 1972), but occasionally may be composed of blood or cerebrospinal fluid (Paradise, 1976; Paparella, 1976). It may result from multiple factors. In children, bacterial infections are the most common causes of middle ear fluid (Klein and Teele, 1976; Sloyer et al., 1977). Infections may cause inflammation of the nasal mucosa and enlargement of the adenoids, which disrupt eustachian tube function and produce a sterile effusion; or they may involve the middle ear directly and produce a purulent effusion. Allergic rhinitis also is a common cause of chronic nasal congestion in children (Chan et al., 1967; Bierman et al., 1970; Dees and Lefkowitz, 1972). It may cause dysfunction of the eustachian tube and induce a serous effusion or may alter the local defense system of the middle ear, making it more susceptible to recurrent infections, and

predispose it to mucoid effusion (Frady et al., 1977).

The middle ear appears to have an elaborate local immune defense mechanism to control infection. In the lamina propria of the middle ear mucosa are mast cells, plasma cells, lymphocytes, macrophages and PMN's (Sade, 1978). There is evidence of local secretory antibody production of the IgA and IgE classes (Mogi, 1976; Mogi et al., 1976). The mucociliary system also plays an important role in middle ear defense. Its effectiveness depends upon the quantity and viscosity of secreted mucus and on ambient CO_2 tension (Sade et al., 1975a). Hypersecretion of mucus or inefficient mucociliary clearance may lead to middle ear fluid accumulation (Sade et al., 1975b). Chronic inflammation of the middle ear appears to stimulate secretory cell proliferation, complement activation, PMN and monocyte chemotaxis, and increased numbers of mast cells in the middle ear (Bernstein, 1976).

ACUTE SUPPURATIVE OTITIS MEDIA

Diagnosis. Clinical presentation of acute suppurative otitis media may vary from the typical symptoms of otalgia, aural fullness, and fever, to otorrhea from rupture of the tympanic membrane without antecedent symptoms. Signs and symptoms are delineated in Table 38–1. As the disease progresses, middle ear effusions may lead to

TABLE 38–1 DIAGNOSIS OF MIDDLE EAR DISEASE

	Suppurative	Serous	Secretory
Etiology	Infection	Eustachian tube dysfunction	Mucociliary/immune dysfunction
Pneumatic otoscopy Appearance Mobility	Red; central/diffuse ±	Amber; no injection ±	Gray; peripheral injection −
Nasal cytology	Polys; lymphs; bacteria	Eosinophils, Polys	Polys; bacteria
Screening audiometry	Conductive loss (intermittent)	Conductive loss (intermittent)	Conductive loss (persistent)
Tympanogram	Flat or peak compliance at positive or negative pressure (intermittent)	Flat or peak compliance at negative pressure (intermittent)	Flat (persistent)

hearing loss (Olmstead et al., 1964). The effusion may persist for several weeks or months Klein, 1976. Physical examination often reveals an erythematous and bulging tympanic membrane, particularly posteriorly and superiorly. Conductive hearing loss can be identified by audiometry or simple tuning fork tests. The Weber test lateralizes to the involved ear, and the Rinne test is negative (bone conduction > air conduction). A 256 Hz tuning fork is recommended for these tests because this is the lowest frequency that will not cause confusion between hearing and feeling. When symptoms are typical and the tympanic membrane has reached the bulging erythematous state, the diagnosis is not difficult, though early diagnosis may be extremely difficult in an irritable small child. Differentiation between bacterial and viral infections is not always possible. Generally, cultures of fluid aspirated from the middle ear fluid in acute otitis media show a predominance of *Streptococcus pneumoniae* (30 to 40 percent), followed by *Hemophilis influenzae* in 20 to 25 percent. *Neisseria*, group A beta hemolytic streptococci, and coliform organisms appear in a few cultures. However, *H. influenzae* is cultured in 50 percent of children between 3 to 6 years of age (Liu et al., 1976). One-fourth to one-third of patients have sterile effusions (Bluestone et al., 1974). Viruses or *Mycoplasma pneumoniae* organisms have been rarely isolated, suggesting that effusions associated with viral illnesses probably result from nasal mucosal swelling and eustachian tube dysfunction rather than from direct infection of the middle ear.

The isolation of bacterial pathogens from the middle ear is complicated by the local immune defense system. All classes of immunoglobulins are present, in addition to lysozymal enzymes probably derived from PMN's (Mogi, 1976). These all act to destroy invading bacteria, to inhibit their growth on culture medium or may act to do both (Branefors et al., 1979).

Therapy. Treatment is noted in Table 38–2. Most acute suppurative otitis media responds well to a 10- to 14-day course of appropriate antimicrobial treatment. Frequently, an antihistamine-decongestant is used in connection with the antimicrobial agent, but its contribution to successful treatment has not been documented; and some believe that it may be detrimental (Olson et al., 1978). Aspiration cultures can

TABLE 38–2 TREATMENT OF MIDDLE EAR DISEASE

	Suppurative	Serous	Secretory
Antimicrobials	+++	±	+
Antihistamines	−	++	+
Decongestants			
Oral	±	++	±
Topical	+	+++	+
Steroids			
Oral	−	±	−
Topical	−	++	−
Insufflation	−	+	±
Myringotomy (without tubes)	For relief of pain Neonate − Dx	−	−
Myringotomy (with tubes)	−	+*	+++*

Key:
− Not effective
± Possibly effective
+Probably effective
+++ Highly effective

*Upon failure of medical therapy

be useful to help identify causative organisms in neonates. However, in older children, this generally is not necessary. Myringotomy can be helpful in relieving pain, but it does not otherwise influence the course of the disease or change the frequency of residual middle ear fluid.

Intracranial complications (meningitis, brain abscess) and acute mastoiditis may follow acute suppurative otitis media, but these are rare. The most frequent complications of acute otitis media involve the middle ear itself and include damage to the lenticular process of the incus, adhesions, tympanosclerosis, and residual middle ear fluid. Recent studies have shown that recurrent bouts of acute suppurative otitis media induce an increased number of mucous glands in the mucosa of the middle ear (Tos and Bak-Pedersen 1977). If appropriate treatment is continued until the tympanic membrane appears normal, and hearing and impedance audiometry (tympanometry) return to normal, complications are minimal.

SEROUS MIDDLE EAR EFFUSION (SEROUS OTITIS MEDIA)

Etiologic and Pathogenetic Factors. Serous middle ear fluid can be caused by dys-

function of the eustachian tube (Sade, 1966; Senturia, 1970). Conditions leading to dysfunction of the eustachian tube include congenital anomalies (such as cleft palate), obstructing adenoids and/or lymphoid tissue surrounding the torus or cartilaginous portion of the eustachian tube, tumors of the nasopharynx, abnormal nasal mucosa occurring in vasomotor rhinitis, rhinitis medicamentosa resulting from excessive use of nose drops, and infections (especially respiratory viral infections).

Allergic factors in the pathogenesis of middle ear effusions have been overlooked in children for the most part. However, allergic children have a high incidence of serous otitis with conductive hearing loss (Bierman and Furukawa, 1978). A prospective study of 480 children with allergic rhinitis diagnosed on the basis of a positive family history of allergy, predominance of eosinophils in nasal secretions, and positive skin tests to suspected environmental allergens revealed a significant incidence of hearing loss. Thirteen percent of these children had effusions with ≥25 db hearing loss at 500, 1000, and 2000 Hz. In addition, 36 percent had negative middle ear pressures of ≥150 mm of water, as determined by impedance audiometry. Half of these patients developed persistent effusion or acute otitis media during the follow-

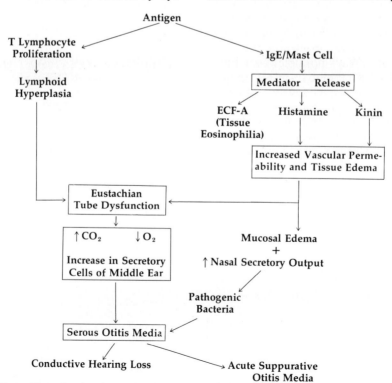

FIGURE 38–1. The role of antigen stimulation in the pathogenesis of middle ear disease in children.

ing 6 months — an incidence of middle ear disease characteristic of this high risk group.

A possible pathogenetic mechanism by which allergic rhinitis may lead to serous effusions is noted in Figure 38–1. Extrinsic allergens reacting with specific IgE antibodies fixed to mucosal mast cells cause secretion of chemical mediators into the nasal mucosa (Kaliner and Austren, 1975). Histamine, kinins, and ECF-A have been identified in nasal secretions. They can induce mucosal edema in the nose and presumably within the lining of the eustachian tube. Extrinsic allergens may stimulate lymphocyte replication, which may lead to hyperplasia of the adenoids and islands of submucosal lymphoid tissue. Nasal mucosal edema and lymphoid hyperplasia can lead to both functional and mechanical obstruction of the eustachian tube, predisposing to development of serous otitis. Once dysfunction of the eustachian tube occurs, interference with eustachian tube function results in decreased ventilation of the middle ear, with decreased oxygen and increased CO_2 tensions, followed by serous fluid accumulation (Sade and Weissman, 1977).

Diagnosis. The diagnosis is readily established by history of symptoms, physical examination, audiometry, and impedance audiometry (tympanometry) (see Table 38–1). Figure 38–2 shows a simplified pneumatic otoscope for use in children.

Serous middle ear fluid is associated with symptoms of aural plugging, fluctuating hearing loss, and sometimes tinnitus. Pain may occur in the absence of infection, owing to rapid development of a negative middle ear pressure.

Physical examination reveals a retracted, amber-colored tympanic membrane. The short process of the malleus is prominent, and the handle appears shortened. In 85 percent of the patients, the middle ear is filled with fluid. In the others, a shifting fluid level with change in head position is pathognomonic of fluid in the middle ear. With pneumatic otoscopy there is decreased motion of the tympanic membrane, and at times a crinkling reaction occurs. In some instances, the tympanic membrane will appear normal, but mobility will be decreased when it is examined by pneumatic otoscopy. All infants and children should be examined with

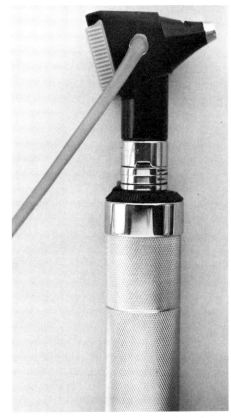

FIGURE 38–2. Modification of closed-head otoscope for pneumatic otoscopy with pipette tubing (see text).

a pneumatic otoscope to avoid misinterpretation of a normal-appearing but dysfunctional tympanic membrane (Bierman et al., 1970).

Impedance audiometry has greatly increased the precision of detecting and following the course of middle ear disease and especially of serous otitis media. In serous otitis, tympanograms are flat when fluid is present or have a peak compliance curve at negative pressures greater than 150 mm H_2O (see Chapter 37).

Treatment. The treatment of serous otitis media can be divided into medical and surgical categories (Table 38–2). Patients with significant allergy to environmental factors or with reactions to respiratory irritants such as tobacco smoke should avoid exposure to such agents as completely as possible. Therapy with antihistamines, decongestants (topical, systemic), topical steroids, and antibiotics can be helpful in selected

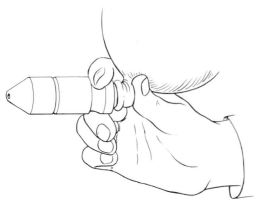

FIGURE 38-3. Mathes Inflator. Using an inflated balloon as a pressure source, air is introduced into the nose during swallowing.

patients. Nonsurgical methods for ventilating the middle ear include training in the Valsalva maneuver, and the use of a balloon insufflator, which inserts air into the nostril during swallowing (Fig. 38-3). Although any of these treatment modalities appear intuitively to be beneficial, few have been subjected to controlled study. In fact, in the area of nonsurgical therapy for serous otitis media, there is only one controlled study that showed benefit from an orally active decongestant preparation (carbinoxamine maleate with pseudoephedrine) (Miller, 1970). However, appropriately controlled studies have shown that oral medication was beneficial in allergic rhinitis, sinusitis, and vasomotor rhinitis (Connell, 1969; McLaurin et al., 1961; Benson, 1971).

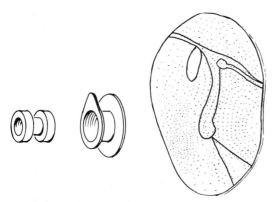

FIGURE 38-4. Examples of middle ear ventilating tubes. They are drawn to the same scale as the tympanic membrane.

When fluid persists in spite of 3 or 4 months of medical management, a myringotomy may be necessary to remove it. If the myringotomy becomes necessary, ventilation of the tympanic cavity with a tympanostomy tube is desirable until normal eustachian tube function has been restored (Fig. 38-4).

There is no evidence that serous fluid becomes thick over a period of time in the absence of infection. However, since serous otitis is associated with hearing loss, the prolonged presence of middle ear fluid may lead to intellectual handicaps. Therefore, surgical treatment should be carried out to restore normal hearing if a limited trial of medical management is not successful. The long-term prognosis is excellent for normal hearing, no matter which type of treatment is employed.

SECRETORY (MUCOID) OTITIS MEDIA (GLUE EAR)

Etiologic and Pathogenetic Factors. Secretory or mucoid otitis is associated with marked changes in structure and function of the middle ear mucosa (Sade, 1978). There is an abundance of immunocompetent and supporting cells in the middle ear mucosa, which includes immunoglobulin-producing plasma cells, epithelial cells, lymphocytes, and macrophages (found in the lamina propria) (Sade and Weissman, 1977; Sipila et al., 1976). The mucoid fluid contains elevated levels of IgG and IgA antibody, decreased total hemolytic complement (CH50) with normal or increased C3, as well as C3 proactivator and C3 activator (Juhn et al., 1973). These findings suggest that a toxic complex reaction may be occurring within the middle ear and contiguous air cells (Veltri and Sprinkle, 1976; Maxim et al., 1977). In toxic complex diseases, the activation of the complement cascade by the classic or alternative pathway rleases chemotactic factors for monocytes and for polymorphonuclear leukocytes and leads to tissue injury.

IgE antibodies responsible for antigen-induced mediator release (type I reactions) also may be important in secretory otitis media. IgE-containing plasma cells have been identified in human middle ear mucosa by immunofluorescence. Fivefold elevations of IgE in secretions, as compared to serum, have been described in some patients with secretory otitis, suggesting active IgE synthesis by plasma cells (Mogi et al., 1976). Middle ear biopsies from patients with secretory otitis have shown an increased number of mast cells in the lamina propria, with many undergoing degranulation. In infants with acute otitis media, IgE antibodies specific for pneumococcal capsular polysaccharide antigens have been identified (Sloyer et al., 1976). Other morphologic changes observed in secretory otitis involve the cilia and the goblet cells. In secretory otitis the number of globet cells increases as does the number of ciliated cells, apparently in response to inflammation (Tos and Bak-Pedersen, 1977). Hypersecretion of viscid mucus coupled with inefficient ciliary activity could lead to defective mucociliary clearance of the middle ear.

Secretory otitis media may occur as a residual of acute suppurative otitis media, as a consequence of a low-grade infection that has never reached the stage of acute suppurative otitis media, or from mucus hypersecretion in the middle ear.

Diagnosis. The symptoms produced by thick, mucoid fluid in the middle ear are hearing loss, ear fullness and, occasionally, tinnitus (see Table 38–1). Physical examination is less likely to reveal evidence of negative pressure in the middle ear (e.g., retracted tympanic membrane) but the membrane usually appears lusterless (partially opaque) and gray and frequently has fine vessels radiating from its periphery, though not sufficient to make the membrane appear erythematous. This resembles the "spoke wheel sign" of secretory otitis. Since the tympanic membrane has a lusterless appearance, fluid itself usually is not observed, but pneumatic otoscopy detects a marked decrease in mobility. The drum "crinkles" with changes in pressure, if it moves at all.

Pure tone audiometry reveals mild to moderate conductive hearing loss in the range 250–2000 Hz. The tympanogram usually is flat, with poor or noncompliant curves with little pressure gradient. This type of tympanogram usually is persistent, and in follow-up evaluations this will aid in distinguishing it from serous otitis media.

Treatment. Management consists of a trial of systemic antibiotics, a one-month course of inflation techniques as mentioned for serous middle ear effusion (see Fig. 38–3), and finally, myringotomy with insertion of ventilating tubes if the first two steps are unsuccessful (see Fig. 38–4). In the middle ear with thick fluid, eustachian tube function usually normalizes after about 4 months of ventilation by tympanostomy tubes.

The outlook for patients with thick middle ear fluid is poor. If thick fluid is allowed to remain, adhesions may result. When a significant amount of thick fluid is present, hearing usually is decreased. It is important to be certain that predisposing factors such as allergic rhinitis have been treated optimally, that adenoids have been removed if they are sufficiently large to obstruct the nasopharynx, and that sinusitis, if present, is adequately treated.

THE USE OF MIDDLE EAR VENTILATING TUBES

The use of ventilation tubes is based on the following chain of events that can cause persistent middle ear disease. In response to eustachian tube dysfunction, the pars flaccida may become indrawn, forming an attic retraction pocket. If this retracted pocket of skin actively and vigorously desquamates and becomes infected, it is known as an *attic retraction cholesteatoma.* A similar pocket may form in the pars tensa, but this is less likely. If the pars tensa is retracted onto the promontory for a prolonged period of time, it may become adherent to the promontory, resulting in middle ear atelectasis and obliterating all or part of the middle ear space. Thick fluid can result in formation of middle ear adhesions that, in turn, limit the motion of the tympanic membrane and ossicles. The presence of thick middle ear fluid appears to increase the suceptibility of the patient to acute suppurative otitis media. Unfortunately, it is not possible to predict accurately which child with persistent middle ear fluid will develop local complications. The complications, which can be irreversible, appear substantially more significant than the risks related to obtaining middle ear ventilation with a tube when necessary. Studies increasingly demonstrate the importance of good hearing to optimal utilization of educational opportunities (Goetzinger, 1962). Thus, when middle ear fluid persists in spite of adequate medical management, it is desirable to remove the fluid and to ventilate the tympanum.

Ventilating tubes are essentially devices that maintain the patency of a perforation and consequently keep the middle ear ventilated in instances in which the eustachian tube fails to accomplish this. They are available in many sizes, shapes, and material. Basically, the two basic types are long tubes with a flange that is placed medial to the tympanic membrane and short tubes that are doubly flanged. One flange is placed medial to the tympanic membrane, and the other flange rests lateral to the membrane. Materials may be polyethylene, vinyl, silicone rubber, or stainless steel. They may be transparent or colored blue or green for easier identification. The larger the diameter of the inner flange, the longer it tends to stay in place. The longer the tube remains in place, the greater the chance that the perforation will remain open after removal or extrusion of the tube. For this reason, many surgeons prefer to use a small flange tube initially and reserve the larger flange tubes for those patients requiring multiple tube insertions.

When the tubes are in place, the patient must avoid getting water into his or her ear. Responsible patients can do this by using lamb's wool or petrolatum-impregnated cotton in the meatus when washing their hair and by using custom-molded ear plugs or "Silly Putty" in the meatus during swimming. *None of these techniques provide complete protection, however.* Patients with ventilating tubes in place should refrain from nose-blowing during an upper respiratory infection, since infected material is more likely to be drawn up the eustachian tube to the tympanum with a tube in place.

The main complications of ventilating tubes are the introduction of infection through the tube, the persistence of a perforation in the tympanic membrane after the tube is removed and, rarely, the development of cholesteatoma following removal of the tube.

Most ventilating tubes extrude spontaneously. When tubes have not extruded after a year, a decision must be made regarding the tube removal. Tympanometry to monitor the pressure-equalizing aspect of the eustachian tube may be utilized to help determine the appropriate time for removal, but this has never been validated. It is necessary to consider tympanometry, physical findings, and clinical course in deciding when to remove ventilating tubes. Removal is particularly desirable in the late spring to permit the tympanic membrane to heal, allowing the patient to swim through the summer.

DISEASES OF THE INNER EAR AND EXTERNAL AUDITORY CANAL

Objective tinnitus can be perceived by the examiner using a stethoscope over the area of the ear. The main objective forms of tinnitus are those due to vascular anomalies or to a tic of the tensor tympani muscle. The latter also can be observed by watching the tympanic membrane jerk medially as the tensor contracts. *Subjective tinnitus* usually indicates damage to the hair cells of the inner ear and may be the result of head trauma, noise trauma, or the effects of toxins or drugs (i.e., aspirin or aminoglycosides) on these cells.

Cerumen often must be removed because it occludes the ear canal and interferes with

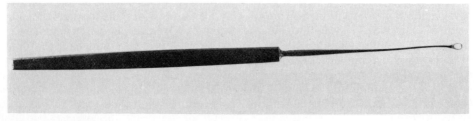

FIGURE 38–5. Shapleigh Cerumen spoon. This model has fine serrations which help manipulate the cerumen, together with a narrow shaft to allow maximum visibility and manipulation.

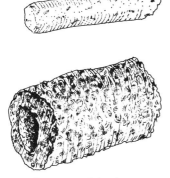

FIGURE 38–6. Pope Ear Wick. The compressed wick is inserted into the external auditory canal and moistened. It then expands to fill the canal holding medication against the entire circumference.

removed by irrigation with body temperature water. At times it is necessary to fill the ear canal with baby oil and allow this to soak overnight prior to irrigation.

Foreign bodies frequently present a difficult challenge. It is important to avoid forcing the foreign body further into the ear canal. Frequently a small right-angled instrument can be passed beyond the foreign body, rotated, and then removed, bringing the foreign body with it.

Otitis externa may represent an acute circumscribed furunculosis or a diffuse contact dermatitis of the skin of the external auditory canal. The most common organisms of diffuse otitis externa are *Pseudomonas* species, which respond well to cleaning the ear canal with suction, introducing an ear wick (Fig. 38–6) together with the use of acidifying drops (VoSol, five drops q.i.d.) or an antibiotic steroid drop. Many commercial combinations include the antibiotic neomycin, which is a frequent contact sensitizer; these should be used with caution. The ear wick should be removed in 3 to 6 days, after which the canal should be thoroughly cleaned with suction or irrigation.

hearing or because it obstructs the physician's view of the tympanic membrane. This usually can be accomplished with a cerumen spoon (Fig. 38–5). If the cerumen is soft and tympanic membrane is intact, it may be

References

Benson, M. K.: Maximum nasal inspiratory flow rate: Its use in assessing the effects of pseudoephedrine in vasomotor rhinitis. Eur. J. Clin. Pharmacol. *3*:182, 1971.

Bernstein, J. M.: Biological mediators of inflammation in middle ear effusions. Ann. Otol. Rhinol. Laryngol. *85*(Supp):90, 1976.

Bierman, C. W., and Pierson, W. E.: The role of the pediatric allergist in the care of patients with eustachian tube dysfunction. Otolaryngol. Clin. North Am. *3*:79, 1970.

Bierman, C. W., Pierson, W. E., and Donaldson, J. A.: The evaluation of middle ear function in children. Amer. J. Dis. Child. *120*:233, 1970.

Bierman, C. W., and Furukawa, C. T.: Medical management of serous otitis in children. Pediatrics *61*:768, 1978.

Bluestone, C. D., Paradise, J. L., and Beery, Q. C.: Physiology of the eustachian tube in the pathogenesis and management of middle ear effusions. Laryngoscope *82*:1654, 1972.

Bluestone, C. D., and Shuris, P. A.: Middle ear disease in children: pathogenesis, diagnosis, and management. Pediatr. Clin. North. Am. *21*:379, 1974.

Branefors, P., Dahlberg, T., and Nylen, O.: A study of the antibody levels against the capsular antigens of *H. influenzae* type B and S. Pneumoniae types 3, 6, 19, and 23 in a group of children with frequent episodes of purulent otitis media. Abstract of the Second International Symposium: Recent Advances in Otitis Media with Effusion (Supplement). Ohio State University, College of Medicine, Columbus, Ohio, May 1979.

Brannon J. B., and Murray, T.: The spoken syntax of normal, hard of hearing and deaf children. J. Speech Hear. Res. *69*:604, 1966.

Connell, J. T.: Effectiveness of topical nasal decongestants. Ann. Allergy *27*:541, 1969.

Chan, J. C. M., Logan, G. B., and McBean, J. B.: Serous otitis media and allergy. Am. J. Dis. Child. *114*:684, 1967.

Dees, S. C., and Lefkowitz, D.: Secretory otitis media in allergic children. Am. J. Dis. Child. *124*:364, 1972.

Frady, R. P., Parker, W. A., and Jackson, R. T.: Studies in permeability of the middle ear mucosa. Arch Otolaryngol. *103*:47, 1977.

Goetzinger, C. P.: Effects of small perceptual losses on language and on speech discrimination. Volta Rev. *64*:408, 1962.

Holm, V. A., and Kunze, L. H.: Effect of chronic otitis media on language and speech development. Pediatrics. *43*:833, 1969.

Juhn, S. K., Huff, J. S., and Paparella, M. M.: Lactate dehydrogenase activity and isoenzyme patterns in serous middle ear effusions. Ann. Otol. Rhinol. Laryngol., *82*:192, 1973.

Kaliner, M., and Austren, K. F.: Immunologic release of chemical medicators from human tissues. Ann. Rev. Pharmacol. *15*:177, 1975.

Klein, J. O., and Teele, D. W.: Isolation of viruses and mycoplasmas from middle ear effusions. *85*(Supp 25):140, 1976.

Lim, D. J., Viall. J., Birck, H., and Pierre, R. S.: The morphological basis for understanding middle ear effusions. Laryngoscope *82*:1625, 1972.

Liu, Y. S., Lim, D. J., Lang, R., and Birck, H. G.: Microorganisms in chronic otitis media with effusion. Ann. Otol. Rhinol Laryngol. *85*(Supp):245, 1976.

Lloyd, L. L., Rolland, J. C., and McManis, D. L.: Performance of hearing impaired and normal hearing retardation selected language measures. Am. J. Ment. Defic. *71*:904, 1967.

Lupovich, P., and Harkins, M. H.: The pathophysiology of effusion in otitis media. Laryngoscope *82*:1647, 1972.

Maxim, P. E., Veltri, R. W., Sprinkle, P. M., and Pusateri, R. J.: Chronic serous otitis media: An immune complex disease. Am. Acad. Ophthalmol. and Otolaryngol. *84*:234, 1977.

McLaurin, J. W., Shipman, W. F., and Rosedale, R.: Oral decongestants. Laryngoscope *71*:54, 1961.

Miller, G. F.: Influence of oral decongestant in eustachian tube dysfunction in children. J. Allergy *45*:187, 1970.

Mogi, G.: Secretory IgA and antibody activities in middle ear effusions. Ann. Otol. Rhinol. Laryngol. *85*(Supp. 25):97, 1976.

Mogi, G., Maeda, S., Yoshida, T.: Radioimmunoassay of IgE studies in middle ear effusions. Acta Otolaryngol. *82*:26, 1976.

Olmstead, R. W., Alvarez, M. D., Moroney, J. D., and Eversden, M.: The pattern of hearing following acute otitis media. J. Pediatr. *65*:252, 1964.

Olson, A. L., Klein, S. W., Charney, E., et al.: Prevention and therapy of serous otitis media by an oral decongestant: A double-blind study in pediatric practice. Pediatrics *61*:679, 1978.

Paparella, M. D.: Blue ear drum and its management. Ann. Otol. Rhinol. Laryngol. *85*(Suppl 25):293, 1976.

Paradise, J. L.: Pediatricians' view of middle ear effusions: More questions than answers. Ann. Otol. Rhinol. Laryngol. *85*(Supp 25):20, 1976.

Sade, J.: Pathology and pathogenesis of serous otitis media. Arch. Otolaryngology. *84*:79, 1966.

Sade, J., Weissman, Z., Nevo, A. C., and Drucker, I.: Effect of environmental factors on respiratory epithelium. Proc. of the Int. Symposium on Respiratory Disease and Air Pollution.

1975 (Ed. A. B. David Klinberg. A. Aharonson). London, John Wiley, 1975*a*.

Sade, J., Meyer, F. A., King, M., and Silberberg, A.: Clearance of middle ear effusions by the mucociliary system. Acta Otolaryngol. *79*:277, 1975*b*.

Sade, J., and Weissman, Z.: Middle ear mucosa and secretory otitis media. Arch. Otol. Rhinol. Laryngol. *215*:195, 1977.

Sade, J.: Secretory and serous otitis media (S.O.M.). Adv. Otol. Rhinol. Laryngol. *22*:1, 1978.

Senturia, B. H.: Classification of middle ear effusions. Ann. Otol. Rhinol. Laryngol. *79*:358, 1970.

Shurin, P. A., Pelton, S. I., Donner, A., and Klein, J. O.: Persistence of middle-ear effusion after acute otitis media in children. New Engl. J. Med. *300*(20):1121, 1979.

Sipila. P., Pyhanrn, P., and Karna, P.: T lymphocytes in effusions of secretory otitis media. Arch. Otol. Rhinol. Laryngol. *220*:108, 1976.

Sloyer, J. L., Jr., Ploussard, J. H., and Howie, V. M.: Immunology and microbiology in acute otitis media. Ann. Otol. Rhinol. Laryngol. *85*(Supp 25):130, 1976.

Sloyer, J. L., Howie, V. M., Ploussard, J. M., Bradac, J., Habercorn, M., and Ogra, P. L.: Immune response to acute otitis media in children. J. Immunol. *118*:248, 1977.

Tos, M., and Bak-Pedersen, K.: Goblet cell population in the pathological middle ear and eustachian tube of children and adults. Ann. Otol. *86*:209, 1977.

Veltri, R. W., and Sprinkle, P. M.: Secretory otitis media. An immune complex disease. Ann. Otol. Rhinol. Laryngol. *85*(Supp):135, 1976.

C. Warren Bierman, M.D.
William E. Pierson, M.D.
James A. Donaldson, M.D.

39

Diseases of the Nose

Chronic nasal obstruction is a prevalent disorder in children. It is manifested by mucosal edema, hypersecretion of mucus, and often by adenoidal hypertrophy. These pathophysiologic changes represent final common pathways of nasal diseases. Table 39–1 lists characteristics of common noninfectious causes of nasal obstruction. The cause of some of these conditions is well known, while that of others still is obscure. For example, eosinophils may be present in secretions signifying allergic rhinitis but may appear also for unknown reasons in pseudoallergic rhinitis (nonallergic rhinitis with eosinophilia).

Since a variety of conditions can result in similar symptoms, chronic nasal obstruction poses a diagnostic and therapeutic challenge. Hyperreactivity to a variety of physical and emotional stimuli or obstruction by mechanical factors such as congenital anomalies or foreign bodies in infants and nose drop abuse or deviated septum in adolescents also may produce symptoms similar to allergic or pseudoallergic rhinitis.

Chronic nasal obstruction can present in a variety of ways, from obvious symptoms of chronic mouth breathing or hayfever to subtle symptoms of hearing loss, chronic fatigue, or recurrent headache, reflecting the frequent coexistence of middle ear or sinus disease. Since the mucosa of the upper airway is continuous and extends into the middle ear and sinuses, diseases of the nasal mucosa may lead directly to sinus or ear disease or indirectly to obstruction of ventilation or compromise of mucociliary clearance. This chapter will consider allergic, pseudoallergic, vasomotor, and obstructive rhinitis. Chapters 38 and 40 discuss sinusitis and middle ear diseases. Acute or chronic upper respiratory infections, which may be primary conditions or may be secondary to underlying nasal disease, are discussed in Chapter 56.

ALLERGIC RHINITIS

Allergic rhinitis is estimated to occur in 10 percent of the population under 20 years of age. Broder and colleagues (1974) found the incidence to be somewhat higher in subjects over 16 years of age; seasonal allergic rhinitis (hayfever) was twice as common as perennial allergic rhinitis.

Etiology and Pathogenesis

Two factors are required for the development of allergic rhinitis: the heritable atopic state and the development of sensitivity to allergens present in the patient's environment. Exposure to allergens such as house dust, mold spores, animal danders, pollens, or even foods in small children may induce development of specific IgE antibodies, which become fixed to nasal mast cells.

511

TABLE 39–1 NONINFECTIOUS RHINITIS IN CHILDREN AND ADOLESCENTS

	Allergic Rhinitis	Pseudoallergic Rhinitis	Vasomotor Rhinitis
Age of Onset	*Infancy to Adulthood*	*Adolescence to Adulthood*	*Childhood to Adulthood*
History Allergy	Common	Rare	Rare
Symptoms			
Congestion	Moderate	Marked	Moderate
Sneezing	Frequent	Occasional	Rare
Itching (nose and eyes)	Marked	Infrequent	Infrequent
Rhinorrhea	Thin to mucoid	Mucoid to mucopurulent	Thin
Postnasal drip	Moderate	Marked	Marked
Aspirin sensitivity	Rare	Common	Rare
Physical Examination			
Turbinates	Mild to marked edema	Edematous	Slightly edematous
Color of mucosa	Pale gray to red	Pale to red	Red; occasionally pale
Polyps	Rare	Common (33%) of patients)	Rare
Laboratory Findings			
IgE	Normal to elevated	Normal	Normal
Positive STs	Usually	Rarely	Rarely
Nasal Cytology	Eosinophils	Many eosinophils	Few PMN's
Sinus disease	±	±	±
Response to Treatment			
Antihistamines	Good	Poor	Poor
Oral decongestants	Moderate	Moderate	Fair
Topical decongestants	Slight	Moderate	Good
Cromolyn	Moderate	Poor	Poor
Steroids	Good	Good	Poor
Immunotherapy	Good	Poor	Poor

Repeated exposure to those allergens results in immune release of mediators and subsequent tissue injury.

Though histamine appears to be the most important mediator in seasonal allergic rhinitis, others such as eosinophilic chemotactic factor of anaphylaxis (ECF-A) and kinins also have been identified in nasal secretions. Histamine dilates postcapillary venules to induce vascular engorgement and mucosal edema and stimulates goblet cells to secrete mucus. ECF-A induces chemotaxis of eosinophils, which appear to ingest antigen-antibody complexes and may inactivate histamine and other mediators.

Nasal mucosal biopsies show marked edema of the submucosal tissue, infiltration by eosinophils and granulocytes, distended Goblet cells, and congested enlarged mucous glands. Intercellular spaces are widened, and the basement membrane is thickened. Rappaport (1953) described a shift in the colloidal balance of the ground substance surrounding cells and blood vessels in allergic rhinitis in which the mucoproteins and mucopolysaccharides change from a relatively semisolid state to a relatively fluid state. The changes appear to be proportional to the duration and severity of the allergic reaction. However, even in long-standing allergic rhinitis the mucosa remains intact with no evidence of tissue destruction, though the basement membrane thickens progressively.

Altered autonomic reflexes are manifested by a lower sneezing threshold as the disease progresses. Paroxysms of sneezing and rhinorrhea may result from changes in air temperature or head movement, odors, irritants, and exposure to small quantities of antigen (Seebohm, 1978).

A "priming effect" to allergens occurs with continued exposure. A much larger dose of allergen is required when the nasal mucosa has been unchallenged for months than after a week or more of daily exposure (Connell, 1966). This may explain the progression of symptoms noted in many patients at the end of a season when pollen counts are dropping. The priming effect also increases the response to nonallergic stimuli such as changes in head position. For example, the supine position may increase nasal resistance threefold in patients with allergic rhinitis due to loss of nasal vascular tone (Rundcrantz, 1964). This may be reduced with hyposensitization treatment (Rundcrantz, 1969).

Exercise also alters nasal congestion in allergic rhinitis. Strenuous exercise will reverse nasal congestion for minutes to hours (Richerson and Seebohm, 1968). This response to exercise can be abolished by blocking the stellate ganglion, suggesting that the reaction is mediated by the sympathetic nervous system and that autonomic imbalance plays a role in allergic rhinitis (Chap. 14).

Clinical Presentation and Manifestation

In susceptible young children, perennial exposure to environmental factors, such as house dust, mold spores, or animal danders, may induce year-round symptoms, often with exacerbations during winter months. Alternatively, hypersensitivity to dietary proteins may induce similar symptoms, especially in the first year or two of life. Perennial rhinitis often is difficult to associate with specific exposure to allergens because of the presence of constant symptoms, but symptoms may vary when the child changes environment temporarily, e.g., on vacation. Also, the "priming effect" of prior antigen exposure or respiratory viral infections further clouds the relationship between cause and effect. A discrete seasonal symptom pattern due to exposure to airborne pollens emerges at about five to six years of age. Its striking seasonal variation is recognized more clearly by parents and physicians. However, pollinosis may be superimposed on perennial rhinitis and may obscure the recognition of the cause of symptoms of nasal obstruction that are constant with no apparent relationship to season of the year. Signs and symptoms of allergic rhinitis

include nasal obstruction, itching, rhinorrhea, sneezing, mouth breathing, snoring, headache, and "stopped up" or "popping" ears. Epistaxis is common. Rhinorrhea may vary from a thin, watery secretion to large quantities of thick white or yellowish mucus. Postnasal mucus drainage may induce coughing and may be associated with mild hoarseness. Often small children will have paroxysmal nocturnal coughing spells with vomiting. Children with allergic rhinitis frequently sleep restlessly, snore, and wake in the morning complaining of a sore throat and fatigue. Loss of smell, a frequently unrecognized complication, may lead to poor eating habits and decreased appetite, which increases family tension at mealtimes.

On physical examination, the child with perennial rhinitis often appears pale with dark circles or "allergic shiners" under the eyes related to periorbital edema due to obstruction of venous drainage. Prolonged nasal obstruction in childhood and persistent mouth breathing can cause flattening of the malar eminences of the maxillary bones, causing an appearance referred to as "adenoidal facies" (Marks, 1973). The lower eyelid also may have an accentuated line from the medial epicanthus extending laterally, which is known as an atopic pleat or Denne's line. The gingivae can be hypertrophic from persistent mouth breathing. Often hyperplasia of the posterior pharyngeal lymphoid tissue can be noted, perhaps secondary to frequent upper respiratory infections or to chronic postnasal drainage.

Unlike the child with perennial rhinitis, the child with seasonal rhinitis (hayfever) has thin watery rhinorrhea, injection of the conjunctivae, and edema of the eyelids. The nasal mucosa often has been described as pale and swollen, but this is not a constant finding, and many children with allergic rhinitis may have inflamed mucosa. The "allergic salute," an upward rubbing of the nose to relieve nasal itching, results in a transverse nasal crease.

One third to one half of children with allergic rhinitis may have abnormal eustachian tube function, serous otitis, or sinusitis resulting from obstruction induced by edematous nasal mucosa. Therefore, special attention should be focused on the examination of the middle ears and sinuses. Pneumatic otoscopy should be performed on all patients presenting with possible allergic rhinitis.

Laboratory Findings

Helpful laboratory tests may include a cytologic examination of nasal secretions, pure tone audiometry, impedance audiometry, sinus radiographs, pulmonary function testing with exercise tests, properly selected skin tests, and, occasionally, serum IgE levels.

Nasal Secretion Cytology. A specimen of nasal secretions can best be obtained by having the patient blow his or her nose onto a plastic wrap. In small children, aspiration of secretions with a rubber bulb syringe is preferable to the use of a cotton-tipped applicator. Table 39–2 lists a simple office technique for microscopic examination of secretions.

Eosinophils are readily identified by their red-staining granules from PMN's, lymphocytes, and macrophages. Ten percent to 90 percent of eosinophils may be present in allergic rhinitis. However, absence of eosinophils does not rule out the diagnosis. During upper respiratory infections, PMN's and lymphocytes may predominate. Eosinophils may be absent also when the patient has not had recent exposure to offending allergens.

Ear Testing. Pure tone audiometry is the test of choice for examining hearing. It can be carried out with ease in an office setting. Children under three or four years of age, however, have difficulty understanding and cooperating with the test condition; at this age, impedance audiometry does not require cooperation and is a valuable screening test for middle ear function. Since impedance audiometry provides information on the compliance of the tympanic membrane and ossicular chain, it also should be performed on children with abnormal pure tone audiograms.

Sinus Radiographs. Sinus abnormalities on radiographs may range from mucosal edema to total opacification. Patients with allergic rhinitis who have superimposed infectious sinusitis frequently have severe persistent night coughing, chronic mucopurulent rhinorrhea, or both. Sinus radiographs are useful to confirm the diagnosis of sinusitis (Chap. 36).

Pulmonary Function Testing. Patients with allergic rhinitis frequently have unrecognized lower respiratory involvement. Spirometry may identify abnormalities in small airway function in the absence of wheezing. Even when resting pulmonary function tests are normal, exercise tolerance tests may be abnormal in up to 40 percent of children with allergic rhinitis tested by free running (Kawabori et al., 1975). These tests may be useful to identify patients at risk of developing asthma or who are handicapped by physical activity.

Quantitative IgE Levels. IgE serum levels generally correlate well with the presence of allergic rhinitis and are elevated in about 45 percent of affected patients. A normal level does not eliminate the possibility of allergy. However, a normal level can be useful in confirming the absence of allergy if other relevant specific skin tests also are negative. (Measurement of IgE serum concentration rarely is needed.)

Allergy Skin Testings. Allergy skin testing is helpful in identifying specific allergens in patients with allergic rhinitis who fail to respond to simple environmental control measures, nonsteroidal drug therapy, or both; or in patients who have complicating serous otitis or sinusitis. Tests should be based on detailed personal, family, and environmental history. A positive skin test provides evidence for allergic (IgE) sensitivity to which special therapeutic attention should be directed. Skin testing is discussed in detail in Chapter 21.

TABLE 39–2 TECHNIQUE OF STAINING NASAL SECRETION

1. Transfer the specimen to a glass slide, dry, and fix with heat.

2. Stain for 30 seconds with Hansel's stain (1:500 eosin and 1:200 methylene blue in alcohol).

3. Add distilled water to take up the stain for 30 seconds.

4. Wash with water.

5. Decolorize with methanol or 95% ethyl alcohol (do not over-decolorize).

6. Dry and examine under oil immersion.

Treatment. Treatment of allergic rhinitis consists of avoidance of allergens and irritants, use of appropriate drugs, and immunotherapy (hyposensitization), when the patient is allergic to dust, mold, and pollens. Each patient's treatment program should be individualized on the basis of the severity and duration of symptoms, associated complications (e.g., serous otitis), and the response to nonsteroidal drugs.

Avoidance of respiratory allergens and irritants can be carried out most effectively in small children since their symptoms are determined largely by the indoor environment in which they spend most of their time. Environmental control becomes progressively more difficult as the environmental exposure expands and as allergy develops to outside aeroallergens (Dockhorn, 1977). Specific details of environmental control measures are discussed in Chapter 22. Effective environmental control will enhance drug management and immunotherapy. If foods are considered potential allergens, a trial elimination diet may be carried out.

Pharmacologic Management

Drugs that may be useful in treating allergic rhinitis include antihistamines, oral decongestants, topical vasoconstrictors, cromolyn sodium, and aerosolized corticosteroids.

Antihistamines. The use of antihistamines is discussed in depth in Chapter 23. Antihistamines compete with histamine for specific histamine receptors located on end organs, such as blood vessels in nasal mucosa and mucosal goblet cells. Antihistamines are more effective if used before exposure to an allergen and should be prescribed in that way whenever possible. The patient will receive far more benefit by taking medication one hour before going outside in the morning during the pollen season or before visiting a friend who has a cat to which he or she may be allergic than by waiting to do so after symptoms have occurred.

Antihistamines are effective in the management of hayfever, seasonal conjunctivitis, and perennial allergic rhinitis if given regularly in effective dosage. Table 39–3 lists suggested antihistamine dosages. Antihistamines, while effective in controlling itching, sneezing, and rhinorrhea, appear to be less effective in controlling nasal obstruction. For instance, in a double-blind trial of hydroxyzine in adults with ad lib pseudoephedrine use, patients on placebo medication who took more pseudoephedrine had a lower incidence of nasal obstruction but significantly more hayfever symptoms than did the hydroxyzine-treated group (Schaaf, 1979).

The patient or parent should be warned about potential side effects of antihistamines, especially sedation. Patients should take a trial dose to test such side effects before driving a car, riding a bicycle in traffic, or working with machinery where alertness is essential. The parents and teachers of children should be aware that these side effects can affect school work. Often it is desirable to offer the patient several different antihistamines on a trial basis, letting the patient decide which one is most effective with the least number of side effects.

Oral Decongestants. Pseudoephedrine and phenylpropanolamine are the two oral alpha-adrenergic agents most frequently employed as decongestants. They act by constricting small blood vessels, thereby reducing mucosal edema. Both may cause CNS stimulation, which can result in insomnia or personality change. Employed in combination with antihistamines, their CNS activity may balance the sedation of the antihistamine. A double-blind crossover trial of pseudoephedrine, triprolidine, and the combination against placebo showed superior therapeutic results for the combination of antihistamines and decongestants (Empey, 1975). This study combined with that of Schaaf et al. (1979) suggests increased effectiveness of combined antihistamine-decongestant treatment of allergic rhinitis. A number of combinations are marketed and widely prescribed as listed in Table 39–4. Whether the relative contents of the two agents are appropriate in such fixed dose combinations has not been established.

Topical Vasoconstrictors. A variety of nose drops and nasal sprays that contain alpha-adrenergic agonists are available for over-the-counter use. Phenylephrine hydrochloride (Neo-synephrine) is the most common short-acting agent in 0.125 percent, 0.25 percent, and 0.51 percent solutions. Oxymetazoline hydrochloride (Afrin) in a 0.025 percent and a 0.05 percent solution and

Test continued on page 520.

TABLE 39–3 DOSAGE RECOMMENDATIONS OF ANTIHISTAMINES IN CHILDREN

Class	Generic	Proprietary	Formulation	Recommended Dose		
				CHILDREN	ADOLESCENT/ADULT	
Ethanolamine	diphenhydramine hydrochloride	Benadryl	Elixir 12 mg/5 ml Capsule 25, 50 mg Parenteral 10 mg/ml	5 mg/kg/24 hours—Administer in 4 divided doses	25–50 mg 3 or 4 times daily	Most widely used parenterally for acute allergic reactions. May be given with epinephrine (*Not a substitute*)
	carbinoxamine maleate	Clistin	Elixir 4 mg/5 ml Tablets 4, 8 mg Timed-released 8, 12 mg	0.8 mg/kg/24 hours—Administer in 4 divided doses	4 to 8 mg 3 or 4 times daily	Low incidence of drowsiness
	doxylamine succinate	Decapryn	Syrup 6.25 mg/5 ml Tablets 12.5, 25 mg	2 mg/kg/24 hours—Administer in 4 divided doses	12.5 to 25 mg 4–6 times daily	High incidence of drowsiness
Ethylenediamine	tripelennamine citrate	Pyribenzamine citrate	Elixir 25 mg/5 ml (HCl salt equivalent)	5 mg/kg/24 hours—Administer in 4 divided doses		
	tripelennamine hydrochloride	Pyribenzamine hydrochloride	Tablets 25, 50 mg Timed-release 50, 100 mg	5 mg/kg/24 hours—Administer in 4–6 divided doses (Timed-release: 2 doses)	25–50 mg every 4–6 hours or 100 mg every 8–12 hours	Less drowsiness, but mild G.I. irritation common
Alkylamine	chlorpheniramine maleate, brompheniramine maleate	Chlor-Trimeton Teldrin Dimetane	Syrup 2 mg/5 ml Tablets 4 mg Timed-release 8, 12 mg Parenteral solution 10 mg/ml in 1 ml ampules	0.35 mg/kg/24 hours—Administer in 4 divided doses	2–4 mg every 4–6 hours 8–12 mg every 8–12 hours (timed-release)	Low incidence of side effects. Some drowsiness May be administered I.V., I.M. or S.C. in adults; S.C. only in children

	Generic	Brand	Preparations	Pediatric dose	Adult dose	Remarks
	tiprolidine hydrochloride	Actidil	Syrup 1.25 mg/5 ml, Tablets 2.5 mg	<2 yrs: 0.6 mg, 2–3 times daily; >2 yrs; 1.25 mg 2–3 times daily	2.5 mg 2–3 times daily	May cause mild drowsiness
Phenothiazines	promethazine hydrochloride	Phenergan	Syrup 6.25 and 26 mg/5 mg, Tablets 12.5, 25, 50 mg, Solution for injection 25 and 5 mg/ml	0.5 mg/kg at bedtime; 0.13 mg/kg in morning	12.5 mg every 4 hrs. in day; 25 mg at bedtime	Pronounced sedation, Photosensitization
	methdilazine	Tacaryl	Tablets (chewable) 3.6 mg, Syrup 4 mg/5 ml, Tablets 8 mg	0.3 mg/kg – Administer in 2 divided dosages (>3 years only)	16–32 mg daily divided into 2–4 doses	Drowsiness not prominent. Recommended as antipruritic
	trimeprazine tartrate	Temaril	Syrup 2.5 mg/5 ml, Tablets 2.5 mg, Timed-release 5 mg	6 mos–2 yrs: 3.75 mg/day, divided into 3 doses; 3–12 yrs: 7.5 mg divided into 3 doses	10 mg/day divided into 4 doses or 2 doses (timed-release)	Drowsiness common. Recommended as anti-pruritic
Piperazine	hydroxyzine hydrochloride	Atarax, Vistaril	Syrup 10 mg/5 ml, Tablets 10, 25, 50, 100 mg, I.M. solution 25 mg/ml, 50 mg/ml, 100 mg/ml	2 mg/kg/24 hours divided into 4 doses	10–20 mg every 4–6 hours	Drowsiness is usually transient
Miscellaneous	cyproheptadine hydrochloride	Periactin	Syrup 2 mg/5 ml, Tablets 4 mg	0.25 mg/kg divided into 3 or 4 doses	4–20 mg daily in divided doses. Do not exceed 0.5 mg/kg/24 hours	Useful for cold urticaria. Drowsiness common. Causes increased appetite and increased growth rate in children

(From AMA Drug Evaluations, 3rd ed., 1977.)

TABLE 39–4 SELECTED ANTIHISTAMINE-DECONGESTANT PREPARATIONS

Antihistamine	Decongestant	Preparation	Infants	Suggested Dosage* Children 1–6 yrs	6–12 yrs	Older Children and Adults
brompheniramine maleate	phenylpropanolamine hydrochloride phenylephrine hydrochloride	Dimetapp				
12 mg each	15 mg each					
4 mg	5 mg each/tsp	extentabs**				1
		elixir		1 tsp	2 tsp	2
carbinoxamine maleate	pseudoephedrine hydrochloride	Rondec				
4 mg	60 mg	T (tablets)				1
4 mg	60 mg	C (chewables)		½	1	1
4 mg/tsp	60 mg/tsp	S (syrup)		½ tsp	1	1
2 mg/ml	25 mg/ml	D (drops)	½–1 ml			
chlorpheniramine maleate	d-pseudoephedrine hydrochloride	Isoclor				
8 mg	120 mg	capsules**				1
4 mg	60 mg	tablets			½	1
2 mg/tsp	30 mg/tsp	elixir		½ tsp	½–1 tsp	2 tsp
chlorpheniramine maleate	phenylephrine hydrochloride	Demazin				
4 mg	20 mg	repetabs**			1	1–2
1 mg/tsp	2.5 mg/tsp	syrup		½–2 tsp	2 tsp	2–3 tsp
chlorpheniramine phenyltoloxamine citrate	phenylpropanolamine hydrochloride phenylephrine hydrochloride	Naldecon				
5 mg	15 mg / 40 mg	10 mg	tablets**			1	1
2.5 mg	7.5 mg / 20 mg	5 mg	syrup		½ tsp	2
0.5 mg/tsp	2.0 mg/tsp / 5 mg/tsp	1.25 mg/tsp	pediatric syrup & drops		1 tsp	2 tsp	
0.5 mg/ml	2.0 mg/ml / 5 mg/ml	1.25 mg/ml		½–1 ml			

Antihistamine		Decongestant	Trade name / form	Dose (drops)	Dose (syrup)	Dose
dexbrompheniramine maleate	6 mg	d-isoephedrine sulfate 120 mg	Drixoral tabs**			1
dexbrompheniramine maleate	6 mg 2 mg	d-isoephedrine sulfate 120 mg 60 mg	Disophrol chronotabs tabs		½–1	1 1–2
pyrilamine maleate (pheniramine maleate) 25 mg / 25 mg 12.5 mg / 12.5 mg 6.25 mg/tsp / 6.25 mg/tsp 10 mg/ml / 10 mg/ml		phenylpropanolamine HCL 50 mg 25 mg 12.5 mg/tsp 20 mg/ml	Triaminic tablets** juvulets** syrup infant drops	5–10 drops	½–1 tsp	1 2 tsp
pyrrobutamine phosphate 15 mg 7.5 mg 7.5 mg/tsp		cyclopentamine hydrochloride 12.5 mg 6.25 mg 6.25 mg/tsp	Co-Pyronil pulvules pediatric pulvules suspension		(1) 1–2 1–2 tsp	1–2 ½–1 tsp 2 tsp
triprolidine HCL 2.5 mg 1.25 mg/tsp		pseudoephedrine hydrochloride 60 mg 30 mg/tsp	Actifed tabs syrup		1 tsp	1 2 tsp

*Suggested average starting dose. (Closely resembles manufacturer's recommendations, generally.) Dosage for syrups and tablets = 3 times a day; sustained release tabs (**) = q12h up to q8h.

(From Pearlman, D. S.: Antihistamines useful in allergic disorders. *In* Miller, R. R., and Greenblatt, D. J. (eds.): Handbook of Drug Therapy. Chap. 59. New York, Elsevier-North Holland, 1979, p. 992.)

xylometazoline hydrochloride (Otrivin) in a 0.05 percent and 0.1 percent solution are most commonly employed agents with a long duration of action. Topical therapy avoids the systemic effects that follow oral administration, but prolonged therapy may be followed by increased nasal congestion after initial improvement. This rebound increase in mucosal edema and vasodilation and the potential for abuse are potential problems with the use of topical decongestants. Adolescents and adults are particularly likely to abuse such agents and develop rhinitis medicamentosa. *Use of topical long-acting drugs should be restricted to no more than twice daily use for short time periods (three to four days) for any single course.*

Cromolyn sodium is a topically active agent that inhibits antigen-induced histamine release from mast cells. In 4 percent solution, it has been moderately effective in the treatment of seasonal rhinitis in double-blind trial (Handelman, 1977), but has the disadvantage of a relatively short duration of action and must be used up to six times daily (Cohen et al., 1976). It is not available in this form in the United States, though it is marketed for nasal and conjunctival use in both Canada and Europe.

Topical Corticosteroids. When obstruction is severe and unrelieved by other agents, a short course of steroids is indicated, preferably as topical therapy. Aerosolized dexamethasone (Turbinaire) can be safely used in short courses (for less than three weeks) without adrenal suppression (Shapiro et al., in press). Once symptoms are suppressed the improvement can be sustained with less frequent use (once or twice daily). Other topically active steroidal agents with better benefit/risk ratios are in clinical trials in the United States, including beclomethasone dipropionate, triamcinolone acetonide, and flunisolide. These agents are highly effective in patients with severe allergic rhinitis who have debilitating sneezing and nasal obstruction. With chronic use, however, they can induce nasal congestion. Perforation of the nasal septum (Miller, 1975) and blunting of adrenal responsiveness have been reported with prolonged use. Systemic corticosteroids are indicated only when symptoms are extreme and cannot be relieved by topical steroids.

Immunotherapy (hyposensitization). This treatment has been demonstrated to be effective in both children and adults with allergic rhinitis caused by air-borne pollens or seasonal molds whose symptoms have not been controlled by other measures (Sadan, 1969; Norman, 1978). Immunotherapy for house dust and indoor molds also may be helpful in patients with severe allergic rhinitis not adequately controlled by environmental control measures and drugs or with complications such as serous otitis or sinusitis. The mechanism of action and methods of administration are discussed in detail in Chapter 24.

Complications

These include serous otitis media, sinusitis, abnormal facial development (adenoidal facies), and eustachian tube dysfunction. Orthodontic problems including malocclusion are common with prolonged allergic rhinitis and mouth breathing (Steele, 1968). Sinusitis is characterized by inflammatory involvement of the mucosal lining of the paranasal sinuses and mucopurulent exudate, which may cause an air–fluid level in the sinus cavity. The incidence of sinusitis may be as high as 60 percent of allergic children with rhinitis and abnormal middle ear function. These conditions are discussed in Chapters 38 and 40.

PSEUDOALLERGIC RHINITIS (NONALLERGIC RHINITIS WITH EOSINOPHILA)

Pseudoallergic rhinitis is a condition often mistaken for allergic rhinitis because of clinical presentation and the presence of eosinophils in nasal secretions. Table 39–1 lists the major differential points between the two conditions.

Etiology and Pathogenesis

Pseudoallergic rhinitis rarely is cyclic and mimics perennial allergic rhinitis. Although its true cause remains unknown, it does not appear to be an IgE-mediated disorder. Immediate wheal skin tests to inhalants are negative, serum IgE levels are normal or low, and immunotherapy with allergens, avoidance of inhalants, and elimination of suspect foods have failed to improve the disease. Its association with infection has led to periodic attempts to establish hypersensitivity to bacteria as the etiologic mechanism, but to date this has not been proved (Seebohm, 1977).

History and Physical Examination

Pseudoallergic rhinitis usually begins in adulthood but may start in adolescence. It rarely is observed prior to this age in contrast to allergic rhinitis, which commonly begins early in childhood. A family history of allergic disease is no more common than that of the general population in comparison to a 35 to 65 percent incidence of positive family history of allergy in patients with allergic rhinitis. Symptoms are primarily those of marked nasal obstruction with only occasional sneezing and little or no nasal or conjunctival itching, in contrast to frequent sneezing with marked itching in allergic rhinitis. Aspirin sensitivity is common in pseudoallergic rhinitis, while it is rare in allergic rhinitis.

On physical examination, the two conditions may appear similar with the exception of nasal polyps, which virtually never occur with uncomplicated allergic rhinitis in children but may occur in up to 30 percent of patients with pseudoallergic rhinitis. Sinusitis also occurs more commonly in the pseudoallergic patients (Seebohm, 1977).

Laboratory Findings

Nasal cytology is similar in the two conditions. In fact, patients with pseudoallergic rhinitis may even have more eosinophils in their nasal secretions (as well as a higher blood eosinophilia). IgE levels generally are normal or low, however, and allergy skin tests are negative or fail to correlate with symptoms.

Treatment

Patients with pseudoallergic rhinitis respond poorly to antihistamines or cromolyn sodium and only minimally to oral or topical decongestants. Many also have rhinitis medicamentosa because of their abuse of nose drops or sprays in an effort to relieve symptoms. Aerosolized topical steroids, such as beclomethasone dipropionate or triamcinolone acetonide, are remarkably effective in controlling symptoms (Mallarkey et al., 1979).

Complications

Nasal polyps (33 percent), paranasal sinusitis (50 percent), and aspirin sensitivity (15 percent) are common and should be sought in these patients.

VASOMOTOR RHINITIS

Vasomotor rhinitis is a condition of nasal hyperresponsiveness to a variety of stimuli. It characteristically responds poorly to drug therapy. Changes in the environment or immunotherapy are of little benefit.

Etiology and Pathogenesis

Vasomotor rhinitis usually is perennial. The nose appears to be in a state of physiologic imbalance, which suggests neurogenic factors are involved (Seebohm, 1978). Histologic examinations have noted a significant increase in the number of mast cells, though the significance of this finding is not clear (Connell, 1969). The vascular control of blood flow may be abnormal and as a result may predispose to stasis within sinusoids and nasal obstruction.

History and Physical Examination

Vasomotor rhinitis can begin in early childhood but occurs more frequently in adolescence and adulthood. Differentiating points from allergic rhinitis include the fact that family or personal history of allergy occurs no more frequently than in the general population. Patients often note many factors that affect them, such as temperature and humidity changes, air conditioning, smoke, odors, and emotional factors. They have an acute awareness of their symptoms and appear to complain disproportionately to findings observed on physical examination. Sneezing and nasal and conjunctival itching can occur but rarely are intense, and there may be a thin rhinorrhea. The nasal mucosa often is inflamed without edema, and polyps occur rarely.

Laboratory Findings

IgE levels are in the normal range, allergy skin tests rarely are positive, and nasal secretions show a few PMN's and bacteria with only rare eosinophils.

Treatment

Success is difficult since these patients respond poorly to antihistamines, oral decongestants, cromolyn sodium, or steroids. Because topical nasal sprays afford some relief, many present with advanced cases of rhinitis medicamentosa. A combination of environmental measures designed to eliminate irritants, such as tobacco smoke, and oral decongestants will give partial benefit. Some patients may find saline nose drops helpful. Topical or systemic steroids are not usually of proven value.

MECHANICAL NASAL OBSTRUCTION

Mechanical factors that cause nasal obstruction include congenital malformations, foreign bodies, enlarged adenoids and tumors, nasal polyps, deviated septum, and iatrogenic disease resulting from abuse of nasal sprays and nose drops.

Congenital Malformations. The most common malformations involving the nose include cleft palate and choanal atresia. Cleft palate and cleft lip usually are obvious from birth and result in feeding difficulties, aspiration of food with respiratory distress, and recurrent otitis because of the reflux of food and secretions into the middle ear. Less obvious is the submucosal cleft palate, which is also associated with eustachian tube dysfunction and recurrent otitis. A submucous cleft palate is associated with a bifid uvula, which is the key to its diagnosis (Smith, 1977).

Posterior Choanal Atresia. This may mimic tracheoesophageal fistula in the neonate and is a surgical emergency. Unilateral choanal atresia may be overlooked at birth, and the symptoms of mouth breathing, unilateral rhinorrhea, and otitis may suggest allergic rhinitis. The diagnosis is made by a soft, flexible catheter that will pass down only one nostril and by confirmatory radiography. Therapy is surgical restoration of the choanal orifice.

Foreign Bodies. Objects in the nose are common in children. A persistent foul odor from the nose associated with a unilateral rhinorrhea indicates a foreign body until proven otherwise (DeWeese, 1977). On physical examination the mucosa of the involved nostril often is inflamed and edematous. Therapy is removal of the foreign body. The most serious complications involve fistula formation into the adjoining sinuses and rarely through the cribriform plate.

Adenoidal Enlargement and Nasopharyngeal Tumors. Although rare, enlarged adenoids in the infant can result in respiratory distress or difficulty with nursing (Eichenwald, 1976). The diagnosis can be made by indirect visualization of the adenoids or by a lateral radiograph of the nasopharynx.

The most frequent nasopharyngeal tumor of childhood is a benign angiofibroma, which can be locally invasive, eroding the bone of the paranasal sinus or upper nasopharynx as it grows. Rare malignant tumors include lymphomas, rhabdomyosarcomas, and primary carcinomas.

Nasal Polyps. These occur rarely in children. When they do occur, cystic fibrosis should be suspected. Polyps are seen more commonly, although still infrequently, in adolescents and in adults with chronic rhinitis, where they occur more commonly in women than men. Nasal polyps most frequently arise from within the ethmoid or maxillary sinuses and project into the nasal cavity. The mass of the polyps is made up chiefly of edema fluid with sparse fibrous cells and few mucous glands. There is infiltration by eosinophils, mononuclear and plasma cells, and PMN's are sparse (Sherman, 1968). Symptoms of nasal polyps can vary from nasal congestion, headaches, and intermittent fever to "chronic colds."

The diagnosis is made with ease on nasal examination, though the edematous nasal mucosa may have to be treated with an adrenergic spray in order to visualize the polyp adequately. Patients with polyps may be uniquely sensitive to aspirin. For example, 29 of 108 patients with nasal polyps gave a history of acute asthma or urticaria on ingesting aspirin (Grove and Farrior, 1939). At polypectomy or sinus irrigation, 85 to 95 percent of cultures of sinuses show bacterial growth. Streptococcus, staphylococcus, or pneumococcus occurs most frequently.

Therapy of nasal polyps includes the use of antibiotics if there is evidence of chronic sinusitis. Aerosolized corticosteroids used two or three times daily over a four week period (and continued once every day for longer periods) may be helpful in reducing the size of polyps and may remove the need for polypectomy. Cromolyn sodium by nasal insufflation has been reported to benefit some patients with polyps associated with nasal allergy. Polypectomy to reduce the degree of nasal obstruction often results only in temporary relief, since polyps tend to recur if the underlying disease is not adequately treated.

Rhinitis Medicamentosa. This condition results from abuse of nose drops and nasal sprays. On physical examination, the nasal mucosa is edematous and spongy. The nasal secretions contain many PMN's and also may have eosinophils if the patient also has allergic or pseudoallergic rhinitis. Rebound congestion of nasal mucosa is common after more than 5 to 10 days of topical treatment with vasoconstrictor drugs. Careful questioning is necessary to make the diagnosis, since patients may forget to mention the use of nose drops or sprays.

Therapy is to stop their use in one nostril at a time until it recovers and then in the opposite nostril. Aerosolized steroids may also facilitate recovery.

TONSILS AND RESPIRATORY ALLERGY

The pharyngeal tonsils are made up of lymphoid tissue supported by fibrous stroma. Lymphocytes of both T and B type have been demonstrated in palatine tonsillar tissues (Ostergaard, 1977a). The tonsils synthesize immunoglobulins of all classes (IgM, IgG, IgA, IgD, IgE) and play a role in local immunity (Curran, 1977) to viruses and pathogenic bacteria (Drucker, 1979). Tonsillectomy reduces the antibody response to polio virus (Ogra, 1971). Tonsillectomy in IgA-deficient children may be associated with an increased incidence of viral infections and a further drop in IgA levels (Donovan and Soothill, 1973). Childhood tonsillectomy has also been reported to be related to the development of Hodgkin's disease in adolescence (Vianna et al., 1971).

Clinical Manifestations

Tonsillar hypertrophy, chronic infection, or both have been associated most commonly with recurrent viral and bacterial infections, with respiratory allergy, and, less frequently, with other systemic diseases and neoplasms (Howard, 1971). Tonsillar hypertrophy may be associated with nasophyarngeal obstruction and persistent mouth breathing, problems in swallowing, and infrequently with cor pulmonale and alveolar hypoventilation. The relationship of tonsillar hypertrophy to recurrent sore throat has been controversial. In a prospective study of a group of children with histories of recurrent tonsillitis, a majority experienced few episodes after coming under close scrutiny, and most of the episodes that developed were mild (Paradise et al., 1978).

The relationship of tonsillar hypertrophy and the effect of tonsillectomy on atopic diseases remains controversial. Cernelc and colleagues (1978) studied T and B lymphocytes in peripheral blood and palatine tonsils removed at operation of 28 atopic and 5 nonatopic children. Although the percentage of T lymphocytes was significantly higher in peripheral blood than in tonsils of all subjects, the mean percentage of B lymphocytes in the tonsils of atopic children was significantly higher than in those of nonatopic children. Hypertrophic tonsils had a higher percentage of B and T lymphocytes than did small tonsils, suggesting that tonsillar hypertrophy is associated with increased numbers of B cells. Ostergaard (1977a) studied serum and salivary immunoglobulin levels in 27 children before and 3 years after tonsillectomy. Serum IgA, which had been low preoperatively in many, decreased further over the next 3 years, as did serum IgG and IgM levels. By contrast, mean salivary IgA did not change with tonsillectomy. Three of the five patients who did not improve and continued to be colonized by pathogenic bacteria had a progressive rise in IgE levels that paralleled the development of atopic disease. Whether there was a cause-and-effect relationship of tonsillectomy to the development of atopic disease in these patients is not clear (Ostergaard, 1977b). Prospective studies of the relationship of tonsillectomy to the course of allergic disease are clearly needed.

Indication for Tonsillectomy

On the basis of current knowledge, allergic disease per se represents neither an indication nor a contraindication to tonsillectomy. Tonsillectomy clearly is indicated in children with peritonsillar abscess or malignancy or when massive hypertrophy of tonsils or adenoids or both results in alveolar hypoventilation or cor pulmonale. It probably is indicated when dysphagia or extreme difficulty in breathing (Paradise, 1977) exists. The American Academy of Pediatrics (1975) also lists four or more documented episodes of tonsillitis with cervical adenitis within a one year period as an indication for tonsillectomy. The question is whether the benefits of removal outweigh the risks of anesthesia, postoperative hemorrhage, or palatal scarring. In the allergic child, it would be wise to defer surgery until underlying allergy is treated, since such treatment may decrease or eliminate indications for surgery.

References

Broder, I., Higgins, M. W., Mathews, K. P., and Keller, J. B.: Epidemiology of asthma and allergic rhinitis in a total community. Tecumseh, Michigan. IV. Natural history. J. Allergy Clin. Immunol. 54:100, 1974.

Černelč, P., Kvalj, J., and Černelč, D.: Immunological function of tonsils in atopic and nonatopic children. Allergie v Immunol. 24:287, 1978.

Cohan, R. H., Bloom, F. L., Rhoades, R. B., et. al.: Treatment of perennial allergic rhinitis with cromolyn sodium. J. Allergy Clin. Immunol. 58:121, 1976.

Committee on Hospital Care, American Academy of Pediatrics: Pediatric Model Criteria Sets. Evanston, Ill., page 32, 1975.

Connell, J. T.: An instrument for measuring the effective cross-sectional nasal airway. J. Allergy 37:127, 1966.

Connell, J. T.: Quantitative intranasal pollen challenges. III. The priming effect in allergic rhinitis. J. Allergy 43:33, 1969.

Curran, R. C., and Jones, E. L.: Immunoglobulin-containing cells in human tonsils as demonstrated by immunohistochemistry. Clin. Exp. Immunol. 21:103, 1977.

Dockhorn, R. J.: Otolaryngologic allergy in children. Otolaryngol. Clin. North Am. 10:103, 1977.

Donovan, R., and Soothill, J. F.: Immunological studies in children undergoing tonsillectomy. Clin. Exp. Immunol. 14:347, 1973.

Drucker, M. M., Agatsuma, Y., Drucker, I., Neter, E., Bernstein, J., and Ogra, P. L.: Cell-mediated immune response to bacterial products in human tonsils and peripheral blood lymphocytes. Infect. Immun. 23:347, 1979.

Eichenwald, H. F.: Respiratory Infections in Children. Hosp. Pract. 11:81, 1976.

Empey, D. W., Bye, C., Hoodes, M., et al.: A double-blind crossover trial of pseudoephedrine and triprolidine alone and in combination for the treatment of allergic rhinitis. Ann. Allergy, 34:41, 1975.

Grove, R. C., and Farrior, J. B.: Chronic hyperplastic sinusitis

in allergic patients: A bacteriologic study of two-hundred operative cases. J. Allergy 11:271, 1939.

Handelman, N. I., Friday, G. A., Schwartz, H. J., et. al.: Cromolyn sodium nasal solution in the prophylactic treatment of pollen-induced seasonal allergic rhinitis. J. Allergy Clin. Immunol. 59:237, 1977.

Howard, W. A.: Tonsillitis and adenoiditis. In Kendig, E. L., and Chernick, V. (eds.): Disorders of the respiratory tract in children. Philadelphia, W. B. Saunders Co., p. 347, 1977.

Kawabori, I., Pierson, W. E., Conquest, L. and Bierman, C. W.: Incidence of exercise-induced asthma in children. J. Allergy Clin. Immunol. 58:447, 1976.

Kjellman, M., Harder, H., Hansson, L., and Lindwall, L.: Allergy, otitis media and serum immunoglobulins after adenoidectomy. Acta Paediatr. Scand. 67:717, 1978.

McCurdy, J. A., Jr.: The tonsillectomy-adenoidectomy dilemma. Am. Fam. Physician 16:137, 1977.

Marks, M. B.: Unusual signs of respiratory tract allergy. Ann. Allergy 31:611, 1973.

Miller, F. F.: Occurrence of nasal septal perforation with use of intranasal dexamethasone aerosol. Ann. Allergy 34(2):107, 1975.

Mullarkey, M. F., Hill, J. S., and Webb, D. R.: Allergic and nonallergic rhinitis. J. Allergy Clin. Immunol. 63:201, 1979.

Norman, P. S., and Lichtenstein, L. M.: The clinical and immunologic specificity of immunotherapy. J Allergy Clin. Immunol. 61:370, 1978.

Ogra, P. L.: Effect of tonsillectomy and adenoidectomy on nasopharyngeal antibody response to polio virus. N. Engl. J. Med. 284:59, 1975.

Ostergaard, P. A.: B- and T-cells and intracellular Ig-synthesis of peripheral lymphocytes in children with asthma and/or previous adeno-tonsillectomy. Acta Path. Microbiol. Scand. Sec C 85:454, 1977a.

Ostergaard, P. A.: IgA levels, bacterial carrier rate, and the development of bronchial asthma in children. Acta Path. Microbiol. Scand. Sec C *85*:187, 1977*b*.

Paradise, J. L.: More on T and A. Pediatrics *59*:641, 1977.

Paradise, J. L., Bluestone, C. D., et al.: History of recurrent sore throat as an indication for tonsillectomy. N. Engl. J. Med. *298*:409, 1978.

Pearlman, D. S.: Antihistamines: Pharmacology and clinical use. Drugs *12*:258, 1976.

Rappaport, B. Z., Samter, M., Catchpole, H. R., and Schiller, F.: The mucoproteins of the nasal mucosa of allergic patients before and after treatment with corticotropin. J. Allergy *24*:35, 1953.

Richerson, H. B., and Seebohm, P. M.: Nasal airway response to exercise. J. Allergy *41*:269, 1968.

Rundcrantz, H.: Posture and congestion of nasal mucosa in allergic rhinitis. Acta Otolargynol. *58*:283, 1964.

Rundcrantz, H.: Postural variations of nasal patency. Acta Otolaryngol. *68*:1, 1969.

Ryan, R. E.: *In* Ryan, Ogura, Biller, and Pratt (eds.): Synopsis of Ear, Nose and Throat Disease, 3rd ed. St. Louis, The C. V. Mosby Co., p. 155, 1970.

Sadan, N., Rhyne, M. B., Melitis, E. D., et. al.: Immunotherapy of pollenosis in children. N. Engl. J. Med. *280*:623, 1969.

Schaaf, L., Hendeles, L., and Weinberger, M.: Suppression of seasonal allergic rhinitis symptoms with daily hydroxyzine. J. Allergy Clin. Immunol. *63*:129, 1979.

Seebohm, P. M.: Allergic and non-allergic rhinitis. In Middleton, E., Jr., Reed, C., and Ellis, E. F. (eds.): Allergy, Principles and Practice. St. Louis, The C. V. Mosby Co., p. 868, 1978.

Shapiro, G. G., Furukawa, C. T., Pierson, W. E., et al.: Double-blind study of aerosolized dexamethasone phosphate in children with eustachian tube dysfunction. In press.

Sherman, W. B.: Hypersensitivity: Mechanisms and Management. Philadelphia. W. B. Saunders Co., pp. 210–217, 1968.

Smith, D. W., Lemli, L., and Oputz, J. M.: A new recognized syndrome of multiple congenital anomalies. J. Pediatr. *64*:210, 1964.

Steele, C. H., Fairchild, R. C., and Ricketts, R. M.: Forum on the tonsil and adenoid problem in orthodontics. Am. J. Orthodont. *54*:485, 1968.

Vianna, N., Greenwald, P., and Davies, J. N. P.: Tonsillectomy and Hodgkin's disease: The lymphoid tissue barrier. Lancet *1*:431, 1971.

40

Gary S. Rachelefsky, M.D.
Gail G. Shapiro, M.D.

Diseases of Paranasal Sinuses in Children

Sinusitis, or inflammation of the paranasal sinuses, is a common problem in children, though its true incidence is unknown. Sinus disease includes inflammatory disease, cysts, tumors, and foreign bodies. The major emphasis in this chapter is on infectious and allergic sinus disease.

DEVELOPMENT OF THE PARANASAL SINUSES

The paranasal sinuses form as evaginations of the mucous membrane of the nasal meatuses and are lined by the same mucosa as the nose. During embryonic development the origin of the ethmoid and maxillary sinuses is apparent by the third to fourth month of intrauterine life. The frontal sinuses become recognizable anatomically by the sixth to twelfth month of extrauterine life, while the sphenoid sinus appears later (Bernstein, 1971). While the maxillary and ethmoids are evident by radiography in infancy, the sphenoid sinuses appear by about the third year of life and the frontal sinuses between the third and seventh years. Developmental variants include hypoplasia of frontal sinuses, with partial or complete absence of the sinuses on radiography. Relative hypoplasia of the maxillary antra can be seen. Occasionally, the maxillary antra is subdivided by

septa and ridges into several small cavities. The ethmoid sinuses are a somewhat variable labyrinthine network of air spaces. Although they are grouped as anterior, middle, and posterior, there is considerable individual variation in structure (Caffey, 1972). Sinus abnormalities are common in patients with cleft lip and palate and in those with midfacial hypoplasia (e.g., Treacher Collins syndrome). Frontal and sphenoidal sinuses are absent and maxillary sinuses are hypoplastic in over 90 percent of children with Down's syndrome. Other syndromes associated with absent or hypoplastic sinuses include pyknodysostosis, McCune-Albright syndrome, thalassemia major, osteodysplasia, and familial microcornea.

LOCAL DEFENSE MECHANISMS

Mucociliary. The paranasal sinuses are lined by pseudostratified ciliated epithelium and bathed in a mucus layer produced by mucosal glands and goblet cells. Projecting from the border of each columnar cell are cilia, the ends of which are in contact with the overlying mucus. Microorganisms and foreign particles that enter the sinuses are removed by the constant motion of the mucus layer, propelled by the underlying

526

cilia. Mucus is carried to the ostium of the sinus in this manner.

Mucus secretions and saliva contain substances (including lysozymes and a lactoperioxidase-thiocyanate system) that decrease bacterial attachment, inhibit bacterial or viral replication, and destroy specific bacteria (Hoffman, 1966). Interferon in the nasal passages decreases the multiplication of viruses. The constant shedding of cells replaces bacterial or viral colonized cells with noncontaminated epithelial cells. Bacterial-epithelial attachment is not well understood but probably plays a role in determining the rate of bacterial multiplication.

Secretory Immune System. The secretory immune system is the first immune line of defense against invading organisms. Local exposure of mucous membranes to antigens induces the formation of secretory antibodies that provide protection against the infecting organisms. Secretory IgA (Tomasi and Bienenstock, 1968) is the predominant immunoglobulin in secretions that bathe mucous membranes that possess antibody activity against viral agents (Artenstein et al., 1964). Secretory IgA antibodies protect against parainfluenza type I (Smith et al., 1966), rhinovirus, influenza virus, and poliovirus (Hanson et al., 1971).

Secretory IgA antibodies against bacteria have been demonstrated to inhaled tetanus toxoid (Hanson et al., 1971), diphtheria toxoid (Newcomb et al., 1969), and to parenterally administered *Salmonella typhi* vaccine (Tourville and Tomasi, 1969). Secretory antibody has been shown to interfere with the attachment of oral streptococcal strains to buccal mucosal cells (Williams and Gibbons, 1972). Although secretory IgA antibodies appear to play an important role in protecting the upper respiratory tract against various kinds of infection, some individuals who lack IgA antibodies do not have an increased number or more severe respiratory infections, possibly because of increased quantities of IgG and IgM in the secretions of many of these patients.

Nonspecific Surface Defenses. Mechanisms that act to clear organisms and debris from the nasal passages include the following: a flow of free fluid that tends to wash away organisms, movement of air currents, coughing, sneezing, and possibly chewing.

FACTORS THAT PREDISPOSE TO SINUS DISEASE

Defense mechanisms of paranasal sinuses function effectively only when there is no obstruction of sinus ostia. Nasal allergy is frequently associated with sinus disease, since the allergic reaction increases mucus production and causes nasal mucosal edema. Swollen mucosal surfaces occlude the sinus ostia and inhibit normal ciliary cleansing action, thus facilitating mucus retention and bacterial sinus infection. Respiratory infections induce similar changes. When viral infections or overuse of topical nasal decongestants is superimposed on obstruction due to allergy, sinus infection becomes even more likely.

Other factors that functionally obstruct sinuses and interfere with sinus drainage include large adenoids, imperforate choanae, deviated nasal septi, nasal polyps, nasal foreign bodies, and tumors. Swimming and diving can force pathogenic bacteria into paranasal sinuses, where they induce sinusitis if normal defense mechanisms are compromised. Chronic parasinusitis, a characteristic finding in children with cystic fibrosis, probably is related to poor ciliary action and viscid secretions. In Kartagener's syndrome, sinusitis appears at least in part to be due to abnormal ciliary function. Down's syndrome and various other immune deficiency disorders frequently are associated with chronic sinusitis. There is a subgroup of asthmatic patients who have aspirin sensitivity, nasal polyps, and sinusitis, although the reason for the association is unknown.

SIGNS AND SYMPTOMS OF SINUSITIS IN CHILDREN

In 106 nonallergic children examined with acute sinusitis, 52 percent showed cough, headache and fever, while postnasal drip, pharyngitis, and paranasal sinus area pain were present in most (Herz and Gfeller, 1977). Half had elevated erythrocyte sedimentation rates and one-third had leukocytosis ($>10,000/mm^3$). Schmid (1972) found similar signs and symptoms in a group of nonallergic children with acute sinus disease, while Bjonnes and Gugler (1973) emphasized abdominal pain as a frequent symptom.

Smith (1964) and Jaffe (1974) observed chronic nasal obstruction with a mucopurulent nasal and posterior pharyngeal discharge as the most common findings in sinusitis; sinus tenderness and fever were unusual in their study. Mucoid or mucopurulent nasal discharge and cough were commonly present in 25 children with sinusitis, whereas fever, sinus pain, and posterior pharyngeal pus rarely occurred (McLean, 1970).

Of 100 consecutive children who had sinusitis diagnosed clinically, the most frequent complaints were rhinorrhea, occurring in 77 percent, persistent cough in 48 percent, and otitis media in 43 percent (Kogutt and Swischuk, 1973). Pain, headache, and fever were found less commonly; 96 percent had abnormal x-rays, with the maxillary sinus most frequently involved. Thirty-eight of the patients had respiratory allergy, and they tended to have "more severe and widespread" involvement.

SINUSITIS IN ALLERGIC CHILDREN

Allergic children with chronic respiratory symptoms have a surprisingly high incidence of sinus disease (Rachelefsky et al., 1978). Sinus x-rays were taken of 70 consecutive children and adolescents between 3 and 16 years of age (mean age 7.9 years) who were referred for chronic allergic rhinitis (70) and for asthma (60). Thirty-seven (53 percent) had abnormal sinus x-rays: nineteen (27 percent) had opacification or marked thickening of sinus membranes (> 6 mm) of one or more maxillary sinuses, while the remainder had lesser degrees of mucosal thickening. The patients with the marked changes tended to be younger (average age 6.5 years vs. 9.2 years) and had more severe complaints of rhinorrhea and both night- and daytime coughing. Asthma was equally distributed among all groups. Nasal smears contained a greater proportion of polymorphonuclear leukocytes and fewer eosinophils in the patients with marked radiographic changes as compared with those with mild changes. With therapy, the number of eosinophils in nasal secretions increased and the number of PMN's decreased. The majority of patients with severe sinus involvement responded favorably to 2 weeks of therapy with ampi-cillin and pseudoephedrine and 5 days of oxymetazoline hydrochloride (0.25 percent) nasal spray, with a decrease of mucosal thickening to 2 mm or less, decreased rhinorrhea, and decreased coughing and/or wheezing. Several patients failed to improve and required maxillary antral punctures, which yielded thick purulent material.

A second study involved 91 atopic children who had chronic coughing refractory to bronchodilator drugs, chronic rhinorrhea, chronic fatigue, irritability, and nasal smears containing predominantly PMN's with ingested bacteria (Shapiro et al., 1980). Many complained of headaches or sleepless nights related to chronic coughing. Twenty-six patients (29 percent) also had middle ear abnormalities, including effusion, marked negative pressure, or ventilating tubes. Sinus radiographs revealed marked mucosal thickening (>6 mm) or opacification of one or more sinuses in 64 patients (70 percent). Most patients responded well to a medical regimen of antibiotics, oral antihistamine, decongestant, intermittent oxymetazoline hydrochloride (0.25 percent) nasal spray for 2 to 3 weeks, and postural drainage twice daily. Some, however, required up to 6 weeks of antibiotics before symptoms resolved. Two patients did not respond to medical therapy and required antral irrigation. The nasal smear was useful in following the course of sinusitis: generally a decrease in PMN's and an increase in eosinophils paralleled clinical improvement.

Chronic allergic rhinitis appears to predispose the patient to sinus disease. *The hallmarks of sinus disease are persistent cough, especially at night, and purulent rhinorrhea—sometimes associated with sore throat or middle ear disease.* Therapy must be aimed at controlling allergic disease as well as infection.

Chronic sinus disease, with persistent postnasal drainage, may induce bronchitis and asthma (McLaurin, 1943), since sinus secretions have been shown to accumulate in the lung. Possible mechanisms by which paranasal sinus disease may induce chronic bronchitis and/or asthma include:

1. Persistent bronchitis due to chronic bacterial seeding from infected sinuses.

2. "Hypersensitivity" to bacterial products that originate in the sinuses.

3. Reflex bronchospasm from paranasal sinus inflammation.

4. Induction of adrenergic blockade and refractory asthma by bacterial endotoxins originating in the sinuses (Phipatanakul and Slavin, 1974).

DIAGNOSTIC CONSIDERATIONS – ACUTE, SUBACUTE AND CHRONIC SINUSITIS

The physician should consider the possibility of sinusitis whenever symptoms are more severe or more protracted than expected for infectious or allergic rhinitis. Acute sinusitis often accompanies or follows viral-induced rhinitis and may present simply as a severe "bad cold." Acute sinusitis is usually caused by bacterial rather than viral infection and is characterized by fever, suppurative rhinitis, and a dull to intense throbbing pain over the affected sinus. Ethmoid sinuses are most commonly involved in younger children, and maxillary sinuses become involved with greater frequency in older children; frontal and sphenoid sinuses are involved least frequently (Gallagher, 1977).

Subacute sinusitis is characterized by a persistent, purulent discharge after an initial "cold." Patients complain of a persistent rhinorrhea and postnasal drip accompanied by a chronic cough which has not responded to cough medicine. Subacute sinusitis usually requires treatment with antibiotics.

Chronic sinusitis, that is, persistent sinus disease that fails to respond to even several months of intensive medical management, may require surgical intervention (Strome, 1976). In chronic sinusitis, permanent mucosal changes result in hypertrophy and in submucosal fibrosis, which lead to nasal polyps, micro-abscesses, areas of osseous resorption and thinning along sinus margins, with other areas of periosteal reaction and sclerotic new bone growth. It is important to recognize that most children with sinusitis rarely have pain to pressure over sinuses, or symptoms of headache and fever which are commonly associated with acute sinusitis in adults. They usually present with such symptoms as chronic rhinorrhea and cough of several weeks' duration (especially when supine), fatigue, headaches, stomach aches, ear plugging or pain, and generalized malaise and irritability (Kogutt and Swischuk, 1973; Rachelefsky et al., 1978).

On physical examination, facial pallor and edema and discoloration of the lower orbito-palpebral grooves ("circles under the eyes") often are impressive. The nasal mucosa is hyperemic, and purulent discharge frequently is seen on the floor of the nose or beneath the middle turbinate. There is a likelihood of coexisting serous otitis media or negative middle ear pressures (Nickman, 1978). The chest may be clear, may have rhonchi reflecting bronchitis secondary to drainage of purulent sinus secretions, or may be wheezy.

The most valuable laboratory tool for evaluating sinusitis is the cytologic examination of fresh nasal secretions obtained by having the patient blow his or her nose on plastic wrap. A large number of polymorphonuclear cells, especially with intracellular bacteria, is a frequent finding in the patient with sinusitis. While PMN's may predominate during a viral upper respiratory tract infection, their presence in large numbers in a profuse rhinorrhea of several weeks' duration suggests sinusitis. The peripheral white cell count and differential and the erythrocyte sedimentation rate usually are of little value.

The use of transillumination to detect sinusitis in children may be helpful, but it is not always reliable. Transillumination may be valuable for following a patient's course once the diagnosis of sinusitis has been confirmed by x-rays (Dawes, 1966).

Paranasal sinuses are visualized best radiographically by using a Waters view (occiput-mental) skull film for optimal maxillary sinus visualization, Caldwell view (occiput-frontal) for ethmoid and frontal sinus visualization, and lateral view for visualization of the sphenoid sinus. The diagnosis of sinusitis is made if one or more sinuses show opacification, an air-fluid level, or marked membrane thickening (see Figs. 40–1 through 40–5). Sinus opacification may occur from bacterial infection, severe allergic mucosal edema with or without secretions, or viral acute respiratory infections. There is a high correlation of culture-proved infection from antral irrigations with the above radiographic findings (Axelsson et al., 1970; Evans et al., 1975). Although there may be active infection with less prominent mucous membrane thickening, the correlation with culture evidence for infection is weaker. In these instances, the total clinical picture and clinical judgment should dictate therapy.

Text continued on page 532.

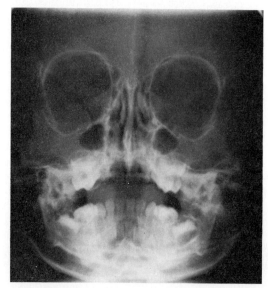

FIGURE 40–1. A normal Waters' view.

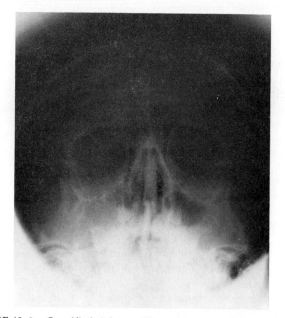

FIGURE 40–2. Opacified right maxillary sinus in a 10-year-old male.

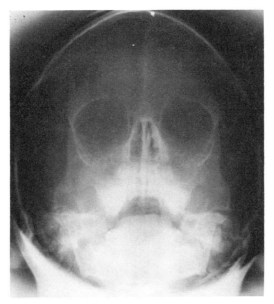

FIGURE 40–3. Opacified maxillary and left ethmoid sinus in a 3-year-old male.

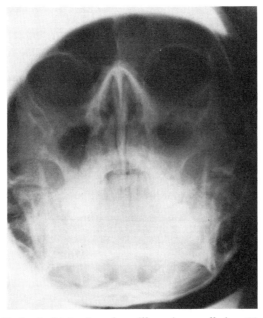

FIGURE 40–4. Moderate thickening of maxillary sinus walls in a 14-year-old female.

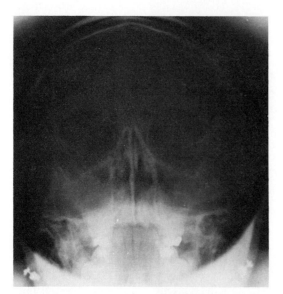

FIGURE 40–5. Marked thickening of maxillary sinus walls in a 16-year-old male. Note air fluid level in right cavity.

Mild membrane thickening rarely requires antibiotic therapy. In a child with recurrent sinusitis, repeated sinus films are not necessary if the clinical picture makes the diagnosis obvious. However, it is helpful to repeat the film in such a patient after medical treatment to be certain that the sinuses are clear. A Waters' view alone may suffice.

PATHOGENS IN SINUS DISEASE

Since maxillary sinusitis occurs most commonly and because the maxillary sinus is most easily cultured, the bacteriology of maxillary sinusitis has been studied extensively. The healthy maxillary sinus is sterile. Kessler (1968) compared the bacteriology of the middle meatus of the nose and the maxillary sinus at operation for chronic maxillary sinusitis. He found poor correlation between nasal and sinus organisms. Nasal organisms were *Staphylococcus aureus, Staphylococcus albus,* and diphtheroids, whereas those cultured from the sinuses were alphahemolytic streptococci and pneumococci, or else the cultures were sterile. In only 9 percent was there complete correlation. In acute sinusitis, the correlation between nasal and sinus cultures is better. Axelsson and Brorson (1973) found that nasal cultures from patients with acute maxillary sinusitis were most commonly bacteriologically sterile or showed *Haemophilus influenzae,* pneumococcus, and *Staphylococcus aureus,* in that order. Aspirated sinus secretions contained a predominance of pneumococcus or *Haemophilus influenzae,* or were sterile. Staphylococci were uniquely limited to the nose. These authors found the same organisms in nasal and sinus cultures in 64 percent of their patients. Aspiration of fluid from the maxillary sinus is the most reliable means of identifying bacterial pathogens. If a sinus culture is not obtained, patients should be treated on the basis of the likely infecting organisms.

Specimens obtained directly from sinuses in adults with acute sinusitis most commonly grow *Haemophilus influenzae,* pneumococcus, *Streptococcus viridans,* and *Staphylococcus aureus* (Evans et al., 1975). *Haemophilus influenzae* organisms either have not been typed or have been reported as nontypeable (Evans et al., 1975). Cultures from chronic sinusitis (more than 1 year) frequently yield anaerobes, such as alpha-hemolytic streptococci, bacteroides, veillonella, and corynebacteria (Frederick and Braude, 1974). In children, pneumococcus, *Haemophilus influenzae,* and beta-hemolytic streptococcus are most commonly cultured from acute maxillary sinusitis, though up to 40 percent of patients may have negative cultures (Nylen, 1972). *Haemophilus influenzae* infections occur at all ages; beta-hemolytic streptococcus occurs in children under 6 years; and pneumococcus becomes more common in older children. Positive bacteriologic cultures are more frequently obtained from sinuses that are opacified or have marked mucosal thickening (Evans et al., 1975). The role of viral infections in acute sinusitis has not been studied in depth. Rhinovirus has been cultured (Evans et al., 1975), and adenovirus was isolated from a patient with chronic sinusitis (Spector et al., 1973). Twenty-one percent of a series of patients with chronic sinusitis in India had L forms (Bhattacharyya, 1972), and L-phase variants of *Haemophilus influenzae* were isolated in Scandinavia from one out of ten cases of acute maxillary sinusitis in adults (Gnarpe and Lundberg, 1971). The implied role of *Mycoplasma pneumoniae* in sinusitis needs to be explored. Sporadic cases of fungal sinusitis have been reported, but appropriate techniques for culturing fungi have not been employed in most previous studies.

TREATMENT OF SINUSITIS

Treatment of sinus disease in children should be aimed at promoting drainage, controlling infection, and providing symptomatic relief.

Ampicillin (100 mg/kg/day), amoxicillin (40 mg/kg/day) or erythromycin (50 mg/kg/day) is administered for 2 to 3 weeks. Sinus drainage is encouraged by use of topical decongestants and antihistamine-decongestant combinations. The former should not be used for more than 5 days because of potential rebound and because of adverse effects on ciliary function. If the patient fails to have complete resolution of symptoms after completing antibiotic treatment, repeat roentgenograms should be obtained. A second antibiotic course may be used if disease persists. Otolaryngologic consultation should be obtained if sinusitis does not respond to treatment. Therapy of chronically opacified maxillary sinuses with associated chronic otitis media, difficult-to-control asthma, or chronic pain may require antral irrigation or needle aspiration of the sinuses. Antral irrigation can be performed in the cooperative child as an office procedure, under local anesthesia. The young child will require general anesthesia. Surgery is indicated when there is evidence of spread of infection outside the sinus cavity (into the orbit or intracranially).

Chronic thickening (less than 6 mm) of the maxillary mucosal wall frequently is secondary to chronic nasal allergy. Environmental control measures to avoid allergens when possible should be stressed. In addition, treatment consists of chronic antihistamine usage with or without decongestants. Topical dexamethasone (Turbinaire Decadron) is helpful in resistant cases. Since some degree of systematic absorption does occur, administration is generally short term (2 to 4 weeks in decreasing dosage) and chronic administration is discouraged. Topical administration of halogenated hydrocortisones, beclomethasone dipropionate (Vanceril) (Tarlo et al., 1977), and flunisolide (Siegel et al., 1978), with potent local effects and weak systemic effects, has potential in the treatment of chronic allergic rhinitis with associated sinusitis. These compounds presently are not available in the United States for nasal usage. Topically administered cromolyn sodium (Cohen et al., 1976) has been used for allergic rhinitis; what effect it may have on preventing sinusitis remains to be determined.

Antral Surgery. Antral puncture and lavage is adequate treatment for the majority of patients with chronic maxillary sinusitis who have failed to respond to medical therapy. In the rare patient with the persistently symptomatic empyema, intranasal antrostomy will function as a means of extended drainage. Healing usually is complete. The Caldwell-Luc operation is rarely indicated and should be avoided in children because of its adverse effect on the growing facial bones and unerupted and recently erupted teeth.

COMPLICATIONS OF SINUSITIS

Unrecognized sinusitis often leads to chronic malaise, irritability, headache, cough, and worsened asthma, which result in school absenteeism and poor school performance.

In addition, unresolved sinus disease may result in other complications. The continual drip of infected sinus secretions may lead to chronic bronchitis and pneumonia. An extension of sinusitis into the orbit may lead to cellulitis and subperiosteal and orbital abscess; 60 percent of orbital cellulitis is secondary to sinusitis (Chandler et al., 1970). Intracranial complications of sinusitis include meningitis, brain abscess, extradural and subdural abscesses, and cavernous sinus thrombosis. Although the incidence of complications from sinusitis has been reduced by antibiotic therapy, sequelae of untreated sinusitis may be grave.

References

Artenstein, M. S., Bellanti, J. A., and Buescher, E. L.: Identification of antiviral substances in nasal secretions. Proc. Soc. Exper. Biol. Med. *117*:558, 1964.

Axelsson, A., Grebelius, N., Chidekel, N., and Jensen, C.: The correlation between the radiological examination and the irrigation findings in maxillary sinusitis. Acta Otolaryngol. 69:302, 1970.

Axelsson, A., and Brorson, J. E.: The correlation between bacteriological findings in the nose and maxillary sinus in acute maxillary sinusitis. Laryngoscope *83*:2003, 1973.

Bernstein, L.: Pediatric sinus problems. Otolaryngol. Clin. North Am. 4:127, 1971.

Bhattacharyya, T. K., Mehra, Y. N., and Agarwal, S. C.: Incidence of bacteria, L-form and mycoplasma in chronic sinusitis. Acta Otolaryngol. 74:293, 1972.

Bjonnes, H., and Gugler, E.: Zur behand lung der sinusitis in kindersalter. Ther. Umsch. 30:452, 1973.

Caffey, J.: *Pediatric X-Ray Diagnosis*. Chicago, Year Book Medical Publications, Inc., 1972, pp. 104–111.

Chandler, J. K., Lagenbrunner, D. J., and Steven, E. R.: The pathogenesis of orbital complications in acute sinusitis. Laryngoscope 8:414, 1970.

Cohen, R. H., Bloom, I. L., Rhoades, R. B., Wittig, H. J., and Haugh, L. D.: Treatment of perennial allergic rhinitis with cromolyn sodium. J. Allergy Clin. Immunol. 58:121, 1976.

Dawes, J. D. K.: Diagnosis and treatment of sinusitis. Br. Med. J. 2:843, 1966.

Evans, F. O., Sydnor, J. B., Moore, W. E. C., Moore, G. R., Manwaring, J. L., Brill, A. H., Jackson, R. T., Hanna, S., Skaar, J. S., Holdeman, L. V., Fitz-Hugh, G. S., Sande, M. A., and Gwaltney, J. M.: Sinusitis in the maxillary antrum. New Engl. J. Med. 292:735, 1975.

Frederick, J., and Braude, A. I.: Anaerobic infection of the paranasal sinuses. N. Engl. J. Med. 290:135, 1974.

Gallagher, T. M.: Nasal discharge. In *Differential Diagnosis in Pediatric Otolaryngology*. Boston, Little, Brown and Co., 1977.

Gnarpe, H., and Lundberg, C.: L-phase organisms in maxillary sinus secretions. Scand. J. Infect. Dis. 31:257, 1971.

Hanson, C. A., Borssen, R., Holmgren, J., Jodal, U., Johansson, B. G., and Kaijser, B.: Secretory IgA. In Kagan, B., and Stiehm, E. R. (eds.): *Immunologic Incompetence*. Chicago, Year Book Medical Publishers, 1971, pp. 39–59.

Herz, G., and Gfeller, J.: Sinusitis in paediatrics. Chemotherapy 23:50, 1977.

Hoffman, H.: Oral microbiology. Adv. Appl. Microbiol. 8:195, 1966.

Jaffe, B. F.: Chronic sinusitis in children. Clin. Pediatr. 13:944, 1974.

Kessler, L.: Bacterienflora der nasenhaupt and nassenebenhohlen bei chronischen sinuitiden and ihre bcziehung zvenander. Hals-Nos-Ohrenartz 16:36, 1968.

Kogutt, M. S., and Swischuk, L. E.: Diagnosis of sinusitis in infants and children. Pediatr. 52:121, 1973.

McLean, D. C.: Sinusitis in children. Lessons from twenty-five patients. Clin. Pediatr. 9:342, 1970.

McLaurin, J. G.: Interrelationship of upper and lower respiratory infections emphasizing routes of infection. Ann. Otol. Rhinol. Laryngol. 52:589, 1943.

Newcomb, R. W., Ishizaka, K., and DeVald, B. L.: Human IgG and IgA diphtheria antitoxins in serum nasal fluids and saliva. J. Immunol. 103:215, 1969.

Nickman, J. N.: Sinusitis, otitis and adenotonsillitis in children: A retrospective study. Laryngoscope 88:117, 1978.

Nylen, O., Jeppsson, P. H., Branefors-Helander, P.: Acute sinusitis. Scand. J. Infect. Dis. 4:43, 1972.

Phipatanakul, C. S., and Slavin, R. G.: Bronchial asthma produced by paranasal sinusitis. Acta Otolaryngol. 100:109, 1974.

Rachelefsky, G. S., Goldberg, M., Katz, R. M., Boris, G., Gyepes, M. T., Shapiro, M. J., Mickey, M. R., Finegold, S. M., and Siegel, S. C.: Sinus disease in children with respiratory allergy. J. Allergy Clin. Immunol. 61:310, 1978.

Schmid, F.: Die sinobronchitis. Padiat. Prax. 7:555, 1972.

Shapiro, G. G., Pierson, W. E., Furukawa, C. T., and Bierman, C. W.: Sinusitis in allergic children. 1980. (In press.)

Siegel, S. C., Katz, R. M., Rachelefsky, G. S., and Crepea, S.: Flunisolide aerosol treatment of perennial allergic rhinitis in children. J. Allergy Clin. Immunol. 61:152, 1978.

Smith, C. B., Purcell, R. H., Bellanti, J. A., and Chanock, R. M.: Protective affect of antibody to parainfluenza type 1 virus. New Engl. J. Med. 275:1145, 1966.

Smith, C. H.: Sinusitis in children. Clin. Pediatr. 3:489, 1964.

Spector, S. L., English, G. M., and McIntosh, K.: Adenovirus in the sinuses of an asthmatic patient with apparent selective antibody deficiencies. Am. J. Med. 55:227, 1973.

Strome, M.: Rhino-sinusitis and mid-facial pain in adolescents. Practitioner 217:914, 1976.

Tarlo, S. M., Cockcroft, D. W., and Hargreave, F. E.: Beclomethasone dipropionate aerosol in perennial rhinitis. J. Allergy Clin. Immunol. 59:232, 1977.

Tomasi, T. B., and Bienenstock, J.: Secretory immunoglobulins. Advances Immunol. 9:1, 1968.

Tourville, D. R., and Tomasi, T. B.: Selective transport of gamma A. Proc. Soc. Exper. Biol. Med. 132:475, 1969.

Williams, R. C., and Gibbons, R. J.: Inhibition of bacterial adherence by secretory immunoglobulin A. A mechanism of antigen disposal. Science 177:697, 1972.

F. Estelle R. Simons, M.D.
Victor Chernick, M.D.

41

Principles of Diagnosis and Treatment of Lower Respiratory Tract Disease

DEVELOPMENT OF THE RESPIRATORY TRACT

Laryngeal structures, including the epiglottis, develop as an outgrowth from the floor of the pharynx, with contributions from the fourth and sixth branchial arches. They are well defined by the twelfth week of gestation. The position of the larynx changes with increasing postnatal age, with the adult position being approximately two vertebral bodies lower than in infancy.

Before birth, the lung passes through four stages of development: (1) an embryonic phase culminating in the presence of lobar buds, (2) a pseudoglandular stage during which the buds divide by dichotomous branching until all the conducting airways in the tracheobronchial tree are formed, (3) a canalicular phase characterized by proliferation of mesenchyme, development of blood supply, and thinning of the epithelium, and (4) a terminal sac phase during which terminal bronchioles give rise to nonalveolar respiratory bronchioles that terminate in pairs of delicate clusters of thin-walled saccules (Chernick, 1976). At birth, only rudimentary alveoli are present. In the early months of postnatal life, peripheral bronchioles enlarge and alveoli appear in a centripetal direction. Alveolar multiplication is rapid in the first year of life and probably continues at least until about age 8 years. Respiratory surface area doubles by age 18 months and trebles by age 3 years, so it is evident that there is a smaller reserve for gas exchange in the very young child.

Conducting airways increase in size, but not in number, from the 16th or 17th week of gestation to adulthood. Until age 5 years, the resistance of peripheral airways accounts for a higher proportion of total airways resistance than in older children and adults, because peripheral airways are relatively narrower in young children (Fig. 41-1) (Hogg, 1977).

In infants and young children, there are fewer and smaller interalveolar communications (pores of Kohn), fewer communications from bronchi to alveoli (Lambert's canals), and fewer openings between alveolar ducts of different acini (portions of the lung supplied by the terminal bronchioles). Mechanical obstruction from edema, mucus, and cellular infiltrates has a greater adverse effect in the infant and young child because of disproportionately narrow peripheral airways, increased peripheral resistance to airflow, and poorly developed collateral ventilation.

The relative amount of smooth muscle in the wall of peripheral airways increases throughout childhood. There also is a decrease in the proportion of mucus glands from birth through adulthood.

As the anatomy and the mechanical properties of the lung change progressively

535

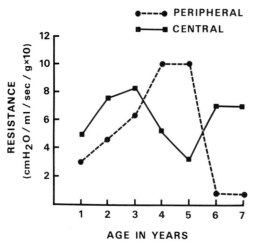

FIGURE 41–1. Comparison of peripheral and central resistance as a function of age in normal human lungs. (Adapted from Hogg, J. C., Williams, J., Richardson, J. B., et al.: Age as a factor in the distribution of lower airway conductance and in the pathologic anatomy of obstructive lung disease. New Engl. J. Med. *282*:1283, 1970.)

through infancy and childhood, the manifestations of nonprogressive pulmonary diseases also change, generally becoming milder with increasing age (Hogg, 1977).

ANATOMY OF THE RESPIRATORY TRACT

Gross Anatomy. The larynx consists of four major cartilages (the cricoid ring, the thyroid cartilage, and the arytenoids, and various accessory cartilages, including the epiglottic cartilage at the base of the tongue and the paired cuneiform and corniculate cartilages) all united by various ligaments, membranes, and muscles. The larynx safeguards the lower airway from aspiration of foreign substances and also is important in phonation, coughing, respiration, and deglutition. The epiglottis deflects food boluses from the airway and shields the false vocal cords.

The patency and shape of the conducting airways is maintained by cartilaginous plates. In the trachea and main bronchi, these are horseshoe shaped; in the lobar and segmental bronchi they are arranged in a jigsaw pattern, and distally they are replaced entirely by bronchial smooth muscle.

Gross anatomic relationships of lung lobes and segments are relatively constant from patient to patient (Fig. 41–2). During physical examination of the chest, the physician should be aware of the surface anatomy of the lobes and segments in order to accurately localize pulmonary pathology (Waring, 1977).

Microscopic Anatomy (Breeze and Wheeldon, 1977). In the epithelium of the pulmonary airways, many cell types are recognized, of which the most numerous are ciliated columnar cells and goblet cells. In the adult, these are present in a ratio of about 5 to 1. The ciliated cells line the

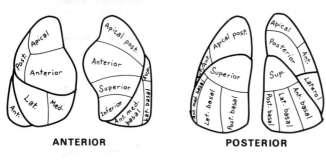

ANTERIOR

POSTERIOR

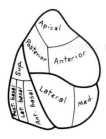

RIGHT LATERAL

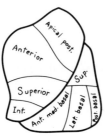

LEFT LATERAL

FIGURE 41–2. Pulmonary lobes and segments.

respiratory tract from the middle nares to the region of the bronchioles, apart from squamous epithelium in the pharynx and larynx. Ciliated cells have a broad luminal surface covered with microvilli and about 250 to 300 cilia per cell. Most of the cilium shaft is bathed in a watery high-shear fluid, but the tip of the cilium penetrates the mucous layer, which is a low-shear gel. By coordinated rhythmic movement, mucus is propelled by the cilia towards the oral pharynx. Goblet cells lack cilia and may be tall and slender when not secreting glycoproteins (mucus).

Additional important cell types include K-cells (Kultschitzsky-like), present at all levels of the tracheobronchial and bronchiolar epithelium. These contain neurosecretory granules and intraepithelial nerve axons. They are similar in type to the amine precursor uptake, decarboxylation, and storage cells (APUD cells) found elsewhere in the body and may regulate the pulmonary circulation, govern smooth muscle tone in the bronchial wall, function as air chemoreceptors, or play a part in the production of amines such as histamine and serotonin. Oncocytes are large cells with eosinophilic granular cytoplasm, which appear after exposure to high oxygen concentrations and have high concentrations of mitochondrial oxidative enzymes. Nonciliated cells (Clara cells), found in the epithelium of the terminal bronchioles, also secrete glycoprotein and may provide a surface active layer, a watery medium for cilia, or even contribute to the hypophase (thick basal layer underlying the single molecular film of surface active material in the alveoli). Globule leukocytes or intraepithelial mononuclear cells are derived from the subepithelial mast cell. Neuroepithelial bodies also are present in bronchial, bronchiolar, and alveolar lining epithelium. Their structure, position, blood supply, and innervation suggest they are neuroreceptor organs with local intrapulmonary secretory activity.

Underlying the epithelium is a basement membrane that appears as a well defined homogenous hyaline structure by light microscopy, but consists of electron-dense bands and interwoven fibrillar structures and translucent zones when viewed by electron microscopy. The submucosa is composed of loose connective tissue rich in capillaries and lymphatics. Bronchial mucosal glands are compound tuboacinar structures connected to the lumen by a short excreting duct. Mast cells are located in the bronchial mucosa, in the alveolar wall, around small blood vessels, and in the pleura. They are target cells in immediate hypersensitivity reactions and are filled with metachromatic electron-dense granules that contain heparin and various amines and enzymes.

Smooth muscle is present as a spiraling network throughout the tracheobronchial tree, including alveolar walls where interstitial cells contain contractile elements.

Alveoli are lined by a continuous layer of epithelial cells. The more numerous Type I epithelial cell, which has long thin cytoplasmic extensions and few cytoplasmic organelles, is incapable of mitotic division, has no known metabolic activity, and is vulnerable to the toxic effects of high oxygen concentration and inhaled irritants. Regeneration of this cell type occurs by division of Type II cells and subsequent transformation to Type I cells. Type II pneumocytes, on the other hand, have abundant endoplasmic reticulum, cytoplasm rich in mitochondria, and lamellar bodies, in which surfactant, the alveolar-stabilizing substance that reduces surface tension, is stored. Type II cells proliferate if the alveoli are injured. Blood gas exchange is assumed to take place in the thinnest part of the alveolar unit, where the barrier consists of a Type I pneumocyte, endothelial cell, and basement membrane.

BASIC CONCEPTS IN PULMONARY PHYSIOLOGY

General Considerations. Classically, human tracheobronchial smooth muscle is said to be controlled directly by the parasympathetic and the sympathetic nervous systems. Stimulation of parasympathetic fibers releases acetylcholine and causes constriction, whereas stimulation of sympathetic fibers results in relaxation, either by direct action on beta adrenergic receptors of smooth muscle or indirectly through alpha adrenergic receptors of the ganglia, which decrease acetylcholine output. Receptors are those components of responsive target cells with which hormones and drugs interact. A nonadrenergic inhibitory system also may act on human tracheobronchial smooth muscle, but its chemical mediator has not yet been identified (Richardson, 1977).

Major metabolic and endocrine functions of endothelial cells of the lung include activation of angiotensin I, and inactivation of bradykinin, serotonin, prostaglandins E and $F_{2\alpha}$, norepinephrine, and possibly histamine.

Pulmonary defense mechanisms include mechanical barriers, physical clearance of foreign particles, and detoxification within the lung (Davis and Green, 1976). Foreign particles, including infectious agents, greater than 10 μ in diameter are cleared by mucociliary or aerodynamic transport. Particles of about 1 μ in diameter may reach the respiratory unit and are phagocytosed by alveolar macrophages whose lysosomal membranes fuse around the particles, which are then digested by hydrolytic enzymes. In addition, an abundant lymphatic network, located in the peribronchial and perivascular connective tissue sheets and in the bronchial walls and underlying the pulmonary pleura, forms a plexiform network with valves that direct the flow of lymph centripetally. Lymphoid aggregates are located along the bronchi, especially at sites of branching. Locally secreted IgA also plays a vital role in neutralizing viral antigens.

Pulmonary Mechanics (Chernick and Avery, 1977). An understanding of static lung volumes is important in assessing the influence of disease on the mechanical properties of the lung and chest wall, and in evaluating the effects of therapy.

The lung volume at which the outward recoil of the chest wall is equal to the inward recoil of the lung is called the *functional residual capacity* (FRC) and is the sum of the *residual volume* (RV) and *expiratory reserve volume* (ERV). FRC or resting lung capacity (a capacity is the sum of two or more lung volumes) is determined by the compliance of the lung and chest wall. It is reduced when lung compliance decreases or chest wall compliance increases and is increased when lung compliance increases or chest wall compliance decreases. FRC is increased with partial lower airway obstruction; this leads to an increase in diameter of intrathoracic airways, which aids in relieving the obstruction and decreasing the work of breathing. (See Chapter 42 for discussion of measurements of pulmonary functions.)

Airway Resistance. The pressure required to generate a given flow of gas through a tube is directly proportional to the length of the tube and the viscosity of the gas, and is indirectly proportional to the radius of the tube raised to the fourth power ($1/r^4$). The resistance (R) to airflow is calculated as the ratio of driving pressure to airflow. Thus

$$R = \frac{\text{driving pressure}}{\text{flow (cm } H_2O/1/\text{sec)}}.$$

The driving pressure for airflow in the lower respiratory tract is the difference in pressure between the alveoli and the mouth. The measurement of alveolar pressure requires special techniques such as body plethysmography. In practice, therefore, an estimate of airway resistance is obtained by measuring the *peak expiratory flow rate* (PEFR), or the amount of air exhaled during the first second of the forced vital capacity maneuver (FEV_1). Since these tests depend on the subject's effort in performing the test, interpretation of the results may be difficult in young children.

In children above the age of about 5 years and in adults, 80 percent of the airway resistance lies in airways larger than 2 mm in diameter. In younger children, the small airways account for about 50 percent of the airway resistance, and any change in small airways resistance, such as that which occurs in bronchiolitis or asthma, seriously affects the small infant. In older children and adults, considerable change in small airways resistance may occur without symptomatology, and usual office tests which indirectly reflect airway resistance (PEFR, FEV_1) may be normal. Several approaches to measuring the contribution of small airways to airway resistance have recently been introduced (Chernick, 1977).

Expiratory flow rates are greatly influenced by lung volume. At high lung volume there is a "tethering" effect of the lung that tends to keep airways widely patent; this tethering effect diminishes or disappears at low lung volumes. Thus, flow is measured continuously during the vital capacity maneuver and related to the volume of air expired, the so-called flow-volume curve. For example, the flow at 75 percent, 50 percent and 25 percent of the vital capacity may be reported. In small airway disease, the flow may be markedly diminished at 25 percent of the vital capacity.

The contribution of small airways to airway resistance also may be measured by comparing the flow-volume curve during air breathing with that obtained during breathing an 80 percent helium – 20 percent oxygen mixture. Since gas flow in small airways is laminar or streamlined, gas flow will not be affected by gas density. Gas flow in large airways is turbulent, so there will be less resistance on breathing a low density gas. Normally, air and helium flow-volume curves appear identical near residual volume. When small airways contribute significantly to the overall airway resistance, the point at which the air and helium flow-volume curves become identical will occur at a higher lung volume.

Airway resistance depends to a very great extent on airway diameter. Forces that tend to narrow airways include smooth muscle contraction and an increase in peribronchial (pleural) pressure. Forces that tend to open airways are increased intraluminal pressure and the tethering action of the surrounding lung, particularly at high lung volumes. Airway closure tends to occur at low lung volumes even in the healthy individual. The lung volume at which airway closure occurs may be determined by measuring the washout of nitrogen from the lung following the inspiration of 100 percent oxygen from RV. Those airways that are open at RV receive less oxygen than those that are closed and, therefore, have a higher nitrogen concentration. During expiration, nitrogen concentration rises sharply at the point of airway closure. The volume at which this occurs is called the *closing volume*; the closing volume plus residual volume is called the *closing capacity*. Closing volume is high in young children and may exceed FRC in children under the age of 6 years. The closing volume decreases to a nadir during the late teenage years and then gradually increases with age. Above the age of about 50 years, closing volume is again above FRC.

Gas Exchange

Carbon Dioxide. The primary function of the lung is to excrete carbon dioxide and to oxygenate the pulmonary capillary

blood. Carbon dioxide, produced in the tissues as a result of aerobic metabolism, is transported to the lung by the blood. Two-thirds of the CO_2 in blood is in the plasma, chiefly as bicarbonate; one-third is in the red cell as bicarbonate and hemoglobin carbonate. When pulmonary capillary blood is exposed to fresh alveolar air containing little CO_2, CO_2 diffuses from the blood into the alveolar air and is eliminated during expiration. In the lung, carbonic anhydrase rapidly converts blood bicarbonate to CO_2 and H_2O, facilitating rapid equilibration with alveolar gas.

The concept of alveolar ventilation ($\dot{V}_A$), therefore, is an important one. The term refers to that proportion of minute ventilation that is involved with gas exchange in the lung, principally CO_2. The relationship between $\dot{V}_A$ and carbon dioxide production ($\dot{V}CO_2$) and alveolar PCO_2 (equivalent to arterial PCO_2 [$PaCO_2$]) is described as:

$$\dot{V}CO_2 = \dot{V}_A (PaCO_2) \times k$$

$$\text{or} \quad PaCO_2 \; \alpha \; \frac{1}{V_A}$$

Thus, for a steady rate of CO_2 production, when alveolar ventilation doubles, $PaCO_2$ must halve, and when $\dot{V}_A$ halves, $PaCO_2$ must double. The measurement of $PaCO_2$ thus is an indication of the adequacy of alveolar ventilation for a given CO_2 production.

In the blood, carbon dioxide is in equilibrium with bicarbonate, and their relationship (Henderson-Hasselbach equation) is:

$$pH = \log pK + \log \frac{HCO_3^-}{\alpha PCO_2}$$

where α is the solubility coefficient for CO_2.

A clinically useful form of this equation is:

$$H^+ \text{ concentration (nanomoles/1)} =$$

$$24 \times \frac{PaCO_2}{HCO_3^-}$$

When HCO_3^- concentration is normal (24 mEq/L), a $PaCO_2$ of 40 is equivalent to a H^+ concentration of 40 nm/l (pH = 7.40).

H^+ concentration at pH's of 7.00, 7.10, 7.20, 7.30, and 7.50 are 100, 80, 62.5, 50, and 32 nm/l, respectively.

The lung excretes about 300 mEq/kg per day of acid in the form of carbon dioxide, while the kidney excretes 1 to 2 mEq/day.

Oxygen. Carbon dioxide in the lung diffuses nearly 21 times faster than oxygen. The transfer of oxygen from alveoli to the red blood cell in the capillary is dependent on the driving pressure (alveolar Po_2 minus capillary Po_2) and the resistance of the alveolar tissue and red blood cell barriers. About half of the resistance to diffusion exists in the alveolar membrane, the other half in the red cell.

Clinically, a reduced arterial Po_2 rarely is the result of a diffusion barrier to oxygen. The most common cause of hypoxemia in patients with lower respiratory tract disease is ventilation-perfusion inequality, which may be treated by increasing inspired oxygen concentration (Fio_2). Another cause is hypoventilation, which also may require an increase in alveolar ventilation, often by mechanical means, as well as an increase in Fio_2. In patients with extrapulmonary right to left shunting, neither method of therapy is successful in raising Pao_2 significantly.

When the patient breathes room air at sea level, the sum of alveolar Po_2 (Pao_2) and Pco_2 cannot exceed 150 mm Hg, since the rest of the total pressure is occupied by nitrogen and water vapor. $Paco_2$ normally is 40, so that Pao_2 is about 110 mm Hg. The alveolar-arterial oxygen tension difference ($A\text{-}aDo_2$) is a useful concept clinically and can be approximated by the following equation:

$$A\text{-}aDo_2 = \text{inspiratory } Po_2 - (Paco_2 + Pao_2)$$

For example, if inspiratory Po_2 is 150 mm Hg, $Paco_2$ is 40 mm Hg and Pao_2 is 40 mm Hg, then $A\text{-}aDo_2$ is 70 mm Hg. This equation assumes a Respiratory Quotient of 1. This calculation is useful in following the progress of patients who require oxygen therapy and is the only way one can detect changes in the ability to oxygenate the blood in the face of a changing $Paco_2$ or changing Fio_2. The normal $A\text{-}aDo_2$ should be less than 20 mm Hg while the patient is breathing room air.

In contrast to carbon dioxide, over 98 percent of the oxygen in the blood is carried in the red cell as oxyhemoglobin, the rest being dissolved oxygen. The relationship between Po_2 and hemoglobin oxygen saturation is curvilinear (oxyhemoglobin dissociation curve) and affected by blood pH, temperature, 2,3-diphosphoglycerate (2,3 DPG), and the type of hemoglobin present. 2,3 DPG binds to hemoglobin and reduces its affinity for oxygen, thus shifting the curve to the right, as does an increase in temperature or a reduction in pH.

Ventilation: Perfusion ($\dot{V}/Q$) Relationships. The fact that mismatched $\dot{V}/Q$ in the lung is a common cause of hypoxemia already has been mentioned. Normally the ratio $\dot{V}/Q$ is about 0.8. If ventilation is disproportionately low in relation to blood flow in an area of the lung, then $Paco_2$ will be disproportionately high, and Pao_2, low. The blood leaving the area of lung will have a low Pao_2 and will mix with blood from relatively normal areas of the lung. This so-called venous admixture may be corrected by letting the patient breathe high oxygen concentrations. Thus, if hypoxemia is present when the patient is breathing room air, Pao_2 will rise to 500 mm Hg or higher when he is given 100 percent oxygen to breathe, if hypoxemia is a result of mismatched $\dot{V}/Q$. If the hypoxemia is caused by true right to left shunting of blood, such as with a transposition of the great vessels, 100 percent oxygen breathing will not reverse the hypoxemia.

When there are low $\dot{V}/Q$ areas, an increase in alveolar ventilation to the other areas of the lung will easily compensate for low CO_2 excretion in the affected area but will not result in additional oxygen uptake by the red cells, which already are virtually 100 percent saturated. $\dot{V}/Q$ abnormality is commonly found in patients with pulmonary disease and usually requires only an inspired oxygen concentration of 25 to 30 percent to provide an arterial Pao_2 of 50 mm Hg or greater, which is adequate for tissue oxygenation. Higher concentrations of oxygen are not necessary and are known to be toxic to the lung with prolonged use.

DIAGNOSTIC PRINCIPLES

History. In contrast to the adult, in the infant and toddler with respiratory disease, history of symptoms referable to the respiratory tract may be nonspecific (Waring, 1977). Refusal to suck or eat, fussiness, and rapid or labored breathing or cough may herald significant respiratory tract disease. It is important to establish whether the episode is acute, recurrent, or chronic, the rate of progression of symptoms, and the effect of prior treatment on symptoms.

If cough is present, it is helpful to know its characteristics. Is it *paroxysmal* (a series of explosive expirations following a single inspiration), indicative of a foreign body or pertussis; *productive,* suggesting pneumonia, bronchiectasis, or cystic fibrosis; *associated with wheezing*, as in tracheobronchial obstruction; "*barking*," indicative of involvement of glottic and subglottic areas, as in croup; *associated with aphonia or dysphonia,* suggesting a laryngeal foreign body or other involvement of the larynx? Cough associated with swallowing suggests aspiration of material into the tracheobronchial tree due to a congenital anomaly such as tracheoesophageal fistula, or to incoordination of swallowing and breathing.

Infants and young children usually do not expectorate sputum but swallow it instead, hence it may be found in vomitus and stools. Mucus plugs may be coughed up in asthma and aspergillosis. If hemoptysis occurs, blood may be coming from the oropharynx, but the possibility of foreign body injury to the respiratory mucosa or the presence of inflammation and erosion of the mucosa, as in cystic fibrosis, must be considered.

Chest pain is not a common complaint in children. It may be associated with prolonged or frequent coughing. It also may occur in diseases of the chest wall such as costochondritis, with rib fractures, in patients with inflammation of the diaphragmatic pleura as in pneumonia, in disorders of the esophagus such as ulceration or the presence of a foreign body, or in pericarditis. Severe chest pain also may be produced by myositis or intercostal neuralgia.

Respiratory distress associated with hoarseness suggests laryngeal involvement; that associated with drooling and muffling of the voice suggests involvement of the epiglottis.

If labored breathing is present, its suddenness of onset and rate of progression must be noted. Provoking factors such as choking, exercise, or a "cold" or exposure to irritants such as smoke or potential allergens should be noted. Associated symptoms such as grunting, cyanosis, stridor, or wheezing must be ascertained.

Chronic halitosis may be noted in patients with bronchiectasis, lung abscess, sinusitis, nasal foreign body, and infectious or allergic rhinitis.

Presence of symptoms in other systems and presence of respiratory symptoms in other family members should be ascertained.

Physical Examination. Physical signs vary with age and, in obstructive disease, depend on air entry.

Inspection. Nonspecific signs of respiratory disease in the child include failure to gain weight or stature, weight loss, pallor, and lethargy. Clubbing commonly occurs in bronchiectasis, cystic fibrosis, pulmonary abscess, empyema, and various chronic pneumonias and neoplasms, as well as in cardiac, hepatic, and gastrointestinal disease.

The upper airway is examined indirectly by listening to the speech and cry of the patient, by noting whether inspiratory stridor or barking cough are present and whether hoarseness or aphonia are present. Inspiratory retractions, particularly in the supraclavicular region, often point to upper airway obstruction. The examiner should palpate the trachea and larynx for tenderness, masses, and distortion of contour. The upper airway also should be examined directly, with care taken not to insert a tongue blade if epiglottitis is suspected.

Cyanosis is most reliably observed in the lips, but also in other mucous membranes, the skin, and the nailbeds. It usually is related to the absolute amount of unoxygenated hemoglobin (deoxyhemoglobin) in the capillaries, which in turn may be due to decreased oxygen in the blood or to diminished blood flow through an area.

The resting rate of respiration varies with age, with the normal respiratory rate at 1 year averaging 30 per minute; the normal average adult rate of 18 per minute is reached at about age 14 years. Hyperpnea (deep breathing) may occur in the absence of respiratory disease in the child with fever, severe anemia, salicylism, metabolic acidosis, or respiratory alkalosis. Hypopnea (shallow breathing) occurs with metabolic alkalosis, as in pyloric stenosis, and with respiratory acidosis.

Dyspnea in the infant or child may be evidenced by flaring of the alae nasi, head bobbing due to contraction of the accessory muscles of inspiration (including the scalene and sternocleidomastoid muscles), and grunting. In the older child, grunting usually is associated with pneumonia or chest pain.

Retractions usually indicate increased inspiratory effort. They may be localized to the lower intercostal areas in infants in whom the diaphragm is the major muscle of respiration. Intercostal bulging may be a sign of great expiratory effort.

The round chest of the term infant flattens ventrodorsally with age. Overinflation of the lung affects the anteroposterior diameter of the thorax more than other dimensions. In severe obstructive disease of the lung, the thoracic index (depth-width ratio obtained by dividing the anteroposterior diameter by the transverse diameter) may be equal to or greater than 1.

Palpation. Tracheal palpation of the suprasternal notch can indicate whether there has been a volume or pressure change in the thoracic cavity. For example, a foreign body in the right main stem bronchus that completely occludes the bronchus and produces atelectasis of the right lung will cause the mediastinum and the trachea to shift to the right. A pneumothorax or any space-occupying lesion on the left also will cause the trachea to shift to the right.

Percussion. Indirect percussion of the chest should be performed in order to localize areas of dullness (atelectasis or consolidation) or to detect hyperinflation. In infants and young children, it is preferable to leave percussion until the end of the physical examination.

Auscultation. Auscultation over each bronchopulmonary segment should be performed using a stethoscope head of appropriate size. The relative duration of expiration to inspiration, normally 2:1, should be noted. The quality of breath sounds should be described, that is: *tracheal* (high-pitched tubular sounds evident throughout both phases of respiration), *vesicular* (soft, low-pitched inspiration and soundless expiration), *bronchovesicular* (soft, low-pitched expiratory note heard in the early part of expiration), and *bronchial* (tubular note throughout all of expiration). Diminished ventilation in a given segment or through the entire lung is significant, since a child with severe airways obstruction may have little stridor or wheezing, owing to the poor air exchange.

Rhonchi are continuous high- or low-pitched musical sounds produced by air moving rapidly past a fixed obstruction in the airway. Rales (crackles) are discontinuous, nonmusical, crackling or bubbling sounds produced when closed airways snap open or produced by air bubbling through secretions. Rales may be fine, medium, or coarse.

In a young child who cannot perform a forced expiration maneuver, manual compression of the chest wall during the expiratory phase may be performed by an assistant to facilitate auscultation. Infants should be auscultated when they are prone, as well as upright or supine. In the prone position the intensity of transmitted rhonchi caused by excessive secretions in the upper respiratory tract is diminished. Infants also should be auscultated when placed on the side with the neck flexed, in order to accentuate any inspiratory stridor present.

The cardiovascular system should be examined carefully; a loud snapping second heart sound in the second and third left interspace may be evidence of pulmonary hypertension.

Evidence of impending *respiratory failure* includes: change in level of consciousness such as agitation, restlessness, or inability to be aroused; extreme respiratory distress and diminished or absent air entry (a "silent chest"); or cyanosis (Downes et al., 1972). Older children may complain of headache or even dimness of vision. Tachycardia or hypertension or (late) hypotension may be present. If hypoxemia is chronic, polycythemia may be present. In hypercapnia, engorgement of the fundal veins, muscular twitching, depressed tendon reflexes and extensor plantar responses, papilledema, and miosis may be present.

Differential Diagnosis. Respiratory disorders are best classified according to the predominant functional abnormality, as this forms a basis for rational approach to therapy. A useful functional classification of respiratory disorders in infancy and childhood is presented in Table 41–1 (Pagtakhan and Chernick, 1977).

In the differential diagnosis of obstructive airways disease, it is important to note the effect of the phase of respiration on increasing or decreasing the obstruction. *Extrathoracic* obstruction is primarily manifest in the *inspiratory* phase, because in forced inspiration the pressure in the main

TABLE 41–1 FUNCTIONAL CLASSIFICATION OF LOWER RESPIRATORY TRACT DISORDERS

Disturbance	Disease Conditions
	OBSTRUCTIVE DISEASE
Upper Respiratory Tract	
Anomalies	Tracheal stenosis, vocal cord paralysis, vascular ring, laryngotracheomalacia
Aspiration	Foreign body,* vomitus
Infection	Laryngitis*, laryngotracheobronchitis*, epiglottitis*, peritonsillar or retropharyngeal abscess
Tumor	Papilloma, hemangioma, lymphangioma, teratoma, gross hypertrophy of tonsils and adenoids
Other	Laryngospasm from local irritation (aspiration, intubation, drowning), tetany, hereditary angioedema, anaphylaxis
Lower Respiratory Tract	
Anomalies	Bronchostenosis, bronchomalacia, lobar emphysema, aberrant vessels
Aspiration	Tracheoesophageal fistula, foreign body*, vomitus, pharyngeal incoordination (Riley-Day syndrome), drowning
Infection	Pertussis*, bronchiolitis*, tuberculosis (endobronchial, hilar adenopathy), cystic fibrosis
Tumor	Bronchogenic cyst, teratoma, atrial myxoma
Allergic	Asthma*
	RESTRICTIVE DISEASE
Parenchymal	
Anomalies	Hypoplasia, congenital cyst, pulmonary sequestration
Atelectasis	Viscous secretions (e.g., postoperative state)
Infection	Pneumonia, cystic fibrosis, bronchiectasis, pleural effusion, pneumatocele
Alveolar rupture	Pneumothorax (trauma, asthma)
Others	Allergic alveolitis, pulmonary edema, lobectomy, chemical pneumonitis
Chest Wall	
Muscular	Amytonia congenita, poliomyelitis, diaphragmatic hernia, eventration, myasthenia gravis, muscular dystrophy, botulism
Skeletal malformations	Kyphoscoliosis, hemivertebrae, absent ribs
Others	Obesity, flail chest
	INEFFICIENT GAS TRANSFER
Pulmonary Diffusion Defect	
Increased diffusion path between alveoli and capillaries	Pulmonary edema, pulmonary fibrosis, collagen disorders, *Pneumocystis carinii* infection, sarcoidosis
Decreased alveolocapillary surface area	Pulmonary embolism, sarcoidosis, pulmonary hypertension, mitral stenosis, fibrosing alveolitis
Inadequate number of erythrocytes	Anemia
Respiratory Center Depression	
Increased cerebrospinal fluid pressure	Cerebral trauma, intracranial tumors, central nervous system infection (meningitis, encephalitis, sepsis)
Excess central nervous system depressant	Oversedation, overdosage with barbiturates or morphine

Common causes of pulmonary disease in childhood.

airways is negative (less than atmospheric) and the normal pressure in surrounding tissues tends to compress the airway and increase the obstruction. *Intrathoracic* obstruction is generally manifest in the *expiratory* phase, because in forced expiration all intrathoracic airways decrease in diameter due to a decrease in the tethering force of the lung as the lung volume decreases. Airways that are between the mouth and the equal pressure point, but still in the thorax, also tend to collapse as pleural pressure exceeds intra-airway pressure, and only the structural rigidity of the airways resists the collapse.

Diagnostic Laboratory Procedures

Radiologic Procedures. Plain posteroanterior and lateral radiographs of the chest should be systematically reviewed with regard to appropriateness of the views; technical variations; the chest wall (congenital or acquired defects of ribs, sternum, or spine); diaphragm (lines intact and domes in normal position); pleura (costophrenic angle, presence or absence of pneumothorax, position of fissures); mediastinum (normal position, heart size, position of aortic arch, clarity of heart borders); clarity of cervical airways, hila, and pulmonary vessels (normal position, size, and caliber); and, finally, pulmonary parenchyma (presence of abnormal densities, air bronchogram, Kerley's lines, areas of hyperaeration, atelectasis, or consolidation) (Poznanski, 1976).

Radiographs of the neck and thoracic inlet may be helpful in investigation of masses such as cellulitis in the retropharyngeal soft tissue and tumors or foreign bodies in the cervical esophagus or the upper airway; in investigating epiglottitis, and also vascular rings such as double aortic arch and right aortic arch with aberrant right subclavian artery.

Esophagrams are particularly important in young patients with airflow obstruction, to define any mediastinal mass that might cause esophageal displacement, and to define disorders such as tracheoesophageal fistula and gastroesophageal reflux. Preferably, these studies are performed under fluoroscopic control using colloidal barium, which is less irritating than water-soluble contrast media, should it enter the tracheobronchial tree.

Bronchography is valuable in the demonstration of bronchiectasis and certain congenital abnormalities such as bronchomalacia and vascular ring.

In children who are old enough to voluntarily suspend respiration, tomography is valuable particularly for investigation of nodules.

Angiography is used for investigation of anomalies of the pulmonary vasculature and for localization of sites of hemoptysis in patients in whom bronchoscopy is not feasible.

Isotope scan may be helpful if perfusion defects are suspected and can be useful in identifying foreign bodies in patients in whom plain films and fluoroscopic assessment are not definitive.

Non-Radiologic Tests

Blood Count. The complete blood count should be checked for evidence of anemia, polycythemia, leukocytosis, esoinophilia, and lymphopenia.

Pulmonary Function Tests. Pulmonary function tests are useful for diagnosis and follow-up (see Chapter 42). In patients under age 6 years, techniques requiring cooperation frequently cannot be used, and special tests, for example, measurement of total respiratory resistance by a forced oscillation technique, may be required (Mansell, 1972).

Blood Gases. Arterial puncture of the radial vessel is a safe and simple procedure at all ages if the ulnar collateral arterial supply is assured (by compressing the radial artery and noting that the palm does not blanch). Use of the femoral artery should be avoided. Use of arterialized capillary blood (Davis et al., 1975) for measurement of Pco_2 and pH is preferable to not measuring these values at all, but serious underestimation of Po_2 may result, particularly if peripheral perfusion is poor, or if the extremity is not vasodilated by warmth or iontophoresis using a histamine-containing cream. Respiratory failure, suspected on the basis of clinical findings, is confirmed if $Paco_2$ is greater than 60 torr or is rising rapidly (> 10 torr per hour) in an exhausted child, or if Pao_2 is less than 55 or 60 torr when the patient is breathing 100 percent oxygen.

Cultures. Infants and young children seldom produce sputum for Gram stain and culture. A sample of tracheal secretions may be obtained by passing a sterile catheter by mouth, but unless a single species is isolated, results may be misleading. Documentation of specific viral infections by means of cultures for viruses, fluorescent antibody studies, and by paired acute and convalescent sera is useful but often impractical.

Lung puncture with a 20 to 22 gauge needle is used to obtain aspirates for histologic study or culture (for example, in severe pneumonia of unknown etiology) and requires only local anesthesia. Complications include pulmonary hemorrhage, empyema, and pneumothorax (Klein, 1969).

Open lung biopsy may be necessary if an organism has not been discovered by less invasive techniques (Roback et al., 1973).

Laryngoscopy. Indirect laryngoscopy is difficult or impossible to perform in most infants and young children. Direct laryngoscopy, usually under general anesthesia, must be performed to identify congenital abnormalities (e.g., laryngomalacia, webs, atresias, paralysis) and tumors and cysts of the larynx.

Bronchoscopy. Bronchoscopy permits visualization of the larger branches of the tracheobronchial tree. Bronchoscopy is performed to identify, localize, and remove foreign bodies and in other situations when less invasive procedures have failed, e.g., when the origin of bleeding or purulent secretions must be ascertained. Anomalies and site of compression may be identified. *In inexpert hands bronchoscopy is hazardous. Timing of the procedure and premedication may be critical* (Sahn, 1976). *In patients with hyperirritable airways (for example, in asthma), bronchoscopy may trigger massive vagal reflex and severe bronchospasm.*

Sweat Chloride Test. Quantitation of sweat chloride by the pilocarpine iontophoresis method (Gibson and Cooke, 1959) should be performed to rule out cystic fibrosis in any child with wheezing or a history of cystic fibrosis in a sibling or first cousin, or of recurrent pneumonia, or pulmonary disease associated with gastrointestinal symptoms or failure to thrive.

Other Laboratory Investigations. Quantitation of immunoglobulins G, A, and M is necessary in patients with recurrent pneumonia and bronchiectasis, to rule out immunodeficiency. Quantitation of IgA may be of interest in asthmatic patients since the incidence of selective IgA deficiency is claimed by some investigators to be increased in this group. Quantitation of IgE may be of prognostic value in bronchiolitis

(Polmar, 1972) and is of interest in asthma (McNicol and Williams, 1973).

Alpha-1-antitrypsin should be measured to rule out deficiency in patients with a clinical picture suggesting emphysema (Talamo, 1975).

Esophageal manometrics, esophagoscopy, and the acid reflux test (intraluminal pH test) are helpful in documenting gastroesophageal reflux in patients with chronic pulmonary disease (Christie et al., 1978).

Open lung biopsy also may be necessary in order to arrive at a specific diagnosis (Roback, 1973).

THERAPEUTIC PRINCIPLES

Goals of treatment of respiratory diseases are the following: preservation of life; facilitation of normal life style, including regular school attendance and participation in normal physical activity; minimizing morbidity from chronic pulmonary disorders; maintenance of normal physical and psychosocial growth and development; prevention of complications such as thoracic deformity, bronchiectasis, and cor pulmonale; and prevention of iatrogenic disease.

Severe late sequelae of acute respiratory disease in childhood have long been known; for example, bronchiolitis may be followed by asthma, bronchiectasis, or hyperlucent lung syndrome (Wohl and Chernick, 1978). Less obvious pulmonary sequelae probably occur much more frequently than recognized. For instance, croup or bronchiolitis may result in residual pulmonary abnormalities years later, even in patients who appear to be symptom-free (Fig. 41–3) (Kattan et al., 1977; Burrows et al., 1977).

General principles of treatment of respiratory disorders are summarized below.

Hydration. Removal of mucus from the airways is aided by adequate fluid intake. Children with acute respiratory disorders often develop fluid and electrolyte deficits because of hyperpnea, tachypnea, vomiting, and fever. Fluid balance must be restored, but fluids should never be "forced" by mouth in the dyspneic infant or toddler because of the high risk of aspiration. Intravenous fluid therapy should be adequate for maintenance and repair of dehydration, but *overhydration and its complication of pulmonary edema must be avoided.*

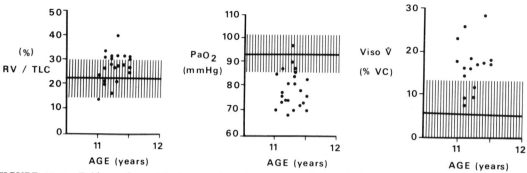

FIGURE 41–3. Evidence for residual parenchymal or airways lesion following bronchiolitis: asymptomatic patients with abnormal residual volume/total lung capacity ratio, PaO_2 and volume of isoflow about 11 years after uncomplicated bronchiolitis. Individual data points and mean and 2 standard deviations above and below mean are shown. (Reprinted with permission from Kattan, M., Keens, T. G., Lapierre, J. G., Levison, H., Bryan, A. C., and Reilly, B. J.: Pulmonary function abnormalities in symptom-free children after bronchiolitis. Pediatrics, *58*:683, 1977.)

Mist treatment, delivered by ultrasonic nebulizer, jet nebulizer, or natural fog generator, may be useful for treatment of croup. In lower respiratory tract disease such as bronchiolitis or asthma, benefits from mist treatment are not clear since particles that pass beyond the major airways tend to deposit in the least obstructed airways (Taussig, 1974), and adverse effects, such as reflex bronchoconstriction, may occur from stimulation of irritant receptors.

Chest Physiotherapy. Chest physiotherapy in its simplest form consists of encouraging a child to cough and breathe deeply. Balloons, blow bottles, and rebreathing tubes may be used. However, forced inspiration and forced expiration maneuvers may provoke further bronchospasm in patients with irritable airways. Postural drainage, accomplished by positioning the patient so that the involved segment of lung is uppermost, is useful in removal of mucus and other foreign material from the lung. Percussion with cupped hands and vibration may be performed over the involved area. Oxygen and suction should be readily available. These measures are more useful in bronchiectasis and cystic fibrosis (Wood, 1976) than in other respiratory disorders. They may be helpful in asthma when atelectasis or excessive secretions predominate over bronchospasm (Huber et al., 1974). Chest physiotherapy is necessary in patients being mechanically ventilated for any reason.

Bronchoscopy. Bronchoscopy may be of fundamental importance in restoring airway patency if a foreign body has been inhaled into the tracheobronchial tree or in the rare instance when tenacious mucous plugs must be removed, as in bronchopulmonary aspergillosis. *It should be used with care in patients with hyperreactive airways.*

Oxygen. Oxygen deprivation leads to clouding of the sensorium, unconsciousness, cardiac arrhythmias, and decreased mental function. The physician dealing with respiratory disease in children must ensure adequate oxygenation. Dependence on a hypoxic drive to ventilation is so rare in childhood that for practical purposes, the physician need not worry about "turning off" ventilation by increasing inspired oxygen. The occurrence of oxygen toxicity depends on the inspired oxygen tension and duration of treatment and does not develop in patients breathing 100 percent oxygen for 24 hours or less. Therefore, oxygen toxicity is never a consideration in transport or resuscitation procedures or in the emergency treatment of tension pneumothorax pending insertion of a chest tube with underwater seal.

In acute respiratory distress, all children should receive oxygen that has been fully saturated with water and warmed to body temperature, initially in a concentration of 30 to 40 percent by face mask and nebulizer, with the concentration later adjusted as needed to maintain an arterial oxygen tensions of 50 to 80 torr. An oxygen analyzer should be used to monitor inspired oxygen concentration.

In infants and young children, administration of oxygen by head box may be necessary if a mask is not tolerated. Nasal prongs cannot be used if nasal obstruction is present; they are poorly tolerated by children. Administration of oxygen by a mist tent is possible in concentrations up to 30 percent if the tent is opened infrequently. However, tents interfere with observation of the patient and with nursing care and are not generally recommended.

If a patient requires mechanical ventilation for respiratory failure over several days, attempts should be made to reduce inspired oxygen concentration by institution of positive end-expiratory pressure (PEEP) and to maintain optimal fluid and electrolyte balance, since use of concentrations of even 60 to 70 percent oxygen for 4 or 5 days may be harmful.

Symptoms of oxygen toxicity include substernal pain, paresthesias, and cerebral symptoms resulting from vasoconstriction. No radiologic or pathologic features of oxygen toxicity are pathognomonic, although collapse of alveoli occurs, especially at low lung volumes in the presence of airway closure. Surfactant activity may be decreased and there may be intra-alveolar, interstitial, and perivascular edema, also hyaline membrane formation and destruction of Type I cells. In the chronic phase, hyperplasia of Type II cells, septal thickening, capillary hyperplasia, and interstitial fibroelastic proliferation occur (Winter and Smith, 1972).

Pharmacologic Treatment. *Bronchodilators* and other drugs are important in restoration and maintenance of airway patency in asthma, laryngotracheobronchitis, and cystic fibrosis, and possibly also in bronchiolitis. These drugs are discussed in Chapter 23.

Anticholinergic drugs such as atropine and ipratropium bromide and antihistamines such as chlorpheniramine should be used with caution in patients with acute respiratory disease as their bronchodilator effect may be outweighed by their drying effect on secretions.

Expectorants such as guaifenesin (guaiacol glycerol ether), ammonium chloride, and iodide are without demonstrable benefit. Some beta adrenergic drugs such as terbuta-line may increase tracheal mucus velocity, however. Cough suppressants such as codeine, dextromethorphan, and noscapine may depress spontaneous respiration and should be used with extreme caution during acute respiratory disease. Diphenhydramine and beta adrenergic drugs may have some antitussive action.

Antimicrobials are of primary importance in the treatment of tonsillitis, epiglottitis, pertussis, bacterial and mycoplasma pneumonias, mycoses and psittacoses, bronchiectasis and cystic fibrosis, and pulmonary abscess and tuberculosis, in which a susceptible organism is involved. There is no justification for "prophylactic antibiotics" in respiratory diseases in children who have a normal immune system (see Chapter 19 for further discussion of antimicrobial therapy).

Alkali Therapy. Respiratory acidosis is treated by establishing adequate ventilation in the patient. For correction of *metabolic acidosis* (pH less than 7.3, base deficit greater than 5 mEq/L), sodium bicarbonate (7.5 percent solution) is the drug of choice. It is given in a dose of 2–5 mEq/kg (maximum 45 mEq) and may be repeated every 10 or 15 minutes.

Sedatives and tranquilizers are contraindicated in the conscious, spontaneously breathing child with acute respiratory disease, no matter how anxious or irritable the patient appears. Anxiety is almost always associated with hypoxia and is treated by ensuring the airways are patent and by administration of supplemental oxygen. Sedatives are necessary in patients being mechanically ventilated for respiratory failure.

Intermittent Positive Pressure Breathing (IPPB). IPPB probably is contraindicated in spontaneously breathing patients who have normal muscles of respiration. IPPB does not enhance peripheral deposition of aerosols in the lungs and tends to deliver medication to least obstructed areas. It also may increase airway resistance and in diseases such as asthma may induce or aggravate pneumomediastinum or pneumothorax (Moore and Cotton, 1972). Currently its only recommended use is for delivery of epinephrine to patients with croup (Westley et al., 1978; also see Chapter 43).

Surgical Therapy. Management of a tension pneumothorax requires aspiration of air and placement of a chest tube in the second intercostal space in the midclavicular line, connected to an underwater seal. Suction will be required if the leak is large. Accumulation of liquid in the pleural space also necessitates tube drainage, but in this instance, the tube is placed in the dependent part of the pleural space. Thoracotomy is required for evacuation of purulent thick pleural fluid and for control of massive pulmonary hemorrhage or persistent air leak.

The infant or child with respiratory symptoms requires a unique diagnostic and therapeutic approach, based on understanding of the influence of normal growth and development of anatomy and physiology of the respiratory tract. In any patient, but especially in the very young patient, the risk versus the benefit of any diagnostic or therapeutic procedure should be carefully weighed.

Management of Respiratory Failure

Intubation should be performed using a polyvinyl chloride tube of appropriate size (Pagtakhan and Chernick, 1977). To prevent aspiration of gastric contents, the stomach must be emptied before, by wide-bore tube. Oral tracheal intubation is simpler to perform than nasal tracheal intubation and therefore often is used in establishing an airway in an emergency. If intubation is necessary for more than 10 or 12 hours, a nasotracheal tube should be inserted in order to facilitate oropharyngeal hygiene and minimize risk or accidental extubation. Placement of the tube should be confirmed by auscultation and chest radiographs; the tip of the tube should be at least 1 cm above the carina. Children weighing less than 20 kg do not require a cuffed tube. Larger children should have cuffed tubes inflated to a minimum volume sufficient to provide a seal. The cuff should be deflated hourly for a few minutes in order to minimize the development of pressure necrosis.

Intubation is used without mechanical ventilation in disorders such as epiglottitis (Rapkin, 1975), laryngotracheobronchitis, and lymphoid airway obstruction (Kravath et al., 1977).

Ventilators may be classified on the basis of control of cycling mechanisms. Volume cycled instruments are suitable for use in patients with markedly increased airway resistance and decreased lung compliance. In these situations, delivery of a fixed volume of gas terminates the inspiratory phase. Pressure cycled instruments (flow rate limited) are those in which attainment of a preselected pressure setting initiates the expiratory phase. Both types of ventilators can control and/or assist a patient's respiratory effort (Pagtakhan and Chernick, 1977).

Frequent or continuous monitoring of vital signs, vigilant monitoring of fluid balance, and frequent auscultation of the chest and measurement of ventilatory indices are important. Suctioning and positioning should be performed frequently. Pao_2, $Paco_2$, pH, urine specific gravity, and serum electrolytes also should be monitored frequently.

Potential complications of mechanical ventilation include mechanical failure of the instrument or power source, improper warming or humidification of inspired air, oxygen toxicity, introduction of pathogens into the respiratory tract, atelectasis, pneumothorax (manifested by sudden increase in peak pressure developed by a volume-preset machine), pneumomediastinum, and subcutaneous emphysema. Complications of endotracheal intubation include intubation of a bronchus, kinking of the tube, obstruction by mucus plug, accidental extubation, and nasal hemorrhage. Hoarseness may occur after extubation and when extubation has been prolonged or the cuff overinflated. The formation of ulcers or granulomas, paralysis of small muscles of the larynx, and subglottic stenosis also may occur. Hyertension, hypotension, and cardiac arrhythmias may occur.

References

Breeze, R. G., and Wheeldon, E. B.: The cells of the pulmonary airways. Am. Rev. Respir. Dis. *116*:705, 1977.
Burrows, B., Knudson, R. J., and Lebowitz, M. D.: The rela-

tionship of childhood respiratory illness to adult obstructive airway disease. Am. Rev. Respir. Dis. *115*:751, 1977.
Chernick, V.: The development of the lung and the onset of

respiration. *In* Goodwin. J. W.. Godden. J. O. and Chance, W. G. (eds.): *Perinatal Medicine.* Toronto, Longman Canada Limited, 1976, page 517.

Chernick, V.: The vulnerable small airway. Pediatrics *59*:783, 1977.

Chernick, V., and Avery, M. E.: The functional basis of respiratory pathology. *In* Kendig, E. L., and Chernick, V. (eds.): *Disorders of the Respiratory Tract in Children,* 3rd Ed. Philadelphia, W. B. Saunders Co., 1977, page 3.

Christie, D. L., O'Grady, L. R., and Mack, D. V.: Incompetent lower esophageal sphincter and gastroesophageal reflux in recurrent acute pulmonary disease of infancy and childhood. J. Pediatr. *93*:23, 1978.

Davis, G. S., and Green, G. M.: Lung defense in asthma. *In* Weiss, E. B., and Segal, M. S. (eds.): *Bronchial Asthma Mechanisms and Therapeutics.* Boston, Little, Brown and Company, 1976, page 439.

Davis, R. H., Beran, A. V., and Galant, S. P.: Capillary pH and blood gas determinations in asthmatic children. J. Allergy Clin. Immunol. *56*:33, 1975.

Downes. J. J., Fulgencio, T., and Raphaely, R. C.: Acute respiratory failure in infants and children. Ped. Clin. North Am. *19*:423, 1972.

Gibson, L. E., and Cooke, R. E.: A test for concentration of electrolytes in sweat in cystic fibrosis of the pancreas utilizing pilocarpine iontophoresis. Pediatrics *23*:545, 1959.

Hogg, J. C.: Age as a factor in respiratory disease. *In* Kendig, E. L., and Chernick, V. (eds.): *Disorders of the Respiratory Tract in Children,* 3rd Ed. Philadelphia, W. B. Saunders Co., 1977, page 177.

Huber, A. L., Eggleston, P. A., and Morgan, J.: Effect of chest physiotherapy on asthmatic children. J. Allergy Clin. Immunol. *53*:109, 1974.

Kattan, M., Keens, T. G., Lapierre, J. G., Levison, H., Bryan, A. C., and Reilly, B. J.: Pulmonary function abnormalities in symptom-free children after bronchiolitis. Pediatrics *59*:683, 1977.

Klein, J. O.: Diagnostic lung puncture in the pneumonias of infants and children. Pediatrics *44*:486, 1969.

Kravath, R. E., Pollak, C. P., and Borowiecki, B.: Hypoventilation during sleep in children who have lymphoid airway obstruction treated by nasopharyngeal tube and T and A. Pediatrics *59*:865, 1977.

Mansell, A., Levison, H., Kruger, K., and Tripp, T. L.:

Measurement of respiratory resistance in children by forced oscillations. Amer. Rev. Respir. Dis. *106*:710, 1972.

Moore, R. B., and Cotton, E. K.: The effect of intermittent positive-pressure breathing on airway resistance in normal and asthmatic children. J. Allergy Clin. Immunol. *49*:137, 1972.

McNicol, K. N., and Williams, H. E.: Spectrum of asthma in children. II, allergic components. Br. Med. J. *11*:12, 1973.

Pagtakhan, R. D., and Chernick, V.: Intensive care of respiratory disorders. *In* Kendig, E. L., and Chernick, V. (eds.): *Disorders of the Respiratory Tract in Children,* 3rd Ed. Philadelphia, W. B. Saunders Co., 1977, page 191.

Polmar S. H., Robinson, L. D., and Minnefor, A. B.: Immunoglobulin E in bronchiolitis. Pediatrics *50*:279, 1972.

Poznanski, A. K.: *Practical Approaches to Pediatric Radiology.* Chicago, Year Book Medical Publishers, Inc., 1976.

Rapkin, R. H.: Nasotracheal intubation in epiglottitis. Pediatrics *56*:110, 1975.

Richardson, J. B.: The neural control of human tracheobronchial smooth muscle. *In* Lichtenstein, L. M., and Austen, K. F. (eds.): *Asthma Physiology, Immunopharmacology, and Treatment.* New York, Academic Press, 1977, page 237.

Roback. S. A., Weintraub. W. H.. Nesbit. M.. Spanos, P. K.. Burke. B., and Leonard. A. S.: Diagnostic open lung biopsy in the critically ill child. Pediatrics *52*:605, 1973.

Sahn, S. A., and Scoggin, C.: Fiberoptic bronchoscopy in bronchial asthma. Chest *69*:39, 1976.

Talamo, R. C.: Basic and clinical aspects of the alpha$_1$-antitrypsin. Pediatr. *56*:91, 1975.

Taussig, L. M.: Mists and aerosols: New studies, new thoughts. J. Pediatr. *84*:619, 1974.

Waring, W. W.: The history and physical examination. *In* Kendig, E. L., and Chernick, V. (eds.): *Disorders of the Respiratory Tract in Children,* 3rd Ed. Philadelphia, W. B. Saunders Co., 1977, page 77.

Westley, C. R., Cotton, E. K., and Brooks, J. G.: Nebulized racemic epinephrine by IPPB for the treatment of croup. Am. J. Dis. Child. *132*:484, 1978.

Winter, P. M., and Smith, G.: The toxicity of oxygen. Anesthesiology *37*:210, 1972.

Wohl, M. E. B., and Chernick, V.: Bronchiolitis. Am. Rev. Respir. Dis. *118*:759, 1978.

Wood, R. E., Boat, T. F., and Doershuk, C. F.: Cystic fibrosis. Am. Rev. Respir. Dis. *113*:833, 1976.

42

J. F. Souhrada, M.D., Ph.D.
J. M. Buckley, M.D.

Value and Use of Pulmonary Function Testing in the Office

Pulmonary function testing is an integral and crucial step in the basic evaluation of patients with asthma and other chronic pulmonary disorders. This chapter discusses the value of pulmonary function tests in the diagnosis and assessment of airway disease, with particular reference to bronchial asthma, the performance of pulmonary function tests in the office, and the indications for more sophisticated lung function evaluations.

SIGNIFICANCE OF MEASURING PULMONARY FUNCTIONS

There are several reasons for employing pulmonary function tests in bronchial asthma: to assist in establishing the presence and degree of airway obstruction; to measure the degree of airway reactivity; to determine which bronchodilator drug or drugs are most effective; to follow the course of disease objectively (Bouhuys, 1974).

Pulmonary function measurements must be interpreted in a clinical context, as pulmonary function abnormalities may or may not have clinical significance. Thus, the clinical history is an important aspect of the assessment of pulmonary functions. Historical points indicative of pulmonary obstruction may be subtle (see other chapters on pulmo-

nary disease). Similarly, the physical examination plays an important role in evaluating the significance of results of pulmonary function tests. It is essential to determine each individual's "normal" pulmonary function values because pulmonary function test results may appear to be within predicted limits when compared to published normal values, while actually being abormally low for the particular child. This often is seen if tests are performed in the "asymptomatic" period shortly after an acute attack (Tooley et al., 1965). In addition, evidence is accumulating that asthma, long regarded as a "reversible" disorder, can be associated with significant irreversible pulmonary changes. It is not difficult to imagine that maintenance of partial airway obstruction (which occurs frequently in asthmatic children whose chronic asthma is not treated vigorously), with local inflammation, recurrent infection, and chronic alveolar overdistension, can lead to a chronic, irreversible element of airway obstruction. *Preventing chronicity* of asthmatic episodes would seem to be critical in minimizing the degree of permanent lung injury (Goddard, 1961). Pulmonary function tests provide information important in assessing airway function, which cannot always be obtained clinically in the long-term evaluation of bronchial asthma.

CHILDREN'S LUNGS VERSUS ADULTS' LUNGS

The major portion of our knowledge regarding postnatal development of the lung is based on anatomic studies. There are several important anatomic and functional differences between the child's and adult's lung that directly influence lung function tests and their interpretation. As the mean number of airway generations and the airway diameter increases from 3 months to 8 years, the airway resistance decreases (Souhrada and Buckley, 1976). The number of alveoli increases more than tenfold between birth and adult life, mainly in the first 8 years (Dunnill, 1962). Thereafter, any increase in lung volume is due to an increase in the linear dimensions of existing alveoli. The alveolar diameter at 8 years of age is 230 microns, and it increases to 280 microns in adulthood. Thus, adverse factors such as chronic respiratory infections or chronic drug therapy (especially steroids) occurring during this critical time, from birth to age 25 (but particularly in the first 8 years), could have profound effects on "normal" lung growth (Kotas et al., 1974). Wide variations are seen in certain pulmonary function tests in the normal population, owing to significant anatomic variations between normal individuals. For instance, the number of alveoli in the normal lung ranges from 2×10^8 to 6×10^8 and is largely related to body size (Angus and Thurlbeck, 1972).

There are more mucus glands in the major bronchi in normal children than in normal adults (Matsuba and Thurlbeck, 1972). By contrast, there seems to be no difference between children and adults in the distribution of airway smooth muscle. In both, the proportion of the muscle is larger in the small airways than in the large airways (Charnock and Doershuk, 1973). These morphologic characteristics may be responsible for a greater involvement of small airways in diseases such as bronchial asthma.

NORMAL LUNG FUNCTION VALUES

Evaluation of pulmonary functions requires comparison with values from a normal reference population. When comparing actual pulmonary function measurements with normal or "predicted" values, it is common to accept measurements within a certain range (usually defined as ± 2 standard deviations of the mean) as normal, unless it can be demonstrated at some point that function in that range is abnormal for the individual. It

TABLE 42–1 PREDICTED EQUATIONS FOR OFFICE SPIROMETRY

Test	Sex	Group	Prediction Equation	S.D.	Normal Range
FVC (1)	*M	≤170 cm	$4.4 \times 10^{-6} \times (Ht\ cm)^{2.67}$	13%	Pred. ± 0.26
	F	≤170 cm	$3.3 \times 10^{-6} \times (Ht\ cm)^{2.72}$	13%	Pred. ± 0.26
	†M	>170 cm, <19 yrs	0.174 Age + 0.0646(Ht cm) − 9.425	0.354	Pred. ± 0.708
	F	>170 cm, <19 yrs	0.102 Age + 0.0461(Ht cm) − 5.869	0.297	Pred. ± 0.594
FEV$_1$ (1)	*M,F	≤170 cm	$2.1 \times 10^{-6} (Ht\ cm)^{2.80}$	10%	Pred. ± 0.20
	†M	>170 cm, <19 yrs	0.121 Age + 0.0563(Ht cm) − 7.864	0.303	Pred. ± 0.606
	F	>170 cm, <19 yrs	0.085 Age + 0.0394(Ht cm) − 4.939	0.290	Pred. ± 0.59
FEV$_1$/FVC (%)	*M,F	<19 years	86%	14%	72% → 100%
FEF$_{25-75\%}$ (1/sec)	†M	<150 cm	0.0370(Ht cm) − 2.614	0.388	Pred. ± 0.776
	F	<150 cm	0.0343(Ht cm) − 2.289	0.347	Pred. ± 0.694
	†M	>150 cm, <19 yrs	0.126 Age + 0.0531(Ht cm) − 6.498	0.612	Pred. ± 1.224
	F	>150 cm, <19 yrs	0.083 Age + 0.0366(Ht cm) − 3.499	0.621	Pred. ± 1.242
PEFR (1/sec)	*M,F	≤170 cm	0.0874(Ht cm) − 7.093	12.8%	Pred. ± 0.256

*Polgar and Promadhat (1971).
†Dickman et al. (1971).

also should be kept in mind that there may be significant variation in normal values between pulmonary function laboratories, based on variations in equipment and techniques utilized in obtaining data. It is a useful rule to test the validity and reproducibility of measured pulmonary functions in the physician's office by comparing pulmonary functions of several normal subjects measured in the office with the established predicted values to be used. Since the majority of pulmonary function tests require patient cooperation, pulmonary function testing in children less than 5 to 6 years of age usually is not practical, though simple airway function tests can be obtained in younger children through use of innovative techniques (see Chapter 45).

In healthy young adults the variation in lung function among indiviuals is due in part to differences in stature (Cotes, 1974). This is the primary reason why the majority of equations used to predict normal lung functions relate to standing height (usually expressed in cm). It has been suggested that, after allowing for body size, the most important factor determining lung function is the level of habitual activity during childhood and early adult life; environmental factors such as altitude also are of importance (Cotes, 1974). Reliable equations for predicting various normal pulmonary functions can be found in Polgar and Promadhat (1971) as well as in a recent publication of the Intermountain Thoracic Society (Kanner and Morris, 1975). Table 42–1 summarizes equations of predicted normal pulmonary functions commonly measured in the physician's office.

STATIC LUNG VOLUMES

Definition of Lung Volumes. In childhood there is a progressive increase in various lung volumes, correlating with body size. Static lung volumes reflect the anatomic dimensions of the lungs. With the exception of functional residual capacity (FRC), all static lung volumes are dependent on the subject's maximal inspiratory or expiratory effort during the test. Figure 42–1 includes a normal spirometric tracing, with static lung volumes illustrated. Vital capacity (VC), defined as the total amount of air that can be exhaled by the patient, can be determined readily by spirometry (discussed later). The amount of air contained in the chest at the

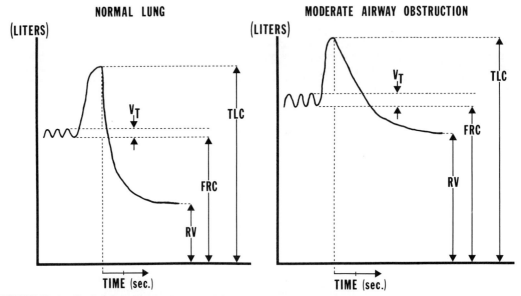

FIGURE 42–1. Static lung volumes in normal lung (left) and lung with moderate airway obstruction (right) as related to spirogram (forced expiratory maneuver). V_T = tidal volume; RV = residual volume; FRC = functional residual capacity; and TLC = total lung capacity. Note that in the lung with airway obstruction tidal volume occurs at higher lung volume (FRC), and lung is thus hyperinflated.

completion of full expiration (residual volume = RV), the amount of air in the chest at the end of quiet expiration (functional residual capacity = FRC), and the amount of air in the chest at the end of maximal inspiration (total lung capacity = TLC) all can be assessed by special techniques such as helium or nitrogen washout and body plethysmography. These techniques are described and summarized in a recent monograph by Cherniack (1977); they are usually performed in specialized pulmonary function laboratories. Sometimes these tests are necessary to confirm suspected hyperinflation.

Hyperinflation. "Barrel chest" is a typical physical finding in children with severe bronchial asthma. This condition is a direct result of chronic lung hyperinflation. The various factors and sequence of events which lead to hyperinflation are discussed below.

At the end of a quiet expiration, forces that inflate and forces that deflate the thorax are in balance. This balance is represented as the resting respiratory level at the end of quiet expiration. It is this position at which the functional residual capacity (FRC) begins (see Fig. 42–1). The deflationary forces that affect resting respiratory level are: the elastic recoil of the lungs (pulling inward), the inward pull of the expiratory muscles, and the weight of the thorax and its contents. In bronchial asthma, the work of breathing during expiration is significantly increased due to airway obstruction. Even in the asymptomatic state, there usually is some degree of airway obstruction. As bronchial obstruction increases, there is an inability to expel the normal tidal volume with each expiration, leading to air-trapping and hyperinflation. However, hyperinflation of the asthmatic lung partially compensates for airway obstruction by increasing the outward pull on the bronchial walls and thus enlarging their caliber. Hyperinflation results in increased effort in breathing, and as hyperinflation progresses, the accessory respiratory muscles must be called into use (Cherniack, 1977). In chronic obstructive airway disease (such as chronic asthma and emphysema), the elastic recoil (pulling inward) of the lung frequently decreases, thus creating an imbalance in inspiratory and expiratory forces and decreasing the amount of air exhaled relative to the amount inhaled. This soon affects the resting

respiratory level, the lungs gradually become hyperinflated, and the thorax expands particularly in anteroposterior diameter.

Hyperinflation can be determined in specialized laboratories by measuring static lung volumes (FRC, RV, and TLC). A practical definition of hyperinflation is based on at least a 20 percent increase above predicted values in two different ratios, RV/TLC and FRC/TLC. Under normal conditions, the normal value for RV/TLC ($\times$ 100) is 24 $\pm$ 5%; for FRC/TLC ($\times$ 100), it is 47 $\pm$ 5%. Static lung volumes also are used to determine the presence of "enlarged lungs." Unlike hyperinflation, enlarged lungs are not an abnormal entity. Usually a 20 percent or more proportional increase is seen above the predicted range in all static volumes (VC, RV, TLC), so that the ratios discussed above are maintained within the normal range. Some teenagers, as well as other physically active people such as professional athletes, will frequently have enlarged lungs.

Restrictive Ventilatory Defect. Measurement of lung volumes also is used to determine a restrictive ventilatory defect. A restrictive defect is characterized most frequently by a decrease in lung volume, such as vital capacity (VC) and total lung capacity (TLC). A decrease of more than 20 percent from mean predicted values usually is considered clinically significant. It must be remembered that, due to a simultaneous decrease in FVC (forced vital capacity) and FEV_1 (volume at 1 second of forced expiration), the ratio of these two volumes can be maintained at the normal level or frequently even increased above the predicted range in the presence of restrictive disease. (This contrasts with changes of FEV_1/FVC in chronic obstructive airway disease, in which this ratio usually is decreased.) Also, in restrictive disease the spirographic breathing pattern at rest shows a decreased tidal volume with an increased respiratory rate. In children and young adults, this most often is seen in kyphoscoliosis and usually persists following corrective surgery. Since the incidence of kyphoscoliosis is the same in asthmatic and nonasthmatic children, this problem frequently complicates pulmonary function testing for obstructive disease. Pectus excavatum, another frequent childhood chest deformity, can produce a similar defect.

DETECTION OF OBSTRUCTIVE DISEASE

Airway obstruction is the leading pathologic abnormality in lung disease, including bronchial asthma. The obstructive process contributes to shortness of breath, limits physical performance in exercise, and leads to labored breathing. It also is responsible for a decrease in maximum expiratory flow rates, as measured by spirometry or flow-volume relationship. Airway obstruction also affects ventilatory patterns and the distribution of inspired air, which leads to disturbance of alveolar ventilation. Alveolar hypoventilation affects ventilation-perfusion relationships and results in hypoxemia and eventually in carbon dioxide retention and respiratory acidosis. Most frequently, airway obstruction involves the peripheral airways (small airways diameter less than 1 or 2 mm) (Macklem, 1971), which may be the earliest site of significant airway involvement and is the last site from which airway obstruction disappears. During the early development of asthma involving predominantly the small airways, "routine" pulmonary function tests (FVC, FEV_1, PEFR) will not demonstrate significant abnormalities. Measurement of other flow rates, however (e.g., $FEF_{25-75\%}$ (MMEF), see below), can be more helpful in detecting early obstructive airway disease.

Detection of Airway Disease in Its Early Stages

In general, the clinical picture of obstructive airway disease is characterized by a slowly decreasing ability to expel air from the lung. At present the principal effort of many investigators is toward establishment of a reliable, sensitive, and simple test to detect airway disease in its early stages. From the standpoint of therapeutic and prognostic considerations, the value of detecting chronic obstructive airway disease in its early stages is obvious.

Small (peripheral) airways comprise the twelfth to twenty-third generations of the bronchial tree of the Weibel lung model. The small airways represent the majority of the airways in the lung, far exceeding in number the first ten to twelve generations or central (large) airways. However, owing to the relatively large total area of the small airways (sum of the squares of their diameters), peripheral airways contribute only about 20 percent of the total resistance to airflow in all airways. Thus, *it is likely that complete occlusion of up to one-half of all peripheral airways may be undetected by the conventional means of pulmonary function testing* (Macklem, 1971). Appropriately, these airways also have been called the "silent zone" or the "quiet zone." As indicated above, the usual office pulmonary function tests (FVC, FEV_1, PEFR) are too insensitive to detect early airway obstruction of small airways. Chronic obstructive disease may start with selective involvement of small airways (Macklem, 1971). Since at that point there are no typical clinical manifestations of disease, the disease may remain unsuspected and may progress for many years.

The following tests are currently used in detecting early airway disease: maximal midexpiratory flow (MMEF or $FEF_{25-75\%}$) obtained from spirometry; $\dot{V}_{max\,50\%}$; or $\dot{V}_{max\,60\%}$ derived from the maximal expiratory flow-volume curve; partial flow–volume curve (PEFV); volume of isoflow (V iso $\dot{V}$); closing volume (CV); slope of alveolar plateau; residual volume (RV); and end-tidal FEV_1. Of these techniques, some can be considered "office procedures," while others generally are not.

Tests that Require Only a Spirometer. The assessment of early disease of the small (peripheral) airways can be made when measurement of the forced midexpiratory flow ($FEF_{25-75\%}$) is done. The principal aspects of $FEF_{25-75\%}$ determination are shown in Figure 42–2. At the same time, however, the values of FEV_1 must be normal (McFadden et al., 1974). Another sensitive test revealing small airway disease that was recently introduced is called end-tidal FEV_1. During this test, the subject performs a maximal expiratory effort from his resting tidal volume position. This can be done easily in the physician's office with standard office spirometry (Lim, 1973).

Tests Requiring an X-Y Plotter. The maximum expiratory flow–volume curve (MEFV curve) represents the graphic relationship between forced vital capacity (FVC) and maximal expiratory flows ($\dot{V}$max) during performance of the forced expiratory maneu-

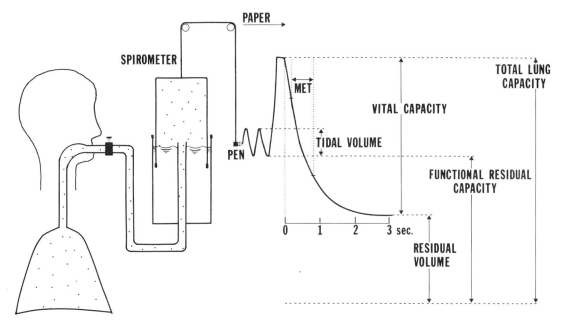

Figure 42–2. Principles of spirometry. Water sealed spirometer is shown on the left side. Movements of light bellow are transmitted and recorded so that tidal volume and forced expiratory maneuver (relationship of time [in sec.] vs. volume [in 1]) can be seen. $FEF_{25-75\%} = \dfrac{1/2\ VC}{MET}$. For comparison, spirographic tracing is shown related to static lung volumes.

ver. A maximal expiratory flow appears to be independent of effort over the lower half to two-thirds of the vital capacity (i.e., at lower lung volumes). This relatively effort-independent descendant portion of the flow-volume curve is affected mostly by small airway diameter, airway compressibility, and lung elastic recoil (Zapletal et al., 1969). The majority of advanced spirometers are equipped to measure flow-volume curves. Reproducibility, however, is relatively poor. The partial expiratory flow–volume curve (PEFV curve) also has been introduced recently as a relatively sensitive indicator of small airway dysfunction (Bouhuys, 1974).

Tests Requiring Special Gas Mixtures. If helium, a less dense gas than nitrogen, is substituted for the normal 80 percent nitrogen of room air and the patient breathes this mixture, higher flow rates during forced expiration are achieved than with the MEFV curve obtained with room air. In the absence of small airway obstruction, the flow-volume curve obtained with room air and the flow-volume curve obtained with a helium mixture meet at a point which is within 10 percent of vital capacity (volume of isoflow or V iso $\dot{V}$). However, in early air-

way obstruction, after breathing the helium-oxygen mixture, the increased expiratory flow ($\dot{V}_{max}$) achieved in the normal lung is not seen, and the intercept occurs at a higher lung volume. This phenomenon increases the volume of isoflow (Hutcheson et al., 1974).

An increase in residual volume is one of the most sensitive indications of airway obstruction, especially in the small airways (McFadden et al., 1974). Often, symptom-free asthmatic patients who are in complete clinical remission have an increased residual volume (Weng and Levison, 1969). RV can be measured by helium or nitrogen washout methods or by utilizing body plethysmography. A relatively simple determination of residual volume can be obtained from routine radiography (Shephard and Seliger, 1969). One disadvantage of residual volume determination, however, is the relatively large range in normal values.

Closing volume is the volume of air in the lung at which the smaller airways (probably terminal bronchioles) start to close during expiration. In early airway obstruction, these airways close even earlier in expiration. With airway obstruction, residual air increases, resulting in a larger lung volume, loss of elastic recoil at the higher lung volumes, subsequent earlier collapse of small airways, and an earlier point of closing volume. Currently, the single breath nitrogen method (Buist et al., 1973) appears to be the most suitable method to use in screening for early small airway disease. This test has relatively good reproducibility when expiration is sufficiently slow (with flow not exceeding 0.5 L/sec). This technical procedure has been described and standardized in an NIH Heart and Lung Institute Report (NIH Report, 1971). As with the determination of residual volume, this technique, which requires special equipment, will identify subjects with early airway obstructive disease.

Established Airway Obstruction

At present, several "routine" pulmonary function tests can produce important information concerning the presence of airway obstruction. Some pulmonary function tests also can indicate the approximate location of airway obstruction, i.e., large vs. peripheral airways. The selection and interpretation of the tests should take into account the fact that tests differ in their sensitivity of detection of airway obstruction. Table 42–2 summarizes available methods detecting airway obstruction. Spirometry and maximal expiratory flow-volume (MEFV) curves determine airway obstruction indirectly. Measurement of airway resistance using body plethysmography, or of respiratory resistance using an oscillatory method, represents attempts to measure changes of airway diameter directly.

In a physician's office the most convenient way to measure the airway obstructive process is by spirometry. Spirometry is as important and routine a test for airway obstruction as determination of blood pressure for hypertension or urine analysis for renal disease. Spirometry consists of recording the volume of air expired by the patient, usually during a maximal expiratory effort, and recording it against time. The advantages of spirometry are its reproducibility, relative ease of performance, and the fact that, properly performed, it generally can readily detect obstructive or restrictive defects. However, it should be kept in mind that spirometry is not a diagnostic test in itself. Measurement of forced expiratory flow variables (such as FEV_1) offers a relatively sensitive measure of obstructive impairment, and a decrease in flow rates during forced expiration correlates with clinical disability. Maximal forced expiration is recorded as displacment of air on a kymograph (see Fig. 42–2) or electronic device. Successful spirometry requires the patient's full cooperation in and understanding of the procedure, but it usually can be performed by children 5 or 6 years old and occasionally by younger children. Pulmonary function measurements that can be obtained from spirometry are summarized in Table 42–3.

The dynamic volume used most often is forced expiratory volume at one second (FEV_1). This is a relatively reproducible and sensitive test, despite the fact that it is large-

TABLE 42–2 DETECTION OF AIRWAY OBSTRUCTION

Test	Physiologic Interpretation	Sensitivity	Equipment
Spirometry (Flow vs. time) FVC FEV_1 $FEF_{25-75\%}$ (MMEF) PEFR	Overall mechanical functions of lung and thorax 1. Airway obstruction 2. Elastic recoil 3. Airway collapse	Good to moderate; Effort-dependent test	Low resistance spirometer
Maximum expiratory flow–volume curve (MEFV curve) (Flow vs. volume)	Same as for spirometry	Same as for spirometry	X-Y plotter Electronic display of flow and volume signal*
Airway resistance (R_{aw})	Flow resistance of large airways (1–12 generations)	Good Requires panting	Body plethysmograph†
Respiratory resistance (Rrs)	Lung and thoracic cage resistance	Good to moderate (not for office use)	Forced oscillator

*For detailed information: Med. Science or Vanguard Spirometer DS-500 with X-Y Plotter may be used.
†For detailed information: W. Collins, Inc., 200 Wood Road, Braintree, Mass. 02184.

TABLE 42–3 PULMONARY FUNCTION VARIABLES DERIVED FROM A FORCED EXPIRATORY MANEUVER (SPIROGRAM)*

Abbreviation	Synonym	Calculation	Definition
FVC (liters)	Fast Vital Capacity		*Forced Vital Capacity.* The maximum inspiration is followed by maximum expiration performed as fast and forcefully as possible.
FEV_1 (liters)	Timed Vital Capacity		*Forced Expiratory Volume.* The volume expired during one second during performance of FVC.
$FEF_{25-75\%}$ (liters/sec.)	MMEF MMF MMER	$\dfrac{1/2 \text{ VC}}{\text{MET}}$	*Forced Mid-Expiratory Flow.* The average flow rate during expiration of the middle 50% of VC.
MET (sec.)	MMT		*Mid-Expiratory Time* (Maximum Mid-Expiratory time). The time required to expel the middle half of the VC during FVC (used in calculation of $FEF_{25-75\%}$).
$FEV_{200-1200}$ (liters/sec.)	MEFR MMFR	$\dfrac{1 \text{ liter}}{\text{time (sec.)}}$	*Forced Expiratory Flow Rate.* The mean expiratory flow rate for that part of the FVC exhaled between 200 and 1200 ml.

*Adapted from Kory, R. C. et al.: Clinical spirometry: Recommendation of the section on pulmonary function testing. Dis. Chest *43*:214, 1963.

ly effort-dependent. A relatively effort-independent test is forced mid-expiratory flow (MMEF or $FEF_{25-75\%}$). As mentioned above, this test may be abnormal in airway disease when the FEV_1 is normal. In such instances, this is a reflection of obstruction predominantly in small airways. Peak expiratory flow rate (PEFR) usually is measured with a Wright peak flow meter. Since peak flow occurs during the effort-dependent portion of the expiratory maneuver, this test is not as precise or reproducible as the $FEF_{25-75\%}$. It also is comparatively insensitive in detection of airway obstruction (Buckley et al., 1974; Steiner and Phelan, 1978). On the other hand, it is an easy test to perform and one which patients can perform and record at home. In general, it should be used only when other pulmonary function tests are not available, or as a supplement to other tests.

PRACTICAL ASPECTS OF SPIROMETRY

Since measurement of expiratory flow rates is effort-dependent, it is critical that the patient be instructed thoroughly in performance of the test and in proper techniques for using the pulmonary function equipment. During the test, the patient should be seated and wear a noseclip. The test results should

be accepted only if the patient developed a maximal expiratory effort following full inspiration. Maximal effort usually is achieved best when the technician first demonstrates how to perform the test and then strongly encourages the patient to use maximal effort during testing. Individual motivation in addition to proper technique is important in obtaining reliable spirometric data. Maximal expiratory effort is not achieved when the patient has pain or a coughing spasm (or when the patient malingers to establish a case for disability). Frequent errors in the test are glottis closure (Valsalva maneuver) and premature termination of expiration. The forced expiratory maneuver should be recorded for at least 6 seconds. Other problems such as an air leak, obstructed mouthpiece, or poor start of the test, warrant repeating the test.

A deep expiratory maneuver, as performed during spirometry, can induce significant bronchial obstruction in patients with bronchial asthma. This may be reflected in progressive decrease in flow rates with subsequent blows. A similar maneuver, i.e., deep expiration, performed by nonasthmatic subjects, results in reflex bronchodilation. These factors could artificially increase the differences between normal and asthmatic subjects. Consequently, no more than three consecutive spirometry tests are advisable for measuring pulmonary functions at a given time, and the highest values should be selected.

Technical details of office spirometry are described in a recent publication of the Intermountain Thoracic Society (Kanner and Morris, 1975).

Peak Flow Meter. At an early phase of forced expiration, the expiratory flow achieves maximal values. This highest flow is known as the peak expiratory flow rate (PEFR). Wright and McKerrow (1959) introduced a relatively simple and inexpensive device, the Wright peak flow meter, to measure PEFR. This instrument has been useful in patient care, as a tool in epidemiologic studies and as a simple monitoring device. Since this equipment is easily operated, after proper training it also can be used by the patient at home. However, there are limitations of peak expiratory flow rate measurements by the peak flow meter. Since peak flow occurs during the effort-dependent portion of the expiratory maneuver, such measurements cannot deliver reproducible and effort-independent information concerning lung function. Also, the relatively normal values for peak flow frequently seen in patients with bronchial asthma do not necessarily indicate lack of significant airway obstruction. "Falsely high" values of PEFR can occur because of airway collapse during high expiratory effort, with initial rapid acceleration of expiration of air. It also should be remembered that no single pulmonary function test can be as informative in detecting ventilatory dysfunction as a complete analysis of a flow-volume curve. In addition, regular calibration of the Wright peak flow meter is mandatory for accurate measurement of PEFR, a procedure unfortunately too often neglected.

Peak expiratory flow rates also can be readily detected from maximal expiratory flow–volume curves (MEFV curves). Usually a more precise procedure and display are used in this method, and the peak expiratory flow so measured is a more accurate assessment of air flow. Since this test requires relatively expensive equipment, however, few offices utilize this procedure.

Choice of Spirometer. An important aspect of pulmonary function testing is the selection of proper equipment. Huge errors (up to 200 percent) can be generated even with simple spirometric measurements if the proper equipment is not used (Fitzgerald et al., 1973). The spirometer chosen for a physician's office should be capable of measuring flows in the range of 0 to 12 liters per second and volumes up to at least 6 liters. This spirometer should be capable of accumulating volumes for at least 6 seconds.

The detection of flows and volumes should be relatively accurate. Accuracy is satisfactory when the volume measured is within ± 3 per cent of the reading or 50 cc, whichever is greater. It is important that weekly calibration be done with a 3-liter syringe to check for correct volume readings. If the Stead-Wells (water-sealed) spirometer is used, the technician should check weekly for deformities in the bell, air leaks in the system, and speed of the kymograph. The water level in the spirometer should be one-half inch below the metal margin. A waterless wedge type spirometer, the Vitallograph spirometer, has the advantage that is more portable and requires less maintenance. It has the disadvantage that if it needs recalibration it must be returned to the manufacturer.

One of the most important requirements for a spirometer in a practitioner's office is the availability of a tracing (spirogram). Graphic documentation will serve for future records and longitudinal evaluation of the patient. Another important requirement is rapid production of data. Reliable, relatively inexpensive spirometers, such as the Stead-Wells or the Vitallograph, produce tracings that require graphic analysis that may be time-consuming. Quick delivery of data can be achieved when an "electronic spirometer" is used. However, reliable electronic equipment tends to be expensive (approximately $5,000). Some of the available electronic "gadgets" do not offer a graphic record option, and their precision is poor.

MEASUREMENT OF REVERSIBILITY OF OBSTRUCTIVE AIRWAY DISEASE

One of the uses of pulmonary function tests is to determine the degree of reversibility of pulmonary obstruction. There is no standardized procedure for ascertaining whether ventilatory dysfunction is "reversible" or "irreversible." Conventionally, however, reversibility is assessed by measuring pulmonary functions before and after inhalation of an aerosolized bronchodilating agent. A recommended technique of aerosol administration is nebulization of isoproterenol (Isuprel) or isoetharine (Bronkosol) through a standard commercial device such as those manufactured by the DeVilbiss Co., using intermittent air pressure (from a cylinder of compressed air). It is recommended that other bronchodilating medications be avoided for at least 5 to 6 hours before this test, and that spirometry be repeated 15 minutes after administration of these drugs. In normal subjects, little change is observed in pulmonary function after inhalation of a bronchodilating drug, but in some healthy subjects a consistent increase of up to 15 percent in certain pulmonary variables may be seen. In patients with reversible obstructive airway disease such as bronchial asthma, significant improvement (more than 20 percent) in abnormal flow rates is observed. In some patients with asthma, only partial reversibility of airway obstruction is demonstrable (see Chapter 45). Restrictive pulmonary disease and emphysema are irreversible by definition, although some patients with irreversible lung disease may in fact have a small but significant reversible component.

In general, reversibility implies a better prognosis than fixed impairment of expiratory flow rates. On the other hand, the interpretation of test results should be made cautiously, since a course of round-the-clock bronchodilator, or a course of steroid therapy sometimes can at least partially reverse obstructive pulmonary disease that appears irreversible with inhaled bronchodilators.

PULMONARY FUNCTIONS AND DETECTION OF AIRWAY HYPERREACTIVITY IN BRONCHIAL ASTHMA

Wheezing, the classic hallmark of hyperreactive airway disease, is not always present in asthma. As with an iceberg of which only a small portion usually is visible, symptoms and physical signs in asthma are only the tip of a large mass of abnormal pulmonary physiology. Indeed, symptoms and signs in asthma may be minimal or not apparent in significant pulmonary disease. Figure 42–3

(A through D) graphically lists four different clinical presentations of patients with bronchial asthma. The figures demonstrate bronchial asthma with and without overt wheezing (examples A and B vs. C and D). Example B illustrates that during the "asymptomatic" period of a patient with asthma or shortly after an asthmatic paroxysm, pulmonary functions may remain abnormal for hours, days, weeks, or months. Asthma also may exist in children in whom overt wheezing never occurs but in whom some evidence of obstructed air flow can be obtained by pulmonary function tests (Example C). These individuals may have significant clinical lower respiratory tract problems as a result of an acute upper respiratory infection, airway irritants, or severe exercise. While hesitancy on the part of the physician to diagnose asthma in the absence of overt wheezing is understandable, nevertheless nonwheezing asthma does exist, and diagnosis is essential to appropriate therapy. It is here that pulmonary function testing can be especially helpful in aiding diagnosis.

Examples B and C in Figure 42–3 depict asthmatic patients whose pulmonary function is always abnormal even though symptoms may never be obvious or may present only sporadically. In both examples, pulmonary function testing provides important information for diagnosis and follow-up that cannot be obtained on clinical grounds alone. In Example C, suspicious historical points which might suggest pulmonary function testing may include complaints (volunteered or elicited) that "all colds go to his (her) chest," "colds are associated with prolonged coughing," and a "tendency to bronchitis and pneumonia."

When the patient does not have have abnormal pulmonary function during an asymptomatic period (examples A and D), but has a nondiagnostic history of respiratory difficulties suggestive of asthma, bronchial provocation tests (bronchial challenge) can be helpful aids in diagnosis (Aas, 1970). Histamine or methacholine (Mecholyl) bronchial challenge tests can be used to demonstrate hyperreactivity manifested as bronchial obstruction with or without wheezing. Bronchial challenge with histamine and methacholine (and exercise challenge tests in the occasional child with cardiac or other abnormalities) are potentially dangerous and

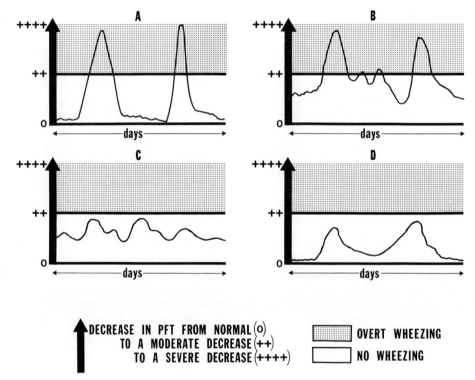

FIGURE 42–3. "Iceberg" concept of bronchial asthma. For explanation, see text.

should be left to appropriate consultants. They are outlined briefly for background information, however, to facilitate both the decision for referral and interpretation of test results. With a history suggestive of exercise-induced asthma, an exercise that constitutes a more "physiologic" bronchial provocation test is preferred.

Asthmatic airways are approximately 10- to 100-fold more sensitive to the bronchoconstrictive effects of histamine than are normal airways (Cade and Pain, 1972), and even more hyperresponsive to methacholine by aerosol. When histamine or methacholine challenges are performed, baseline pulmonary functions are obtained and the response to diluent alone assessed to identify any irritant effect unrelated to the test chemical. Graded doses of histamine or methacholine are then administered using standardized methods, described by Chai et al. (1975). A bronchodilating aerosol or adrenaline always is on hand to reverse any bronchoconstriction that occurs. Histamine challenge tests will elicit bronchoconstriction in approximately 90 percent of patients with bronchial asthma (Mellis et al., 1978), whereas methacholine administration will identify at least 89 percent and up to 100 percent, depending on the sensitivity of pulmonary function tests utilized (Kiviloog, 1973). Although histamine and methacholine have been widely used in bronchial challenge testing, there is little information on their side effects. Evidence obtained in animal studies suggests that *repeated* exposure to methacholine may result in irreversible lung injury (Binns et al., 1975).

Exercise testing is an extremely useful technique for demonstrating airway hyperreactivity (Cropp, 1975) and to assess the effects of medication in preventing exercise-induced bronchospasm (EIB). Exercise testing compared with the tests described above is less sensitive in the identification of patients with hyperreactive airways. However, it is considered safer and of particular value in attempting to reproduce and assess the significance of symptoms related to exercise. It is of additional value in convincing certain patients (especially competitive teenagers) that medications prescribed, if taken properly, are efficacious and can ameliorate or completely abort exercise-induced bronchospasm (Bierman et al., 1977). In order to demonstrate EIB, the patient's pulse rate should reach and be maintained during exercise at a level equal to 80–85 percent of predicted maximum. With a history of EIB, it is seldom necessary "to push" a patient to get an adequate objective response, especially if sensitive measures such as $FEF_{25-75\%}$ are used. Suggestions for standardized exercise tests have been made (Buckley et al., 1974; Sly, 1970; Eggleston and Guerrant, 1976), but agreement on these sugggestions is not universal.

A note of caution about these tests already has been voiced, especially with regard to methacholine and histamine challenge tests, which can provoke serious and even fatal bronchoconstriction. It is emphasized that such testing should be left in the hands of experienced specialists. This also applies to the use of allergens in bronchoprovocation tests. The technique for this procedure has been described in detail elsewhere (Chai et al., 1975). The bronchoprovocation test using an allergen (e.g., animal dander) can be used to provide proof of clinical significance of allergen exposure, but generally is not necessary for intelligent diagnosis and treatment of allergic disorders.

PULMONARY FUNCTIONS IN VARIOUS CLINICAL STAGES OF ASTHMA

As pointed out by Bates et al. (1971), asthmatic patients may be seen in various clinical states: in complete remission; in partial remission; with moderate bronchial obstruction; with severe bronchial obstruction; and in status asthmaticus.

Period of Complete Remission (Symptom-Free Period). In this symptom-free period, all available pulmonary function test results often are found to be normal. It is a frequent observation that the morning after a patient has had an asthmatic attack, the dynamic pulmonary functions such as those tested by spirometry will be normal; however, little data exist indicating whether hyperinflation (increased RV) is present. One abnormality still present in this period of remission is persistent bronchial hyperreactivity.

Period of Partial Remission. In this stage an asthmatic child may be regarded by the physician as in complete remission.

However, there are persistent abnormalities in pulmonary functions. Weng and Levison (1969) studied 30 asthmatic children during a symptom-free period. Vital capacity was normal, but other static volumes such as RV and TLC were elevated. An increase in the resting respiratory level toward inspiration also was found. The increase in RV and the trapped air volume are responsible for lung hyperinflation. In Weng and Levison's study, the only dynamic volume found to be abnormal was $FEF_{25-75\%}$, which, as indicated previously, is a relatively sensitive measure of airway obstruction.

Moderate to Severe Airway Obstruction. In these two clinical stages the most frequent pulmonary functions demonstrate air flow abnormalities. Significant decreases are found in FEV_1, $FEF_{25-75\%}$ and FEV_1/FVC. These changes often can be suspected from the history or by auscultation, but are easily quantified in the office by spirometry. As expected, body plethysmography measurements are markedly abnormal, indicating hyperinflation. Increases in airway resistance and FRC usually are found.

Status Asthmaticus. During initial therapy of status asthmaticus, the most valuable technique for determining the clinical status of the patient is by blood gas analysis rather than pulmonary function tests. Once blood gas measurements stabilize, spirograms become useful for follow-up measurements. Little attention has been given to testing pulmonary functions immediately after acute attack. The duration of the recovery period often is surprisingly long when pulmonary function tests are used when compared to reliance on the patient's history and physical examination alone.

PRACTICAL USE OF PULMONARY FUNCTION TESTS IN THE OFFICE

Cases have been chosen to illustrate the value and use of pulmonary function tests in the care of patients with asthma. These are intended to demonstrate how the patient's clinical history and the physician's findings alone, without pulmonary function tests, may mislead the physician into prescribing inappropriate therapy or stopping therapy too quickly, or may encourage the physician

to use more aggressive therapy (e.g., steroids) to prove or disprove reversibility of the condition. Pulmonary function tests can aid the physician in deciding when to curtail such aggressive therapy or to refer the patient for further tests if reversibility is not easily demonstrated. To the physician treating chest diseases, especially those associated with hyperreactive airways, pulmonary function tests are as important as the stethoscope.

CASE 1

Clinical History. S.D., the 13-year-old brother of a patient with well-established bronchial asthma, presented with a history of chronic coughing for 2 months, associated with "throat drainage" and "chest tightness" that was most pronounced with exercise. Symptoms were worse at night and were unassociated with fever. The cough was unresponsive to decongestants, expectorants, and cough suppressants.

Findings on Physical Exam. Intermittent, thick pharyngeal mucus. Rhonchi by auscultation, but no wheezing.

Results of Pulmonary Function Tests (PFT's):

Baseline PFT's. FVC, FEV_1, and PEFR all within normal range.
Post-Bronchodilator. Insignificant increase in FVC, FEV_1 and PEFR.
Post-Exercise. No decrease in pulmonary function tests.
Methacholine Bronchoprovocation. No decrease in pulmonary function tests.

Sinus X-Ray Film. Both maxillary antra diffusely clouded.

Comments. Because of the noted family history of asthma (brother) and the nocturnal and post-exercise coughing problem, the presence of hyperreactive airways was suspected, but ruled out by the appropriate pulmonary function and bronchoprovocation tests. The correct diagnosis was then made from the sinus x-ray films. Treatment of sinusitis resulted in complete resolution of symptoms and physical findings, as well as clearing of the sinus films.

CASE 2

Clinical History. C.P. was a 7-year-old girl who had a history of asthma in infancy, with frequent severe attacks of asthma despite administration of regular, appropriate-dose, round-the-clock bronchodilators; intermittent, short-term oral steroids; and inhaled steroids. At no time in her 18-month record of treatment in the physician's office had she had normal or close to normal pulmonary function test findings. The obvious question was, how much of her airway obstruction was reversible?

Findings on Physical Exam. Non-cushingoid patient with no dyspnea or retractions, but with a moderately hyperinflated chest with increased anteroposterior diameter. On chest auscultation, she demonstrated symmetrically decreased breath sounds with inspiratory and expiratory wheezing and a prolonged expiratory phase.

Chest X-Ray Film. Moderate hyperexpansion only.

Results of Pulmonary Function Tests (PFT's). FVC and FEV_1 were 43 percent of predicted, PEFR and MMEF were 15 percent of predicted. Minimal changes in pulmonary function test results were seen after epinephrine injection and isoetharine inhalation. After a 4 week course of oral steroids, she showed a marked improvement with nearly complete reversal (100 per-

cent of predicted) in all pulmonary function test results, except 90 percent for PEFR and 88 percent for MMEF. The pulmonary functions remained normal as steroids were slowly tapered and discontinued over an additional 4 weeks while oral bronchodilators were continued.

Comments. In treating patients with obstructive airway problems, whether child or adult, it is necessary to verify the amount of reversibility. When a patient's pulmonary function tests return to the normal range, the patient's asthma often becomes more stable, and in some cases, all oral steroids and inhaled bronchodilators can be stopped. The pulmonary function tests were used as an objective method first to monitor the effectiveness of the treatment and, second, to guide the physician in timing the tapering and discontinuation of oral steroids. If significant (not necessarily complete) reversal of pulmonary obstruction is not demonstrated by aggressive therapy for asthma, the diagnosis of asthma (reversible obstructive airway disease) is suspect. Additional diagnostic tests are indicated to establish the proper diagnosis.

References

Aas, K.: Bronchial provocation tests in asthma. Arch. Dis. Child. *45*:221, 1970.

Angus, G. E., and Thurlbeck, W. M.: The number of alveoli in the human lung. J. Appl. Physiol. *32*:483, 1972.

Bates, D. V., Macklem, P. T., and Christie, R. V.: *Respiratory Function in Disease.* Philadelphia, W. B. Saunders Co., 1971.

Bierman, C. W., Pierson, E., and Shapiro, G. G.: Effects of drugs on exercise-induced bronchospasm. *In* Dempsey, A., and Reed, E. (eds.): *Muscular Exercise and the Lung,* University of Wisconsin Press, 1977, pp. 289–300.

Binns, R., Clark, G. C., and Hardy, C. J.: Methacholine: A 7-day inhalation toxicity study with primates. Toxicology *4*:117, 1975.

Bouhuys, A.: *Breathing: Physiology, Environment and Lung Disease.* New York, Grune and Stratton, 1974, pp. 187–191.

Buckley, J. M., Souhrada, J. F., and Kopetzky, M. T.: Detection of airway obstruction in exercise-induced asthma. Chest *66*:244, 1974.

Buist, S. A., van Fleet, D. L., and Ross, B. R.: A comparison of conventional spirometric tests and the test of closing volume in an emphysema screening center. Am. Rev. Respir. Dis. *107*:735, 1973.

Cade, J. F., and Pain, M. C. F.: Lung function in provoked asthma: Responses to inhaled urea, methacholine, and isoprenaline. Clin. Sci. *43*:759, 1972.

Chai, H., Farr, R. S., Froehlich, L. A., Mathison, O. A., McLean, J. A., Rosenthal, R. R., Sheffer, A. L., Spector, S. L., and Townley, R. G.: Standardization of bronchial inhalation challenge procedures. J. Allergy Clin. Immunol. *56*:323, 1975.

Charnock, E. L., and Doershuk, C. F.: Development aspects of the human lungs. Pediatr. Clin. North Am. *20*:275, 1973.

Cherniack, R. M.: *Pulmonary Function Testing.* Philadelphia, W. B. Saunders Co., 1977.

Cotes, J. E.: Genetic factors affecting the lung. Bull. Physiol. Pathol. Respir. *10*:109, 1974.

Cropp, G. H. A.: Exercise-induced asthma. Pediatr. Clin. North Am. *22*:63, 1975.

Dickman, M. L., Schmidt, C. D., and Gardner, R. M.: Spirometric standards for normal children and adolescents (age 5 years through 18 years). Am. Rev. Respir. Dis. *104*:680, 1971.

Dunnill, M. S.: Postnatal growth of the lung. Thorax *17*:329, 1962.

Eggleston, P. A., and Guerrant, J. L.: A standardized method of evaluating exercise-induced asthma. J. Allergy Clin. Immunol. *58*:414, 1976.

Fitzgerald, M. X., Smith, A. A., and Gaensler, E. A.: Evaluation of "electronic" spirometers. N. Engl. J. Med. *289*:1283, 1973.

Goddard, R.: Pre-emphysema in children. Its recognition and treatment. Ann. Allergy *19*:1125, 1961.

Hutcheson, M., Griffin, P., Levison, H., and Zamel, N.: Volume of isoflow. A new test in detection of mild abnormalities of lung mechanics. Am. Rev. Respir. Dis. *110*:458, 1974.

Kanner, R. E., and Morris, A. H. (eds.): *Clinical Pulmonary Function Testing.* Salt Lake City, Intermountain Thoracic Society, 1975.

Kiviloog, J.: Bronchial reactivity to exercise and methacholine in bronchial asthma. Scand. J. Respir. Dis. *54*:347, 1973.

Kory, R. C., Rankin, J., Snider, G. L., and Tomashefski, J. F.: Clinical spirometry: Recommendation of the section on pulmonary function testing. Dis. Chest *43*:214, 1963.

Kotas, R. V., Mims, L. C., and Hart, L. K.: Reversible inhibition of lung cell number after glucocorticoid injections into fetal rabbits to enhance surfactant appearance. Pediatrics *53*:358, 1974.

Lim, T. P. K.: Airway obstruction among high school students. Am. Rev. Respir. Dis. *108*:985, 1973.

Macklem, P. T.: Airway obstruction and collateral ventilation. Physiol. Rev. *51*:368, 1971.

Matsuba, K., and Thurlbeck, W. M.: A morphometric study of bronchial and bronchiolar walls in children. Am. Rev. Respir. Dis. *105*:908, 1972.

McFadden, E. R., Kiker, R., Holmer, B. and deGrott, J. W.: Small airway disease. An assessment of the tests of peripheral airway function. Am. J. Med. *57*:171, 1974.

Mellis, C. M., Kattan, M., Keens, T. G., and Levison, H.: Comparative study of histamine and exercise challenges in asthmatic children. Am. Rev. Respir. Dis. *117*:914, 1978.

NIH Report: Suggested standard procedures for closing volume determination (nitrogen method), Division of Lung Disease, National Institute of Heart and Lung, 1971.

Polgar, G., and Promadhat, V. (eds.): *Pulmonary Function Testing in Children.* Philadelphia, W. B. Saunders, 1971.

Shephard, R. J., and Seliger, V.: On the estimation of total lung capacity from chest x-rays. Radiographic and helium dilution estimates on children aged 10–12 years. Respiration *26*:327, 1969.

Sly, R. M.: Exercise-related changes in airway obstruction: Frequency and clinical correlates in asthmatic children. Ann. Allergy *28*:1, 1970.

Souhrada, J. F., and Buckley, J. M.: Pulmonary function testing in asthmatic children. Pediatr. Clin. North Am. *23*:249, 1976.

Steiner, N., and Phelan, P. D.: Physiological assessment of severe chronic asthma in children. Respiration *35*:30, 1978.

Tooley, W. H., DeMuth, M. D., and Nadel, J. A.: The reversibility of obstructive changes in severe childhood asthma. J. Pediatr. *66*:517, 1965.

Weng, T. R., and Levison, H.: Pulmonary fubction in children with asthma at acute attack and symptom-free status. Am. Rev. Respir. Dis. *99*:719, 1969.

Wright, B. M., and McKerrow, C. B.: Maximum forced expiratory flow rate as a measure of ventilatory capacity. Br. Med. J. *2*:1041, 1959.

Zapletal, A., Motoyama, E. K., Van de Woestinjne, K. P., and Bouhuys, A.: Maximal expiratory flow-volume curves and airway conductance of children and adolescents. J. Appl. Physiol. *26*:308, 1969.

Peyton A. Eggleston, M.D.
Edwin L. Kendig, Jr., M.D.

43

Obstructive Diseases of the Larynx and Trachea

Obstructive lesions of the larynx and trachea frequently present with stridor and spasmodic cough; thus they may be confused with asthma occasionally. This especially is true of those that are recurrent, such as croup, or those that produce chronic cough. This chapter describes the more common obstructive conditions of the larynx and trachea and identifies important clinical points that help distinguish these conditions from asthma.

EPIGLOTTITIS

Epiglottitis is a "cellulitis" of the larynx, pharynx, and epiglottis induced by a specific organism, *Haemophilus influenzae,* type b. Although other organisms such as the streptococci may infect the pharynx, *H. influenzae* seems uniquely capable of producing rapidly progressive, diffuse cellulitic involvement of both the laryngeal and pharyngeal structures. Fortunately, children rapidly develop immunity to the causative organism, thus making this an uncommon disease.

The anatomy of the larynx is illustrated in Figure 43–1 to facilitate an understanding of why cellulitis may cause obstruction. The cricoid cartilage encircles the larynx. The posteriorly located epiglottis serves as a flap valve to limit inspiration of food and water. The mucosa of the epiglottis, vocal cords, and the peritonsillar tissue are continuous anteriorly and are enveloped in loose areolar tissue, which allows freer movement and aids in phonation. Obstruction may follow rapidly when cellulitis involves the larynx or cord in this loose areolar tissue, or when a swollen epiglottic flap valve obstructs the laryngeal inlet.

The onset of epiglottitis is abrupt (8 to 24 hours), and the child develops stridor with or without a croupy cough. Characteristically, the patient is febrile, toxic, and lethargic and complains of marked pharyngeal pain, frequently so severe that the child will drool rather than swallow. There is marked leukocytosis and frequent occurrence of bacteremia (80 percent) with *Haemophilus influenzae.*

The combination of croup, dysphagia, and severe toxicity should alert the physician to the possibility of epiglottitis. Any attempt to confirm the diagnosis by visualization of the epiglottis should be approached with extreme caution since in a large proportion (10 to 40 percent) of children with this syndrome abrupt occlusion of the larynx will occur. If epiglottitis is suspected, an anesthesiologist, otolaryngologist, or surgeon accustomed to emergency resuscitation should be present, with equipment for intubation ready, before the child is examined.

An alternative method of confirming the diagnosis is a lateral neck roentgenogram to identify the swollen, bulbous epiglottis. This is not the procedure of choice when the diagnosis is highly suspect since acute obstruction may occur while the roentgenogram is being taken. It is used more appropriately to rule out the syndrome in less well-defined

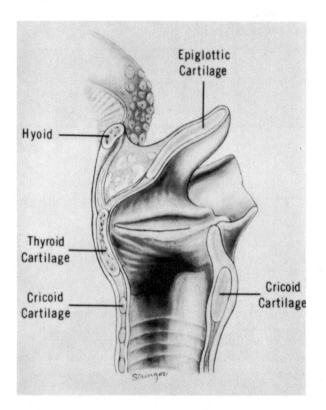

Epiglottic
Cartilage

Hyoid

Thyroid
Cartilage

Cricoid
Cartilage

Cricoid
Cartilage

FIGURE 43–1. Sagittal view of the larynx showing normal anatomic relationships.

cases. Even in these conditions, a physician should be present while the x-ray examination is made.

Other diseases usually considered in the differential diagnosis of epiglottitis are spasmodic croup and laryngotracheobronchitis. Neither of these two syndromes is associated with extreme toxicity. In borderline situations in which fever and leukocytosis are present, a lateral neck roentgenogram to demonstrate the presence or absence of an enlarged epiglottis is appropriate.

Epiglottitis is an emergency, and the child so affected should be hospitalized promptly. Because of the high mortality rate (30 percent) and because death usually results from abrupt obstruction, it generally is accepted that emergency creation of an artificial airway, either insertion of a nasotracheal tube (Milko et al., 1974) or tracheostomy (Margolis et al., 1972) should be performed as soon as the diagnosis is made. Intravenous antibiotic treatment with ampicillin, 150 mg per kg of body weight per day, and chloramphenicol, 50 to 100 mg per kg of body weight per day, should be instituted immediately. Treatment with both ampicillin and chloramphenicol should be instituted because ampicillin-resistant organisms are being encountered now with increasing fre-

quency. Once appropriate measures are undertaken, the syndrome subsides rapidly, and extubation usually is possible after 1 to 2 days.

CROUP
(LARYNGOTRACHEOBRONCHITIS)

Croup occurs most commonly between 3 months and 3 years of age and is characterized by a barking cough and inspiratory obstruction, apparently the result of widespread infection of large airways.

In the majority of cases, the infecting agent is viral. Characteristically, this is a parainfluenza virus, most often type 3, but many other viruses also have been found, including influenza, adenovirus, rhinovirus, and enterovirus (Glezen et al., 1971). These viruses are associated with croup only when younger children are infected. Infection with these viruses in older children and adults usually is associated with nonspecific upper respiratory symptoms. It thus appears that an unusual host response rather than a specific organism is necessary to produce the syndrome in these age groups.

Several mechanisms may be involved in causing laryngeal and tracheal obstruction. Edema and inflammation of the larynx, trachea, and bronchi may narrow the lumen. These changes usually are seen in the rare cases that have been autopsied. Since the resistance to nonturbulent air flow relates to the fourth power of the radius, the decreased luminal area in the narrower airways of young children will be reflected in large changes in flow.

Muscular spasm also appears to be responsible for some part of the obstruction. Although this is most likely to be on the basis of reflex laryngospasm, tracheobronchial smooth muscle spasm resulting from inflammation also may contribute. In some children, the abrupt onset and resolution of obstruction suggest that this mechanism is the predominant cause; these children are more prone to recurrence of the syndrome. Excessive or viscid secretions also may be a problem.

Even though much of the obstruction is in the extrathoracic airway, high intrathoracic pressures generated during a cough may cause the flexible trachea of the young child to collapse, increasing the obstruction.

Typically, the sequence in a child with croup begins with an upper respiratory infection or "cold," without unusual toxicity or fever. The croup syndrome may begin with hoarseness, then progress to a dry, hacking cough that becomes brassy as inspiratory stridor and hoarseness develop. Alternatively the brassy cough, hoarseness, and stridor may develop abruptly. Croup occurs usually at night, most often reaching a peak at about 10 to 11 o'clock. Depending on the severity of obstruction, the child may be anxious, air-hungry, and dyspneic. Crying and agitation may lead to frequent spasms of coughing, which increase obstruction.

Although fever may be present, the child usually is afebrile and hoarse. Lethargy and toxicity are not noteworthy usually, but some stridor and sternal and lower rib retractions are present. In severe cases, children are anxious, agitated, and cyanotic. Chest examination reveals only stridor and transmitted sounds of upper airway secretions.

There is no specific therapy, and the most important aspect of management is careful, expectant observation. Hospitalization is indicated if close observation is not possible at home, if there is any question about the severity, or if the process appears to be worsening.

The usual treatment at home consists of the use of a vaporizer, increased oral intake of fluids, and bed rest. Syrup of ipecac in sub-emetic doses (1 drop per month of age up to 2 years) is believed to help resolve spasmodic croup syndrome. Caution should be exercised when using ipecac in any child with severe obstruction to avoid aspiration of the vomitus.

After examination in the emergency room has determined that the child does not have epiglottitis, inhalation of 2.25 percent racemic epinephrine nebulization may be tried (Adair et al., 1971). Even if the patient shows improvement after such inhalation, response may be temporary (Westley, 1978). The patient therefore should be retained in the emergency room for at least 4 hours after satisfactory response.

In the hospital, the respiratory rate, sternal retractions, and the degree of stridor and cyanosis should be monitored carefully. The patient should be placed in a room close to a nursing station. At the same time, every effort must be made to keep the child quiet and undisturbed since agitation and apprehension may exacerbate obstruction. The use of blood gas determinations, which would otherwise be an extremely helpful method of assessing severity, therefore should be limited.

Moisture and increased inspired oxygen tension can be provided in a mist tent. However, the potential benefits must be balanced against the disadvantages of increasing the child's anxiety and making observation more difficult. Effective drug treatment is limited. If symptoms respond to racemic epinephrine, treatment may be continued with doses given every 1 to 2 hours; however, the patient should be observed carefully for marked or persistent tachycardia. A recent publication (Leipzig et al., 1979) suggests that corticosteroid therapy may be helpful.

The chief complication of the syndrome is respiratory failure and cardiorespiratory arrest. This is uncommon, and tracheostomy is required in only 2 to 8 percent of cases. Recurrences are more likely to occur in children who have a clearly spasmodic component.

The most important differential diagnosis is epiglottitis. The appearance of a toxic, febrile child, sometimes with dysphagia and drooling, should alert the physician. Such a child should have a careful examination of the epiglottis visually or by lateral neck roentgenogram, observing the same precautions noted earlier.

Asthma may be confused with croup, especially recurrent croup. One should be suspicious if there is a suggestion of wheezing, if the response to epinephrine is impressive, or if there is a strong family history of asthma.

Both pertussis and croup are characterized by a tight, spasmodic cough and both occur in younger children. Immunization history, peripheral lymphocytosis, and the duration of illness should make differentiation easy. The possibility of aspirated foreign body should be considered whenever the croup syndrome begins abruptly without preceding upper respiratory tract infection, especially if localized obstruction or pneumonia is seen on chest roentgenogram.

TRACHEOMALACIA AND BRONCHOMALACIA

Tracheomalacia and bronchomalacia are syndromes caused by excessive flexibility of the trachea and exacerbated by respiratory infection involving that area. They are characterized by signs of obstruction, chiefly during expiration, and by noisy breathing and recurrent infections. The conditions occur predominantly in infancy, usually early infancy, and spontaneous resolution occurs with age.

Expiratory obstruction occurs with tracheomalacia because intrathoracic airways are affected by pressures generated during respiration. During quiet respiration, with normal, compliant lungs, minor negative intrathoracic pressures are generated to expand the lungs. Expiration occurs as the elasticity of the lungs and thorax restores expiratory volume, and little positive pressure is developed. However, during a cough with normal lungs, intrathoracic pressure may briefly rise to 300 cm of water; with obstructive lung disease, quiet respiration may induce pressures of 10 to 20 cm of water.

The shape of the trachea and bronchi normally are maintained by cartilage rings and by the elastic properties of the lung. Obviously, any factors that increase elasticity of the trachea or bronchi, or decrease elasticity of the lungs, will cause airway compression during normal respiration and coughing. At the same time, more widespread lung disease may increase intrathoracic pressures and cause normal airways to collapse.

However, expiratory compression forces do not occur throughout the tracheobronchial tree. In the very small airways at the periphery of the lung, pressure changes occur almost simultaneously with those elsewhere in the lung. At the upper trachea, airway pressure is near atmospheric level (zero), until expiratory air flow progresses to that point. Since expiratory pressure in the surrounding lung is higher, maximal collapsing forces are generated at the upper trachea. Progressing from the trachea toward the alveoli, pressure inside airways approaches that in the surrounding lung. At some point, airway and lung pressures are equal, and there are no collapsing forces in the more distal airways. This *equal pressure point* occurs in segmental bronchi in the normal lung.

Since autopsied cases rarely demonstrate absent cartilage (Baxter and Dunbar, 1963) and since tracheomalacia usually is most apparent in the upper trachea (Wittenborg et al., 1967), it is felt by some that tracheomalacia almost always is due to coincident lung disease and secondary tracheal compression. An obvious exception is the localized deformity of the trachea or bronchi that follows removal of an extrabronchial mass.

The onset of symptoms associated with tracheomalacia usually is abrupt, beginning with a respiratory infection in early infancy, but the syndrome may have a more insidious beginning. A barking, croupy cough is prominent and resolves more slowly than with the usual croup. There may be an associated stridor, but evidence of loose, moist expiratory obstruction and wheezing is more common. Crying or exertion may promote obstruction and thus precipitate bouts of coughing. Recurrent infections are common, and with each one the pattern of respiratory distress with obstruction, brassy cough, and slow resolution repeats itself.

In the rare case of localized absence of bronchial cartilage, the chest roentgenogram may show localized hyperinflation of a lobe or lung. More commonly one sees only peribronchial or interstitial infiltrates and generalized hyperinflation. Inspiratory and expiratory radiograms show excessive motion in the trachea, just under the glottis. This excessive motion is even more apparent with cinefluoroscopy. In the occasional case in which bronchoscopy is performed, the tracheal and bronchial walls may be seen to flex inward during expiration.

In general the prognosis is good. Mortality is low, and most children improve spontaneously by 3 to 4 years of age.

Treatment is nonspecific and supportive.

Humidified oxygen may be necessary, and chest percussion and postural drainage may be helpful. Bacterial infections should be treated aggressively with antibiotics. Above all, careful follow-up should be maintained in order to detect any significant increase in respiratory difficulty. Surgical therapy rarely is indicated. In general, even the localized deformity associated with extrabronchial obstruction is too extensive for successful resection. Lobar resection for localized bronchomalacia may improve oxygenation by removing hyperinflated lung that may be compressing adjacent normal lung. It is important to investigate and manage any suspected associated lung disease.

A number of diseases should be considered in the differential diagnosis. As mentioned previously, the syndrome may occur secondary to pulmonary diseases that diffusely decrease compliance (viral interstitial pneumonia, desquamative interstitial pneumonitis, pulmonary hemosiderosis), to cardiac disease that decreases lung compliance, or to pulmonary diseases with generalized obstruction of the airway (e.g., asthma, bronchiolitis obliterans). Differential diagnosis from asthma may be especially difficult since wheezing, hyperinflation, coughing, and upper respiratory infection–related exacerbations can be seen with either.

OBSTRUCTIVE LESIONS — MASSES

Many lesions in and around airways present with symptoms that mimic croup or asthma, and that must be considered in a differential diagnosis. These may be categorized into extrabronchial, intrabronchial, and intramural lesions.

Extrabronchial Lesions

Neoplasms may involve intrathoracic structures and thus impinge on airways (Whittaker and Lynn, 1973). The most common include: lymphoid tissue (Hodgkin's disease, lymphosarcoma, leukemia, lymph node metastases); neural crest tissue (neuroblastoma, ganglioneuroma, ganglioneuroblastoma); thymus (thymoma, lymphosarcoma, teratoma); and miscellaneous tissues (teratoma, cystic hygroma).

Lymphoid tissue may be involved in nonneoplastic, inflammatory processes. The thymus characteristically is large in infants and may sometimes impinge on the airway if placed high in the thoracic outlet. Similarly, lymphadenopathy associated with tuberculosis, fungal, or bacterial lung disease may compromise the airway. Primary pulmonary tuberculosis almost invariably presents with hilar adenopathy; in most instances a parenchymal lesion cannot be demonstrated, even though one necessarily exists. Sarcoidosis occasionally involves paratracheal nodes and almost always produces bilateral hilar lymphadenopathy; parenchymal lesions are present in about half the cases.

Bronchogenic cysts are uncommon. They are usually single and occur more commonly in the area of the right mainstem bronchus and to the right of the trachea.

A variety of vascular anomalies can compress the airways. They most commonly produce a vascular ring syndrome (right aortic arch with persistent ductus or ligamentum arteriosis, double aortic arch), with compression of both the esophagus and trachea. In addition, a pulmonary sling may be produced by an aberrrant left pulmonary artery arising from the right and crossing the trachea and left mainstem bronchus to supply the left lung, or by an innominate artery arising to the left of the trachea. Finally, hemangiomas may compress the airways.

It should be apparent that most lesions causing extrabronchial compression are located in the mediastinum. The anterior mediastinum contains the thymus and the anterior aspect of the heart. The most common anterior mediastinal masses are hyperplastic thymus and teratomas; when enlarged, they frequently cause respiratory symptoms. The posterior mediastinum contains principally neural tissue and the esophagus. The most common posterior mediastinal masses are neurogenic tumors; respiratory symptoms are encountered only late in the course. The middle mediastinum contains the heart, airways, great vessels, and lymph nodes. The most common middle mediastinal masses are hyperplastic or neoplastic lymph nodes, or bronchogenic cysts; respiratory symptoms occur early.

Certain lesions are most commonly found at a particular age. Bronchogenic cysts, cystic hygromas, and teratomas are most commonly encountered before 2 years of age. Lymphomas, leukemic adenitis, and fungal adenitis are more commonly seen in older school-age children and adolescents.

Symptoms are produced either by direct compression of the airway or by secondary complications. Compression may lead to a persistent wheeze, to atelectasis, or to air-trapping and hyperinflation. Stridor is unusual unless the lesion is high in the superior mediastinum. Vagal reflexes may lead to more widespread wheezing. Secondary problems may arise when secretions cannot be cleared and become infected, or when a vessel eroded by the mass bleeds into the airway or mediastinum.

Symptoms begin insidiously unless bleeding or infection occurs or unless a cyst ruptures into the airway. Usually an irritative cough, stridorous respiration, and wheezing or dysphagia constitute the earliest symptoms. Chest discomfort, pain, fever, and weight loss usually occur later.

Routine posterior-anterior and lateral chest roentgenograms usually will localize the lesion to a particular mediastinal section. Examination of the tracheobronchial air columns may demonstrate local compression. A barium esophagram may further help define the extent and location of the mass. Tomograms are useful. Computerized axial tomography may be helpful, but its exact role in evaluation is not yet defined.

Laboratory studies furnish supporting evidence. A hemogram may demonstrate anemia or leukocytosis, or the sedimentation rate may be elevated. Skin tests for tuberculosis and serology for fungal infections should be performed in all cases. Sputum or tracheal aspirates may be examined for cytology and fungal cultures. Urinary vanillylmandelic acid (V. M. A.) and hydrovanillylmandelic acid (H. V. A.) will be elevated with neuroblastomas.

Bronchoscopy may be extremely helpful, especially with the availability of the flexible bronchoscope: the site of the lesion can be identified and cultures, cytology, and biopsy obtained as appropriate. Although major technical problems still exist with use of bronchoscopy in smaller children, rapid progress is being made so that bronchoscopy may be a reasonable diagnostic procedure even in young children in the near future.

The treatment of most lesions is surgical. Prognosis depends on the specific lesion.

Intrabronchial lesions, which will be discussed below, and asthma constitute the major problems in differential diagnosis. It is well to recognize that a common disease such as asthma may coexist with one of these lesions and may further complicate diagnosis and treatment. For this reason, every child with severe asthma should have a chest roentgenogram, and any abnormalities should be defined.

Intrabronchial Lesions

Intrabronchial obstructive lesions usually are due to foreign bodies or neoplasms. Foreign bodies consist most often of particles of food, which usually lodge in the trachea or mainstem bronchi. However, anything may be aspirated and may lodge anywhere. Intrabronchial neoplasms most often reported in childhood are bronchial adenomas and papillomas. Papillomas may be multiple and recurrent and frequently are associated with laryngeal papilloma.

Obstruction from intrabronchial lesions may be partial, leading to localized wheezing and distal hyperinflation, or may be complete, leading to absorptive atelectasis. Infection frequently occurs, usually localized to the involved bronchus or to the lobe subserved by that bronchus. Generalized wheezing may occur, presumably mediated by vagal reflexes, and can confuse the picture of localized obstruction.

Intrabronchial obstruction usually presents with cough, which may be irritative at first and then productive, with dyspnea and with wheezing. Foreign bodies should be suspected when symptoms begin abruptly, especially when associated with gagging and apneic episodes, and particularly when symptoms occur in children 6 months to 6 years of age. Usual radiographic findings are localized hyperinflation or atelectasis. This is associated with a visible foreign object if the foreign body is radiopaque. Localized air-trapping may be suggested in expiratory films or fluoroscopy, by marked deviation away from the involved lobe on expiration. Alternatively, decubitus films may demonstrate that mediastinal structures will shift toward the normal lung when it is dependent but not toward the hyperinflated lung.

If an intrabronchial lesion is suspected, bronchoscopy should be performed as soon as possible but should be carried out only if an experienced bronchoscopist and an anesthesiologist are available, and the hospital is equipped for the study of infants. Occasionally, pneumonia or severe respiratory distress must be treated prior to bronchoscopy. The foreign body usually can be removed at bronchoscopy. Excisional biopsy specimens of tumors may be obtained in this way as well. Only bronchial adenomas require lobectomy.

Intrabronchial lesions should be suspected in any child with sudden onset of wheezing that resists the usual therapy for asthma, especially if there is anything in the history, physical examination, or laboratory evaluation to suggest a bronchial lesion. It is well to remember that wheezing may be generalized and may respond briefly or partially to bronchodilator therapy.

Intramural Lesions

Intramural lesions include neoplasms and postinflammatory mural thickenings. Purely intramural neoplasms are rare, and include hamartomas, bronchial adenomas, fibromas, leiomyosarcomas, and angiomas. In general, most lesions expand into the airway to produce intraluminal obstruction, rather than infiltrate the bronchial wall. Postinflammatory intramural obstruction occurs most often after prolonged intubation or after removal of a foreign body or tumor. An acute obstruction may be related to a reversible process (edema and inflammation), which may become both irreversible and more severe as a cicatrix forms.

Depending on the level of obstruction, illness may begin with stridor or wheezing observed chiefly during expiration. In general,

cough is not prominent and when present is productive. With upper respiratory infections or anything that increases tracheal secretions and inflammation, respiratory distress becomes more severe and may lead to acute respiratory failure.

Chest roentgenograms may show a localized constriction in the air bronchogram. Neoplasms are almost invariably associated with masses apparent in nodes around the airways or in the lung parenchyma. Barium esophagrams, tomograms, and computerized axial tomography may be helpful in defining the nature and extent of the lesion. Bronchoscopy may be helpful but should be employed with particular caution when significant obstruction is present.

Treatment is nonspecific in the case of inflammatory lesions. Humidification may be helpful. It is appropriate to use bronchodilators to relieve any bronchospastic component and to vasoconstrict local vessels; epinephrine and phenylephrine aerosols may accomplish both. Steroids may be helpful in preventing or treating postintubation obstruction. Surgical dilation, resection, or tracheostomy has been the only recourse in chronic cases.

The major lesions to be differentiated are other mass-obstructive lesions. For this reason, bronchoscopy, careful radiologic examination, and exploratory thoracotomy should be considered when the diagnosis is in question.

References

Adair, J. C., Ring, W. H., Jordan, W. S., et al.: Ten-year experience with IPPB in the treatment of acute laryngotracheo bronchitis. Anesth. Analg. 50:649, 1971.

Baxter, J. D., and Dunbar, J. S.: Tracheomalacia. Ann. Otol. Rhinol. Laryngol. 72:1013, 1963.

Glezen, W. P., Loda, F. A., Clyde, W. A., Jr., et al.: Epidemiologic patterns of acute lower respiratory disease of children in a pediatric group practice. J. Pediatr. 78:397, 1971.

Leipzig, B., Oski, F. A., Cummings, C. W., et al.: A prospective randomized study to determine the efficacy of steroids in treatment of croup. J. Pediatr. 94:194, 1979.

Margolis, C. Z., Ingram, D. L., and Meyer, J. H.: Routine tracheostomy in *Hemophilus influenzae* type b epiglottitis. J. Pediatr. 81:1150, 1972.

Milko, D. A., Marshak, G., and Striker, T. W.: Nasotracheal intubation in the treatment of acute epiglottitis. Pediatrics 53:674, 1974.

Westley, C. R., Cotton, E. K., and Brooks, J. G.: Nebulized racemic epinephrine by IPPB for the treatment of croup: A double-blind study. Amer. J. Dis. Child. 132:484, 1978.

Wittenborg, M. H., Gyepes, M. T., and Crocker, D.: Tracheal dynamics in infants with respiratory distress, stridor and collapsing trachea. Radiology 88:563, 1967.

Whittaker, L. D., Jr., and Lynn, H. B.: Mediastinal tumors and cysts in the pediatric patient. Surg. Clin. North Am. 53:893, 1973.

44

Howard Faden, M.D.
Elliot Ellis, M.D.

Acute Bronchopulmonary Infections

BRONCHITIS

Bronchitis is a frequently diagnosed but poorly characterized condition in childhood. It is scarcely mentioned in recent American pediatric textbooks (Rudolph, 1977; Hoekelman et al., 1978) and is, in a sense, an obsolete diagnostic term which reflects a concept that various disease states affect anatomically distinct divisions of the respiratory tract. Although signs and symptoms referable to one portion may predominate, the entire tract is usually involved when inflammation is induced by infections (especially viral) or toxins (e.g., chemical fumes, smoke). Even patients who are diagnosed as having a "cold" have evidence of peripheral airway dysfunction (Cate et al., 1973; Picken et al., 1972), and children with viral croup have evidence of lower respiratory tract involvement (Newth et al., 1972). Since the term "bronchitis" is so firmly implanted in medical practice, however, it will be used, even though the reader must recognize its limitations.

Acute Bronchitis. Acute bronchitis is a common manifestation of viral respiratory tract infection. All the major viral agents of childhood, including respiratory syncytial virus, parinfluenza virus, adenovirus, rhinovirus and influenza virus, may act as etiologic agents. There is little evidence that bacterial agents, other than *B. pertussis* and *M. tuberculosis,* have a primary role in acute bronchitis in children. The role of bacteria in chronic bronchitis will be discussed below.

Cough is the principal symptom of bronchitis and is due to stimulation of afferent vagal receptors in the airway. During the early stage of the illness, the cough is dry and irritative in character and adventitious sounds in the chest characteristically are absent. After 3 to 4 days, the cough becomes moist and looser, and at this time rhonchi and rattling sounds may be heard on auscultation. Sputum generally is not produced in significant quantities, and that which is usually is swallowed by young children. Typically, the chest roentgenogram is normal.

Asthmatic bronchitis or "wheezy bronchitis" is a diagnostic term applied to children, particularly those under 5 years of age, who wheeze with each respiratory infection but who are essentially free of respiratory symptoms in between. Williams and McNicol (1969), in a careful, long-term epidemiologic study, were unable to separate "wheezy bronchitis" as a distinctive entity from asthma during early life. There were no discernible differences in clinical features nor in outcome of children diagnosed as having wheezy bronchitis from those with asthma. Asthmatic bronchitis is a euphemism used by physicians who do not fully comprehend the spectrum of asthma in childhood (see Chapter 45). The

572

young child who has recurrent episodes of wheezing with viral respiratory infections should be considered as having asthma until proven otherwise.

Pertussis, which represents the most severe and best example of bacterial bronchitis in children, is due to a gram-negative rod, *Bordetella pertussis.* Other agents such as *Bordetella parapertussis* and adenovirus also have been reported to cause a similar clinical picture (Connor, 1970; Krugman and Ward, 1977). The illness begins with a highly infectious catarrhal stage which lasts 1 to 2 weeks, followed by several weeks of severe paroxysmal coughing. Coughing episodes may be severe enough to cause cyanosis and apnea. The greatest morbidity and mortality occurs in children less than 1 year of age.

When pertussis was prevalent in the past, the disease was noted to be the provocateur of the initial attack of asthma in some children. This observation is of particular interest because of the ability of *B. pertussis* to produce beta adrenergic blockade in animals that persists for many weeks. Furthermore, airway irritability in individuals recovering from pertussis appears to persist for many months. Children who have had pertussis recently may respond to subsequent viral illnesses with paroxysms of coughing similar to those observed during the pertussis illness. The frequency of asthma does not appear to be higher in pertussis-immunized children compared to those who have not received the pertussis vaccine, and thus there is little to suggest that pertussis immunization may predispose children to asthma.

The characteristic whooping cough suggests a diagnosis of pertussis. An additional aid includes the peripheral white blood cell count, which usually demonstrates an absolute lymphocytosis; but this finding may be absent in the very young child. The lymphocytosis is due to a disturbance in the normal pattern of lymphocyte recirculation, in which the rate of entry of lymphocytes from the blood into the lymphoid tissue is substantially decreased (Morse, 1976). Although culture of the nasopharynx is an excellent method to establish the diagnosis, most clinical bacteriology laboratories do not maintain the special (Bordet-Gengou) media needed to isolate the organism. Fluo-

rescent antibody staining of nasopharyngeal secretions is the most rapid and reliable diagnostic technique.

Primary tuberculosis with endobronchial involvement may produce a true bronchitis with signs and symptoms of large airway involvement. *Fungal involvement* of the bronchi is rarely encountered in children on a primary basis. *Bronchopulmonary aspergillosis* is not often diagnosed in children in the United States. This disorder is discussed in Chapter 47. With the increasing use of potent surface-active corticosteroids in children with asthma, monilial bronchitis due to local depression of cell-mediated immunity may be anticipated.

Chemical causes of acute bronchitis in children include aspiration of gastric contents in infants with functional deficiency of the cardioesophageal sphincter, smoke inhalation from burning buildings, cigarette smoke in teenagers who use tobacco, and perhaps air pollution in heavily polluted areas.

Acute infectious bronchitis of *viral etiology* is best treated symptomatically. During the acute stage of the disease, when the cough is irritative and nonproductive, a codeine-containing cough preparation may be prescribed.

Several antibiotics demonstrate *in vitro* activity against *B. pertussis,* but erythromycin is currently the drug of choice (Bass et al., 1969). It appears to limit the period of communicability and may prevent the appearance of clinical symptoms when used early in the incubation period (Altemeier and Ayoub, 1977). Unfortunately, treatment does not appear to shorten the course of the disease once significant clinical symptoms are manifested. Despite the prolonged illness, pulmonary sequelae are uncommon after pertussis. The treatment of primary tuberculosis with endobronchial involvement requires more aggressive therapy than that of uncomplicated primary tuberculosis (Kendig, 1977). Therapy of noninfectious acute bronchitis initially is symptomatic and subsequently is directed toward treatment or avoidance of the causative factor.

Chronic Bronchitis. In contrast to adult populations in whom chronic bronchitis is a reasonably well defined clinical condition with characteristic pathologic findings, the disorder is distinctly rare as a primary entity in children. Chronic bronchitis almost always occurs as a manifestation of an underlying disorder such as cystic fibrosis, humoral immune deficiency states (most often in those with panhypoimmunoglobulinemia, but perhaps in some children with isolated IgA deficiency), and Kartagener's syndrome. The organisms isolated from sputum cultures of the above patients vary with the disease. For example, in cystic fibrosis, staphylococci and *Pseudomonas* organisms are recovered most often, while in immune deficiency states, *Haemophilus influenzae* and *Streptococcus pneumoniae* predominate. Sputum production may be significant, particularly in older children. Typically, the sputum consists of polymorphonuclear leukocytes, mononuclear cells, and debris. Eosinophils are not present, a finding in contrast to the more or less regular presence of eosinophils in sputum from asthmatics. Many children who are labeled as having chronic bronchitis on the basis of chronic cough and perhaps some wheezing will be found, on careful study, to be suffering from asthma. In true chronic bronchitis due to underlying disease, clubbing of the extremities is common; it is extremely rare in asthma, a useful differential diagnostic feature.

Treatment of chronic bronchitis is principally directed toward the underlying disease. Pulmonary hygiene is most important and the full use of doses of antimicrobial agents on a regular basis in many patients seems to reduce sputum production and improves general well being. The fear of overwhelming infection due to emergence of resistant pathogens seems to be unfounded on the basis of clinical experience.

PNEUMONIA

Pneumonia is one of the most frequent and serious infections of childhood. Infants less than 1 year of age are prone to develop the most severe illness. Almost every class of microorganism has been shown to produce pneumonia in children. During the neonatal period, bacterial infections predominate. Viruses account for most of the illness thereafter in infancy, while myco-plasmas cause a significant proportion of disease in school-age children.

Identification of the infectious agents that cause pneumonia in children is frequently difficult. There are, however, certain features of bacterial pneumonias that help to differentiate them from viral or mycoplasma-caused disease (Table 44–1). The onset of bacterial illness usually is sudden, and the child appears toxic. In the infant, examination of the chest may be normal, but in the older child evidence of consolidation is present. The white blood cell count usually is in excess of 15,000/mm^3. Radiographs of the chest often demonstrate lobar or segmental consolidation, and pleural effusions frequently are present.

There is no simple method to identify the specific bacteria that may be etiologic in a given child. Sputum generally is unavailable and throat cultures are of little value in establishing the diagnosis since pathogenic bacteria such as *Streptococcus pneumoniae* inhabit the nasopharynx of healthy children (Loda et al., 1975). Blood cultures yield the causative agent in only about 25 percent of cases (Smith, 1977). Lung aspiration represents the most direct method to establish the diagnosis, but it usually is reserved for the seriously ill child or for the child who fails to respond to therapy.

Streptococcus pneumoniae remains the most common bacterial cause of pneumonia. The clinical picture of pneumococcal pneumonia is similar in children and adults; however, abdominal pain often is present in children and may lead to the mistaken diagnosis of appendicitis. Children with pneumococcal pneumonia respond rapidly to penicillin therapy. Small pleural effusions when present often resolve without drainage.

Staphylococcus aureus causes a severe, rapidly progressive pneumonia in the young infant. Empyema and pneumatoceles are common. The diagnosis often is established when the empyema fluid is drained and yields the organism. Unlike pneumococcal disease, staphylococcal pneumonia is slow to resolve despite effective treatment with a penicillinase-resistant penicillin. Ultimately, the pneumatoceles and pleural changes disappear, leaving no sequelae (Ceruti et al., 1971).

TABLE 44–1 CHARACTERISTIC FINDINGS IN BACTERIAL AND VIRAL PNEUMONIA

Findings	Bacterial	Viral
Onset	Sudden	Gradual
Progression	Rapid	Slow
Toxicity	Severe	Mild-moderate
Cough	Productive	Nonproductive
Fever	High	Low
Physical findings	Unilateral evidence of consolidation	Bilateral rales
X-ray findings	Lobar or segmental infiltrate; pleural effusions common	Diffuse, patchy bronchopneumonia; pleural effusions uncommon.
WBC	>15,000/mm³	≤15,000/mm³
Response to antibiotics	Good	None

Group A streptococcus may cause pneumonia in children. Effusions also occur with this organism. The diagnosis may be difficult to establish without the presence of empyema fluid. A rise in one of the streptococcal antibodies such as ASO may corroborate the diagnosis.

Haemophilus influenzae type b is becoming more important as a cause of pneumonia in children. Unfortunately, there are no distinctive signs or symptoms which suggest *H. influenzae* as the etiologic agent. However, it should be suspected in the young child who fails to respond to penicillin therapy. Unlike pneumococcal disease, haemophilus tends to produce a subacute process with lobar or bronchopneumonic infiltrates. The illness is slow to respond to appropriate therapy. Effusions occur in 50 percent of cases (Honig et al., 1973). The diagnosis may be established by blood culture or demonstration of the organism in pleural fluid. Recently developed diagnostic tests, such as countercurrent immunoelectrophoresis, may prove helpful in establishing the diagnosis. Since the appearance of ampicillin-resistant *Haemophilus influenzae*, chloramphenicol has become the drug of choice in the seriously ill child. The true incidence of this disease remains to be established, but recent reports suggest it is on the increase (Faden and Overall, 1976).

Mycobacterium tuberculosis is an infrequent cause of pneumonia in children today. The diagnosis often is considered only after the child fails to respond to routine antibiotic therapy. The presence of hilar adenopathy on the chest roentgenogram suggests the diagnosis, and a positive skin test with PPD provides supportive evidence. Isolation of the organism from sputum, gastric washings or urine confirms the diagnosis. Prolonged treatment with isoniazid in combination with para-aminosalicylic acid and streptomycin has been the traditional therapeutic regimen; however, the use of either rifampin or ethambutol with isoniazid may prove more effective (Lincoln and Sewell, 1977).

Mycoplasma pneumoniae accounts for 10 to 20 percent of all cases of pneumonia in childhood and is the primary cause of pneumonia among teenagers and young adults. It characteristically produces headache, low-grade fever, pharyngitis and a dry cough. Young infants may acquire the infection, but they manifest little or no disease (Fernald et al., 1975). Physical examination of the chest demonstrates rales. A chest radiograph shows a patchy infiltrate which often is more impressive in extent than the physical examination suggested. The diagnosis is suggested by the presence of serum cold agglutinins. Seventy to 90 percent of patients with mycoplasma develop elevated cold agglutinins (Chanock, 1965). Other infectious agents also have been shown to induce cold agglutinins, however (Sussman et al., 1966). Culture, which requires 2 to 3 weeks, and a specific complement fixation test remain the best methods to definitely establish the diagnosis. Numerous antibiotics have been used but only erythromycin and tetracycline seem effective. Despite treatment, patients continue to excrete the organism (Foy et al., 1966). Immunity to mycoplasma is not long lived, and repeated infections occur (Foy et al., 1977). The role of mycoplasma in chronic lung disease is not known.

Recently, *Chlamydia trachomatis,* an organism known to be a cause of urethritis in adults, has been identified as a significant cause of respiratory tract disease in children. Estimates of incidence range as high as 30 percent of all pneumonias in infants hospitalized during the first 6 months of life. Respiratory symptoms appear at 2 to 3 weeks of age, with the diagnosis made typically at 6 weeks. There is conjunctivitis by history in 50 percent of the affected infants. Systemic signs are minimal and the affected infants are not febrile. Nasal obstruction and mucoid discharge are common. Tachypnea in the range of 50 to 60 per minute is the most prominent finding. A staccato-like cough is present, similar to that of pertussis but without a whoop. On examination of the chest, hyperinflation is evident, breath sounds are not diminished, and crepitant rales are heard throughout. Expiratory wheezing is absent or minimal. Chest x-ray shows hyperinflation and diffuse interstitial and patchy alveolar infiltrates. Blood gases show a decreased Pao_2, with a normal or low $Paco_2$. IgG and IgM are increased, and there is a mild absolute eosinophilia. The course of the illness is protracted. Cough and tachypnea may last for several weeks, and rales and x-ray findings for a month or more (Beem and Saxon, 1977; Harrison et al., 1978). The organism requires special culture techniques, which few clinical laboratories are able to provide at present. The illness is of particular interest because of its many similar features to bronchiolitis and asthma in infancy.

At the present time, viruses are believed to be the most common cause of pneumonia in children. The clinical picture of viral pneumonia helps to distinguish it from bacterial disease (Table 44–1). Most often, viral pneumonia is found concurrently with upper respiratory illness. The illness progresses gradually over several days. Although the majority of children are not very ill, severe disease does occur, especially in the very young. Tachypnea is a common finding as are other signs of pneumonia, such as crepitant rales.

The total white blood cell count may be normal or minimally elevated. Chest roentgenograms demonstrate interstitial patchy infiltrates. Pleural effusions are uncommon.

Respiratory syncytial virus is the single most important agent that causes lower respiratory tract disease in children. It may be responsible for as much as 25 percent of all pneumonias in hospitalized patients (Kim et al., 1973). It tends to occur in outbreaks in mid-winter and early spring. Very young children are likely to develop severe disease. The reason (or reasons) for such severe disease in the young is (are) not well understood. Initially, it was believed that maternal antibody played a direct role in the pathogenesis of the disease (Chanock et al., 1970), but currently it is believed that cell-mediated immunity developed by the infant or child is associated in some way with the evolution of the disease (Scott et al., 1978).

Parainfluenza is the second most frequent viral cause of pneumonia in children. It cannot be distinguished clinically from other viral pneumonias.

Although *adenoviruses* 1 and 5 commonly produce disease in children, types 7 and 21 have been reported to cause severe disease (Lang et al., 1969; Brown et al., 1973). Children less than 2 years of age are the most susceptible. Hospital outbreaks of adenovirus have resulted in mortality rates approaching 25 percent (Brown et al., 1973). Among survivors, significant sequelae, including pulmonary fibrosis, bronchiectasis and obliterative bronchiolitis, have been observed (Lang et al., 1969).

Influenza virus has the potential to produce croup and bronchiolitis as well as pneumonia in children. Fever may be the only clinical sign in very young infants. In a single report, fever greater than 39° C occurred in more than 50 percent of infected children (Wright et al., 1977). Pneumonitis may be severe and lead to death. Secondary bacterial pneumonia is not uncommon. Chronic pulmonary changes have been reported in children developing disease in the first 4 years of life. These changes include radiographic evidence of fibrosis, bronchiectasis, and obliterative bronchiolitis. Obstructive and restrictive pulmonary function defects also have been observed during long-term follow-up (Laraya-Cuasay et al., 1977; Winterbauer et al., 1977).

Although no specific treatment for influenza exists, amantadine has been effective in preventing and possibly modifying the disease in adults; it has not been extensively studied in children. Influenza vaccine also prevents disease, but it is recommended only for children who are at high risk for severe disease (Report, 1977). Recent trials of influenza vaccine in children demonstrate significant febrile responses to whole virus vaccines (Gross et al., 1977). In contrast, split virus preparations produce less fever, but are less immunogenic and require more than one injection (Gross et al., 1977).

Pneumonia may occur as part of the clinical picture in such common childhood viral diseases as measles, varicella-zoster, and rubella. *Measles* produces a giant cell pneumonia which is seen during large outbreaks of disease, especially in malnourished populations. As with influenza, secondary bacterial pneumonia may complicate the clinical picture. *Varicella* pneumonia is uncommon in normal children but is seen with increasing frequency in immunosuppressed patients, such as those with leukemia. Normal adults who acquire varicella also are susceptible to developing primary varicella pneumonia. Pneumonia due to *rubella* is unusual; however, congenitally infected infants may develop a chronic form of pneumonia due to the virus.

Occasionally, parasites are responsible

for pneumonias in children. In the United States, *Ascaris lumbricoides* and *Toxocara canis* both produce a picture in which wheezing, pulmonary infiltrates and eosinophilia occur. Helminthic infestation has been suggested as a cause of asthma, but evidence for this is weak (Tullis, 1970).

BRONCHIOLITIS

Bronchiolitis is an acute inflammatory disease of airways that range in caliber from 300 μ to approximately 75 μ. The principal pathologic features of acute bronchiolitis are necrosis of the bronchiolar epithelium which sloughs into the lumen, increase in mucous secretions, and an inflammatory exudate, all of which combine to form dense plugs. A peribronchial infiltrate composed principally of lymphocytes occurs with some involvement of plasma cells and macrophages as well. There is edema of the submucosa and adventitial tissues but no damage to smooth muscle or elastic fibers. The degree and extent of bronchiolar obstruction determines whether acute obstructive emphysema (hyperinflation) or atelectasis occurs. Collateral ventilation is less well developed in the immature lung, and the small airways are disproportionately narrow. Both factors make the infant particularly vulnerable to bronchiolar inflammatory disease.

Infants affected with bronchiolitis show clinical findings that have been correlated physiologically in adults with small airway disease, namely tachypnea, hypoxemia (often profound), and hyperinflation. Limited studies of mechanics of breathing in infants with bronchiolitis have shown an FRC of about twice normal, decreased dynamic compliance, and increased total respiratory resistance. The abnormal physiologic findings revert to normal within 2 weeks after the acute illness. Bronchiolitis is principally a disease of the winter and spring months, affects males predominantly, and has its peak incidence during the first 6 months of life, at which time morbidity and mortality are higher. Epidemic bronchiolitis most often is due to respiratory syncytial virus and, to a lesser extent, parainfluenza virus. *M. pneumoniae* can cause the bronchiolitis syndrome in older children.

Signs, Symptoms, and Laboratory Findings. The illness commonly presents with signs and symptoms of a cold which usually has been transmitted from another member of the family. Low-grade fever usually not exceeding 39° C is present in the majority of patients. Tachypnea with respiratory rates of 50 to 60 breaths per minute, but sometimes as high as 80 breaths per minute, develops rapidly and is accompanied by cough, wheezing, and retractions. The infant appears dyspneic. Hyperinflation of the chest, which sometimes is extreme, is evident upon inspection and hyperresonance is noted upon percussion. Rales may be heard in addition to diffuse wheezing. The liver often is palpable as a result of diaphragmatic depression by the overinflated lungs. X-ray examination of the chest shows hyperlucency with increase in the anteroposterior diameter of the chest, retrosternal air, and flattening of the diaphragm. Small areas of increased density may be seen, representing atelectasis, and lung markings commonly are increased. Blood gas analysis almost always shows arterial hypoxemia as a result of $\dot{V}_A/\dot{Q}$ abnormality. The Pa_{CO_2} is variably altered as is the pH, depending upon the severity and stage of the illness. When acidosis is present, a metabolic component (due to accumulation of organic acids) may cause a substantial base deficit. The white blood cell count usually is moderately elevated.

Differential Diagnosis. Various causes of airway obstruction in infancy in addition to congestive heart failure must be considered. Asthma is the disorder with which bronchiolitis most often is confused. If respiratory syncytial (RS) virus is prevalent in the community and the infant is less than 6 months of age, the diagnosis of bronchiolitis is most likely. However, in the older infant, there is no way to distinguish with certainty between the two conditions. Actually, there are more similarities than differences between the two entities, and physicians spend too much time for little purpose at the bedside trying to distinguish between the two disorders. Symptoms and physical, radiographic, physiologic, and blood gas findings are virtually identical. The response to epinephrine, which often is used by clinicians as a differential point, can be minimal in severe asthma. On the other hand, infants with bronchiolitis due to RS virus can have a good response to epinephrine; thus, the test is of little diagnostic value. The argument that airway obstruction in bronchiolitis is due to infection while in asthma it is due to an allergic reaction is not tenable. Asthma during infancy, like bronchiolitis, is most often due to viral infection. Measurement of total IgE may be of some value in older infants in distinguishing between those who have infectious bronchiolitis without asthma and those who will subsequently be shown to have asthma. In a single study of this nature, it was observed that only 6 percent of infants with epidemic bronchiolitis had serum IgE concentrations increased over the 95th percentile, while 35 percent of infants with nonepidemic (sporadic) bronchiolitis had such an increase (Polmar et al., 1972). Studies that associate bronchiolitis with the subsequent development of asthma are difficult to interpret. Eisen and Bacall (1963) and Wittig and Glaser (1959) showed that 25 and 32 percent of infants with bronchiolitis developed asthma, but these are retrospective reports. Thus, one is unable to determine how many of the infants diagnosed as having bronchiolitis actually were suffering from their first episode of asthma. Similarly, the question whether RS-positive bronchiolitis is more or less likely to result in the subsequent development of asthma cannot be resolved on the basis of published data. Simon and Jordan (1967) in a study of children with RS-positive and RS-negative bronchiolitis, concluded (with little follow-up data) that those with RS virus–induced bronchiolitis were not at risk of subsequent asthma. To the contrary, Rooney and Williams (1971), in a follow-up of infants with RS-positive bronchiolitis, found a significant incidence of subsequent wheezing and a positive personal and family history of atopic disease. Of additional concern is the recent report that 10 of 15 older asymptomatic children who had been hospitalized under 18 months of age with bronchiolitis had physiologic evidence of persistent small airway disease (Kattan et al., 1976).

Treatment. The treatment of acute bronchiolitis is largely supportive. Oxygen sufficient to maintain the Pao_2 between 70 and 90 must be administered since hypoxemia is almost invariably present. Hydration *(with great care not to overhydrate)* also is indicated. Despite the fact that adrenergic aerosols were not shown in one study (Phelan and Stocks, 1974) to be helpful in relieving the airway obstruction of bronchiolitis, the question is not resolved and isoetharine or isoproterenol administered by Maxi-myst or other compressed air device is worth trying. A trial of intravenous aminophylline also is advisable. Corticosteroid usage is more controversial because of older studies which showed no benefit in bronchiolitis (Leer et al., 1969). However, in the extremely ill infant, the short-term use of high-dose steroids does no harm; and their use would seem prudent. Since there is little to suggest significant bacterial superinfection in infants with viral bronchiolitis, the routine administration of antimicrobial agents is not indicated (Aherne et al., 1970).

References

Aherne, W., Bird, T., Court, S. D. M., Gardner, P. F., and McQuillin, J.: Pathological changes in virus infections of the lower respiratory tract in children. J. Clin. Pathol. 23:7, 1970.

Altemeier, W. A., Jr., and Ayoub, E. M.: Erythromycin prophylaxis for pertussis. Pediatrics 59:623, 1977.

Bass, J. W., Klenk, E. L., Kotheimer, J. B., Linnemann, C. C., and Smith, M. H. D.: Antimicrobial treatment of pertussis. J. Pediatr. 75:768, 1969.

Beem, M. O., and Saxon, E. M.: Respiratory tract colonization and a distinctive pneumonia syndrome in infants infected with *Chlamydia trachomatis*. New Engl. J. Med. 296:306, 1977.

Brown, R. S., Nogrady, M. B., Spence, L., and Wiglesworth,

F. W.: An outbreak of adenovirus type 7 infection in children in Montreal. Canad. Med. Assoc. J. 108:434, 1973.

Cate, T. R., Roberts, J. S., Russ, M. A., and Pierce, J. A.: Effects of common colds on pulmonary function. Am. Rev. Respir. Dis. 108:858, 1973.

Ceruti, E., Contreras, J., and Neira, M.: Staphylococcal pneumonia in childhood. Am. J. Dis. Child. 122:386, 1971.

Chanock, R. M.: Mycoplasma infections in man. New Engl. J. Med. 273:1199, 1257, 1965.

Chanock, R. M., Kapikian, A. Z., Mills, J., Kim, H. W., and Parrott, R. H.: Influence of immunological factors in respiratory syncytial virus disease of the lower respiratory tract. Arch. Environ. Health 21:347, 1970.

Connor, J. D.: Evidence for an etiologic role of adenoviral

infection in pertussis syndrome. New Engl. J. Med. *283*:390, 1970.

Eisen, A. H., and Bacal, H. L.: The relationship of acute bronchiolitis to bronchial asthma. A 4- to 14-year followup. Pediatrics *31*:859, 1963.

Faden, H. S., and Overall, J. D.: *Hemophilus influenzae* empyema — two cases. Clin. Pediatr. *15*:1143, 1976.

Fernald, G. W., Collier, A. M., and Clyde, W. A.: Respiratory infections due to *Mycoplasma pneumoniae* in infants and children. Pediatrics *55*:327, 1975.

Foy, H. M., Grayston, J. T., Kenny, G. E., Alexander, E. R., and McMahon, R.: Epidemiology of *Mycoplasma pneumoniae* in families. J.A.M.A. *197*:859, 1966.

Foy, H. M., Kenny, G. E., Sefi, R., Ochs, H. D., and Allan, I. D.: Second attacks of pneumonia due to *Mycoplasma pneumoniae*. J. Infect. Dis. 135:673, 1977.

Gross, P. A., Ennis, F. A., Gaerlan, P. F., Denson, L. J., Denning, C. R., and Schiffman, D.: A controlled double-blind comparison of reactogenicity, immunogenicity, and protective efficacy of whole-virus and split-product influenza vaccines in children. J. Infect. Dis. *136*:623, 1977.

Harrison, H. R., English, M. G., Lee, C. K., and Alexander, E. R.: *Chlamydia trachomatis* infant pneumonitis. Comparison with matched controls and other infant pneumonitis. New Engl. J. Med. *298*:702, 1978.

Hoekelman, R. A., Blatman, S., Brunell, P. A., Friedman, S. B., and H. M. Seidel: *Principles of Pediatrics*. New York, McGraw-Hill Book Co., 1978.

Honig, P. J., Pasquariello, P. S., and Stool, S.: *H. influenzae* pneumonia in infants and children. J. Pediatr. *83*:215, 1973.

Kattan, M. Keens, T., LaPierre, J. G., Levison, H., and Reilly, B. J.: Pulmonary function abnormalities in symptom-free children ten years after bronchiolitis. Pediatr. Res. *10*:457, 1976.

Kendig, E. L., Jr.: Tuberculosis. *In* Kendig, E. L., Jr. (ed.): *Disorders of the Respiratory Tract in Children,* 3rd ed. Philadelphia, W. B. Saunders Co., 1977, p. 821.

Kim, H. W., Arrobio, J. O., Brandt, C. D., Jeffries, B. C., Pyles, G., Reid, J. L., Chanock, R. M., and Parrott, R. H.: Epidemiology of respiratory syncytial virus infection in Washington, D.C. I. Importance of the virus in different respiratory tract disease syndromes and temporal distribution of infection. Am. J. Epidem. *98*:216, 1973.

Krugman, S., and Ward, R.: Pertussis (whooping cough). *In* Krugman, S., and Ward, R. (eds.): *Infectious Diseases of Children and Adults,* 6th ed. St. Louis, C. V. Mosby Co., 1977, pp. 173–181.

Lang, W. R., Howden, C. W., Laws, J., and Burton, J. F.: Bronchopneumonia with serious sequelae in children with evidence of adenovirus type 21 infection. Br. Med. J. *1*:73, 1969.

Laraya-Cuasay, L. R., DeForest, A., Huff, D., Lischner, H., and Huang, N. N.: Chronic pulmonary complications of early influenza virus infections in children. Am. Rev. Respir. Dis. *116*:617, 1977.

Leer, J. A., Green, J. L., Heimlich, E. M., Hyde, J. S., Moffet, H. L., Young, G. A., and Barron, B. A.: Corticosteroid treatment in bronchiolitis. A controlled, collaborative study

in 297 infants and children. Am. J. Dis. Child. *117*:495, 1969.

Lincoln, E. M., and Sewell, E. M.: Tuberculosis. *In* Krugman, S., and Ward, R. (eds.): *Infectious Diseases of Children and Adults,* St. Louis, C. V. Mosby Co., 1977, pp. 389–450.

Loda, F. A., Collier, A. M., Glezen, W. P., Strangert, K., Clyde, W. A., Jr., and Denny, F. W.: Occurrence of *Diplococcus pneumoniae* in the upper respiratory tract of children. J. Pediatr. *87*:1087, 1975.

Morse, S. I.: Biological activities of *Bordetella pertussis*. Adv. Appl. Microbiol. *20*:9, 1976.

Newth, C. J. L., Levison, H., and Bryan, A. C.: The respiratory status of children with croup. J. Pediatr. *81*:1068, 1972.

Phelan, P. D., and Stocks, J. G.: Management of severe viral bronchiolitis and severe acute asthma. Arch. Dis. Child. *49*:143, 1974.

Picken, J. J., Niewoehner, D. E., and Chester, E. H.: Prolonged effects of viral infections of the upper respiratory tract upon small airways. Am. J. Med. *52*:738, 1972.

Polmar, S. H., Robinson, L. D., and Minnefor, A. B.: Immunoglobulin E in bronchiolitis. Pediatrics *50*:279, 1972.

Report of the Committee on Infectious Diseases of the American Academy of Pediatrics, 18th edition, 1977; Influenza, pp. 227–229.

Rooney, J. C., and Williams, H. E.: The relationship between proved viral bronchiolitis and subsequent wheezing. J. Pediatr. *79*:744, 1971.

Rudolph, A. M. (ed.): *Pediatrics,* 16th ed. New York, Appleton-Century-Crofts, 1977.

Scott, R., Kaul, A., Scott, M., Chiba, Y., and Ogra, P.: Development of *in vitro* correlates of cell-mediated immunity to respiratory syncytial virus infection in humans. J. Infect. Dis. *137*:810, 1978.

Simon, G., and Jordan, W. S.: Infectious and allergic aspects of bronchiolitis. J. Pediatr. *70*:533, 1967.

Smith, M. H. D.: Bacterial pneumonias. *In* Kendig, E. L. (ed.): *Disorders of the Respiratory Tract in Children.* Philadelphia, W. B. Saunders Co., 1977, p. 381.

Sussman, S. J., Magoffin, R. L., Lennette, E. H., and Schieble, J.: Cold agglutinins, Eaton agent, and respiratory infections of children. Pediatrics *38*:571, 1966.

Tullis, D. C. H.: Bronchial asthma associated with intestinal parasites. New Engl. J. Med. *282*:370, 1970.

Williams, H., and McNicol, K. N.: Prevalence, natural history and relationship of wheezy bronchitis and asthma in children. An epidemiological study. Br. Med. J. *4*:321, 1969.

Winterbauer, R. H., Ludwig, R. W., and Hammar, S. P.: Clinical course, management, and long-term sequelae of respiratory failure due to influenza viral pneumonia. Johns Hopkins Med. J. *141*:148, 1977.

Wittig, H. J., and Glaser, J.: The relationship between bronchiolitis and childhood asthma. J. Allergy *30*:19, 1959.

Wright, P. F., Ross, K. B., Thompson, J., and Karzon, D. T.: Influenza A infections in young children. Primary natural infection and protective efficacy of live-vaccine–induced or naturally acquired immunity. New Engl. J. Med. *296*:829, 1977.

David S. Pearlman, M.D.
C. Warren Bierman, M.D.

45

Asthma (Bronchial Asthma, Reactive Airways Disorder)

Asthma is a chronic obstructive disorder of the tracheobronchial tree characterized by paroxysmal episodes of respiratory distress generally interspersed with prolonged periods of apparent complete well-being. Typically, there are wide variations in the degree of obstruction over relatively short periods of time; the obstruction may subside spontaneously or only as a result of therapy. The hallmark of the disease is *wheezing,* a squeaky sound made by air rushing through the larger but narrowed airways. Cough also is a characteristic part of the disorder and may constitute the major symptom with which asthma presents. Asthma may even present with "croup" and/or other subtle symptoms of bronchopulmonary obstruction *without wheezing,* a fact not fully appreciated until relatively recently (McFadden, 1975*a* and *b*; Corrao, et al., 1979). The more subtle symptoms and signs of asthma often are unappreciated, and asthma is a commonly underdiagnosed disorder. Because of this, and the prevalence of erroneous concepts of the etiology of asthma, its course and prognosis, asthma also tends to be a greatly undertreated disorder in childhood.

PATHOLOGY (see Reid, 1977)

Examination of postmortem lung specimens of patients dying of asthma show smooth muscle hyperplasia of bronchial and bronchiolar walls, thick tenacious mucus plugs often completely occluding airways, a markedly thickened basement membrane, and variable degrees of mucosal edema and denudation of bronchial and bronchiolar epithelium. Eosinophilia of the submucosa and secretions is prominent whether or not allergic (IgE-mediated) mechanisms are present. Plasma cells that contain IgG, IgM, and IgA may be seen, and in some patients plasma cells that contain IgE also are observed. Occasionally in children there is an inflammatory response indicative of infection, a finding more common in adults, especially those with concurrent chronic bronchitis. Mucous plugs contain layers of shed epithelial cells and eosinophils, and may contain PMN's, lymphocytes, and plasma cells. The mucosal edema with separated columnar cells and stratified nonciliated epithelium, which replace ciliated epithelium, results in abnormal mucociliary clearance. Mast cells often are absent, possibly reflecting degranulation and discharge of the chemical mediators. Submucous gland hypertrophy and increased goblet cell size are not a constant feature of asthma, being more characteristic of chronic bronchitis.

The thickened basement membrane is a striking feature of asthma and has been reported even in "mild" asthmatics, sometimes associated with deposition of various immunoglobulins. Basement membrane thickening is thought to occur early in the disease, but its pathogenetic significance remains to be determined. All of these findings have been observed in symptom-free asthmatic individuals following accidental death. Although an occasional patient may show localized bronchiectasis and small focal areas of alveolar destruction, this is not characteristic of asthma, and there is little evidence that asthma leads to destructive emphysema. On the other hand, "distensive emphysema," clinically significant diminution in pulmonary elasticity, may be a concomitant of long-standing alveolar hyperinflation. Bronchiectasis may be seen in asthma associated with allergic bronchopulmonary aspergillosis and in a small number of patients with similar disorders.

EPIDEMIOLOGY

Asthma commonly begins in childhood and has been considered mistakenly to be a disorder confined largely to early life. Much childhood asthma persists through adulthood, and almost half of all asthma in adults begins in childhood. The vast majority of childhood asthma begins before the age of 8 years, most begins before age 6 years, and about half begins before age 3 years. Until puberty, males are affected twice as frequently as are females. In the teens and in early adulthood, there is a reversal of this trend, so that by mid to late adult life, females are affected more frequently than are males.

Asthma is a deceptively common disorder of childhood; the exact figures on incidence and prevalence vary from study to study, related at least in part to different criteria for diagnosis and different methodologies used in the studies (see Chapter 13). At any given time, approximately 3 percent of a population is considered to have asthma, but this undoubtedly is a gross underestimate. It is probable that the true prevalence is at least two to three times this figure. The mortality rate among asthmatics is approximately 0.1 percent per year, a relatively low yet significant rate. However, the morbidity in asthma is extraordinarily high. It is a source of chronic fatigue that may interfere with sleep, with school performance, and with normal exercise and physical development. It may affect the child's psychologic growth and development and his or her interactions with family and peers, disturbing family life and often causing economic hardship — because of direct medical costs as well as time lost from work by the parent who cares for the child.

NATURAL COURSE

It is a common belief that childhood asthma generally is "outgrown" by adulthood. Indeed, in various studies, 30 to 50 percent of asthmatic children have been reported to be symptom-free at puberty. Remissions occur somewhat earlier in girls than in boys, as do pubertal changes. However, many children who have "outgrown" asthma in puberty develop recurrent asthmatic symptoms in later adult life, as is clearly shown in a series of studies by Flensborg (1944) and Ryssing (1959). Flensborg reported initially that at the end of a 5- to 18-year follow-up of children with asthma, approximately 40 percent were free from overt asthma "attacks" but that less than 30 percent were completely free of symptoms. Fifteen years later, Ryssing reexamined the subjects in Flensborg's study and again found that approximately 29 percent were completely symptom-free and attack-free. However, half of those who were asthma-free in 1944 had again developed symptoms of asthma.

Asthmatic children and adults examined during "symptom-free" periods frequently have clinically significant evidence of obstruction by objective testing. In addition, pharmacologic hyperactivity of the airways in asthmatic individuals generally persists for many years even in the absence of overt asthmatic attacks (Townley et al., 1975), and pathologic evidence of pulmonary obstruction can be found in patients many years after the apparent cessation of asthmatic symptoms. Thus, many asthmatic children improve significantly by puberty; a small subpopulation may actually develop more severe asthma with puberty, however. It is clear also that only in a relatively small proportion does asthma completely disappear. More often it is the pediatrician rather than the disease that is outgrown (Levison et al., 1974).

ETIOLOGY

An extraordinary tracheobronchial hyperreactivity to acetylcholine and to other neurotransmitters and mediators of inflammation, such as prostaglandin $F_{2\alpha}$, SRS-A, histamine, and kinins, is a basic characteristic of asthma, and occurs irrespective of the presence or absence of demonstrable allergic mechanisms (see Chapter 14). This pharmacologic hypersensitivity is the basis of a diagnostic test for asthma (methacholine bronchial challenge). The fact that the chemical mediators to which the tracheobronchial tree is hypersensitive can be liberated by various mechanisms, both immune and nonimmune, may explain the observation that in most asthmatic individuals, numerous factors such as inhalant irritants, allergens, exercise, infection, and psychologic factors act as triggers of bronchoconstriction. Recently, Szentivanyi has proposed that this hypersensitivity to pharmacologic mediators in asthma is due to an imbalance in the autonomic nervous system concerned with counterbalancing the effects of various chemical mediators (see Chapter 14). Heightened tracheobronchial sensitivity can be demonstrated also in chronic bronchitis, following some viral respiratory tract infections, and in family members of asthmatic patients without asthmatic symptoms, but generally not to the degree observed in asthma.

The basis for this pharmacologic hypersensitivity of asthma appears to be genetic. There is a familial association of the clinical asthmatic state and of tracheobronchial hypersensitivity and, separately, a familial association of IgE hyperimmunoglobulinemia. The coexistence of asthma and of increased IgE antibody production is far greater than in the population at large, but each is separable and seems to be genetically independent. Within a given family constellation, some family members may have asthma and also manufacture large amounts of IgE; others may have asthma but produce little IgE; and still others may manufacture IgE antibody extraordinarily well, but have no evidence of tracheobronchial hypersensitivity (Townley et al., 1976). The exact mode of inheritance of asthma is still not clear. Although in twin studies, concordance for asthma generally has been greater for identical twins compared to nonidentical twins or other non-twin siblings, concordance nevertheless is lower than 50 percent (Bias, 1973).

Though most children with asthma have specific skin-sensitizing (IgE) antibody, the proportion of asthmatic adults with demonstrable IgE antibodies is much lower. The presumption that all asthma was "allergic" or had an immune basis led to the concept of "extrinsic" asthma, due to exogenous allergens, and "intrinsic" asthma, due to "normal" bacterial allergens from the respiratory tract (Rackemann, 1940). However, in many individuals with asthma, no evidence can be found that allergic mechanisms are operative in the disease. Moreover, even when "allergy" is present, it rarely is the only important factor, and sometimes the IgE antibody present may be irrelevant to the asthma (Aas, 1970).

Environmental factors play a critical role in the expression of asthma in "susceptible" individuals. In childhood and in adult life, the onset of asthma frequently is associated with a (viral) respiratory tract infection. Certain viruses, such as respiratory syncytial virus and adenovirus, parainfluenza and possibly corona virus, influenza, and mycoplasma, are particularly important (Ellis, 1977; also see Chapter 44). In addition, inhalation of allergens and irritants can increase tracheobronchial reactivity further in asthmatic patients, possibly acting through the parasympathetic (vagal) system.

PRECIPITATING AND AGGRAVATING FACTORS IN ASTHMA

Allergens. In some individuals with asthma, it is possible to induce an asthmatic reaction to substances to which IgE and possibly other skin-sensitizing antibody can be demonstrated. In others, allergens may play only an ancillary or a negligible role. Allergic reactions may induce bronchoconstriction directly or may increase tracheobronchial sensitivity in general. Although "immediate" responses to allergens via IgE antibody-induced mediator release are striking, it is probable that "late" reactions (which occur 6 to 12 hours after antigen contact and may be mediated also in part by IgE-antibody related mechanisms) are more important in the disease. Allergens that may induce asthma include foods (mainly in early life), dusts, animal danders, mold spores, pollens, insects (mainly by inhalation but also by sting), infectious agents (especially fungi), and, occasionally, drugs.

Irritants. Numerous upper and lower respiratory tract irritants have been implicated as precipitants of asthma. These include odors from paints, hairsprays, perfumes, chemicals, air pollutants, cigarette smoke (also cigar and pipe smoke), cold air, cold water, cough, and positive ions. Some allergens may act also as irritants.

Weather Changes. Atmospheric changes commonly are associated with an increase in asthmatic activity. The mechanism of this effect has not been defined (see Chapter 18).

Infection. By far the most common infectious agents responsible for precipitating or aggravating asthma are viral respiratory pathogens. In some instances, however, fungal infections (e.g., bronchopulmonary aspergillosis), bacterial infections (pertussis), and parasitic infestations (*Toxocara* infestation or ascariasis) can be important triggers.

Exercise. Strenuous exercise ordinarily associated with breathlessness, such as running, bicycle riding and cross-country skiing (downhill skiing generally is not a problem), all may induce bronchial obstruction in the vast majority (about 70 to 80 percent) of individuals with asthma. In some instances, exercise is a major asthmatic precipitant, whereas in others it is minor or insignificant altogether (see Chapter 46). It can be a subtle though significant problem.

Emotional Factors. The influence of the psyche on asthma is unquestioned, and in some instances, suggestion has been shown to alter airway resistance significantly. To be certain, emotional upsets clearly aggravate asthma in some individuals. However, there is no evidence indicating that psychologic factors are the *basis* for asthma. The elegant studies of Kinsman et al. (1977) strongly indicate that coping styles of patients, their families, and their physicians can intensify or lead to more rapid amelioration of asthma. Conversely, denial of asthma by patients, parents (or doctor) may delay therapy to the point that reversibility of obstruction is more difficult. The influence of psychosocial factors on compliance and the effect of hostility or fear on the ability or propensity to comply

is yet another important facet of treatment failure or success.

Just as psychologic factors may influence the course of asthma in a given individual, however, it is important to recognize that asthma itself can strongly influence the emotional state of the patient, of the family, and of other individuals associated with the patient. That is, asthma probably is more frequently "somatopsychic" than it is "psychosomatic" (see Chapter 26).

Gastroesophageal Reflux (GER). Reflux of gastric contents into the tracheobronchial tree has been associated with aggravation of asthma in some children as well as in adults (see Chapter 27).

Allergic Rhinitis, Sinusitis, and Upper Respiratory Tract Inflammation. Acute or chronic sinusitis can be associated with aggravation of asthma, and it is probable that allergic rhinitis also can aggravate asthma through irritant or "reflex" mechanisms. Irritation of the upper respiratory tract by any of a variety of mechanisms appears capable of triggering asthmatic symptoms.

Nonallergic Hypersensitivity to Drugs and Chemicals. Though allergic sensitivity to aspirin has been reported on occasion with manifestations that include asthma, aspirin and other nonsteroidal antiinflammatory drugs (such as indomethacin) are more likely to exacerbate asthma on a nonallergic basis. Aspirin ingestion may diminish pulmonary functions in up to one third of children and adolescents with severe asthma (Rachelefsky et al., 1975). In many instances, this effect may be subtle. Consequently, as a general rule, it is wise to restrict aspirin and aspirin-containing products for all individuals who have asthma. A small proportion of aspirin-sensitive asthmatics also are sensitive to tartrazine (FD&C yellow dye No. 5), a common dye found in many foods and drugs.

Endocrine Factors. Aggravation of asthma occurs in some patients in relation to the menstrual cycle, beginning in such cases shortly before menstruation. Whether this reflects changes in water and salt balance, irritability of bronchial smooth muscle, or other factors is unknown. The use of birth control pills occasionally also aggravates asthma. Hyperthyroidism has been reported to aggravate (or precipitate) asthma severely in an occasional patient, with disease amelioration following treatment of hyperthyroidism (also see Chapter 50). Relationships between pregnancy and asthma are discussed in Chapter 51. (See also Weinstein, 1979.)

Interaction of Various Precipitating Factors. Not infrequently, concurrent exposure to various precipitating or aggravating factors may induce additive effects in asthma. For example, some individuals experience exercise-induced asthma only when exercising in cold air, or when exercising during a pollen allergy season. Others recognize increased symptoms from specific allergen exposure after a respiratory infection.

ASTHMATIC PATTERNS

In some asthmatic children, most of the factors listed above appear to play an important role in asthma, whereas in others only some are of importance. Table 45–1 provides examples of various reaction patterns in patients with asthma. For example, patient A's asthma may be precipitated by each of the factors listed, while for patient B, allergic triggers are of predominant importance in the disease, with other factors being of minor influence. Patient C is a child with "nonallergic" asthma. The estimated importance of each of the precipitating factors in the pediatric population is noted in the table. Table 45–2 relates the importance of various asthmatic precipitants to age. For example, viral infections are of great importance in precipitating asthma early in life, but become relatively less important as the child grows older, only to assume a major role again in adulthood.

TABLE 45–1 REACTIVE AIRWAYS DISORDER – PATTERNS

Precipitant	Example A	B	C	Estimated Involvement (% of cases)
Viral infections	+	(+)	+	90%
Irritants	+	(+)	(+)	100%
Exercise	+	(+)	(+)	70%
Allergens	+	+	–	65%
Emotions	+	(+)	–	?

+ = Major importance
(+) = Minor importance
– = No importance

Since the development of allergy is dependent on duration and intensity of exposure to allergens, allergy to foods in infancy generally precedes allergy to inhaled substances. Thereafter, inhaled allergens become progressively more important, as prolonged exposure to such perennial factors as danders from domestic animals, housedust, and airborne mold spores results in allergic sensitization. As the child grows older, repeated pollen exposure results in pollen asthma. Exercise becomes a more important trigger factor in later childhood and adolescence, when exercise tends to be more strenuous and prolonged and the patient participates in competitive sports.

THE PRESENTATION OF ASTHMA

Asthma may present with any or all of a variety of symptoms, which can include wheezing, cough, shortness of breath, complaints of "chest congestion," "tight chest,"

TABLE 45–2 PRECIPITANTS OF ASTHMATIC SYMPTOMS IN VARIOUS AGE GROUPS

	Infancy	Early Childhood	Later Childhood	Adulthood
Viral infection	++++*	+++	+(+)	+++
Exercise	+	++	+++	++
Irritants	+	++	+++	++
Foods	++	+	(+)	(+)
Indoor Inhalants	+(+)	+++	+++	+++
Pollens		++	+++	+++
Emotions	(+)†	(+)	(+)	(+)

*Denotes relative importance
†See text

exercise intolerance, and recurrent "bronchitis" or recurrent "pneumonia." Often it presents subtly as coughing without overt wheezing, especially in conjunction with colds or during pollen seasons. The adage attributed to Chevalier Jackson that "not all that wheezes is asthma" has been well publicized and, indeed, causes for wheezing other than asthma are numerous (see Table 45–3). On the other hand, it has become apparent also that "not all asthma wheezes" (at least not overtly). In many instances, cursory physical examination fails to reveal evidence of obvious pulmonary obstruction (although careful examination might have done so), and obstructive disease of the lower respiratory tract may be overlooked unless pulmonary function is tested. Thus the physician should be suspicious of asthma not only when the patient has recurrent wheezing, but even in the absence of wheezing when there are recurrent complaints referable to the lower respiratory tract.

"Wheezing" may be a late sign in asthma. It is caused by air rushing past a narrowed area in sufficient force to generate air vibrations perceived as sound, and it occurs only in the larger airways. The small airways are "silent," since the air moves too slowly to generate sound. Consequently, marked small airway obstruction can be present that may not be identified on physical examination. In most instances, airway narrowing in asthma is sufficiently generalized that large and small airway obstruction coexist, so that wheezing is audible either overtly or by auscultation. Before wheezing is perceptible to patient or parent, however, there generally are more subtle symptoms of obstruction, such as cough or a feeling of chest discomfort.

This phenomenon may be more readily appreciated using as an analogy the concept of an iceberg (Figure 45–1). By this analogy, the ocean floor represents completely normal pulmonary function, and the ocean surface the point at which pulmonary obstruction is obvious clinically. Wheezing, in other words, is the tip of the iceberg. Just as most of the iceberg is not evident, pulmonary obstruction begins well before wheezing is heard. In some instances, the slope to the tip of the iceberg is slight, obstruction progressing slowly (days); but in others it is steep, with pulmonary obstruction advancing rapidly to overt symptoms in minutes to hours. Auscultation may detect wheezing or prolonged expiration before wheezing is overt, and

CLINICAL PRESENTATIONS OF ASTHMA

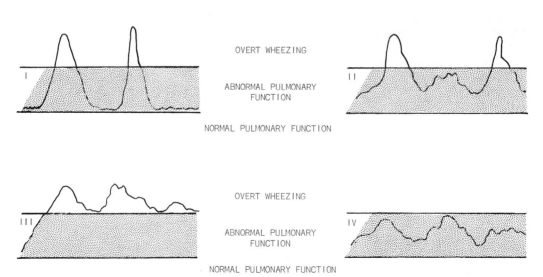

FIGURE 45–1.   Iceberg concept of asthma. The "ocean floor" represents pulmonary normality; the surface of the ocean, the point at which asthmatic symptoms (e.g., wheezing) are obvious.

sensitive pulmonary function measurements may detect obstruction before wheezing can be heard by auscultation.

Figure 45–1 contains various examples of asthma patterns, selected for illustrative purposes. In some instances, as illustrated in example I, the obstructive phenomenon is short-lived, beginning and ending over a period of hours to days. In other instances, obstruction may be constant, surfacing periodically as wheezing and apparent paroxysms of asthma interspersed with minor or no obvious symptoms (example II), or associated with virtually constant wheezing of varying intensity (example III). Example IV is an illustration of the patient who never wheezes despite significant pulmonary obstruction; the obstruction may not be recognized unless the examiner is alert enough to perform pulmonary function tests. Figure 45–1 also illustrates the point that there are two sides to the asthma iceberg. Although overt asthmatic symptoms may cease after a relatively short period of time, there is a prolonged phase of diminishing but significant pulmonary obstruction. This has been well documented by various investigators, including McFadden in adults (McFadden, 1973), and by Levison and coworkers (1974), in children who showed that days to weeks

after an asthma attack, at a time when patients claim to be completely asymptomatic, abnormal flow rates, and/or hyperinflation, remain.

This concept of asthma may be developed into a classification of disease severity that considers frequency of asthmatic attacks, severity of attacks, functional impairment between attacks, and overall functional disability. Such a classification is useful in defining therapy as well as following the course of the disease (see table).

Recognition of the varied patterns has important therapeutic implications. First, early treatment of asthma is more successful than is late treatment, and even subtle signs of pulmonary obstruction should be a signal to institute therapy. In the child who wheezes with upper respiratory tract infections, the characteristic cough that precedes overt wheezing should be a signal to initiate therapy. In addition, pharmacologic therapy should be continued even when overt symptoms of asthma have cleared and until pulmonary obstruction has reversed or pulmonary functions have become stable at an acceptable functional level for the child.

In asthmatic children who have chronic pulmonary obstruction, pharmacologic treatment must be continuous or "round-the-

Classification	Definition
(Examples in Fig. 45–1) Mild (Example I)	Less than six mild attacks per year *and* asymptomatic between attacks, *and* no functional impairment between attacks *and* no medication used between attacks
Moderate to moderately severe (Examples II, IV)	Up to eight severe attacks per year *and* mild to moderate symptoms between attacks *and* mild to moderate functional impairment between attacks *and* on continuous medication
Severe (Example III)	More than eight severe attacks per year while on continuous medication *and* moderate to severe functional impairment between attacks, steroid dependent, *or* at least 2 episodes of status asthmaticus per year

Continuous medication is defined as medication used on more than 25% of the days in the past year.
Functional impairment is defined as:
Normal functional activity—on par with peers
Minimal functional impairment—1 or 2 disability days/quarter
Moderate functional impairment—1 or 2 disability days/month
Severe functional impairment—1 or more disability days/week
A *disability day* is defined as a day on which a person stays in bed most of the day for asthma or a work or school day loss.

clock." *Asthma is a chronic disorder that may surface periodically, but in which chronic obstruction may be more severe than frequently is appreciated.*

PROGNOSIS

In children and adolescents, asthma frequently is a completely "reversible" obstructive airway disease and, indeed, no abnormalities in pulmonary function can be detected in many asthmatic children when they become symptom-free. However, there is a subpopulation of asthmatic children (and adults) who, even in the absence of symptoms for prolonged periods of time, have persistent abnormalities in pulmonary functions, with chronic hyperinflation and/or decreased pulmonary flow rates, with or without mild hypoxemia. The potential reversibility of abnormal pulmonary functions — even in severely asthmatic children — towards or to normal by intensive therapy was demonstrated by Tooley et al. (1965). However, it is clear that in many children with severe asthma normal pulmonary functions cannot be maintained without continuous intensive therapy, including corticosteroids. Reversibility of pulmonary function abnormalities with therapy is transient in that withdrawal of constant therapy usually leads to the return of pulmonary functions to initial abnormal baselines (Cade and Pain, 1973).

As noted previously, even severe asthma generally does not progress to emphysema. However asthma appears to progress to chronic nonreversible obstructive disease in a small proportion of individuals with the disorder. Chronic mucus plugging, tracheobronchial ciliary dysfunction, smooth muscle hyperplasia, and persistent hyperinflation possibly may lead to pulmonary abnormalities in adult life. Recent findings of residual pulmonary function abnormalities following respiratory viral infection early in life (Kattan et al., 1977), and the fact that viral respiratory tract infection occurs more commonly in asthmatic children than in their nonasthmatic siblings (Minor et al., 1974), further confuse the issue.

Since the natural course of continued bronchial obstruction is not known, a therapeutic dilemma arises about the extent to which asthma should be treated. Should the child be treated until pulmonary function is totally normal, or to the point that the child can function reasonably normally even though pulmonary functions are abnormal? Whether intensive therapy early in the course of asthma or persistent therapy to achieve constant pulmonary normality can prevent any irreversible changes later, in childhood or adult life, needs to be determined.

Information on the relationship between age of onset, severity of asthma, and ultimate prognosis is conflicting. It appears, however, that asthma that begins before 6 months of age may have a worse prognosis in terms of severity and longevity than asthma that begins later in childhood. *Severe* asthma earlier in life also appears to have a less favorable prognosis than does mild asthma. The onset of asthma after the age of 6 months, but before the age of 2 or 3 years does not imply a worse prognosis than does asthma that begins later in childhood. Asthma tends to be more severe and/or is less likely to become symptom-free if allergic mechanisms are involved in the disease. Conversely, there is some suggestion that nonallergic asthma precipitated mainly by viral respiratory tract infection ("wheezy bronchitis" or "asthmatic bronchitis") more likely will become symptom-free in later childhood. Nonallergic asthma in adulthood, on the other hand, has a significantly worse prognosis than does allergic asthma. Asthma tends to be more severe in general and occur earlier if there is a family history of atopic disease in close relatives, or if there is a personal history of other atopic disorders (atopic dermatitis or allergic rhinitis). Patients who are not symptom-free during puberty are unlikely to outgrow their symptoms as young adults (Blair, 1977).

DIAGNOSIS

Clinical Diagnosis

History and Physical Examination. Though patients with asthma may present in a variety of ways, most share certain common historical features, and asthma often can be diagnosed by history alone. The wheezing associated with asthma characteristically is expiratory; in severe obstruction, it may be heard both in inspiration and expiration. Wheezing only in inspiration suggests obstruction high in the airway (e.g., laryngeal area) and is uncharacteristic of asthma. On history taking, it is essential that parent or patient understands the meaning of the term "wheezing." Wheezing usually is accompanied by cough; occasionally cough may be the only symptom. Asthmatic attacks are episodic at first, with intervals of symptom-free periods between, but as the disease becomes more chronic, the number of symptom-free intervals tend to diminish progressively.

Symptoms usually are more severe at night or in the early morning and improve through the day. A history of symptomatic improvement after an injection of epinephrine, inhaled or oral adrenergic drugs, or oral theophylline, suggests the diagnosis. A typical "attack" usually lasts 5 to 7 days and may clear spontaneously (though lung function abnormalities often persist between attacks).

Symptoms vary with age. The infant and young child may have a history of recurrent bronchitis, bronchiolitis, or pneumonia, persistent coughing with colds, recurrent "croup," or just a chronic chest "rattle." Older children often develop a "tight" chest with colds, recurrent "chest congestion," or persistent coughing or wheezing. Respiratory symptoms may be precipitated or exacerbated also by exposure to animals, moldy or dusty areas, tobacco smoke, or cold air or by exercise.

Physical examination of a child whose history suggests asthma should focus on overall growth and development, on respiratory mechanics, a careful examination of the chest, and on associated signs of allergic disease.

Growth. Weight and height should be recorded and plotted on a growth grid. Asthma itself as well as therapy with steroids can affect growth. Growth retardation may be caused by chronic hypoxemia, and under such circumstances, control of asthma may be associated with a growth spurt. The blood pressure should be recorded, since steroids, adrenergic agents and possibly theophylline prescribed for asthma may elevate blood pressure.

Respiratory Mechanics and Chest Examination. The physician should observe respiratory rate, color of lips and nail beds, evidence of clubbing of the fingers (*not* a concomitant of asthma), dyspnea or prolongation of expiration, retractions, or use of accessory muscles by which the patient lifts his shoulders in breathing. A round-shouldered posture with an increase in anterior-posterior diameter results from hyperinflation. In children who develop asthma in early childhood there may be a "pseudo-rachitic" chest deformity from long-standing airway obstruction. In the small child, the lungs are best examined first when the child is cooperative, before he or she has been frightened by a flashlight or otoscope.

Examination of the lungs frequently reveals rhonchi, which clear on changing position or coughing, or unequal breath sounds. Compression of the chest during expiration may produce latent wheezes. Though wheezing can be elicited frequently with a forced expiratory maneuver, occasionally there is only prolongation of expiration, without wheezing. Frequently it is difficult to persuade the older child or adolescent to exhale forcefully to induce latent wheezes, because the patient has discovered intuitively that such a maneuver may induce coughing that can increase bronchospasm. It is important to note air exchange, for some patients with severe asthma do not wheeze — because too little air is exchanged to generate a wheezing sound. With marked hyperinflation, the heart and liver both may be displaced downward as the diaphragm is depressed, shifting the point of cardiac maximal impact, decreasing precardiac dullness, and making the liver palpable. Though examination of the heart may be difficult when heart sounds are obscured by wheezing, it is important, since both asthma and its therapy may alter cardiac rate and rhythm.

Associated Signs of Allergy. The recognition of signs of upper respiratory allergy that coexist frequently with asthma may aid in achieving better control of asthma, by identifying aggravating factors (e.g., sinusitis) or decreasing coexistent physical disability (e.g., serous otitis with conductive deafness). If nasal polyps are present, they should suggest cystic fibrosis in the young child or paranasal sinusitis with aspirin sensitivity in the adolescent. Polyps occur rarely in children with uncomplicated asthma. Eardrums should be examined with a pneumatic otoscope for serous otitis. The conjunctivae should be examined for edema, inflammation, and tearing. A slit lamp examination for cataracts also is indicated in the child who is receiving chronic treatment with corticosteroids. Note also the texture of the skin and subcutaneous tissue as it relates to nutrition and fluid balance, and examine flexor creases and other areas of skin for active or healed atopic dermatitis.

Differential Diagnosis

Table 45–3 notes common conditions to be differentiated from asthma at various ages of childhood. Almost all can coexist with asthma. A comprehensive list of conditions associated with wheezing is found elsewhere (Siegel et al., 1978).

Laryngo-tracheo-bronchomalacia. A congenital disorder of cartilage, laryngo-tracheo-bronchomalacia can coexist with asthma. Symptoms increase with respiratory infections. The condition usually subsides spontaneously by age 2 years (see Chapter 43).

Cystic Fibrosis. Cystic fibrosis should be suspected in any infant who has recurrent bronchial infection with poor growth. A diagnosis of cystic fibrosis does not rule out asthma, since the two may coexist in the same patient (see Chapter 48).

Chronic Disease due to Respiratory Viral Infections. Both adenovirus and respiratory syncytial virus infections may cause chronic pulmonary disease in infants. The ultimate prognosis for such children is not known at present, though several prospective studies are now in progress (see Chapter 44).

Foreign Body. The presence of a foreign body must be distinguished from asthma at any age. *The sudden onset of persistent nonremitting wheezing is due to a foreign body until proven otherwise.* Some foreign bodies may not induce immediate symptoms, however, depending on their composition and the regions in which they lodge. For instance, an aspirated peanut may cause progressive symptoms not only because it induces progressive inflammation per se but also because it may induce allergic sensitization that may lead to a progressive allergic reaction to peanut antigens. Inflammation caused by a foreign body may progress to localized bronchiectasis. If foreign body is suspected, chest x-rays should be taken in inspiration and expiration, followed if necessary by fluoroscopy and/or bronchoscopy (see Chapter 43).

Croup and Acute Epiglottitis. Croup is a common condition due to a respiratory virus; acute epiglottitis is a fulminating infection due to *Hemophilus influenzae* infection (Chapter 43). Often, children with asthma have a history of recurrent croup. In both, "wheezing" is mainly inspiratory.

Hyperventilation Syndrome. This condition is more likely to occur in the adolescent age group than in childhood; it may be mistaken for asthma or may coexist with it. Typically, the patient is anxious, complains

TABLE 45–3 DIFFERENTIAL DIAGNOSIS OF ASTHMA

Condition	Relative Frequency of Occurrence		
	INFANCY	CHILDHOOD	ADOLESCENCE
Laryngomalacia-tracheomalacia-bronchomalacia	++	±	—
Cystic fibrosis	+++	+	—
Chronic viral infection	+++	++	
Foreign body	++	+++	±
Croup	++	+	—
Epiglottitis	+++	+	—
Pertussis	+++	+	—
Congenital anomalies	+++	+	—
Hyperventilation syndrome	—	+	+++
Bronchiectasis	+	+	+
Mitral valve prolapse	—	—	+

of marked dyspnea and difficulty getting her or his breath in the face of excellent air exchange on auscultation and in the absence of wheezing. Often, there are associated complaints of headache and tingling of fingers and toes. Pulmonary function tests are helpful in differentiating hyperventilation syndrome from asthma if the patient's cooperation can be obtained. (The patient sometimes will refuse to perform them because of fear of "smothering.") Immediate therapy consists of reassurance, and possibly rebreathing into a paper bag to elevate $PaCO_2$ levels. Long-term therapy involves evaluation of the cause of anxiety and psychotherapy as appropriate.

Mitral Valve Prolapse. Mitral valve prolapse occurs in slender asthenic adolescents and is more frequent in females than males. Patients with this condition have symptoms of chest pain during or following strenuous exercise; it is this symptom which could be confused with asthma induced by exercise. On physical examination, diagnosis may be suspected by hearing systolic "clicks" in the mitral area and may be confirmed by echocardiography (Devereux et al., 1976). An exercise test would rule out exercise-induced asthma, but should be performed only with a cardiac monitor.

Laboratory

Table 45–4 lists laboratory tests useful in asthma.

CBC. The *complete blood count* often is normal. Eosinophilia, if present, does not indicate an allergic etiology, since eosinophil counts may vary with adrenal function and severity of asthma (see Chapter 63); nor does a leukocytosis greater than 15,000/mm^3 necessarily indicate infection, since both epinephrine administration and the "stress" of acute asthma can induce a leukocytosis.

Sputum and Nasal Mucus. Examinations of sputum and nasal mucus are simple, noninvasive tests. Asthma in older children and adults is characterized by abundant, thick, tenacious sputum. In young children, sputum rarely is observed since they ordinarily swallow it. When obtained, it usually is white or "clear"; it may be interspersed with small yellow plugs (often containing eosinophils), even when infection is not present.

On microscopic examination, eosinophils usually are present, along with other findings listed in Table 45–4. Sputum eosinophilia is present in both nonallergic and allergic asthma.

By contrast, nasal secretions are obtained readily in children. When eosinophils predominate, they suggest accompanying nasal allergy in children, though adolescents and adults can have nasal eosinophilia in the absence of proven allergy. A predominance of PMN's and lymphocytes occurs with viral respiratory infections; and PMN's and ingested bacteria are seen frequently in patients with sinusitis.

Serum Tests. Quantitative immunoglobulin levels of G, M, and A are useful only to rule out immunodeficiency syndromes in children with recurrent or chronic infection. In children with asthma, IgG levels usually are normal, IgA levels occasionally are low, and IgM levels may be elevated. IgE levels rarely are needed. *A normal IgE level does not rule out allergy, and an elevated one does not diagnose it.* They may be useful occasionally in infancy in the child with recurrent bronchitis or in the occasional patient in whom there is a question of "allergy." In the child with shifting pulmonary infiltrates, tests for precipitating antibody to *Aspergillus* species and agents causing hypersensitivity pneumonitis are indicated (see Chapter 47).

Sweat Test. A sweat test should be carried out on infants and children with chronic respiratory symptoms to rule out cystic fibrosis. However, cystic fibrosis and asthma (or at least a large reactive airways component) may coexist.

X-Rays. All children with asthma should have a chest x-ray at some time to rule out parenchymal disease, congenital anomaly, and foreign body. A chest x-ray should be obtained or at least considered on every child admitted to a hospital with asthma. Chest x-rays in asthma may range from normal to hyperinflation with peribronchial interstitial infiltrates and atelectasis. In a 3-year study of children hospitalized for asthma, the following abnormalities were seen: 76 percent had hyperinflation with increased bronchial markings (Fig. 45–2A); 20 percent had infiltrates, atelectasis, pneumonia, or a combination of the three (Fig. 45–2B); 5.4 percent had pneumomediastinum (Fig.

Text continued on page 594.

TABLE 45–4 LABORATORY TESTS IN ASTHMA

Test	Possible Abnormalities in Asthma	Comments
Complete blood count	Leukocytosis (occasionally)	Induced by infection, epinephrine administration, "stress" (?)
	Eosinophilia (frequently)	Varies with medication, time of day, adrenal function; not necessarily related to "allergy." (Often higher in "intrinsic" than "extrinsic" asthma.)
Sputum Exam White or "clear" and small yellow plugs	Eosinophils	In both "intrinsic" and "extrinsic" asthma.
	Charcot-Leyden crystals	Derived from eosinophils.
	Creola bodies	Clusters of epithelial cells.
	Curschmann's spirals	Threads of glycoprotein.
Nasal smear	Eosinophils	Suggests concomitant nasal allergy in children.
	Lymphocytes, PMN's, macrophages	Replace eosinophils in URIs.
	PMN's with ingested bacteria	Bacterial rhinitis or sinusitis
Serum tests	IgG, IgA, IgM	Often normal. May be abnormal — various patterns seen.
	IgE	Sometimes elevated in "allergic" asthma. Often normal.
	Aspergillus-precipitating antibody	Suggestive, not diagnostic of bronchopulmonary aspergillosis
Sweat test	Normal in asthma Perform to rule out cystic fibrosis	Cystic fibrosis and asthma can coexist.
Chest x-ray	Hyperinflation, infiltrates, pneumomediastinum, pneumothorax	Indicated once in all children with asthma. Indicated on hospitalization for asthma.
Lung function tests	$\downarrow FEV_1, \downarrow FVC, \downarrow FEF_{25\text{-}75\%}, \downarrow PEFR$; $FEV_1/FVC < 75\%$	Useful for following course of disease, response to treatment.
Response to bronchodilators	$> 15\%$ improvement FEV_1; PEFR	Safest diagnostic test for asthma.
Exercise tests	Decreased lung function after 6 minutes of exercise PEFR and $FEV_1 > 15\% \downarrow$ $FEF_{25-75\%} > 25\% \downarrow$	Useful to diagnose asthma in children. Often abnormal when resting lung function is normal.
Methacholine inhalation test (Mecholyl test)	20% fall in lung function with dose tolerated by "normal" subjects.	Should be performed only by specialists.
Antigen inhalation test	20% fall in lung function immediately after challenge; may cause delayed response 6–8 hrs. later	Potentially dangerous; specialist only.
Allergy skin tests	Identifies allergic factors which *might* be causative factors	Test only likely factors — selected by history.
RAST	Same significance as skin tests	More expensive than skin tests.

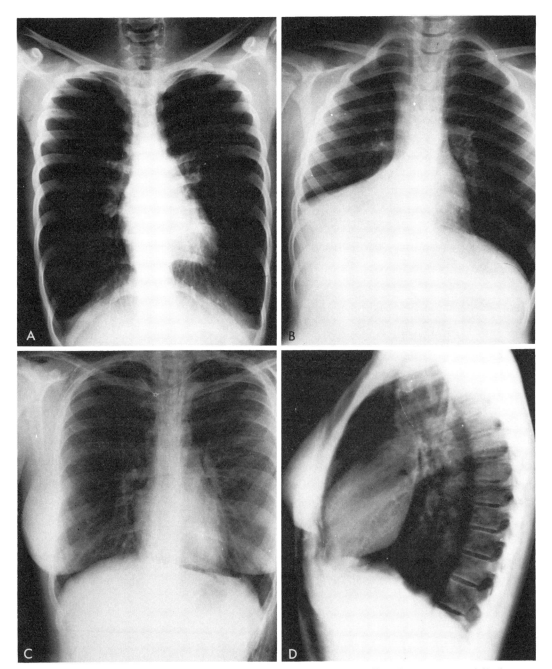

FIGURE 45–2.   *A,* Severe asthma evidenced by extreme hyperaeration, "scalloped" appearance of diaphragm as insertions are visualized, and mediastinal air seen along right heart border.

B, There is almost complete collapse of right middle and right lower lobes with considerable shift of the mediastinum and elevation of the right hemidiaphragm.

C, Extensive mediastinal and subcutaneous emphysema is present without pneumothorax. The lungs are hyperexpanded and diaphragm is flattened, consistent with the clinical diagnosis of asthma.

D, Lateral view of *C* showing extensive mediastinal air.

Legend and illustration continued on the next page.

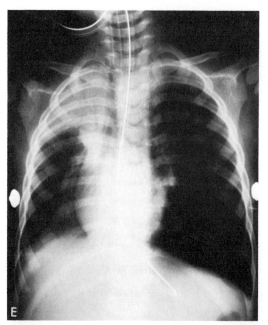

FIGURE 45–2 Continued. *E,* Marked right pneumothorax with shift of pneumomediastinum to the right and hyperaeration of left lung.

45–2*C* and *D*), often with infiltrates (Eggleston et al., 1974). Pneumothorax occurs rarely (Fig. 45–2*E*). Paranasal sinus x-rays also should be considered in children with persistent nocturnal coughing and headaches (see Chapter 40).

Lung Function Tests. Lung function tests are objective and noninvasive and are cost-effective in diagnosing and following the patient with asthma (see Chapter 42). A simple mechanical spirometer from which an FEV_1 and FVC can be calculated or a Wright Pediatric Peak Flow Meter for younger children is useful in office practice. Children as young as 2 years can be taught to perform pulmonary function maneuvers with a birthday party favor (Fig. 45–3). Results can be compared with normal standards (Chapter 42).

Response to Bronchodilators. The safest diagnostic test for asthma is to observe for improvement in lung function before and after administration of bronchodilators such as epinephrine (epinephrine hydrochloride 1:1000–0.01 ml/kg up to a maximum dosage 0.3 ml subcutaneously), inhalations of isoproterenol (0.25 percent) by pressurized aerosol or equivalent or 5 to 10 minutes aerosolized isoproterenol solution (0.05 percent) or equivalent. A greater than 15 percent improvement is virtually diagnostic of asthma.

Exercise Tolerance Tests. In older children and adolescents, a free-running exercise tolerance test is simple to perform and requires little equipment (see Chapter 46). A fall of greater than 15 percent in FEV_1 and in PEFR, or 25 percent in $FEF_{25-75\%}$ is diagnostic of asthma.

Bronchial Challenge Tests. Extreme airway sensitivity characterizes the patient with

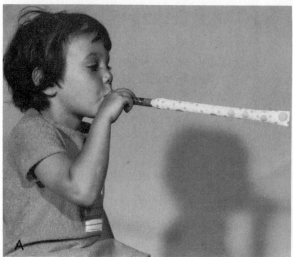
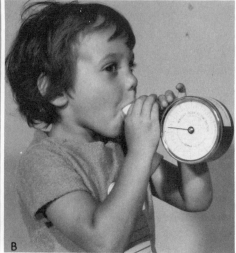

FIGURE 45–3. Illustration of use of party favor to teach young children technique applicable to use of equipment for measuring pulmonary functions.

asthma, whose airways are 50 to 1000 times more sensitive to methacholine than are those of the normal person. This has been developed as a diagnostic test for asthma (Chai et al., 1975).

Another challenge test involves the inhalation of allergens in various concentrations to determine the patient's bronchial sensitivity to them (bronchial provocation test). Often this test induces a biphasic reaction, an initial fall in lung function followed in 6 to 8 hours by more severe protracted bronchospasm. *All bronchial challenge testing (both methacholine tests and allergen challenges) are potentially dangerous; they should be performed only by specialists who have special training in their use.*

Allergy Testing. Allergy testing (skin testing or RAST) is indicated in patients in whom specific allergic factors are believed to be important factors. Testing is done for selective allergens based on history and known or potential allergen exposures (see Chapter 21).

THERAPEUTIC CONSIDERATION

Philosophy of Management

A comprehensive approach to treatment of asthma in children requires an understanding of the disease, the manner in which it presents in children, and how it may affect physical and psychologic growth and development. *The ultimate goal is to prevent disability and to minimize physical and psychologic morbidity.* This includes facilitating social adjustments of the child with the family, school, and community, including normal participation in recreational activities and sports. This is achieved in steps and should begin with early diagnosis and appropriate management of acute episodes. Irritant and allergic factors should be identified and eliminated from the child's environment. *Education of the parents and child to the long-term course of asthma and in how to manage exacerbations is an essential part of asthma therapy.* Unnecessary and illogical restrictions of the child's and family's life styles should be avoided. Associated conditions that exacerbate asthma and predispose to school absenteeism or inter-

fere with school performance must be recognized and treated. The ultimate goal should be "functional" normality — in which maximal benefit is achieved from total therapy, with the fewest detrimental effects from treatment.

Achieving these goals requires time, knowledge and experience. The demands on the physician will vary depending on the severity of the disease, the age of the patient, and the resources of the family. The family physician or pediatrician *who is willing to devote the time* can care adequately for the child with mild or moderate asthma. However, the patient with severe asthma and chronic obstructive pulmonary changes will benefit by referral to a physician who has the knowledge, experience, and time to initiate appropriate therapy, follow the child longitudinally, and act as an advisor to the primary care physician. Such a referral should emphasize prompt and effective treatment of acute attacks to minimize the need for hospitalization (or, when hospitalization is necessary, to reduce length of hospital stay). A team approach that includes regular communication between the referring physician and the specialist is essential for consistent and comprehensive long-term care.

Compliance by patient and family is the keystone of any therapy. Compliance is influenced by many factors — by the physician's attitude, by the family and/or patient's understanding of the disease, and by peer pressures. It is in *compliance* that psychologic factors are of overwhelming importance. The child's attitude toward asthma and willingness to comply with recommendations reflect the parents' attitude toward the disease. The physician's guidance can prevent overprotection or neglect by helping the family of the younger child to cope with such aspects of asthma as the inconvenience of round-the-clock medication schedule and environmental control. As the child grows, the physician and family should give the patient the responsibility for his or her own medication, though the physician should help by providing the most convenient medication schedule possible — ideally one which avoids the need to take medication in school. When medication is needed at school, the patient should be permitted to take it privately without embarrassment. The physician should aid patient and family in making decisions on such activities as sports, overnight visits, and camping trips, taking care to avoid overprotection while ensuring appropriate control of asthma. The physician also can help to change attitudes of teachers, principals, and coaches (and in some cases, school nurses) by educating them to the needs of the individual child and by showing them how the school program can be adjusted to the child's physical capacity, so that the child is not penalized or singled out for ridicule.

Finally, when a child or parents fail to comply, the physician should try to find out the reasons for noncompliance and work out a reasonable solution, acceptable to the patient and the family.

Office Management of Asthma

The means available for office management of asthma include pharmacologic therapy; identification and elimination of exacerbating or aggravating factors; immunotherapy (hyposensitization) when appropriate for major allergens that cannot be eliminated or avoided; provision for optimal physical exercise; and *education of the patient and family about the disease.*

Avoidance. Allergic and irritant factors that exacerbate asthma should be identified and removed from the child's environment. Major allergic or irritant factors in the home or school suggested by a detailed history and confirmed when applicable by skin tests should be eliminated or avoided to the extent possible within the framework of normal physical and psychologic growth and development (Chapter 22). Though the removal of important allergic and irritant factors from the home is essential, the physician also must be flexible and reasonable. Often, effective environmental control may involve a compromise between what is desirable medically and what is acceptable emotionally to the family and child.

Maximum Exercise Function. Participation in normal family, school, and community functions requires reasonably normal exercise tolerance. Regular exercise should be encouraged. The child with asthma does particularly well in such sports as swimming, downhill skiing, or gymnastics, and in soccer, in which acceptance as a normal team member strengthens the ego and builds self-respect. Pretreatment with appropriate medication and a "warm-up" consisting of a short period of mild exercise before more active exercise are especially helpful (see Chapter 46).

Allergy Injection Therapy. Hyposensitization (immunotherapy) is indicated for major environmental allergens that cannot be avoided, such as pollen antigens. Many children and adolescents have allergic rhinitis, for which hyposensitization has proved efficacious (see Chapter 24). Hyposensitization also can ameliorate the allergic component of asthma in children (Warner, 1978).

Management of the Acute Attack. Acute asthma in children can occur as a mild illness that responds promptly to bronchodilators, or it can develop into a medical emergency over a matter of a few hours, especially in the young child who is unable to retain oral medication and fluids. In such a child, decreasing wheezing may be ominous, signaling increasing obstruction of airways with concomitant decrease in air exchange. If the child's asthma fails to respond to home treatment, he or she should be seen on an emergency basis in the physician's office or in a hospital emergency room.

In treating acute asthma, drugs of choice are epinephrine by injection or aerosolized adrenergic agents (Table 45–5). Epinephrine may be repeated up to three times at 15-minute intervals if necessary, or aerosolized agents administered by oxygen-driven nebulizer or ultrasonic nebulizer for 5 to 10 minutes at 30-minute intervals. Pulse rates should be monitored during aerosol treatment, and the treatment should be discontinued if the pulse rate exceeds 200 beats/minute. *IPPB should not be used,* because it might induce or worsen pneumomediastinum or pneumothorax (*Lancet,* 1978). If the child can and will cooperate, pulmonary function testing employing measurement of peak expiratory flow or spirometry before and after therapy is quite helpful, since apparent improvement by stethoscope may be misleading in the presence of severe bronchial obstruction. If the patient responds to initial therapy, an injection of Sus-Phrine may maintain bronchodilation until oral medication becomes effective. Pressurized adrenergic hand nebuilizers are used with

TABLE 45–5 TREATMENT OF ACUTE ATTACK

Drug	Administration	Dosage	Frequency	Notes
Epinephrine aqueous, 1:1000 solution	Subcutaneously	0.01 ml/kg (max. 0.3 ml)	15 min × 3	
Isoproterenol HCl Solution, 0.05%	Aerosol by nebulizer*	5 ml for 10 min	30 min × 3	Monitor pulse
Isoetharine HCl. 0.25%	Aerosol by nebulizer**	5 ml for 10 min	30 min × 3	>12 years only
Salbutamol or terbutaline, 0.5%	Aerosol by nebulizer***	5 ml for 10 min	30 min × 3	Not available in USA
Suspension epinephrine, 1:200 (Sus-Phrine®)	Subcutaneously	0.005 ml/kg (max. 0.2 ml)	Single dosage	To follow initial treatment if appropriate (see text)

*Made up as 1 part drug to 9 parts saline
**Made up as 1 part drug to 3 parts saline
***Made up as 1 part drug to 9 parts saline

TABLE 45-6 TREATMENT OF MILD ASTHMA

Drug*	Formulation	Dosage	Frequency	Notes
Theophylline	Liquid or tablet	4–6 mg/kg	6 hours	May need to begin at 1/2 dosage
Metaproterenol	Liquid or tablet	0.6 mg/kg	4–6 hours	
Terbutaline	Tablet	0.75 mg/kg	6 hours	>12 yrs only
Cromolyn sodium	Inhaled powder	20 mg	4 times daily	Prevention only

* See Chapter 23.

particular caution in children because of abuse potential; they should be used only as an adjunct to oral therapy. When they are prescribed, the parent or patient should be warned of the dangers of overuse. If an adequate trial of epinephrine or aerosolized adrenergic drug fails to produce a significant response, the patient should be admitted to the hospital and treated for status asthmaticus.

Management of Mild Asthma. Mild asthma, in which the patient has only intermittent episodes of asthma but is completely symptom-free between episodes, can often be managed by oral theophylline or oral adrenergic drugs administered only for attacks (Table 45–6)

For the child unable to retain medication, theophylline or aminophylline administered by rectal solution (4–6 mg/kg) is reliably absorbed, but *aminophylline suppositories should be avoided* because of erratic and slow absorption and potential overdosage. Cromolyn sodium may be effective if used before anticipated exposure to known allergens (such as cats) or prior to exercise, but it should be discontinued during acute attacks.

Management of Moderately Severe Asthma. When asthma interferes with activity,

sleep, or exercise and is characterized by persistently abnormal lung function, round-the-clock oral theophylline is the drug of choice (Table 45–7). The theophylline dosage that provides a round-the-clock therapeutic serum concentration ("optimal" concentration = 10–20 μg/ml) for the individual child is best established by therapeutic monitoring. Conversion to an 8-hour or 12-hour timed-release formulation makes a round-the-clock schedule more convenient and increases compliance. Theophylline dosages and formulations are discussed more fully in Chapter 23. Adrenergic agents such as terbutaline or metaproterenol may be added for acute exacerbations or employed in place of theophylline on a round-the-clock basis. Pressurized adrenergic aerosols, believed by some to be useful adjuncts to oral therapy, should be employed only if physicians and parents can assure against abuse. Cromolyn sodium administered four times daily by Spinhaler should be tried for at least 1 month in those patients with an inadequate response to theophylline or oral adrenergic drugs. For acute exacerbations, a short course of prednisone or prednisolone may be necessary, beginning with 30 to 40 mg/day administered as a single or two divided doses the first day, then tapered by

TABLE 45-7 TREATMENT OF MODERATE ASTHMA

Drug*	Formulation	Dosage	Frequency	Notes
Anhydrous theophylline	Liquid or tablet	4–6 mg/kg	6 hours ⎫	Check theophylline level*
Timed-release theophylline	Tablet or Spansule	16–24 mg/kg/day	8–12 hours ⎭	
Terbutaline	Tablet	2.5–5 mg	6–8 hours	>12 yrs: may be used with theophylline
Metaproterenol	Tablet, liquid	5–20 mg	4–6 hours	May be used with theophylline
Cromolyn Sodium (preventive only)	Inhaled powder	20 mg	4 times daily	Discontinue during attacks
Short course of prednisone	Tablets	30–40 mg initially (see text)	Once daily	Taper over 5–7 days to 0

* See Chapter 23.

TABLE 45-8 TREATMENT OF SEVERE ASTHMA

Theophylline, adrenergic drugs, cromolyn: as outlined in Table 45-7 for moderately severe asthma.

Prednisone—40 mg/day: *Taper to lowest possible dose which maintains adequate lung function.* Shift to every second day (q.o.d.) using 2½ times the lowest daily dose which achieved asthma control. Give before 8:00 A.M.

Beclomethasone dipropionate—2 to 4 sprays, 4 times daily or 3-4 sprays 3 times daily.

Reduce prednisone or beclomethasone to lowest possible dosage; eventually discontinue altogether if possible. Dosage reductions of q.o.d. prednisone and beclomethasone should be attempted at 2-week intervals. Use prednisone course for acute asthma, surgery, trauma, and acute illnesses (see text).

---

administering the drug daily in the early morning, discontinuing it in 5 to 7 days.

Management of Severe Asthma. In severe asthma, the patient continues to have incapacitating dyspnea, cough, and obstructed airways in spite of treatment as described for moderate asthma. Long-term corticosteroid therapy is essential to the treatment of such patients. Therapy is outlined in Table 45-8.

When a patient has received oral steroids for a prolonged period, prednisone should be tapered slowly when attempting to replace by aerosolized steroids, since the hypothalmic-pituitary-adrenal axis may take up to a year to recover normal responsiveness. Oral candidiasis, the major complication of aerosolized steroid therapy, can be minimized by rinsing the mouth with water after each treatment. If the patient is on alternate-day or aerosolized steroid therapy, short courses of daily steroids should be considered for acute exacerbations of asthma, major surgery (see Chapter 62), and for acute severe illness in general.

Other Drugs. Other agents sometimes prescribed for asthma include expectorants, antibiotics, sedatives, tranquilizers, and antihistamines. All expectorants depend upon adequate hydration for effective action. Iodides, the traditional expectorants of the past, should be avoided in children because their many adverse effects make their use unacceptable (A.A.P. Committee on Drugs, 1976). Other expectorants such as glyceryl guaiacolate add little at best to adequate hydration. Antibiotics are indicated only when there is substantial evidence of bacteri-

al or mycoplasma infections (see Chapter 19). Troleandomycin (TAO), sometimes prescribed in severe chronic asthma, should be left to the specialist. *Sedatives and tranquilizers are contraindicated in asthma.* Agitation is related to airways obstruction, dyspnea, and hypoxemia. It is most effectively relieved by adequate asthma therapy. Antihistamines may be useful for therapy of allergic rhinitis in asthmatic patients but *they are not effective for the treatment of asthma itself.*

Comment on Drug Therapy. Recommendations given here are intended as guidelines only (see also Chapter 23). Drug therapy must be individualized to the child's age, disease severity, and ability to tolerate the drug. It must be readjusted regularly for growth and changes in severity, using the lowest dosage and least toxic drugs compatible with "functional normality."

Hospital Management of Asthma

Status asthmaticus, or acute severe asthma refractory to nonsteroid drugs, may be a life-threatening medical emergency that requires prompt, systematic, and aggressive management. Young children can progress from acute asthma to status asthmaticus in a matter of hours. The sooner status asthmaticus is recognized and treated, the shorter the hospital stay and fewer the complications.

Pathophysiology. Status asthmaticus results from a respiratory triad of bronchial and bronchiolar smooth muscle spasm, mucosal inflammation and edema, and increased secretion of mucus. In the infant and young child, mucosal edema and mucus plugging predominate (Field, 1968), whereas in the older child bronchospasm becomes a major cause of obstruction (Matsuba, 1971). As airway obstruction increases, PEFR falls while the FRC and RV increase. A progressive imbalance between lung perfusion and ventilation and increased rate of breathing cause a fall in both arterial oxygen tension ($\downarrow$ Pao_2) and carbon dioxide tension ($\downarrow$ $Paco_2$). Increased work of breathing, fever, and vomiting all superimpose a metabolic acidosis, *at first* compensated, but eventually with a decreasing pH. As fatigue and progressive pulmonary obstruction occur, the $Paco_2$ (which should be decreased by the "hyperventilation" associated with severe asthma) may rise. *Hence, an elevated* *or even "normal"* $Paco_2$ *is an ominous sign.* This may progress to frank respiratory failure, cardiac arrhythmias, and cardiorespiratory arrest with irreversible hypoxic brain damage or death.

Initial Evaluation

1. Begin humidified oxygen by mask or nasal prongs.
2. Begin intravenous infusion — 5 percent glucose in 0.2 percent saline. Obtain urine for specific gravity.
3. Perform history and physical examination.
4. Obtain arterial or arterialized blood gases, serum electrolytes, serum theophylline level.
5. Perform baseline pulmonary function tests — if patient can cooperate (FVC and/or flow rates).
6. Obtain chest x-ray.

The patient should be admitted to the intensive care unit or equivalent for close observation, and *humidified oxygen* administered at once by nasal prongs or Venturi mask. *Every patient with severe asthma has significant hypoxemia.* Hypoxemia occurs far in advance of hypercapnea and often is present when cyanosis is not detectable. Thus, *cyanosis is a late and unreliable clinical index for administration of oxygen.*

Chest x-rays should be obtained on admission to rule out infection and complications such as pneumomediastinum, pneumothorax, atelectasis, and large airway mucus plugging.

Intravenous Therapy to Ensure Proper Hydration and for Drug Administration. An intravenous infusion should be initiated early with 5 percent dextrose in 0.2 percent saline for hydration, with subsequent fluids for maintenance and repair of fluid deficit. Patients with severe asthma are frequently dehydrated on admission. Care should be taken not to *overhydrate,* however, since overhydration in the face of negative pulmonary pressures associated with severe asthma may lead to pulmonary edema. Use urine specific gravity measurements to help in assessment of state of hydration, both initially and during on-going therapy.

Drug Therapy. Aminophylline should be administered intravenously, the initial dos-

GUIDELINES FOR INTRAVENOUS FLUIDS IN STATUS ASTHMATICUS

1. *Hydration.* 12 ml/kg or 360 ml/m² for first hour, 5% glucose in 1/4 normal saline.
2. *Maintenance.* 50–80 ml/kg/24 hours, depending on age, or 1500 ml/m², 5% glucose with 2mEq potassium and 3mEq sodium/100 ml fluids.
3. *Depletion Repair.* 20–30 ml/kg or 300 to 500 ml/m² of 1/2 normal saline depending on age.
4. *Correction of Acidosis.* If pH is below 7.30 and neg base excess >5mEq/l, correct to normal range using the formula:

mEq bicarbonate = (neg) base excess × 0.3 × body wt. (kg)

Administer one-half initially and remainder after repeat blood gas and pH determinations.

Note: If patient is in severe distress, administer sodium bicarbonate 2mEq/kg intravenously without delay over 10 minutes. Obtain pH and correct acidosis further as appropriate.

age depending upon prior therapy. Ideally, aminophylline should be administered by constant infusion (Pierson, 1971), but it can be administered over a 20-minute period every 4 to 6 hours. If theophylline blood levels can be measured, therapy should be aimed at achieving a level between 10 and 20 µg theophylline/ml serum.

Corticosteroid therapy should be initiated intravenously immediately in *severely ill patients who are already on steroids or who have been on prolonged oral steroid therapy (greater than 2 weeks) or who have been on aerosolized steroid therapy in the previous 6 weeks.* Corticosteroids reduce inflammation, increase rate of recovery from hypoxemia,

AMINOPHYLLINE ADMINISTRATION

Loading dose. 7 mg/kg diluted in saline. Administer over 15 minutes by Volutrol or constant infusion pump. Modify loading dose on basis of medication history or initial serum theophylline level.

Maintenance dose. Average, but modified by serum theophylline levels obtained by measurement:

<10 kg body weight: 0.65 mg/kg/hr (15 mg/kg/24 hr)
>10 kg body weight: 0.9 mg/kg/hr (21 mg/kg/24 hr)

Administer by continuous drip infusion (preferred) or give every 4 to 6 hours over a 15 to 20 minute period.

CORTICOSTEROID THERAPY

Dexamethasone or betamethasone phosphate, 0.3 mg/kg stat and 0.3 mg/kg/24 hrs.
  or
Hydrocortisone hemisuccinate, 7 mg/kg stat and 7 mg/kg/24 hrs (divide maintenance dosage into four 6-hr. doses).
  or
Methylprednisolone sodium succinate, 2 mg/kg stat and 2 mg/kg/24 hrs.

---

and may aid in restoring responsiveness to beta-adrenergic agents (Pierson, 1974).

Adrenergic Agents. After fluid, drug, and oxygen therapy has been initiated, another trial of adrenergic agents is appropriate, by low-pressure ultrasonic or wall nebulizer (Garra, 1977) or by injection. During a treatment, the child's pulse rate should be monitored, and a treatment should be discontinued if the pulse exceeds 200 beats/minute.

Antibiotics. Antibiotics should be administered if there is specific evidence of bacterial infection, or if there is any question of bacterial infection when the asthma appears to be life-threatening.

There are no special indications for the use

ADRENERGIC AGENTS

Drugs
  Aerosol
Isoproterenol sol.†	0.05%
Metaproterenol sol.**	0.5%
Isoetharine sol.††	0.25%
Salbutamol sol.*	0.5%
Terbutalone sol.*	

  Injection
  Epinephrine aqueous 1:1000, administer 0.1 to 0.25 cc sc q 20 min × 2.

Administration
  Low-pressure ultrasonic or wall nebulizer for 5 to 10 minutes every half-hour × 4, then as indicated by patient's condition. Follow pulse during each treatment. Discontinue if ≥ 200/minute.

---

  *Not available in United States.
  **Possibly available in United States in 1980.
  †1 part drug to 9 parts saline.
  ††1 part drug to 3 parts saline.

of antibiotics in asthma or in other allergic disorders (Shapiro, 1974). Antibiotics have been used frequently in asthma when no clear indication of infection exists, and their excessive use has been partly responsible for the frequent sensitization of allergic patients to penicillin and other antibiotics and/or chemotherapeutic agents. It is well to remember that (1) asthma frequently is accompanied by patchy atelectasis which often is misinterpreted as bronchopneumonia on x-ray; and (2) leukocytosis of 15,000 or even higher may be seen in severe asthma in the absence of demonstrable bacterial infection, particularly after epinephrine administration, and is not an indication per se for antibiotic therapy.

Sedation. CAUTION: Patients with severe asthma have good reason to be extremely anxious, and more often than not, their anxiety is an expression of the severity of respiratory distress rather than the main cause of it. *Sedatives that depress the respiratory center, such as barbiturates, are contraindicated in asthma.* If sedation is considered necessary, use chloral hydrate (200 to 500 mg p.o. or by rectum) *with caution. Tranquilizers,* particularly members of the phenothiazine group (e.g., chlorpromazine), should not be used since they may have a depressant effect on respiration and on bronchial reflexes, especially in the face of hypoxemia; and they exert multiple effects on the CNS that are poorly understood. The use of adrenergic agents in a patient on phenothiazines also may precipitate profound hypotension.

Further Therapy in Hospital. Oxygen therapy should be continued until asthma is adequately controlled and the patient's Pao_2 is stable and "adequate" in room air. Monitoring airways function in the hospital when possible provides a further guide to therapy. After 24 to 48 hours, theophylline, corticosteroids, and antibiotics usually can be administered orally.

Outpatient Treatment. Though status asthmaticus often can be controlled sufficiently to discharge the child from hospital in 48 to 72 hours, full control of asthma and optimal pulmonary functions may not return for many days to weeks. *As the patient improves, do not wean from therapy too rapidly.* Patients should be discharged on round-the-clock bronchodilators and on prednisone administered as a single 8 A.M. dosage, to be tapered over one week. *Follow-up is important.*

Complications of Asthma

Respiratory Failure. Respiratory failure occurs in a small but significant number of children admitted to hospital with status asthmaticus. It often occurs because the physician has failed to recognize the severity of the child's asthma. *The best treatment of respiratory failure is prevention by effective early treatment of asthma.* Signs of overt respiratory failure include decreased or absent pulmonary breath sounds, severe intercostal retraction, pulsus paradoxicus, use of accessory muscles of respiration, cyanosis in 40 percent oxygen, decreased response to pain, poor skeletal muscle tone, and diaphoresis.

Respiratory failure is characterized by an elevated Pa_{CO_2} (>40 Torr) and a decreased Pa_{O_2} (<55 Torr).

The consultant allergist, chest physician, and anesthesiologist should be notified early about any child at risk of impending respiratory failure. Treatment is intravenous isoproterenol, or mechanical ventilation.

1. *Intravenous isoproterenol.* If this therapy is tried, it should be in a well-equipped intensive care unit, with ready provision for mechanical ventilation since 10 to 20 percent of such patients will still require mechanical ventilation (Wood, 1972). The patient should receive isoproterenol by calibrated constant infusion pump, beginning with 0.1 $\mu g/kg/min$, increasing the dosage 0.1 $\mu g/kg/min$ every 15 to 30 minutes until clinical improvement or tachycardia (>200/min) develops. Hazards of this therapy include cardiac arrhythmias and myocarditis. *Treatment may be unsuccessful and means for mechanical ventilation must be available immediately.* Adults and probably older children are particularly susceptible to cardiac overstimulation, and treatment with IV isoproterenol is discouraged in children who are past their early teens.

2. *Mechanical ventilation.* Endotracheal intubation, neuromuscular blockage, sedation and mechanical ventilation with a volume ventilator with constant monitoring of ECG and frequent blood gas determinations may be necessary. Once the asthma has been controlled, the patient can be shifted to intermittent mandatory ventilation, and generally can be extubated in 24 to 48 hours (Simons, 1978).

Atelectasis. Atelectasis is a common finding in acute asthma and may be present in up to 20 percent of children hospitalized for asthma (Eggleston, 1974). Frequently perihilar interstitial infiltrates are mistaken for "bronchopneumonia" and treated with antibiotics. Atelectasis may involve a major pulmonary segment or an entire lobe. The right middle lobe is involved most frequently, possibly because the right main stem bronchus tends to twist with hyperinflation, though it is unclear why this lobe is involved more commonly in girls than in boys (Dees, 1966). Therapy of asthma and physical therapy with postural drainage and clapping is sufficient to induce expansion in most cases. Persistent atelectasis may result from foreign body, anatomic defect, or obstructing peribronchial lymph nodes. *Only rarely is bronchoscopy or bronchography necessary.* When these are performed, especial caution must be exercised because of the hyperirritable tracheobronchial tree of asthmatics. It is unusual for chronic atelectasis to progress to localized bronchiectasis needing surgical treatment.

Pneumomediastinum and Pneumothorax. Pneumomediastinum is a relatively common complication of severe asthma in children and may occur in up to 6 percent of those admitted to hospital with severe asthma. It occurs more commonly in older children and is rare under 2 years of age (Eggleston, 1974). Pneumomediastinum occurs when air ruptures alveolar bases and dissects along pulmonary vascular sheaths to the mediastinum. From there, air usually dissects along fascial planes into the subcutaneous tissue of neck and axilla. This condition will resolve spontaneously with control of asthma. However, air in the mediastinum rarely may rupture the parietal pleura and induce pneumothorax (Bierman, 1967). Pneumothorax also may occur in longstanding severe asthma from rupture of a pulmonary "bleb," which can result in sudden death if not recognized and treated promptly (Jorgensen, 1963).

Inappropriate ADH Response. The "inappropriate" secretion of antidiuretic hormone may complicate intravenous fluid therapy in status asthmaticus. A fall in serum sodium concentration or decreased plasma urine osmolality can lead to water intoxication. ADH secretion is probably stimulated by left atrial receptors with decreased left atrial filling due to asthma (Baker, 1976).

Flaccid Paralysis. Flaccid paralysis of an arm or leg following severe asthma has been reported from widely separated geographic areas. In most patients a lag between asthma and onset of paralysis with constitutional symptoms and pleocytosis in the CSF suggest a viral infection. To date viral studies in such patients have been negative for poliomyelitis and other neurotropic viruses (Hopkins, 1974; Shapiro, 1979).

Irreversible Pulmonary Changes. An increasing number of patients with severe asthma in childhood are recognized as having chronic non-reversible obstructive disease in adulthood (see Prognosis of Asthma). The pathogenetic mechanism which leads to irreversibility is unknown.

Psychologic Problems. In chronic asthma, various psychologic problems may require specialist referral. The type of problems requiring consultation include the child or family whose denial of asthma leads to treatment delays or noncompliance and repeated hospitalization; estranged parents who use the child's asthma in their quarrels; parents who overprotect their children into adult life and are unable to allow them to grow up; parents who are overcontrolled by the child who has asthma; and patients who use their asthma consistently to avoid responsibility or uncomfortable situations such as tests at school (see Chapter 26).

Allergic Bronchopulmonary Aspergillosis. A rare complication of chronic childhood asthma in North America, allergic bronchopulmonary aspergillosis is characterized by progressive fatigue, weight loss, night sweats, and coughing. Clubbing of the fingers may occur. Expectorated sputum may contain brownish plugs from which *Aspergillus fumigatus* can be cultured. Chest x-rays show lobular infiltrates. The serum contains precipitating antibodies to *A. fumigatus*, and skin tests show a dual response of an immediate wheal and flare in 10 to 15 minutes and a delayed response 6 to 8 hours later. Prolonged corticosteroid therapy may be necessary to prevent development of proximal bronchiectasis (see Chapter 47).

References

A. A. P. Committee on Drugs: Adverse reactions to iodide therapy of asthma and other pulmonary diseases. Pediatrics 57:272, 1976.

Aas, K.: Bronchial provocation tests in asthma. Arch. Dis. Child. 45:221, 1970.

Baker, J. D., Yerger, S., and Segar, W. E.: Elevated plasma antidiuretic hormone levels in status asthmaticus. Mayo Clinic Proc. 51:31–34, 1976.

Bias, W. B.: The genetic basis of asthma. In Austen, K. F., and Lichtenstein, L. M. (eds.): Asthma. N.Y., Academic Press Inc., pp. 39–48, 1973.

Bierman, C. W.: Pneumomediastinum and pneumothorax complicating asthma in children. Am. J. Dis. Child. 114:42, 1967.

Blair, H.: Natural history of childhood asthma. Arch. Dis. Child. 52:613, 1977.

Cade, J. F., and Pain, M. C. F.: Pulmonary function during clinical remission of asthma. How reversible is asthma? Aust. N.Z.J. Med. 3:545, 1973.

Chai, H., Farr, R. S., Froehlich, L. A., Mathison, D. A., McLean, J. A., Rosenthal, R. R., Sheffer, A. L., Spector, S. L., and Townley, R. G.: Standardization of bronchial inhalation challenge procedures. J. Allergy Clin. Immunol. 56:323–327, 1975.

Corrao, W. M., Braman, S. S., and Irwin, R. S.: Chronic cough as the sole presenting manifestation of bronchial asthma. N. Engl. J. Med. 300:633, 1979.

Dees, S. C., and Spock, A.: Right middle lobe syndrome in children. J.A.M.A. 197:8, 1966.

Devereux, R. B., Perloff, J. K., Reichele, N., and Josephson, M. F.: Mitral valve prolapse. Circulation 54:3, 1976.

Editorial: Alveolar rupture. Lancet II:137, 1978.

Eggleston, P. A., Ward, B. H., Pierson, W. E., and Bierman, C. W.: Radiographic abnormalities in acute asthma in children. Pediatrics 54:442, 1974.

Ellis, E. F.: Role of infection in asthma. Adv. Asthma, Allergy Pulmonary Dis. 4:28, 1977.

Field, W. E.: Mucous gland hypertrophy in babies and children aged 15 years or less. Br. J. Dis. Chest 62:11, 1968.

Flensborg, E. W.: The prognosis for bronchial asthma arisen in infancy after the nonspecific treatment hitherto applied. Acta Paediatrica 33:4–23, 1945.

Garra, B. J., Shapiro, G. G., Pierson, W. E., Dorsett, C. S., et al.: A double-blind evaluation of the use of nebulized metaproterenol and isoproterenol in hospitalized asthmatic children and adolescents. J. Allergy Clin. Immunol., 60:63–68, 1977.

Hopkins, I. J., and Shield, L. K.: Poliomyelitis-like illness associated with asthma in childhood. Lancet 1:760, 1974.

Jorgensen, J. R., Falliers, C. J., and Bukantz, S. C.: Pneumothorax and mediastinal and subcutaneous emphysema in children with bronchial asthma. Pediatrics 31:824–832, 1963.

Kattan, C. M., Keens, T. G., Lapierre, J-G., Levison, H., Bryan, C., and Reilly, B. J.: Pulmonary function abnormalities in symptom-free children after bronchiolitis. Pediatrics 59:683–688, 1977.

Kinsman, R. A., Dahlein, N. W., Spector, S., and Staudenmayer, H.: Observations on subjective symptomatology, coping behavior, and medical decision in asthma. Psychosomat. Med. 39:102–119, 1977.

Levison, H. S., Collins-Williams, C., Bryan, A. C., Reilly, B. J., and Orange, R. P.: Asthma. Current Concepts. Ped. Clin. N. Amer. 21:951–965, 1974.

Matsuba, K., and Thurlbeck, W. M.: The number and dimensions of small airways in non-emphysematous lungs. Am. Rev. Respir. Dis. *104*:516–524, 1971.

McFadden, E. R., Jr.: Exertional dyspnea and cough as preludes to acute attacks of bronchial asthma. N. Engl. J. Med. *292*:555–559, 1975*a*.

McFadden, E. R., Jr.: The chronicity of acute attacks of asthma–mechanical and therapeutic implications. J. Allergy Clin. Immunol. *56*:18–26, 1975*b*.

McFadden, E. R., Jr., Kisser, R., and DeGroot, W. J.: Acute bronchial asthma: Relations between clinical and physiological manifestations. N. Engl. J. Med. *288*:221–228, 1973.

Minor, T. E., Baker, J. W., Dick, E. C., DeMeo, A. N., Oulette, J. J., Cohen, M., and Reed, C. E.: Greater frequency of viral respiratory infections in asthmatic children as compared with their nonasthmatic siblings. J. Pediatr. *85*:472, 1974.

Pierson, W. E., Bierman, C. W., and Kelley, V. C.: A double-blind trial of corticosteroid therapy in status asthmaticus. Pediatrics *54*:282, 1974.

Pierson, W. E., Bierman, C. W., Stamm, S. J., and Van Arsdel. P. P., Jr.: Double-blind trial of aminophylline in status asthmaticus. Pediatrics *48*:642, 1971.

Rachelefsky, G. S., Coulson, A., Siegel, S. C., and Stiehm, E. R.: Aspirin intolerance in chronic childhood asthma: detected by oral challenge. Pediatrics *56*:443, 1975.

Rackemann, F. M.: Intrinsic asthma. J. Allergy *11*:147, 1940.

Reid, L.: Pathological changes in asthma. *In* Clark, T. J. H., and Godfrey, S. (eds.): Asthma. Philadelphia, W. B. Saunders Co., 1977, pp. 79–95.

Ryssing, E.: Continued follow-up investigation concerning the fate of 298 asthmatic children. Acta Pediatr. *48*:255, 1959.

Shapiro, G. G., Eggleston, P. A., Pierson, W. E., Ray, C. G., and Bierman, C. W.: Double-blind study of the effectiveness of a broad-spectrum antibiotic in status asthmaticus. Pediatrics *53*:867, 1974.

Shapiro, G. G., Furukawa, C. T., Bierman, C. W., and Pierson, W. E.: Poliomyelitis-like illness after acute asthma. J. Pediatr. *94*:767, 1979.

Siegel, S. C., Katz, R. M., and Rachelefsky, G. S.: Asthma in infancy and childhood. *In* Middleton, E., Reed, C. E., and Ellis, E. F. (eds.): Allergy: Principles and Practice. Pages 722–723, C. V. Mosby Co., St. Louis, 1978.

Simons, F. E. R., Pierson, W. E., and Bierman, C. W.: Respiratory failure in childhood status asthmaticus. Am. J. Dis. Child. *131*:1097, 1977.

Tooley, W. H., DeMuth, C., and Nadel, J. A.: The reversibility of obstructive changes in severe childhood asthma. J. Pediatr. *66*:517, 1965.

Townley, R. G., Guirgis, H., Bewtra, A., Watt, G., Burke, K., and Carney, K.: IgE levels and methacholine inhalation responses in monozygous and dizygous twins. J. Allergy Clin. Immunol. *57*:227, 1976 (abstract).

Townley, R. G., Ryo, U. Y., Kolokin, B. M., and Kang, B.: Bronchial sensitivity to methacholine in current and former asthmatic and allergic rhinitis patients and control subjects. J. Allergy Clin. Immunol. *56*:429, 1975.

Warner, J. O., Price, J. F., Soothill, J. F., and Hey, E. N.: Controlled trial of hyposensitization to dermatophagoides pteronyssimus in children with asthma. Lancet *II*:912, 1978.

Weinstein, A. M., Dubin, B. D., Podleski, W. K., Spector, S. L., and Farr, R. S.: Asthma and pregnancy. J.A.M.A. *241*:1161, 1979.

Wood, D. W., Downes, J. J., Schemkoph, H., and Lecks, H. I.: Intravenous isoproterenol in the management of respiratory failure in childhood status asthmaticus. J. Allergy Clin. Immunol. *50*:75, 1972.

Peyton A. Eggleston, M.D. 46

Exercise-Induced Asthma

Most children with asthma have some degree of bronchoconstriction when they exercise. This may be manifested by wheezing, coughing, or symptoms which may be less obvious. Parents, teachers, and physicians may confuse this characteristic manifestation of asthma with the dyspnea that normally follows exercise, or with the increased dyspnea that would be expected with any lung disease or with an attack of hyperventilation.

The asthma attack that follows exercise is brief but indistinguishable from asthma from other causes. As shown in Figure 46–1, pulmonary functions begin to diminish after exercise, reach a nadir 3 to 20 minutes after completion of typical exercise, then spontaneously return to resting levels within 2 hours. The pulmonary function changes seen are similar to those seen with any acute asthma attack and indicate responses by both large and small airways. The attack may be severe, as in the case illustrated in Figure 46–1, in which FEV_1 decreased into the range in which significant hypoxia might be expected. Depending upon the severity of the attack, patients may complain of mild chest tightness, irritation and cough, or they may wheeze overtly and become severely dyspneic and disabled. Often patients will experience slight bronchodilatation during and immediately after exercise, prior to developing the characteristic postexercise bronchoconstriction.

Exercise-induced asthma can have an important impact on the physical and mental well being of an asthmatic child, and optimal control of asthma must include control of this commonly overlooked condition. Beyond this, there also are unique psychosocial and long-term health considerations. Childhood is a peculiarly physical time of one's life (picture a school yard), a time when physical prowess is rewarded and nonconformity is penalized. The child

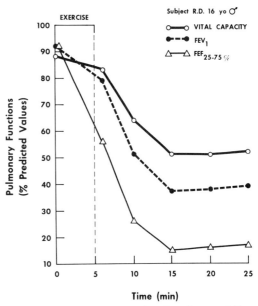

FIGURE 46–1. Pulmonary function changes following treadmill exercise by a 16-year-old boy with lifelong severe asthma. VC (Vital capacity), FEV_1 (Forced expiratory volume in first second), and $FEF_{25-75\%}$ (Mid-expiratory flow rate).

who coughs and wheezes at play has a handicap particularly ill-suited to this time in life. A child may avoid exercise, but at the cost of exclusion from his peer group, and at the risk of establishing sedentary habits that may increase health risks later in life.

MECHANISMS OF EXERCISE-INDUCED ASTHMA

To understand the pathophysiology of exercise-induced asthma, the physiologic response to exercise must first be appreciated. Normally, exercise requires adaptive responses of many systems. Cardiac output increases, by increasing heart rate and, to a lesser extent, stroke volume. Ventilation increases chiefly by increasing tidal volume. Blood is shunted from the viscera to skeletal and cardiac muscle and to skin; only cerebral and renal flow remain undiminished. Epinephrine, norepinephrine, ACTH, and cortisol secretion increase while insulin secretion decreases; in response, levels of plasma free fatty acids and glucose increase, and provide increased substrate for energy metabolism to muscle.

Maximal work capacity is determined primarily by the limits of oxygen transport and utilization at the cellular level. As work loads increase, oxygen consumption rises from resting levels of approximately 3.5 ml per kg per min to a maximum of about 50 ml per kg per min, and then plateaus; these maximal levels can be maintained only for short periods. Cardiovascular reserve does not appear to be the limiting factor, since heart rate and cardiac output are able to rise in parallel to levels of maximal oxygen consumption. Similarly, ventilation increases 30-fold, so that arterial Pao_2 is normal until maximal work loads are reached.

Maximal work capacity seems to be determined primarily by the limits of intracellular oxygen transport and utilization, and the consequences of cellular hypoxia. At about 70 percent of maximal work loads, the limits of mitochondrial pyruvate metabolism are reached, and lactate accumulation begins. Above this level, intolerable lactic acidosis quickly develops, with diminution in arterial pH to less than 7.30.

When exercise stops, acidosis decreases slowly and increased oxygen consumption continues for up to several hours to balance what is termed the "oxygen debt."

Maximal working capacity, maximal oxygen consumption, and maximal cardiac output all are at their greatest in children in their mid-teens, and diminish in later years. Maximal working capacity may be increased by physical conditioning, but maximal oxygen consumption and cardiac output are relatively fixed limits that can be increased only by prolonged strenuous training. In other words, training seems to diminish the response to a given exercise load and to increase the amount of work needed to reach one's limits of oxygen consumption and cardiac output, but has little effect on the limits themselves.

Many theories have been proposed to explain how normal adaptive responses to exercise stress induce asthma (Table 46–1). While none of these mechanisms completely explains why asthma follows exercise, each may contribute. Similarly, resting pulmonary function abnormalities, i.e., the severity of a child's asthma at the time he or she exercises, contribute to the severity of the exercise response. This effect may not be a direct one on the response itself. Instead, patients who begin exercise with partial airway obstruction need only have a minimal response to exercise to become severely obstructed.

The theory that best fits the known experimental observations is that chemical mediators such as histamine, SRS-A, or acetylcholine are released in the lungs during exercise, perhaps in response to mechanical stresses in the lung during hyperventilation, or in response to mucosal heat and moisture losses related to warming and humidifying the markedly increased volumes of inspired air. These mediators then act on the hyperresponsive bronchi of asthmatics to induce asthma. Four pieces of evidence support the mediator release theory: exercised-induced asthma is inhibited by cromolyn sodium, the principle action of which is inhibition of mediator release; histamine concentrations in blood but not plasma are elevated during exercise; the severity of exercise-induced asthma correlates with the degree of bronchial sensitivity to mediators; the degree of asthma diminishes

TABLE 46–1 SUMMARY OF PROPOSED THEORIES OF THE ETIOLOGY OF EXERCISE-INDUCED ASTHMA

Theory	Evidence For	Evidence Against
Lactic acidosis	Peak airway response coincides with peak lactic acidosis	Lactate infusion does not cause asthma Prevention of acidosis during exercise does not prevent asthma
Hypocapnia	Hypocapnia causes bronchospasm Hypocapnia is seen during exercise-induced asthma	Isocapneic hyperventilation causes bronchospasm
Abnormal adrenergic response	Marked increase in cathecholamines during exercise	Response similar in normals, asthmatics
Vagal reflex	Irritant receptors in nasopharynx and airway can be stimulated by cold, dry, polluted air	Atropine does not abolish exercise-induced asthma
Release of allergic mediators from the lung	Airway reaction can be fatigued with repeated exercise at 1 hour intervals, will return to pre-exercise levels after 2 to 3 hours.	Not blocked by antihistamine or anti SRS-A drugs. Increased serum histamine or SRS-A levels similar in normals, asthmatics

with repeated exercise periods if carried out at hourly intervals but not at 3-hour intervals, when mediators would have had a chance to build up again.

CLINICAL IMPORTANCE AND IDENTIFICATION

Exercise is not a unique trigger of asthma, but only one of many. To illustrate this point, 71 asthmatic children and their parents were given a list of nine possible precipitants of an acute asthma attack and were asked to indicate which they thought they could relate to the children's condition. Most picked five or more factors. As seen in Table 46–2, exercise was included most of the time. More importantly, 71 percent ranked exercise as one of the three most important causes of attacks.

Every child suspected of having asthma should be asked if he or she wheezes, coughs, has chest tightness after exercise, or has gross exercise intolerance. For instance, a child with a chronic cough or with recurrent bronchitis who also has a history of coughing or wheezing after exercise probably has asthma, and should be further evaluated with this in mind. Similarly, children at risk of developing asthma, such as relatives of asthmatics or children

with allergic rhinitis or eczema should be questioned about exercise-related symptoms. Those with convincing histories should be screened by an exercise-tolerance test.

While a history is helpful, it must depend on the patient's awareness and recollection. The limited reliability of the history alone is illustrated by the fact that history correlated with exercise testing only 57 percent of the time in a study by Kawabori et al. (1976). The incidence of exercise-induced asthma detected by testing was similar whether or not asthmatic patients gave a history of exercise-induced asthma. Persons who said they did not wheeze fol-

TABLE 46–2 FACTORS RELATING TO ACUTE ASTHMA ATTACKS*

Factor	Number Ranking No. 1	Number Times in Top Three
Infection	22	49
Weather changes	20	45
Exercise	10	40
Inhalant allergen	14	35
Irritant	2	14
Emotions	3	9
Time of day	0	2
Foods/drugs	0	2
Other physical factors	0	3

*71 patients; 59 mentioned over 3 factors (mean 4.8).

lowing exercise apparently mistook wheezing for dyspnea, while those who thought they did wheeze were probably misinterpreting dyspnea and hyperventilation. A second observation from this study should be emphasized: 41 percent of patients with no previous history of asthma and no physical evidence of asthma, had significant pulmonary function changes after exercise, although few of them had really severe attacks. Thus, the most sensitive and reliable method to evaluate exercise-induced asthma is an exercise challenge. Although testing sounds formidable, it can be done easily in a clinical practice setting.

EXERCISE TESTING

The equipment may be as simple as a sidewalk or stairway, and a stethoscope or inexpensive peak flow gauge. The figures in Table 46–3 should serve as guidelines to allow selection of appropriate exercise conditions. They have been adapted from figures for the 600-yard walk-run event of the President's Physical Fitness Test and represent average figures that most children can meet when running on level ground. It should be stressed that these are guidelines and not rigid figures for minimum distances to be run. If the sidewalk is on a grade, the distance should be adjusted downward. The 5 to 8 minute exercise period was chosen because significantly less asthma results from shorter periods of exercise, and many children cannot run for longer periods.

A stairway provides an alternative exercise surface if a sidewalk is not convenient or safe. To provide the same work load, a school-aged child should ascend and descend the equivalent of one to two flights

each minute for 5 to 8 minutes. The pulmonary response should be assessed frequently for at least 15 minutes after exercise. Although auscultation while the child forcibly exhales is the simplest method, measurement of simple pulmonary functions with an inexpensive peak flow gauge or wedge spirometer will increase the sensitivity and usefulness of the procedure.

Pulmonary functions are usually measured before exercise and at 1, 5, 10, 15, and 20 minutes after exercise. The response is usually expressed as the maximum percent change from baseline, calculated as follows:

$$\frac{\text{(pre-exercise PFT)}-\text{(lowest PFT after exercise)}}{\text{(pre-exercise PFT)}} \times 100$$

In general, a decrease of 15 percent in either FEV_1 or peak flow rate (PEFR) is considered abnormal. A change of 30 to 45 percent is considered a moderately severe response, and greater than 45 percent a severe response.

While these procedures are helpful for clinical evaluation, they are inadequate for research purposes. For such purposes, a method of controlling exercise (treadmill or cycloergometer) is required, as well as equipment to quantitate a subject's response to exercise stress through effects on heart rate, ventilation, or oxygen consumption. Equipment for more accurate assessment of pulmonary functions also is essential. References are given at the end of the chapter which describe these methods in detail.

Even though children exercise every day and the exercise test does not constitute a severe stress, certain safety procedures should be followed. The running should be

TABLE 46–3 RECOMMENDED WORK LOAD FOR EXERCISE TESTING— BASED ON HEIGHT

Height (Approximate)		Speed		Distance (to be covered in approx. 6 min)	
INCHES	cm	mph	kph	FEET	METERS
47	120	3.0	4.8	1600	480
59	150	3.5	5.6	1850	555
71	180	4.2	6.8	2200	660
78	200	4.7	7.6	2500	750

supervised by a nurse or physician, and the child be allowed to stop if overly tired. Children with severe asthma or other significant lung or heart disease should be exercised cautiously, as should sedentary children. Adequate equipment for resuscitation (including epinephrine and oxygen) should be readily available, and all personnel instructed properly in its use. Though no major problems have occurred in centers where these tests are performed frequently, the physician should be prepared for rare emergencies.

THERAPEUTIC CONSIDERATIONS

Exercise-induced asthma may be prevented by pretreatment with many of the medications usually employed in asthma therapy. Those most useful are included in Table 46–4. (Note that corticosteroids, either inhaled or oral, generally are not helpful, nor are antihistamines.) Some of these medications can be obtained without a prescription, such as epinephrine aerosols (e.g., Primatene Mist, Bronkaid Mist) and tablets which contain theophylline, ephedrine, and phenobarbital (e.g., Primatene tablets, Tedral).

To be effective, medications must be given before exercise. Most inhaled drugs may be used immediately before, although effects may last for several hours. Drugs administered orally, on the other hand, should be taken 1½ to 2 hours before exercise to attain therapeutic drug levels when exercising. Dosage should be adjusted to achieve optimal effects without toxicity.

Drug selection is influenced both by practical and pharmacologic considerations. In a patient already using appropriate medication, that medication should be used initially and the dosing time simply adjusted for optimal effect. If the patient is not taking other medications for asthma, oral theophylline in a dose adequate to modify exercise-induced asthma would be the first choice, cromolyn sodium the second choice, and inhaled adrenergic agents the third choice. Cromolyn has few side effects, but it is not effective for some patients and should be inhaled shortly before exercise, which may expose some patients to ridicule by their peers. Aerosolized adrenergic agents are most effective inhibitors, in general have fewer side effects than oral preparations, and in fact are used as the drug of first choice by some physicians. However, the physician and patient should be aware of the potential for occasional paradoxical effects and for abuse with these agents. Certain drugs (ephedrine, isoproterenol, and metaproterenol) are not allowed in international competition, although college and high school rules generally allow any drug prescribed by a child's physician to be used.

TABLE 46–4 SUGGESTED DRUG THERAPY FOR EXERCISE-INDUCED ASTHMA

Drug	Dosage	Route of Administration	Time of Administration Prior to Exercise
Theophylline			
tablets	5–8 mg/kg	oral	2 hours
liquid	5–8 mg/kg	oral	1 hour
Isoproterenol			
100 μg/puff	1–2 puffs	inhalation	0–30 min
Isoetharine			
500 μg/puff	1–2 puffs	inhalation	0–30 min
Epinephrine			
100 μg/puff	1–2 puffs	inhalation	0–30 min
Metaproterenol			
tablets, liquid	0.3 mg/kg	oral	1–2 hours
aerosol 650 μg/puff	1–2 puffs	inhalation	0–2 hours
Terbutaline			
tablets	0.075 mg/kg	oral	1–2 hours
Cromolyn sodium	20 mg	inhalation	0–30 min

With the exception of cromolyn, all of these drugs have inotropic and chronotropic cardiac effects, and there is a possibility of inducing tachyarrhythmias with their use. If a child has a coincident cardiovascular abnormality or participates in strenuous competitive athletics, these effects constitute a potential risk. In these circumstances, cromolyn sodium would be the drug of first choice; an inhaled selective beta$_2$ adrenergic agent would be the second choice. Of the adrenergic aerosols available in the United States, metaproterenol has slightly fewer cardiac effects than isoproterenol or epinephrine and has a longer duration of action. Other adrenergic aerosols may be marketed soon.

In addition to prescribing medication to prevent an asthma attack and providing thorough instruction in its use, the physician should advise the patient and the family that coughing and wheezing after exercise is related to asthma, and is not the normal response to exercise. This should be emphasized especially when the child does not have the symptoms at any other time, since it will be less obvious to the child and family under this circumstance. The implications of having exercise-induced asthma and potential for more severe asthma should be explained, but at the same time, it should be emphasized that physical activity is a major part of normal development. *Activity should be encouraged,* including normal participation in school gym classes. An easily treated physical limitation should not be allowed, untreated, to interfere with normal physical and psychosocial development.

In many children, however, certain exercise restrictions may need to be imposed, either as a general rule, or from time to time when extraneous factors dictate. For example, on days when asthma at rest is more severe, some exercise restrictions are wise, since the resulting asthma will be significantly more severe. Similarly, on cold days or on days when ambient pollution or pollen load is heavy, exercise or premedication may need to be adjusted.

If there is an interest in competitive athletics, the child should be encouraged to select sports which are least likely to induce asthma, so as to minimize any physical disadvantage compared to nonasthmatic children. Swimming is the most appropriate. At the Munich Olympics, the only asthmatics winning gold medals were swimmers. Sports that emphasize coordination to a greater extent than exertion, such as gymnastics, baseball, downhill skiing, tennis or golf also are appropriate. Football, basketball, track, soccer, field hockey or lacrosse are sports that require extended periods of running and are least appropriate.

The child, family, and coach should be familiar with general measures to limit exercise-induced asthma. Individualized graded physical conditioning in which running is emphasized over calesthenics is important since the stress of a given exercise is lessened with physical (cardiopulmonary) training. It has been suggested that breathing through the nose rather than the mouth may prevent asthma; considerable training may be required to do this when dyspneic. It has been found that when a person exercises twice within an hour or less, milder bronchoconstriction follows the second exercise; the more severe the first exercise and degree of bronchospasm, the milder the bronchospasm after the second exercise load (Edmunds, 1978). Thus, if warming up is done an hour or so before competition, the asthmatic athlete should be able to compete in a more "normal" state. A similar phenomenon is described by asthmatic athletes as "running through" their asthma (with periods of exercise longer than 6 minutes, less severe asthma attacks follow; apparently bronchoconstriction with recovery can occur during exercise itself). Be cautious when discussing the phenomenon of "running through" asthma. Although this may be useful to persons competing in events with continuous moderate activity, it takes a considerable degree of insight to tread the path between recovery and inappropriate activity during a severe attack.

All concerned — child, family, and coach — should understand that there will be times when athletic activity will be ill-advised, as well as times when the young athlete will have to drop out to recover from asthma. The dangers of using aerosol sprays *during* events to try to ameliorate attacks, or trying to "tough it out" in order to continue cannot be overemphasized.

Finally, the school and community in

general should be made more aware of the problem of exercise-induced asthma. They should know that it is an abnormal response to exercise and that effective treatment is available. The asthmatic child should be encouraged to exercise, to participate in gym class, and even to enter competitive athletics. At the same time, the restrictions mentioned above should be understood and applied. The parent, physician, teacher, and coach should work toward a common goal: to allow the asthmatic child safely to lead as unrestricted a life as possible.

References

Edmunds, A. T., Tooley, M., and Godfrey, S.: The refractory period after exercise-induced asthma: its duration and relation to the severity of exercise. Am. Rev. Resp. Dis., *117*:247, 1978.

Kawabori, I., Pierson, W. E., Longquest, L. L., et al.: Incidence of exercise-induced asthma in children. J. Allergy Clin. Immunol., *58*:447, 1976.

GENERAL REFERENCES

The Asthmatic Athlete: Report of the Committee on the Medical Aspects of Sports. American Medical Association, 535 N. Dearborn St., Chicago, Ill., 1977.

Astrand, P., Rodahl, K.: *Textbook of Work Physiology: Physiologic Bases of Exercise,* 2nd ed. New York, McGraw Hill Book Co., 1977.

Cropp, G. J. A.: Exercise-induced asthma. Pediatr. Clin. North Am. *22*:63, 1975.

Eggleston, P. A., and Guerrant, J. L.: A standardized method of evaluating exercise-induced asthma. J. Allergy Clin. Immunol., *58*:414, 1976.

Godfrey, S.: *Exercise Testing in Children.* London, W. B. Saunders, Co. Ltd., 1974.

Lange-Andersen, K., Shephard, R. J., Denolin, H., et al.: *Fundamentals of Exercise Testing.* Geneva, World Health Organization, 1971.

Sly, R. M.: Exercise-induced asthma. In Weiss, E. B., and Segal, M. S.: *Bronchial Asthma: Mechanisms and Therapeutics.* Boston, Little, Brown and Co., 1976.

Strauss, R. H., McFadden, E. R., Jr., Ingram, R. H., Jr., et al.: Influence of heat and humidity on the airway obstruction induced by exercise in asthma. J. Clin. Invest. *61*:433, 1978.

Symposium on Exercise and Asthma. (Edited by Bierman, C. W., and Pierson, W. E.) Pediatrics *56*(5), Part 2, 1975.

47

F. Stanford Massie, M.D.

Hypersensitivity Pneumonitis and Pulmonary Reactions to Drugs and Chemicals

Hypersensitivity pneumonitis (HP) presents with fever, cough, malaise, and severe nonwheezing dyspnea several hours after inhalation of organic dust that contains any of a wide variety of antigenic materials from thermophilic organisms, bird proteins, chemicals, or drugs (Table 47–1). It occurs primarily in nonatopic individuals. Pulmonary reactions resembling asthma or diffuse pulmonary disease also may be induced by drugs and chemicals and occur in atopic and nonatopic individuals with equal frequency. Because there is a delay in onset of symptoms following exposure to the causative agent, the patient and physician may fail to notice a relationship. Early diagnosis and prompt therapy are essential in order to prevent irreversible lung damage, with fibrosis and progressive pulmonary disability (Bierman et al., 1977).

HYPERSENSITIVITY PNEUMONITIS

Hypersensitivity pneumonitis, also called extrinsic allergic alveolitis, involves the distal airways and pulmonary parenchyma. It can occur as an acute intermittent systemic and respiratory illness or as an insidious, chronic-progressive pulmonary disease. Table 47–2 (Fink et al., 1976) lists charac-teristics of the two forms of the disease. It occurs in 5 to 20 percent of persons regularly exposed to etiologic agents.

The Acute Form. Chills, fever, malaise, cough and dyspnea, basilar rales, leukocytosis, pulmonary infiltrates, and restrictive-type pulmonary function test defects usually begin 4 to 6 hours after exposure to the causative organic dust. Symptoms and signs are frequently mistaken for infectious pneumonitis. Temperature may be as high as 40° C (104° F). Rapid respirations and moist crepitant rales may be heard predominantly at the lung bases, and there usually is no wheezing and minimal hyperinflation. These abnormalities usually resolve within 12 to 18 hours, but occasionally may persist for several days, unless terminated by corticosteroid therapy.

The Insidious Form. With prolonged and continuous exposure to the offending dust, cough and dyspnea may be progressive without acute episodes. Dyspnea on exertion, anorexia, weight loss, and fatigue may occur without fever, and positive findings may be limited to fine basilar rales and, rarely, clubbing of the fingers.

Laboratory Features. In the acute form, leukocytosis may be as high as 25,000 white blood cells per mm^3, with a predominance of segmented polymorphonuclear leukocytes

TABLE 47–1 CLASSIFICATION OF HYPERSENSITIVITY PNEUMONITIS

Type of Exposure	Disease	Source	Antigen
Environmental	Humidifier lung	Home humidifiers and air conditioning systems	Thermophilic actinomycetes
	Humidity tent lung	Home humidity tents	*Bacillus subtilis* enzymes (?)
Hobbies — pets	Pigeon breeder's disease	Pigeon, parakeet or parrot droppings	Avian protein antigen
Occupational	Bagassosis	Moldy sugar cane	*Micropolyspora faeni*
	Cheese worker's disease	Cheese mold spores	*Penicillium caseii*
	Enzyme worker's lung	Bacterial products inhalation	*B. subtilis* enzymes
	Farmer's lung	Moldy hay	*Micropolyspora faeni* and
	Mushroom worker's disease	Compost	*Thermoactinomyces vulgaris*
	Malt worker's lung	Germinating barley	*Aspergillus clavatus*
	Maple bark disease	Moldy maple bark	*Cryptostroma corticale*
	Mill worker's disease	Mill dust	*Sitophilus granarius*
	Poultry worker's disease	Poultry sheds	Chicken dander
	Sequoiosis	Moldy redwood sawdust	*Graphium pullularia* Alternaria species
	Suberosis	Moldy cork dust	*Penicillium frequentans*
Medication	Pancreatic extract lung	Pancreatic enzymes inhalation	Pig pancreatic protein
	Pituitary snuff–taker's lung	Pituitary powder inhalation	Ox or pig protein

Modified from Bierman, C. W., et al.: *Disorders of the Respiratory Tract in Children,* Kendig, E. L. Jr. Ed., Philadelphia, W. B. Saunders. Co., 1977, p. 671.

TABLE 47–2 DIAGNOSTIC CLINICAL AND LABORATORY FEATURES IN EIGHT PATIENTS WITH INTERSTITIAL LUNG DISEASE

	Acute Form	Insidious Form
Dyspnea	4/4	4/4
Cough	4/4	3/4
Weight loss	3/4	2/4
Abnormal chest roentgenogram	4/4	4/4
Abnormal pulmonary functions	4/4	4/4
Thermophiles in environment	3/4	2/4
Serum precipitins to thermophiles	4/4	4/4
Serum precipitins to other dusts	4/4	2/4
Biopsy evidence of interstitial lung disease	4/4	3/4
Thermophiles detected in biopsy	ND	3/3
Response to challenge with antigen	4/4	ND
Relief by environmental alteration	4/4	2/4
Intermittent respiratory symptoms related to environmental exposure	4/4	0/4
Intermittent chills and fever	4/4	0/4
Progressive respiratory symptoms without acute episodes	0/4	4/4

From Fink, J. N., et al.: Ann. Intern. Med. *84:*410, 1976.

and up to 10 percent eosinophils, in association with chills and fever. These findings return to normal as symptoms subside, usually 12 to 18 hours after onset. As in other chronic pediatric pulmonary disorders, such as those in cystic fibrosis and chronic granulomatous disease, serum immunoglobulins may be elevated. IgE is usually normal, however, except coincidentally in individuals with atopic disease. This has been reported most frequently with bird fancier's lung disease. Nonspecific serologic findings such as the presence of rheumatoid factor and positive mononucleosis spot test may be seen in the acute illness. The erythrocyte sedimentation rate occasionally is elevated. Smears and cultures of the throat, sputum, and blood are negative for pathogenic organisms. Leukocytosis and other nonspecific abnormal findings are usually absent in the chronic intermittent exposure form of the disease (Fink, 1978).

Roentgenographic Features. In the acute form, the chest x-ray film shows a diffuse interstitial infiltrate with fine reticular densities, multiple small nodules, and patchy infiltration at the lung bases. In the chronic phase, diffuse interstitial fibrosis with coarsening of the bronchovascular markings, and contraction of lung tissue is seen. Hyperinflation is uncommon but can occur (Figure 47–1).

Pulmonary Function Tests. Restrictive impairment of pulmonary function, with reduced forced vital capacity (FVC), is the primary abnormality of HP. This may return to normal between acute episodes; but in the chronic phase of the disease, FVC is reduced irreversibly due to pulmonary fibrosis. Increased stiffness of the lung, with decreased compliance, may be accompanied by an alveolar-capillary blockade with reduced gas transfer and diminished carbon monoxide diffusion. Functional residual capacity and total lung capacity are low. Arterial blood gases reveal diminished Po_2, decreased oxygen saturation, and diminished Pco_2. The pH is slightly elevated, with a mild respiratory alkalosis during acute episodes. Airways resistance as measured by plethysmography, forced expiratory volume at one second (FEV_1), and other flow rates are usually normal unless the patient has significant bronchiolitis or has superimposed asthma (as in bird fancier's lung). In the insidious form of the disease, increased residual volume and decreased flow rates may be seen, indicating loss of pulmonary elasticity, as is found in emphysema.

Immune Responses. Antigens that induce HP appear to be of appropriate size ($<10 \mu$) for reaching the bronchial tree, where they are processed by pulmonary macrophages. They are nondigestible by lysosomal enzymes, are particulate in nature, are capable of directly activating complement, and have an adjuvant effect on pulmonary immune responses (Schatz et al., 1977). In the serum of patients with HP, precipitating IgG antibodies characteristically are found to suspect organic dust-containing fungal antigens, thermophilic actinomycetes, or avian proteins. These antibodies may be detected in up to 50 percent of asymptomatic similarly exposed individuals and therefore, their presence per se is not indicative of disease. Epidemiologic studies have suggested that they simply reflect predominant antigen exposure. Early studies postulated that they were responsible for a type III or local Arthus hypersensitivity reaction in the lung. Although type III reactions appear to occur in these diseases, recent experimental and human studies have implicated monocytes and lymphocytes (and presumably type IV reactions) in the pathogenesis of the pulmonary reaction. Precipitating antibodies may play a protective role in antigen-clearing mechanisms. Antibody titers generally are higher in symptomatic individuals. Cross-reactions have been noted between various organic dust antigens and are believed to indicate a wide degree of exposure to the antigens capable of inducing HP in patients with the disease. Patients with farmer's lung disease have been found to have a broad immune response with elevated specific antibodies to a panel of respiratory viruses and mycoplasma, compared to normal individuals, perhaps indicating wide antigenic exposure or unknown peculiarities in host reponsiveness.

Serum complement has been reported to be decreased in asymptomatic, but not in symptomatic, pigeon breeders upon inhalation challenge with pigeon antigens; however, in other studies, alveolar-fluid levels of complement from patients with hypersensitivity lung disease did not differ from levels in patients with idiopathic pulmonary fibro-

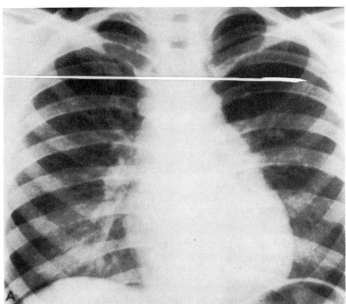

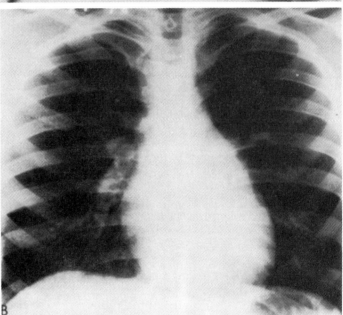

FIGURE 47–1. Acute (*A*) and convalescent (*B*) chest films of child with hypersensitivity pneumonitis due to exposure to doves in the home. (From Cunningham, A. S., Fink, J. N., and Schleuter, D. P.: Pediatrics *58*: 436, 1976.)

sis or normal controls. Furthermore, extracts of *Micropolyspora faeni*, important in farmer's lung disease, have been found to consume complement *in vitro* in the absence of detectable antibodies. The immunopathogenic role of complement activation directly by causative antigens (alternative pathway?) or through antigen-antibody interaction (classic pathway) requires further elucidation.

Cellular Immune Studies. Peripheral blood lymphocytes from patients with HP undergo blast transformation and release macrophage migration inhibition factor (MIF) when cultured *in vitro* with appropriate fungal or avian antigens. In contrast, lymphocytes from asymptomatic individuals do not react in this manner even though there may be serum-precipitating antibodies present to the antigens. In animals models of

HP, lymphocytes appear to be of prime importance. Animal transfer experiments with infusion of sensitized lymphocytes were followed by pulmonary lesions on antigen challenge by inhalation. In most studies, serum transfer was less likely to induce typical HP lesions after inhalation challenge.

Genetic control of the pulmonary response is suggested by studies in animals and humans. Pulmonary damage appears to develop after an immune response that combines both antigen-specific humoral antibodies and cellular hypersensitivity, with mononuclear cells releasing lymphokines. Complement activation in the lung and irritant effects of the thermophilic agents also may be important. Cellular hypersensitivity to organic dusts may lead to HP, after being triggered by a nonspecific inflammatory process, such as a respiratory infection.

Skin Tests. Scratch, prick, or intradermal tests are useful with bird-derived antigens in pigeon-breeder's disease or bird-fancier's lung disease. Extracts of thermophilic actinomycetes are irritating and cannot be used for testing in farmer's lung and other related HP. The usual skin response is erythema and edema at 4 to 8 hours. Biopsy of the skin reveals a perivascular infiltrate consistent with an immune complex or Arthus reaction.

Inhalation Challenge Studies. All the signs and symptoms of HP can be reproduced when appropriate extracts of causative agents are used for inhalation challenge. Care must be taken in performing these tests, since reactions may be severe. Re-exposure to suspect environmental areas, such as pigeon coops, may be necessary.

Histologic Studies. Lung biopsies from patients with acute HP reveal interstitial pneumonitis with involvement of alveolar walls, spaces, and bronchioles. Infiltrations with lymphocytes, plasma cells, foamy histiocytes, and increased numbers of alveolar macrophages are seen with an alveolar proteinaceous exudate. Focal granulomas and minimal vasculitis may be present. In the chronic phase, fibrosis with destruction of lung parenchyma is seen. A "honeycomb" pattern of cystic changes, and obliteration of bronchioles by deposition of collagen and granulation tissue are associated with severe interstitial fibrosis.

Experimental Studies. Many different animal models of HP have been reported in which all features of the human disease have been reproduced. Detailed information on immunopathogenesis has recently been reviewed (Schatz et al., 1977; Roberts et al., 1977).

Diagnosis. A high index of suspicion and a detailed history of the patient's home environment, hobbies, and work are necessary for diagnosing HP. Infectious pneumonia is frequently misdiagnosed in the acute form, but attention should be paid to recurrence of symptoms on returning to the previous environment. Symptoms may occur 5 nights of the week after work. Cultures of the environment for airborne fungi and serologic tests for precipitins should be considered. Lung biopsy and inhalation challenge with pulmonary function tests may be necessary, particularly in the insidious form.

Therapy. Careful avoidance of re-exposure to causative agents, and corticosteroid therapy will achieve remission in the acute form. Steroid therapy in children should begin with a single early morning dose of 40 mg of prednisone with gradual daily dose reduction. Chest x-ray films and lung function should be carefully monitored. If long-term steroid therapy is necessary, an alternate-day regimen should be tried. Avoiding re-exposure may be difficult since occupation or life styles may need to be changed. Lack of compliance may be followed by recurrence or progression of pulmonary disease. In one experimental model, clinical improvement followed desensitization with injection of thermophilic antigens. This approach may provide additional therapy in the future (Wilkie, 1977) *but is not currently recommended.*

Specific Syndromes

Disease Related to Home Environment

Interstitial Lung Disease due to Contamination of Forced Air Systems. Home and office air conditioning systems present specific hazards of HP. It has been reported after exposure to office air conditioners, home furnace humidifiers, room humidifiers, air conditioners, and cool mist vaporizers. Etiologic agents have been identified as *Thermoactinomyces candidus, T. vulgaris,* and *T. sacchari.* The thermophilic agents contaminated the air conditioning or humidifying equipment and led to sensitization. Thermo-tolerant bacteria and amebae also may be involved in some cases. In one report the source of such agents was a contaminated water supply delivered to the humidifier. In children with persistent respiratory problems, long-term use of humidifiers, vaporizers or tents, as in cystic fibrosis, should be suspected as a possible cause of lung disease.

Disease Due to Hobbies

Pigeon-Breeder's Disease. Pigeon-breeder's disease (PBD) is the most common and best studied pediatric hypersensitivity pneumonitis (Cunningham et al., 1976). It has been reported after long-standing exposure to avian antigens from pigeons, parrots, doves, parakeets (budgerigars), and chickens. HP also has been reported after exposure to mice, rats, gerbils, and guinea pigs. There usually is an insidious onset with a prolonged course. Weight loss is a common sign. Clinical features include cough, dyspnea, basilar rales, absence of wheezing, abnormal chest x-rays with infiltrates, and restrictive lung disease with reduced forced vital capacity and diffusing capacity. There is a history of exposure to avian antigens, with variable duration from 6 weeks to 7 years. Skin testing with pigeon serum or extracts of feathers and droppings may reveal both an immediate and a late onset skin reaction. Precipitating antibodies to avian proteins are present in the serum. Careful inhalation challenge in hospitalized patients with bird-derived extracts will be followed by an acute syndrome with cough, dyspnea, and rales 4 to 8 hours after exposure with abnormal pulmonary function studies. Lung biopsy reveals a chronic interstitial mononuclear infiltration. Therapy consists of elimination of birds and a course of corticosteroids. This is followed by clearing of the abnormal signs and chest x-ray films, providing exposure has not been sufficient to produce pulmonary fibrosis.

Occupational Lung Disease. As outlined in Table 47–1, HP may be seen in workers exposed to organic dust containing thermophilic actinomycetes or other fungi from sugar cane (Bagassosis), cheese, laundry detergent enzymes (*Bacillus subtilis*), moldy hay (Farmer's lung disease), mushroom compost, wood dust, and medications containing pig or cow proteins. Clinical features of HP have been reported in mothers caring for their children with cystic fibrosis (pancreatic enzymes), or in patients with diabetes insipidus (pituitary snuff). Synthetic pitressin has significantly reduced the incidence of this latter problem.

A high index of suspicion and a careful environment history are essential in diagnosis of any individual with chronic cough and interstitial pneumonitis. Failure to recognize a relationship between environmental exposure to causative agents and preventable chronic lung disease may lead to insidious pulmonary deterioration, with fibrosis as the end result.

DRUG AND CHEMICAL-INDUCED PULMONARY DISEASE

Numerous industrial materials and drugs are known to produce pulmonary disease. The types of reactions have been obstructive, with asthma-like syndromes (aspirin, industrial chemicals); restrictive, with diffuse pulmonary disease suggesting pneumonitis (nitrofurantoin); and combined obstructive and restrictive (metal fumes). Mediastinal and hilar changes have been reported from phenytoin and corticosteroids, and respiratory muscle paralysis from a number of antibiotics has been reported.

Table 47–3 lists some of the major causes of chemical- and drug-induced hypersensitivity lung diseases (Bierman et al., 1977). Pulmonary reactions to chemical substances are an increasing problem in industry. Occupational asthma has been estimated to have a worldwide prevalence of 2 percent. Higher regional incidence has been reported. While it is primarily a problem in adults, children and adolescents are also at risk for later overt pulmonary disease following intense exposure to diverse chemicals used in hobbies, without the safety monitoring employed in industry.

In vitro laboratory tests have not been helpful in most drug- or chemical-induced lung disease (Rosenow, 1976). Recently, increasing numbers of positive bronchial provocation tests with suspected offending agents have been reported in industrial workers. In some instances these have been correlated with positive skin tests, passive transfer tests to man or monkey, and specific IgE in the serum with the radioallergosorbent test

TABLE 47–3 CAUSES OF CHEMICAL- AND DRUG-INDUCED
HYPERSENSITIVITY LUNG DISEASE

Disease	Source	Substance(s)	Type of Reaction
CHEMICALS			
Cedar worker's disease	Western red cedar sawdust	Plicatic acid	Obstructive, restrictive or both
Metal fume fever	Metal refining, plating	Zinc, nickel, or platinum salts	Obstructive and restrictive
Occupational asthma	Industry	Many	Obstructive
Meat wrapper's asthma	Plastic wrap	Copolymers of polyvinyl chloride	Obstructive
Coffee worker's asthma	Coffee bean dust	Green coffee bean	Obstructive and restrictive
Polymer fume fever	Industry	Polytetrafluoroethylene	Obstructive
TDI	Polyurethane	Toluene diisocyanate	Obstructive
Veterinarians and workers	Animal, bird, fish and insect	Serum, dander secretions	Obstructive
DRUGS			
Aspirin asthma	Oral medication	Acetylsalicylic acid	Obstructive
Blood transfusion lung	Multiple transfusions	Donor HLA antigens	Restrictive
Cromolyn sodium	Inhaled medication	Cromolyn sodium	Obstructive and restrictive
Diffuse pulmonary disease	Oral medication	Nitrofurantoin	Restrictive and pleural effusion

Modified from Bierman, C. W., et al.: Nonasthmatic allergic pulmonary disease. *In* Kendig, E. L., Jr. (ed.): *Disorders of the Respiratory Tract in Children*. Philadelphia, W. B. Saunders Co., 1977, p. 689.

(RAST). In most pulmonary reactions following chemical or drug exposure, the causative antigens, antibodies, and mechanisms of tissue damage are unknown. Reactions develop in only a small number of exposed individuals, and to a number of agents, they appear to be specifically acquired.

Specific Syndromes

Chemicals

Cedar Worker's Disease. Exposure to plicatic acid from the dust of western red cedar (*Thuja Plicata*) may induce a syndrome of asthma and rhinitis or hypersensitivity pneumonitis. Lumbermen may develop symptoms up to 20 years after initial contact. Bronchial inhalation challenge may be followed by a dual response with immediate obstructive airway disease and chest pain, chills, fever, and lassitude 4 to 8 hours later. Avoiding exposure to dust usually affords recovery.

Metal Fume Fever and Asthma. Restrictive and obstructive lung disease may occur in workers exposed to metallic salts in industry. High particulate metallic oxide fumes with zinc, copper, iron, magnesium, cadmium, or antimony may induce delayed febrile pneumonitis with influenza-like symptoms in steel workers. Platinum salts commonly induce respiratory symptoms in photographic workers. Immediate asthmatic symptoms may be followed by late onset asthmatic attacks in some. Bronchial provocation and positive prick skin tests to platinum salts confirm the diagnosis. Hyposensitization has been reported to be helpful in symptomatic platinum workers. Less common occupational asthma from chrome and nickel salts has been reported in workers in the plating industry. Reactions may be immediate or late in onset (Editorial, Lancet, 1978; Pepys et al., 1978).

Occupational Asthma. Obstructive airway disease may be seen from exposure to a wide variety of industrial materials. The constantly enlarging list includes gases in the chemical and petroleum industry; urea and formalin in metal foundry workers and medical personnel; castor bean, green coffee bean, papain, pancreatic and *Bacillus subtilis* enzymes in the oil, food and detergent industries; ethylenediamine, phthalic anhydride, trimellitic anhydride from exposure to industrial plastics, rubber, or resin; phenylglycine acid chloride, ampicillin and others in pharmaceutical workers; flour and grain in bakers and farmers; wood dusts in mill workers and carpenters; soldering fluxes in electricians and sheet metal workers; and cotton dusts in textile and vegetable oil industries. Many of these reactions appear to be IgE-mediated and positive bronchial provocation tests, skin tests and *in vitro* radioallergosorbent tests (RAST) have been reported (Karr et al., 1978).

Meat Wrapper's Asthma. Cutting and sealing polymeric polyvinyl chloride plastic film with a hot wire can induce sneezing, rhinorrhea, and coughing. Symptoms occur immediately or four to five hours after exposure and are most common in smokers. Wheezing and other signs of obstruction are ameliorated by bronchodilators. Heat-activated pyrolysates from the wrapping material and price labels appear to be the etiologic agents. Immunopathogenetic mechanisms have not been identified.

Coffee Worker's Disease. Hypersensitivity pneumonitis of insidious onset may be seen in workers exposed to coffee bean dust. A maculopapular rash may be seen, with infiltrative chest disease evident on x-ray examination. Green coffee bean dust also can induce obstructive airway disease with asthmatic symptoms of both immediate and delayed onset types. Bronchial provocation tests, skin tests, and RAST may be found positive. Castor bean dust may contaminate coffee bean sacks and, in some instances, may act as an occult etiologic agent. Exposure to this substance also causes asthma in individuals who produce castor bean oil, fuel, and fertilizer.

Polymer Fume Fever. Episodes of chest tightness, dry cough, and high fever occur in some workers several hours after exposure to heat degradation products of polytetrafluoroethylene plastic (Teflon). Heated Teflon degradation products appear when above-normal cooking temperatures are reached. Pulmonary function studies have shown a mild obstructive disorder (Kuntz et al., 1974).

TDI and TMA Diseases. Industrial chemicals and plastics place 40,000 workers in the United States at risk for developing pulmonary hypersensitivity disease. Toluene diisocyanate (TDI) is used to manufacture polyurethane, an important component of paint, varnish, plastics, wire coating, and foam insulation. It is a strong respiratory irritant at 0.5 parts per million, and at lower levels about 5 percent of regularly exposed individuals develop occupational asthma. An atopic "predisposition" does not appear to be an important determinant for developing this form of asthma. As an allergen, TDI may complex to protein of bronchiolar mucosal cells and induce an immune reaction with IgE, IgG, or both. However, it is not clear whether it is an immune, pharmacologic (altered cAMP metabolism), or irritant reaction. The clinical features are variable — some patients experience immediate-onset sneezing and chest tightness, whereas others have a delayed onset syndrome of cough, chest tightness, low-grade fever, and wheezing. Complement-dependent, TDI-latex agglutination responses may be seen in the latter. Another group of patients who are initially symptomatic develop tolerance on continued exposure. This is coupled with developing anti–TDI-IgG precipitating antibodies. Positive bronchial provocation testing with polyurethane varnish and activator TDI confirm sensitivity. Asthma may be recurrent in highly sensitive workers even after exposure is terminated, and "safe" industrial levels below 0.01 to 0.02 ppm may induce disease. Bronchodilators and cromolyn sodium may be helpful.

Trimellitic anhydride (TMA) is widely used in the manufacture of plasticizers, alkyl resin in surface coatings, and as a curing agent for epoxy resins. Zeiss and co-workers have described TMA inhalation with immediate onset asthma and rhinitis; late onset asthma with systemic symptoms ("TMA flu"); and airway irritation (Zeiss et al., 1977). Laboratory studies included skin tests with TMA-human serum albumin conjugate, measurement of TMA-specific IgG antibodies by polystyrene tube radioimmunoassay, lymphocyte stimulation, passive cutaneous anaphylaxis in monkeys (PCA), histamine release assays, and rheumatoid factor analysis. TMA-IgE appeared to mediate the immediate asthma syndrome, whereas TMA-IgG antibodies were highest in late onset asthma with "flu-like" symptoms. This study established the immune nature of this occupational lung disease. Similar studies are needed in all the occupational pulmonary diseases.

Animal, Bird, Fish and Insect Asthma. Veterinarians, laboratory workers, fish processors, animal and poultry breeders, and silk producers are at risk for developing obstructive airway disease from sensitizing proteins in serum, dander, and dusts. This problem is a common one. It is estimated that there are 4000 occupational-asthmatic laboratory workers in the United States. Individuals exposed to birds and to pigeon proteins may develop either hypersensitivity pneumonitis or immediate and late respiratory reactions that are asthmatic in nature. In many of these conditions, atopic individuals appear to be at greater risk of developing asthma from industrial materials than do nonatopic persons. Industrial selection of employees by screening for atopy (history, skin tests, and IgE levels) has been suggested to prevent sensitization and disease. Criteria for monitoring respiratory function in cotton workers have been developed and should have wide future application in other industries.

Drugs

Aspirin Asthma. The triad of aspirin intolerance, nasal polyps, and sinus disease associated with asthma has been extended from recognition in 3 to 26 percent of adults with intrinsic asthma to children with chronic asthma. Twenty-eight percent of 50 children were found to have asthmatic reactions following aspirin ingestion but did not have nasal polyps or sinus disease (Rachaelefsky et al., 1975). A 13 percent incidence of adverse pulmonary reaction to aspirin has been reported in another group of chronic asthmatic children (Vedanthan et al., 1977). Inhibition of the microsomal enzyme system responsible for the production of prostaglandins and thromboxanes is believed responsible for the obstructive airway disease. Unrelated drugs including indomethacin, ibuprofen, mefenamic acid, and the yellow food dye, tartrazine, also may initiate wheezing episodes, presumably through similar mechanisms. Children with chronic asthma should avoid aspirin-containing drugs. Acetaminophen is a suitable alternative, although a rare patient may wheeze after exposure to this drug.

Asthma also may be induced by aerosolized penicillin, polymyxin B, enzymes, isoproterenol, and cromolyn sodium. Mechanisms are probably both allergic and irritant in nature.

Blood Transfusion Lung. Noncardiac pulmonary edema with acute dyspnea and diffuse pulmonary disease may occur in individuals given transfusions from multiparous women donors with high titers of anti–human leukocyte antigen antibodies or in patients who have received multiple transfusions and have become sensitized to donor HLA leukocyte antigens. It may occur during the course of transfusion with as little as 50 cc of blood and may resemble anaphylaxis, but there is no bronchospasm. The reaction may be fatal. At autopsy massive hemorrhagic pulmonary edema with hemosiderin-laden phagocytes, dilated vessels, and alveoli filled with RBC's and granulocytes are seen. Minimizing extraneous leukocyte antigens in RBC preparations should be the goal in preventing this pulmonary disease.

Cromolyn Sodium and Aerosolized Steroids. In addition to acute irritant bronchospasm, pulmonary infiltrates with eosinophilia may occur in a few patients inhaling cromolyn sodium for asthma. Immune mechanisms have been suggested by the demonstration of both humoral and lymphocytic (in vitro MIF production) factors in sensitive patients. Recently beclomethasone dipropionate aerosol has been associated with the development of eosinophilic pneumonia in asthmatics. Hypersensitivity to the drug probably is not of clinical importance. Both entities respond to oral corticosteroid therapy.

Nitrofurantoin Lung Disease. Nitrofurantoin is the most common antibiotic associated with pulmonary reactions. Acute and chronic syndromes are seen, and a third type of pulmonary reaction with pure bronchospasm has been reported. There are over 200 case reports of pulmonary reactions to this drug, with an incidence of one in 400 patients.

The acute form is most common, with dyspnea, cough, fever, and bronchospasm within a few hours to 10 days after beginning therapy with the drug. A diffuse pulmonary infiltrate suggesting noncardiac pulmonary edema is seen on chest x-ray films, and there may be pleurisy with effusion. Rapid clearing usually occurs when the drug is stopped. The problem may be confused with infectious pneumonitis.

In the chronic form, a diffuse interstitial pneumonitis with fibrosis may present like the Hamman-Rich syndrome. There is a history of slowly progressive cough and dyspnea in individuals taking nitrofurantoin for 6 months to several years. Desquamative interstitial pneumonia has been seen on lung biopsy in some patients on long-term nitrofurantoin therapy. The acute form of the disease has not been reported to progress to the chronic. Cessation of the drug and treatment with corticosteroids has a better outcome in this disease than in idiopathic fibrosing alveolitis (Hamman-Rich). Immune mechanisms are probably causative in the chronic form, with cell-mediated immune responses to the drug being demonstrable in some patients (Rosenow 1977). Lymphocytes from patients may produce MIF and cytotoxic factors to human alveolar cells when cultured with nitrofurantoin (Pearsall et al., 1974). *In vitro* studies of this type are needed in delineating immune mechanisms in all drug-induced pulmonary reactions.

References

Bierman, C. W., Pierson, W. E., and Massie, F. S.: Non-asthmatic allergic pulmonary disease. *In* Kendig, E. L., Jr. (ed.): *Disorders of the Respiratory Tract in Children.* Philadelphia, W. B. Saunders Co., 1977. pp. 670–969.

Cunningham, A. S., Fink, J. N., and Schleuter, D. P.: Childhood hypersensitivity pneumonitis due to dove antigens. Pediatrics 58:436, 1976.

Editorial: Inhalation fevers. Lancet *I (8058)*:249, 4 February 1978.

Fink, J. N., Banaszak, E. F., Barboriak, J. J., Hensley, G. T., Kurup, V. P., Scanlon, G. T., Schlueter, D. P., Sossman, A. J., Thiede, W. H., and Unger, G. F.: Interstitial lung disease due to contamination of forced air systems. Ann. Intern. Med. 84:406, 1976.

Fink, J. N.: Hypersensitivity pneumonitis. *In* Middleton, E., Jr., Reed, C. E., and Ellis, E. F. (eds.): *Allergy: Principles and Practice.* St. Louis, C. V. Mosby Co., 1978, pp. 855–867.

Karr, R. M., Davies, R. J., Butcher, B. T., Lehrer, S. B., Wilson, M. R., Dharmarajan, V., and Salvaggio, J. E.: Occupational asthma. J. Allergy Clin. Immunol. 61:54, 1978.

Kuntz, W. D., and McCord, C. P.: Polymer fume fever, J. Occup. Med. 16:480, 1974.

Pearsall, H. R., Ewalt, J., Tsoi, M., Sumida, S., and Backus, D.: Nitrofurantoin lung sensitivity. J. Lab. Clin. Med. 83:728, 1974.

Pepys, J., and Davies, R. J.: Occupational asthma. *In* Middleton, E., Jr., Reed, C. E., and Ellis, E. F. (eds.): *Allergy: Principles and Practice.* St. Louis, C. V. Mosby Co., 1978, pp. 812–842.

Rachaelefsky, G. S., Coulson, A., Siegel, S. C., and Stiehm, E. R.: Aspirin intolerance in chronic childhood asthma: Detected by oral challenge. Pediatrics 56:443, 1975.

Roberts, D. C., and Moore, V. L.: Immunopathogenesis of hypersensitivity pneumonitis. Am. Rev. Respir. Dis. *116*:1075, 1977.

Rosenow, E. C., III: Drug induced hypersensitivity disease in the lung. *In* Kirkpatrick, C. H., and Reynolds, H. Y. (eds.): *Immunologic and Infectious Reactions in the Lung.* New York, Marcel Dekker, Inc., 1976, pp. 261–287.

Rosenow, E. C., III: Drug induced pulmonary disease. Clinical Notes on Respiratory Diseases 16:3, 1977.

Schatz, M., Patterson, R., and Fink, J.: Immunopathogenesis of hypersensitivity pneumonitis. J. Allergy Clin. Immunol. 60:27, 1977.

Vedanthan, P. K., Menon, M. M., Bell, T. D., and Bergin, D.: Aspirin and tartrazine oral challenge: Incidence of adverse response in chronic childhood asthma. J. Allergy Clin. Immunol. 60:8, 1977.

Wilkie, B. N.: Experimental hypersensitivity pneumonitis: Reduced severity of clinical response following repeated injections of *Micropolyspora faeni* antigen. Int. Arch. Allergy Appl. Immunol. 53:389, 1977.

Zeiss, C. R., Patterson, R., Pruzansky, J. J., Miller, M. M., Rosenberg, M., and Levitz, D.: Trimellitic anhydride–induced airway syndromes: Clinical and immunologic studies. J. Allergy Clin. Immunol. 60:96, 1977.

48

Robert H. Schwartz, M.D.

Nonallergic Chronic Pulmonary Disease

A partial listing of the entities to be considered in the differential diagnosis of chronic pulmonary diseases in children and adolescents is found in Table 48–1. It is important to recognize that lower respiratory tract insult by different pathogenetic mechanisms can result in similar manifestations of pulmonary disease. On the other hand, similar insults may induce different host pulmonary responses, some of which may evolve into "atypical" clinical patterns. Months and years after etiologic clues are irretrievable, some of these conditions can only be termed "idiopathic." From the time of insult, pulmonary changes may be reversible, static or progressive. Functionally, they are obstructive, restrictive or both.

Cough, labored breathing, wheezing, sputum production, chest pain, and hemoptysis — alone and in combination — are the cardinal signs and symptoms of pulmonary disease. These may be associated with abnormal pulmonary function and roentgenographic findings. Acute illnesses usually subside spontaneously or with therapy within 3 weeks. Illnesses that last from 3 weeks to 3 months can be considered subacute. Chronicity is implied when abnormal signs and symptoms last 3 or more months. When separated by periods of health, the respiratory condition can be considered recurrent. Recurrent (or persistent) pneumonia should alert the physician to a chronic underlying disorder.

Bronchial asthma with its various modes of onset, severity and complications can fulfill any of the above temporal designations. Indeed, it remains the most common chronic pulmonary disease of childhood and adolescence. Prior to the eras of public health sanitation measures, respiratory pathogen immunization, and antibiosis, the bulk of the remainder of recognized chronic childhood lung disease consisted of tuberculosis and postinfectious complications of pertussis, measles, and bacterial pneumonias. Today we are confronted with a number of chronic pulmonary diseases whose etiologies are unknown, pathogeneses incompletely understood, natural histories yet to be determined, and therapies only palliative. Their apparent increasing numbers can be accounted for by better diagnostic methods, case finding, and reporting; partial therapeutic breakthroughs; and successful management of other pre-existing diseases. Also, hereditary risk factors, such as for alpha-1-antitrypsin deficiency, either alone or in combination with environmental factors (air pollution and smoking) and/or common viral infections (RSV, influenza, adenovirus) are being recognized as predisposing to the development of chronic lung disease in young people and adults.

The constellation of nonallergic chronic pulmonary disease of childhood and adolescence can be seen only in large university centers. Familiarity with these conditions is necessary so that they be diagnosed correctly and not confused with bronchial asthma, so that more can be learned about their etiology, pathogenesis and natural history,

TABLE 48–1 CHRONIC PULMONARY DISEASES IN CHILDREN AND ADOLESCENTS

Allergic
  Bronchial asthma
  Hypersensitivity pneumonitis
  Allergic bronchopulmonary aspergillosis
  Hypersensitivity reactions to drugs and chemicals
Infectious
  Chronic tuberculosis and atypical mycobacteria
    infection
  Histoplasmosis
  Other mycoses
  Cytomegalic inclusion disease
  Chlamydia, including psittacosis and ornithosis
  Pneumocystis carinii
  Visceral larva migrans
Postinfectious
  Bronchiectasis
  Bronchiolitis obliterans
  Unilateral hyperlucent lung syndrome
  Interstitial fibrosis
Congenital and Hereditary
  Anomalies of the lung (cysts and sequestration)
  Congenital lobar emphysema
  Cystic fibrosis
  Immune deficiency disorders
  Alpha-1-antitrypsin deficiency
  Immotile cilia syndrome and Kartagener's syndrome
  Ectodermal dysplasia
  Familial dysautonomia
Associated with underlying systemic disease
  Sarcoidosis
  Collagen diseases
  Malignancy
  Reticuloendothelioses
    Liporeticuloses
      Gaucher's disease
      Niemann-Pick disease
    Histiocytosis-X
      Letterer-Siwe disease
      Hand-Schüller-Christian disease
      Eosinophilic granuloma
  Wegener's granulomatosis
Complicating management of pre-existing disease
  Bronchopulmonary dysplasia
  Radiation pneumonitis
  Musculoskeletal disorders
  Central nervous system disorders
Idiopathic
  Pulmonary hemosiderosis
  Fibrosing alveolitis (usual interstitial pneumonia—
    UIP)
  Desquamative interstitial pneumonia—DIP
  Lymphoid interstitial pneumonia—LIP
  Giant cell interstitial pneumonia—GIP
  Bronchiolitis obliterans with interstitial pneumonia—
    BIP
  Pulmonary alveolar microlithiasis

and so that the most effective therapy can be provided. When hereditary factors are recognized, prevention and genetic counseling can be offered.

This chapter discusses the more important nonallergic chronic pulmonary diseases of infancy, childhood and adolescence which either share some signs and symptoms of allergic pulmonary disease or may be encountered in its evaluation.

CYSTIC FIBROSIS

Cystic fibrosis (CF) often has been confused with both upper and lower respiratory tract allergy. Nasal polyposis (15 percent of CF cases), chronic sinusitis, and rhinitis (100 percent of cases), chronic cough (eventually all patients), wheezing and hyperirritable airways (25 percent and in more severe cases), atelectasis, and allergic bronchopulmonary aspergillosis (2 percent to 5 percent of cases) are associated both with respiratory allergic disorders and CF. In early life the diarrhea of CF can mimic gastrointestinal allergy. Therefore, when considering "allergy" in a child or adolescent with these findings, there should be a high index of suspicion for CF. Allergy skin testing also can be misleading since 40 percent or more of CF patients exhibit immediate wheal and flare reactions to common inhalant allergens. These usually are to mold spore allergens, including *Aspergillus fumigatus* (40 percent of cases), which probably reflects sensitization to antigens derived from germinating mold spores in bronchiectatic lesions. To make the issue more complicated, allergic rhinitis and asthma can coexist with CF; there is evidence both for more and for less favorable prognoses when the combination occurs. When CF is confused with gastrointestinal milk allergy, the substitution of soybean milk preparations has led to a syndrome of severe failure to thrive, edema, anemia and panhypoproteinemia, especially in the first year of life, since soybean proteins are poorly utilized by the untreated child with CF.

The sweat test done by pilocarpine iontophoresis (to stimulate local sweating), finding sodium and chloride greater than 60 mEq/L, is the sine qua non for diagnosis. A sweat test should be considered in any child or adolescent with nasal polyps no matter how well he or she appears, since nasal polyps due to respiratory allergy are rare in this age group. Similarly, since digital clubbing is so rare in chronic asthma but common in CF, this finding should prompt a sweat test. Adrenal insufficiency, diabetes insipidus, glycogen storage disease, and the hypohidrotic form of ectodermal dysplasia can produce false positive sweat tests. As discussed later, ectodermal dysplasia frequently has both chronic respiratory and allergy manifestations. A sweat test is indicated in any infant with wheezing if the cause of wheezing is not readily apparent.

Incidence. Cystic fibrosis is the most common lethal genetic disease of Caucasian children, adolescents, and young adults. Transmission follows an autosomal recessive mode of inheritance, and its incidence is estimated at between 1:1600 and 1:2500 live births. Although the incidence in nonwhites is low, its described occurrence in blacks, Orientals and American Indians should alert one to the possibility of diagnosis in any race. There are 13,000 known living patients in the United States and 30,000 presumed to exist. It is estimated that 5 percent of the white population are carriers (heterozygotes). Heterozygote detection with genetic counseling and CF prenatal diagnosis with abortion are regarded as future options for eliminating the disease. Neither of these now is possible.

Pathophysiology, Diagnosis, and Complications. No cellular or subcellular biochemical inherited defect has been described to account for the pathophysiology of CF. Progress in this direction has been hampered by various factors: the wide spectrum of disease severity, which suggests modifying genetic influences and raises the possibility that CF is more than one disease; the systemic nutritional-metabolic derangements and chronic pulmonary infection that create secondary laboratory observations far removed from the basic genetic defect; and the lack of an animal model.

The pathophysiologic and diagnostic hallmarks of CF are: (1) pancreatic enzyme deficiency, (2) progressive chronic obstructive, infective (usually *Staphylococcus* and eventually *Pseudomonas*), and destructive pulmonary disease, and (3) elevated sweat sodium, chloride, and potassium concentrations. The first two have been attributed to the production of abnormal and thick mucus secretions. The third is the result of abnormal reabsorption of electrolytes by sweat ducts. When these are considered together, CF is thought to be a generalized disease of exocrine glands. Elevated calcium levels in salivary gland and tracheobronchial secretions also have been described. A pathophysiologic link between thick mucus secretions and abnormal electrolytes has not been established. Indeed, each may be the independent result of a more basic defect in secretion and transport at the membrane surface of cells.

Common indications for suspecting CF and for quantitative sweat testing include: failure to thrive in infancy, meconium ileus, steatorrhea, malabsorption, recurrent rectal prolapse, childhood cirrhosis, hypoprothrombinemia with purpura beyond the newborn period, heat prostration, hyponatremia and hypochloremia (in infants), and metabolic alkalosis (in older children). Sweat tests should also be performed on children with unexplained chronic cough, recurrent or chronic pneumonia, when *Staphylococcus* or *Pseudomonas* is responsible for pulmonary infections, and in young people with nasal polyps. Methods of diagnostic testing, including neonatal screening of meconium for elevated concentrations of albumin and rapid sweat test analyses by conductivity or chloride electrode methods, are still in an investigative stage and cannot be relied upon

Cystic fibrosis is a generalized disease with numerous unusual complicating features affecting practically every organ system of the body. An exhaustive review of these can be found in the recent literature (Wood et al., 1976).

Approach to Management and Prognostic Considerations. The natural history of CF has changed in the past 40 years. A disease formerly lethal in the first years of life is now one in which the mean age of survival has surpassed 16 years. There are many patients in their twenties and thirties who are leading productive lives with minimal disability. Improvement in morbidity and mortality has been made possible by medical and public awareness with earlier diagnosis facilitated by the sweat test; by the use of oral pancreatic enzymes to control steatorrhea and azotorrhea and minimize maldigestion; by the intensive and aggressive use of new antibiotics to control acute and chronic bronchial infections and the chronic colonization of the respiratory tract with staphylococcus and pseudomonas organisms; by the daily therapeutic and prophylactic modality of postural drainage and cupping to the chest followed by coughing to facilitate mobilization of mucus from all segmental bronchi; by the establishment of over 120 CF care centers in the United States, which has facilitated access to experienced medical care. Despite progress, generally the prognosis remains grim. The extent and rate of progression of the pulmonary disease is the limiting factor. Both are now impossible to determine for the individual patient, especially early in the course of the disease. Lung function usually is normal at birth. The first sign of pulmonary involvement is hyperexpansion or increased radiolucency of lung fields on chest x-ray. This is due to the earliest lesion of CF — bronchiolar obstruction with mucus. This predisposes to infection and inflammation, progressing with time to the larger airways and destruction of airway walls. Mucociliary clearance is impaired. Bronchiolitis, bronchitis, bronchiectasis, peribronchial fibrosis, and large cystic bronchial dilatation occur that may involve all subsegmental bronchi. Alveolar destruction ensues, with infection of atelectatic areas or with episodes of patchy pneumonia and hemorrhagic pneumonia. There is progressive loss of pulmonary function, which may be complicated by massive hemoptysis, recurrent pneumothorax, hypoxia and cor pulmonale, all of which are poor prognostic signs. The presence of mucoid strains of *Pseudomonas* in CF sputum also seems to separate the more severe from the milder cases. Mucoid *Pseudomonas* organisms are almost unique to CF. If mucoid strains of *Pseudomonas* are isolated from a patient with a chronic productive cough, a sweat test is indicated.

Proper management of patients with CF requires a broad understanding of the pathology of CF, a knowledge of its variable patterns of onset, expression and complications, and an appreciation of the psychologic, social, and financial stresses imposed. Even the most capable physician can no longer be the sole provider of the multiple services needed. The Cystic Fibrosis Foundation (6000 Executive Blvd., Suite

TABLE 48–2 SERVICES PROVIDED BY CYSTIC FIBROSIS CENTERS

Sweat testing and confirmation of diagnosis
Evaluation and outline of therapeutic and prophylactic programs
Education of the patient and the entire family
Instruction in pulmonary physiotherapy and inhalation therapy
Instruction in nutrition and diet
Genetic counseling
Vocational counseling
Financial counseling
Teenage and parent discussion groups
Other consultative services, including otolaryngology, surgery, allergy, psychiatry
Hospitalization and treatment for complications
Voluntary research by patients and relatives

309, Rockville, Maryland 20852) serves as a clearinghouse of medical information and recent advances in the understanding and management of CF. The medical director and his staff are equipped to triage all inquiries and to direct the health care professional to his or her nearest cystic fibrosis center. Personnel at CF centers are trained to confirm the diagnosis and to coordinate contemporary care of patients with this chronic illness in the context of family and community life styles. An informed case manager, whether the primary physician, cystic fibrosis specialist, nurse practitioner, family counselor, or other health professional, is a necessity. The goal in therapy is not only to increase life span but also improve the quality of life.

Relationship Between the Primary Care Person and the Cystic Fibrosis Specialist. A team effort by the primary care person and CF center provides the most comprehensive care. The extent of responsibility of each should be spelled out at the beginning of the relationship and made clear to the patient and family so that lines of communication will remain open. Table 48–2 summarizes services that CF centers provide. In most states, financial assistance for center visits and hospitalization are available through crippled children's programs. This aid usually terminates at age 21 years. When the clinical situation dictates frequent visits, evaluation is aimed at assessing the patient's state of health and at the detection of complications of CF.

Genetic Counseling. Although there are specialists who provide genetic counseling,

TABLE 48–3 RISKS OF PRODUCING A CHILD WITH CYSTIC FIBROSIS

One Parent	Other Parent	Risk of CF in Each Pregnancy
With no CF history	With no CF history	1:1600
With no CF history	With first cousin having CF	1:320
With no CF history	With aunt or uncle having CF	1:240
With no CF history	With sibling having CF	1:120
With no CF history	With CF child by previous marriage	1:80
With no CF history	With parent having CF	1:80
With no CF history	With CF	1:40
With sibling having CF	With sibling having CF	1:9
With CF child	With CF child	1:4

these functions are best initiated and performed by the health professional who understands the patient and the family most thoroughly. The process begins at the time of diagnosis, when parents learn that cystic fibrosis is an inherited disease and that mother and father each are carriers of a single autosomal recessive CF gene. Various issues, including misplaced guilt and blame, must be dealt with from the beginning in order to preserve family harmony and cohesiveness, especially around the time of diagnosis. Table 48–3 outlines the risks of producing a child with CF. Once a couple has a child with CF, the risk of each subsequent pregnancy resulting in CF is 1:4. Prenatal diagnosis by amniocentesis is not now possible. Although the sweat test cannot identify the heterozygote (carrier), all siblings should be tested. They may have CF and may have been overlooked because the diagnosis had not been previously considered or because the extent of the disease was at the mild end of the CF spectrum. Each sibling's chance of being a carrier is 2:3 or 66 percent, and the chance of the same parents producing a carrier with each subsequent pregnancy is 2:4 or 50 percent.

As the teenage and young adult years approach for the patient with CF, genetic and vocational counseling is an integral part of their guidance. The horizons depend greatly upon the physical condition of the patient. Limitations are imposed by the pulmonary status and rate of deterioration. When severe, puberty is delayed; many but not all males are sterile due to ablation of the ductus deferens system. Males of reproductive age contemplating marriage should have sperm analyses. The difference between sterility and virility (not impaired) should be made clear. Many females with CF have had children of their own, although their fertility may be impaired due to thick cervical mucus. Their chance of having a child with CF is 1:40 when the carrier status of the father is unknown (assuming a 1:20 carrier rate for the general white population). All non-CF children of a mother with CF will be carriers. Other realistic concerns are whether the female with CF can survive a pregnancy and whether her health will permit her to raise her child.

ECTODERMAL DYSPLASIA

Ectodermal dysplasia has certain similarities to CF, which include heritability, abnormalities of sweating, abnormalities of respiratory mucus production, increased susceptibility to upper and lower respiratory infection, a high frequency of wheezing, and an increased incidence of allergic sensitization as defined by multiple positive immediate skin tests to common inhalant allergens (Vanselow et al., 1970; Beahrs, 1971). Similarly, the spectrum of disease is great; probably the mildest forms never seek medical attention and therefore remain undiagnosed. A positive sweat test (elevated sodium and chloride concentrations) may occur in the hypohidrotic form, presumably because of shortened sweat ducts and their inability to reabsorb sodium and chloride elaborated from sweat coils as an isotonic solution. This type is associated with sensorineural deafness. Confusion with CF thus can occur, and it seems likely that some patients with the hypohidrotic form of ectodermal dysplasia have been misdiagnosed as having CF, having both chronic pulmonary disease and a positive sweat test.

Major Forms of Ectodermal Dysplasia

Anhidrotic Type. This disease is inherited as an X-linked recessive disorder. Males inherit the complete form, whereas the females usually inherit a partial form. Anhidrosis (no sweating) or severe hypohidrosis, anodontia or severe hypodontia, and hypotrichosis are the cardinal features that should lead directly to this diagnosis. Other physical findings include prominent frontal bossing, saddle-shaped nose, protruding or deformed ears, thin wrinkled eyelids with prominence of the supraorbital ridge, thick and protruding lips, delayed or absent dentition. When present, the incisors are widely spaced and the canines have a conical shape. Anodontia and hypodontia affect both the deciduous and permanent teeth. Other abnormalities found in most patients include sparse, fine, blonde hair and absent eyebrow, eyelash, body, axillary and pubic hair. The skin is smooth and dry; fingernails are dystrophic. Flexural eczema typical of atopic dermatitis has been reported in several cases (Reed et al., 1970; Vanselow et al., 1970).

The external manifestations are the result of absent or decreased numbers of skin appendages — hair follicles, and sweat, sebaceous and apocrine glands. Mammary, salivary, and lacrimal glands also may be absent in some cases. The cutaneous pathology produces an inability to regulate body temperature in warm weather, resulting in high fevers. Involvement of entodermal elements accounts for both chronic upper and lower respiratory tract disease. Mucous glands of the respiratory tract often are atrophied. Absence of seromucous glands in the pharynx, larynx, trachea, and large and small bronchi have been reported (De Jager, 1965). Virtual absence of seromucous glands but presence of goblet cells have been observed in two infants with this disorder (Capitanio et al., 1968). Deficiency of seromucus interferes with mucociliary clearance in the respiratory tract and leads to dryness, bronchitis, and infection, especially with staphylococci. Allergen sensitization via the respiratory tract may be due to increased permeability. Allergic rhinitis and asthma (both seasonal and perennial) have been described.

Hidrotic Type. In contrast to the anhidrotic type of ectodermal dysplasia, the hidrotic type is inherited as an autosomal dominant with complete penetrance. Males and females are equally affected. Female carriers of the X-linked form may have similar clinical findings. These include sparse, thin, fragile hair with reduced tensile strength on the head, eyebrows, and body and dystrophic thick nails with subungual infections. The skin of the palms and soles is thick, with

brownish pigmentation. There may be generalized hypopigmentation, with hyperpigmentation present on the extensor surfaces of the elbow, areolar area of the breasts, umbilicus, and interphalangeal joints. Fingernails may be dystrophic, occasionally absent, thin, or thickened with striations. It has been said that there is no aplasia or hypoplasia of the sweat, sebaceous, and mucous glands. Some patients have decreased sweating, elevated sweat sodium and chloride levels, sensorineural deafness, and hypodontia. Studies of mucus-secreting glands of the respiratory tract have not been reported. A molecular abnormality of keratin with increased amount of reactive sulfhydryl groups has been described (Scriver et al., 1965).

Treatment of Ectodermal Dysplasia. Genetic counseling is the only preventive measure. Those anhidrotic patients with respiratory abnormalities require proper environmental humidification and temperature regulation. Patients should be advised to limit exercise in hot weather. Although there is no evidence for efficacy of postural drainage for those patients with chronic cough, postural drainage probably is beneficial since mucociliary clearance is impaired. Patients should be treated promptly with appropriate antibiotics when upper and lower respiratory infections occur. They are strong candidates for both viral and bacterial vaccine prophylaxis. Dentures should be made for those with anodontia and hypodontia.

KARTAGENER'S SYNDROME AND THE IMMOTILE-CILIA SYNDROME

Kartagener's syndrome consists of a triad of dextrocardia with situs inversus totalis, chronic sinusitis and/or agenesis of the frontal sinuses, and bronchiectasis. The incidence of Kartagener's syndrome has been estimated at one per 50,000 population, whereas the incidence of situs inversus is one in 8,000 (Adams and Churchill, 1937). Bronchiectasis, which occurs in less than 0.5 percent of the general population, is found in as high as 25 percent of patients with situs inversus (Olsen, 1943). Dextrocardia with or without situs inversus may include other anomalies such as single ventricle, arterial transposition, pulmonary stenosis, ventricular and atrial septal defects, and asplenia. Other associated manifestations and conditions have included nasal polyps, conductive hearing loss, transient deficiency of immunoglobulin A and mesangiocapillary glomerulonephritis with hypocomplementemia (Egbert et al., 1977).

Kartagener's syndrome has been reported among family members and the mode of inheritance is thought to be autosomal recessive. Penetrance is variable, as siblings may have bronchiectasis without situs inversus. Vertical transmission from an affected parent to a child has not been reported. An important component of this syndrome is male infertility. Women with Kartagener's syndrome have borne children.

Pulmonary Manifestations. Symptoms of rhinitis, wheezing, and respiratory difficulty may begin in the first year of life. Recurrent pneumonias are due to *Hemophilis influenzae* and *Streptococcus pneumoniae,* in contrast to staphylococcus and pseudomonas organisms, which are the common pathogens of CF. Chronic pulmonary changes resemble postinfectious interstitial pneumonitis and cylindrical, follicular, and saccular bronchiectasis. Persistent cough, sputum production, and recurrent fevers ensue when bronchiectasis becomes severe.

Pathogenesis and Immotile Cilia. The finding of bronchiectasis without situs inversus in family members is compatible with both partial expression of a genetic trait and with exogenous factors such as infection producing an acquired pulmonary lesion. Immune deficiency and abnormal mucous glands and/or ciliary dysfunction have been proposed as alternative explanations for a basic abnormality. The most convincing mechanism is based on electron microscopic studies which indicate that respiratory cilia are structurally abnormal and functionally nonmotile (Afzelius, 1976; Pederson and Mygind, 1976; Eliasson et al., 1977). Dynein arms — normal structures of nine microtubular filaments responsible for generating the movement of sperm tails and cilia — have been found to be lacking in sperm and decreased in number or shorter than normal in cilia. Corresponding to this, tracheobronchial mucociliary transport is markedly diminished or absent. Ciliated epithelia are present in the respiratory tract, paranasal sinuses, eustachian tubes, oviducts, and vas

efferentia. Ciliary dysfunction could explain upper and lower respiratory tract pathology and other abnormalities in this syndrome. Additionally, immotile cilia may account for situs inversus (Afzelius, 1976). Since unidirectional embryonic ciliary beating determines organ spiral orientation, in the absence of ciliary movement, there is an even chance of rotation to either side. Thus, situs inversus occurs by chance. This also is compatible with the finding of immotile cilia and sperm in patients without situs inversus as, by chance, 50 percent of people with this defect will have normal organ orientation. Similar and various other cilial abnormalities have recently been identified in Polynesian patients with bronchiectasis (Waite et al., 1978).

Treatments. Situs inversus should be diagnosed in the newborn period. As indicated previously, as many as 25 percent of these infants will develop bronchiectasis. Anticipatory and preventive measures should be started at the time of diagnosis. These should include immunization against respiratory pathogens — rubeola, pertussis, influenza, pneumococci and *Hemophilis influenzae* Type B — according to age and dosage recommendations, early detection of bacterial infection by culture and early treatment with antibiotics, and regular postural drainage to prevent pooling of secretions.

BRONCHIECTASIS

Bronchiectasis means dilatation of bronchi; bronchial wall destruction also is implied. Cylindrical, tubular or pseudobronchiectasis (absence of normal bronchial tapering) frequently follows acute lower respiratory infections and is reversible. Saccular bronchiectasis (irregular bronchial dilatations and narrowings) is irreversible. Large dilatations are referred to as cystic bronchiectasis. Proximal or central bronchiectasis is associated with allergic bronchopulmonary aspergillosis.

Bronchiectasis usually is acquired, although there may be familial occurrence based on genetic susceptibilities to infection and inflammation. The Williams-Campbell syndrome is a congenital deficiency of bronchial cartilage (Wayne and Taussig, 1976), leading to bronchiectasis. Bronchiectasis occurs commonly in disorders such as CF, immune deficiency states, Kartagener's syndrome, alpha-1-antitrypsin deficiency, and occasionally in severe chronic asthma. Postinfectious bronchiectasis is seen less frequently than in former years. The decreased incidence (Nemir, 1977) is due to a decline in measles and pertussis infections, former common precursors of bronchiectasis; the effective use of antibiotics in lower respiratory infections; the decreased occurrence of primary tuberculosis in infancy and early childhood; and better management of atelectasis and chronic bronchial inflammation by bronchial drainage and physiotherapy. Most acquired postinfectious bronchiectasis may now be the sequelae of infections with viruses such as influenza (Laraya-Cuasay et al., 1977) and adenovirus, particularly Types 3, 7, and 21 (Becroft, 1971). Acute adenoviral infections induce a necrotizing bronchiolitis, which may proceed to bronchiolar obliteration (bronchiolitis obliterans). Consequences of this include atelectasis (absorption of gas, collapse, and fibrosis) and inflammation in areas of stagnant secretions, both thought to be the main causes of bronchiectasis. Bronchial obstruction also follows mucus plugging, foreign body aspiration, and compression or erosion of bronchi by tuberculous lymph nodes.

Clinical Features and Diagnosis. Bronchiectasis should be anticipated when acute lower respiratory illnesses are slow to resolve, when there is a history of recurrent pulmonary infections, or when there is persistent atelectasis. Lesions may be localized or diffuse. Localized lesions most commonly involve the left lower lobe except with foreign body aspiration, which most commonly involves the right middle lobe. For unknown reasons, the right upper lobe commonly is the first and most severely involved in CF.

The cardinal clinical feature of bronchiectasis is chronic cough productive of mucopurulent sputum, which on culture usually yields *Hemophilus influenzae* or *Streptococcus pneumoniae*. Gram negative organisms such as *E. coli*, *Proteus* and *Klebsiella* also may be cultured after multiple courses of antibiotics. *Staphylococcus* and *Pseudomonas* are the predominant organisms in cystic fibrosis. Bronchiectasis frequently is associated with chronic maxillary sinusitis

and each may contribute to the chronicity of the other. *Staphylococcus, Streptococcus* and anaerobic *Bacteroides* organisms may infect the sinuses. Wheezing may occur in the absence of bronchial asthma. Hemoptysis in advanced cases is due to erosion of bronchial blood vessels. The spectrum of bronchiectasis is large, ranging from almost asymptomatic localized disease to full-blown chronic diffuse disease. Malnutrition, clubbing, hypoxemia, pulmonary hypertension, and cor pulmonale are late complications. Clubbing may occur with localized lesions and has been noted to disappear when these are resected. Emphysema, broncho-pleural fistula, and metastatic brain abscess are less common complications since the advent of antibiotics. Pneumonia and atelectasis are frequent complications.

Chest roentgenograms may appear normal or may exhibit increased linear markings in mild disease. If disease is allowed to progress, small cystic and nodular lesions show a "honeycomb" pattern. Large cysts and bullae occur with most advanced disease. These may be filled with air or air-fluid and predispose to aspergillomas. Bronchography can be used to diagnose both tubular and saccular bronchiectasis. It is reserved for those cases in which a localized lesion is suspected or when surgical resection of a localized lesion is contemplated. It should be done first on the suspected side and then at another time on the "unaffected" side to rule out more generalized disease. Medical management should include physiotherapy, bronchodilators and appropriate antibiotics for 2 to 4 weeks prior to bronchography to eliminate obstructing bronchial secretions, minimize infection, and to allow time for resolution of reversible lesions.

Treatment. Nemir (1977) has discussed the medical and surgical treatment of childhood bronchiectasis. Medical management is preferred for patients who are asymptomatic with minimal disease, patients with early disease that may be reversible, and patients with advanced diffuse disease who are unable to tolerate surgery because of greatly impaired pulmonary function. Surgical treatment is reserved for those symptomatic patients whose disease is localized to one segment or lobe with either persistent or recurrent obstruction, infection uncontrolled by antibiotic therapy, recurrent hemoptysis from a localized source, or foreign body that cannot be removed by bronchoscopy. In cystic fibrosis, prognosis may be improved by resection when one segment or lobe has far advanced bronchiectasis and the remaining lung involvement is mild. Resection always should be an elective procedure, done after optimal medical management has failed. Regular pulmonary physiotherapy with strong emphasis on positioning to drain all segmental bronchi or with concentration of one or two positions to drain localized lesions is of utmost importance in medical management.

ALPHA-1-ANTITRYPSIN (AAT) DEFICIENCY AND DISEASE

Alpha-1-antitrypsin is a glycoprotein synthesized by the liver and is a major inhibitor of several proteolytic enzymes. It migrates with the alpha-1 region on electrophoresis, and accounts for 90 percent of the protein in this region. Alpha-1-antitrypsin deficiency was discovered by Laurell and Eriksson in 1963. In 1965, Eriksson established the association of AAT deficiency with an inherited form of panacinar emphysema by observing that 22 of 33 homozygous-deficient patients had emphysema. It soon became apparent that only a minority of patients with emphysema have homozygous AAT deficiency, and that some homozygous AAT-deficient adults and even aged relatives of AAT-deficient emphysema patients were completely free of clinical disease.

In 1969, Sharp et al. reported the association of familial juvenile cirrhosis with the homozygous deficiency. Since then, it has been learned that many cases of "idiopathic neonatal hepatitis" that progressed to cirrhosis were associated with AAT deficiency, and that cirrhosis in combination with emphysema and/or chronic obstructive lung disease (COLD) occurs in children and adults. The risk of the newborn with AAT deficiency developing neonatal hepatitis and cirrhosis has been estimated at 20 percent. Several studies indicate that 25 percent of children previously thought to have idiopathic neonatal hepatitis have had AAT deficiency. Approximately 12 percent of adult emphysema patients have AAT deficiency.

AAT is found in all body fluids and plays a role in the homeostatic mechanisms of inflammation. It is hypothesized that lung disease occurs in the homozygous deficient individual when proteolytic enzymes (especially elastase) — released from inflammatory cells by natural decay, toxic or infectious insult — are unchecked because of a deficiency of AAT. Therefore, excessive tissue destruction is induced at the site of insult (especially of elastin present in alveolar septae). The variable course of deficiency in children and adults and the finding of asymptomatic AAT-deficient adults suggest, however, that other endogenous (protective-genetic) and exogenous (toxic-infectious) factors also are important in modulating the course of disease.

The incidence of homozygous AAT deficiency is 1:2000, which is almost identical to the incidence of CF. The prevalence of the heterozygote is 3 percent of most Caucasian populations studied. These "carriers" have been considered to be "partially deficient" or to have a "low intermediate deficiency" and have serum AAT levels which are 60 percent of normal. The finding of a significant aggregation (11 percent) of "carriers" in a population of patients with COLD (Mittman et al., 1974) suggests that individuals with "partial AAT deficiency" also are at risk in developing COLD.

Genetics and Electrophoretic Variants. AAT migrates as a series of electrophoretic bands moving towards the anode. The entire pattern, called Pi-type (protease inhibitor), represents the sum of the genetic input of two inherited alleles. Family studies indicate a multi-allelic co-dominant mode of inheritance, with over 30 patterns described. AAT serum levels vary in quantity and activity and are regulated by the Pi-type. Pi ZZ's are severely deficient, with serum AAT levels 10 to 15 percent of the common "normal" Pi MM type. Pi ZZ occurs in an incidence of 1:2000. Pi MZ has about 60 percent (low intermediate deficiency) of Pi MM quantity and Pi MS (high intermediate deficiency) about 80 percent (Table 48–4). A Pi^{null} (Pi$^-$) variant with completely absent AAT has been described in one family. The severe deficiency (ZZ and SZ) can be detected by finding a flat alpha-1 region on a serum protein electrophoresis pattern. Pi-typing of family members is nec-

TABLE 48-4   ALPHA-1-ANTITRYPSIN SERUM CONCENTRATIONS*

Pi Type	Males (mg ± 1 SD/100 ml)	Females (mg ± 1 SD/100 ml)	+ B.C. (mg ± 1 SD/100 ml)	− B.C. (mg ± 1 SD/100 ml)
Pi MM	207 ± 38	238 ± 55	284 ± 50	223 ± 48
Pi MS	178 ± 31	204 ± 41	231 ± 49	193 ± 31
Pi MZ	138 ± 27	147 ± 22	175 ± 14	137 ± 15

*Values obtained from a random sample of 950 (half males, half females) adults — Monroe County, New York.
B.C. = Birth control pills.

essary to confirm the type and inheritance pattern.

Pulmonary Manifestations. The classic form of emphysema associated with AAT deficiency occurs with equal frequency in men and women. Emphysema in general is more common in men. Progressive dyspnea without cough or sputum production usually begins in the third decade of life, which is significantly earlier than with emphysema in general. Panacinar emphysema may be evidenced by increased basilar lucency of chest roentgenogram at this time. As the disease progresses, chronic cough, chronic bronchitis, and bronchiectasis may add to the clinical picture. The variability of clinical course in AAT (Pi Z) deficiency has been stressed (Black and Kueppers, 1978). Avoidance of respiratory irritants also can significantly improve prognosis.

Children may also have severe AAT deficiency and chronic progressive respiratory disease (Talamo, 1977). Symptoms include chronic cough, progressive dyspnea, and wheezing. Digital clubbing may occur when respiratory disease is severe or with the juvenile cirrhosis, which also is a manifestation of AAT (Pi ZZ and Pi SZ) deficiency in childhood. Panacinar emphysema and emphysema complicated by chronic bronchitis and bronchiectasis may occur. Both liver and lung disease may co-exist in children (Fig. 48-1).

Several epidemiologic studies have implicated an association of partially deficient AAT variants in adults and children with asthma (Fagerhol and Hague, 1969; Katz et al., 1976). Others studied perennial allergic asthmatic children and were not able to find such an association (Schwartz et al., 1977). The prevalence of Pi variants is increased (46 versus 11 percent) in nonallergic asthmatic children (Arnaud et al., 1976). Functional abnormalities of peripheral airways also have been described in Pi MZ asymptomatic nonasthmatic children (Vance et al., 1977).

PULMONARY HEMOSIDEROSIS

Pulmonary hemosiderosis is the result of intra-alveolar hemorrhage (hemorrhagic alveolitis) and deposition of iron as hemo-

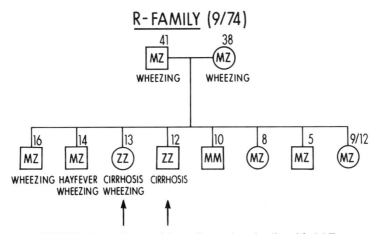

FIGURE 48-1. Liver and lung disease in a family with AAT.

siderin in the interstitium of the lung. Though these patients may exsanguinate, they more frequently develop iron deficiency anemia because of recurrent hemoptysis and/or sequestration of iron in the lung. After repeated bleeding, pulmonary hemosiderosis and fibrosis ensue, with impairment of lung function including decreased diffusion, decreased compliance, and airway obstruction. Initially, roentgenograms show diffuse perihilar infiltrates and patchy alveolar densities. Later, diffuse reticular markings and septal thickening are seen with pulmonary fibrosis. Pulmonary hemosiderosis may be secondary to mitral stenosis with increased pulmonary venous pressure, collagen disease vasculitis, and other chronic bleeding diatheses. In all other cases, the etiology is unclear. Most of these occur in infants and children except for Goodpasture's syndrome (Proskey et al., 1970), which usually afflicts young male adults. In Goodpasture's syndrome, the initial acute respiratory episode is soon followed by glomerulonephritis, progressing to renal failure and death.

Diagnosis. The disease should be suspected in any young child with chronic pulmonary symptoms, especially with hemoptysis, associated with iron deficiency anemia and typical roentgenographic findings. Many children have chronic rhinitis, recurrent otitis media and failure to thrive, persistent cough, wheezing, tachypnea, pallor, and cyanosis. Others have been described with cor pulmonale secondary to adenoidal upper airway obstruction, alveolar hypoventilation especially during sleep, and pulmonary hypertension (Boat et al., 1975). The diagnosis of intra-alveolar bleeding is confirmed by the finding of hemosiderin-laden alveolar macrophages in sputum, tracheobronchial washings, or lung biopsy specimens. Since needle biopsies have resulted in massive pulmonary hemorrhage, open lung biopsies should be done only after repeated efforts have been made to find these cells in other fluids.

Pulmonary Hemosiderosis in Children Associated with Immune Phenomena. Heiner and Sears (1960) reported the association of chronic respiratory disease with multiple circulating precipitins to cow milk. Heiner et al. (1962) implicated hypersensitivity to cow milk proteins as the basis of the chronic disease and added pulmonary hemosiderosis to a syndrome consisting of poor growth, pulmonary and gastrointestinal symptoms, and iron deficiency anemia. Symptoms resolved with substitution of evaporated milk for fresh milk or with the complete removal of cow milk from the diet. Pulmonary hemosiderosis without milk precipitins has also been observed (Heiner, 1977). Some of these cases also have shown response to milk withdrawal.

Inconstant immunologic features of childhood idiopathic pulmonary hemosiderosis include peripheral eosinophilia, elevated serum levels of IgE, LE or tart cells, positive direct Coombs' test, circulating cold agglutinins, and increased lymphocyte incorporation of tritiated thymidine on stimulation with cow milk protein. The types of hypersensitivity reactions which may contribute to the development of pulmonary lesions has yet to be elucidated, however. A unique immune mechanism has not been demonstrated for cow milk–induced pulmonary hemosiderosis (Stafford et al., 1977).

Many investigators believe that milk sensitivity accounts for the pulmonary disease and that sensitization occurs via the gastrointestinal tract. Serious consideration also must be given to the respiratory route for both sensitization and elicitation of the pulmonary lesions. Milk precipitins have been found in children with defects in swallowing (Peterson and Good, 1962) and in association with other pathologic phenomena in which there is an increased likelihood of aspiration, e.g., in children with esophageal atresia or stenosis (Handleman and Nelson, 1964), Down's syndrome (Nelson, 1964), and profound mental retardation (McCrea et al., 1968). Animal experiments further support this aspiration hypothesis (Richerson, 1974; Hensley et al., 1978; Scherzer and Ward, 1978). Acute hemorrhagic alveolitis with inflammation of capillaries can be induced in actively or passively immunized animals by respiratory insufflation of animal proteins or by endotracheal instillation of preformed immune complexes. The reaction has characteristics both of immune complex disease and of the Arthus reaction.

Treatment. In view of the above considerations, milk should be eliminated from the diet in children with chronic or recurrent lower respiratory disease in whom multiple milk precipitins are found. The physician should ask about possible aspiration and should observe the infant feed. He or she may need to pursue dynamic radiologic studies of swallowing (deglutition) for evidence of subtle aspiration and gastroesophageal reflux. If such evidence is found, elimination of milk, the use of small, frequent and thickened feedings, and positioning the child in an upright position during and after feeding may prevent aspiration and sensitization. Steroids, azathioprine, and a combination of the two have been used empirically to suppress the pulmonary inflammatory process (Heiner, 1977).

PULMONARY FIBROSIS

Pulmonary fibrosis, also called Hamman-Rich syndrome, interstitial fibrosis, cryptogenic fibrosing alveolitis, and honeycomb lung, is probably the end stage of several different inflammatory processes of the alveolar wall (interstitial pneumonitis), initiated by known and unknown etiologic agents. It also is associated with a variety of underlying diseases (see below).

Alveoli, their lining cells, basement membrane, capillaries, and connective tissue become involved in an inflammatory reaction. A cellular exudate or inflammatory reaction occurs in the early stages in alveolar spaces. When interstitial pneumonia resolves incompletely, alveolar fibroplasia and organization follow that obliterate alveoli and induce compensatory dilatation of remaining alveoli, alveolar ducts, and bronchioles. This results in the characteristic honeycomb lung seen on x-ray films. The course can be rapid, as in the Hamman-Rich syndrome, with dry cough and severe progressive dyspnea ending in respiratory failure and cor pulmonale within months of the onset of symptoms. The course also can be slower, incomplete, or nonprogressive. Pulmonary fibrosis is a restrictive lung disease: pulmonary function studies demonstrate a decrease in lung volumes, diffusion capacity, and compliance. Hypoxemia which becomes more severe with exercise also is a common feature.

Etiology. Some cases may be genetically determined (Bonnani et al., 1965). Pulmonary fibrosis and interstitial pneumonitis occur with connective tissue diseases (systemic lupus erythematosus, dermatomyositis, scleroderma, rhumatoid arthritis),

other diseases with immune features (Sjögren's syndrome, Hashimoto's thyroiditis, chronic active hepatitis, hypergammaglobulinemic renal tubular acidosis, ulcerative colitis, sarcoidosis), chronic hypersensitivity pneumonitis, the use of cytotoxic drugs (hexamethonium, pentolinium, mecamylamine, busulfan, bleomycin, cytoxan, melphalan, hydralazine, hydantoin), drug sensitivity (nitrofurantoin) (Rosenow, 1972), and viral infections (Laraya-Cuasay, 1978).

Classification. Liebow (1975) has classified the interstitial pneumonias on the basis of the type and location of the inflammatory process: usual interstitial pneumonia (UIP), desquamative interstitial pneumonia (DIP), lymphoid interstitial pneumonia (LIP), giant cell interstitial pneumonia (GIP), and bronchiolitis obliterans with interstitial pneumonia (BIP). These descriptions give little etiologic information but provide prognostic and therapeutic information that may justify open lung biopsy. When viral cultures are positive, an etiologic diagnosis can be established.

Prognosis and Treatment. Alveolar wall fibrosis implies a poor prognosis (Patchefsky et al., 1973). Desquamative interstitial pneumonias in infants, children and adults respond to steroid therapy. These patients may present with a variable clinical picture (including cough, tachypnea, cyanosis and failure to thrive) which develops over one day to several weeks after a viral respiratory infection. Chest x-ray shows a diffuse ground glass appearance, accentuated perihilar markings, and patchy infiltrates. Children who have protracted symptoms with suggestive x-ray findings should be considered for open lung biopsy and possibly for steroid therapy to halt progression of disease (Harwood et al., 1977).

An association of circulating immune complexes and interstitial pneumonias responsive to steroid therapy recently has been described (Dreisin et al., 1978). Immune complexes may play a pathogenetic role in the cellular (UIP, DIP, LIP) interstitial pneumonias. Immune complex assays may identify patient populations that are potentially steroid-responsive. Circulating immune complex assays are investigative, however; and until they are validated and routinely available, the use of steroids to prevent progression of the inflammatory cellular response to fibrosis or to stabilize the fibrosing process will have to remain a clinical decision based upon change in symptoms, serial pulmonary function tests, and chest roentgenograms.

SARCOIDOSIS

Although fewer than 200 cases of sarcoidosis have been reported in children, it is possible that sarcoidosis would be diagnosed more commonly in children if this diagnosis was considered more commonly (Kendig, 1977). In childhood, diagnoses are made most commonly in the 9 to 15 year age group, but sarcoidosis has been seen even as early as 2 months of age. In the United States, sarcoidosis appears more frequently among the black population than any other racial group; but elsewhere in the world, there are comparable attack rates among white populations.

Clinical Manifestations. Sarcoidosis may affect any organ or part of the body. Symptoms at first may be protean, the most common being lassitude, apathy, and malaise. Symptoms referrable to the respiratory tract often consist of dry, hacking cough, and mild to moderate shortness of breath. Other presenting complaints are fever, weight loss, adenopathy, and vision loss. Other diseases that produce granulomatous lesions which should be considered in the differential diagnosis include tuberculosis, histoplasmosis, coccidioidomycosis, chronic granulomatous disease, berylliosis, farmer's lung (hypersensitivity pneumonitis), and aspergilloma. The chest roentgenogram of advanced sarcoidosis may be indistinguishable from advanced CF, but bilateral hilar adenopathy is of particular importance as a diagnostic point in sarcoidosis.

The following are also seen in sarcoidosis: enlarged lymph nodes (54 percent of cases); eye involvement with uveitis and iritis (42 percent of cases); skin lesions (45 percent of cases), consisting of small, discrete nodules, large conglomerate masses, or large flat plaques varying in color from waxy to reddish-blue; and uveoparotid fever (12 percent of cases) with uveitis, parotid gland swelling, and fever frequently associated with facial nerve palsy; and hepatic (18 percent of cases) and splenic (23 percent of cases) involvement, leading to portal hypertension, hypersplenism and, in some cases, massive sarcoid splenomegaly. In addition, bone lesions (24 percent of cases) are found in patients with chronic skin lesions and consist of either single or multiple punched out areas in metacarpals or metatarsals. Hypercalcemia and hypercalcuria caused by increased absorption of dietary calcium as a result of increased sensitivity to vitamin D result in nephrocalcinosis, nephrolithiasis, and chronic renal disease. Sarcoid granulomas may involve the myocardium, central nervous system, and endocrine glands. Cardiac arrhythmias, seizures, hypopituitarism, diabetes insipidus, adrenal insufficiency, and thyroiditis have been reported in both adults and children.

Etiology. The etiology of sarcoidosis is unknown. Immune features of sarcoidosis include depressed cell-mediated immunity and raised or abnormal immunoglobulins, but the relationship of these abnormalities to etiologic factors is unclear.

The Kveim Test. This is the best assay for confirming the diagnosis of sarcoidosis; it is positive in 80 percent of cases. The antigen, however, is not available commercially and can be obtained only from individuals who are engaged in research on sarcoidosis. Skin test antigen is prepared from extracts of spleen from patients with active sarcoidosis. The material is injected intradermally as with the tuberculin test. The site is observed for six weeks. If a nodule forms, this is biopsied; the test is considered positive if granuloma typical of sarcoid is seen.

Prognosis and Treatment. Since so few cases of sarcoidosis have been described in children, the long-term prognosis is difficult to determine as is the efficacy of steroid therapy. Prognosis may be better in children than in adults. The prognosis is most favorable in children with early stage sarcoid, in whom the disease may resolve spontaneously. Cutaneous lesions, bone lesions and pulmonary fibrosis are associated with a poor prognosis. Steroids are the principal drug of choice and generally cause prompt resolution of clinical manifestations (Kendig and Brummer, 1976).

CHLAMYDIA INFECTIONS

Infections caused by Chlamydia organisms include trachoma, inclusion conjunctivitis, urethritis, and lymphogranuloma venereum. Chlamydiae also cause respiratory infections including psittacosis (acquired from parrots and parakeets), ornithosis (acquired from most wild and domestic birds), and a pneumonia syndrome in infants.

Psittacosis and ornithosis are acquired from handling birds, feathers, inhaling bird droppings, or from contact with an infected person. The incubation period is a few days to 2 weeks, followed by the abrupt onset of a flu-like illness with fever, chills, myalgias, photophobia, and cough. Fever initially is high and disappears by the end of the third week. Diffuse rales are heard throughout both lungs. Chest roentgenograms show diffuse bronchopneumonia or interstitial pneumonia similar to that seen with viral infections. Diagnosis is made by history and confirmed by culture (not generally available) and serologic tests. Treatment consists of general supportive measures and the use of tetracycline or sulfonamides.

The chlamydia syndrome in infants may last weeks and months. Infection is acquired at birth from a mother whose cervix or vagina is colonized with the organism. Colonization of the newborn is common. Postnatal inclusion conjunctivitis, a diagnostic clue, appears 5 to 7 days after birth. However, eye involvement is not always seen; the reason for the variability between infants, both in tissue involvement and susceptibility to infection, is not clear (Beem and Saxon, 1977). At about 2 to 3 weeks of age there is a gradual onset of progressive respiratory symptoms mimicking pertussis, such as increased nasopharyngeal secretions, tachypnea, and repetitive staccato coughing. Unlike pertussis, there is no post-tussic inspiratory whoop. Fever and malaise are conspicuously absent. Follicular conjunctivitis and secretory otitis media may be present. Chest roentgenograms show diffuse interstitial infiltrates and areas of patchy alveolar densities. Symptoms may persist for weeks, and roentgenogram changes may last for months. Laboratory findings include an absolute peripheral eosinophilia, elevated immunoglobulins (IgG and IgM), and an elevated antibody titer to lymphogranuloma venereum, Type 1. Conjunctivitis can be treated with sulfacetamide ointment or with tetracycline ointment or solution. Pneumonias and respiratory shedding of organisms respond to sulfisoxazole or erythromycin.

BRONCHOPULMONARY DYSPLASIA

Bronchopulmonary dysplasia (BPD) occurs in infants who have had idiopathic respiratory distress syndrome (IRDS) or recurrent apnea, who have been treated with prolonged mechanical ventilation with high oxygen concentration. The smaller the infant is, the greater is the likelihood of its developing BPD. Mechanical ventilation produces airway damage that creates edema, increased secretions, and disruption of elastic tissue. High oxygen tensions produce interstitial edema and epithelial necrosis. All lead to airway obstruction, air trapping, bleb formation, decreased compliance, and disturbances in gas exchange. The process may be slowly or rapidly progressive or may resolve spontaneously. Surviving infants frequently exhibit roentgenographic findings of hyperaeration, coarse interstitial markings, atelectasis, and bilateral cystic changes, which may persist for months. Chronic or recurrent tachypnea, retractions and wheezing are not unusual, and periodic respiratory exacerbations with wheezing, especially with viral respiratory tract infections, are common especially in infancy.

Children with BPD require close follow-up. Persistent roentgenographic changes, if unappreciated, may erroneously appear to be "acute" and, in the presence of a febrile illness, may lead to excessive antibiotic therapy. Mild chronic symptoms can be managed with chest physiotherapy and bronchodilators to create an optimal pulmonary toilet and minimize atelectasis. Minor residual roentgenographic and pulmonary function abnormalities have been observed 5 to 10 years after the initial illness (Lamarre et al., 1973). Because of the pulmonary growth potential early in life, however, sufficient recovery from BPD to minimize development of chronic obstructive lung disease is possible.

PULMONARY MYCOSES

Histoplasmosis, coccidioidomycosis, actinomycosis, blastomycosis, cryptococcosis, sporotrichosis, aspergillosis, nocardiosis, and mucormycosis should be suspected in any child with chronic localized pneumonia. Each can produce areas of chronic pneumonitis with or without cavitation and calcification. Exposure to organisms causing histoplasmosis and coccidioidomycosis is common in certain areas of the United States. The vast majority of primary histoplasmosis and coccidioidomycosis infections are benign, self-limited and do not require therapy. However, progressive, disseminated forms with acute and chronic complications do occur. In both diseases, acute and chronic forms may resemble tuberculosis. Heavy exposure to fungal spores produces acute influenza-like syndromes.

Histoplasmosis

In the United States, exposure to *Histoplasma* organisms is most likely in areas bordered by the western Appalachians and the tributaries of the Ohio, Mississippi, and Missouri Rivers (Ohio, Indiana, southern Illinois, Missouri, Arkansas, Kentucky, and Tennessee). The soil is the natural habitat of the yeast phase of *H. capsulatum,* which is distributed throughout the temperate zones of the world. Infection is inevitable in highly endemic areas, with histoplasmin skin tests positive in 25 percent of children by 1 year of age in such areas, reaching a peak of 87 percent reactivity at 10 to 14 years of age. Infection with airborne spores occurs by the respiratory route. Unlike tuberculosis, human-to-human spread does not occur. Avian and bat excrement encourages fungus growth. Intense exposure to spores may occur in chicken houses, starling and pigeon roosts, and in bat-infested caves, attics, and lofts. Cleaning old chicken houses, bulldozing starling roosts, and exploring caves or handling dirt or bats in dry caves promote development of acute infections.

Classification and Description. A clinical classification of histoplasmosis is based upon extent of exposure or re-exposure, age, status of immune responsiveness, and preexisting pulmonary structural abnormalities (Goodwin and Des Prez, 1978). Primary infections from mild exposure usually are asymptomatic. Symptomatic primary infections occurring in children are self-limited and generally do not require treatment. Variable fever begins 5 to 18 days after exposure and may last up to 3 weeks. Brassy cough, sometimes with wheezing, is due to compression of the trachea and bronchi by mediastinal and hilar lymph nodes. Roentgenographic findings are similar to tuberculosis, with patchy or clustered parenchymal infiltrates, streaky lymphangitis to the regional lymph nodes, and hilar and mediastinal adenopathy.

Pulmonary and extrapulmonary complications after primary histoplasmosis occur in children, infants, and immunocompromised hosts. Organisms spread via the blood stream and lymphatics to other areas of the lungs and the liver and spleen. Pulmonary hematogenous dissemination results in a "snow storm" appearance to the chest roentgenogram. Hepatosplenomegaly also occurs. Depending upon the host's ability to mount an immune inflammatory response, lesions of the lung, lymph nodes, liver, and spleen progress or localize. When contained, cellular immune inflammatory reactions result in caseous necrosis, fibrous encapsulation, and calcification. Caseous and enlarged lymph nodes compress bronchi and lead to atelectasis or obstructive symptoms. Calcifications of histoplasmosis are larger than those associated with tuberculosis. Paratracheal "mulberry" and hepatic and splenic calcifications constitute presumptive evidence of previous primary histoplasmosis. Thoracic calcifications also may be seen, however, with granulomatous reactions of varicella, atypical measles and coccidioidomycoses, with hamartomas and teratomas, and in idiopathic pulmonary alveolar microlithiasis.

Severe dissemination is associated with extrathoracic complications, including chorioretinitis, uveitis, carditis, ulcerative colitis, oropharyngeal ulcers, meningitis, Addison's disease, and anemia, leukopenia and thrombocytopenia. The majority of cases of disseminated histoplasmosis occur in the first year of life and usually are fatal. Short courses (7 to 14 days) of amphotericin B have been suggested for infants with continuing spiking fevers, spreading pulmonary infiltrates, massive adenopathy and enlarging liver and spleen, failure to gain weight, falling white blood cell count, decreasing hematocrit, and decreasing platelet count (Fosson and Wheeler, 1975). Christie (1977) has recommended triple sulfonamides as the drugs of choice in severe symptomatic forms other than the progressive disseminated variety.

Reinfection acute histoplasmosis occurs in patients who have maintained some immunity by recent or repeated contact with histoplasmosis antigens and are then heavily exposed to *H. capsulatum*. It differs from primary infections in that it has a shorter incubation period (3 to 7 days) and disseminated pulmonary granulomatosis similar to those of miliary tuberculosis. Also, pulmonary nodules are smaller and usually clear within 3 months without residual calcification, and hilar adenopathy is not observed. Symptoms are similar to primary histoplasmosis, with abrupt onset of fever, headache, malaise, and cough.

Chronic pulmonary histoplasmosis occurs as an opportunistic infection in persons with pre-existing chronic obstructive pulmonary disease, such as centrilobular and bullous emphysema. Emphysematous areas, commonly in the posterior apical regions, become colonized with *H. capsulatum,* producing necrotic cavities. Antigenic material from infected cavities is spilled in the bronchial tree, inducing a hypersensitivity pneumonitis with a picture of interstitial pneumonitis. Spontaneous contraction of pneumonitic areas occurs over a period of months, leaving linear fibrous remnants similar to healing pulmonary infarcts. Symptoms are similar to but less severe than those in pulmonary tuberculosis: malaise, fever, cough, night sweats, and weight loss. Hemoptysis occurs in a third of cases. Pneumonic episodes respond to rest and to limited physical activity. Amphotericin B is used for persistent cavities. The prognosis and course with or without specific therapy is difficult to determine, since the outcome depends on the underlying pulmonary disease.

Diagnostic Tests. *H. capsulatum* grows well in yeast form on Sabouraud's agar at 30°C and in mycelial form on enriched cysteine blood agar at 37°C. The yeast phase can be identified in mononuclear phagocytes in biopsy specimens of granulomatous inflam-

mation or smears of bone marrow, lymph node, liver, and spleen. Oropharyngeal ulcers can be scraped for these cells, which can be seen easily when stained by Wright's or methenamine silver methods. As with tuberculosis, skin sensitivity to histoplasmin appears 4 to 6 weeks after the infection has started and may be absent in progressive and disseminated infections. Active or current infection is indicated only when there is recent positive skin test conversion. Serologic tests (agar gel precipitin test, yeast phase complement fixation test, and latex particle agglutination test) are available also. Blood should be drawn for these tests prior to skin testing, since the skin test may produce a rise in titers. High titers or rising titers (greater than 1:32) indicate recent or primary infection.

Coccidioidomycosis

Coccidioidomycosis, also known as San Joaquin fever and valley fever, is caused by inhalation of arthrospores of *Coccidioides immitis*. It is endemic to the area of the United States limited to what is known as the Lower Sonoran Life Zone (southern California, southwest Texas, Arizona, New Mexico, parts of Utah and Nevada), which also includes part of Mexico, Guatemala, Honduras, Argentina, Venezuela and Paraguay (Seabury, 1977). Infection usually occurs at the end of the wet desert season, with drying of the topsoil. Children have milder disease than adults. Dissemination is more likely to occur in pregnant females and nonwhites. On rare occasions, the disease may be transmitted from person to person when arthrospores are inhaled from draining skin lesions or from fomites from patients with chronic pulmonary coccidioidomycosis with cavities.

The primary disease is similar to histoplasmosis with mild, transient, or severe variations. Extrapulmonary lesions and dissemination similarly may occur. Pleurisy and erythema nodosum are more common than in histoplasmosis or tuberculosis. The chest roentgenogram shows parenchymal infiltrates or a miliary pattern, with or without hilar adenopathy. Most primary lesions resolve over a period of months. Chronic pulmonary coccidioidomycosis occurs when the primary lesion fails to resolve (approximately 5 percent of cases). Chronic pneumonitis, and cavitary lesions that appear as densely fibrotic thin-walled structures occur. These may rupture into the pleural space and produce empyema. Hemoptysis is a common complication of coccidioidomycosis.

History and suspicion in endemic areas are the main factors leading to diagnosis. Infection often is asymptomatic. Diagnosis can be confirmed by serologic conversion and delayed-type hypersensitivity skin test conversion. Serum precipitins appear early; complement fixation titers rise between 1 and 3 months after onset; and skin test positivity develops 3 to 6 weeks after exposure.

Amphotericin B therapy is reserved for severe and disseminated lesions. Surgical removal of pulmonary lesions may be indicated.

TUBERCULOSIS

The number of new cases and deaths from tuberculosis has dramatically decreased, to the point that new physicians are at risk of complacency in considering its diagnosis. In the United States, the death rate has decreased from 400 per 100,000 population in the early 19th century to 1.5 per 100,000 in 1976 (Anastasiades, 1977). The new case rate has dropped from 76.7 per 100,000 in 1932 to 15 per 100,000 in 1976; and the prevalence of tuberculin sensitivity among children entering the first grade of school has reached a plateau of less than 0.2 percent (Edwards, 1974). Infection rates are higher in slum areas and racial "ghettos," and among American Indians and Eskimos, migrant farm workers, and recent immigrants into the United States from areas of high prevalence. It is important to remember that tuberculosis caused by *Mycobacterium tuberculosis* is almost entirely acquired by inhalation of organisms (except for rare infections with the bovine strain). Close, frequent, and/or prolonged exposure to tubercle bacilli from a coughing patient with reinfection (adult-type) active tuberculosis and a susceptible host result in transmission and primary infection in children. Adults and adolescents with active disease are the main contact sources of infection for children. Only 5 percent of newly infected individuals develop clinical disease within a year of infection and 15 percent within 5 years of infection. The remainder are a part of a "reservoir of infection" who are at risk of developing active disease at any time in later life (Farer, 1978).

The onset of primary tuberculosis usually is symptomless or may resemble an upper respiratory tract infection, with mild cough, fever, and fatigability. At this time, disease may or may not be demonstrable by chest roentgenogram. The sequence of events in primary infection is as follows: tubercle bacilli gain access to alveoli (usually in the lower lobes), multiply, invade local tissue, and are carried by the lymphatics to regional hilar and paratracheal lymph nodes. Generally, the infection localizes here but, in rare situations, the disease progresses, with development of tuberculous pneumonia and parenchymal cavitary formation. There also may be extension from tuberculous lymph nodes through bronchial walls, creating edematous, granulomatous, ulcerative lesions, and causing bronchial obstruction with hyperinflation, atelectasis and bronchiectasis. Post-primary hematogenous spread of infection may occur to the meninges, brain, kidneys, epiphyses of bones, and upper lobes of the lungs.

Acquired immunity, manifested by a positive tuberculin test, usually develops between 2 and 10 weeks after initial infection. During this time, primary lesions generally heal through granuloma formation in which the cell-mediated immunity developed to tubercular organisms plays an important role. This inflammatory response results in localization and containment of bacterial foci and eventual calcification of the lesion. This process is imperfect, however, and viable bacilli can persist in focal lesions with the potential for reactivation of infection any time thereafter. The reader is referred to Farer (1978) for an excellent extensive review article on tuberculosis.

Chronic Pulmonary Tuberculosis. This often has been described as "reinfection" or "adult" tuberculosis and occurs primarily in adolescents and adults. Ninety percent of cases occur by spread of previously contained tuberculous infection. Known contributing risk factors to reactivation include pertussis and measles infection; hormonal changes, especially those associated with adolescence; immunosuppressive therapy, including corticosteroids; diabetes mellitus; silicosis; and hematologic and reticuloendothelial disease, such as leukemia or Hodgkin's disease. It also occurs more frequently in the geriatric age group, in the postpartum period, and after gastrectomy. Lesions usually appear in the apices of the lung. From there, bronchial dissemination may occur, resulting in diffuse or multifocal tuberculous bronchopneumonia. Symptoms may vary from low-grade fever, slight cough, and anorexia to high fever, considerable weight loss, anorexia, cough with hemoptysis, and production of sputum containing large numbers of viable organisms. X-ray changes may consist of linear densities and small or large parenchymal infiltrates and cavitary lesions.

Tuberculin Testing. The Committee on Infectious Diseases of the American Academy of Pediatrics ("Red Book" Report, 1977) recommends that initial tuberculin testing be performed at 1 year of age. The test should be done at the time of, or preceding, measles (rubeola) immunization, currently recommended at 15 months of age. The frequency of repeated tuberculin tests depends on risk of exposure and on the prevalence of tuberculosis in the population group. For office practice or outpatient clinic, an annual or biennial tuberculin test generally is appropriate (Kendig, 1977). The diagnosis of new cases of tuberculosis is directly related to physicians' awareness of its prevalence in the community (Edwards, 1974). When the prevalence of tuberculin sensitivity exceeds 1 percent (10 per 1000) in the school-age population, benefits of more frequent routine tuberculin testing outweigh its costs.

The tine test is a quick screening method. Suspicious and definitely positive reactions are confirmed by intradermal tests using five tuberculin units (5 TU) of PPD (purified protein derivative) stabilized with Tween 80.

The skin test is read at 48 to 72 hours. Sensitization to *M. tuberculosis* is indicated by erythema and palpable induration measuring 10 mm or more in diameter. A positive reaction indicates only that infection with mycobacteria has occurred; infectious contact may have taken place years before or may be of recent origin. Chest x-rays and bacterial cultures may be needed in these instances. Reactions 4 mm or less are considered negative. Induration measuring 5 to 9 mm is considered a doubtful reaction except when there is known contagious contact. Doubtful reactions should be followed by chest x-ray and a repeat tuberculin test within 1 to 2 months, since tuberculin sensitivity may take 2 to 10 weeks to develop fully.

Doubtful reactions in children also may indicate infection with atypical mycobacteria. These organisms resemble *M. tuberculosis* on microscopic examination and can be distinguished from *M. tuberculosis* only by culture. Clinically the distinction can be facilitated by comparative simultaneous skin testing with PPD and atypical mycobacteria antigens (PPD-Y, G, B, F). The larger reaction indicates the probable source of infection. In adults, the main focus of infection with atypical mycobacteria is the lung. In children, atypical mycobacteria infection most frequently is characterized by lymphadenitis involving cervical, submandibular and/or preauricular lymph nodes.

Malnutrition, overwhelming tuberculous infection, administration of corticosteroids and immunosuppressive agents, and disorders associated with T cell immune deficiency may be associated with an inability to develop a tuberculin response. Viral illnesses (such as measles, varicella, rubella, mumps, and influenza) and vaccination against measles, rubella, and mumps may suppress the skin test for as long as 4 weeks.

References

Adams, R., and Churchill, E. D.: Situs inversus, sinusitis, bronchiectasis: Report of five cases including frequency statistics. J. Thorac. Surg. 7:206, 1937.

Afzelius, B. A.: A human syndrome caused by immotile cilia. Science 193:317, 1976.

Anastasiades, A. A.: Tuberculosis in children: Current concepts. Pediatr. Ann. 6:797, 1977.

Arnaud, R., Chapuis-Cellier, C., Souillet, G., Carron, R.,

Creyssel, R., and Fudenberg, H. H.: High frequency of Pi deficient phenotypes of alpha-1-antitrypsin in nonatopic asthma. Clin. Res. 24:488A, 1976.

Beahrs, J. O., Lillington, G. A., Rosa, R. C., Russin, L., Lindgren, J. A., and Rowley, P. T.: Anhidrotic ectodermal dysplasia: Predisposition to bronchial disease. Ann. Int. Med. 74:92, 1971.

Becroft, D. M. O.: Bronchiolitis obliterans, bronchiectasis and other sequelae of adenovirus type 21 infection in young children. J. Clin. Pathol. 24:72, 1971.

Beem, M. A., and Saxon, E. M.: Respiratory tract colonization and a distinctive pneumonia syndrome in infants infected with C. trachomatis. New Engl. J. Med. 296:306, 1977.

Black, L. F., and Kueppers, F.: Alpha-1-antitrypsin deficiency in nonsmokers. Am. Rev. Respir. Dis. 117:421, 428, 1978.

Boat, T. F., Polmar, S. H., Whitman, V., Kleinerman, J. I., Stern, R. C., and Doershuk, C. F.: Hyperreactivity to cow milk in young children with pulmonary hemosiderosis and cor pulmonale secondary to nasopharyngeal obstruction. J. Pediatr. 87:23, 1975.

Bonnani, P. P., Frymoyer, J. W., and Jacox, R. F.: A family study of idiopathic pulmonary fibrosis: A possible dysproteinemic and genetically determined disease. Am. J. Med. 39:411, 1965.

Capitanio, M. A., Chen, J. T. T., Arey, J. B., and Kirkpatrick, J. A.: Congenital anhidrotic ectodermal dysplasia. Am. J. Roentgen. 103:168, 1968.

Christie, A.: Histoplasmosis. In Kendig, E. I., and Chernick, V. (eds.): Disorders of the Respiratory Tract in Children. Philadelphia, W. B. Saunders Co., 1977, Chap. 49.

De Jager, H.: Congenital anhidrotic ectodermal dysplasia: Case report. J. Path. Bacteriol. 90:321, 1965.

Dreisin, R. B., Schwartz, M. I., Thiophilopoulos, A. N., and Stanford, R. E.: Circulating immune complexes in the interstitial pneumonias. New Engl. J. Med. 298:353, 1978.

Edwards, P. Q.: Tuberculin testing of children. Pediatrics 54:628, 1974.

Egbert, B. M., Schwartz, E., and Kempson, R. L.: Kartagener's syndrome: Report of a case with mesangiocapillary glomerulonephritis. Arch. Pathol. Lab. Med., 101:95, 1977.

Eliasson, R., Mossberg, B., Camner, R., and Afzelius, B. A.: The immotile-cilia syndrome. New Engl. J. Med. 297:1, 1977.

Erikkson, S.: Studies in alpha-1-antitrypsin deficiency. Acta Scand. (Suppl. 432) 177:1, 1965.

Fagerhol, M. K., and Hauge, H.E.: Serum Pi types in patients with pulmonary disease. Acta Allergol., 24:107, 1969.

Farer, L. S.: All about TB — what the practicing physician must know and can do about tuberculosis. Clinical Notes on Respiratory Diseases. Vol. 16, No. 4, 1978 pp. 3–14. American Thoracic Society, Medical Section of the American Lung Association.

Fosson, A. R., and Wheeler, W. E.: Short-termed amphotericin B treatment of severe childhood histoplasmosis. J. Pediatr. 86:32, 1975.

Goodwin, R. A., and Des Prez, R. M.: State of the art: Histoplasmosis. Am. Rev. Respir. Dis. 117:929, 1978.

Handleman, N. I., and Nelson, T. L.: Association of milk precipitins with esophageal lesions causing aspiration. Pediatrics 34:699, 1964.

Harwood, I. R., Olmstead, N., and Giammona, S. T.: Desquamative interstitial pneumonia in infancy and childhood. Pediatr. Res., 11:572, 1977.

Heiner, D. C.: Pulmonary hemosiderosis. In Kendig, E. L., and Chernick, V. (eds.): Disorders of the Respiratory Tract in Children. Philadelphia, W. B. Saunders Co., 1977, Chap. 36.

Heiner, D. C., Sears, J. W., and Kniker, W. T.: Multiple precipitins to cow's milk in chronic respiratory disease. Am. J. Dis. Child. 103:40, 1962.

Heiner, D. C., and Sears, J. W.: Chronic respiratory disease associated with multiple circulating precipitins to cow's milk. Abstract and Discussion. Am. J. Dis. Child. 100:500, 1960.

Hensley, G. T., Fink, J. N., and Barboriak, J. J.: Hypersensitivity pneumonitis in the monkey. Arch. Pathol. 97:33, 1974.

Katz, R. M., Lieberman, J., and Siegel, S. C.: Alpha-1-antitrypsin levels and prevalence of Pi variant phenotypes in asthmatic children. J. Allergy Clin. Immunol. 57:41, 1976.

Kendig, E. L.: Chronic lung disease in children. Hosp. Pract. 87–98, 1977.

Kendig, E. L., and Brummer, D. L.: Prognosis of sarcoidosis in children. Chest 70:351, 1976.

Lamarre, A., Linsao, L., Reilly, B. J., Swyer, P. R., and Levison, H.: Residual pulmonary abnormalities in survivors of idiopathic respiratory distress syndrome. Am. Rev. Respir. Dis. 108:56, 1973.

Laraya-Cuasay, L. R.: Pulmonary sequelae of acute viral infection. Pediatr. Ann. 7:21, 1978.

Laraya-Cuasay, L. R., DeForest, A., Huff, D., Lischner, H., and Huang, N. N.: Chronic pulmonary complications of early influenza virus infection in children. Am. Rev. Respir. Dis. 116:617, 1977.

Laurell, C. B., and Erikkson, S.: The electrophoretic alpha-1-globulin pattern of serum in alpha-1-antitrypsin deficiency. Scand. J. Clin. Lab. Invest. 15:132, 1963.

Liebow, A. A.: Definition and classification of interstitial pneumonias in human pathology. Hum. Pathol. Prog. Respir. Res. 8:1, 1975.

McCrea, M. G., Heston, J. F., Wood, H. F., and Sullivan, J. E.: Milk precipitins: A serologic survey of 932 individuals. J.A.M.A. 203:557, 1968.

Mittman, C., Lieberman, J., and Rumsfeld, J.: Prevalence of abnormal protease inhibitor phenotypes in patients with chronic obstructive lung disease. Am. Rev. Respir. Dis. 109:295, 1974.

Nelson, T. L.: Spontaneously occurring milk antibodies in mongoloids. Am. J. Dis. Child. 108:494, 1964.

Nemir, R. L.: Bronchiectasis. In Kendig, E. L., and Chernick V. (eds.): Disorders of the Respiratory Tract in Children. Philadelphia, W. B. Saunders Co., 1977, Chap. 25.

Olsen, A. M.: Bronchiectasis and dextrocardia: Observations on aetiology of bronchiectasis. Am. Rev. Tuberc. 47:435, 1943.

Patchefesky, A. S., Fraimow, W., and Hoch, W. S.: Desquamative interstitial pneumonia: Pathologic findings and follow-up in thirteen patients. Arch. Int. Med. 132:222, 1973.

Pedersen, H., and Mygind, N.: Absence of axonemal arms in nasal mucosa in Kartagener's syndrome. Nature 262:494, 1976.

Peterson, R. D. A., and Good, R. A.: Antibodies to cow's milk proteins — their presence and significance. Pediatrics 31:209, 1962.

Proskey, A. J., Weatherbee, L., Easterling, R. E., et al.: Goodpasture's syndrome: A report of five cases and review of the literature. Am. J. Med. 48:162, 1970.

Reed, W. B., Lopez, D. A., and Landing, B.: Clinical spectrum of anhidrotic ectodermal dysplasia. Arch. Dermatol. 102:134, 1970.

Richerson, H. B.: Varieties of acute immunologic damage to the rabbit lung. Ann. N.Y. Acad. Sci. 221:340, 1974.

Rosenow, E. C.: The spectrum of drug-induced pulmonary disease. Ann. Int. Med. 77:977, 1972.

Scherzer, H., and Ward, P. A.: Lung and dermal vascular injury produced by preformed immune complexes. Am. Rev. Respir. Dis. 117:551, 1978.

Schwartz, R. H., Van Ess, J. D., Johnstone, D. E., Dreyfuss, E. M., Abrishami, M. A., and Chai, C.: Alpha-1-antitrypsin in childhood asthma. J. Allergy Clin. Immunol. 59:31, 1977.

Scriver, C. R., Solomons, C. C., Davies, E., et al.: A molecular abnormality of keratin in ectodermal dysplasia. J. Pediatr. 67:946, 1965.

Seabury, J. H.: The mycoses (excluding histoplasmosis). In Kendig, E. L., and Chernick, V. (eds.): Disorders of the Respiratory Tract in Children. Philadelphia, W. B. Saunders Co., 1977, Chap. 50.

Sharp, H., Bridges, R. A., Krivit, W., and Freier, E. F.: Cirrhosis associated with alpha-1-antitrypsin deficiency; A previously unrecognized inherited disorder. J. Lab. Clin. Med. 73:934, 1969.

Stafford, H. A., Polmar, S. H., and Boat, T. F.: Immunologic studies in cow's milk–induced pulmonary hemosiderosis. Pediatr. Res., 11:898, 1977.

Talamo, R. C.: Emphysema and alpha-1-antitrypsin deficiency.

In Kendig, E. L., and Chernick V. (eds.): *Disorders of the Respiratory Tract in Children*. Philadelphia, W. B. Saunders Co., 1977, Chap. 39.

Vance, J. C., Hall, W. J., Schwartz, R. H., Hyde, R. W., Roghmann, K. J., Mudholkar, G. C.: Heterozygous alpha-1-antitrypsin deficiency and respiratory function in children. Pediatrics *60*:263, 1977.

Vanselow, N. A., Yamate, M., Adams, M. S., and Callies, Q.: The increased prevalence of allergic disease in anhidrotic congenital ectodermal dysplasia. J. Allergy *45*:302, 1970.

Waite, R. W., Steele, J. J., Ross, L., et al.: Cilia and sperm tail abnormalities in Polynesian bronchiectasis. Lancet *2*:132, 1978.

Wayne, K. S., and Taussig, L. M.: Probable familial congenital bronchiectasis due to cartilage deficiency (Williams-Campbell Syndrome). Am. Rev. Respir. Dis. *114*:15, 1976.

Wood, R. E., Boat, T. F., and Doershuk, C. F.: State of the art: Cystic fibrosis. Am. Rev. Respir. Dis. *113*:833, 1976.

49

S. Lance Forstot, M.D.

Diseases of the Eye

The eye and ocular adnexae are the sites of allergic reactions in the infant, child, and adolescent. The function of the eye may be affected critically by minor alterations in structure generated by the allergic response; therefore, the eye is an exquisitely sensitive responder to allergic inflammation. The visibility of the ocular structures also makes signs of allergic disease easily observed. Because of certain anatomic and physiologic peculiarities, the eye may respond slightly differently to allergic reactions than do many other tissues.

ANATOMIC AND PHYSIOLOGIC CONSIDERATIONS

In contrast to most other tissues in which allergic reactions take place, the cornea, lens, and vitreous normally are avascular structures. The cornea is nourished by contents of the tear film, aqueous humor, and limbal circulation. The lens possesses a capsule that further isolates it from the aqueous and vitreous. The globe (corneo-scleral shell) and its contents also have no lymphatic drainage. In addition, there is a blood-aqueous barrier which is selective in that contents of the aqueous are not proportional to the contents of blood.

The conjunctiva, as an exposed epithelial surface, comes in contact with a variety of microorganisms and noninfective allergens. The ability of the conjunctiva to mount an inflammatory response is relatively limited: the inflamed "red" eye reflects dilation of conjunctival blood vessels; chemosis (edema) of the conjunctiva occurs with transudation of fluid through vessel walls; cellular elements may exude with transudation and, together with glandular mucus secretion and tears, may produce an ocular "discharge."

With acute inflammation, the palpebral conjunctiva may develop follicles and papillae. Follicles are collections of lymphoid cells (lymphocytes, macrophages, and plasma cells) in the conjunctiva (Fig. 49–1). Conjunctival lymphoid tissue develops in the first months of life. The intensity (size and number) of the follicular response is determined by the stimulus. As follicles form, they displace vessels and appear to have a vascular coat. These most often occur in the inferior palpebral conjunctiva and lower fornix. The papilla is a vascular structure more often seen on the upper palpebral conjunctiva (Fig. 49–2A). A papilla has a vessel in the central core and is composed of various "acute" inflammatory cells (polymorphonuclear leukocytes, basophils, and eosinophils).

As will be discussed later, examination of the type of conjunctival response (follicular or papillary) as well as examination of the cellular makeup (conjunctival smears) of the discharge (exudate) can aid in the diagnosis of disease etiology.

The cornea normally is clear and transparent. Corneal inflammation is characterized by stromal infiltrates that produce a granular opacity. If these opacities originate in avascular corneas, they often are of limbal vessel origin and marginal in location. In vascularized (inflamed) corneas, stromal infiltrates

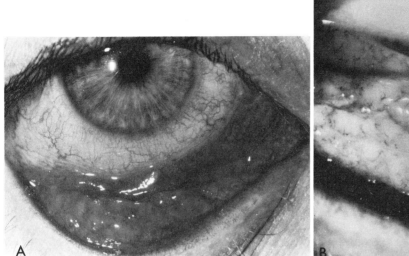
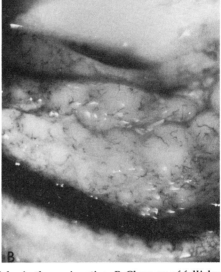

FIGURE 49-1.   *A,* Chlamydial inclusion conjunctivitis with follicles in the conjunctiva. *B,* Close-up of follicles.

originate near the new vessels and can occur more centrally. In acute inflammation, these infiltrates are composed of polymorphonuclear leukocytes that come from vessels, either limbal or more central new vasculature.

Another important physiologic consideration in ocular allergy is the "lymph node" phenomenon. Since the eye itself has no lymphatic drainage, it is believed that antigen is processed at a distant site and that sensitized lymphocytes return to the site of origin. The uveal tract (iris, ciliary body, and choroid) is the vascular coat of the eye and is the principal site of lymphoid cell supply in the eye. The vascular watershed area of the cornea, the limbus, also may be a site of sensitized cells in diseases in which the antigen is of corneal origin. Repeated exposures to antigen, either at the eye or in a more remote area of the body, could trigger local antibody formation and local "lymph node" activity with the production of recurrent uveitis or keratitis (Silverstein, 1968).

GENERAL DIAGNOSTIC AND THERAPEUTIC CONSIDERATIONS

Diagnostic Considerations. In dealing with conjunctival disease, cytologic smears, microbial smears (Gram stain for bacteria, Giemsa stain for various organisms) and microbial cultures for bacteria or fungi are of paramount diagnostic importance. In atopic conjunctivitis and vernal conjunctivitis, eosinophils are abundant in epithelial scrapings. In viral conjunctivitis (herpes or adenovirus), lymphocytes are predominant, whereas in bacterial conjunctivitis and chlamydial infections, a polymorphonuclear response is present. In addition, conjunctivitis of viral or chlamydial origin is characterized by a predominantly follicular conjunctival reaction; in vernal and atopic conjunctivitis the reaction is mainly papillary.

In uveal tract disease, serologic tests may be helpful. Systemic-onset juvenile rheumatoid arthritis (JRA) and polyarticular JRA usually are not associated with iridocyclitis. However, one type of pauciarticular JRA may be associated with the presence of antinuclear antibody in as many as 50 percent of cases and has severe morbidity from a chronic anterior uveitis, whereas another type of pauciarticular JRA is antinuclear antibody negative and is associated with an acute iritis and with HLA-B27 histocompatibility antigen (Wedgwood and Schaller, 1977). Posterior uveitis due to toxoplasmosis may be diagnosed both on morphologic grounds and with a positive serologic test for antibody to the organism.

Therapeutic Considerations. Both lid inflammation and exudative conjunctivitis require good lid hygiene. The lid may become encrusted with exudate or inflammatory scaling that can hinder antibiotic effectiveness. Removal of this encrustation is important in therapy. A mild soap, such as a baby shampoo, diluted from full strength, is an effective lid cleanser, applied either with a washcloth or cotton-tipped applicator to the lid margin and eyelash base.

Both acute and chronic allergic conjunctivitis respond symptomatically to oral antihistamines. Topical vasoconstrictors (decongestants) (Table 49-1) and topical antihistamines (Table 49-2) may be of value as adjunctive therapy. Topical steroids also may be required to relieve more severe symptoms, especially in vernal conjunctivitis. However, the chronic use of topical steroids can lead to the development of cataracts. In susceptible patients, intraocular pressure may rise, causing a secondary glaucoma. Topical steroids also can potentiate herpes simplex keratitis and secondary bacterial infection. Because of this, *chronic* use of topical steroids is best managed in conjunction with an ophthalmologist. The choice of a topical steroid preparation involves a decision on the type of steroid compound (solution versus suspension) (Table 49-3). If profuse epiphora is prominent, the efficacy of drops may be diminished through dilution by tears. An ointment may be required in vernal conjunctivitis with severe epiphora.

Prednisolone acetate is a particularly effective therapeutic steroid preparation (Leibowitz and Kupferman, 1975). However, this suspension can be irritating because of its particulate nature; the importance of shaking such preparations before administration is emphasized.

In patients with uveitis, the intraocular inflammation may cause both cataract and glaucoma. It may be difficult to distinguish between drug-induced and disease-induced problems. Chronic topical steroids may induce local problems, and systemic steroids in children with uveitis also may cause severe systemic side effects. Periocular injections may circumvent these, but systemic adsorption of drugs by this route occurs and can be associated with systemic steroid side effects.

Antibiotic therapy is indicated in diagnosed bacterial disease. Though often self-limited, topical antibiotic therapy will shorten the course of bacterial conjunctivitis as well as decrease the opportunity for patient-

TABLE 49-1 VASOCONSTRICTORS (DECONGESTANTS)

Preparation	Vasoconstrictor	Preservative
Albalon	NZ 0.1%	BAC, EDTA
Collyrium w/Ephedrine	E 0.1%	TM
Clear Eyes	NZ 0.012%	BAC, EDTA
Degest	NZ 0.012%	BAC, EDTA
Efrical	PE 0.12%	BAC
Murine	THZ 0.05%	BAC, TM
Naphcon	NZ 0.012%	BAC
Naphcon Forte	NZ 0.1%	BAC
Neozin	PE 0.12%	BAC
Optised	PE 0.12%	BAC
Prefrin Liquifilm	PE 0.12%	BAC
Soothe Eye Drops	PE 0.15%	TM, EDTA
Vasocon Regular	NZ 0.1%	PMA
Visine	THZ 0.05%	BAC, EDTA
Zincfrin	PE 0.12%	BAC

Key:

E	= ephedrine		BAC	= benzalkonium chloride
NZ	= naphazoline		EDTA	= disodium edetate
PE	= phenylephrine		PMA	= phenylmercuric acetate
THZ	= tetrahydrozoline		TM	= thiomerisol

TABLE 49–2 ANTIHISTAMINES

Preparation	Antihistamines	Vasoconstrictor	Preservative
Albalon-A	AZ 0.5%	NZ 0.05%	BAC, EDTA
Prefrin-A	PM 0.1%	PE 0.12%	BAC, EDTA
Vasocon-A	AZ 0.05%	NZ 0.05%	PMA

Key:

AZ = antazoline
PM = pyrilamine maleate
NZ = naphazoline
PE = phenylephrine

BAC = benzalkonium chloride
EDTA = disodium edetate
PMA = phenylmercuric acetate

to-patient spread. As most bacterial conjunctivitis is due to gram-positive cocci, the use of sulfacetamide or erythromycin (drops or ointment) will be of value. Topical drops combining gramicidin, neomycin, polymyxin B (or ointments combining bacitracin, neomycin, polymyxin B) provide broad-spectrum coverage in acute conjunctival disease. These drugs treat both gram-positive and gram-negative organisms. Initially a drop every 1 to 4 hours may be required, depending on severity; after a therapeutic response, this may be tapered to 4 times a day. Therapy should be continued 24 to 48 hours beyond cessation of signs and symptoms or after a negative culture. Because neomycin has a high rate of sensitization, preparations containing it should be used acutely and not chronically.

Antiviral therapy is required for herpes simplex keratitis and frequent intensive treatment is needed. Idoxuridine (0.1 percent solution or 0.5 percent ointment) and vidarabine (3 percent ointment) are currently available, while trifluorothymidine (1 percent solution), which appears in clinical trials to be more potent, may soon be on the U.S. market.

DISEASES OF EYELIDS

The lids may be involved in a generalized acute allergic reaction, with urticaria or angioedema. Foods, drugs, insect bites, and contact allergens can initiate the reaction (see Chapter 33).

Contact dermatitis and blepharoconjunctivitis may occur with ocular drug therapy. This may be due to the active drug, the preservative, or the ointment base. Over-the-counter preparations cannot be excluded as offending agents. Compilations of artificial tear preparations and ocular lubricants, including their preservatives, are found in Tables 49–4 and 49–5. Preservatives found in topical vasoconstrictor and antihistaminic preparations are included in Tables 49–1 and

TABLE 49–3 RELATIVE ANTI-INFLAMMATORY ACTIVITY
(DECREASING ORDER – CORNEA WITH INTACT EPITHELIUM)

Compound	Strength	Preparation
Prednisolone acetate	1.0%	Suspension
Dexamethasone alcohol	1.0%	Suspension
Fluorometholone	0.1%	Suspension
Prednisolone sodium phosphate	1.0%	Solution
Prednisolone acetate	0.125%	Suspension
Prednisolone sodium phosphate	0.125%	Solution
Dexamethasone phosphate	0.1%	Solution
Dexamethasone phosphate	0.05%	Ointment

Modified from Leibowitz, H. M., and Kupferman, A.: Bioavailability and therapeutic effectiveness of topically administered corticosteroids. Trans. Am. Acad. Ophthalmol. Otolaryngol. *79:*OP-78, 1975.

TABLE 49–4   ARTIFICIAL TEAR SOLUTIONS

Preparation	Polymer	Preservative
Adsorbotear	PVP, HEC	TM, EDTA
Hypotears	Lipiden	BAC, EDTA
Isoptotears	HPMC 0.5%	BAC
Lacril	HPMC	CB
Liquifilm Forte	PVA 3%	CB
Liquifilm Tears	PVA 1.4%	CB
Lyteers	HEC 0.2%	BAC, EDTA
Methulose	MC 0.25%	BAC
Tearisol	PVP, HEC	BAC, EDTA
Tears Naturale	Duasorb	BAC, EDTA
Visculose ¼% or 1%	MC 0.25% or 1.0%	BAC

Key:

HEC   = hydroxyethyl cellulose
HPMC = hydroxypropyl methylcellulose
MC   = methylcellulose
PVA   = polyvinyl alcohol
PVP   = polyvinyl pyrrolidone

BAC   = benzalkonium chloride
CB   = chlorobutanol
EDTA = disodium edetate
TM   = thiomerisol

49–2. Cosmetics may also cause a contact dermatitis (see Chapter 32). Therapy consists of withdrawal of the contact allergen and symptomatic treatment. Topical steroid ointment may be used as well as oral antihistamines. Chronic steroid ointments used on the lids carry the same risks as topical steroids in the eye — cataract formation, induced glaucoma, and suprainfection.

Blepharitis is either microbial or seborrheic in origin. *Staphylococcal blepharoconjunctivitis* is the most common form of bacterial blepharitis. The lid margin may be red, with ulceration and crusting around the lashes. A concomitant superficial punctate keratitis may exist. Therapy consists of good lid hygiene, with lid scrubs using a mild soap. Antibiotic therapy such as sulfacetamide or erythromycin ointment on the lids will help. In severe inflammation, a mild topical steroid used for a short period may be helpful. Acute recurrent hordeola (styes) are of staphylococcal origin and also require good lid hygiene and antibiotic therapy. In recalcitrant cases, systemic antibiotics may be beneficial. In adults, oral tetracycline is helpful; but, because of developing dentition, other antibiotics such as erythromycin are preferred in children.

Seborrheic blepharitis occurs in patients with seborrhea of the scalp and eyebrows. The lids characteristically have dandruff-like deposits known as "scurf." Treatment consists of good lid hygiene and control of seborrhea on the scalp and brow with appropriate shampoo (see Chapter 35).

TABLE 49–5   LUBRICATING OINTMENT

Preparation	Ingredients	Preservative
LacriLube s.o.p.	White petrolatum Mineral oil Nonionic lanolin derivatives	Chlorobutanol
Duratears	White petrolatum Anhydrous liquid lanolin Mineral oil	Methylparaben Propylparaben

DISEASES OF CONJUNCTIVA

Ophthalmia Neonatorum. Ophthalmia neonatorum is any conjunctivitis that occurs within the first month of life. The cause with the earliest onset is "chemical conjunctivitis," due to silver nitrate instillation for gonococcal prophylaxis. This mild conjunctivitis begins in 24 hours with hyperemia and watery discharge. It usually is self-limited and requires no specific treatment. Gonococcal conjunctivitis is a purulent conjunctivitis beginning usually between the third and fifth day of life. It is associated with chemosis and lid edema. The cornea may be involved. Because corneal ulceration can be devastating, both systemic and topical penicillin is used in treatment. Diagnosis is made by cultures and smears showing gram-negative intracellular diplococci. Chlamydiae are the most common cause of microbial ophthalmia neonatorum. "Inclusion conjunctivitis" (blenorrhea) usually has an onset 5 days or more after birth. Follicles are not present, as the infant has no lymphoid tissue. Late untreated disease may progress to follicular conjunctivitis after 6 weeks. Basophilic cytoplasmic inclusions can be seen in over 90 percent of Giemsa-stained conjunctival scrapings. Therapy consists of topical tetracycline or sulfa. Systemic therapy often is indicated, since there is a high association with systemic chlamydial disease acquired at birth, e.g., pneumonitis, rhinitis, and otitis. Systemic erythromycin usually is employed. Other causes of bacterial ophthalmia neonatorum include staphylococci, streptococci, *E. coli,* and *Haemophilus* species; each requires specific topical antibiotic therapy. Pseudomonas conjunctivitis may occur in premature newborn infants.

Atopic conjunctivitis. Atopic conjunctivitis may be acute, subacute, chronic, or seasonal in nature. The conjunctivitis of hay fever is characterized by conjunctival injection and edema. The discharge is watery, occasionally with a mucoid component. The most prominent symptom is itching. Cytology of conjunctival scrapings reveals eosinophils. Treatments consist of topical vasoconstrictors and oral antihistamines to relieve itching. Topical steroids occasionally are necessary for symptomatic relief. Recurrent bouts of atopic conjunctivitis can lead to chronic conjunctival change, which predispose to a keratitis (atopic keratoconjunctivitis) (Hogan, 1953). Corneal vascularization and opacification can occur. When corneal changes cause abnormal tear patterns with rapid tear film breakup, wetting agents such as artificial tears may be helpful in preventing further scarring.

Vernal conjunctivitis. A bilateral, recurrent inflammation of the conjunctiva, vernal conjunctivitis derives its name from the fact that it occurs in the spring and summer months. The tarsal (palpebral) form is characterized by cobblestone (flat-topped) papillae (Fig. 49–2A), and the limbal form (Fig. 49–2B) by limbal papillary hypertrophy often associated with white dots (Trantas' spots). Both forms may co-exist. Symptoms include itching, tearing, and photophobia. Excess mucus production is common. Patients also may complain of foreign body sensation. The diagnosis can be made clinically on the appearance of the giant cobblestone papillae or limbal Trantas' dots. Cytologic smears reveal numerous eosinophils.

The disease occurs most commonly between the ages of 5 and 20 years and spontaneously disappears in 5 to 10 years. In children, it is more common among males. More than 50 percent of children with vernal conjunctivitis also have an atopic disorder (asthma, eczema, allergic rhinitis) and concentrations of IgE in tears have been found to be high by some investigators. However, an immune basis for this disorder has not been established.

The mainstay of therapy in vernal conjunctivitis is topical corticosteroids; systemic steroids are almost never necessary. Soluble steroids may be of greater benefit than suspensions, because suspensions contain particles that may become caught between papillae and cause irritation. Occasionally, ointments may be helpful when tearing is profuse, since steroid drops may be diluted to the point of ineffectiveness. Because of side effects of topical steroids, the dose should be titrated to the minimum required to control the disease.

The thick lardaceous mucus produced in vernal conjunctivitis often contributes to irritation. Mucolytic agents, such as acetylcysteine made in a 10 or 20 percent solution, may be helpful in decreasing symptoms (Rice et al., 1971). This drug presently is not avail-

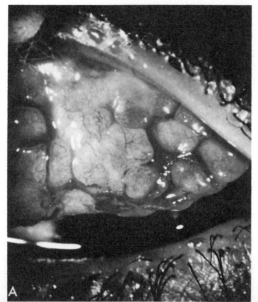

FIGURE 49–2. Vernal conjunctivitis. *A,* Tarsal (palpebral) form. Everted upper lid with giant "cobblestone" papillae. *B,* Limbal form. Gelatinous conjunctival hypertrophy.

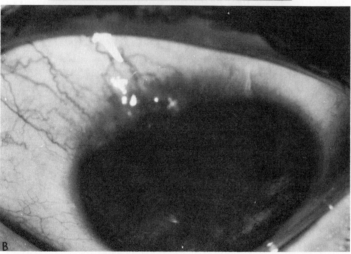

able in the United States for ophthalmic use. Antibiotic therapy usually is not needed. If a vernal ulcer develops, prophylactic antibiotics to prevent secondary infection are indicated, however. Topical cromolyn sodium has been evaluated and found to be effective in decreasing symptoms and decreasing the need for topical steroids (Easty et al. 1971).

The cornea may become involved with a superficial punctate keratitis. Occasionally a large shallow oval ulcer occurs in the upper one-third of the cornea; the ulcer tends to be indolent but eventually heals, often leaving a corneal opacity at the level of Bowman's membrane and anterior stroma. Occasion-

ally, therapeutic soft contact lenses may help in protecting the eroded cornea from the trauma of the papillae.

Giant Papillary Conjunctivitis in Contact Lens Wearers. Allansmith et al. (1977) have described a syndrome of conjunctival inflammation characterized by giant papillae on the upper tarsal conjunctiva, with increased mucus production, mild itching, and decreased tolerance to contact lenses, in wearers of hard and soft contact lenses. The clinical picture resembles that of vernal conjunctivitis. However, all patients affected were wearers of contact lenses, had no seasonal variation in symptoms, did not tend to have atopic disease, and had resolution of symptoms with discontinuation of lens wear. All lenses had deposits on them. Conjunctival scrapings revealed eosinophils. Histology of the conjunctiva revealed basophils, eosinophils, and mast cells in the epithelium. In the stroma, lymphocytes and plasma cells were seen in large numbers. Eosinophils and basophils also were seen in the stroma. An immune etiology is postulated, with material in the lens deposits suspected as constituting the antigenic stimulus. Because of the character of the cellular infiltrate, delayed hypersensitivity of the cutaneous basophilic type is suspected. Therapy, as noted, consists of removal of the old contact lens, with almost immediate cessation of symptoms expected within 5 days.

Phlyctenular Keratoconjunctivitis. Nodule formation (phlyctenule), 1 to 2 mm in size, of the conjunctiva, cornea, or limbus characterizes phlyctenular keratoconjunctivitis. The nodules evolve as microabscesses with ulceration but leave no scarring. It has been suspected as being an allergic reaction to tuberculoprotein, but sensitivity to staphylococci also has been implicated. Symptoms include irritation and itching when the phlyctenules are conjunctival. Corneal phlyctenules produce pain, tearing, and photophobia. Treatment for corneal phlyctenular disease consists of the use of topical steroids. A cycloplegic may be necessary if the keratitis is severe. If there also is staphylococcal conjunctival infection with purulent discharge, antibiotics should be employed. Conjunctival phlyctenules may not need treatment if symptoms are minimal, as they resolve spontaneously. Children also should be evaluated for tuberculosis with skin tests and chest x-ray.

Erythema Multiforme. An acute bullous inflammation of the skin and mucous membranes, erythema multiforme in its mild form may involve only the skin. In the more severe form, extensive skin and mucous membrane involvement can occur. This latter form, in toxic patients who are febrile and who have severe ocular involvement, is known as Stevens-Johnson syndrome (Baum, 1973). The etiology is unknown, but inciting factors have included systemic bacterial and viral infections as well as drugs (see Chapter 35). Ocular involvement occurs with a mucopurulent conjunctivitis. Mucosal blistering occurs. As the disease progresses, pseudomembranous or membranous conjunctivitis is common. It may become purulent if a secondary infection occurs. The conjunctiva heals with progressive cicatrization and symblepharon formation. Conjunctival scarring causes a secondary aqueous tear deficiency. Corneal drying and scarring may occur with eventual corneal vascularization. Conjunctival scarring also may lead to lid deformity and trichiasis with secondary corneal scarring. Conjunctival smears early in the disease show polymorphonuclear lymphocytic response with some eosinophils. Ocular therapy is supportive and involves the use of systemic steroids. Topical steroids may be helpful in relieving ocular symptoms but usually do not change the cicatrizing course and may predispose to secondary infection. Mechanical lysis of adhesions of the conjunctiva may be necessary. Topical antibiotics are used if secondary infections occur. Artificial tears will be required if tear deficiency ensues. Often, "bandage" soft contact lenses may aid in protecting and moistening the cornea.

Viral Conjunctivitis. Usually caused by adenovirus, viral conjunctivitis is characterized by an acute follicular inflammation with serous discharge. It usually is bilateral and has preauricular node enlargement. Symptoms include eye itching, a feeling of grittiness, and a foreign body sensation in the eye. Signs include redness, chemosis, and marked follicular conjunctival response. A syndrome in children may include fever and pharyngitis (pharyngeal-conjunctival fever — PCF). Conjunctival smears show predominantly mononuclear cells. The disease is self-limited and benign, unless more severe corneal keratitis ensues (typically with Type 8 or 19 adenovirus). Initially, it is a punctate epithelial keratitis, which may progress to subepithelial opacities. The epithelial lesions often cause severe photophobia; occasionally, the late subepithelial opacities may decrease vision. Steroids may be of symptomatic benefit in these patients. Antibiotics do not alter the course. If the late subepithelial opacities are visually handicapping, topical steroids can be used to dissolve these infiltrates, although 50 percent will return with discontinuance of the steroid. These lesions spontaneously resolve without therapy over months.

A mild, self-limited viral conjunctivitis may be associated with both measles and chickenpox infection. The conjunctivitis is catarrhal with serous discharge. Symptoms are minor and usually require no treatment.

Chlamydia. Chlamydiae presently are the most common cause of oculogenital disease in the neonate, child, and adolescent (Ostler, 1976a). The disease in children is somewhat different from ophthalmia neonatorum. It manifests itself as a mucopurulent follicular conjunctivitis, most prominent in the lower fornix and tarsal conjunctiva (see Fig. 49–1). Neonates have no lymphoid tissue to manifest this follicular reaction. In addition, older children have less of a tendency to form pseudomembranes from the exudate. Preauricular adenopathy is present. A superficial epithelial keratitis may develop, with small peripheral subepithelial infiltrates. Conjunctival smears show a polymorphonuclear leukocytic response, and inclusion bodies may be seen on Giemsa stain. The conjunctivitis may be self-limited in older children and young adults, but responds well to topical tetracycline or sulfa drugs. Systemic therapy also should be employed because of the oculogenital transmission of the conjunctival disease.

Trachoma. Though not common in the United States, trachoma is an extremely prevalent chlamydial conjunctivitis in children throughout the world and a leading cause of blindness. It is characterized by a chronic follicular conjunctivitis, with follicular hypertrophy more prominent in the upper tarsus. Some papillary reaction to the conjunctiva is present. With progression of the disease, conjunctival scarring occurs. Late sequelae of the scarring include tear deficiency and lid deformity with trichiasis leading to progressing corneal scarring. Direct corneal involvement may develop with an epithelial keratitis and later subepithelial keratitis, with subsequent development of corneal vascularization and pannus formation. The diagnosis is made on the basis of the clinical picture and conjunctival smears for inclusion bodies. Treatment is with topical tetracycline or topical sulfonamides.

Parinaud's Oculoglandular Conjunctivitis. Parinaud's oculoglandular conjunctivitis is a syndrome of unilateral focal granulomatous lesion and follicular conjunctival reaction associated with prominently enlarged preauricular, cervical, and submandibular lymph nodes. The etiologic agent in most cases is unknown, though there often is a history of an association with cats. This entity may be related to cat scratch fever, as fever and malaise may accompany the other features of the syndrome. There is no specific therapy.

DISEASES OF THE CORNEA

Thygeson's Superficial Punctate Keratitis. SPK is characterized by multiple, discrete, epithelial corneal opacities, occurring bilaterally. These small lesions usually require a slit lamp for accurate diagnosis — allowing good visualization of the pathognomonic epithelial lesions. The conjunctiva is not affected. The disease has a chronic course, usually lasting 6 months to 4 years with waxing and waning symptomatic periods of photophobia, tearing, and foreign body sensation. These symptoms are caused by microerosions of the corneal epithelium overlying these elevated opacities. The etiology of this disease is unknown. Attempts at viral isolation or identification with electron microscopy have been fruitless. Topical steroids usually induce remission of symptoms. Therapeutic soft contact lenses have also been used to alleviate symptoms due to the microerosions.

Keratoconjunctivitis Medicamentosa. Keratoconjunctivitis medicamentosa is characterized by superficial punctate erosions. The desquamated epithelial cells give rise to symptoms of foreign body irritation and photophobia. This reaction can be caused by almost any ocular drug or by its preservative when used frequently. Therapy consists of discontinuation of the drug. Patching the eye and cycloplegia may provide symptomatic relief until the epithelium heals.

Catarrhal Marginal Ulcers. Catarrhal marginal ulcers are peripheral corneal infiltrates often associated with chronic staphylococcal blepharoconjunctivitis. Coagulase-positive staphylococci are often but not always isolated from the conjunctiva. The lesions begin as small infiltrates close to the limbus. The infiltrates break down and may coalesce to form crescentic ulcers. The etiology of the marginal ulcers is believed to be hypersensitivity to staphylococcal toxins. Therapy with topical steroids usually is effective. Antibody therapy is indicated if bacteria are isolated.

Herpes Simplex Virus. HSV infections can cause a self-limited follicular conjunctivitis with preauricular adenopathy. However, primary infection with herpes simplex usually is asymptomatic, involving vesicular lesions of the lip or buccal mucosa. This infection occurs in infancy when protection from maternal antibodies has declined. Most children have antibodies to HSV by the age of 10 years (Ostler, 1976*b*). Recurrent ocular herpetic disease may be in the form of blepharitis or blepharoconjunctivitis but most commonly is a dendritic keratitis. This dendritic keratitis is a linear branching epithelial ulcer. The adjacent epithelial tissue is abnormal and usually has viral infection. This can be demonstrated with rose bengal vital stain. Corneal sensation often is decreased or lost. Most dendritic ulcers will heal spontaneously in 7 to 14 days, though some persist longer. Occasionally the linear dendritic ulcer will progress to a large broad area of ulceration with borders resembling a map (geographic) or amoeba (amoeboid). These ulcers have a longer clinical course and often follow prior inadvertent use of topical corticosteroids in dendritic disease. Topical corticosteroids generally are contraindicated in ocular herpetic disease.

Another form of keratitis is the indolent ulcer or metaherpetic disease. In this entity, the ulcer has a protracted course unresponsive to antiviral therapy. There usually is marked corneal anesthesia. These ulcers do not culture virus and are believed to be related to recurrent epithelial erosions that fail to heal because the epithelium poorly attaches to Bowman's membrane.

Herpes virus also can invade the corneal stroma. These lesions may or may not be associated with epithelial keratitis. They may become progressively necrotic, with ultimate corneal thinning and perforation.

An additional form of stromal keratitis is a disciform lesion characterized by a central round stromal opacity with corneal thickening and edema. The opacity is a fine granular infiltrate. Descemet's membrane may have striae. A uveitis is usually a concomitant finding, with keratic precipitates on the endothelium behind the disc of edema. Rarely, an immune ring is seen surrounding the central lesion (Fig. 49–3). The vision usually is blurred, with some tearing and photophobia.

Therapy of the lesions with active viral epithelial disease (dendritic and geographic ulcers) requires antiviral therapy (idoxuridine, vidarabine, or trifluorothymidine). Debridement may be of benefit. Antiviral therapy also is indicated in active stromal disease. In the disciform stromal disease and uveitis, the etiology is thought to be an immune response to viral antigen without active viral replication occurring. Judicious use of topical steroids in conjunction with antiviral coverage is employed. A similar disciform stromal keratitis with edema may occur following chickenpox (varicella) conjunctivitis with corneal epithelial keratitis and is thought to represent an immune response to viral antigen. As in HSV disciform keratitis, topical steroid therapy is indicated; but antiviral therapy is not required.

Keratoconus. Keratoconus is a corneal degeneration of unknown etiology that usually is bilateral and manifests itself with apical corneal thinning, scarring and conical ectasia of the central cornea. It is noninflammatory and results in a painless, progressive visual loss, owing to slowly developing irregular myopic corneal astigmatism. It usually becomes manifest during puberty. Patients with a previous history of atopic conjunctivitis or vernal conjunctivitis may develop it. There is a high incidence of prior atopic disease in general in patients with keratoconus. The irregular corneal astigmatism usually can be corrected with contact lenses to provide good vision. If the disease progresses, a corneal transplant may be necessary. Because the disease occurs in an avascular cornea, success rates for corneal transplant are greater than 90 percent.

DISEASES OF THE LENS

Atopic Cataract. Cataract formation usually is related to congenital developmental problems, senile changes, or trauma, or it may be drug-induced (steroid), or secondary to intraocular inflammation. However, patients with atopic dermatitis have an increased incidence (8 to 10 percent) of cataracts in early adult life. Typically the cataract develops as an irregular plaque located in the posterior cortex, although anterior cortical changes may occur. Another form of cataract is located in the posterior subcapsular epithelial region. The exact link between atopic disease and the cataract formation is not known, but steroid use in the atopic disease probably is not the cause of the characteristic type of "atopic" cataract.

Lens-Induced or Phacogenic Uveitis. Following traumatic or surgical rupture of the lens capsule, a sterile inflammation of the iris and ciliary body may occur owing to the release of lens material into the aqueous.

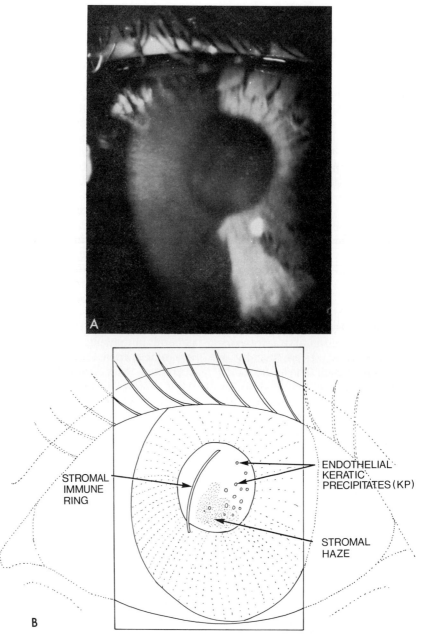

FIGURE 49–3. Herpes simplex keratouveitis. Disciform stromal infiltrates with keratic precipitates on endothelium and immune ring surrounding the stromal opacity.

This uveitis develops between 1 and 14 days following insult to the lens. Lid and corneal edema may ensue. The anterior chamber is clouded with inflammatory debris. The inflammation is an immune response to the liberated lens protein, which is "foreign" to the immune system since the lens is isolated both structurally and anatomically. Keratic precipitates are seen on the endothelium. They are actually accumulations of inflammatory cells on the corneal endothelium. The "mutton-fat" types, as seen in phacogenic uveitis, are large precipitates consisting of macrophages, monocytes, and histiocytes. (The precipitates in more acute inflammations with polymorphonuclear leukocytes are more granular and punctate.) Posterior synechiae from iris to lens and even a cyclitic membrane may develop. The histologic picture reveals polymorphonuclear leukocytic infiltration of the disrupted remnant lens material; these cells are then surrounded by a zone of mononuclear cells, with some epithelioid and multinucleate giant cells. The iris and ciliary body are primarily involved (with the choroid secondarily affected) and are infiltrated with mononuclear cells, lymphocytes, and plasma cells.

Rarely the opposite, uninjured eye may develop a uveal inflammation at a later time. This uveitis also is characterized by a cellular exudation in the anterior chamber, keratic precipitates, and often a hazy cornea. This phenomenon usually occurs if this second lens is traumatized or develops a cataract. The mechanism is thought to be related to restimulation of previously primed lymphoid tissue. This is similar to sympathetic ophthalmia, discussed later.

DISEASES OF THE UVEAL TRACT

Inflammation of the uveal tract (iris, ciliary body, or choroid) is relatively uncommon in children and adolescents and almost nonexistent in infants. In infants, two entities may mimic an anterior uveitis. One is juvenile xanthogranuloma of the iris, with recurrent hyphema. The second condition is retinoblastoma, in which free-floating cells from tumor form a pseudo-hypopyon in the anterior chamber.

Uveitis Associated with Juvenile Arthritis. The most common type of uveal inflammation in children and adolescents is associated with arthritis. The arthritic entities are discussed in Chapter 64. Associated with pauci- or monoarticular arthritis is a chronic iridocyclitis. It may present as a red eye with decreased vision or develop as a quiet uveitis with few symptoms. If unilateral, the episode may pass unnoticed because vision is only unilaterally affected. Examination often will reveal a dense flare in the anterior chamber and few keratic precipitates. Posterior synechiae can occur with the iris adherent to the lens. Long-term changes include posterior subcapsular cataract and band keratopathy. Retinal edema, cystoid macular edema, and hypotony can also occur. Three-quarters of the cases are bilateral. Females are affected five times more often than males. Serologically, the patients are rheumatoid factor–negative, but about 50 percent will have antinuclear antibody (ANA).

A second type of pauciarticular juvenile arthritis is associated with a more acute symptomatic iridocyclitis. Males greatly outnumber females in those affected. Serologically, these patients do not have rheumatoid factor or ANA. Characteristically, they have an HLA-B27 haplotype. The spine usually is affected, and a pattern of early ankylosing spondylitis is present. The acute iridocyclitis is marked by a red eye with ciliary injection, and the anterior chamber has marked flare. The aqueous may look thickly proteinaceous and synechiae may form. The acute iridocyclitis of pauciarticular (ankylosing spondylitis–like) arthritis often will resolve with topical steroid therapy. In therapy of juvenile uveitis, the use of systemic steroids should be avoided as much as possible. Occasionally, a short course of oral steroids is necessary, however. The chronic iridocyclitis poses a more difficult therapeutic problem. It may not be controlled totally with topical steroids. Systemic steroids administered chronically cause severe side effects, including growth and hormonal problems, and must be used with caution. Periocular steroid injections can be used, but they are less well tolerated by children than by adults.

Uveitis Associated with Infection. Uveitis may occur on an infectious or allergic (immune) basis. Even in uveitis associated with known infection, it is not clear whether the uveitis is due to active infection or due to the immune response to the organism and uveal antigens present. An anterior iridocyclitis may be seen with viral corneal disease or as a sequela of it. This is true for both herpes simplex and varicella-zoster virus. A posterior uveitis is associated with toxoplasmosis. This usually is congenitally acquired when parasites reach the fetus via the placenta. The initial inflammation may leave residual organisms encysted in the retina. Periodically these cysts may rupture and give rise to clinically recurrent attacks of a retinochoroiditis. This inflammation usually is suppressed with systemic steroids; antiparasitic therapy consists of sulfadiazine in conjunction with pyrimethamine, with folic acid supplement used to circumvent the folic acid block in humans. (Toxoplasma organisms cannot utilize it.) Clinically, the picture is a characteristic retinochoroiditis. The diagnosis can be confirmed by a positive serologic test. The classic Sabin-Feldman dye test is positive, but this test is less frequently used since it requires live parasites. Most commonly, an indirect fluorescent antibody test is used in which IgA antibodies and IgM antibodies can be detected. Indirect hemagglutination and complement fixation tests also detect antibodies to the organism. The serologic test is considered significant at any titer if associated with a retinal lesion morphologically compatible with toxoplasmosis.

Sympathetic Ophthalmia. Sympathetic ophthalmia is a rare granulomatous uveitis that follows an ocular perforating injury involving the uveal tract. The onset of the uveitis is at least 2 weeks and usually 4 to 8 weeks after the injury. The anterior chamber develops a leukocytic reaction and serous exudation. Inflammation spreads through the entire uveal tract — iris, ciliary body, and choroid. The sympathizing eye develops a similar inflammation simultaneously or after the one in the exciting eye. It is postulated that the inflammation arises due to an autoimmune phenomenon, with the uveal pigment acting as the antigenic stimulus. Treatment in the past required enucleation of the potentially exciting eye within 2 weeks following the injury to prevent the sympathetic uveitis. With the advent of steroids to suppress inflammation, enucleation of the exciting eye probably is not indicated except in eyes traumatized beyond repair.

References

Allansmith, M. R., Korb, D. R., Greiner, J. V., Henriquez, A. S., Simon, M. A., and Finnemore, V. M.: Giant papillary conjunctivitis in contact lens wearers. Am. J. Ophthalmol. 83:697, 1977.

Baum, J. L.: Systemic disease associated with tear deficiencies. Int. Ophthalmol. Clin. 13(1):154, 1973.

Easty, D., Rice, N. S. C. and Jones, B. R.: Disodium chromoglycate (Intal) in the treatment of vernal keratoconjunctivitis. Trans. Ophthalmol. Soc. U.K., SCI:491, 1971.

Giles, C. L.: Uveitis in childhood. In Duane, T. D. (ed.): Clinical Ophthalmology, Vol. 4. Hagerstown, Md., Harper and Row, 1975.

Hogan, M. J.: Atopic keratoconjunctivitis. Am. J. Ophthalmol. 36:937, 1953.

Leibowitz, H. M., and Kupferman, A.: Bioavailability and therapeutic effectiveness of topically administered corticosteroids. Trans. Am. Acad. Ophthalmol. Otolaryngol. 79:OP-78, 1975.

Ostler, H. B.: Oculogenital disease. Surv. Ophthalmol. 20:233, 1976a.

Ostler, H. B.: Herpes simplex: The primary infection. Surv. Ophthalmol. 21:91, 1976b.

Rice, N. S. C., Esty, D., Gerner, A., Jones, B. R. and Tripathi, R.: Vernal keratoconjunctivitis and its management. Trans. Ophthalmol. Soc. U.K., XCI:483, 1971.

Silverstein, A. M.: Allergic reactions of the eye. In Gell, P. G. H., and Coombs, R. R. A. (eds.): Clinical Aspect of Immunology. London, Blackwell Scientific Publications, 1968, pp. 1160–1175.

Wedgwood, R. J., and Schaller, J. G.: The pediatric arthritides. Hosp. Practice. 83, 1977.

GENERAL REFERENCES

Bron, A. J., and Tripathi, R. C.: Corneal disorder. In Goldberg, M. G. (ed.): Genetic and Metabolic Eye Diseases. Boston, Little, Brown and Co., 1974, pp. 281–323.

Dawson, C. R., and Togni, B.: Herpes simplex eye infections: Clinical manifestations, pathogenesis and management. Surv. Ophthalmol. 21:121, 1976.

Duane, T. D. (ed.): External diseases and the uvea. Clinical Ophthalmology. Vol. 4. Hagerstown, Md., Harper and Row, 1976.

Rahi, A. H. S., and Garner, A.: Immunopathology of the Eye. Oxford, Blackwell Scientific Publications, 1976.

Theodore, F. H., and Schlossman, A.: Ocular Allergy. Baltimore, William and Wilkins Co., 1958.

Helen G. Morris, M.D.
John C. Selner, M.D.

50

Endocrine Aspects of Allergy

REGULATION OF ENDOCRINE FUNCTION

The Neuroendocrine System

The endocrine system consists of specialized tissues which are dispersed throughout the body but function as an integrated unit to regulate cellular metabolism and to maintain internal homeostasis. By definition, endocrine tissues exert their effects on the internal environment by humoral (hormonal) mechanisms. Hormones are specialized molecules that are synthesized by endocrine tissues, secreted into the blood stream, and transported in the blood to their sites of action in other tissues. The endocrine system operates in concert with the autonomic nervous system, and the two systems function as an integrated neuroendocrine unit.

Figure 50–1 illustrates some of the major constituents of the neuroendocrine system. The brain has a central role in perceiving changes in the internal and external environment and in initiating the neural and endocrine responses that are needed to preserve homeostasis.

One of the principal sites for integration of neural and endocrine function is the hypothalamus, which regulates "autonomic" functions by hormonal as well as by neural mechanisms. Certain areas of the hypothalamus regulate function at distant sites, including endocrine organs, via neural impulses that release neurotransmitters such as acetylcholine and norepinephrine at nerve endings. Neurons in other areas of the hypothalamus synthesize small peptide molecules that regulate function by hormonal mechanisms. Sometimes, as in the case of vasopressin, the hormone synthesized by a neuron is transported to a storage area in the posterior pituitary via neuronal axons and later released into the blood. In other instances, the peptides synthesized by hypothalamic neurons (hypothalamic releasing hormones) are released directly into the blood.

Neural and endocrine functions also are integrated by other tissues that serve as "neuroendocrine transducers" and transform neural messages to a hormonal output. For example, adrenergic neurons release norepinephrine at nerve endings throughout the body, but in the adrenal medulla, neural impulses evoke release of epinephrine and norepinephrine, which circulate as hormones. Similarly, adrenergic neurons from the cervical sympathetic chain regulate synthesis and release of the hormone melatonin by the pineal gland. Autonomic neurons also participate in the regulation of insulin release by pancreatic islet cells and control secretion of aldosterone by the adrenal cortex through regulation of the synthesis of the enzyme renin by renal juxtaglomerular cells. Other, less well-characterized pathways serve as further links between the brain and the endocrine system and are responsible for many of the adaptive changes in endocrine function.

In addition to the components of the endocrine system shown in Figure 50–1, there are a number of other short-lived substances that also fulfill the criteria for a hormone in that they are synthesized by one tissue, can

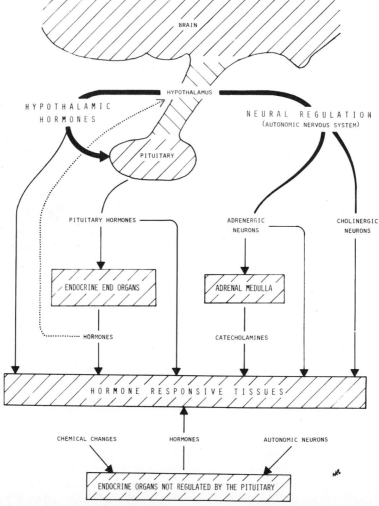

FIGURE 50–1. The neuroendocrine system. Neural and endocrine functions are integrated in the hypothalamus. Neural mechanisms influence function of endocrine glands and hormone responsive tissues. Some endocrine functions are regulated by the hypothalamic-pituitary axis, with three levels of hormone secretion:

(1) Hypothalamic hormones: CRH—corticotropin releasing hormone; TRH—thyrotropin releasing hormone, gonadotropin releasing factor, vasopressin, oxytocin; (2) Pituitary trophic hormones: ACTH, TSH, gonadotropins, GH, prolactin; (3) Hormones produced by endocrine end organs: Cortisol, thyroid (T_4), estrogens, progesterone, androgens.

Other endocrine functions are *not* controlled by the pituitary: Hormones include PTH, calcitonin, insulin, glucagon, gastrointestinal hormones, renin, angiotensin, erythropoietin, and thymosin.

Hormone response tissues: All tissues with receptors for specific hormones.

be found in the circulation, and affect function in other tissues. These substances include the "humoral mediators of allergy," such as histamine, serotonin, SRS-A, bradykinin, and the prostaglandins. As in the case of certain other hormones, the humoral mediators, particularly prostaglandins, modulate function of cells at or near the site of synthesis. These locally active "tissue hormones" integrate the function of individual cells within a multicellular tissue in a manner

analogous to the integrated function exerted by the endocrine system in the organism as a whole.

Regulation of Hormone Secretion

As shown in Figure 50–1, several endocrine organs, such as the thyroid, gonads, and adrenal cortex, are under direct hypothalamic-pituitary control. The sequence of events that regulates hormone secretion by these organs is as follows: Neural impulses from the brain activate particular neurons in the hypothalamus, which secrete specific peptide releasing hormones such as TRH (thyrotropin releasing hormone) and CRF (corticotropin releasing factor). The releasing factors act on particular cells in the anterior and median lobes of the pituitary to regulate synthesis and release of trophic hormones (TSH — thyroid stimulating hormone; ACTH — adrenal cortical stimulating hormone). Finally, the trophic hormones act on the corresponding endocrine organs to regulate synthesis and release of hormones such as thyroid, sex, and adrenal cortical hormones. An appropriate level of hormone secretion therefore requires the functional integrity of the brain, hypothalamus, pituitary and target endocrine gland.

The secretion of hormones by endocrine organs that are governed by the hypothalamic-pituitary axis also is regulated in part by a negative feedback system, which adjusts the secretory activity of the gland in accordance with the concentration of hormone in the circulation. Elevations in the concentration of hormones such as thyroid or cortisol inhibit release of the corresponding hypothalamic releasing factor, whereas low concentrations of hormone enhance release of the appropriate hypothalamic factor and lead to increased secretion of hormone. The negative feedback system thus senses and responds to changes in specific hormone concentration. Other hormones also interact with the hypothalamic-pituitary axis and further modify the secretory activity of endocrine organs controlled by this pathway.

Some endocrine organs are not under hypothalamic-pituitary control but are regulated instead by changes in chemical components of the internal environment. Changes in glucose concentration regulate secretion of insulin and influence secretion of growth hormone and glucagon. Calcium concentrations regulate secretion of parathyroid hormone (PTH) and calcitonin (CT). The release of vasopressin (antidiuretic hormone — ADH) is responsive to changes in osmotic tension. Sodium concentrations regulate synthesis of renin by renal juxtaglomerular cells and influence secretion of aldosterone by the adrenal cortex. The common feature in the regulation of these hormones is that the endocrine tissue or a closely integrated component of the nervous system senses the change in chemical environment and initiates release of the hormone that preserves homeostasis. Other hormones also interact with endocrine tissues which are responsive to changes in internal environment and further modify hormone secretion.

In some instances multiple factors participate in the regulation of hormone secretion. For example, the primary stimulus for insulin secretion is an elevation of blood glucose concentration, but secretion is enhanced by cholinergic stimuli and inhibited by adrenergic stimuli. Secretion of insulin also is regulated in part by glucagon, which is synthesized by alpha cells in pancreatic islets, and by several gastrointestinal hormones that are secreted into the blood in response to ingested food.

Mechanisms of Hormone Action

Hormones may be broadly classified into two major categories: (1) peptide or amine hormones that serve as extracellular messengers and (2) steroid hormones that enter cells and exert their effects on gene expression. The first category encompasses the majority of hormones, including hypothalamic releasing factors, pituitary hormones, parathyroid hormone, calcitonin, insulin, and glucagon. This category also includes catecholamines, which have a mode of action similar to the peptide hormones. The second category includes steroid hormones such as glucocorticoids, mineralocorticoids, androgens, and estrogens — as well as the thyroid hormones.

Peptide and amine hormones do not enter cells; instead, they transmit their messages by binding to specific receptor proteins on the cell surface. There is a unique receptor for each hormone in responsive cells. Even when a cell is capable of responding to several hormones, the binding of each hormone occurs at a separate site and can be selectively blocked. The majority of peptide and amine hormones, with the notable exception of insulin, are thought to exert their effects through cAMP, which serves as the intracellular messenger. Binding of the hormone by the receptor is coupled to activation of the membrane-bound enzyme adenylate cyclase, which catalyzes the conversion of ATP to cAMP. The increase in cAMP leads to activation of one or more protein kinases, which in turn catalyze the phosphorylation of specific proteins (enzymes) that mediate the intracellular effects of the hormone (Sutherland, 1972). The increase in cAMP also is associated with redistribution of intracellular calcium, which modifies enzyme activity and also affects membrane permeability (Rasmussen et al., 1972).

The mechanism of action of the steroid hormones differs from the above in that the hormone molecules enter cells and are bound to specific protein receptors in the cell cytosol. Binding of the hormone induces a conformational change in the receptor, which activates the protein. The entire hormone-receptor complex is then translocated to the cell nucleus, where it becomes attached to nuclear chromatin DNA and affects gene expression. The association of the hormone-receptor complex with DNA leads to transcription of messenger RNA (mRNA) and eventually to the synthesis of new enzyme protein (Baxter and Forsham, 1972). In contrast to the effects of the peptide and amine hormones, which are relatively rapid, hormonal effects induced by steroid and thyroid hormones occur more slowly and in part reflect the lag in time required for synthesis of new protein. Steroid-induced effects do not require the mediation of a second messenger such as cAMP; instead the effects are produced directly by activation or suppression of key intracellular enzymes.

Despite the differences in initial mechanisms of action exhibited by the two categories of hormones, there are many similarities. All hormone action depends on the availability of specific receptors in target tissue that are capable of recognizing and responding to the hormone. Receptors for some hormones — such as glucocorticoids, thyroid hormone, catecholamines, and insulin — are widely distributed and are associated with hormonal effects in many tissues. Conversely, receptors for other hormones — such as hypothalamic releasing factors, ACTH, and TSH — have a more limited distribution, and hormonal action is largely limited to a single target organ.

Hormonal action results in changes (usually increases) in energy utilization by the target cell and in changes in permeability of the cellular membrane to water, ions, and various energy substrates. Additionally, hormones affect the rate at which specialized functions, which are characteristic of the particular target cell, are carried out. In every instance, the reactions are dependent on the particular enzymatic machinery within the cell. Hormones do not initiate chemical reactions; rather, they alter the rate of such reactions by enhancing or inhibiting the activity of key enzymes that catalyze the reactions. In some instances the effect of the hormone is to activate pre-existing enzyme, whereas in other instances the hormone also stimulates synthesis of new enzyme protein.

In addition to affecting cellular activity, hormones may induce proliferation or maturation of cells. Thus, ACTH stimulates synthesis of corticosteroids by the adrenal cortex and also causes proliferation and hypertrophy of adrenal cortical cells. Parathyroid hormone stimulates the activity of the bone-resorbing osteoclasts and, over a longer period of time, increases the formation of osteoclasts from osteoprogenitor cells. As shown by the effects of the sex hormones on responsive tissue, steroid hormones also increase the number of target cells.

MECHANISMS OF ENDOCRINE DYSFUNCTION

Endocrine function is determined in part by the quantitative availability of biologically active hormone. Excessive quantities of hormone usually are due to hyperplasia or neoplasia of hormone-secreting tissues. Deficient quantities of hormone may be due to congenital or acquired loss of hormone-secreting cells by infectious or toxic agents, neoplasms or autoimmune mechanisms. In both instances *abnormal quantities of hormone* may result from primary alterations in the hormone-secreting cells or from disturbances in the pathways that regulate hormone synthesis.

In some instances the availability of active hormone may be diminished even when glandular secretion is normal. Certain hormones are synthesized and released as relatively inactive precursors, which require further modification before full hormonal action can occur. For example, most of the hormone secreted by the thyroid gland is tetraiodothyronine (T_4), which is subsequently converted to T_3, the active form of the hormone. Depending on the position of the iodine atom that is deleted from the T_4 molecule, either T_3 or "reverse T_3", which has little biologic activity, may be formed. Another example of a secreted hormone that must be modified for biologic activity is testosterone, which must be converted to dihydro-testosterone in responsive tissues. A different type of modification is required for biologic activity of growth hormone (GH). Although the secreted hormone has some direct effects, most of the actions are due to an intermediary hormone, somatomedin, which is synthesized in the liver under the influence of GH.

Endocrine dysfunction also may be due to *alterations in the responsiveness of target tissues* to available hormone. As indicated previously, all hormonal action depends on specific receptors in target tissue, which are capable of recognizing and binding the hormone, and on the subsequent activation of key enzymes that mediate the intracellular effects of the hormone. Although all tissues are exposed to the hormone via the circulation, hormonal action occurs only in those tissues that possess specific hormone receptors. An important concept is that the number of receptors in target tissue is not fixed but instead varies in relation to metabolic events within the cell; in turn, the availability of receptors determines the responsiveness of target tissue to biologically active hormone (Roth et al., 1975).

Diabetes mellitus is an example of a common endocrine disease that may be due to abnormal tissue responsiveness to available hormone. Although some patients have an absolute deficiency of insulin, in many instances the disease is due to tissue "resistance" to available insulin. In comparison with those of normal subjects, cells from obese diabetics and other patients with insulin resistance have decreased numbers of insulin receptors. Correction of the metabolic problem is associated with restoration of the number of insulin receptors toward normal and improved responsiveness to insulin.

Alterations in tissue responsiveness may also stem from a process of hormone-induced desensitization. There is evidence that continued exposure of cells to peptide or amine hormones results in desensitization of the cell to further stimulation by that hormone (Roth et al., 1975; Mukherjee et al.,

1975). The most extensive investigations have involved adrenergic agents, but similar effects are seen with other stimuli that operate through the cAMP system. The process appears to involve reduction in the number of receptors for the stimulating hormone and/or inhibition of an intermediary step between hormone receptor binding and adenyl cyclase activation (Mukherjee et al., 1975; Lamprecht et al., 1977).

Autoimmune Mechanisms of Endocrine Dysfunction

Defective immune surveillance often contributes to the pathogenesis of endocrine dysfunction. The underlying mechanism involves the failure of suppressor T lymphocytes to prevent survival of "forbidden," self-directed clones of lymphocytes. Such lymphocytes are thought to arise from random mutation or, in some instances, may stem from viral-induced alterations of lymphocyte DNA. The "forbidden" clones of organ-specific, self-reactive T lymphocytes interact with antigens that are produced normally by the organ and cause morphologic and functional changes in the tissue via humoral and cell-mediated immune mechanisms (Volpe, 1977).

The thyroid gland has served as a prototype for studies of autoimmune disease of endocrine and nonendocrine tissues. Initial studies involved Hashimoto's thyroiditis, a disease associated with lymphocytic infiltration of the thyroid gland and eventual loss of thyroid hormone–producing cells. Patients with this disease were found to have circulating antibody to components of thyroid tissue, and a similar disease could be produced experimentally by immunization of animals with autologous thyroid tissue. Subsequently, evidence was obtained that cell-mediated immune mechanisms also contribute to the pathogenesis of Hashimoto's thyroiditis. The exact mechanisms responsible for the cytotoxic effects on thyroid cells are unclear. Current evidence suggests that the most likely mechanism involves antibody-dependent lymphocyte-mediated cytotoxicity and that either antibody or immune complexes activate "killer" lymphocytes or macrophages to produce tissue damage (Volpe, 1977).

Graves' disease is another autoimmune

TABLE 50–1   AUTOIMMUNE DISORDERS OF ENDOCRINE
AND NON-ENDOCRINE TISSUES

Endocrine Disorders	Nonendocrine Diseases
Hashimoto's thyroiditis	Rheumatoid arthritis
Graves' disease	Systemic lupus
Diabetes mellitus (insulin deficiency)	Pernicious anemia
Addison's disease	Idiopathic thrombocytopenia purpura
Idiopathic hypoparathyroidism	Vitiligo
Autoimmune oophoritis	Myasthenia gravis
Autoimmune orchitis	Sjögren's syndrome
(?) Autoimmune hypophysitis	Chronic active hepatitis

The spectrum of autoimmune disease encompasses endocrine and nonendocrine disorders. In some instances, the disease involves a single organ, whereas in other instances, various combinations of endocrine and nonendocrine disturbances are present. Endocrine disorders are listed in order of frequency.

disease of the thyroid gland that is associated with hyperplasia of thyroid tissue and excessive production of thyroid hormone; the disease also may be associated with an infiltrative ophthalmopathy. Patients with Graves' disease have many of the same antibodies and cell-mediated immune factors found in Hashimoto's disease. However, a unique feature of Graves' disease is the presence of a circulating immunoglobulin that is specifically directed against the TSH receptor of thyroid cell membrane and mimics the effect of TSH. Thus, Graves' disease is characterized by the presence of an anti-receptor antibody. In contrast to other anti-receptor diseases such as myasthenia gravis, however, the antibody of Graves' disease is unique in that it is capable of stimulating cells (Brown, 1978).

As shown in Table 50–1, the spectrum of autoimmune disease encompasses a variety of endocrine disorders as well as disorders of nonendocrine tissue. In some instances the disturbance involves a single tissue and may be due to an isolated defect in immune surveillance. Other patients exhibit multiple endocrine disturbances or a combination of endocrine and nonendocrine disease, suggesting a more profound alteration in surveillance. The predisposition to autoimmune disease appears to be genetically determined, since there is an increased frequency of anti-organ antibodies in asymptomatic relatives of propositi and also a higher incidence of clinical autoimmune disease involving the same or a different organ. In addition to the genetic predisposition, unknown trigger mechanisms seem to be necessary for the development of overt disease. One of the factors relates to the influence of sex and sex hormones. The frequency of autoimmune disease is greater in females than in males, and experimental studies in animals have suggested that the development of autoimmune disease and its subsequent course can be modified by castration or administration of sex hormones (Roubinian et al., 1977; Duvic et al., 1978). In recent years, with the decreasing frequency of endocrine dysfunction due to other causes, particularly destruction of hormone-secreting cells by infectious agents, there has been increasing recognition of the role of autoimmune mechanisms in the pathogenesis of endocrine dysfunction.

Endocrine Dysfunction Due to Pharmacotherapy of Allergic Disease

Many of the agents used in the therapy of allergic disease have direct hormonal actions or have metabolic effects that alter hormone balance. The most frequent manifestations of endocrine dysfunction in patients with allergy, therefore, stem from the effects of pharmacotherapy rather than primary endocrine disease.

The most widespread effects are those caused by corticosteroid therapy, which mimics the effects of endogenous cortisol and may be associated with manifestations of hormone excess. Steroids also suppress the hypothalamic-pituitary axis and may induce adrenal cortical insufficiency. Corticosteroids also influence growth, sexual maturation and function, utilization of energy substrates, bone metabolism, and many other bodily functions. The widespread effects of corticosteroids include alterations of hormone synthesis and release, changes in hormone metabolism, and alterations in tissue responses to hormones.

Other medications used in the treatment of allergy also influence endocrine function. Sputum liquefiers containing iodides may cause hypothyroidism and goiter formation. Theophylline affects secretion and action of parathyroid hormone. At least three of the agents used in the treatment of asthma, i.e., steroids, theophylline, and catecholamines, have potent effects on glucose metabolism and are diabetogenic. Table 50–2 summarizes the major hormonal effects of agents used in the treatment of asthma.

HORMONAL EFFECTS ON THE IMMUNE RESPONSE

Multiple lines of evidence demonstrate that hormones have potent effects on cells that participate in the immune response. The evidence is derived in part from clinical observations, studies in animals, and more recently from examination of specific hormonal effects on immune responses in human cells. In conjunction with current interest in "hormonal receptors," it has been found that lymphocytes, thymocytes, and monocytes possess receptors for a number of hormones, including steroids, thyroid hormones, catecholamines, histamine, insulin, growth hormone, and probably thymosin. The number of receptors and binding kinetics in lymphoid cells are comparable to those in other target organs for the respective hormones. Furthermore, hormone binding is associated with demonstrable change in metabolic activity of the cells and in functional changes in immune responsiveness. The recognition that lymphoid tissues are responsive to hormones has begun to explain the association between certain endocrine deficiency syndromes and immune suppression and has suggested that hormones may have an important role in the development of "nonendocrine" malignancies. Similarly, as noted above, hormonal influences on immunity may account for the striking sex incidence of autoimmune disorders.

Table 50–3 summarizes current information about hormonal effects on immunity. It can be anticipated that this list will be expanded as further studies define the interaction of various hormones on specific immune functions and particularly on the alterations that lead to disturbances in immune surveillance.

INTERRELATIONSHIPS BETWEEN FUNCTIONS OF ENDOCRINE ORGANS AND ALLERGIC DISEASE

Hypothalamus

Several lines of evidence suggest that asthma is associated with an autonomic imbalance, with relatively enhanced cholinergic activity or diminished beta adrenergic activity (Szentivanyi, 1968; see also Chapter 14). Although mechanisms responsible for the autonomic imbalance have not been defined fully, similar manifestations could result from disturbances at any point in the autonomic pathway from the hypothalamus to the release of neurotransmitters or to altered responsiveness of the target tissues.

Recent studies have focused on the function or quantitative availability of beta adrenergic receptors in target tissue. It is noteworthy, however, that in his early studies, Szentivanyi demonstrated that stimulation or ablation of specific areas of the hypothalamus could influence bronchial reactivity to a wide variety of chemical mediators. Studies in our own laboratory have indicated that patients with asthma have diminished hormonal responses to the stress of asthma. Despite the ability of the adrenal gland to respond appropriately to other stresses, such as hypoglycemia, during symptomatic asthma the adrenal glands release only small quantities of the hormones (cortisol, epinephrine) which might alleviate asthmatic symptoms (Kumar et al., 1971; Morris et al., 1972). When hormone release is evoked by another stress such as hypoglycemia, symptomatic patients exhibit spontaneous amelioration of asthma (Morris et al., 1972). Thus, the influence of the hypothalamus and autonomic nervous system on the clinical manifestations of allergic disease remains an open question.

Text continued on page 664.

TABLE 50–2 HORMONAL EFFECTS OF PHARMACOLOGIC AGENTS USED IN THE TREATMENT OF ASTHMA

Drug	Biochemical Mechanism	Clinical Effect
Corticosteroids	Excess availability of glucocorticoid	Cushing's syndrome
	Suppression of HPA axis ↓ ACTH ↓ Adrenal steroid production	Adrenal insufficiency
	↑ availability β-adrenergic receptor ↓ neuronal uptake catecholamines	Synergism with catecholamines
	↑ Gluconeogenesis ↓ Insulin action	Diabetes mellitus
	↓ Formation somatomedin	Growth retardation
	↓ Release pituitary gonadotropins	Retardation of sexual maturation Delayed maturation of epiphyses (?) ↓ Sexual function
	↑ Parathyroid hormone ↑ Calcitonin Loss of calcium in urine and stool	Demineralization of bone
ACTH	Similar to corticosteroids except:	
	↑ Production of glucocorticoids ↑ Production of androgenic steroids by adrenal cortex	Hirsutism Closure of epiphyses
TAO	Mechanism unknown	↑ Steroid action
Adrenergic agents	↑ cAMP synthesis	Synergism with corticosteroids
	Desensitization of β-adrenergic receptors	Beta adrenergic blockade
	↑ Gluconeogenesis ↓ Insulin secretion ↓ Insulin action	Diabetogenic
	↓ Counter-regulation to hyperglycemia	Reactive hypoglycemia
Theophylline	↓ cAMP degradation	Synergism with epinephrine
	↑ Release of epinephrine	Cardiac arrhythmia
	↓ Insulin action	Diabetogenic
	↑ Insulin release	Reactive hypoglycemia
	↑ PTH	Demineralization of bone
Iodides	↓ Formation thyroid hormone secondary ↑ TSH	Hypothyroidism Goiter
Cromolyn sodium	No known endocrine effect	None known
Antihistamines	No known endocrine effect	None known

TABLE 50–3   HORMONAL EFFECTS ON IMMUNE RESPONSES

Hormone	Immune Effect	Reference
Glucocorticoids	Suppress all aspects of inflammation Redistribution of leukocytes in body ↓ leukocyte accumulation at inflammatory site ↓ release of inflammatory mediators ↓ macrophage response to inflammatory mediators Protect target cells from T lymphocyte killer activity (?) ↓ lymphocyte proliferation	Fauci et al., 1976; Schreiber, 1977
	↓ serum immunoglobulins	Berger et al., 1978; Settipane et al., 1978
	↓ serum complement levels	Atkinson and Frank, 1973
Catecholamines	Suppress all leukocyte functions ↑ leukocyte cAMP ↓ mediator release (histamine, SRS-A, MIF) ↓ antibody formation ↓ phagocytosis	Bourne et al., 1974
Thymosin	↑ Maturation of T lymphocytes ↑ number of lymphocytes in thymus, spleen, lymph nodes ↑ cell-mediated immunity	Schulof and Goldstein, 1977
Insulin	Receptors present on monocytes, macrophages Appearance of receptors on T lymphocytes associated with ↑ cGMP or immune activation	Helderman and Strom, 1977
Growth hormone	Immunogenic. Dwarfed Snell-Bagg mice have atrophy of thymus, spleen, lymph nodes; GH corrects dwarfism, causes repopulation of thymus and spleen with lymphocytes. ↑ number of plaque forming cells ↑ uptake of 3H-thymidine into lymphocyte DNA ↑ metabolic activity of thymus medulla	Talwar et al., 1975
Thyroid hormone	Immunogenic. Peripheral lymphocytes possess nuclear binding sites for T_3 ↑ leukocyte response to PHA	Bernal et al., 1976; McKenzie and Zakarija, 1977
Parathyroid hormone	Stimulates mitotic division in thymic lymphoblasts in presence of Ca^{++}	Rasmussen, 1971; Rasmussen et al., 1972
Calcitonin	Inhibits mitotic division in thymic lymphoblasts, blocks PTH effect	Rasmussen, 1971; Rasmussen et al., 1972
Stress hormone (non-traumatic shock)	Crowding ↑ lymphocyte response to PHA stimulation; more apparent in females Various stresses (e.g., swimming, cold) alter lymphocyte response to PHA and pokeweed mitogen	McKenzie and Zakarya, 1977

Table continued on next page.

663

TABLE 50–3 HORMONAL EFFECTS ON IMMUNE RESPONSES *(Continued)*

Hormone	Immune Effect	Reference

Sex steroids	In animals, estrogens enhance:
	↑ immune responses
	↑ serum immunoglobulins
	↑ specific antibody
	↑ cell-mediated immunity
	↑ rejection of tumors and homografts
	Androgens (or anti-estrogens) decrease
	    immune response through an effect
	    on thymocytes
		Roubinian et al., 1977

	Sex hormone important in autoimmunity Androgens and anti-estrogens inhibit manifestation of autoimmunity	Duvic et al., 1978

Pituitary

Patients with allergic disease have no evidence of primary pituitary dysfunction. However, patients with allergy may present as diagnostic problems which require differentiation from pituitary disease. In particular, "failure to thrive" or problems in growth and development may be the presenting complaints in children with *either* endocrine or allergic disease. Additionally, agents used in the pharmacotherapy of allergy, particularly corticosteroids, may alter pituitary function.

Disturbance in Growth and Allergy. Over 90 percent of children with delayed growth have no endocrine disease. Delayed growth may be associated with any systemic illness and is particularly apt to occur in situations associated with hypoxemia or disturbances of sleep and nutrition. Experience gained during the pre-steroid era indicated that asthma was associated with an incidence of dwarfism which was two to three times greater than that seen in the general population. The frequency and severity of dwarfism increased in relation to the severity of asthma, consistent with the importance of tissue oxygenation and nutrition on growth.

Following introduction of corticosteroids for treatment of severe asthma, there was a further sharp increase in frequency of dwarfism—which was directly attributable to the effects of corticosteroids and was dose-dependent. As many as 35 percent of asthmatic children who received daily steroids (10 to 15 mg prednisone) for 2 or more years had significant growth retardation with heights more than 2 standard deviations below those expected for age and sex (Morris, 1975). The use of alternate-day steroid therapy decreased the frequency of growth retardation but the effects still are related to corticosteroid dose (Reimer et al., 1975).

Although acute administration of corticosteroid may inhibit synthesis and release of growth hormone, most asthmatic children have normal quantities of plasma GH during sleep and normal growth hormone responses to hypoglycemic stress (Morris et al., 1968). The major block induced by corticosteroids results from interference with GH-induced synthesis of the intermediary hormone, somatomedin. Unfortunately, there is no way at present to overcome this steroid effect other than by reducing the dosage or discontinuing corticosteroid therapy. Administration of growth hormone to steroid-treated patients will not promote growth, and somatomedin is not available for clinical use.

The initial evaluation of a child with a growth problem should focus on identification of an underlying systemic illness or a nutritional problem. The possibility of a relatively common hormonal deficiency, such as hypothyroidism, also should be considered.

If the above approach is unrevealing, the next step is to obtain a lateral skull film to rule out the presence of a pituitary tumor, which is not common but accounts for many of the cases of true growth hormone (GH) deficiency. A random plasma sample containing measurable quantities of growth hormone rules out an absolute deficiency of growth hormone, but since values often are low in the absence of stimulation, random specimens may not be diagnostic. In such instances, one or more plasma samples obtained 2 hours after onset of night sleep should reveal measurable GH levels. If further diagnostic studies are indicated, these are best carried out under the direction of an experienced endocrinologist, since subtle abnormalities of hypothalamic-pituitary function may be involved.

Delayed Sexual Maturation and Allergy. In most instances, delayed sexual maturation is not due to primary endocrine disease. Systemic illnesses may delay the maturation of the pituitary-gonadal axis, but complete maturation usually occurs eventually. Retardation of growth often precedes the delay in sexual maturation, but patients may not present until adolescence, when the delay of the normal growth spurt and development of secondary sexual characteristics makes the problem strikingly apparent. As with growth suppression, corticosteroids may further delay the onset of puberty.

The delayed appearance of secondary sexual characteristics is due to delay in maturation of the hypothalamic-pituitary-gonadal axis and the consequent reduced synthesis of gonadal steroids (androgens and estrogens). However, in contrast to the situation with growth hormone, tissues are fully responsive to exogenously supplied gonadal steroids. Therefore, treatment with such hormones may accelerate development of secondary sexual characteristics; unfortunately, such therapy also may stimulate rapid maturation and closure of long bone epiphyses and lead to greater suppression of height than might occur spontaneously. Gonadal steroids should *not* be used to stimulate growth in pre-adolescent or adolescent children. Occasionally such therapy may be considered for treatment of delayed sexual maturation associated with severe emotional problems. In such instances, the patient and family should be fully appraised of the risks before hormone therapy is initiated.

Adrenal Cortex

The frequency of an association between clinical allergy and adrenal disease is not known with certainty. In a review of the experience at the Mayo Clinic, Carryer

(1960) reported that approximately 10 percent of patients with documented Addison's disease (primary adrenal insufficiency) also had allergic symptoms, including asthma, hay fever, allergic rhinitis, urticaria and drug allergy. Approximately two-thirds of the patients with associated allergic disease developed evidence of allergy at about the time of onset of the Addison's disease. There are also several recent case reports of patients in whom Addison's disease and asthma occurred simultaneously. Although the presenting symptoms may relate to either condition, the prognosis is poor unless both problems are recognized and treated simultaneously. Unfortunately, in many instances the diagnosis was not made until postmortem examination (Green and Lim, 1971; Harris and Collins, 1971).

The possibility of associated disease should be borne in mind since Addison's disease is one of the more frequent autoimmune endocrinopathies. As the frequency of Addison's disease secondary to tuberculosis or meningococcemia decreases, an increasing proportion of the patients with this disease are found to have antibodies directed against adrenal cortical tissue.

In the majority of patients with allergic disease, the abnormality in adrenal function is due to pharmacotherapy with corticosteroids rather than to primary disease of the adrenal gland. Patients receiving corticosteroids often exhibit the clinical signs of Cushing's syndrome (adrenal cortical excess), the severity of which is dependent upon the dose and duration of steroid therapy. At the same time, steroid therapy results in suppression of the hypothalamic-pituitary-adrenal (HPA) axis. Initially, the suppression is largely functional and withdrawal of steroid therapy is associated with rapid recovery of normal function. When therapy is continued for a longer period, pathologic changes occur in the pituitary and adrenal glands and the recovery period is considerably longer. Withdrawal of corticosteroids may be associated with frank evidence of adrenal insufficiency. Manifestations of adrenal insufficiency also may occur during treatment with small doses of exogenous steroids, if the patient is subjected to a severe stress, since the adrenal is unable to synthesize the additional steroid needed in such situations.

Effects of Corticosteroids in Patients

with Allergic Disease. The use of corticosteroids in allergic disease stems from empiric evidence of the beneficial effects of these agents on allergic symptoms, but the precise mechanisms have not been fully defined. Some of the mechanisms which contribute to the anti-inflammatory effects of corticosteroids are summarized in Table 50–3. The most likely explanations for the therapeutic effectiveness of corticosteroids relate to their ability to suppress accumulation of leukocytes at the site of injury and to suppress the release of and response to allergic mediators of inflammation. Although steroids suppress the total quantity of circulating antibody in animals and are associated with a measurable decrease in the circulating levels of IgG and, to a lesser extent, IgA immunoglobulins in humans, there is little evidence that the synthesis of specific antibody is inhibited.

Another factor that contributes to the anti-inflammatory effect of corticosteroids is their synergism with catecholamines. The suppressive effects of adrenergic agents on release of inflammatory mediators results in part from an increase in intracellular cAMP. Corticosteroids inhibit an enzyme concerned with degradation of cAMP. Corticosteroids also affect the metabolism of catecholamines. A major mechanism that contributes to the termination of catecholamine action is a reuptake process that removes catecholamine from the extracellular environment. By inhibiting this process, corticosteroids increase the availability of catecholamines at the site of release and prolong their action. In addition, corticosteroids inhibit desensitization of beta adrenergic receptors, perhaps by inhibiting synthesis of an intermediary protein between receptor binding of catecholamine and adenyl cyclase activation, and thereby further enhance the action of catecholamines.

The mechanism of the anti-asthmatic effect of corticosteroids is conjectural. Since corticosteroids do not have direct bronchodilator activity, the anti-asthmatic effects of corticosteroids may result from suppression of edema or inflammation in bronchi or pulmonary tissue. Another possibility is that steroids in some way suppress the activity of a neural reflex arc that mediates bronchial reactivity. The latter is a more plausible explanation for the effectiveness of aerosol corticosteroids, which are administered in minute quantities and have relatively little systemic (hence pulmonary tissue) effect.

Although *in vitro* studies demonstrate that the initial biochemical events in corticosteroid action begin within minutes after exposure of the cell to corticosteroid, alterations in cellular metabolism are not detectable clinically for several hours. Specifically, changes in glucose metabolism and redistribution of leukocytes are not apparent until 2 hours after steroid administration. The improvement in pulmonary function after administration of steroids to asthmatic patients requires an even longer time; the maximal effects of the steroid dose may not occur until 6 to 9 hours after treatment, although the synergism with catecholamines may begin somewhat earlier (Ellul-Micallef et al., 1974; Ellul-Micallef and Fenech, 1975). The lag time in corticosteroid action is of importance therapeutically and emphasizes a need for concomitant use of other, more rapidly acting agents in acute situations such as anaphylaxis, shock, or status asthmaticus.

Side Effects of Corticosteroid Treatment. The side effects of corticosteroid therapy result from exposure of tissues to supra-physiologic quantities of hormone and are identical to those observed in spontaneous Cushing's syndrome. Since steroids affect virtually all tissues in the body, the side effects encompass multiple bodily functions. The major hormonal effects induced by corticosteroids are listed in Table 50–2. The widespread effects include alterations of hormone synthesis and release, changes in hormone metabolism, and alterations in tissue responses to hormones.

The effects of ACTH administration are similar to those resulting from corticosteroids. There are, however, several notable differences.

Steroids used therapeutically are primarily glucocorticoids and have little androgenic effect, whereas some of the steroid molecules synthesized by the adrenal cortex have potent androgenic activity. Under the influence of ACTH, synthesis of all steroid molecules produced by the adrenal cortex is increased, including those with androgenic activity.

Side effects of ACTH, therefore, include

both glucocorticoid effects and androgenic effects such as hirsutism, acne and, in children, maturation of epiphyses. The latter effect is particularly important in preadolescent children. Although the initial effects of ACTH administration may be associated with less retardation of growth than that seen during steroid therapy, the accelerated maturation of the epiphyses ultimately may lead to greater stunting of growth. ACTH also differs from steroids in that it causes hyperplasia of adrenal cortical cells rather than adrenal cortical atrophy, which occurs secondary to corticosteroid-induced suppression of the HPA axis.

If corticosteroid therapy can be withdrawn, there is amelioration of many of the side effects. This includes recovery of the functional integrity of the HPA axis. Suppression of adrenal cortical secretion is not an indication for continued steroid therapy in patients with allergic disease. HPA function invariably returns to normal when corticosteroid therapy is discontinued; in some instances, however, particularly when steroid therapy is used intermittently during recovery, the process may be prolonged. There is no documentation of permanent adrenal atrophy after a period of corticosteroid treatment except in patients with primary adrenal disease. Certain steroid side effects such as stunting of growth, however, may be permanent.

Assessment of Pituitary-Adrenal Function. Because of the number of ways in which steroid therapy may mimic primary adrenal disease and because of the rare possibility of an association between adrenal disease and asthma, the following guidelines may be useful in assessing function of the HPA axis:

The simplest and most useful method for assessment of HPA function is the determination of plasma cortisol concentrations. The two methods used most commonly for cortisol measurement are competitive protein binding assays and radioimmunoassay. A problem with both methods is that certain steroids (notably prednisone and prednisolone) cross-react with cortisol in the assays (Morris et al., 1973 and 1974). To avoid erroneous assessment of HPA function, it therefore is necessary that blood samples be obtained 12 to 24 hours after administration

of exogenous steroid. Alternatively, the same assays can be used to monitor the concentrations of exogenous steroid in the circulation. If the patient has been treated with ACTH, at least 24 to 48 hours should elapse between treatment and assessment of endogenous function.

Plasma cortisol concentrations normally exhibit a circadian rhythm, with the highest concentrations in the early morning and lower levels at all other times. Measurement of early morning plasma cortisol concentrations therefore provides the best index of endogenous adrenal function. As cortisol secretion is episodic, individual samples may contain relatively low concentrations, but if several early morning samples are obtained from the same individual or a group of individuals, the values should approximate the normal mean of 12 to 15 μg/dl. Values that are consistently below 10 are indicative of at least partial suppression of adrenal function. Studies in our laboratory have demonstrated that in patients with allergic disease in whom there is no disturbance of CNS function, early morning cortisol concentrations adequately reflect the functional integrity of the pituitary adrenal system and show good correlation with response to stress (Morris and Jorgensen, 1971).

Although measurement of cortisol response to administered ACTH is used by some physicians to evaluate function of the adrenal cortex, this is a poor test for HPA function in patients who have received corticosteroid therapy. The response to administered ACTH provides no indication of steroid-induced suppression of endogenous ACTH secretion and may override the adrenal cortical suppression that results from deficiency of endogenous ACTH. Additionally, administration of ACTH (including the synthetic materials) has been associated with anaphylactic reactions.

Adrenal Medulla

There is no evidence of a primary disturbance in adrenal medullary function in patients with allergic symptoms. Most patients secrete normal quantities of epinephrine and norepinephrine and respond to stimuli such as exercise, hypoglycemia, and hypotension with appropriate increases in catecholamine secretion. As indicated in the section dealing with the hypothalamus, however, there is a peculiarity in the expected catecholamine response to symptomatic asthma, suggesting an abnormality in the ability of the nervous system to sense and respond to such symptoms by evoking catecholamine release. Studies by Mathé and Knapp (1969) suggest that asthmatic patients also respond to emotional stress with a smaller increase in catecholamine release than normal subjects. These observations point to an abnormality in the activation of a neural signal that evokes catecholamine release.

Influence of Catecholamines on Allergic Disease. Adrenergic agents have been found to be useful in the treatment of allergic symptoms. The mode of action of these agents appears to be mediated by an increase in cAMP, which is associated with suppression of mediator release by inflammatory cells. All leukocyte functions are affected. In addition, catecholamines alter the distribution of leukocytes in the body and have direct effects on bronchial smooth muscle and pulmonary vasculature. Although there is no doubt about the effectiveness of adrenergic agents in reducing allergic manifestations, current information on "receptor desensitization" and reduced cAMP responses following exposure of cells to catecholamines suggests that mechanisms other than an increase in cAMP may contribute to the therapeutic effectiveness of these agents.

In recent years there has been considerable interest in the possibility that asthma might be associated with "blockade" of beta adrenergic receptors. This possibility was suggested initially by observations that patients with asthma exhibited reduced metabolic responsiveness (e.g., changes in blood glucose, free fatty acids) to administered adrenergic agents; responses of asthmatic patients were similar to those observed in individuals who had been treated with beta adrenergic antagonists. The subsequent observation that leukocytes obtained from asthmatic subjects had reduced cAMP responses to adrenergic stimulation *in vitro* further suggested that an alteration in beta adrenergic receptor function might be a central feature of asthma (Parker and Smith, 1973).

More recently, however, it has become apparent that alterations in beta adrenergic receptor responses can stem from effects of previous adrenergic therapy (Conolly and Greenacre, 1976; Morris et al., 1978; see also Chapter 14). Multiple lines of evidence indicate that following the initial binding of catecholamine by the receptor and activation of the adenylate cyclase system, cells enter a refractory period during which they are unable to respond to further adrenergic stimulation with an increase in cAMP; the refractory period persists for a number of hours. The mechanisms responsible for the refractory period are still controversial, but may involve an absolute decrease in the number of available beta adrenergic receptors or synthesis of a protein that inhibits subsequent activation of adenyl cyclase. Recent studies have suggested a decrease in maximal bronchodilator response during continued treatment with an adrenergic agent (Nelson et al., 1977). Nevertheless, the persistence of therapeutic benefit during continued treatment with adrenergic bronchodilators when other parameters indicate suppression of cAMP response suggests that factors other than cAMP my contribute to the therapeutic action of adrenergic agents.

Influence of Medications for Asthma on Adrenal Medullary Function. The synergism between corticosteroids and catecholamines has been discussed previously. Another type of interaction between these substances is exerted at the level of epinephrine synthesis. The enzyme phenylethanolamine methyl transferase, which catalyzes the conversion of norepinephrine to epinephrine in the adrenal medulla, is induced by corticosteroids. Through the portal circulation adrenal cortical hormones reach the adrenal medulla in high concentration. Epinephrine synthesis requires high concentrations of glucocorticoid and occurs only in those tissues which are exposed to elevated steroid concentrations. However, studies in our laboratory have indicated that the pharmacologic doses of steroid used for treatment of asthma are sufficient to maintain epinephrine synthesis even in the presence of suppressed cortisol synthesis (Morris et al., 1973).

Theophylline influences catecholamines in two ways. Acute administration of theophylline is associated with enhanced release of epinephrine from the adrenal medulla (Atuk et al., 1967). It is not clear whether this effect persists during continued administration of theophylline. However, the acute effects on catecholamine release may account for some of the early side effects of theophylline therapy and may be responsible for the cardiac arrhythmia or death that sometimes occurs after bolus administration of theophylline. A second interaction produced by theophylline relates to its ability to serve as an inhibitor of the enzyme phosphodiesterase, thereby potentiating the action of epinephrine on cAMP.

Pancreas (Insulin Secretion and Action)

Good statistics are not available concerning the association between allergic disease and diabetes mellitus. In part, there is a problem in definition. Since allergic disease and diabetes are common conditions, with susceptibility for each disease in up to 25 percent of the population, and since both conditions encompass a wide range of clinical severity, it is difficult to define the criteria that would be necessary for statistical evaluation. Nevertheless, because of the frequency of the two conditions, associated disease is not uncommon. The association occurs more frequently in adults (when diabetes is also more common in the general population) than in children. As indicated previously, diabetes (particularly insulin-dependent diabetes) is one of the autoimmune endocrinopathies and may be associated with anti–islet cell antibodies.

Although a considerable amount of folklore suggests an association between hypoglycemia and allergic disease, statistics are unavailable and in most instances adequate documentation has not been obtained. Such an association, if it exists at all, is unlikely to involve a primary abnormality in islet cell function (Merimee, 1977). A more likely possibility is that there is a defect in one of the counter-regulatory mechanisms which defend against hypoglycemia (Morris, 1971; Morris et al., 1973).

Glucose Metabolism and Allergic Disease. A variety of neuroendocrine mechanisms normally contribute to the main-

tenance of blood glucose homeostasis. The hyperglycemia following ingestion of food evokes the release of insulin, which fosters removal of glucose from the circulation by enhancing glucose entry into peripheral tissues and by storage of excess glucose in the form of glycogen or fat. As the blood glucose concentration returns to the normal range, it sometimes dips below normal. The trend toward hypoglycemia stimulates a number of counter-regulatory mechanisms that antagonize the effects of insulin and help to maintain the glucose concentration within fairly narrow limits. The role of the counter-regulatory mechanisms is more apparent when frank hypoglycemia is induced by an excess of insulin. Such mechanisms include release of epinephrine, cortisol, glucagon, and growth hormone — all of which inhibit insulin action and exert hyperglycemic effects. The crucial role of the nervous system in evoking hormonal release has been demonstrated in animal studies in which the responses to hypoglycemia were investigated after ablation of neural tissue.

Patients with asthma may show poor counter-regulation to insulin-induced hypoglycemia and also may exhibit secondary (reactive) hypoglycemia after a hyperglycemic stimulus. The frequency of this abnormality is such that some years ago the changes in blood glucose concentration were used as a diagnostic test in patients with allergic disease. At that time it was suggested that the abnormal glucose response might be indicative of relative adrenal insufficiency. It is now known, however, that the poor counter-regulation to hypoglycemia occurs in the presence of normal cortisol, growth hormone, and epinephrine responses; glucagon concentrations have not been examined (Morris 1971; Morris et al. 1973). The abnormality may involve altered tissue responsiveness to available hormone. One such mechanism relates to the disturbance of beta adrenergic receptor function that follows administration of adrenergic bronchodilators. Whether abnormalities of response to other hormones also contribute to the hypoglycemia is not known.

Influence of Medications Used in the Treatment of Asthma on Glucose Metabolism. Several of the agents used in the treatment of asthma are diabetogenic in that they induce hyperglycemia and complicate management of patients with overt diabetes. The effectiveness of corticosteroids in promoting gluconeogenesis and inhibiting insulin action in peripheral cells is such that these agents are used as a diagnostic test in patients with suspected latent diabetes. In patients with normal pancreatic reserve, the initial hyperglycemic effects of corticosteroid are followed by enhanced secretion of insulin and preservation of normal glucose homeostasis. In patients with diminished reserve, hyperglycemia or frank diabetes may occur. Corticosteroids usually do not induce ketotic diabetes unless the patient has underlying diabetes mellitus. Corticosteroids, however, may induce hyperosmotic coma which occurs even in the absence of ketosis when blood glucose concentration is markedly elevated. Hyperglycemia or diabetes mellitus may be an early complication of corticosteroid therapy. Because of the frequency of blood glucose abnormalities during steroid therapy, glucose concentrations (plasma or urine) should be monitored periodically in all patients who receive steroid therapy.

Corticosteroids complicate the management of patients with diabetes mellitus and often increase the requirements for insulin treatment. When patients receive an alternate day program of steroid therapy, it may be necessary to employ an alternate day program of insulin therapy as well. When both treatments are given on alternate-day schedules, the pattern of hyperglycemia and/or glocusuria is indicative of the onset and duration of corticosteroid action; glucosuria begins 4 to 10 hours after steroid administration, persists for 18 to 24 hours and then abates.

The hyperglycemic effects of adrenergic agents have been mentioned previously. Mechanisms by which these agents induce hyperglycemia include enhanced gluconeogenesis by the liver, suppression of insulin secretion, and inhibition of insulin action on peripheral glucose uptake. The result of these effects is to make more glucose available for tissues (such as the brain) that are totally dependent on glucose as a source of energy. In the presence of beta adrenergic blockade, failure of inhibition of peripheral glucose uptake results in a lower blood glucose response to administered epinephrine and poor counter-regulation to hypoglycemia.

Theophylline has dual and somewhat antagonistic effects on glucose metabolism. One action involves enhancement of insulin secretion. The other involves inhibition of insulin action in peripheral tissue. Thus, administration of theophylline may be associated with reactive hypoglycemia if the patient has considerable pancreatic reserve and can synthesize increased quantities of insulin. Alternatively, the primary effect of theophylline may be diabetogenic if pancreatic reserve is decreased. In most patients, glucose homeostasis is normal, but plasma insulin levels are elevated.

Insulin Allergy. (See also Chapter 54.) Administration of insulin for diabetes mellitus may be associated with clinical insulin hpersensitivity. Most of the insulin used therapeutically is derived from beef or pork pancreas and contains an amino acid sequence that differs slightly from human insulin. Administered insulin therefore is perceived as a foreign protein, and the majority of patients treated with exogenous insulin have circulating anti-insulin antibodies. Additionally, methods used to complex insulin to provide longer-acting forms of therapy may further alter the protein and enhance antibody formation. In most patients, the presence of insulin antibodies does not appear to be of clinical significance except that the amount of insulin required for therapeutic purposes often is greater than that produced by the normal pancreas. The possibility that insulin antibodies or insulin-antibody complexes contribute to the development of the late vascular complications of diabetes, however, has not been excluded.

In some patients, insulin administration is associated with hypersensitivity reactions at the site of injection or, rarely, with systemic allergic reactions. Patients with insulin allergy may exhibit extraordinary insulin "resistance" and require enormous quantities of insulin for control of blood glucose concentrations. Hypersensitivity reactions can be modified sometimes by switching to a different insulin preparation (e.g., beef vs. pork, monocomponent insulin, "regular" non-complexed insulin), a change in the technique used for insulin injection, desensitization procedures, or in some instances, administration of corticosteroids. Fortunately, in many patients, diabetes can be controlled with non-insulin forms of therapy such as the oral hypoglycemic agents. This problem has been reviewed recently (Mattson et al., 1975; deShazo, 1978).

Thyroid

Disorders of the thyroid gland are relatively frequent causes of endocrine dysfunction. An association between primary thyroid disease and allergy therefore is not uncommon. As indicated previously, autoimmune mechanisms operate in a significant proportion of thyroid disease and may be associated with either hormone excess or hormone deficiency. Additionally, anti-thyroid antibodies are found in a considerable number of asymptomatic individuals. There is no evidence, however, that patients with allergic disease have an unusual frequency of autoimmunity.

In addition to autoimmune forms of thyroid disease, which may represent an incidental association in patients with allergy, therapy for asthma may be associated with other mechanisms of thyroid dysfunction. Pharmacologic quantities of iodide that are included in many antiasthmatic preparations or are administered as therapeutic adjuncts may inhibit synthesis of biologically active thyroid hormone. This phenomenon occurs commonly after acute administration of iodides, but in most individuals escape occurs during continued administration and normal quantities of thyroid hormone are synthesized. Occasionally the inhibition of synthesis persists and may give rise to clinical hypothyroidism and/or goiter secondary to compensatory TSH stimulation.

Formerly, local radiation of the tonsils, adenoids, cervical lymph nodes or thymus was used as a form of therapy in patients with allergic disorders. It now is known that such treatment, particularly in children, may be responsible for subsequent development of thyroid malignancy. Recent publicity about this association undoubtedly has de-creased the use of radiation to the head and neck. Patients who have received such therapy previously should be followed carefully with measurement of TSH and thyroid hormone levels, thyroid scan and, when indicated, thyroidectomy and/or administration of thyroid treatment in doses which suppress further hyperplasia of the gland.

Thyroid Function and Allergy. A number of case reports have suggested an adverse relationship between thyroid hormone excess and clinical asthma (Settipane et al., 1972; Bush et al., 1977). The exact mechanisms are poorly understood, since thyroid hormone usually enhances tissue responses to endogenous or exogenous catecholamines, possibly by increasing the availability of adrenergic receptors. These effects would be expected to improve the course of asthma rather than exacerbate the disease. Several factors may contribute to deleterious effects on asthma. One relates to the emotional lability which is a frequent component of hyperthyroidism. Dyspnea is another frequent manifestation of hyperthyroidism even in the absence of pulmonary disease and may result in part from the increased tissue requirements for oxygen and the associated increased work of breathing. Additionally, the increased rate of metabolism in hyperthyroidism is associated with enhanced clearance of a variety of substances, including therapeutic agents. Thus increased requirements for asthma medications may be due in part to the faster clearance of therapeutic agents and their consequent reduced duration of effect.

Because of the adverse effects on asthma it is particularly important that hyperthyroidism be controlled in asthmatic patients. However, beta adrenergic antagonists such as propranolol should not be used in patients with asthma. These agents are employed frequently to suppress signs and symptoms of hyperthyroidism, such as tachycardia and tremor, which are due to enhanced sensitivity to catecholamines. However, the use of these agents has been associated with exacerbations of asthmatic symptoms and may cause slight increases in airway resistance even in normal individuals (Beumer, 1974).

Hypothyroidism decreases tissue oxygen

requirements and in some instances decreases the need for medications in patients with asthma. However, hypothyroidism suppresses respiratory drive. When hypothyroidism is associated with goiter, symptoms due to pressure effects in the neck and mediastinum are tolerated particularly poorly by patients with respiratory disease.

Parathyroid

DiGeorge's syndrome is a rare form of associated endocrine and immune deficiency due to congenital aplasia of the thymus and parathyroid glands, both of which are derived from the third and fourth pharyngeal pouches. Patients with this disorder usually exhibit tetany during the neonatal period, as a result of the hypoparathyroidism. The thymic aplasia is associated with absence of cell-mediated immunity and an inability to defend against viral, bacterial, or fungal infections. Patients rarely survive beyond one year of age, but thymic implants or administration of thymosin may restore cellular immunity (see Chapter 6).

Some of the features of DiGeorge's syndrome also are seen in patients with hypoparathyroidism developing beyond the postnatal period or during childhood. In this instance, the pathogenesis of the disease appears to result from an autoimmune disorder and may be associated with autoimmune adrenal disease and/or mucocutaneous candidiasis. Candidiasis may be the presenting feature of the disease. Some of these patients have disturbances of cell-mediated immunity and may be benefited by thymic implants or thymosin (Schulof and Goldstein, 1977; Goldstein, 1978).

Asthma Medications and Bone Disease. One of the most disturbing complications of asthma therapy relates to the induction of osteopenia by chronic corticosteroid therapy. Corticosteroids have numerous effects on substances concerned with bone metabolism, including vitamin D, parathyroid hormone, and calcitonin. Corticosteroids interfere with hydroxylation of vitamin D to form the active metabolites, 1,25-dihydroxycholecalciferol and 24,25-dihydroxycholecalciferol, which are needed for absorption of calcium from the gastrointestinal tract and mineralization of bone. Corticosteroids also increase the release of PTH and CT but may interfere with their action in target tissue. The overall effect is to cause negative calcium balance, demineralization of bone, enhanced bone resorption, and decreased bone formation, resulting in osteopenia and fractures with minor trauma. Theophylline also enhances secretion of PTH and contributes further to the demineralization of bone and negative calcium balance.

At present there is no satisfactory way of correcting the osteopenia other than by discontinuing corticosteroid therapy to stop progression of the bone disease. Preliminary studies of vitamin D and calcium administration suggest that this therapy is not helpful and may sometimes result in vitamin D intoxication (Swedlund, 1978). The value of additional therapy with large doses of sodium fluoride is still unclear. Similarly, there is little experience about the potential usefulness of therapy with the active metabolites of vitamin D that are most concerned with bone formation.

Thymus

In part, thymic effects on immune function are mediated by a humoral factor (hormone). This factor, called thymosin, is synthesized by thymic epithelial cells, which contain typical endocrine secretory granules. The chemical properties of thymosin have not been fully characterized but a peptide-rich preparation derived from calf thymus has been utilized for clinical trials in patients with DiGeorge's syndrome and other disorders associated with thymic hypoplasia with suggestive improvements in immunocompetence (Goldstein, 1978).

References

Atkinson, J. P., and Frank, M.: Effect of cortisone therapy on serum complement components. J. Immunol. *111*:1061, 1973.

Atuk, N. O., Blaydes, M. C., Westervelt, F. B., and Wood, J. E.: Effect of aminophylline on urinary excretion of epinephrine and norepinephrine in man. Circulation *35*:745, 1967.

Baxter, J. D., and Forsham, P. H.: Tissue effects of glucocorticoids. Am. J. Med. *53*:573, 1972.

Berger, W., Pollock, J., Kiechel, F., et al.: Immunoglobulin levels in children with chronic severe asthma. Ann. Allergy *41*:67, 1978.

Bernal, J., DeGroot, L. J., Refetoff, S., et al.: Absent nuclear thyroid hormone receptors and failure of T_3-induced TRH suppression in the syndrome of peripheral resistance to thyroid hormone. *In* Robbins, J., and Braverman, L. E. (eds.): *Thyroid Research.* Elsevier, Excerpt. Medica, 1976, p. 316.

Beumer, H. M.: Adverse effects of beta-adrenergic receptor blocking drugs on respiratory function. Drugs *7*:130, 1974.

Bourne, H. R., Lichtenstein, L. M., Melmon, K. L., et al.: Modulation of inflammation and immunity by cyclic AMP. Science *184*:19, 1974.

Brown, J., Solomon, D. H., Beall, G. N., et al.: Autoimmune thyroid diseases — Graves' and Hashimoto's. Ann. Int. Med. *88*:379, 1978.

Bush, R. K., Erlich, E. N. and Reed, C. E.: Thyroid disease and asthma. J. Allergy Clin. Immunol. *59*:398, 1977.

Carryer, H. M., Sherrick, D. W., and Gastineau, C.: Occurrence of allergic disease in patients with adrenal cortical hypofunction. J.A.M.A. *172*:1356, 1960.

Conolly, M. E., and Greenacre, J. K.: The lymphocyte-adrenoceptor in normal subjects and patients with bronchial asthma. J. Clin. Invest. *58*:1307, 1976.

deShazo, R. D.: Insulin allergy and insulin resistance: Two immune reactions. Postgrad. Med. *63*:85, 1978.

Duvic, M., Steinberg, A. D., and Klassen, L. W.: Effect of the antiestrogen, nafoxidine, on NZB/W autoimmune disease. Arthritis and Rheumatism *21*:414, 1978.

Ellul-Micallef, R., Borthwick, R. C., and McHardy, G. J. R.: The time-course of response to prednisone in chronic bronchial asthma. Clin. Sci. Mol. Med. *47*:105, 1974.

Ellul-Micallef, R., and Fenech, F. F.: Effect of intravenous prednisolone in asthmatics with diminished adrenergic responsiveness. Lancet *2*:1269, 1975.

Fauci, A. S., Dale, D. C., and Balow, J. E.: Glucocorticosteroid therapy: Mechanisms of action and clinical considerations. Ann. Int. Med. *84*:304, 1976.

Goldstein, A. L.: Thymosin: Basic properties and clinical potential in the treatment of patients with immunodeficiency diseases and cancer. Antibiot. Chemother. *24*:47, 1978.

Green, M., and Lim, K. H.: Bronchial asthma with Addison's disease. Lancet *1*:1159, 1971.

Harris, P. W. R., and Collins, J. V.: Bronchial asthma with Addison's disease. Lancet 1:1349, 1971.

Helderman, J. H., and Strom, T. B.: Emergence of insulin receptors upon alloimmune T cells in the rat. J. Clin. Invest. *59*:338, 1977.

Kumar, L., Miklich, D. R., and Morris, H. G.: Plasma 17-OH corticosteroid concentrations in children with asthma. J. Pediatrics *79*:955, 1971.

Lamprecht, S. A., Zor, U., Salomon, Y. et al.: Mechanism of hormonally induced refractoriness of ovarian adenyl cyclase to luteinizing hormone and prostaglandin E_2. J. Cyclic Nuc. Res. *3*:69, 1977.

McKenzie, J. M., and Zakarija, M. LATS in Graves' disease. Rec. Progr. Horm. Res. *33*:29, 1977.

Mathe, A. A. and Knapp, P. H.: Decreased plasma free fatty acids and urinary epinephrine in bronchial asthma. New Engl. J. Med. *281*:234, 1969.

Mattson, J. R., Patterson, R., and Roberts, M.: Insulin therapy in patients with systemic insulin allergy. Arch. Int. Med. *135*:818, 1975.

Merimee, T. J.: Spontaneous hypoglycemia in man. Adv. Int. Med. *22*:301, 1977.

Morris, H. G.: Delayed recovery of blood glucose after insulin hypoglycemia in asthma: A manifestation of beta-adrenergic blockade? J. Allergy *47*:110, 1971.

Morris, H. G.: Growth and skeletal maturation in asthmatic children: Effect of corticosteroid treatment. Pediatric Res. *9*:579, 1975.

Morris, H. G., DeRoche, G., and Caro, C. M.: Detection of synthetic corticosteroid analogs by the competitive protein-binding radioassay. Steroids *22*:445, 1973.

Morris, H. G., DeRoche, G., and Earle, M. R.: Urinary excretion of epinephrine and norepinephrine in asthmatic children. J. Allergy Clin. Immunol. *50*:138, 1972.

Morris, H. G., DeRoche, G., and Earle, M.: Effect of corticosteroid treatment on urinary epinephrine response to induced hypoglycemia in asthmatic children. J. Pharm. Exp. Therap. *184*:180, 1973.

Morris, H. G., DeRoche, G., Winkler, S. M., and Caro, C. M.: Effect of oral prednisone on the measurement of plasma steroid concentrations by the competitive protein-binding radioassay. J. Pediatrics *85*:248, 1974.

Morris, H. G., and Jorgensen, J. R.: Recovery of endogenous pituitary-adrenal function in corticosteroid-treated children. J. Pediatrics *79*:480, 1971.

Morris, H. G., Jorgensen, J. R., and Jenkins, S. A.: Plasma growth hormone concentration in corticosteroid-treated children. J. Clin. Invest. *47*:427, 1968.

Morris, H. G., Rusnak, S. A., Selner, J. C., and Barnes, J.: Diminished leukocyte cAMP responses to adrenergic stimulation after therapeutic administration of beta-adrenergic agonists. Chest 73:Suppl. 973, 1978.

Mukherjee, C., Caron, M. G., and Lefkowitz, R. J.: Catecholamine-induced subsensitivity of adenylate cyclase associated with loss of β-adrenergic receptor binding sites. Proc. Nat. Acad. Sci. *72*: 1945, 1975.

Nelson, H. S., Raine, D. Jr., Doner, H. C., and Posey, W. C.: Subsensitivity to the bronchodilator action of albuterol produced by chronic administration. Am. Rev. Respir. Dis. *116*:871, 1977.

Parker, C. W., and Smith, J. W.: Alterations in cyclic adenosine monophosphate metabolism in human bronchial asthma. I. Leukocyte responsiveness to β-adrenergic agents. J. Clin. Invest. *52*:48, 1973.

Rasmussen, H.: Ionic and hormonal control of calcium homeostasis. Amer. J. Med. *50*:567, 1971.

Rasmussen, H., Goodman, D. B. P., and Tenenhouse, H.: The role of cyclic AMP and calcium in cell activation. CRC Crit. Rev. Biochem. *1*:95, 1972.

Reimer, L. G., Morris, H. G., and Ellis, E. F.: Growth of asthmatic children during treatment with alternate-day steroids. J. Allergy Clin. Immunol. *55*:224, 1975.

Roth, J., Kahn, R., Lesniak, M. A., et al.: Receptors for insulin, NSILA-S, and growth hormone: Applications to disease states in man. Rec. Progr. Horm. Res. *31*:95, 1975.

Roubinian, J. R., Papoian, R., and Talal, N.: Androgenic hormones modulate autoantibody responses and improve survival in murine lupus. J. Clin. Invest *59*:1066, 1977.

Schreiber, A. D.: Clinical immunology of the corticosteroids. Progr. Clin. Immunol. *3*:103, 1977.

Schulof, R. S., and Goldstein, A. L.: Thymosin and the endocrine thymus. Adv. Int. Med. *22*:121, 1977.

Settipane, G. A., Pudupakkam, R. K., and McGowan, J. H.: Corticosteroid effect on immunoglobulins. J. Allergy Clin. Immunol. *62*:162, 1978.

Settipane, G. A., Schoenfeld, E., and Hamolsky, M. W.: Asthma and hyperthyroidism. J. Allergy Clin. Immunol. *49*:348, 1972.

Sutherland, E. W.: Studies on the mechanism of hormone action. Science *177*:401, 1972.

Swedlund, H. A., Van Dellen, R. G., Kelly, P. J., and Jowsey, J. O.: Bone changes in asthmatic patients receiving corticosteroids, calcium, vitamin D, and fluoride. Proc. 34th Annual Meeting American Acad. Allergy, Feb. 1978, Abst. #77.

Szentivanyi, A.: The beta-adrenergic theory of the atopic abnormality in bronchial asthma. J. Allergy *42*:203, 1968.

Talwar, G. P., Pandian, M. R., Kumar, N., et al.: Mechanism of action of pituitary growth hormone. Rec. Progr. Horm. Res. *31*:141, 1975.

Volpe, R.: The role of autoimmunity in hypoendocrine and hyperendocrine function with special emphasis on autoimmune thyroid disease. Ann. Int. Med. *87*:86, 1977.

Harold S. Nelson, M.D.

51

Pregnancy and Allergic Diseases

Pregnancy gives rise to significant physiologic alterations in the mother, many of which have an influence on allergic disorders and their treatment. Circulatory changes and changes in fluid balance, energy metabolism, hormonal levels, immune reactivity, and pulmonary physiology are likely to have the greatest impact on allergic diseases and their management.

CIRCULATION AND FLUID BALANCE

During pregnancy there is retention of sodium and water. Maternal circulating blood volume increases by about one liter, largely owing to an increase in plasma volume. Even in the absence of edema, interstitial fluid increases by 3 to 4 liters. A 30- to 60-percent increase in cardiac output results from greater stroke volume despite little change in heart rate. The increased cardiac output is required to supply the uterine and placental circulations and to supply the metabolic needs of the fetus. The increase in extracellular fluid has been viewed as a reservoir to protect the increased circulating volume against temporary fluid deficits.

Severe attacks of asthma frequently lead to dehydration and reduced plasma volume, and fluid replacement during status asthmaticus is important to ensure adequate cardiac output while avoiding overhydration. If corticosteroids are required to control the patient's asthma, the pregnant woman with already increased extracellular fluid is vulnerable to excess fluid retention and edema, and sodium intake must be monitored carefully.

ENERGY METABOLISM

The net effect of increased levels of estrogens, progesterone, and cortisol, plus placental insulinase and human placental lactogen (HPL), in the pregnant woman is the production of insulin resistance. To compensate for this decreased ability to utilize glucose for energy, free fatty acids are more easily mobilized from fatty tissue through HPL. Fasting may produce maternal hypoglycemia. Since glucose can pass from the fetus to the mother, prolonged maternal fasting can deplete fetal glycogen and promote fetal gluconeogenesis at the expense of its supply of amino acids. In the mother with severe asthma and inadequate caloric intake, it may be advisable to administer parenteral glucose to protect the fetus from the deleterious effects of maternal hypoglycemia.

HORMONAL LEVELS

The predominant hormone of early pregnancy is chorionic gonadotropin, whereas elevated levels of progesterone and estrogen are most prominent in the second and third trimesters. Total plasma cortisol is markedly elevated, owing to a decreased rate of catabolism. However, transcortin, the cortisol binding protein, also is elevated, so that

675

physiologically active, free cortisol is not appreciably altered throughout most of pregnancy. Late in pregnancy, the free cortisol fraction does rise, perhaps due to replacement of cortisol from transcortin by progesterone, but evidence of increased glucocorticoid effect is equivocal.

Since there is no indication of any material alteration in pharmacologic effects of corticosteroids during pregnancy, the usual dosages should be prescribed when corticosteroid therapy is indicated. Diamine oxidase (histaminase) levels often are significantly elevated during pregnancy, but there is no evidence that the catabolism of endogenous histamine is altered significantly.

IMMUNE REACTIVITY

The fetus contains histocompatibility antigens inherited from the father and thus represents a paternal allograft to the mother. Not only does an interface between fetal and maternal tissue exist in the placenta, but fetal leukocytes and erythrocytes penetrate this barrier to the maternal circulation frequently.

Maternal cell-mediated immunity appears to be depressed during pregnancy, and there is evidence for blocking antibodies to fetal antigens. These factors in combination with the placental barrier may account for maternal tolerance of the fetus.

Prolonged skin graft survival and depressed delayed-hypersensitivity skin tests have been reported in pregnancy, but longitudinal study in several hundred tuberculin-positive women found no significant depression of tuberculin skin tests at any stage of pregnancy (Present and Comstock, 1975). An enhanced susceptibility to tuberculosis in pregnancy and to certain viral infections (infectious hepatitis, influenza, smallpox, varicella, and poliomyelitis) also may reflect a depression in cell-mediated immunity. Even though B, T, and null lymphocytes are normal in number during pregnancy, responsiveness of T lymphocytes to PHA stimulation and in mixed lymphocyte reaction is depressed during pregnancy. Suppression of lymphocyte function may be due to suppressive serum factors. Suppressive factors in the maternal circulation during pregnancy include: human chorionic gonadotropin

(HCG), pregnancy zone (PZ) protein, human chorionic somatomammotropin, progesterone, cortisol, alpha feto-protein, alpha-2 macroglobulin, and trophoblast specific antigen. The serum inhibitory effect increases progressively throughout pregnancy but is no longer present by 1 week following delivery. Suppression of T lymphocyte function appears greater in the immediate vicinity of the placenta than in the peripheral blood. This suggests that immunosuppressive substances that play the greatest role in maintaining pregnancy arise in the fetus or uterus (Tomoda et al., 1976). Suppression of maternal immune responses appears to be limited to cell-mediated immunity; humoral antibody responses to specific antigens are intact. There is evidence, in fact, that maternally manufactured IgG antibody, perhaps in complex with placental antigen, coats fetal cells in the placenta, blocking recognition of these fetal antigens by maternal lymphocytes. Circulating immune complexes containing IgG, C3, and probably a fetal or placental antigen appear to occur regularly in pregnancy (Masson et al., 1977). These immune complexes share many features with the circulating blocking factors that have been described in some patients with progressive malignancies.

PULMONARY PHYSIOLOGY

Despite the marked elevation of the resting diaphragm toward term, caused by the gravid uterus, pulmonary function is altered relatively little by normal pregnancy. A decrease in functional residual capacity does occur consistently, with an average reduction of 15 percent by term (Cugell et al., 1953). Inspiratory capacity is increased, probably due to some increased mobility of the ribs, so that vital capacity and total lung capacity are not significantly altered.

Measurements of air flow, such as the maximum breathing capacity and one-second forced expiratory volume, remain unchanged. A more sensitive measurement, specific conductance, has been variously reported to be unchanged or increased.

Beginning in the first trimester, minute ventilation is increased, resulting from an increased tidal volume. Since this increased ventilation consistently exceeds that required to compensate for the increased metabolism of pregnancy, it represents "hyperventilation" and results in a fall in Pa_{CO_2} and mild alkalosis. The Pa_{O_2} is not altered. There is a large gradient between maternal and fetal Pa_{O_2}. The Pa_{O_2} on the maternal side of the placenta ranges from 91 to 96 mm Hg (sea level), whereas the fetal Pa_{O_2} ranges between 21 and 29 mm Hg (Bartels et al., 1962). Compensatory mechanisms allow the fetus to prosper at this low oxygen tension, but there is little margin to tolerate maternal hypoxemia, especially if it is associated with alkalosis, which increases the affinity of maternal hemoglobin for oxygen, further reducing the oxygen supply available to the fetus. It is clear that the normal alkalosis due to the hyperventilation of pregnancy plus the hypoxemia and alkalosis of moderate asthma could result in severe fetal hypoxia.

EFFECT OF PREGNANCY ON THE COURSE OF BRONCHIAL ASTHMA

In reviewing studies of asthma in pregnancy, asthma was found to improve in 36 percent of patients, remain the same in 41 percent, and worsen in 23 percent (Gluck and Gluck, 1976). Information from other studies suggests that in women with mild asthma prior to pregnancy there is likely to be little change or some improvement in asthma during pregnancy. In women with severe asthma, there is likely to be a worsening of symptoms if any change occurs at all. In a majority of women, in general, if asthma worsened during the initial pregnancy, it will worsen during subsequent pregnancies (Williams, 1967). In about a third of women studied by Williams, there was a tendency toward progressive worsening of symptoms with successive pregnancies, which was a reflection of a worsening of their asthma in general.

Effect on Asthma of Drugs Used to Terminate Pregnancy. Recent changes in obstetrical practices require consideration of the possible deleterious effect on asthma of prostaglandins employed to terminate pregnancy. $PGF_{2\alpha}$ is a potent bronchoconstrictor, and asthmatics are many times more sensitive to this effect than are normal individuals. PGE_2 is normally a bronchodilator.

However, both $PGF_{2\alpha}$ and PGE_2, when given intravenously in doses employed for inducing abortion, caused increased airway resistance, even in normal women, indicating that prostaglandin should be used with special caution in women with asthma.

THE EFFECT OF PREGNANCY ON OTHER ALLERGIC DISEASES

Allergic Rhinitis. Nasal congestion is not an uncommon complaint in pregnant women who have no history of nasal complaints when not pregnant. Hyperemia of the nasal mucosa develops by the end of the first trimester and progresses throughout pregnancy. Mucosal edema is prominent particularly in the last 2 months before term. These mucosal changes parallel the increased levels of estrogen and progesterone, which probably cause them.

Women who have allergic or vasomotor rhinitis prior to pregnancy may experience a marked increase in symptoms of rhinorrhea and nasal obstruction due to the additive effect of the nasal changes of pregnancy on their underlying rhinitis. Paradoxically, some women may experience improvement in chronic rhinitis during pregnancy.

Atopic Dermatitis. The effect of pregnancy on atopic dermatitis, if any, is unpredictable. It may improve or exacerbate and may fluctuate during the course of a single pregnancy and between different pregnancies in the same patient. This suggests that pregnancy has little effect on atopic dermatitis.

EFFECT OF BRONCHIAL ASTHMA ON THE COURSE OF PREGNANCY

A significant increase in risks of premature birth (7.4 vs. 5 percent), low birth weight (7.4 vs. 3.7 percent), and neonatal mortality (18.5/1000 vs. 8/1000) have been reported in pregnancy in Norwegian women with asthma (Bahna and Bjerkedal, 1972). Among pregnant patients with bronchial asthma treated in a New York hospital, the incidence of premature birth was 8.9 percent compared to 6.2 percent for nonasthmatic controls (Schaefer and Silverman, 1961). In another study from New York, the asthmatic group as a whole did not have a significantly increased incidence of premature labor or low-birth-weight infants, but women with severe asthma had a 35 percent incidence of low-birth-weight infants and a 28 percent perinatal mortality (Gordon et al., 1970).

EFFECTS OF DRUGS USED TO TREAT ASTHMA ON THE DEVELOPMENT OF THE FETUS AND THE COURSE OF PREGNANCY

A primary concern regarding drugs administered during pregnancy is their possible effect on the development and survival of the fetus. Substances of molecular weight less than 600 daltons readily cross the placenta, whereas those greater than 1000 do not. Since most therapeutic agents are in the range of 250 to 400 daltons, they can be assumed to enter the fetal circulation. This placental transmission is modified somewhat by the extent of protein binding and ionization of the drug, both of which impede movement across the membrane.

Effects on Fetal Development. An adverse effect of a drug on fetal development is most likely to occur during the organ-forming period, which in the human fetus is the thirteenth to the fifty-sixth day of gestation. Following the first trimester, most organs already are formed, but in the urogenital system and the central nervous system maturation continues to occur, making them still susceptible to adverse drug effects.

Documentation of teratogenic effect of drugs currently employed in the United States and Canada is sparse, and the incidence of teratogenesis due to drugs is presumed to be extremely low. However, there is suggestive evidence that women who bear children with congenital abnormalities take more drugs during the first trimester of their pregnancy than do those with normal offspring, and it is prudent to avoid any unnecessary drug during this critical period.

Certain drugs are considered to be contraindicated during pregnancy. *Tetracycline* is capable of retarding fetal skeletal growth and causing dental enamel dysplasia and discoloration. *Iodides* can block fetal organic binding to elemental iodine, leading to decreased thryroid hormone synthesis, increased TSH, and goiter. Goiters have caused respiratory obstruction and death in the newborn. *Live viral vaccines* should be avoided during pregnancy. Not only is there a possibility of harm to the fetus, but there is also a possibility of severe infection in the mother, owing to her compromised cell-mediated immunity.

There is no evidence that suggests adverse fetal effects from antihistamines or bronchodilators (Greenberger and Patterson, 1978). The case with corticosteroid drugs is not so clear. In rodents, corticosteroids produce an increased incidence of cleft palate and also suppress placental growth, resulting in an increased incidence of abortions. An early study of a small group of women who received steroids throughout pregnancy suggested an increased incidence of placental insufficiency, acute fetal distress, and stillbirth associated with their use (Warrell and Taylor, 1968). However, several subsequent studies have failed to confirm this high incidence of fetal effects, though the incidence of cleft palate may increase with corticosteroid use. In general it appears safer to use corticosteroids in mothers with severe asthma which does not respond to non-steroidal bronchodilators than to risk fetal damage associated with severe maternal asthma and resultant hypoxemia (Schatz et al., 1975).

Effects on Uterine Function. In addition to possible effects on fetal development, drugs can influence the fetus indirectly through effects on uterine blood flow or on uterine contractility and the progress of labor.

Beta adrenergic agonists are capable of relaxing uterine as well as bronchial smooth muscle. Beta sympathomimetics recently have been employed by intravenous infusion to control premature labor. No deleterious effects have been reported on the fetus or newborn as a result of this therapy.

A possible deleterious effect that might result from the use of beta$_2$ adrenergic agonists in pregnancy is dilation of the vascular bed supplying the skeletal muscles, with consequent shunting of blood away from the uterus. Evidence suggests that both epinephrine and salbutamol induce this effect, but it is unclear if the changes are clinically significant.

Although beta adrenergic agonists and

theophylline can reduce uterine contractions, neither agent has been shown to slow the progress of labor in doses customarily employed for bronchodilation.

TREATMENT OF BRONCHIAL ASTHMA AND ALLERGIC RHINITIS IN PREGNANCY

Current knowledge does not suggest a need for major alteration in the approach to therapy of bronchial asthma or allergic rhinitis in pregnancy, except for avoidance of tetracycline and those antihistamine preparations and combination bronchodilators that contain iodides (e.g., Ornade, Quadrinal). Recent studies do not confirm the earlier concerns of increased congenital anomalies associated with the use of piperazine antihistamines. Medications employed during the first trimester should be limited to those absolutely required for the patient's well being. Throughout pregnancy, the principal concern should be control of the patient's asthma and avoidance of hypoxemia. Corticosteroids should be used only when absolutely necessary to control asthma adequately. If patients have received systemic corticosteroids during pregnancy, supplemental steroids should be considered at the time of delivery to protect the mother against stress in case her adrenal-pituitary axis is still suppressed. An acceptable schedule is cortisone acetate 100 mg intramuscularly every 8 hours throughout labor and delivery. The infant should be observed carefully, in addition, for the uncommon complication of adrenal insufficiency, but routine administration of steroids to the infant is not indicated at birth.

IMMUNOTHERAPY

Severe systemic reactions to injections of allergy extract can be accompanied by lower abdominal cramping pain and uterine bleeding. Spontaneous abortion has been reported in a few such instances, but several studies attest that administration of allergy immunotherapy throughout pregnancy increases neither the risk of fetal loss, even in the face of systemic reactions, nor the risk of congenital malformation (Metzger et al., 1978). Nevertheless, hyposensitization medication should be administered with particular caution during pregnancy. Dosage should be increased slowly while building to maintenance dosage. During the patient's pollen season, when the possibility of inducing a constitutional reaction is more likely, dosage should be reduced.

There would appear to be no reason to limit immunotherapy while nursing. Although it is possible that antigen may be secreted in milk in trace amounts, absorption by the infant is considered to be clinically unimportant. Allergic sensitivity that occurs in early infancy usually is related to food allergens, which should not be contained in the allergy extract used for hyposensitization.

BREAST FEEDING

Immunology of Breast Milk. Human colostrum and milk contain macrophages, neutrophils, and lymphocytes, which appear to retain their immune or inflammation-promoting properties when ingested by the infant (Beer and Billingham, 1975). Immunoglobulins of all major classes also are present, particularly secretory IgA, which is the predominant immunoglobulin of breast secretions. During the first 4 to 5 days postpartum, levels of IgA are four to eight times as high in breast secretions as in the serum, indicating local production by IgA-secreting plasma cells which have migrated from the gastrointestinal lymphoid tissue (Ogra and Ogra, 1978; see also Chapter 2). The colostrum and breast milk appear to provide important immune defenses for the infant's gastrointestinal tract, particularly during the early neonatal period. Breast feeding during this period should be viewed as a further contribution of the mother to the infant's ability to survive in an extrauterine environment, and not merely as a source of nutrition.

Drug Excretion in Breast Milk. Most drugs can be secreted into the mother's milk, usually in concentrations that may approach those of maternal serum (Stirrat, 1976). Of the drugs frequently used to treat allergic diseases, *tetracycline* and *iodides,* both of which occur in breast secretions in the same concentration as in the serum, should not be taken by nursing mothers.

Unbound *theophylline* is rapidly secreted into the milk, resulting in milk levels about three-quarters of those in the serum at the same time. Infant hyperirritability has been related to maternal theophylline therapy, though in most nursing infants this has not been a problem. Usually the infant will not ingest over 8 mg of theophylline per liter of milk, and this amount will not be sufficient to cause symptoms. If there is any question of drug effect on the nursing infant, the amount of theophylline in the milk can be reduced by postponing ingestion of theophylline until just after nursing. *Beta adrenergic bronchodilators* also are secreted into the milk, but problems have not been reported from their use by nursing mothers.

Corticosteroids are secreted into the breast milk in amounts of less than 1 percent of the administered dose. *Antihistamines* also are secreted into the milk in trace amounts, but no effects other than sleepiness have been associated with their use by nursing mothers.

References

Bahna, S. L., and Bjerkedal, T.: The course and outcome of pregnancy in women with bronchial asthma. Acta Allergol. 27:397, 1972.

Bartels, H., and Moll-Metcalfe, J.: Physiology of gas exchange in the human placenta. Am. J. Obstet. Gynecol. 84:1714, 1962.

Beer, A. E., and Billingham, R. E.: Immunologic benefits and hazards of milk in maternal-perinatal relationship. Ann. Intern. Med. 83:865, 1975.

Cugell, D. W., Frank, N. R., Gaensler, E. A., and Badger, T. L.: Pulmonary function in pregnancy: I. Serial observations in normal women. Am. Rev. Tubercul. 67:586, 1953.

Gluck, J. C., and Gluck, P. A.: The effects of pregnancy on asthma: A prospective study. Ann. Allergy 37:164, 1976.

Gordon, M., Niswander, K. R., Berendes, H., and Kantor, A. G.: Fetal morbidity following potentially anoxigenic obstetric conditions: VII. Bronchial asthma. Am. J. Obstet. Gynecol. 106:421, 1970.

Greenberger, P., and Patterson, R.: Safety of therapy for allergic symptoms during pregnancy. Ann. Intern. Med. 89:234, 1978.

Masson, P. L., Delire, M., and Cambiasco, C. L.: Circulating immune complexes in normal human pregnancy. Nature 266:542, 1977.

Metzger, W. J., Turner, E., and Patterson, R.: The safety of immunotherapy during pregnancy. J. Allergy Clin. Immunol. 61:268, 1978.

Ogra, S. S., and Ogra, P. L.: Immunologic aspects of human colostrum and milk: I. Distribution characteristics and concentrations of immunoglobulins at different times after the onset of lactation. J. Pediatr. 92:546, 1978.

Present, P. A., and Comstock, G. W.: Tuberculin sensitivity in pregnancy. Am. Rev. Resp. Dis. 112:413, 1975.

Schaefer, G., and Silverman, F.: Pregnancy complicated by asthma. Am. J. Obstet. Gynecol. 82:182, 1961.

Schatz, M., Patterson, R., Zeitz, S. O'Rourke, J., and Melam, H.: Corticsoteroid therapy for the pregnant asthmatic patient. J.A.M.A. 233:804, 1975.

Stirrat, G. M.: Prescribing problems in the second half of pregnancy and during lactation. Obstet. Gyn. Surv. 34:1, 1976.

Tomoda, Y., Fuma, M., Miwa, T., Saiki, N., and Ishizuka, N.: Cell-mediated immunity in pregnant women. Gynecol. Invest. 7:280, 1976.

Warrell, D. W., and Taylor, R.: Outcome for the fetus of mothers receiving prednisolone during pregnancy. Lancet 1:117, 1968.

Williams, D. A.: Asthma and pregnancy. Acta Allergol. 22:311, 1967.

James G. Easton, M.D.

52

Anaphylaxis

"Anaphylaxis" is an immunologically mediated systemic reaction often of great severity and potentially always life-threatening. The clinical reaction has its onset usually within a brief period, often within minutes, following exposure to antigen to which sensitization previously has been established. Without adequate treatment, the reaction generally is rapidly progressive. "Anaphylactoid" reactions are clinically identical or similar reactions resulting from nonimmune (or unknown) mechanisms.

PHYSIOPATHOLOGY

Human anaphylaxis is most frequently mediated through IgE antibodies that bind to surface receptors of basophils and tissue mast cells (Freedman, 1976). Such cells are considered to be "sensitized." When antigen combines with this specific cell-bound IgE, a sequence of biochemical events occurs that results in release of chemical mediators from the cell. These mediators in turn bind to specific receptors on smooth muscle and blood vessels and induce smooth muscle contraction, increased small blood vessel permeability and increased mucous gland secretion, which account for the various symptoms of anaphylaxis. Histamine and slow-reacting substance of anaphylaxis (SRS-A) appear to be the most important of these mediators, but several others have also been implicated (Austen, 1971) (see Chapter

11). Anaphylactoid reactions are presumed to occur as the result of release of the same chemical mediators, but through pathways that do not involve antigen and antibody. The specific mechanism whereby certain agents cause this nonimmune release from mast cells and basophils is incompletely understood, but in some instances may be due to complement activation through the alternative pathway or direct facilitation of calcium transport into the mast cell. Since this type of reaction does not require prior sensitization, it may occur without previous exposure to the causative agent. Since different organ systems may be involved to different degrees, a varied spectrum of signs and symptoms may result from the same basic mechanisms.

CLINICAL MANIFESTATIONS

Clinical manifestations of anaphylactic and anaphylactoid reactions may vary considerably in severity, particularly in the early stages. In general, the sooner symptoms occur after antigen exposure, the more rapid and severe the clinical reaction is apt to be. It is important for the clinician to appreciate that even though symptoms may be initially relatively mild, the potential for progression to severe and even irreversible stages is always present. *Thus, prompt and effective treatment must be provided even when initial symptoms appear mild.* Symptoms may be

681

TABLE 52–1 SYMPTOMS OF ANAPHYLAXIS

Skin
Flushing
Pruritus
Urticaria
Angioedema

Respiratory
Stridor and horseness (indicative of upper airway and
  laryngeal obstruction)
Wheezing and chest tightness (bronchial spasm)
Cough and dyspnea (upper or lower airway obstruction)
Possible progress to severe hypoxemia and respiratory failure

Cardiovascular
Rapid weak pulse
Hypotension
Cardiovascular shock (due to fluid loss from increased vascular
  permeability; may also be neurogenic)
Possible cardiac arrhythmias

Gastrointestinal
Dysphagia
Nausea
Vomiting
Diarrhea

Other
Apprehension
Sweating
Incontinence
Convulsions (rarely)

classified by organ systems, as noted in Table 52–1.

Occasionally, it may be difficult to distinguish anaphylaxis from neurogenic shock or vasovagal syncope. Urticaria, angioedema, and airway obstruction do not occur with these syndromes, although apprehension may produce hyperventilation. Generally, the patient is flushed in early stages of anaphylaxis, whereas with the other syndromes the patient is quite pale.

CAUSATIVE AGENTS

The list of substances implicated as causes of anaphylactic or anaphylactoid reactions is extremely large, and it is impractical to attempt to list them all. Discussion is confined to those agents most frequently responsible for these reactions.

Antibiotics. Penicillin and the synthetic penicillin derivatives are the most frequent reported causes of anaphylaxis (Caldwell and Cliff, 1974). Some patients sensitive to penicillin also react to the cephalosporins, although the exact incidence of this cross-reactivity is not clearly established. Other antibiotics have been incriminated less frequently (see Chapter 54).

OTHER DRUGS. ACTH and insulin both may cause anaphylaxis. Aspirin occasionally may be responsible for true anaphylaxis, but the majority of reactions to aspirin occur from nonimmune mechanisms. Dextran, iron-dextran compounds, codeine, morphine, and radiographic contrast media all appear to act through non–antibody-mediated pathways. Gamma globulin injections may induce anaphylactoid or anaphylactic reactions.

HETEROLOGOUS ANTISERA. These are used in the prophylaxis or treatment of tetanus, diphtheria, rabies, botulism, and poisonous snake bites. Immune sera derived from hyperimmunized horses or other animals contain foreign serum proteins to which the patient may be sensitive.

STINGING INSECTS. These belong to the Hymenoptera order and include the bee, wasp, yellow jacket, and hornet. Also belonging to this order of insets are ants, some species of which have a stinging apparatus and may produce anaphylaxis, e.g., the imported fire ant (see Chapter 53).

FOODS. Almost any food may cause anaphylaxis, but those most frequently responsible are eggs, milk, nuts, legumes, fish, and shellfish. Ordinarily, anaphylaxis is caused by food ingestion, but in unusually sensitive patients, inhalation of food particles can induce symptoms.

POLLEN EXTRACTS. Anaphylaxis may occur from allergen injections used in immunotherapy for allergic rhinitis or allergic asthma. In unusually sensitive patients, even skin testing can induce anaphylaxis.

PROPHYLAXIS

Prevention of anaphylaxis and anaphylactoid reactions should be a major concern of all physicians. Although this is not always possible, certain procedures and precautions can minimize its frequency. A carefully obtained history regarding possible previous reactions of this type should be a part of the history of all patients. Avoidance of the offending substance is *the* most important means of preventing severe reactions. It is important to identify "hidden sources" of exposure and to make sensitive patients aware of these sources. For example, aspirin may be found in "cold" or "sinus" preparations, and food additives or colors may be found in a large variety of foods and medicines.

Immunizations should be kept current (or instituted in unimmunized patients) to avoid the potential need for antisera. The indiscriminate use of antibiotics should be avoided, since minimizing exposure to these agents lessens the possibility of sensitization. When antibiotics are indicated, they should be given orally if possible. When penicillin must be used in a presumably sensitive patient or when antisera must be administered, skin testing may rule out or identify the patient likely to react. If there is no alternative agent, a desensitization program may be carried out. This is discussed further in Chapter 54. Skin testing material

that will reliably reflect "allergy" is not available for other antibiotics or other drugs.

Patients known to be sensitive to substances producing anaphylactic or anaphylactoid reactions should be instructed to wear Medic-Alert bracelets or necklaces clearly indicating the substance to which they are at risk. (These can be obtained from Medic-Alert Foundation, Turlock, California.)

TREATMENT

Anaphylaxis represents a medical emergency, and satisfactory treatment depends upon early recognition and prompt institution of therapy. Table 52–2 lists the essential and desired equipment for the treatment of anaphylaxis. These items should be kept together in a quickly accessible "emergency kit" in the physician's office or clinic. Table 52–3 summarizes therapeutic steps discussed below.

Epinephrine is the most important drug in emergency treatment (Weiser, 1972). It is given intramuscularly in doses of 0.2 to 0.5 ml of a 1:1000 aqueous solution as soon as anaphylaxis is recognized. It may be repeated at 15-minute intervals as indicated. Blood pressure should be monitored during this time, since hypotension is an indication for more aggressive therapy. If the initiating agent was given by injection (including insect stings), a tourniquet to retard venous return should be placed proximal to the injection

TABLE 52–2 EQUIPMENT FOR TREATMENT OF ANAPHYLAXIS

Epinephrine for injection, 1:1000, aqueous
Diphenhydramine (Benadryl) for injection
Aminophylline for injection
Oxygen
Tourniquets
Syringes and needles for subcutaneous and
  intravenous administration of medications
Intravenous solutions (normal saline as a starter)
Sphygmomanometer
Metaraminol (Aramine)
Corticosteroid for intravenous administration
Sodium bicarbonate for intravenous injection
Laryngoscope and endotracheal airways
Tracheostomy set

TABLE 52-3 SUMMARY OF TREATMENT OF ANAPHYLAXIS

Initial Therapy of Anaphylaxis

Apply tourniquet above the site of injection if appropriate.

Give epinephrine, 0.2–0.5 ml IM, repeated every 15 minutes if necessary—plus 0.1 ml into site of injection, if applicable.

Establish IV site; use normal saline.

Administer oxygen.

Monitor blood pressure.

Give diphenhydramine (Benadryl), 10–25 mg for infants and younger children and 25–50 mg for older children IV.

Secondary Therapy

Give aminophylline, 5–6 mg/kg diluted in 25–50 ml saline for bronchospasm. Administer IV over 10–15 minutes and repeat every 4–6 hours as appropriate.

Administer hydrocortisone 100–250 mg IV, every 4–6 hours.

Prevent aspiration of vomitus.

Isotonic saline IV for hypotension: albumin or plasma may be appropriate.

Metaraminol (Aramine), 0.4 mg/kg in 500 ml IV fluid for hypotension.

---

site if possible and 0.1 ml of aqueous epinephrine given directly into the injection site to retard systemic absorption. The tourniquet should be removed temporarily every 10 to 15 minutes. Frequently these measures will successfully terminate the reaction, but it is generally advisable to observe the patient until all signs and symptoms of anaphylaxis have cleared.

Antihistamines are given following the initial use of epinephrine and should be continued probably for 24 hours past any symptoms whatsoever. If the reaction appears severe, antihistamines can be administered intravenously. Diphenhydramine (Benadryl) is given slowly (over a 10-minute period) in doses of 10 to 25 mg in infants and younger children and 25 to 50 mg in older children and adolescents. This dose may be repeated at 3- to 4-hour intervals. Hypoxemia with anaphylaxis occurs secondary to hypotension and/or airway edema, and supplementary oxygen should be administered early in the course of treatment. With severe or ques-

tionably severe reactions, it is essential that an intravenous infusion be initiated early, both to administer saline or volume expanders to control hypotension (see below) and to administer medication. Aminophylline, 5 to 6 mg/kg diluted in 25 to 50 ml of isotonic saline solution, is given by intravenous infusion over a 10 to 15 minute period if there are signs of bronchospasm; it is repeated every 4 to 6 hours as needed. Measures to prevent aspiration from vomiting also should be taken; and vital signs, particularly blood pressure, must be monitored frequently. An intubation tray and a tracheostomy tray and personnel expert in their use should be immediately available.

Administration of corticosteroids is thought to be an important adjunct of therapy of anaphylactic reactions. It must be remembered, however, that it may take 4 to 6 hours for pharmacologic effect from these agents. Thus, corticosteroids are considered only after the previously described measures have been instituted. A dose of 100 to 250 mg of hydrocortisone or its equivalent is given intravenously every 4 to 6 hours.

Physiologic studies indicate that an acute loss of plasma volume is primarily responsible for the cardiovascular shock that may occur with anaphylaxis (Hanashiro and Weil, 1967). Restoration of plasma volume with intravenous administration of colloid material, preferably albumin, is indicated in such cases. However, rapid infusion of isotonic saline can be used initially if colloid material is not immediately available, since prompt expansion of the plasma volume is essential. A vasopressor agent such as metaraminol (Aramine) 0.4 mg/kg given slowly in 500 ml of intravenous fluid also may be used as an emergency measure.

Anaphylactic or anaphylactoid reactions that do not respond to the above measures should be managed further in a hospital intensive care unit. Appropriate medical personnel should be contacted to make themselves readily available for anticipated problems associated with severe anaphylaxis. Endotracheal intubation or tracheostomy may be necessary with severe airway obstruction and other late complications such as cardiac arrhythmias, hypoxic seizures, and metabolic acidosis necessitate the use of specialized hospital equipment, including cardiac monitors and a blood gas laboratory.

Patients with known previous anaphylactic reactions from agents that may be encountered where medical care is not immediately available (insect stings, food ingestion, etc.) should be supplied with emergency medication for personal use *and should be properly instructed in its use*. They should also be instructed to go to the nearest medical facility immediately after use of the emergency medication. Injectable epinephrine is the medication of choice and is available in disposable syringes containing a measured dose. Patients who experience upper airway edema and obstruction as their primary manifestation, particularly those in whom there is serious question regarding their ability or willingness to self-administer epinephrine, can be given inhaled epinephrine in the form of a freon-propelled nebulizer such as the Medihalor-Epi. Isoproterenol or other beta adrenergic agents should not be used, since they do not vasoconstrict appreciably and may, in fact, dilate mucosal blood vessels and accentuate mucosal swelling. Oral antihistamines should be readily available. Although they are of some benefit in delaying progression of symptoms, they are not a replacement for epinephrine.

References

Austen, F.: Histamine and other mediators of allergic reactions. *In* Samter, M. (ed.): *Immunological Disease*, 2nd ed. Boston, Little, Brown and Co., 1971, Vol. 1, pp. 332–355.

Caldwell, J.R., and Cliff, L.E.: Adverse reactions to antimicrobial agents. J.A.M.A. *230*:77, 1974.

Freedman, S.O.: Anaphylaxis and serum sickness. *In* Freedman, S.O., and Gold, P. (ed.): *Clinical Immunology*, 2nd ed. Hagerstown, Md., Harper and Row, 1976, pp. 78–91.

Hanashiro, P.K., and Weil, M.H.: Anaphylactic shock in man. Arch. Intern. Med. *110*:129, 1967.

Weiszer, I.: Allergic emergencies. *In* Patterson, R. (ed.): *Allergic Diseases*. Philadelphia, J.B. Lippincott Co., 1972, pp. 327–340.

53

James G. Easton, M.D.

Insect Allergy

The most severe form of insect allergy, anaphylaxis from stings, is caused almost entirely by insects of the order Hymenoptera (bee, wasp, yellow jacket, hornet, and fire ant) and is mediated by IgE antibodies. Stings of these insects are responsible for at least 40 deaths per year in the United States (Barnard, 1973). It is likely that more go unrecognized because insect stings may not be considered as a cause of unexplained sudden death. Reactions to insect stings may be classified as local or systemic. With the immediate systemic type there is a pattern of progression of reaction severity with successive stings, beginning with mild urticaria and progressing to more severe urticaria associated with angioedema, upper (laryngeal) airway obstruction, bronchospasm, and eventually to cardiovascular collapse. It is essential, therefore, that all physicians recognize the potential seriousness of even mild generalized symptoms and make certain that patients with systemic insect sensitivity receive appropriate medical management.

TREATMENT

The treatment of anaphylaxis is discussed in the preceding chapter. Placing a tourniquet proximal to the sting when possible and local application of ice are measures that the patient or parent can institute immediately and which will retard systemic venom absorption. In addition, if a stinger has been left in place (the honey bee is the only insect to do so), "flicking" it out with a knife blade or similar instrument, taking care not to squeeze additional venom into the wound, is advised. Folk remedies such as placing mud or baking soda on the sting are not useful and should not be employed.

Patients with previous systemic reactions should have available at all times emergency medication, preferably injectable epinephrine, for immediate use. In the case of school-age children, especially younger ones, it may be necessary to keep such medication in several locations, e.g., home, school, and baby-sitter's home. All persons responsible for supervising the child should be instructed in the administration of epinephrine. Injectable epinephrine is available by prescription in disposable syringes containing a premeasured dose, usually 0.5 ml. A dose of 0.2 to 0.5 ml should be used, based on the size of the patient. Most frequently the epinephrine comes in a packaged "emergency kit" (e.g., ANAKIT) that also contains a tourniquet and antihistamine tablets. *Antihistamines are not a substitute for epinephrine* but may be of some additional therapeutic value. Freon-propelled epinephrine nebulizers (e.g., Medihaler-Epi, Primatene) may be prescribed for those patients in whom there is question about the ability or willingness of patient or family to administer injectable medication. Several inhalations will minimize or prevent airway obstruction and may result in systemic absorption of sufficient quantity to achieve a therapeutic effect. (Isoproterenol may increase airway edema and obstruction as the result of its dilating effects on mucosal blood vessels, and it should *not* be prescribed.) Instruction in the proper self-administration of emergency medication is particularly important in older children and adolescents who may be stung while fishing or camping or in other situations in which medical care is not readily available. The patient should seek medical attention as quickly as possible after undertaking emergency measures.

PREVENTION

Prevention of insect stings is a crucial part of insect sting therapy. Table 53–1 lists several practical measures to discourage the possibility of insect stings. The patient and parents should be made aware of the importance of these measures and instruction should be repeated periodically in these and emergency medical measures.

Immunotherapy. All patients who have had systemic hypersensitivity symptoms resulting from insect stings, even if mild, are candidates for immunotherapy (hyposensitization). It is necessary, however, to distinguish anaphylactic reactions from toxic reactions resulting from multiple stings, since the

TABLE 53–1 MEASURES TO MINIMIZE INSECT STINGS

1. Do not go barefoot out of doors.
2. Wear light colored clothes when possible. White probably is the least attractant to insects, though dull blue and green seem equally inert.
3. Do not wear scented cosmetics out of doors, e.g., colognes, perfumes, hair sprays.
4. Avoid areas that are likely to harbor stinging insects, such as garbage or trash cans or areas, flower beds, fields of clover, and picnic grounds.
5. Insect nests or hives in the areas of a patient's home or work should be destroyed by professional exterminators.

latter are not indications for this type of treatment. Unusually large local reactions to stings, often defined as those that extend beyond the nearest major joint, occasionally are encountered. The existence of venom-specified IgE antibody has been demonstrated in the serum of 50 percent of patients with this type of reaction, but whether or not immunotherapy is indicated is at present not completely resolved (Reisman and Arbesman, 1975). Recent evidence strongly suggests that immunotherapy with venom extracts is considerably more effective than that with whole body extracts (which have been the major source of antigenic material for Hymenoptera immunotherapy for many years [Lichtenstein, 1974]). With the current availability of venom extracts, the effectiveness of immunotherapy for Hymenoptera sting sensitivity should be improved greatly.

At the time of publication of this text, Hymenoptera venom extracts for skin testing and immunotherapy have been available commercially for several months. General guidelines for their use in children are established, but some questions remain unanswered.

All patients with a history of systemic symptoms following Hymenoptera stings, and probably those who have had large local reactions (as defined previously) should be skin tested using the appropriate venom extract if there has been positive identification of the insect. In those instances in which identification is not conclusive (the majority of cases), testing should be done using all extracts, e.g., honey bee, yellow jacket, yellow hornet, white faced hornet, and wasp. Appropriate positive and negative controls using histamine and diluent should be performed simultaneously. Clearly positive or negative results are obtained in about 95 percent of patients tested, although a positive test is not necessarily indicative of anaphylaxis with a subsequent sting.

Patients with negative skin tests are not treated with immunotherapy; however, those with a clear history of serious systemic manifestations should be advised on the use of emergency medication. Patients with a history of severe reactions (airway compromise, hypotension, or severe urticaria) and positive tests are candidates for immunotherapy. There is some controversy about the most appropriate management of patients with a history of mild to moderate urticaria or large local reactions and positive skin tests. Some of these patients will develop more serious reactions with subsequent stings; however, the exact frequency is not known. It is our current policy to discuss the advantages and disadvantages of immunotherapy with parents of these patients and to proceed with treatment if it is desired. We feel that all patients in this category should be instructed in the proper use of emergency medications since there is no accurate way to determine which patients will develop progressively more severe reactions.

Results of clinical trials using venom immunotherapy indicate at least a 90 percent success rate defined as no reaction other than the normally expected local erythema and pain following a deliberate re-sting under controlled conditions. The necessary length of treatment is unknown at present, but some evidence suggests it may be necessary to continue indefinitely. Possible serious side effects or toxicity from long-term therapy are also unknown at present, although experience with beekeepers who are repeatedly stung (injected with venom) and with patients who have so far received several years of treatment suggests these may not occur.

Further details regarding skin testing and treatment schedules can be found in the package insert (Pharmacia Laboratories, Piscataway, N. J.) and in Lichtenstein, 1979; Reisman, 1979; Yunginger, 1979.

Although the majority of systemic hypersensitivity reactions due to insects are caused by the winged Hymenoptera, it is now recognized that the imported fire ant and the harvester ant, also members of the Hymenoptera order and equipped with a similar stinging apparatus, can be responsible for this type of reaction (James, 1976). Fire ants are found in the Gulf Coast areas while harvester ants have a widespread distribution in the western United States. The venom from these insects also may prove to be superior for diagnostic testing and treatment (Pinnas, 1977).

INHALANT INSECT SENSITIVITY

Our atmosphere is frequently contaminated with debris from a variety of insects, and the debris may produce allergic upper or lower respiratory tract disease when inhaled. The best documented allergies of this type are caused by the May and Caddis flies in the Lake Erie area (Gutman, 1972). Cockroaches have also been implicated. Immunotherapy has been successful in some cases.

LOCAL REACTIONS TO BITING INSECTS

Some patients develop unusually large local reactions to the salivary secretions of biting insects such as flies, mosquitos, and fleas; and at times these appear to be urticarial in nature. The possible immune nature of these reactions has been incompletely investigated, and the use of immunotherapy is not warranted in such cases. However, there are several measures which can be used in the management of such patients to reduce the frequency of bites and/or the inflammatory reaction that results from bites. Avoidance of areas known to be heavily infested, if possible, is an obvious measure, as is the use of insecticides in and around the house. Topical insect repellents also are of some benefit. The use of large doses of oral thiamine hydrochloride (vitamin B_1) has been recommended in the past as a means of reducing the frequency of bites. However, a controlled study in military personnel showed no significant benefit compared to a placebo control; and since studies evaluating side effects from such doses have not been carried out in children, this therapy is not recommended. Local corticosteroid creams are helpful in controlling the pruritus from insect bites; besides the discomfort from pruritus, repeated scratching may lead to secondary infection. Oral antihistaminic agents also are of some value. Perhaps of equal importance is reassurance of the patient and parents that these other insect bites are not associated with the same potential for anaphylactic reactions as are Hymenoptera stings.

References

Barnard, J.H.: Studies of 400 hymenoptera sting deaths in the United States. J. Allergy Clin. Immunol. *52*:259, 1973.

Gutman, A.A.: Allergens and other factors important in atopic disease. *In* Patterson, R. (ed.): *Allergic Diseases*. Philadelphia, J.B. Lippincott Co., 1972, pp. 117–118.

James, F.K., Jr., et al.: Imported fire ant hypersensitivity. J. Allergy Clin. Immunol. *58*:108, 1976.

Lichtenstein, L.M., Valentine, M.D., and Sobotka, A.K.: A case for venom treatment in anaphylactic sensitivity to hymenoptera sting. N. Engl. J. Med. *290*:1223, 1974.

Lichtenstein, L. M., Valentine, M. D., and Sobotka, A. K.: Insect allergy: The state of the art. J. Allergy Clin. Immunol. *64*:5, 1979.

Pinnas, J.L., et al.: Harvester ant sensitivity: In vitro and in vivo studies using whole body extracts and venom. J. Allergy Clin. Immunol. *59*:10, 1977.

Reisman, R.E., and Arbesman, C.E.: Stinging insect allergy. Ped. Clin. North. Amer. *22*:185, 1975.

Reisman, R. E.: Stinging insect allergy. (Editorial). J. Allergy Clin. Immunol., *64*:3, 1979.

Yunginger, J. W.: The sting revisited. (Editorial). J. Allergy Clin. Immunol. *64*:1, 1979.

54

John A. Anderson, M.D.

Drug Allergies

Adverse reactions to drugs are important considerations when choosing therapeutic or diagnostic agents. Comprehensive drug surveillance studies of medical inpatients have shown a 4.8 percent incidence of adverse reactions to drugs prescribed (Jick et al., 1970). In a representative sample (40 percent children) of an American ambulatory prepaid health plan population, 3.2 percent of the total health care was involved with the treatment of adverse drug reactions. Surveillance studies in pediatric inpatients have revealed adverse drug reaction rates of 6.5 percent (Whyte and Greenan, 1977). In a study of adverse reactions in children that led to admission to a university hospital over a 3-year period, 2 percent of hospital admissions were due to adverse drug reactions (McKenzie et al., 1976). Most children with drug reactions were over 6 years of age. Forty percent of the reactions were severe or life-threatening and contributed to four deaths. Drug-related deaths among 26,462 adult inpatients admitted to acute-disease medical wards over a 5-year period were reported to be 0.9 per 1000 patients (Porter and Jick, 1977).

The incidence of drug-induced anaphylaxis in a large group of medical inpatients was 0.6 cases per 1000 patients (Boston Collaborative Drug Study, 1973). Hypersensitivity reaction rates in children have been presumed to be lower than this, since the degree and length of exposure to drugs is generally less in children than adults. However, these rates vary between centers, between inpatients and outpatients, with the severity of illness, and with the number and types of drugs used. In McKenzie and colleagues' (1976) series of drug reactions in children leading to hospitalization, 11 of 3,556 were classified "allergic," giving an incidence rate of 3.1 cases per 1000 patients.

DEFINITION OF ADVERSE REACTIONS TO DRUGS

DeSwarte (1972) has classified adverse reactions to drugs into seven categories:

Drug overdose: An excessive dose taken accidentally or deliberately.

Drug side effect: A therapeutically undesirable but often unavoidable pharmacologic action of a drug.

Secondary drug effect: An effect of a drug which is unrelated to its primary pharmacologic action and which may not occur in every patient.

Drug interaction: The action of an administered drug upon the effectiveness or toxicity of another drug. This may occur through interference with drug metabolism or drug absorption, or competition for protein-binding for drug receptor sites.

Drug idiosyncrasy: A quantitatively abnormal response to a drug, differing from its pharmacologic effects. This response may resemble a hypersensitivity reaction clinically but does not involve immune mechanisms. Enzyme deficiencies may be responsible in some cases.

Drug hypersensitivity: True hypersensitivity, or "allergic" reactions, occur only in some patients and are unrelated to the drug dose and to the pharmacologic action of the drug. Unlike an idiosyncratic reaction, hypersensitivity reactions *are* related to immune mechanisms. Unfortunately, more allergic drug reactions are *suspected* than proven to be on an immune basis. In addition, drug reactions may involve nonimmune mediator release, which may mimic hypersensitivity reactions.

When dealing with children, two additional adverse drug classifications must be considered:

Teratogenicity: Drugs used by the mother during early pregnancy may cause developmental defects in the fetus.
Maternal-fetal or maternal-child toxic drug transfer: Toxic effects upon the newborn from drugs taken by the mother shortly before or after birth. Drugs may be transferred to the fetus through the placenta, and to the newborn through breast milk.

PATHOGENESIS OF HYPERSENSITIVITY DRUG REACTIONS

The pathogenesis of hypersensitivity drug reactions has been reviewed by Parker (1975). Few drugs are "complete" antigens, which produce allergic reactions by virtue of their ability to combine with proteins. Generally it is a metabolic derivative of the drug, rather than the native molecule itself which is able to combine with protein. Thus, antibodies demonstrated in drug reactions usually are directed to the haptenic metabolic breakdown product of the drug, covalently linked to a tissue protein. If the enzymatic reaction involving drug metabolism is located in a specific organ or tissue, antigen will accumulate in that tissue, making the tissue a primary target of the hypersensitivity response. An immune reaction also may develop to the tissue carrier protein, thus creating organ- or tissue-directed autoimmunity. Identification of the metabolic pathways involved in formation of important drug antigens is difficult. Each drug may have numerous metabolites, and in most instances, not all metabolites have been identified.

The role of the protein carrier in promoting the immune response to drugs is not clear. It appears, however, that the carrier protein is able to interact with thymus-derived (T) lymphocytes, which initiate the immune response in a manner similar to initiation of responses to antigens in general.

As with most immune reactions that involve mediator release, drug antigens must be multivalent in order to permit aggregation of antibody molecules, complement activation and/or other mediator release. Univalent haptens (whether free drugs or unconjugated drug metabolites) combine with receptors without bridging and can inhibit antigen-induced mediator release by competing with the multivalent drug antigens for antibody. Univalent metabolites, thus, may protect the host from hypersensitivity reactions to drugs.

MODIFYING FACTORS IN HYPERSENSITIVITY DRUG REACTIONS

The type of drug and frequency of use affects the incidence of adverse reactions. For instance, penicillin and its derivatives, which are among the most frequently used antibiotics, are the drugs most commonly implicated in producing hypersensitivity reactions in children (Jick et al., 1970; Whyte and Greenan, 1977). The route of administration of a drug is an important factor in the development of drug hypersensitivity. Topical administration, for example, is more likely to induce sensitization than drug administration by other routes. Oral drug administration appears to be least sensitizing, whereas parenteral administration lies between these extremes. Intravenous administration is less likely to sensitize than intramuscular or subcutaneous administration. The greater the number of different drugs administered, the more severely ill the patient, or the longer the duration of therapy, the greater is the risk that an allergic drug reaction will develop. Intermittent therapy also is more likely to induce sensitivity than is continuous therapy.

Berkowitz (1953) demonstrated an eight-fold greater incidence in allergic drug reactions in atopic compared with nonatopic children. However, Stember and Levine (1973) studied 1043 adult subjects who were screened for atopic allergy and for penicillin hypersensitivity by history and by aeroallergen and penicillin skin tests. These investigators found no difference in the reaction rate to penicillin: 3.9 percent in the atopic group; 4.5 percent in the non-atopic group. On the other hand, a genetic predisposition to hypersensitivity reactions to specific drugs is suggested by the association between HLA haplotypes and specific drug allergy, such as that between HLA-B7 and allergic reactions to insulin in diabetic patients (Bertrams and Grüneklee, 1977).

Hepatic involvement by infectious and malignant diseases may alter drug metabolism and predispose toward drug reactions. Immunosuppression may increase the sensitization potential of weakly allergenic drugs, possibly by inhibiting suppressor–T cell function and enhancing specific IgE antibody production to drug antigens (VanArsdel, 1978).

The vast majority of patients with infectious mononucleosis treated with ampicillin develop a macular rash. The mechanism by which this viral infection predisposes to an adverse reaction to ampicillin is unclear. Most ampicillin rashes are *not* associated with infectious mononucleosis, but many could be related to other viral infections (Kerns et al., 1973).

CLINICAL MANIFESTATIONS OF HYPERSENSITIVITY DRUG REACTIONS

Hypersensitivity drug reactions can be categorized to a large extent according to the classification of Gell and Coombs. As pointed out in Chapter 10, however, although this classification is an oversimplification of mechanisms of immune tissue injury, it is useful for purposes of discussion.

Anaphylactic Reactions (Type I). Anaphylactic reactions are considered to be mediated by homocytotrophic (mainly IgE) antibody. Urticaria is the mildest manifestation of this reaction. Urticaria may or may not be associated with angioedema, allergic rhinitis, conjunctivitis, and bronchial asthma. In its severest form, airway obstruction, shock, circulatory collapse, coma, and death may occur. Generally, anaphylaxis is less severe in children than adults and is most frequently manifested by urticaria, commonly associated with angioedema.

In the Boston Collaborative Drug Surveillance Program (1973) study of over 11,000 consecutively hospitalized medical patients, anaphylaxis was recorded eight times (0.6/1000 cases). It was found most commonly following blood transfusion (2.4/1000 exposures) and following parenteral administration of drugs such as aqueous penicillin and cephalothin sodium (1.3/1000 exposures). In a series of children (McKenzie et al., 1976) admitted with a drug reaction, four were admitted because of L-asparaginase-induced anaphylaxis (1/1000 admissions) and three were cases of Stevens-Johnson syndrome caused by diphenylhydantoin and antibiotic therapy. The American Academy of Pediatrics, Committee on Drugs (1973), lists drugs and biologicals considered to be major causes of anaphylactic reactions in children (Table 54-1). Penicillins lead the list of offenders.

Cytotoxic Reactions (Type II). Cytotoxic immune reactions to drugs result from antibodies directed against tissue or organs with which drugs have interacted. Tissues or organs that may be involved include the skin, kidney, lungs, heart, liver, muscles, peripheral nerves, and formed elements of the blood. Tissue damage may result from direct drug reaction with tissue, in which tissue-haptenic groups become targets of antibodies or from drug-induced tissue alteration that changes tissue immunogenicity and results in tissue directed antibodies (autoimmunity).

Immune hemolytic anemia can result from adherence of drugs to red cells — exemplifying the first mechanism listed above. Drugs that have been implicated include penicillin, quinine, quinidine, dipyrone, aminosalicylic acid, mephenytoin, stibophen, cephalothin, and phenacetin (Parker, 1975). This type of hemolytic anemia must be differentiated from that of red cell, glucose-6-phosphate dehydrogenase enzyme deficiency which can be triggered by such drugs as primaquine, nitrofurantoin, aspirin in large doses, and sulfonamides (Chan et al., 1976).

In immune thrombocytopenia, anti-platelet drug complex antibodies or anti-drug antibodies are involved. Drugs that may cause this condition include quinine, quinidine, meprobamate, chlorothiazide, thiouracils, chloramphenicol, the sulfonamides, and allyl-isopropyl-acetylcarbomide (Sedormid) (Parker, 1975). Drugs that induce immune granulocytopenia include aminopyrine, phenylbutazone, phenothiazines, the thiouracils, the sulfonamides, anticonvulsants, and tolbutamide (Parker, 1975).

TABLE 54–1 MAJOR DRUG CAUSES OF ANAPHYLAXIS* IN CHILDREN

Antibiotics
  Penicillin and its semisynthetic derivatives
  Cephalosporins (Keflex, Fafocin, Loridine, Keflin)
  Chloramphenicol
  Colymycin
  Kanamycin
  Polymyxin B
  Streptomycin
  Tetracyclines
  Troleandomycin (Cyclomycin, Tao)
  Vancomycin (Vancocin)
  Amphotericin B (Fungizone)

Biologicals
  Foreign serums (antitoxins, antilymphocyte globulins {ALG})
  Chymotrypsin
  Gamma globulin and other blood products
  Asparaginase
  Polypeptide hormones (ACTH, TSH, insulin)
  Influenza vaccine
  Tetanus toxoid
  Measles and other egg-based vaccines

Injectable medications
  Iron dextran (Imferon)
  Dextran
  Methylergonovine maleate (Methergine)
  Nitrofurantoin
  Intravenous narcotics

Local anesthetics

Aspirin (acetylsalicylic acid)

Diagnostic agents
  Radiocontrast media
  Sulfobromophthalein (B.S.P.)

Allergy extracts

*In those cases in which an immune mechanism has *not* been identified, the term "anaphylactoid" (anaphylaxis-like) reaction should be used.

Adapted from Committee on Drugs, American Academy of Pediatrics, 1973.

Immune Complex Reactions (Type III). Serum sickness is a systemic immunologically mediated reaction, in which soluble antigen-antibody complexes are formed and induce tissue damage largely by activating complement. Clinically, the reaction is characterized by fever, urticaria, lymphadenopathy, arthritis and, on occasion, neuritis, vasculitis and glomerulonephritis. In primary serum sickness, a latency period of 7 to 12 days is usual. The drug injection site may become erythematous and swollen 24 to 72 hours before onset of systemic signs. Generally, the symptoms are self-limited, lasting 4 to 5 days. IgG, IgM, and IgE antibodies can be involved. IgE antibodies occur early and are associated with clinical signs, particularly the urticaria and local skin reaction. Drug anti-IgG and anti-IgM complexes probably also are involved in the initial reaction. Complement is activated by the antigen-antibody complex and mediates damage to the vessel walls or glomeruli. The patient recovers when antigen has been cleared from the body.

The incidence of primary serum sickness depends on the amount and source of the serum administered. Studies of reactions to anti-rabies horse serum show a relationship to age in that only 12.3 percent of the children under 5 years had serum sickness, whereas 46.3 percent of those over 15 years had reaction. This increased reaction rate may also be related to an increased dose given because of increased size (Arbesman and Reisman, 1972).

Although the term "serum sickness" originated as a description of reactions to heterologous serum (primarily horse serum), a similar symptom complex can be induced by drugs. The most common drugs that induce serum sickness-like reactions are penicillins, sulfonamides, thiouracils, cholecystographic dyes, diphenylhydantoin, aminosalicylic acid, and streptomycin (Parker, 1975).

Cell Mediated Reactions (Type IV). Cell mediated hypersensitivity is mediated by sensitized lymphocytes. Allergic contact dermatitis is an example of this reaction (see Chapter 32). Following the initial, usually topical, exposure to the drug, lymphocytes become sensitized and induce a dermatitis when the drug is re-administered. Potential contact sensitizers include antihistamines, ammoniated mercury compounds, bacitracin, benzocaine, ethylenediamine, fluorouracil, formaldehyde, glucocorticoids , idoxuridine, lanolin, neomycin, parabens, paraminobenzoic acid, sulfonamides, thimerosal, and iodochlorhydroxyquin. Of particular importance are drugs used in dermatologic preparations — for example, ethylenediamine, a stabilizer and basis of an antihistamine class, which cross-reacts with aminophylline. Topical sensitization to ethylenediamine can result in a systemic reaction when oral or intravenous aminophylline is administered. Patients sensitized to thimerosal or paraben preservatives also can develop a generalized reaction following the use of an injectable containing these preservatives.

The *in vitro* lymphocyte transformation test has been used to identify a long list of "drug reactions." The usefulness of this test in diagnosing cell mediated drug reactions in general is not clear, but it may be helpful in identifying certain drug allergens under specific circumstances (Rocklin, 1974).

CUTANEOUS MANIFESTATIONS OF HYPERSENSITIVITY DRUG REACTIONS

Skin eruptions are the commonest manifestations of drug allergy and can take almost any form, including urticaria and angioedema, maculopapular, morbilliform or erythematous eruptions, erythema multiforme, eczema, and erythema nodosum, photosensitivity and a fixed eruption. In addition, they may present with pruritus without any skin findings. The most severe drug-related reactions are exfoliative dermatitis and such vesicobullous eruptions as Stevens-Johnson syndrome and toxic epidermal necrolysis (Lyell's syndrome). Table 54–2 lists drugs associated with cutaneous reactions and their incidence among 22,227 consecutive medical inpatients (Arndt and Jick, 1976).

Urticaria may occur alone or as part of a serum sickness reaction. Almost any drug can be involved, but in children, the penicillins, aspirin, and injections of allergenic extracts are common causes. Urticaria and maculopapular rashes may occur as a result of viral infections, however, and an antibiotic or other drug may be mistakenly implicated as the cause of the eruption.

Exfoliative dermatitis is an erythematous, scaly eruption causing loss of the superficial layers of skin. It frequently is associated with systemic symptoms; it can follow other types of eruptions and can be fatal. Commonly implicated drugs include penicillin, sulfonamides, barbiturates, hydantoins, and occasionally, aminophylline.

Stevens-Johnson's and Lyell's syndromes. Stevens-Johnson syndrome is characterized by erythema multiforme (target) skin lesions, which may appear to be urticarial but also may enlarge to become

TABLE 54–2 ALLERGIC SKIN REACTIONS TO DRUGS

Drug	Reaction per 1000 Recipients*
Trimethoprim-sulfamethoxazole	59
Ampicillin*	52
Semisynthetic penicillins**	36
Blood, whole human**	35
Corticotropin	28
Erythromycin	23
Sulfisoxazole	17
Penicillin G*	16
Gentamicin sulfate**	16
Practolol	16
Cephalosporins*	13
Quinidine**	12
Plasma protein fraction	12
Dipyrone**	11
Mercurial diuretics**	9.5
Nitrofurantoin	9.1
Packed red blood cells*	8.1
Heparin*	7.7
Chloramphenicol	6.8
Trimethobenzamide HCL**	6.6
Phenazopyridine HCL	6.5
Methenamine	6.4
Nitrazepam*	6.3
Barbiturates*	4.7
Glutethimide	4.5
Indomethacin	4.4
Chlordiazepoxide*	4.2
Metoclopramide HCL	4.0
Diazepam*	3.8
Propoxyphene*	3.4
Isoniazid**	3.0
Guaifenesin and Theophylline*	2.9
Nystatin	2.9
Chlorothiazide**	2.8
Furosemide*	2.6
Isophane insulin suspension**	1.3
Phenytoin**	1.1
Phytonadione*	0.9
Flurozepan HCL*	0.5
Chloral hydrate*	0.2

Key:
*Drugs in series received by at least 1000 patients.
**Drugs in series received by 500–999 patients.
All other drugs listed; received by 100–499 patients.

Adapted from Arndt and Jick, 1976.

vesicular and bullous. The eruption involves not only the skin but also the mucous membranes of the conjunctivae, nose, mouth, and genitalia. Protracted illness, with malaise and even severe prostration, is common. The mortality rate is 2 percent (Böttiger, 1975). Corneal ulcerations may be followed by scarring and blindness.

Toxic epidermal necrolysis (Lyell's syndrome) is characterized by generalized erythema followed by desquamation. Healing without scarring may occur within 2 weeks. Mortality, however, may be up to 36 percent. In a review of 89 cases of Stevens-Johnson syndrome and Lyell's syndrome by Böttiger (1975), 40 percent of the patients were under 20 years of age and 87 percent of the patients had received prior drugs. Females predominated in the drug-treated group. Drugs were believed to have been etiologically important in approximately one-half of the group on drugs—most frequently, the long-acting sulfonamides, the penicillins, and the anti-epileptic drugs. *Mycoplasma pneumoniae* and *Staphylococcus aureus* were the most common infectious agents implicated.

Henock-Schönlein purpura (anaphylactoid purpura) in children occasionally has been reported to result from reactions to drugs, including salicylates (see Chapter 67).

Erythema nodosum is uncommon in children. In addition to infection, drugs have been implicated in causing the disorder and include iodides, bromides, penicillin, sulfonamides, and salicylates (see Chapter 35).

Drug photodermatitis. There are two types of photosensitivity drug reactions: phototoxic and photoallergic (see Chapters 34 and 35). Drugs implicated in causing phototoxic reactions include psoralens, topical coal tar, and demethylchlorotetracycline (VanArsdel, 1978). Drugs implicated in photoallergic reactions include phenothiazines, sulfonamides and griseofulvin. Bacterostatic agents, bithionol, and halogenated salicylamides used in soaps and topical medications also can induce reactions (VanArsdel, 1978).

Fixed drug eruptions present as edematous, round, pigmented, single or multiple skin lesions that may recur at the same location when the implicated drug is readministered. Pruritis is unusual, and there are no systemic symptoms. The reaction is felt to be immune, perhaps of cell mediated type, but this is not proved. Commonly suspected drugs include phenolphthalein, tetracycline, penicillin, barbiturates, sulfonamides, antipyretics, and quinine (DeSwarte, 1972).

Differential Diagnosis of Drug Rash

Children with rashes present a diagnostic dilemma. Although drug reactions may be suspected, other considerations must be kept in mind. In cases of urticarial lesions, urticaria pigmentosa, though uncommon, should be considered. Papular urticaria is a common consideration in children. It usually presents as "small hives" or firm papules or wheals, usually clustered on the extensor surfaces of the arms and legs, which appear as crops and last for 10 to 14 days. Fleas from domestic dogs and cats are responsible in over two-thirds of the cases (Wright, 1972).

Hereditary angioedema should be considered in cases of recurrent angioedema with pain but *without* pruritis and urticaria. The differential diagnosis between allergic contact dermatitis and atopic dermatitis sometimes is difficult.

Infections are the biggest problems in diagnosis. A viral exanthem must be considered, particularly when the presenting rash is maculopapular or erythematous in nature. Acute viral respiratory infections probably cause acute urticaria more frequently than generally appreciated. Viral exanthems in children may develop in sun-exposed areas and thus, may masquerade as "photodermatitis" (Gilchrest and Baden, 1974). Rash is not an uncommon manifestation of mycoplasma infection (Cherny et al., 1975).

Clinically, drug-induced toxic epidermal necrolysis (Lyell's syndrome) and staphylococcus (phage group 2) scalded skin syndrome (Ritter's disease) are indistinguishable (Margileth, 1975). Microscopic examination of freshly peeled skin in the involved area may help differentiate between the two. In staphylococcus-induced lesions, focally adherent granular cells are present in the stratum corneum. In the drug-induced form, one sees all the epidermal layers in various stages of degeneration (Amon and Dimond, 1976). In this group of severely ill children, Leiner's disease, an hereditary deficiency of C_5 (Jacobs and Miller, 1972) and mucocutaneous lymph node syndrome (Kawasaki's disease) also must be considered.

Finally, self-induced skin lesions, or dermatitis factitia, always should be in the differential diagnosis of drug-induced skin rash (Curian, 1973).

DRUG FEVER

Fever can be the single manifestation of an adverse reaction to a drug, or it may be coupled with or precede other manifestations, including dermatitis, vasculitis, or focal necrosis (Cluff and Johnson, 1964; see also Chapter 58). If there has been no previous drug sensitization, fever may begin about 7 to 10 days after initiation of drug therapy. Once sensitization has occurred, the fever may occur immediately after reintroduction of the drug.

The incidence of "drug fever" in children is low (Whyte and Greenan, 1977); however, fever occurs commonly after immunization with biologic materials and occasionally after transfusion of blood products. Common drugs that are associated with fever include aspirin, penicillin and other antibiotics, and hydantoin. Many other drugs have been associated with drug fever, but these ordinarily are used in adults (VanArsdel, 1978).

OTHER DRUG REACTIONS

The role of hypersensitivity in drug-induced inflammation of the liver, kidney, lungs, and small blood vessels is not well defined. Frequently, toxicity is suspected. An *immune mechanism* is suggested by (1) limited frequency of that form of reaction for a given drug, (2) a latent period between initiation of drug therapy and reaction, (3) "typical" immune reaction, signs, symptoms, or pathology, and (4) recurrence of similar symptoms or signs upon readministration of the drug in low dose. Conversely, a *toxic drug reaction* is suggested by (1) frequent association of that form of reaction with a particular drug, (2) rapid induction of signs and symptoms after administration of the drug, (3) absence of known previous exposure to the drug, and (4) no evidence of increasing sensitivity on serial drug exposure in the same patient (Parker, 1975).

Hepatitis. Many drugs have been implicated in inducing either cholestatic or hepatocellular liver changes (VanArsdel, 1978). Most reactions occur in adults. Little direct immunologic evidence exists to prove hypersensitivity. However, of significance in children is the association of aspirin-induced (ASA) hepatotoxicity with acute rheumatic fever, juvenile rheumatoid arthritis, and systemic lupus erythematosus. Hepatitis associated with juvenile rheumatoid arthritis (JRA) has been studied most extensively (Bernstein et al., 1977). Some patients with JRA receiving ASA show clinical signs of hepatic disease. In most cases, liver involvement is detected by serial enzyme determinations. In a series of 102 JRA patients, the serum glutamic oxaloacetic transferase level was elevated in 59 percent of the cases on at least one occasion. Younger children and those with higher ASA blood levels tend to have more liver involvement, but liver enzyme changes can occur at "safe" salicylate blood levels. These patients may metabolize salicylates abnormally or may be uniquely sensitive on some other basis to hepatotoxic effects of a metabolite of ASA. Hepatotoxicity has been reported recently in an 18 year old with Reiter's syndrome, who was treated with aspirin (Ricks, 1976). The association between HLA-B27 and Reiter's syndrome raises the question of a genetic susceptibility in patients with Reiter's syndrome to hepatic sensitivity to salicylates.

Pulmonary "Hypersensitivity" Reactions. A wide variety of drugs have been implicated in inducing an asthmatic type of reaction (Kounis, 1976). Some asthmatic reactions are simply manifestations of an anaphylactic reaction to specific drugs. With the vast majority of drug-induced reactions, however, an immune basis for the reaction has not been established. Aspirin is known to result in bronchospasm in certain individuals, probably by inhibition of prostaglandin synthesis. In a series of 2000 patients, even hydrocortisone acetate injections were observed to cause bronchospasm in 0.09 percent of the cases. Nitrofurantoin can induce hypersensitivity pneumonitis. Signs and symptoms of this reaction include fever, cough, diffuse pulmonary infiltration, pleural effusion, hilar adenopathy, and occasionally, asthma. Cromolyn sodium on rare occasion produces eosinophilic pneumonitis.

Both nitrofurantoin and cromolyn sodium have been shown in some cases to induce MIF production from lymphocytes *in vitro,* lending support to involvement of cell mediated hypersensitivity mechanisms (Van-Arsdel, 1978).

Kidney Disease. Interstitial nephritis appears to be the most typical immune reaction, often accompanied by fever, eosinophilia and skin rash. Hematuria, proteinuria, and azotemia occur. Methacillin, other penicillins, cephalothin, cephaloridine, and polymixin B seem on occasion to be nephrotoxic. In hydantoin-induced interstitial nephritis reported in a 6-year-old child (Sheith et al., 1977), lymphocyte proliferation by diphenylhydantoin could be demonstrated *in vitro.* Anti-IgG, anti-IgM and anti-IgA deposits on Bowman's capsule were found along with focal C_3 deposits in the basement membrane and IgE in plasma cells in the interstitium.

Systemic Lupus Erythematosus-Like Drug Reactions. Hydralazine was reported in 1954 to produce a systemic lupus erythematosus-like reaction in adults. The drug-induced syndrome and idiopathic disease differ in many respects. The idiopathic form occurs seven to eight times more frequently in females than in males, whereas the drug-induced form has less predilection for females. The idiopathic form occurs frequently in blacks; the drug form does not. The idiopathic SLE frequently is associated with kidney involvement; the drug-induced form is associated more frequently with lung involvement. Drug-induced SLE usually improves with the elimination of the causative drug. Other drugs implicated in producing drug-induced lupus-like syndrome include procainamide, hydralazine, phenytoin, isoniazid, and chlorpromazine (Harpey, 1974). In children, the hydantoin anti-convulsants are important (Beernink and Miller, 1973). Although clinical signs were not apparent, antinuclear antibodies were found in 11 of 48 asymptomatic individuals while on drugs. In these patients, the drug appears to alter nuclear proteins, making them immunogenic and inducing the formation of immune complexes. Children who develop a drug-induced lupus erythematosus syndrome do not appear to be at risk of developing "idiopathic" lupus erythematosus.

Vasculitis. Vascular inflammation often accompanies serum sickness, drug fever, drug-induced lupus erythematosus and drug hypersensitivities with hepatitis or glomerulonephritis (Parker, 1975). Pathologically, the vascular changes usually are termed hypersensitivity vasculitis, polyarthritis nodosa, or lymphocytic vasculitis. Drugs that have been implicated include antibiotics (penicillins), anticonvulsants, diuretics, and analgesics. There is no evidence that short-term drug exposure can induce chronic vasculitis.

DRUG REACTIONS THAT ARE NOT DUE TO HYPERSENSITIVITY

Anaphylactoid Reactions. Non-immunologically mediated drug reactions may mimic anaphylaxis. These reactions usually result from mediator release. Drugs known to induce direct histamine release include opiates, 48/80, radiocontrast media, and polymixin B. In some instances, chemical mediators are liberated by drug-induced activation of the alternative complement pathway.

Aspirin. Aspirin may induce severe asthma, urticaria, and nasal polyps. Aspirin-induced asthma may occur more frequently in adolescent children than previously thought (Rachelefsky et al., 1975). Most aspirin reactions are mediated by nonimmune mechanisms. Aspirin probably induces asthma by inhibiting the endogenous biosynthesis of prostaglandins and, thereby, upsetting the "balance" of bronchial reactivity (Toogood, 1977) and possibly by increasing the formation of SRS-A (Parker, 1975).

Hydantoins. Gingival hyperplasia occurs as a direct nonimmune response to anti-convulsant therapy with continuous diphenylhydantoin (phenytoin) (Dilantin). There may be other mucosal effects, including hyperplasia of bronchial mucosa. In addition, gross enlargement of the lips and nose and a generalized thickening of the subcutaneous tissue of the face and scalp may occur with high-dose therapy of this drug (Lefebvre, 1972).

Maternal-Fetal or Newborn Drug Effects. Since the thalidomide tragedy of the 1960s considerable attention has been focused on the effect on the fetus of drugs taken during pregnancy. This has resulted in stricter testing methods in the control of new drugs and often an attitude of therapeutic nihilism among physicians following a pregnancy. In spite of this, a recent survey revealed that during the perinatal period, 93.4 percent of pregnant women took at least two different drug products that may be unsafe to the fetus (Doering and Stewart, 1978). It is difficult to restrict drugs in pregnant women who have chronic diseases. For example, diphenylhydantoin may be needed for women with epilepsy, but it also may be teratogenic (Hill et al., 1974).

Alcohol, barbiturates or opiates to which the mother may be addicted pose special problems for the newborn in terms of acute drug withdrawal. Chronic fetal exposure to these drugs — for example, the fetal alcohol syndrome, characterized by pre-natal and post-natal growth deficiency, developmental delay, microcephaly and mental retardation — is being diagnosed with increasing frequency in infants born to alcoholic mothers (Christoffel and Salafsky, 1975).

Drug Toxicity Reactions. Aspirin in doses ordinarily used in children may induce severe gastrointestinal hemorrhage and anemia (Bergman et al., 1976). It is well recognized that chloramphenicol therapy may cause aplastic anemia and that tetracycline therapy may cause tooth staining and abnormal tooth development in the child. Overdoses of Lomotil prescribed for diarrhea may cause problems because of atropinism or respiratory depression from its opiate content. Commonly used drugs such as digitalis and theophylline require careful therapeutic monitoring because of the relatively narrow range between therapeutic and potentially toxic drug dosages.

DIAGNOSIS OF HYPERSENSITIVITY DRUG REACTIONS

History

As with other allergic disorders, the history of the event surrounding the onset of the adverse drug reaction is most important in making the correct diagnosis. The physician often faces the question whether the patient's symptoms are caused by a drug or by an infectious agent (see earlier discussion of cutaneous manifestations of drug reactions).

The problem is more complicated in the patient who is taking more than one drug. Table 54–2 tabulates the relative risk of drug reactions manifested by skin eruption, for specific drugs (Arndt and Jick, 1976). If the patient is on two or more of these drugs, analysis of relative reactivity rates is helpful in identifying the drug most likely to be responsible for the reaction.

Laboratory Diagnosis

There is no single test for drug allergy. This is not surprising in view of the various mechanisms by which drugs induce allergic symptoms. A basic problem in diagnosing drug reactions by immunologic methods is the fact that most drugs are not complete antigens, but rather are haptenic metabolites of the parent drug, coupled with a carrier tissue protein. Except for penicillin, immunoreactive drug metabolites rarely have been identified.

Two techniques may provide new laboratory methods to help in the diagnosis of drug allergy. The first involves coupling the drug directly to a tissue protein, e.g., serum albumin, and then using this complex in a test system (e.g., RAST) (Dolovich and Bell, 1978). The second approach consists of inducing the formation of the drug metabolite in vitro by exposing the drug to rat liver microsomal fractions. By employing this technique, antigenically active metabolites may be formed that will provide antigen for specific immune tests (Amos et al., 1977).

IgE Mediated Reactions. Immediate skin test reactions are useful in diagnosing penicillin (Green et al., 1977) and insulin (Lamkin et al., 1976) allergy and may possibly be useful for sensitivities to local anesthetics, streptomycin, quinine, chloramine T, and organic mercurials (Parker, 1975). When appropriate antigens become available, the radioallergosorbent test (RAST) should be useful in diagnosing penicillin and other drug hypersensitivity (Jublin et al., 1977). Penicillin allergy also may be identified by the *in vitro* histamine release assay (Parker, 1975).

Cytotoxic Antibody Reactions. Immune hemolytic anemia such as that induced by penicillin may be diagnosed by the indirect Coombs' antihuman globulin test, using normal red cells preincubated with penicillin. (In hemolytic anemia caused by drugs as the result of an "innocent bystander" type of reaction, the direct Coombs' test is positive when an anticomplement test reagent is used, since the adsorbed antibody is present only in low concentrations.) In autoimmune hemolytic anemia, the direct Coombs' test for gammaglobulin on the RBC is strongly positive but may be negative for complement.

Antiplatelet antibodies in immune thrombocytopenia can be detected by complement fixation or by platelet lysis or agglutination. The clot-retraction incubation test is less sensitive. Immune agranulocytosis may be suspected in the presence of drug-dependent leukoagglutination. Passive transfer experiments have identified the presence of antileukocyte antibodies but leukocyte damage may not be demonstrable *in vitro* because of the requirement for a drug metabolite in the reaction (Parker, 1975).

Immune Complex-Mediated Reactions. In serum sickness, hemagglutinating IgG and IgM drug (e.g., penicillin) antibodies usually are present in high titers. High antibody titers may occur in the absence of an allergic reaction, however. Documentation of a fall in total hemolytic complement activity (CH_{50}) or specific complement (C_3 or C_4) is helpful in diagnosing serum sickness, but is not always present, particularly in drug-induced diseases. The identification of circulating complexes by $C1\bar{q}$ binding or Raji cell assays also is helpful.

In penicillin- or methacillin-induced renal lesions, fluorescent staining of kidney biopsy tissue for antigen, IgG, and complement may be diagnostic. (Identification of a linear pattern favors a cytotoxic reaction while a "lumpy-bumpy" pattern favors an immune complex reaction.) (Arbesman and Reisman, 1971).

Cell Mediated Reactions. Drug-induced contact dermatitis may be diagnosed by direct patch testing. In several types of drug allergy, peripheral lymphocytes respond *in vitro* to the drug antigens, either by lymphocyte blastogenesis or the production of a lymphokine (MIF). The reactions may be indicative of the presence of cell mediated hypersensitivity. The specificity and diagnostic significance of these lymphocyte reactions is not yet clear, except possibly for

penicillin, hydantoin, cromolyn sodium, and nitrofurantoin.

DRUG CHALLENGE

In spite of a thorough history and the laboratory tests available, the relationship between a drug and a given set of signs and symptoms often is questionable. When it is therapeutically necessary, a drug challenge may be considered. If the adverse symptom is mild — e.g., nausea — the risk of the challenge is small. If, however, severe anaphylaxis occured, the drug challenge should be done (if at all) only under strictly controlled conditions and with extreme caution, with provision for immediate, emergency treatment if necessary. Drug challenge is used as the sole diagnostic test for aspirin sensitivity and for adverse reactions to radiocontrast media; it also is the preferable means of diagnosing reactions to local anesthetics (*vida infra*).

DRUG REACTIONS FREQUENTLY ENCOUNTERED IN CHILDREN

Penicillin

Penicillin is the most common cause of serious allergic drug reactions in children, as in adults. Hypersensitivity develops frequently because penicillin and its catabolites are highly reactive with serum proteins and form complete antigens. Catabolism has been studied extensively, and immunoreactive determinants have been identified (DeWeck, 1972). Catabolism to a penicilloyl specificity is the major (approximately 85 percent of the drug) degradation product, hence penicilloyl is considered the "major" antigenic determinant. "Minor" determinants (those penicillin catabolites that occur less frequently, *in vivo*) of some allergenic importance include the parent drug, penicillin itself, as well as penicilloate and penilloate specificities (Green et al., 1977).

Penicilloyl coupled with polylysine (PPL — "Pre-Pen", Kremers Urban Co.), a "major" determinant skin test antigen, has been used along with various minor determinants for testing for penicillin allergy. These minor determinant preparations include:

benzyl penicillin (Green et al., 1977), sodium benzyl-penicilloate and sodium benzyl-penilloate minor determinant mixture (Levine and Zolov, 1969), and shelf-aged benzyl penicillin (Bierman and VanArsdel, 1969). In a group of children, ages 9 months to 14 years, admitted with the diagnosis of penicilin allergy, only 10 percent were found to exhibit wheal and erythema skin test reactions to either major or minor determinants (Bierman and VanArsdel, 1969). In a large series of clinically penicillin-sensitive patients, mostly adults (Green et al., 1977), a 19 percent incidence of positive skin tests was found. In clinically penicillin-sensitive, skin test-positive individuals, skin test reactions occurred 79 percent of the time to PPL, 47 percent of the time to penicillin, and 25 percent of the time to both agents. The test more commonly was positive in patients who had systemic anaphylaxis or urticaria within 24 hours of penicillin administration and who were tested within one year of the reaction. Patients having a maculopapular rash (common in children) usually had a negative penicillin skin test.

Minor determinants, other than penicillin G itself, may be associated with immediate anaphylaxis and it is possible that some patients may react only to them. Since these minor determinants are not available for testing, an important subpopulation of penicillin-sensitive patients may be overlooked with currently available commercial skin test materials (Levine and Zolov, 1969). However, the vast majority of penicillin-allergic individuals will be identified by testing with penicillin G and PPL. The testing should be done cautiously, with appropriate emergency equipment available, since the skin test itself can cause anaphylaxis in patients with extreme penicillin allergy.

IgE antibodies to penicillin also can be detected by the *in vitro* RAST procedure, but this test is less sensitive than the skin test, and, as with the skin test, minor determinant antigens are not available commercially for testing.

The semi-synthetic penicillins all contain the six amino-penicillenic acid nucleus, the group responsible for reactivity with body proteins to produce complete penicillin allergens. Patients allergic to penicillin also may be allergic to the semi-synthetic penicillins

and should be considered so until proven otherwise. Specific major and minor skin test antigens to these penicillins will be of further aid in the specific diagnosis of allergy to these drugs (Jublin et al., 1977). The cephalosporins share a common highly reactive beta lactam ring structure with penicillin. While the exact incidence of chemical cross-reactivity between the penicillins and the cephalosporins is unknown, it has been reported to be as high as 50 percent in some patients who are allergic to penicillin (Green et al., 1977).

Penicillin Skin Testing Procedure. Penicillin skin testing should be done by qualified personnel. *Only those patients who are clinically suspected to have reacted to penicillin, (and in whom there is an indication for this antibiotic) should be tested.* If penicillin skin testing is not available and the patient is clinically reactive, the patient should be *assumed* to be allergic to penicillin and, if possible, an alternate antibiotic should be used.

The Penicillin Study Group of the American Academy of Allergy recommends the following skin testing procedures (see Table 54–3):

Reagents

1. Benzyl penicillin (penicillin-G), potassium or sodium — 1,000,000 Units/vial, supplied by E. R. Squibb and Son. This is freshly diluted with normal saline weekly to a concentration of 10,000 units/ml, the usual starting concentration for testing (though others prefer a concentration of 1000 units/ml).

2. Penicilloyl polylysine (PPL) in a single skin test strength supplied by Kremers Urban Co., Milwaukee, Wisconsin.

Procedure. A skin test should first be done by the scratch or prick method and read at 20 minutes for the development of a wheal and erythema. If this is negative, it should be followed by an intradermal test using 0.02 cc of the same strength antigen, comparing the reaction to a saline control. More dilute antigen may be used for intradermal skin testing in patients having a history of severe (anaphylactic) sensitivity. Skin tests may be negative when performed immediately after an acute reaction with penicillin, probably because of consumption of IgE antibodies in the reaction. In this case, the skin test should be repeated in 2 weeks.

TABLE 54–3 PENICILLIN SKIN TEST*

| | Penicillin G† | | |
SKIN TEST	CONCENTRATION	VOLUME	DOSE
Prick or scratch	10,000 μ/ml	1 drop	
Intradermal	(100 μ/ml optional)	0.02 cc	2 units
	(1000 μ/ml optional)	0.02 cc	20 units
	10,000 μ/ml	0.02 cc	200 units

| | Penicilloyl Polylysine‡ | |
SKIN TEST	CONCENTRATION (6×10^{-5} M)	VOLUME
Prick or scratch	Skin test strength	1 drop
Intradermal	Skin test strength	0.02 cc.

*Skin tests are read at 10-minute intervals.
†Squibb and Company, prepared fresh weekly — see text.
‡Kremers Urban Company — supplied in skin test strength.

If the skin test to either penicillin G or PPL is positive, the patient should be considered allergic to penicillin until proven otherwise. A positive PPL reaction correlates well with urticarial penicillin reactions, and a positive-penicillin-G skin test correlates with more serious immediate anaphylaxis; either or both skin tests may be positive.

Interpretation. If the skin tests are negative, the results weigh against significant penicillin hypersensitivity but *do not rule it out,* since the patient may be sensitive only to minor determinant antigens which may not have been present in the skin test preparations. Thus, patients who have negative penicillin skin test results and need penicillin should be challenged cautiously and under controlled conditions with penicillin. Oral challenge is considered safest.

Semi-synthetic Penicillins or Cephalothins. If a semi-synthetic penicillin must be given to a patient with penicillin allergy, skin testing to the parent drug may be done with similar concentrations using the same procedures. "Major determinants" for the semi-synthetic penicillins are not available commercially. Suitable concentrations of cephalothin for skin testing are 0.25 mg/ml, 2.5 mg/ml, and 25 mg/ml (DeSwarte, 1972).

Penicillin Desensitization. Desensitization is necessary in patients hypersensitive to a biologic serum or a drug and who *must* be given the drug when other therapies are not available. The desensitization process involves the administration of increasing amounts of serum or drug over a short period of time. Allergic reactions are controlled with epinephrine, antihistamines, theophylline, and corticosteroids as necessary. As increasing amounts of antigen are administered, corresponding IgE antibodies are

TABLE 54–4 SUBCUTANEOUS* PENICILLIN-G DESENSITIZATION PROGRAM

Drug Concentration (units/ml)	Volume Given (ml)	Dose Given (units)	Cumulative Dose Given (units)
100†	0.05	5	5
	0.1	10	15
	0.2	20	35
	0.4	40	75
	0.8	80	155
1,000	0.15	150	305
	0.3	300	605
	0.6	600	1,205
	1.0	1,000	2,205
10,000	0.2	2,000	4,205
	0.4	4,000	8,205
	0.8	8,000	16,205
100,000	0.15	15,000	31,205
	0.3	30,000	61,205
	0.6	60,000	121,205
	1.0	100,000	221,205
1,000,000	0.2	200,000	421,205
‡	0.4	400,000	621,205

*To be started after intradermal skin testing (200 units).

†Dose to be advanced every 15 minutes. The rate should be modified by anaphylactic reactions.

‡Once top dose is achieved, regular intravenous doses may be given.

Adapted from DeSwarte, 1972.

TABLE 54–5 INTRAVENOUS*
PENICILLIN-G DESENSITIZATION
PROGRAM

Drug Concentration (units/ml)	Volume Given (ml)	Dose Given (units)	Cumulative Dose Given (units)
1	50	50	50
10	50	500	550
100	50	5,000	5,550
1,000	50	50,000	55,550
10,000	50	500,000	555,550
†			

*The rate of infusion of each drug concentration will depend upon occurrence of anaphylactic reactions.

†Once top dose has been achieved, regular IV doses may be safely given.

Adapted from VanArsdel, 1978.

consumed, eventually enabling therapeutic amounts of serum or drug to be given with minimal or no clinical reaction (Gorevic and Levine, 1978).

Various penicillin desensitization procedures have been recommended. When given subcutaneously (see Table 54–4), the dose of penicillin is doubled at 15-minute intervals. Once dose levels reach 500,000 units, it usually is safe to administer therapeutic intravenous doses. Penicillin also may be given intravenously for desensitization (see Table 54–5). Gradually increasing concentrations of penicillin are administered in 50 cc aliquots.The rate of administration is governed by signs of adverse reaction. The intravenous method offers better procedural control than does the subcutaneous method of desensitization. Similar procedures may be used for desensitization to other drugs and biologic sera.

Ampicillin

A maculopapular rash due to ampicillin is one of the most common cutaneous adverse drug reactions, occurring in 3 to 7 percent of children in some reports (Bass et al., 1973). However, the incidence of ampicillin rashes increases in patients receiving allopurinol and in patients with infectious mononucleosis (Boston Collaborative Drug Surveillance Program, 1972). The rash begins 1 to 20 days after the start of therapy and lasts 1 to 7 days after drug treatment is stopped. In patients with a maculopapular rash and negative skin tests to penicillin G and PPL, the rash usually does not recur with readministration of the ampicillin therapy. In these patients, the rash is more likely to be "toxic" and transient, and ampicillin can be continued without risk. Urticarial eruptions due to ampicillin, on the other hand, are more likely to be on an allergic basis and subsequent administration of penicillin or ampicillin in such patients may induce a severe allergic reaction (Bierman et al., 1972).

Aspirin

In children, aspirin is a frequent cause of adverse drug reactions. Urticaria, angioedema, and associated nasal polyposis can occur, as well as other adverse reactions including anaphylactoid reactions, hepatitis, and gastritis. Most cases of aspirin sensitivity are nonimmune in origin (Toogood, 1977). Children usually do not have the complete syndrome of urticaria, bronchial asthma, and nasal polyposis seen frequently in adult women. Such patients may develop severe asthma within minutes or hours after ingesting aspirin.

Although severe asthma associated with aspirin administration is believed to be uncommon in children, Falliers (1972) demonstrated clinical aspirin sensitivity in 5.6 percent of a large number of intractable asthmatic, institutionalized children. In a double-blind challenge study of 50 children with intractable allergic asthma, 28 percent had a significant decrease in the FEF_{25-75} after administration of aspirin (Rachelefsky et al., 1975).

Aspirin intolerance may be familial but does not appear to be linked to HLA haplotype (vonMaur et al., 1974). In aspirin-sensitive patients, asthma also may be induced by other substances, including tartrazine (FD&C yellow dye No. 5), indomethacin, antipyrine, other anti-inflammatory agents, and benzoic acid derivatives.

There is no immunologic test to diagnose aspirin sensitivity. In those few children who are clinically sensitive to aspirin, aspirin challenge usually is considered unnecessary and risky. In children in whom the diagnosis is questionable, an oral aspirin challenge can be done under controlled conditions. In the case of the asthmatic child, a graded challenge (60 mg; 120 mg; 300 mg) may be done by following serial pulmonary function testing over a 4-hour period at each dose. The test is considered positive if there is a 30 percent decline in either the FEV_1 or FEF_{25-75}. Based on Rachelefsky's studies (1975), it would seem advisable to restrict aspirin from all patients with intractable asthma as a precautionary measure.

Insulin

Insulin hypersensitivity and resistance are recognized immune reactions. Although reactions occur more frequently in adults, the condition also is seen in the juvenile diabetic (especially local reactions). There is evidence that insulin hypersensitivity may be linked to the HLA-B7 histocompatibility antigen (Bertrams and Grüneklee, 1977). Three types of reactions may occur: local or systemic hypersensitivity and insulin resistance. Coombs' positive hemolytic anemia and LE cell reaction to insulin also have been reported.

Local Reactions. Immediate reactions begin after the injection of insulin, increase in intensity for 12 to 24 hours, and subside after several days. Occasionally, a dual reaction — immediately followed by delayed response — occurs. The frequency of these reactions is reported to be 14 to 55 percent of patients taking insulin. A local reaction may precede a systemic reaction. Biopsies of local reactions have shown evidence of a cell-mediated, hypersensitivity reaction in some and a combination of IgE-mediated and immune complex reactions in others.

Animal insulin is similar to human insulin; human and porcine (pork) insulin are almost identical. Most diabetic patients receive a mixture of beef and pork insulin. Since pork insulin is closer to the structure of human insulin, most reactions are to the beef fraction. Local reactions may be treated by switching to another less reactive or more purified (single peak, single component) insulin.

Systemic Reactions. In diabetic therapy, 40 percent of patients develop IgE antibodies to foreign insulin and have a positive immediate skin test to insulin (Witters et al., 1977). At the same time, IgG "blocking" antibodies are produced which appear to be protective against IgE-mediated reactions. A few patients have systemic reactions to insulin, and almost all occur when the patient begins insulin therapy again after a break in treatment. In most cases, the reaction is characterized by urticaria with or without angioedema.

Skin Testing for Insulin Sensitivity. The diagnosis of sensitivity to a particular insulin can be made by testing for an immediate skin test reaction, read in 10 minutes. Prick tests are first done with U-10, U-5 or U-2 strength material. If these tests are negative, serial intradermal skin testing is done, beginning with U-0.01 and progressing to U-0.02, U-0.04, U-0.1, U-0.2, U-0.4, U-1 and U-2 strength insulin. Tests should be done to the insulin in question plus other types (beef, pork, beef-pork, human, single peak or single component, or Lente insulins). Specific test antigens can be obtained from Eli Lilly and Company, Indianapolis, Indiana (Lamkin et al., 1976).

Desensitization to Insulin. When desensitization is necessary, a schedule of intradermal testing beginning with 0.00001 units of insulin has been suggested (Mattson et al., 1975). The insulin dose is increased tenfold three times daily, until 1 unit has been given. The subcutaneous route is then used, progressing with twofold increments until the proper dose is reached or a reaction occurs. An alternate program is outlined in the Eli Lilly Insulin Allergy Desensitization Kit.

Insulin Resistance. In insulin resistance, IgG antibodies develop and bind insulin so that it is not pharmacologically active. Treatment involves switching to another insulin source totally different from the one to which antibodies were induced (Mattson et al., 1975).

REACTIONS TO OTHER FOREIGN ANIMAL PROTEIN IMMUNIZATIONS*

Allergy Injection Therapy. Allergic reactions to allergy injections are well docu-

---

*See also Chapters 4 and 24.

mented. Usually, but not always, local reactions precede systemic reactions. The most common cause of such reaction is an error in dosage, but systemic anaphylaxis can occur if a bolus of allergenic extract is administered directly into a vein or capillary plexus.

Reactions to ACTH. ACTH administration is no longer common. Newer, purified synthetic preparations have been developed which reduce (but do not eliminate) the risk of reaction.

Reactions to Horse Serum. At one time, widespread use of horse antiserum constituted a common risk for both anaphylaxis and serum sickness. Such antisera is little used now, and the availability of human rabies and tetanus immune gammaglobulin has further reduced the risk. Snake venom antiserum currently is prepared from horses. Serum sickness is likely to develop in any patient in whom a large amount of foreign serum is administered, and the risk is dose dependent. This applies also to transplantation patients receiving antilymphocyte globulin prepared in horses.

Reactions to Tetanus Toxoid. Hypersensitivity reactions to tetanus toxoid have been documented in a group of children and adults with high tetanus antibody titers, many of whom had not had a booster immunization in 5 years. Sixty-three percent had positive immediate skin test reactions; 32 percent had Arthus reactions; and 74 percent had delayed skin test reactions (Facktor et al., 1973). Reaction rates correlated with serum IgG antibody titers. Atopic children are more prone to develop IgE antitetanus antibodies than are nonatopic children (Nagel et al., 1978). The significance of the presence of tetanus IgE antibodies with regard to subsequent reactions to tetanus toxoid is not clear, however. Subcutaneous administration of aluminum phosphate-absorbed tetanus toxoid preparation induces a local reaction in 2.6 percent of patients in the general population. If reactions occur, further immunization should be given only if the protective level of 0.01 antitoxin units per ml has not been achieved (Bellanti and Frenkel, 1978). Delayed local reactions are common. A skin test with tetanus toxoid may be used as a measure of cell-mediated immunity to a common antigen.

Reactions to Diphtheria Toxoid and Pertussis Vaccine. Adverse reactions to diphtheria toxoid are more frequent than reactions to tetanus toxoid, especially systemic reactions with fever and convulsions in children over 6 years of age. For this reason, adult-type of DT is recommended for primary immunization of children over 6 years of age. The dose of diphtheria toxoid is reduced to a safer level — one third of the diphtheria dose of that in pediatric DPT vaccine).

The pertussis component of the DPT vaccine has been associated with serious neurologic sequelae. In infants over 18 months of age, encephalopathy may develop after the first inoculation, with an incidence as high as 1:600. The reaction probably is not immune system mediated. The vaccine should be withheld from older infants and from children with neurologic disorders (Bellanti and Frenkel, 1978).

Reactions to Preservatives. Paraben (Nagel et al., 1977) and merthiolate (Reisman, 1969) preservatives used in vaccines, other biologicals, and pharmacologic agents have been implicated in IgE-mediated and cell mediated local and systemic reactions to these agents.

Egg Sensitivity in Viral Vaccine Recipients. The safety of administering viral vaccines made in chick embryo to egg-allergic children frequently is questioned. Purification techniques for vaccines used in recent years generally eliminate problematic antigens, and generally, even in egg sensitive individuals, allergic reactions to the vaccine do not occur. Nevertheless, reactions can occur in highly sensitive individuals. A good rule of thumb is if the child can eat eggs without reaction, whether or not he has a positive skin test to egg, it is safe to use an egg-containing vaccine; if the patient does have clinical problems on egg ingestion, skin testing with the vaccine to be used (influenza, mumps, and measles) should be performed. Prick or scratch testing with 1:10 dilution in saline of the vaccine followed, if negative, by intradermal testing with 0.02 ml of a 1:100 dilution and then a 1:10 dilution is advised (Bellanti and Frenkel, 1978). The vaccine should be withheld if there is a significant wheal and erythema reaction greater than a saline control.

Reactions to Human Immune Globulin. Reaction rates to human immune globulin approach 1:500 injections (Medical Research Council 1969). Reactions are due to aggregation of immune globulin, or development by the recipient of antibodies to antigenic markers on genetically different donor immunoglobulin. Patients who have absent or low serum IgA levels develop IgG anti-human-IgA antibodies (Wells et al., 1977). Such patients are liable to become sensitized with the administration of any blood product and are at risk of severe systemic reactions on readministration.

Reactions to Blood Transfusions. Anaphylaxis (2.4 reactions per 1000 recipients — Boston Collaborative Drug Surveillance Program, 1973), skin rash (35 reactions per 1000 recipients — Arndt and Jick, 1976), and fever (Swisher, 1972) are common adverse reactions to blood and plasma transfusions. The reactions to administered foreign proteins usually are immune in nature. Although ABO and Rh typing restrict the number and severity of the reactions, there is a substantial risk of reaction with any transfusion. This risk is increased with multiple transfusions and in the immunodeficient (particularly IgA-deficient) patient.

Reactions to Radiocontrast Media. Reactions to radiocontrast media appear to be non–antibody mediated for the most part, and can result from direct drug-induced release of histamine and other mediator release from tissue mast cells and circulating basophils. Vasovagal reflexes and other (unknown) mechanisms also may be operative. The reaction rate in children is lower than in adults (Yocum et al., 1978), partially reflecting a lower exposure rate in children to radio-opaque dyes.

The risk of a serious anaphylactoid reaction upon reexposure to dye may be successfully predicted by intravenous challenge but *not by skin testing*. After a careful history and informed consent, each specific dye to be used is administered intravenously at 15-minute intervals (Table 54–6). If this "pretest" challenge is negative, the radiologist is advised to use diphenhydramine (Benadryl) 50 mg (adults) or 1 mg per kg body weight, up to 50 mg (children) intravenously, 5 minutes prior to the radiocontrast media injection. If the pretest is positive, the dye should not be used. If, however, radiocontrast media must be used in spite of the risk, the patient should be premedicated with 50 mg of prednisone p.o. q̄ 6 hours for three doses, ending one

TABLE 54–6 RADIOCONTRAST MEDIA INTRAVENOUS PRETESTING

Dilution (w/vol)*	Volume Given (ml)†
1:10,000	0.1
1:1,000	0.1
1:100	0.1
1:10	0.1
full strength	0.1
full strength	1.0
full strength	5.0

*Full-strength RCM is freshly diluted in buffered physiologic saline.

†Dilutions are advanced at 15-minute intervals unless adverse reactions occur.

hour prior to the test study, and 50 mg of diphenhydramine (Benadryl) should be administered intramuscularly one hour prior to dye administration (Kelly et al., 1978). In spite of premedication, a small number of patients may react to the administration of radiocontrast material. Radiocontrast media pretesting is valuable in that it identifies the high-risk patient.

Radiocontrast media pretesting must be done under controlled conditions, and for this reason, it is not always practical. Under these circumstances, in which a patient who has had a significant previous reaction to radiocontrast media must receive the dye again, premedication with diphenhydramine and corticosteroids is advised.

Reactions to Local Anesthetics. Anaphylactoid reactions to local anesthetics are not common, especially in children, but other types of adverse reactions are, especially in adults who undergo multiple dental procedures. Most reactions are due to drug toxicity related to drug overdose or rapid drug absorption. Symptoms include nausea and vomiting, excitation, nervousness, dizziness, disorientation, convulsion, coma, shock, and respiratory and cardiac failure. Contact dermatitis is the commonest allergic reaction. Local swelling also may be the result of a cell mediated hypersensitivity reaction. Urticaria and other allergic signs and symptoms may occur, but an immune reaction has not been clearly identified in these cases.

Local anesthetics may be divided into two groups, based on their chemical structure

TABLE 54–7 LOCAL ANESTHETIC PROVOCATIVE TESTING

Route of Administration	Dilution (w/vol)	Volume Given (ml)
Prick or scratch*	full strength	drop
Intradermal*	full strength	0.02 cc
Subcutaneous†	1:10,000‡	0.1
Subcutaneous	1:1,000	0.1
Subcutaneous	1:10	0.1
Subcutaneous	full strength	0.1
Subcutaneous	full strength	0.3
Subcutaneous	full strength	0.6

*An optional prick and intradermal skin test may be performed prior to subcutaneous provocative testing.

†Dilutions are advanced at 15-minute intervals unless adverse reactions occur.

‡Full strength L.A. is freshly diluted in buffered physiologic saline.

(Incaudo et al., 1978). Group I anesthetics contain para-amino-benzoic ester and frequently are cross-reactive. They include: benoxinate (Dorsacaine), benzocaine, butacaine (Butyn), butethamine (Monocaine), butyl aminobenzoate (Butesin), chloroprocaine (Nesacaine), larocaine, naepaine (Amylsine), procaine (Novocain), and tetracaine (Pontocaine). Group II local anesthetics do not cross-react with each other or with anesthetics of Group I. They include: amydricaine (Alypin), cyclomethycaine (Surfocaine), dibricaine (Nupercaine), dimethisoquin (Quotaine), diperodon (Diothane), dyclonine (Dyclone), hexylcaine (Cyclaine), lidocaine (Xylocaine), mepivacaine (Carbocaine), oxethazine (Oxaine), phenacaine (Holocaine), piperocaine (Metycaine), pramoxine (Tronothane), proparacaine (Ophthaine), and pyrrocaine (Endocaine).

The immediate reacting skin test has been felt by some to be helpful in making a diagnosis of "allergy" to local anesthetics (Aldrete and Johnson, 1970). A more recent study concludes that the immediate skin test is of little value, but that provocative or challenge testing aids in the management of these cases

(Incoudo et al., 1978). Table 54–7 demonstrates the method of provocative or challenge testing, modified by our own experience. Using this method, testing usually is done with at least one anesthetic from Group I and selected drugs from Group II, based on the drug with which the patient may have had an adverse reaction, as well as other drugs that the dentist or physician may wish to use as a substitute anesthetic. Some reactions to local anesthetics may be due to the preservatives (e.g., parabens). Testing may be done for reactions to local anesthetics (lidocaine 1%) with or without paraben preservatives if paraben sensitivity is suspected.

TREATMENT OF ADVERSE DRUG REACTIONS

The best treatment for any type of drug reaction is to discontinue the drug promptly! Tests for identifying the offending drug at the time of reaction are limited. Even with penicillin hypersensitivity in which an immediate reacting skin test to appropriate penicillin reagents can aid greatly in diagnosis, a wait of up to 2 weeks after a clinical drug reaction may be necessary, because of a temporary "anergic" period to the drug. In cases in which many drugs can be suspect, information on reaction rates to various drugs (see Table 54–2) can be of value in narrowing the field of suspects to the most likely candidate(s).

The treatment of anaphylactic and anaphylactoid reactions (Kelly and Patterson, 1974) is covered in Chapter 52. If the offending drug can be identified, parents and children should be warned about further exposure to the same drug and exposure to cross-reacting drugs. Alternative drugs, if necessary, should be prescribed. In the quest for developing new, more specific and safer drugs, unexpected adverse reactions are frequently first encountered in children. It is the responsibility of the physician who prescribes such agents to be alert to possible drug reactions.

References

Ahlstedt, J., Audal, L., Ekstrom, B., Svard, O. P., and Wide, L.: Antibody reactivity in penicillin-sensitive patients determined with different penicillin derivatives. Int. Arch. Allergy Appl. Immunol. 54:19, 1977.

Aldrete, J. A., and Johnson, D. A.: Evaluation of intracutaneous testing for investigation of allergy to local anesthetic agents. Anaesth. Analg. 49:173, 1970.

Amon, R. B., and Dimond, R. L.: Rapid diagnosis of toxic epidermal necrolysis. New Engl. J. Med. 294:55, 1976.

Amos, H. E., Lake, B. G., and Atkinson, H. A. C.: Allergic drug reactions — An in vitro model using a mixed function oxidase complex to demonstrate antibodies with specificity for a practotol metabolite. Clin. Allergy 7:423, 1977.

Arbesman, C. E., and Reisman, R. E.: Serum sickness and human anaphylaxis. In Samter, M. (ed.): Immunologic Diseases, 2nd ed. Boston, Little, Brown and Co., 1972, pp. 405–414.

Arndt, K. A., and Jick, H.: Rates of cutaneous reactions to drugs; A report from the Boston Collaborative Drug Surveillance Program. J.A.M.A. 235:918, 1976.

Bass, J. W., Crowley, D. M., Steele, R. W., Young, F. S. H., and Harden, L. B.: Adverse effects of orally administered ampicillin. J. Pediatr. 83:106, 1973.

Beernink, D. H., and Miller, J. J., III: Anticonvulsant-induced antinuclear antibodies and lupus-like disease in children. J.Pediatr. 82:113, 1973.

Bellanti, J. A., and Frenkel, L. D.: Adverse reactions to immunizing agents. In Middleton, E., Reed, C. E., and Ellis, E. F. (eds.): Allergy, Principles and Practice. St. Louis, C. V. Mosby Co., 1978, pp. 1172–1182.

Bergman, G. E., Phillippidis, P., and Nairman, J. L.: Severe gastrointestinal hemorrhage and anemia after therapeutic doses of aspirin in normal children. J. Pediatr. 88:501, 1976.

Berkowitz, M., Glaser, J., and Johnstone, D. E.: The incidence of allergy to drugs in pediatric practice. Ann. Allergy 11:561, 1953.

Bernstein, B. H., Singsen, B. H., King, K. K., and Hanson, V.: Aspirin-induced hepatotoxicity and its effect on juvenile rheumatoid arthritis. Am. J. Dis. Child. 131:659, 1977.

Bertrams, J., and Grüneklee, D.: Association between HLA-B₇ and allergic reactions to insulin in insulin-dependent diabetes mellitus. Tissue Antigens 10:273, 1977.

Bierman, C. W., and VanArsdel, P. P., Jr.: Penicillin allergy in children — The role of immunological tests in its diagnosis. J. Allergy 43:267, 1969.

Bierman, C. W., Pierson, W. E., Zeitz, S. J., Hoffman, L. S., and VanArsdel, P. P., Jr.: Reactions associated with ampicillin therapy. J.A.M.A. 220:1098, 1972.

Boston Collaborative Drug Surveillance Program: Excess of ampicillin rashes associated with allopurinol or hyperuricemia. New Engl. J. Med. 286:505, 1972.

Boston Collaborative Drug Surveillance Program: Drug-induced anaphylaxis. J.A.M.A. 224:613, 1973.

Böttiger, L. E., Strandberg, J., and Westerholm, B.: Drug-induced febrile mucocutaneous syndrome; With survey of the literature. Acta Med. Scand. 198:229, 1975.

Campbell, W. H., Johnson, R. E., Senft, R. A., and Azevedo, D. J.: Treated adverse effects of drugs in an ambulatory population. Medical Care 15:599, 1977.

Chan, T. K., Todd, D., and Tso, S. C.: Drug-induced haemolysis in glucose-6-phosphate dehydrogenase deficiency. Br. Med. J. 2:1227, 1976.

Cherny, J. D., Hurwitz, E. S., and Welliver, R. C.: Mycoplasma pneumonial infections and exanthems. J. Pediatr. 87:369, 1975.

Christoffel, K. K., and Salafsky, I.: Fetal alcohol syndrome in dyzgotic twins. J. Pediatr. 87:963, 1975.

Cluff, L. E., and Johnson, J. E., III: Drug fever In Kallos, P., and Waksman, B. H. (eds.): Progress in Allergy. Vol. 8. Basel, S. Karger, 1964, p. 149.

Committee on Drugs, American Academy of Pediatrics: Anaphylaxis. Pediatrics 51:136, 1973.

Curian, J. P.: Hysterical dermatitis factitia. Am. J. Dis. Child. 125:187, 1973.

DeSwarte, R. D.: Drug allergy. In Patterson, R.: Allergic Disease, Diagnosis and Management. Philadelphia, J. B. Lippincott Co., 1972, pp. 393–493.

DeWeck, A. L.: Drug reactions. In Samter, M. (ed.): Immunologic Diseases, 2nd ed. Boston, Little, Brown and Co., 1972, pp. 415–440.

Doering, P. L., and Stewart, R. B.: The extent and character of drug consumption during pregnancy. J.A.M.A. 239:843, 1978.

Dolovich, J., and Bell, B.: Allergy to a product (S) of ethylene oxide gas (Demonstration of IgE and IgG antibodies and hapten specificity). J. Allergy Clin. Immunol. 62:30, 1978.

Facktor, M. A., Bernstein, R. A., and Fireman, P.: Hypersensitivity to tetanus toxoid. J. Allerg. Clin. Immunol. 52:1, 1973.

Falliers, C. J.: Late onset asthma linked to aspirin sensitivity. J.A.M.A. 221:244, 1972.

Gilchrest, B., and Baden, H. P.: Photodistribution of viral exanthems. Pediatrics 54:136, 1974.

Gorevic, P. D., and Levine, B. B.: Desensitization for anaphylactic hypersensitivity to penicilloate derivative of carbenicillin. J. Allergy Clin. Immunol. 61:147, 1978.

Green, G. R., Rosenblum, A. H., and Sweet, L. C.: Evaluation of penicillin hypersensitivity — Value of clinical history and skin testing with penicilloyl-polylysine and penicillin-G. J. Allergy Clin. Immunol. 60:339, 1977.

Harpey, J. P.: Lupus-like syndromes induced by drugs. Ann. Allergy 33:256, 1974.

Hill, R. M., Verniaud, W. M., Horring, M. G., McCulley, L. B., and Morgan, N. F.: Infants exposed in utero to antiepileptic drugs — Prospective study. Am. J. Dis. Child. 127:645, 1974.

Incaudo, G., Schatz, M., Patterson, R., Rosenberg, M., Yamamoto, F., and Hamburger, R. N.: Administration of local anesthetics to patients with a history of prior adverse reactions. J. Allergy Clin. Immunol. 61:339, 1978.

Jacobs, J. C., and Miller, M. E.: Fatal familial Leiner's disease — Deficiency of opsonic activity of serum complement. Pediatrics 49:225, 1972.

Jick, H., Miettinen, O. S., Shapiro, S., Lewis, G. P., Siskind, V., and Slone, D.: Comprehensive drug surveillance. J.A.M.A. 213:1455, 1970.

Jublin, J., Ahlstedt, S., Audal, L., Ekstrom, B., Svard, O. P. and Wide, L.: Antibody reactivity in penicillin-sensitive patients determined with different penicillin derivatives, Int. Arch. Allergy Appl. Immunol. 54:19, 1977.

Kamin, P. B., Fein, B. T. and Britton, H. A.: Use of live, attenuated measles virus vaccine in children allergic to egg protein. J.A.M.A. 193:143, 1965.

Kelly, J. F., and Patterson, R.: Anaphylaxis course, mechanisms and treatment. J.A.M.A. 227:1431, 1974.

Kelly, J. F., Patterson, R., Stevenson, D., and Mathison, D.: Radiographic contrast media studies in high-risk patients. J. Allergy Clin. Immunol. 61:147, 1978.

Kerns, D. L., Shira, J. E., Go, S., Summers, R. J., Schwab, J. A., and Plunket, D. C.: Ampicillin rash in children; relationship to penicillin allergy and infectious mononucleosis. Am. J. Dis. Child. 125:187, 1973.

Kounis, N. G.: A Review — Drug-induced bronchospasm. Ann. Allergy 37:285, 1976.

Lamkin, N., Lieberman, P., Hashimoto, K., Morohashi, M., and Sullivan, P.: Allergic reactions to insulin. J. Allergy Clin. Immunol. 58:213, 1976.

Lefebvre, E. B., Haining, R. C. and Labbe, R. F.: Coarse facies, calvarial thickening and hyperphosphatasia associated with long-term anticonvulsant therapy. New Engl. J. Med. 286:1301, 1972.

Levine, B. B., and Zolov, D. M.: Prediction of penicillin allergy by immunological tests. J. Allergy 43:231, 1969.

Margileth, A. M.: Scalded skin syndrome —Diagnosis, differential diagnosis and management of 42 children. So. Med. J. 68:447, 1975.

Mattson, J. R., Patterson, R., and Roberts, M.: Insulin therapy in patients with systemic insulin allergy. Arch. Intern. Med. 135:818, 1975.

McKenzie, M. W., Marchall, G. L., Netzloff, M. L. and Cluff, L. E.: Adverse drug reactions leading to hospitalization. J. Pediatr. 89:487, 1976.

Medical Research Council Working Party: Hypogammaglobulinemia in the United Kingdom. Lancet 1:163, 1969.

Nagel, J. E., Fuscaldo, J. T., and Fireman, P.: Paraben allergy. J.A.M.A. 237:1594, 1977.

Nagel, J. E., White, C., Lin, M. S., and Fireman, P.: Tetanus and diphtheria IgE antibodies in allergy and non-allergic children. J. Allergy Clin. Immunol. 61:177, 1978.

Parker, C. W.: Drug allergy. New Engl. J. Med. 292:511; 732; 957, 1975.

Porter, J., and Jick, H.: Drug-Related Deaths Among Medical Inpatients. J.A.M.A. 237:879, 1977.

Rachelefsky, G. S., Coulson, A., Siegel, S. C., and Stiehm, E. R.: Aspirin intolerance in chronic childhood asthma — Detected by oral challenge. Pediatrics 56:443, 1975.

Reisman, R. E.: Delayed hypersensitivity to merthiolate preservative. J. Allergy 43:245, 1969.

Ricks, W. B.: Salicylate hepatotoxicity in Reiter's syndrome. Ann. Int. Med. 84:52, 1976.

Rocklin, R. E.: Clinical application of in vitro lymphocyte tests. In Schwartz, R. S. (ed.): Progress in Clinical Imunology. Vol. 2, New York, Grune and Stratton, Inc., 1974.

Sheith, K. J., Casper, J. T., and Good, T. A.: Interstitial nephritis due to phenytoin hypersensitivity. J. Pediatr. 91:438, 1977.

Stember, R. H., and Levine, B. B.: Prevalence of allergic diseases, penicillin hypersensitivity and aeroallergen hypersensitivity in various populations. J. Allergy Clin. Immunol. 51:100, 1973.

Swisher, S. N.: Transfusion reactions and blood group substances. In Smater, M. (ed.): Immunologic Diseases, 2nd ed. Boston, Little, Brown and Co., 1972, pp. 441–458.

Toogood, J. H.: Aspirin intolerance of asthma, prostaglandins and cromolyn sodium. Chest 72:135, 1977.

VanArsdel, P. P., Jr.: Adverse drug reactions. In Middleton, F., Reed, C. F., and Ellis, E. F. (eds.): Allergy, Principles and Practice. St. Louis, C.V. Mosby Co., 1978, pp. 1133–1158.

vonMaur, R. K., Adkinson, N. F., Jr., vanMetre, T. E., Jr., Marsh, D. G., and Norman, P. S.: Aspirin intolerance in a family. J. Allergy Clin. Immunol. 54:380, 1974.

Wells, J. V., Buckley, R. H., Schonfield, M. S., and Fudenberg, H. H., Clin. Immunol. Immunopath. 8:265, 1977.

Whyte, J., and Greenan, E.: Drug usage and adverse drug reactions in paediatric patients. Acta Paed. Scand. 66:767, 1977.

Witters, L. A., Ohnan, J. L., Weir, G. G., Raymond, L. W., and Lowell, F. C.: Insulin antibodies in the pathogenesis of insulin allergy and resistance. Am. J. Med. 63:703, 1977.

Wright, G. E.: Domestic pet infestation and papular urticaria. Practitioner, 208:406, 1972.

Yocum, M. W., Heller, A. M., and Abels, R. I.: Efficacy of intravenous pretesting and antihistamine prophylaxis in radiocontrast media-sensitive patients. J. Allergy Clin. Immunol. 62:309, 1978.

Roger M. Katz, M.D. **55**

Chronic Cough

Recurrent or chronic cough constitutes one of the most frustrating diagnostic and therapeutic problems in practice. After days, weeks, and even months of repeated coughing, patients present with fatigue, pain, respiratory tract irritation, difficulty in breathing, headaches, and congestion. Frequently these patients are depressed or anxious. Sometimes asthmatic patients with severe cough seek medical aid after an episode of syncope or a convulsion.

Cough may be of acute onset, paroxysmal, or recurrent in nature. It may be associated with swallowing, aphonia, or dysphonia, with or without sputum production, and may be *brassy, croupy, bovine or hacky* in quality. The diverse etiologies and the complex differential diagnosis of cough require an understanding of the pathophysiology of cough.

PATHOPHYSIOLOGY OF COUGH

Typically cough is preceded by initial inspiration with opening of the glottis. The inflow of air increases lung volume and lengthens the bronchi; this is followed by a compression phase, with closing of the glottis and active contraction of the expiratory muscles. A final opening of the glottis, with a rapid expiratory phase occurs, which expels secretions or other material from the respiratory tree.

The physiology of the cough reflex is not well defined, although it appears to be an intricate response that involves receptor sites, afferent and efferent nerve pathways, integration at a medullary center, and an end organ response. Cough receptors are located in upper, mid, and lower peripheral airways of cats and dogs, and presumably also in man. Those in the upper airways are located in the paranasal sinuses, ear canals, tympanic membranes, nasal airways, and pharynx. In the mid airways, cough receptors are located in the larynx and trachea; in the lower airways they are concentrated in the carina, bronchial bifurcations, and to a lesser extent in the peripheral airways (Widdicombe et al., 1962). Cough receptors also can be found in the pleura, diaphragm, and nonpulmonary receptor sites located in the pericardium and stomach (Nadel, 1973).

Stimulation of cough receptors creates nerve impulses that travel through the afferent pathways to the medullary cough center, which in turn stimulates efferent nerve pathways (the vagus, phrenic, and possibly the spinal motor nerves). Sympathetic nerves innervate the larynx, tracheobronchial tree, heart, and gastrointestinal tracts (Dahlstrom et al., 1966). They apparently act to oppose the action of the parasympathetic nervous system. In dogs, and possibly in man, alpha adrenergic constrictor pathways may not be important in airways (Cabezas et al., 1971).

An alternate but less accepted concept of cough physiology postulates a direct reflex arc from the mucosa to the bronchial smooth muscles. According to this view,

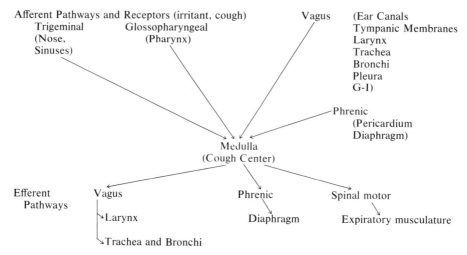

FIGURE 55-1. Cough reflex pathways.

irritation of mucosal receptors initiates bronchospasm, which in turn activates cough receptors in the lungs. Bronchoconstriction dynamically compresses the tracheobronchial tree, which results in the forced expiratory phase of cough. In animals this bronchoconstriction can be blocked by cutting the vagus nerve, and in man by atropine sulfate, indicating that postganglionic cholinergic pathways are involved (Nadel et al., 1962) (Fig. 55-1).

COMMON CAUSES OF COUGH

Causes of cough are numerous and are listed in Table 55-1. Allergy is probably one of the most common causes of chronic cough. Allergens entering the airway may initiate the cough reflex by inducing release of histamine and other mediators, which in turn, stimulate cough or irritant receptors. The resulting cough may begin with a tickling or burning sensation of the mucosa. Such mediator release also may cause bronchospasm. Patients with asthma sometimes present with chronic cough that masks underlying wheezing. Also, cough may be the only symptom of exercise-induced bronchospasm (Katz, 1970a).

Various respiratory irritants (smoke, noxious gases, dust, fumes, scents, and other inhalants) can activate cough receptors directly and also can induce reflex coughing through activation of vagal receptors in the upper airway. Thus, middle ear infections or chronic sinusitis can cause coughing that is severe enough to interfere with sleep. Other physical or environmental factors (such as cold air, high humidity, or dry inhaled air) also stimulate irritant receptors and induce cough (Simonsson et al., 1967).

Cough associated with nasopharyngitis (the common cold) and sinusitis may be related to pharyngeal irritation from drainage. Other infections such as pertussis or respiratory viruses induce coughing over a protracted postinfectious period by sensitizing epithelial cough receptors. Tuberculosis may cause cough by inflammatory airway and parenchymal involvement that impinges upon receptors of the mid and lower airways. Cough is a common feature of bronchiectasis, which is associated with chronic infection of peripheral airways. Chronic atelectasis or foreign body in a lung segment can manifest as chronic cough. In cystic fibrosis, pulmonary involvement often is reflected by a chronic cough.

An extraluminal chest mass (i.e., mediastinal tumor) or intraluminal gastroesophageal lesion can induce a cough symptom complex, presumably through activation of a component of the cough reflex arc. Cough receptors in the large airway can be stimulated by lesions of the cardiovascular system, such as left atrial enlargement or aortic aneurysm, which may initiate a loud and brassy cough. Other extrapulmonary lesions associated with coughing include foreign bodies found in the upper or mid airways and in the esophagus.

Cough tic is seen or associated frequently with psychologic problems and neurologic diseases. This type of cough, usually distress-

TABLE 55–1 CAUSES OF COUGH

General Causative Agents	Causes by Location *(Continued)*
IRRITANTS	Tumor
Smoke (tobacco smoke, fireplace smoke)	Vascular ring
Noxious gases (burning plastics)	Intraluminal obstruction
Organic dusts (house dust)	Foreign body
Fumes (formaldehyde fume resins)	Mucus plugs
Scents (perfume)	Tumor
Aerosols (pressurized household sprays,	Inflammation
deodorants)	Bronchospasm
PHYSICAL FACTORS	**PERIPHERAL AIRWAYS**
Cold	Infections
Humidity	Cysts
Dryness	Sequestration of the lung
INFLAMMATION	Congenital malformation
	Pneumonitis
Causes by Location	Interstitial disease
	EXTRAPULMONARY
UPPER AIRWAY	Congenital heart disease
Sinus and nasal polyps	Congestive heart failure
Sinus, ear, nasal, pharyngeal infections or irri-	Great vessel abnormalities
tation	Central nervous system disorders
Foreign body	Infection
Retropharyngeal and perifaucial infections	Edema
MIDDLE AIRWAY	Hysteria
Epiglottic and laryngeal disorders	Paralysis
Infection	Drug intoxication
Structure abnormalities	**GASTROINTESTINAL**
Vocal cord paralysis—polyp and tumors	Gastroesophageal reflux
Foreign body	Hiatus hernia
CENTRAL AIRWAYS	Inflammation
Tracheomalacia	Tumor
Infection	
Extraluminal compression	
Nodes	

ing to the parents and others, may not seem to affect the individual with the cough. An important diagnostic point is that the tic usually disappears with sleep or other distractions. In such cases, psychologic intervention may be required to alleviate the symptoms.

Gastroesophageal reflux should be considered when the patient's primary problem occurs at night or is associated with complaints of chest fullness, vomiting, recurrent pneumonias, and bronchospasm. Cough and bronchospasm may occur in asthmatic children with gastroesophageal reflux, owing to aspiration of gastric contents (Euler et al., 1978).

COMPLICATIONS OF COUGH

Chronic cough can lead to various complications, some of which are severe. One such complication is cough syncope. This is characterized by paroxysmal coughing spasms associated with facial congestion, turgidity, and cyanosis, which are followed by syncope or a seizure-like episode and unconsciousness that may last from seconds to several minutes. The syndrome most often is seen in individuals who have asthma, with marked decrease in pulmonary compliance. The coughing spasm increases intrathoracic pressure, which results in decreased venous return, decreased cardiac output, and cerebral hypoxia due to diminished cranial blood flow (Katz, 1970b).

Painful muscle strain and even muscle rupture may complicate chronic cough. The Mallory-Weiss syndrome (esophageal bleeding due to tearing of the esophageal mucosa) may be caused by chronic coughing. Rib fractures along the lateral margins of the rib cage rarely occur in children with chronic cough. Pneumomediastinum, pneumothorax, and subcutaneous emphysema, examples of the more severe complications, probably result from sharply increased intrathoracic pressure, which causes rupture of alveolar blebs or shearing of alveolar bases that permits air to enter perivascular spaces. Such constitutional symptoms as fatigue, insomnia, anorexia, vomiting, and headache may be due to chronic cough.

DIAGNOSTIC EVALUATION

A history of present illness should focus not only on onset, type and mucus production related to the cough, but should include a review of the family history of illnesses associated with coughing, and detailed environmental and occupational history.

An abrupt onset of a harsh, barking, and irritative cough associated with respiratory distress and dysphagia with or without wheezing, often is associated with a foreign body in the esophagus or lower respiratory tract; the sudden onset of harsh, barking, and inspiratory stridor usually is associated with partial obstruction of the epiglottis, larynx, or trachea. Hyperinflation with dyspnea, and wheezing and recurrent coughing are more often associated with more peripheral airway obstruction, such as that of asthma or a continuous bronchiolitis. Chronic hacking day and night is characteristic more of upper airway disease, particularly of the sinuses and middle ears; whereas a loud, brassy, deep paroxysmal cough tends to be associated with the lower respiratory tract. Associated fever and green purulent sputum suggests concomitant bronchitis or pneumonia.

The physical examination (Table 55–2) often will provide clues to the underlying cause of cough. Cough in individuals with atopic disorders, for example, is likely to emanate from airways or sinuses in which edema and viscous mucus secretions result in obstruction of the upper as well as lower respiratory tract.

Physical findings of pharyngeal mucus or pus, mucosal inflammation and/or congestion, as well as point tenderness over the paranasal sinuses, are hallmarks of sinusitis. Involvement of the upper portion of the lower airway results in inspiratory stridor, edema and inflammation of the glottis or epiglottis, and hoarseness. Expiratory wheezing, rhonchi or rales, along with hyperinflation or dullness to percussion will help localize the problem to the lower respiratory tract.

Useful tests include a Hansel stained preparation of nasal secretions or sputum for cellular morphology. Large numbers of eosinophils occur with allergy; a predominance of PMN's, lymphocytes, or macrophages occur with viral infections; and PMN's, with large quantities of ingested bacteria occur with a bacterial infection or sinusitis. Examination of nasal secretions is more useful than white blood counts or sedimentation rates in

TABLE 55–2 COUGH–HELPFUL POINTS IN LOCALIZING CAUSE

Respiratory System

UPPER RESPIRATORY TRACT

Sinus—congestion, headache, jaw or tooth pain, point tenderness, postnasal drip, associated with cough during day and night

Nasal—profuse nasal discharge, pharyngeal irritation, dry irritative cough

Otic
　　Middle ear—congestion, pain, hacky cough
　　External ear—hacky cough, local pain

Pharyngeal or tonsillar/adenoidal—nasopharyngeal obstruction and irritation of pharyngeal mucosa; irritative cough

MIDDLE AIRWAYS

Epiglottal—inspiratory stridor

Laryngeal—acute and spasmodic, tight, brassy, barking, hoarse cough; inspiratory stridor

Tracheal—deep and paroxysmal cough

LOWER RESPIRATORY TRACT

Bronchial—deep, paroxysmal, hacky cough, or productive cough, associated with wheeze

Atelectasis (especially right middle lobe)—irritative cough

Peripheral—suppressed cough associated with chest pain and dyspnea, often paroxysmal, accentuated by postural changes

Miscellaneous

Impinging on bronchi (vascular rings, vessel abnormalities, cardiac enlargement, node enlargement, tumor)—loud and brassy

Foreign body—abrupt onset, respiratory difficulty, dysphagia; harsh, hacky, irritative cough; associated respiratory click or slap in airway involved suggesting existence of chronic paranasal sinusitis (Rachelefsky et al., 1978). Skin tests for specific infectious agents such as tuberculosis, coccidioidomycosis, or histoplasmosis should be performed if there is chronic pulmonary infection. Roentgenographic views of the sinuses can be most helpful in delineating abnormalities of the maxillary, ethmoid, frontal, and sphenoid sinuses. Opacification, cloudiness, and blurring of the peripheral margins of one or more of the paranasal sinuses are associated with significant sinus disease (see Chapter 40). Sinus disease may present as chronic cough as early as 2 months of age. Additional x-ray examination of the pharyngeal regions and chest to establish the presence of pharyngeal lymphoid tissue and thymus gland may be important in the differential diagnosis of immune deficiency disease. When suspected, immunodeficiency states should be evaluated as outlined in Chapter 6.

Chest x-ray films can help to differentiate between abnormalities of the pulmonary and extrapulmonary systems. The cineesophagram is helping in establishing the presence or absence of vascular rings or other cardiac abnormalities and tracheoesophageal fistulas. Gastroesophageal reflux often can be determined with the cineesophagram, or Tuttle test (Byrne et al., 1978; Bernoken, 1978). With chronic pulmonary lesions, tomography, bronchoscopy, and bronchography should be considered.

Evaluation of allergic disorders has been discussed in great detail elsewhere. Pulmonary function tests may indicate obstructive and restrictive pulmonary lesions when the auscultatory examination is normal. Consider appropriate referrals for evaluation of congenital heart disease, gastroesophageal reflux evaluation, and allergy or for removal of foreign body.

TREATMENT

Successful therapy depends upon identification of the cause of cough. Treatment for the specific disorders in which cough is a common symptom is covered elsewhere in this book. Symptomatic treatment often is disappointing, especially in patients with severe cough. Antitussives and expectorants, used properly, however, may benefit some with cough syndromes.

Cough preparations can be classified according to their site of action. Central cough suppressants act by depressing the medullary integrative cough center. Peripheral depressants appear to work chiefly on irritant receptors, either by anesthetizing them or otherwise decreasing their activity. Both narcotic and nonnarcotic antitussives are available. Codeine phosphate is the principal antitussive narcotic in clinical use. In the older child or adult, the oral dose ranges from 10 to 60 mg; this should be reduced in younger children if codeine phosphate is used at all. In general, there is little experimental evidence for the effectiveness of nonnarcotic antitussives, although dextromethorphan is claimed to be equally effective as codeine at comparable oral dosage, and clinical complications from excessive dosages are less likely than with codeine. The use of these agents in children has not been studied extensively, however.

Anticholinergic agents such as atropine sulfate and derivatives of atropine may block the cough and irritant receptor responsiveness to acetylcholine. If given in large doses, they may induce side effects such as mouth dryness, blurred vision, and skin flushing. Recent evidence indicates that aerosolized atropine in dosages of 0.5 to 1 mg may be beneficial in patients who have bronchospasm and cough.

Expectorants that include iodides and guaifenesin (glyceryl guaiacolate) are supposed to aid by thinning secretions. Experimental data on their effectiveness is conflicting. Iodides as expectorants have adverse reactions that often outweigh any possible benefit (AAP Committee on Drugs, 1975). Side effects of iodides include parotid swelling, metallic taste, marked exacerbation of acne, skin rash, and goiter. Guaifenesin is made from wood distillate. It appears to act as a respiratory tract secretory gland irritant, but appropriate dosage — and indeed its effectiveness as an expectorant — are still in question. Daily dosage recommended ranges from 100 to 400 mg, divided into four to six doses. Large dosages may cause platelet aggregation. In animal studies, ammonium chloride is effective as an expectorant if given in large doses.

Mucolytic agents such as acetylcysteine, pancreatic dornase, and streptokinase are effective in reducing viscosity of secretions, but must be delivered by aerosol. They are irritating and may induce severe bronchospasm. Adequate oral hydration to thin secretions is important, especially in acute asthma.

References

American Academy of Pediatrics Committee on Drugs: Adverse reactions to iodide therapy of asthma and other pulmonary diseases. Pediatrics 57:272, 1976.

Bernoken, I. L.: Asthma in adults. In Middleton, E., Jr., Reed, C. E., and Ellis, E. F. (eds.): Allergy, Vol. 2. St. Louis, The C. V. Mosby Co., pp. 747–748, 1978.

Cabezas, G. A., Graf, P. D., and Nadel, J. A.: Sympathetic vs. parasympathetic nerve regulation of airway of dogs. J. Appl. Physiol. 31:651, 1971.

Dahlstrom, A., Fuxe, K., Hokfelt, T., and Norberg, R. A.: Adrenergic innervation of bronchial muscles of cat. Acta. Physiol. Scand. 66:507, 1966.

Euler, A. R., Byrne, W. J., Ament, M. E., Fonkalsrud, E. W., Strobe, C. T., Siegel, S. C., Katz, R. M., and Rachelefsky, G. S.: Recurrent pulmonary disease in children: A complication of gastroesophageal reflux. Pediatrics 63:47, 1979.

Katz, R. M.: Exercise induced bronchospasm in childhood. Ann. Allergy 28:361, 1970a.

Katz, R. M.: Cough syncope in children with asthma. J. Pediatrics 77:48, 1970b.

Nadel, J. A.: pp. 29–37 In Austen, K. F., and Lichenstein, J. M. (eds.): Asthma: Physiology, Immunopharmacology and Treatment. New York, Academic Press, 1973.

Nadel, J. A., and Widdicombe, J. G.: Reflex effects of upper airway irritation on total lung resistance and blood pressure. J. Appl. Physiol. 17:861, 1962.

Rachelefsky, G. S., Goldberg, M., Katz, R. M., Boris, G., Gyepes, M. T., Shapiro, M. J., Mickey, M. R., Finegold, S. M., and Siegel, S. C.: Sinus disease in children with respiratory allergy. J. Aller. Clin. Immunol. 61:310, 1978.

Simonsson, B. G., Jacobs, F. M., and Nadel, J. A.: Role of autonomic nervous system and cough reflex in the increased responsiveness of airways in patients with obstructive airway disease. J. Clin. Invest. 46:1812, 1967.

Widdicombe, J. G., Kent, D. C., and Nadel, J. A.: Mechanisms of bronchoconstriction during inhalation of dust. J. Appl. Physiol. 17:613, 1962.

Sheldon C. Siegel, M.D.

56

Recurrent and Chronic Upper Respiratory Infections and Chronic Otitis Media

Acute respiratory infections in children are the most common ailments with which practicing physicians have to deal. They account for nearly two-thirds of the total illnesses in a community (Dingle et al., 1964) and are responsible for over a third of school absences (Saliba et al., 1967). In primary care pediatric practices, respiratory tract infections account for over half of all illness diagnoses. These illnesses also have a tremendous economic impact on society; the dollar cost of respiratory pharmaceuticals alone in the United States has been estimated to exceed $550 million per year. Recurrent (RURI) or chronic respiratory infections also are commonly encountered in childhood; often these infections become challenging diagnostic and therapeutic problems to the physician caring for these children.

Evidence also has been presented suggesting that respiratory allergic disorders may predispose a patient to a primary (usually viral) or secondary (usually bacterial) respiratory infection. Furthermore, it has been well documented that viral infections frequently precipitate asthmatic attacks. The similarity of the symptoms and signs of respiratory allergic diseases to those of infectious respiratory illnesses adds an additional diagnostic dilemma for the physician. In this chapter, an attempt is made to delineate those etiologic and contributing factors (with special emphasis on the role of allergy) that

may relate to the problem of chronic or recurring upper respiratory or ear infections. Practical diagnostic and therapeutic considerations also will be discussed.

What is a recurrent or chronic infection? These terms are extremely difficult to define precisely because of the wide variation in the frequency and severity of respiratory infections that occur in children and because of different criteria used in classifying these infections. For example, a normal 3-year old child attending nursery school, where there is repeated exposure to numerous respiratory viruses, might routinely have as many as ten infections per year. On the other hand, it would be abnormal for an older child to have that many URI's. In addition to increased frequency of infection, an increased susceptibility to infection also should include unusually severe or prolonged infections, infections without a symptom-free period, unexpected manifestations or complications of infection, or an infection with an organism of low pathogenicity.

FACTORS CONTRIBUTING TO RECURRENT OR CHRONIC RESPIRATORY INFECTIONS

Numerous factors contribute to the number and severity of upper respiratory

715

TABLE 56–1 FACTORS CONTRIBUTING TO RECURRENT OR CHRONIC RESPIRATORY INFECTIONS

Etiologic Agents
  Viruses
  Bacteria
  Other organisms

Environmental Factors
  Exposure to infectious agents
    School exposure
    Family size
    Baby sitters
  Seasonal variations
  Air pollution

Variation in Host Susceptibility
  Age and sex
  Nutrition
    Malnutrition
    Obesity
  Microbial factors
    Alteration of cellular and humoral immunity
    Impairment of reticuloendothelial system
    Anatomic alterations
    Facilitating colonization by other organisms
  Disorders leading to increased infections
    Circulatory
    Anatomic obstruction
    Integument defects

Allergy

infections in children. These are listed in Table 56–1.

Etiologic Agents

Clearly, the type of organism infecting the respiratory tract would have some bearing particularly on the chronicity or severity of the infection. The vast majority of respiratory infections are caused by viruses. Over 150 different viruses have been isolated and shown to be associated with both upper and lower respiratory infections. Although it is now realized that a causative agent seldom confines itself to a specific area, it is common practice to separate URI's into clinical syndromes (e.g., common cold, pharyngitis, laryngitis). It also is recognized that certain organisms tend to produce certain types of syndromes. The 90 or more different serologic rhinoviruses, as implied by the name,

primarily infect the nose and are the major etiologic group responsible for the common cold syndrome. The myxoviruses (respiratory syncytial, parainfluenza, influenza viruses) are the predominant pathogenetic agents encountered in serious respiratory infections in infants and children. Respiratory syncytial viruses are accountable for approximately 75 percent of bronchiolitis, whereas parainfluenza viruses more commonly cause laryngotracheobronchitis (croup). Influenza viruses frequently produce febrile illnesses with upper respiratory symptoms in older children and are infrequently implicated as a cause of severe lower respiratory disease in the pediatric age group. Adenoviruses are responsible for outbreaks of fever, pharyngitis, and conjunctivitis. Cornaviruses have been implicated as the etiologic agents in approximately 10 to 24 percent of the common cold syndromes; some enteroviruses (Coxsackie and ECHO viruses) also may be etiologic in producing URI's. Herpes virus can cause ulcerative lesions in the pharynx and mouth; however, herpangina commonly seen in children during the summer months is due to several Coxsackie A viruses. Although the classic illness produced by *Mycoplasma pneumoniae* is atypical pneumonia, this organism also may be etiologic in upper respiratory disease and bullous myringitis. Thus, depending on the type of infecting viral agent, a wide spectrum of clinical upper respiratory syndromes can be observed.

The role of bacteria and other organisms as causative factors in upper respiratory infection is more difficult to define. Unusual causes of common cold-like illnesses are *Coccidioides immitis, Histoplasma capsulatum, Bordetella pertussis, Chlamydia psittaci* and *Coxiella burnetii* (Q fever). As with most URI's, viruses are the major causes of pharyngitis and laryngitis. The only bacterial species commonly encountered as a cause of nasopharyngeal disease is the group A beta-hemolytic streptococcus. In the past, diphtheria and tuberculosis occasionally were responsible for pharyngeal infection, and pertussis in its preparoxysmal catarrhal stage had to be differentiated from other common causes of upper respiratory infections. Occasionally, in children under 3 years of age, *Hemophilus influenzae* may produce a mild nasopharyngitis; this organism also is responsible for the distinctive clinical entity of acute epiglottitis, the course of which can be fulminating and fatal if not recognized and treated promptly. There is little evidence that staphylococcus, non–group A streptococcus, or pneumococcus cause significant pharyngeal disease.

On the other hand, chronic tonsillitis generally is due to streptococci. Once chronic scarring has occurred, the organism is difficult to eradicate with antibiotic therapy. Repeated attacks of nasopharyngitis also may be caused by a chronic adenoiditis. Children with this infection generally have a chronic runny nose, repeated episodes of otitis media, and are chronic mouth breathers. The diagnosis is established on physical examination by finding a purulent postnasal drip or by palpating and expressing pus from the enlarged adenoid mass with a gloved finger. Antimicrobial therapy often is ineffectual, and removal of the hypertrophied tissue sometimes is necessary. It also should be mentioned that secondary bacterial infections in general account for many of the complications arising from the primary viral infections and undoubtedly contribute to the chronicity or recurrences of some infections seen in children. This will be further discussed under complications.

Environmental Factors

Exposure to Infection. The frequency of respiratory infections in children increases sharply when they enter nursery school or kindergarten, owing to exposure to a greater range of viruses. The infection rate in preschool children in a family also rises when an older sibling enters school. In general, the larger the family, the greater the individual attack rate for upper respiratory illnesses.

Seasonal Variations. Although the mechanisms involved are poorly understood, there is an increased incidence of infections during the winter months. This seasonal variation occurs in areas of high mean temperatures in wintertime as well as in locations with colder climates. In the tropics, respiratory infections are more prevalent during the rainy season. However, contrary to popular belief, there is no evidence that cold weather

per se, chilling, wet feet, and drafts cause or increase an individual's susceptibility to upper respiratory infections.

Air Pollution. Atmospheric pollution does not appear to affect the incidence of upper respiratory infections significantly, but has been found to be related to increased lower respiratory tract disease. Air pollutants such as photochemical smog and sulphur dioxide can cause ciliary paralysis, mucus gland hypertrophy, excess secretions with retention in the airways, slow resolution of respiratory infections, and susceptibility to further infections. There also is evidence that parental smoking increases the incidence of respiratory infections in children.

Psychosocial. Boyce et al. (1977) investigated the relationship between social environment and respiratory illness in children. Although life changes had no influence on the frequency of respiratory illnesses, they did correlate highly with the duration and severity of illness. Overcrowding and inadequate clothing also have been reported to increase the incidence and severity of acute and chronic respiratory infections (Brimblecombe et al., 1958).

Variations in Host Susceptibility

There are a number of host factors that can affect the incidence or severity of upper respiratory disease. These include age, sex, immune factors, microbial alterations of host susceptibility, and allergies.

Age and Sex. For reasons that are not clear, boys tend to have more upper respiratory infections than do girls (Badger et al., 1953). Boys under 6 years of age also have twice as many lower respiratory infections as do girls (approximately the same ratio as with asthma).

Nutrition. There is a general agreement that nutritional deficiencies will reduce the host's defense mechanisms to infection (Katz and Stiehm, 1977). In turn, both the infection and the malnutrition interfere with normal immune responses. Humoral antibody responses appear to be little affected, whereas T cell function is profoundly impaired in human malnutrition. Although all lymphoid tissue atrophies, the thymus gland is the most severely affected. It is of interest that despite high levels of IgE in many malnourished children, allergy is uncommon. It has been postulated that the elevated IgE levels reflect diminished thymic influence on IgE synthesis. Though phagocytic function remains intact, complement components decrease in proportion to the degree of malnutrition. Whether this has any practical consequences remains to be determined.

Obese subjects are more susceptible to respiratory infections (Chandra & Newberne, 1977), perhaps due to local factors such as reduced vascularity of adipose tissue, restricted pulmonary function, and/or defective microbicidal activity of granulocytes.

Immune Factors. Both primary and secondary immunodeficiency diseases are associated with recurrent respiratory infections, recurrent diarrhea, and failure to thrive (Stiehm and Fulginiti, 1980). Since they are discussed in detail elsewhere (Chapter 6), they will be mentioned briefly.

The most common of these disorders is selective IgA deficiency. The overall incidence is estimated to be 1 in 500, whereas in an atopic population the incidence is as high as 1 in 200. IgA deficiency may be associated with recurrent upper and lower respiratory infections, autoimmunity, gastrointestinal disorders, and increased risk of neoplasia, though many individuals with this condition may be asymptomatic. IgA deficiency is inherited, the pattern being either autosomal dominant or autosomal recessive. The diagnosis is easily confirmed by demonstrating serum levels less than 5 mg of IgA per deciliter. There is no specific treatment. Gamma globulin injections are contraindicated since they may cause sensitization of the patient by the production of anti-IgA antibodies.

Primary hypogammaglobulinemias also must be considered in children predisposed to respiratory infections, though they are less common than selected IgA deficiency. In both the congenital and the common variable type, the diagnosis is established by quantification of serum immunoglobulins and antibody responses. Replacement therapy with injections of gamma globulin or transfusions of plasma given every 3 to 4 weeks is the treatment of choice in these disorders.

The Wiskott-Aldrich syndrome, Buckley's syndrome (Buckley et al., 1972), and ataxia-telangiectasia also are associated with frequent respiratory infections. Generally the infections are severe compared to those of immunologically normal children.

Microbial Alteration of Host Susceptibility. Microbial alteration of the host may also promote invasion by secondary pathogens (Machowiak, 1978). The diminished ability to resist these secondary invaders is brought about by alterations in cellular or humoral immunity, or in the anatomy of the host. Temporary suppression of cell-mediated immunity has been demonstrated in a wide variety of infections, but the mechanisms responsible are poorly understood. Whether this increases the risk of secondary invasion by organisms is not entirely clear. Reports of a high incidence of reactivated tuberculosis during measles epidemics and adenovirus infections in persons recently immunized with smallpox or typhoid vaccine suggests a clinical association.

Various microorganisms also appear to predispose to secondary infections by altering humoral immunity by inhibiting antibody production, stimulating production of sensitizing antibodies, or inducing blocking antibodies.

Viruses also can impair reticuloendothelial system function and suppress phagocytosis temporarily. Both of these factors could conceivably predispose the host to invasion by secondary pathogens. However, further studies are necessary in man before impairment of the reticuloendothelial system can be implicated as a major factor responsible for bacterial superinfections following such infections as influenza.

Disorders Leading to Increased Infection. In general, recurrent infections at one site, often with the same organism, should make one suspect disorder of circulation, mechanical obstruction, or skin function. In contrast, infections due to a systemic immunodeficiency occur at multiple sites and frequently are caused by many different organisms. Examples of circulatory disorders leading to recurring infections include sickle cell anemia, diabetes, and nephrosis.

Mechanical obstruction frequently causes localized infection of the upper respiratory tract. Infants and children are especially prone to these infections. Because infants are obligatory nose breathers, nasal obstruction in infancy creates significant difficulties.

For example, nasal mucosal edema in a child with prominent lymphoid tissue and a short, straight, horizontal eustachian tube (as compared with the adult's) predispose to obstruction and infection. Obstruction and dysfunction of the eustachian tube and obstruction of the ostia of the sinuses from edema and secretions due to allergy or polyps also frequently give rise to recurrent or chronic ear infections and sinusitis.

Micromechanical problems also have been recently recognized. Abnormalities of clearance mechanisms due to disorganized ciliary movement in cystic fibrosis (due to the "CF factor in serum") and the immobile cilia syndrome in Kartagener's syndrome (chronic sinusitis, situs inversus, and bronchiectasis) are examples (Eliasson et al., 1977).

Skin defects that alter the primary mechanical barrier to organisms can also lead to an increased susceptibility to infection. Such disorders include skull fractures, midline sinus tracts, burns, and eczema.

Allergy. As previously mentioned, a relationship between allergy and respiratory infections has long been recognized. In addition to the well known bronchial hyperreactivity effects produced by various viral infections (McIntosh et al., 1973), asthmatic children have a greater frequency of viral respiratory infections as compared to their nonasthmatic siblings (Minor, 1974). This increased incidence of infection (especially rhinovirus infections) might have been related to increased time spent indoors, increased nasal viral inoculation due to nasal pruritus, and/or defects in antibody-dependent cellular toxicity noted in "infectious asthma" (Flaherty et al., 1976; Reed and Busse, 1978). A reduction of antibody-dependent cytotoxicity might not only make the patient more susceptible to infection but might also result in additional cell damage before the infection is terminated.

How upper respiratory viral infections cause airway hyperreactivity has not been clearly identified. The two most commonly offered explanations, (1) cholinergic sensitization and (2) beta adrenergic blockade, could conceivably play a role in the increased number of infections (primary and secondary) observed in allergic patients. The proponents of the cholinergic theory explain the increased hyperreactivity as due to increased sensitivity of the irritant receptors, owing to virus-induced bronchial epithelial damage. The latter also could be a factor contributing to the increased susceptibility to secondary bacterial infections. The other theory postulates that certain metabolites produced by the virus-infected cells act to interfere with beta adrenergic responses of some cell types, including sensory neurons that maintain normal bronchial tone. Not only is the beta receptor response impaired in neurons, but also in lymphocytes and polymorphonuclear cells. Thus, inflammation could be prolonged by interfering with the normal catecholamine effects on the leukocytes involved in the inflammatory process (see Chapter 14).

Other observations have related upper respiratory infections to allergic reactions. The onset of allergic disease in children has been linked to upper respiratory infections. Frick et al. (1977) found that 12 out of 13 children had their allergic sensitization initiated by upper respiratory infections. They developed increased IgE levels, positive radioallergosorbent tests (RAST), leukocyte histamine release, and lymphocyte transformation following the infection. Ida and co-workers (1977) have shown that virus-induced interferon enhances IgE-mediated histamine release from human basophils, which may be explain further how viral infections precipitate or potentiate allergic reactions.

There also is evidence that the incidence of recurrent otitis media, chronic serous otitis media, and acute and chronic sinusitis may be increased in allergic individuals (Bierman and Furukawa, 1978). Some investigators have contended that secretory otitis media can be a primary allergic response of the middle ear mucosa and contiguous tissues to a specific allergen. I feel, along with most authors, that the secretory otitis media results from abnormal function or mechanical obstruction of the eustachian tube, caused by allergy. Bluestone (1978) recently has postulated several other possibilities: (1) inflammatory swelling of the eustachian tube, (2) inflammatory obstruction of the nose, and (3) aspiration of bacteria-laden allergic nasopharyngeal secretions into the middle ear cavity.

Frequently, both secretory otitis and chronic sinusitis coexist, suggesting a common etiology; one such factor may be underlying allergic respiratory disease (Ho-shaw and Nickman, 1974). Anecdotal data suggest that sinusitis occurs frequently in patients with allergic respiratory disease and that, when present, it may be a precipitating event in bronchial asthma. In a recent study, Rachelefsky et al. (1978) evaluated 70 consecutive children referred for allergic evaluation for the prevalence of sinus disease (see Chapter 40 on sinusitis). Abnormal sinus x-ray results were found in 37 (53 percent) subjects and 15 (21 percent) had complete opacification of one or more sinuses. A purulent nasal discharge associated with cough, postnasal drip, complaints of sore throat, and nasal secretions which contained PMN's predominantly, were the clinical and laboratory findings that suggested this diagnosis. Sinus disease appears to be extremely common in allergic children and often contributes to the chronicity of symptoms.

Finally, the symptoms of upper respiratory allergic disease frequently are mistaken by the patient (and sometimes by the physician) as symptoms of an infection. For example, in a study of several hundred subjects, the incidence of allergic disease was significantly higher in those who had five or more "colds" per year compared to those who had two or fewer "colds" per year (Siegel et al., 1952).

DIAGNOSIS AND TREATMENT

It is evident that there are a vast number of factors that can contribute to recurrent or chronic upper respiratory infections. When the parent says "My child is sick all the time," how does the physician determine whether this is due to a variation of normal or due to a more serious underlying disorder?

History. Foremost among helpful diagnostic procedures is a detailed history. Although emphasis should be placed on the respiratory system, the history should be complete, since symptoms involving the other systems will give clues as to possible underlying disease processes.

Information regarding factors previously discussed that may contribute to the etiology of recurrent or chronic upper respiratory infections should be obtained. It is particu-larly important to differentiate three syndromes that are either frequently misdiagnosed or contribute to these infections in children: *perennial allergic rhinitis, vasomotor rhinitis,* and *recurrent infectious rhinitis.* The salient features of each of these disorders are presented in Table 56–2. Most often the diagnosis of each of these conditions can be established by history alone.

The development of specific therapeutic measures make the early and accurate diagnosis of the immunologically incompetent child more urgent. *The history often will provide the initial clues as to possible defects in host defense mechanisms and may be sufficient to differentiate nonimmune problems.* Usually, immunodeficient children are constantly sick, in contrast to normal children, who are well in between respiratory infections. Multiple sites of infections are the rule, whereas recurrent infections at the same locale (such as otitis media) should suggest an anatomic defect. When infections involve only the respiratory tract, allergy must be suspected. The type of organisms identified may also be of diagnostic significance. Gram-positive organisms often cause infections in children with antibody deficiencies, whereas infections by gram-negative organisms, fungi, protozoa, viruses or mycobacteria occur with cellular deficiencies. A family history of consanguinity, early infant deaths, cancer, or allergic, collagen, or autoimmune diseases also may suggest heritable disorders of host immunity.

Physical Examination. The physical examination may suggest whether the child's infections are "normal" or related to an underlying disease. In addition to distinctive symptoms (especially nasal pruritus and paroxysmal sneezing), the nasal mucous membranes in patients with allergic rhinitis often have a pale, bluish, moist, and glistening appearance (except when secondarily infected). However, the features of the nasal mucous membranes in vasomotor rhinitis are similar, so that the diagnosis cannot be established by physical examination alone. Children with allergies also often exhibit a number of characteristic stigmata. "Allergic shiners," dark and often swollen circles below the eyes, are presumed to be caused by stasis of blood resulting from swollen nasal and paranasal mucous membranes compressing the veins that drain this area.

Chronic nasal pruritus often leads to a transverse crease, a horizontal or hypopigmented groove across the lower third of the nose. A gaping appearance also may be present due to longstanding nasal obstruction and associated mouth breathing. Evidence obtained by history or physical findings of other atopic manifestations in the patient or the family

TABLE 56–2 DIFFERENTIAL DIAGNOSIS OF ALLERGIC, INFECTIOUS, AND VASOMOTOR RHINITIS

Findings	Allergic	Infectious	Vasomotor
HISTORY			
Usual age of onset	Childhood	Childhood	Adulthood, but not uncommon in childhood
Seasonal variations	Recurrent attacks	Single attacks, more frequent during winter months	Perennial, milder during summer months
Symptomatic between exacerbations	Persistent mild symptoms between attacks	Asymptomatic	Persistent symptoms
Nasal, ocular, or palatal pruritus	Marked	Minimal	Minimal
Paroxysmal sneezing	Frequent, especially in A.M.	Occasionally, early in course	Uncommon, mild sneezing can occur
Loss of taste or smell	Occasionally	Rarely	Occasionally
Wheezing and coughing associated	Often	Coincidental	Occasionally
Past history of atopic manifestations	Frequent	Coincidental	Coincidental
Allergens etiologic	Usual	Coincidental	Coincidental
Family history for allergy	Usual	Coincidental	Coincidental
Etiology	Allergens	Viruses	Unknown
Contagiousness	None	Frequently	None
PHYSICAL EXAMINATION			
Appearance of nasal mucous membranes	Usually pale and edematous, but may be erythematous	Hyperemic, red and edematous	Pale and edematous, or erythematous
Nasal discharge	Watery or mucoid	Mucopurulent or purulent	Watery or mucoid
Nasal polyps*	Occasionally	Infrequent	Occasionally
Other manifestations of atopy	Often present	Coincidental	Occasionally wheezing (nonallergic)
Allergic facies: shiners, nasal crease, gaping	Common	Usually absent	Usually absent
Allergic "salute"	Common	Absent	Usually absent, but can occur
LABORATORY TESTS			
Nasal eosinophilia greater than 10%	Usually positive	Negative	Usually negative
Peripheral eosinophilia	Usually positive	Negative†	Negative†
Positive immediate skin tests	Usually positive	Negative†	Negative†
Positive RAST	Usually positive	Negative†	Negative†
Elevated IgE levels	Approximately 60%	Normal†	Normal†
RESPONSE TO THERAPY			
Environmental control measures	Improvement	No improvement	No improvement
Antihistamines	Effective	Minimal effects	Poor
Topical cromolyn sodium	Effective	None	Poor
Topical corticosteroids	Excellent	Poor	Fair

*If present, cystic fibrosis should be ruled out.
†Unless coincidental allergic disease also present.

help to support the diagnosis of allergic rhinitis. If nasal polyps are present in children, the diagnosis of cystic fibrosis always must be ruled out by performing a sweat test.

The physical examination also may reveal important clues in immunodeficiency. Usually immunodeficient children appear pale, irritable, have poor subcutaneous fat, a distended abdomen, and appear chronically ill. Hepatosplenomegaly is common. Cervical nodes may be absent (despite a history of recurrent upper respiratory infections) or may be unduly enlarged or suppurative. Lymphoid tissue often is absent or markedly diminished. Tympanic membranes are frequently scarred or perforated, and there may be purulent ear drainage. Thrush and mouth ulcers are common. Evidence of lower respiratory infection (deep cough, rales, or wheezing) frequently is found. (These findings also suggest the possibility of asthma.) Rashes, abscesses, pyoderma, petechiae, paronychias, alopecia, sparse hair, arthritis, or telangiectasias often are present.

Laboratory Studies. Laboratory tests that are helpful in differentiating allergic, infectious, and vasomotor rhinitis are listed in Table 56–2. Examination of the type of cells in the nasal secretions can be especially helpful. The presence of eosinophils in the nasal secretions (greater than 10 percent of the cells) is highly suggestive of allergic rhinitis (Williams and Gwaltney, 1972). On the other hand, absence or a small number of eosinophils, during quiescent periods of allergic disease or in the presence of a secondary infection, does not rule out the diagnosis. In addition, the ratio of eosinophils to neutrophils can be an important indicator of the role that infection may be playing in patients with rhinitis.

Immediate type skin tests and RAST may not only be of help in pinpointing specific etiologic allergens but are useful in determining whether the patient is an allergic individual. However, elevation of IgE levels in the serum is less useful in determining the presence or absence of allergy since only about 60 percent of patients with allergic rhinitis have elevated serum IgE levels (Yunginger and Gleich, 1975).

Although the precise diagnosis of an immunodeficiency requires special tests normally available only in specialized centers, a number of initial screening tests can be performed easily by the practitioner that may help in resolving the dilemma of how to proceed with the patient presenting with recurrent or chronic infections. They are discussed in Chapter 6.

Differential Diagnosis and Complications. Other disorders that need to be considered in the differential diagnosis of allergic rhinitis, RURI, and chronic URI include adenoiditis or tonsillitis, chemical rhinitis, nasal congestion due to drugs, and foreign bodies. In addition, some of the complications of allergic rhinitis or recurrent infectious rhinitis (see Table 56–3) may contribute further to the chronicity of these infections and add to the diagnostic and therapeutic dilemmas when dealing with children who "are sick all the time." Although these conditions are discussed elsewhere, it should be emphasized that uncontrolled chronic rhinitis may lead to chronic sinusitis or recurrent acute or chronic otitis media.

Treatment. Appropriate management of chronic and recurrent URI requires recognition of the disorder as well as diagnosis of the underlying factors that contribute to it. In the young child with recurrent upper respiratory infections due to unavoidable exposure in nursery school, it may be necessary to remove the child from school temporarily. Antimicrobial therapy is not beneficial in shortening the duration of URI's nor in preventing secondary bacterial complications except perhaps the prophylactic use of sulfonamides for the prevention of recurrent otitis media (Biedel, 1978; Perrin et al., 1974). Once a secondary bacterial infection such as otitis media or sinusitis has been identified, selection of an appropriate antimicrobial agent depends on the patient's age, clinical signs and symptoms, knowledge of the organisms most often involved, and in-

TABLE 56–3 COMPLICATIONS OF ALLERGIC RHINITIS AND RURI

Sinusitis
Bacterial infections
   Adenoiditis and/or tonsillitis
   Pharyngitis
Lower respiratory infections
Triggering asthma
Otitis media

formation regarding penetration of the drug into the infected area (see Chapter 19). In recurrent otitis media, *Staphylococcus aureus* and *Hemophilus influenzae* are more commonly isolated than are *Diplococcus pneumoniae* and Group A streptococcus. If the organism is unknown, the preferred antibiotics at the present are amoxicillin for children and cloxacillin for adults and older children. The predominant organisms in sinusitis usually are *H. influenzae* and pneumococcus. Treatment with amoxicillin usually is effective. Therapy should be given for a minimum of 10 days, because the antibiotic penetrates into the sinuses poorly. One should keep in mind that inadequate treatment with antimicrobial agents also may be a factor in contributing to a chronic or recurrent infection.

Despite the wide usage of over-the-counter remedies containing decongestants and antihistamines, their efficacy has not been demonstrated clearly (Lampert et al., 1975; West et al., 1975). Evidence that these agents may help to maintain eustachian tube patency in children with chronic serous otitis media or recurrent otitis media is derived mainly from two studies (Miller, 1970; Strickler et al., 1967); more definitive studies are badly needed (see Chapter 38).

The therapeutic value of myringotomy in acute otitis remains doubtful other than for relieving severe otalgia (Giebrink and Quie, 1978). Ventilation of the middle ear with tympanostomy tubes does not appear to alter the long-term outcome of chronic and recurrent otitis media. Likewise, the effectiveness of adenoidectomy or tonsillectomy has not been proven.

Numerous other remedies have been ad-vocated for the prevention and management of RURI and chronic respiratory tract infections in children. These include vitamins (especially vitamin C), antiseptic aerosols, ultraviolet irradiation, autogenous and stock bacterial vaccines, transfer factor, and levamisole. None have been proven to be of value, and some may be potentially harmful. Although immunization against specific viral and bacterial agents has been successful in a few instances (e.g., influenza A and pneumococcus), many major problems must be overcome before immunization to the vast majority of upper respiratory infections can be successful. Chemoprophylaxis against viral infections is equally ineffective, with the possible exception of amantadine for influenza.

The management of specific immune disorders was considered briefly and is covered in more detail in Chapters 6 and 7. *The empirical and indiscriminate administration of serum immune globulin to a child with normal immune function (to prevent RURI or chronic respiratory tract infection) is without demonstrated value and may be harmful.*

When confronted with the child with recurrent or chronic respiratory tract infections, the physician should have a high index of suspicion for a possible underlying allergic disorder and should take appropriate measures to reverse the process if it is present. Successful management of upper respiratory allergic diseases consists of avoidance of suspected and known offending allergens, pharmacologic therapy, and allergy injection therapy (hyposensitization). Each of these approaches is discussed in detail in other chapters.

References

Badger, G. F., Dingle, J. H., Feller, A. E., Hodges, R. G., Jordan, W. S., Jr., and Rammelkamp, C. H., Jr.: A study of illness in a group of Cleveland families. II. Incidence of the common respiratory diseases. Am. J. Hyg. *58*:31, 1953.

Beidel, C. W.: Modification of recurrent otitis media by short-term sulfonamide therapy. Am. J. Dis. Child. *132*:681, 1978.

Bierman, C. W., and Furukawa, C. T.: Medical management of serous otitis in children. Pediatrics *61*:768, 1978.

Bluestone, C. D.: Eustachian tube function and allergy in otitis media. Pediatrics *61*:753, 1978.

Boyce, W. T., Jensen, E. W., Cassel, J. C., Collier, A. M., Smith, A. H., and Ramey, C. T.: Influence of life events and family routines on childhood respiratory tract illness. Pediatrics *60*:609, 1977.

Brimblecombe, F. S. W., Cruickshank, R., Masters, P. L., Reid, D. D., and Stewart, G. T.: Family studies of respiratory infections. Brit. Med. J. *1*:119, 1958.

Buckley, R. H., Wray, B. B., and Belmaker, E. Z.: Extreme hyperimmunoglobulinemia E and undue susceptibility to infection. Pediatrics *49*:59, 1972.

Chandra, R. K., and Newberne, P. M.: Nutrition, immunity and infection. In *Mechanisms of Interactions.* New York, Plenum Press, 1977.

Dingle, J. H., Badger, G. F., and Jordan, W. S.: *Illness in the Home: A Study of 25,000 Illnesses in a Group of Cleveland Families.* Cleveland, The Press of Western Reserve University, 1964.

Eliasson, R., Mossberg, B., Camner, P., and Afzelius, B. A.:

The immotile-cilia syndrome, a congenital ciliary abnormality as an etiologic factor in chronic airway infections and male sterility. New Engl. J. Med. 297:1977.

Flaherty, D. K., Storms, W. W., and Kritz, R.: Antibody-dependent cell cytotoxicity in asthmatics. Fed. Proc. 35:790a, 1976.

Frick, O. L., Ashton, F. A., and Mills, J.: Virus infection association with onset of allergic sensitization in infants. The American Congress of Allergy and Immunology, New York (Abstract) No. 162, 1977.

Giebrink, G. S., and Quie, P. G.: Otitis media: The spectrum of middle ear inflammation. Ann. Rev. Med. 29:285, 1978.

Hoshaw, T. C., and Nickman, N. J.: Sinusitis and otitis in children. Arch. Otolaryngol. 100:194, 1974.

Ida, S., Hooks, J. J., Siraganian, R. P., et al.: Enhancement of IgE-mediated histamine release from human basophils by viruses; role of interferon. J. Exp. Med. 145:892, 1977.

Katz, M., and Stiehm, E. R.: Host defense in malnutrition. Pediatrics 59:490, 1977.

Lampert, R. P., Robinson, D. S., and Sozka, L. F.: A critical look at decongestants. Pediatrics 55:550, 1975.

Machowiak, P. A.: Microbial synergism in human infections. New Engl. J. Med. 298:21 and 83, 1978.

McIntosh, K., Ellis, E. F., Hoffman, L. S., Lybass, T. G., Eller, J. J., and Fulginiti, V. A.: The association of viral and bacterial respiratory infections with exacerbation of wheezing in young asthmatic children. J. Pediatr. 82:578, 1973.

Miller, G. F.: Influence of oral decongestant on eustachian tube function in children. J. Allergy 45:187, 1970.

Minor, T. E., Baker, J. W., Dick, E. C., DeMeo, A. N., Ouellette, J. J., Cohen, M., and Reed, C. E.: Greater frequency of viral respiratory infections in asthmatic children as compared with their nonasthmatic siblings. J. Pediatr. 85:472, 1974.

Perrin, J. M., Charney, E., MacWhinney, J. B., Jr., McInerny, T. K., Miller, R. L., and Nazarian, L. S.: Sulfasoxazole as chemoprophylaxis for recurrent otitis media: A double-blind crossover study in pediatric practice. New Engl. J. Med. 291:664, 1974.

Rachelefsky, G. S., Goldberg, M., Katz, R. M., Boris, G., Gyepes, M. T., Shapiro, M.J., Mickey, M. R., Finegold, S. M., and Siegel, S. C.: Sinus disease in children with respiratory allergy. J. Allergym. Clin. Immunol. 61:310, 1978.

Reed, C. E., and Busse, W. W.: The relationship between the autonomic nervous system and respiratory infections in the pathogenesis of asthma. Current Concepts Allergy & Clin. Immunol. 7:1, 1978.

Saliba, G. S., Glezen, W. P., and Chin, T. D. Y.: Etiologic studies of acute respiratory illness among children attending public schools. Am. Rev. Respir. Dis. 95:592, 1967.

Siegel, S. C., Goldstein, J. D., Sawyer, A., and Glaser, J.: The incidence of allergy in persons who have many colds. Ann. Allergy 10:24, 1952.

Stiehm, E. R., and Fudenberg, H. H.: Serum levels of immune globulins in health and disease: A survey. Pediatrics 37:715, 1966.

Stiehm, E. R., and Fulginiti, V. A.: Immunologic Disorders in Infants and Children. Philadelphia, W. B. Saunders Co., 1980.

Strickler, G. B., Rubenstein, M. M., McBean, J. B., Hedgecock, L. L., Hugstad, J. A., and Griffing, T.: Treatment of otitis media. IV. A fourth clinical trial. Amer. J. Dis. Child. 114:123, 1967.

West, S., Brandon, B., Stolley, P., and Rumrill, R.: A review of antihistamines and the common cold. Pediatrics 56:100, 1975.

Williams, R. B., and Gwaltney, J. M.: Allergic rhinitis or virus cold? Nasal smear eosinophilia in differential diagnosis. Ann. Allergy 30:189, 1972.

Yunginger, J. W., and Gleich, G. J.: The impact of the discovery of IgE on the practice of allergy. Ped. Clin. N. Am., 22:3, 1975.

Gilbert A. Friday, M.D.
D. Lee Miller, M.D.
Michael J. Painter, M.D.

57

Headache

Headache is not an uncommon complaint in childhood and is a symptom seen in a great variety of clinical conditions. Although it is difficult to assess the incidence of all types of headache, as many as 4 percent of school children appear to suffer from vascular headaches (Bille, 1962). Even before the age of 6 years, it is not uncommon for a child to complain that his head hurts. In most instances, headache is not associated with allergic disease. Chronic headache may signal the presence of an underlying structural, physiologic, or psychologic disease process that warrants therapy, and all chronic or recurrent headaches demand painstaking consideration of their etiology. The determination of the cause of chronic headache requires careful and systematic history taking, thorough general physical and neurologic examination, and the use of selective laboratory studies. Rational therapy can best be accomplished after a specific etiologic factor(s) is found.

CLASSIFICATION OF HEADACHE

Classifications of headaches are necessarily incomplete, since the etiology and mechanisms in many instances are unknown. It is useful, however, to consider headaches according to pathophysiologic processes of pain production, namely: vascular, sustained muscle contraction, and traction-inflammatory.

Headaches of Vascular Origin. Evidence suggests that the pre-headache phenomena observed in some vascular headaches is related to constriction of cerebral arteries (Bruyn, 1976; Dalessio, 1972 and 1974). The pain in migraine actually is related to subsequent dilatation of cranial arteries, principally in the distribution of the external carotid vessels, but may be due in fact to the associated increased vascular permeability that results in a sterile inflammation. Various vasoactive substances have been implicated in this process. These include histamine, kinins, SRS-A, 5-hydroxytryptamine, prostaglandins, and extraneous vasoactive agents such as tyramine and phenylethylamine.

Headaches Due to Sustained Muscle Contraction. A common factor in the production of headache is sustained contraction of head or neck musculature. Several important mechanisms for muscular spasm have been described. Reflex feedback pathways from the spinal cord impair muscle relaxation. It must be remembered that not only can the pathologic process conduct impulses, which ultimately results in muscle contraction, but also the contracted muscle may send stimuli to the cord that augment the already existing spasm. Finally, muscular spasm is perceived by the cerebral cortex as painful.

Traction-Inflammatory Headaches. The final mechanism responsible for the production of head pain is direct traction, torsion, or inflammation of pain-sensitive structures of the scalp, skull, and intracranial contents. The principal intracranial pain-sensitive structures include the venous sinuses and their tributaries, parts of the dura in the vicinity of the large arteries of the brain leading to and coming from the circle of Willis, and the arteries themselves. In addition, the anterior and middle meningeal arteries of the dura are pain-sensitive. Extracranial structures that possess pain receptors include the periosteum of the skull, the skin of the scalp, and its blood supply, appendages and muscles. Nerves that conduct pain include the trigeminal, facial, vagus, glossopharyngeal, and second and third cervical nerves. Intracranial structures not sensitive to pain include the brain parenchyma, pia mater, arachnoid membrane, parts of the dura mater, the ependyma lining ventricles, and the choroid plexus.

CLINICAL HEADACHE SYNDROMES

Vascular headache syndromes include migraine, cluster headaches, headaches caused by arterio-venous malformations, hypertension, and fever. Sustained muscle contractions are the basis of the common tension headache associated with spasm of scalp and neck musculature, pain in the temporomandibular joint area from malocclusion, and "ophthalmic headaches" from hyperopic refractive errors. Traction-inflammation headaches include head pain associated with meningitis, brain abscesses, inflamed nasal and paranasal structures as well as traction on pain-sensitive structures by tumors, cysts, A-V malformations, hematomas, hydrocephalus, periosteal elevation, and lumbar punctures (Friedman and Harms, 1967).

Migraine. Migraine headaches may be divided into classic and common types. About 10 percent of migraine headaches are of the classic variety, which consist of three phases: pre-headache, headache, and post-headache. During the pre-headache phase, there may be pallor, scotomata, scintillations, tinnitus, and other sensations. This period lasts from minutes to hours. The prodromal phase gives way to a painful headache phase characterized by deep, aching, throbbing pain felt behind the eye on the affected side. This pain will then progress to involve the ipsilateral hemicranium and, at times, the entire head. Photophobia, tearing, and blurred vision are frequent. Edema of the lid and face is not unusual. Duration is from hours to days. Toward the end of the

attack, vomiting may occur. This phase is associated with marked dilatation of the external carotid system, sometimes even observable on the patient's forehead. With the ultimate disappearance of the headache, the third, or post-headache, phase may be accompanied by dehydration, feelings of euphoria, or total apathy. Common migraine may not be characterized by a prodromal stage or localization. "Migrainoid" syndromes may occur with or without headache, presenting as cyclic vomiting or abdominal pain.

Uncommon Vascular Headaches. Uncommon vascular headaches include the following: cluster headache, "malignant migraine," basilar artery migraine, head trauma, and vascular malformations. Cluster headaches, characteristically occurring nocturnally, consist of a series of closely spaced attacks followed by remissions of months or years. Extraocular muscle palsies, hemiplegia, hemiparesis, and confusional states characterize "malignant migraine." Basilar artery migraine (Bickerstaff, 1961; Golden and French, 1975) has been described as a type of migraine occurring primarily in young women and girls, often having a striking relation to menstruation and characterized by vertigo, ataxia, dysarthria, and paresthesias followed by severe, throbbing occipital headache with vomiting. Head trauma may precipitate vascular headaches. Vascular malformations may cause headache clinically indistinguishable from migraine. Convulsions, focal signs outlasting the headache, and continuous cranial bruit are among the associated neurologic findings. Headache of vascular malformations may also be due to subarachnoid hemorrhage. Hypertension is an occasional cause of headache in children. Fever may produce head pain by means of vasodilatation.

Muscle-Tension Syndrome. Muscle-tension headaches are often located in bitemporal or occipital areas and characterized by band-like or constrictive pain of dull quality and moderate intensity. Historically, these headaches are often generated by anxiety-producing events. Disorders of the temporomandibular joint, regardless of the cause (e.g., malocclusion), may produce muscle-tension headache.

Traction-Inflammatory Syndrome. Headaches caused by dural traction or meningeal inflammation, including meningitis, brain abscess, brain tumors, cysts, A-V malformations, hematomas, and hydrocephalus, are varied in quality and severity. Constant, severe, dull headache is the most constant feature of brain abscess, while headache is often inconspicuous in hydrocephalus. Pain on eye movement is often a clue to the meningeal origin of headache. The head pain associated with increased intracranial pressure is dull, of moderate intensity, and tends to be most severe early in the morning. Occasionally, the headache is localized adjacent to structural lesions because of dural traction but may be referred to a distant site.

Rhinocephalgia. The word *rhinocephalgia*, has been coined to describe pain originating from the nasal structures. Headaches, especially those associated with acute disease of the paranasal structures, often become clinically important. Allergic rhinitis with engorgement of the nasal turbinates may block sinus ostia, resulting in sinus infection with subsequent inflammation of the pain-sensitive nasal structures leading to headache. Wolff, through a series of careful experiments identified the pain-sensitive structures in the nasal and paranasal areas (Dalessio, 1972). These are listed in Table 57–1. Stimulation of the pharyngeal tonsillar area and nasal floor induces localized pain of low intensity. Stimulation of nasal turbinates may result in intense pain, depending upon the area stimulated. Stimulation of the ostia of the maxillary sinuses results in severe pain with referral to the nasopharynx, molars, zygoma, and the temple. Stimulation of the duct of the frontal sinuses and the superior nasal cavity also gives significant pain, which is felt locally as well as at the inner canthus of the eye, zygoma, temple, angle of the jaw and molars. It is of interest to note that in these experiments stimulation of the mucosa of the paranasal sinuses produced little discomfort. Stimulation of the cavity of the sphenoid sinus produces referred pain to the vertex of the skull. When the maxillary sinus

TABLE 57–1 EXPERIMENTAL STUDY OF PAIN FROM NASAL AND PARANASAL STRUCTURES*

Structures Stimulated	Sites of Pain	Intensity (1 to 10+)
Pharynx and posterior nasopharynx	Local, deep throat	1–2+
Tonsil	Local, behind ear	1–2+
Nasal floor	Local	1–2+
Nasal septum		
Middle	Zygoma to ear	1–2+
Upper	Inner and outer canthus of eye	1–2+
Turbinates		
Upper	Local, inner canthus, forehead, lateral wall of nose	4–6+
Middle	Local, zygoma, to ear and temple	4–6+
Lower	Local, upper teeth, under eye, zygoma to ear	4–6+
Ostium of maxillary sinus	Local, nasopharynx, back teeth, zygoma, temple	5–8+
Nasofrontal duct	Inner canthus, zygoma, temple, angle of jaw, upper back teeth	5–7+
Sinuses		
Frontal	Local, bridge of nose	1/2+
Sphenoid	Vertex of skull	1–2+
Maxillary	Eye, jaw, back teeth	1/2+
Superior nasal cavity		
Anterior	Over eye, upper canthus, teeth	6+
Posterior (vicinity of ethmoidal sinuses)	Teeth, outer canthus	5–6+

*After Wolff (see Dalessio, 1972).

Structures were stimulated by pressure from a probe and by faradic current. Pain was described as 1+, 2+, etc. The magnitude of the current used for stimulation was based on a scale in which a 1+ pain was the lower limit of pain perception by the tip of the tongue.

is stimulated, discomfort can be felt about the eye, angle of the jaw, and posterior molars.

Thus, inflammation of the sinuses involving the ostia, particularly the maxillary ostia, may result in "sinus headaches," whereas infection of the sinus *per se* may be painless. Pressure in the maxillary and frontal sinuses produces little or no discomfort. Wolff also found that headaches originating in paranasal sinuses are uncommon. When headaches did occur, they were usually deep, dull, aching and nonpulsating. They rarely caused nausea or vomiting and seldom rivaled migraine headaches in intensity. In acute sinus disease, headaches are more intense than in chronic sinus inflammation.

ROLE OF INGESTANTS IN HEADACHE PRODUCTION

It has been claimed that migraine headaches may be caused by food hypersensitivity. There is no correlation between the presence of IgE antibody to a particular food and the appearance of migraine following ingestion of that food, however. Many studies associating food allergy with migraine have been uncontrolled. In the controlled studies by Wolff (Dalessio, 1972), Loveless (1950), and Walker (1960), challenges with disguised foods did not regularly induce a headache to historically "offending" foods. In early infancy, when the gastrointestinal tract is most permeable to food allergens, migraine is least common.

Certain foods do precipitate headaches in some individuals, however (Dalessio, 1972). Alcohol, for example, may produce headaches in subjects prone to migraine. Patients with cluster headaches notoriously are sensitive to small amounts of alcohol. Alcohol is a nonspecific vasodilator, which probably accounts for its precipitation of the vascular headache process. Another example of a vasoactive substance precipitating headaches is unusual sensitivity to sodium nitrate, used in cured meats such as hot dogs, bacon, ham, and salami. Large amounts of ingested monosodium glutamate may produce generalized vasomotor reactions that include headache ("Chinese restaurant syndrome").

PRACTICAL CONSIDERATIONS IN THE EVALUATION OF HEADACHE IN CHILDREN

A careful history should include the location, duration, intensity, quality, and timing of head pain. Sustained contraction headache is usually occipital or bitemporal in location, of moderate severity and is constricting or band-like in quality. A vascular headache is a severe "pounding or throbbing" headache which is associated frequently with vomiting in the pediatric age group. The headache usually is unilateral but usually alternates sides, and may be bilateral. A pounding headache that occurs on the same side and associated with focal neurologic deficit should raise suspicion of an underlying structural abnormality (e.g., an arteriovenous malformation). The subcategory of cluster headache is extremely rare in childhood but has been described in neurofibromatosis. Dull constant headaches, which occur primarily in the morning, should raise the suspicion of elevated intracranial pressure.

A careful dietary history is of value in eliciting inciting agents. As previously mentioned, occasional vascular headache sufferers have headaches precipitated by chocolate, alcohol, or foods with a high content of tyramine or other vasoactive substances.

General physical examination including determination of blood pressure should be performed. Neurologic evaluation must include auscultation of the skull, visual field evaluation by confrontation, funduscopic examination, and evaluation of sensation, gait, and reflexes. Soft systolic bruits are heard on auscultation of the skull in many children between the ages of 3 and 15 years. However, detection of a loud, continuous cranial bruit is an indication for more extensive neurodiagnostic procedures. It must be recognized, however, that angiography is undertaken with great care in the evaluation of individuals with vascular headaches, as they have an increased incidence of angiographic complications, including stroke. An electroencephalogram, skull films, and computerized tomographic scanning should be considered in patients with focal neurologic deficit, headaches at a consistent location, scalp or periosteal tenderness, and refractory headaches. In the presence of fever and meningeal signs, lumbar puncture is indicated. However, if there is a significant possibility that a space-occupying intracranial lesion such as a tumor or abscess is present, lumbar puncture is to be avoided as an initial diagnostic procedure. Referral to a neurologist should be considered if there is reason to suspect headache due to a structural abnormality.

Head pain consistent with rhinocephalgia may require x-ray examination of the paranasal sinuses, allergy evaluation, and possibly further immunologic study. Pale engorgement of the nasal turbinates suggests allergy or vasomotor rhinitis. In chronic purulent rhinitis, abnormalities of the humoral, cell-mediated or phagocytic limb of the immune system must be considered. In this instance, appropriate evaluation of the immune system should be undertaken. Headache due to temporomandibular joint dysfunction and hyperopia are uncommon in children and require the services of an orthodontist or ophthalmologist.

TREATMENT OF HEADACHES

Intelligent therapy of headache in childhood rests upon proper diagnosis. Headaches of inflammatory origin or those due to intracranial space-occupying lesions and arteriovenous malformations will not be further considered, as they are beyond the scope of this text. Muscle contraction headache usually responds to analgesics, muscle relaxants, or mild tranquilizers. In evaluating patients with muscle tension headache, however, signs of depression should be sought and, if present, psychiatric evaluation is indicated. Cluster headache is extremely rare in childhood and will not be further considered here. Various drugs have been advocated for the treatment of childhood migraine. Ergots, because of their unpredictable profound ef-

fects on the cerebral vasculature of children, are not recommended in the treatment of childhood migraine. Anticonvulsants such as phenobarbital and phenytoin have been used for treatment of childhood migraine. However, hirsutism, gingival hyperplasia, and changes in collagen structure and other side effects are associated with the use of phenytoin, and this drug should be avoided in the treatment of childhood migraine.

Propranolol can be an effective prophylactic agent in childhood migraine (Ludvigsson, 1974). Since it must be employed on a daily basis, prophylactic therapy is inconvenient. It may be best to leave the decision regarding daily prophylaxis up to the child. If the headache is of sufficient severity and frequency to warrant daily prophylaxis, propranolol would appear to be the most efficacious agent. *Note:* It is to be avoided in patients with asthma since it can precipitate or intensify bronchospasm. Although cyproheptadine has not been found to be of value for migraine prophylaxis in adults, it occasionally is efficacious in pediatric patients. The side effects of drowsiness and somnolence, which are so troublesome to the adult, are less commonly seen in the pediatric age group. Vascular headaches may respond to treatment with acetaminophen or aspirin. Before embarking on a therapeutic regimen of daily prophylaxis utilizing potent pharmacologic agents, the response of an individual headache to less potent agents such as acetaminophen or aspirin should be evaluated.

Allergic management may include avoidance, drug therapy, and immunotherapy. When sinusitis is found, appropriate treatment of this condition may include nasal decongestants, antihistamines, and broad-spectrum antibiotics (Evans et al., 1975). Since *Hemophilus* species and *Streptococcus pneumoniae* are common pathogenic bacteria found in acute and chronic sinusitis, antibiotics should be chosen to treat these organisms (see Chapter 19).

References

Bille, B.: Migraine in school children. Acta Neurol. Scand. *51*:Suppl. 136.

Bickerstaff, E. R.: Basilar artery migraine. Lancet *1*:15, 1961.

Bruyn, G. W.: Biochemical basis of migraine: a critique. *In*

Klawans, J. R. (ed.): *Clinical Neuropharmacology.* New York, Raven Press, 1976, pp. 185–213.

Dalessio, D. J.: Wolff's Headache and Other Head Pain, 3rd ed. New York, Oxford University Press, 1972.

Dalessio, D. J.: Mechanisms and biochemistry of headache. Postgrad. Med. *56*:55, 1974.

Dalessio, D. J.: Dietary migraine. Am. Fam. Physician *6*:60, 1972.

Evans, F. O., Sydnor, J. D., Moore, W. E., et al.: Sinusitis of the maxillary antrum. New Engl. J. Med. *293*:735, 1975.

Friedman, A. T., and Harms, E.: *Headaches in Children.* Springfield, Ill., Charles C Thomas, 1967.

Golden, G. S., and French, J. D.: Basilar artery migraine in young children. Pediatrics *56*:722, 1975.

Loveless, M.: Milk allergy: A survey of its incidence: Experiments with a masked ingestion test: Allergy for corn and its derivatives: Experiments with a masked ingestion test for its diagnosis. J. Allergy *21*:489, 1950.

Ludvigesson, J.: Propranolol used in prophylaxis of migraine in children. Acta Neurol. Scand. *50*:109, 1974.

Walker, V. B.: Report to the Ciba Foundation's Conference on Migraine. London, Nov. 1960.

Paul P. VanArsdel, Jr., M.D.

58

Fever

Elevation of body temperature may be produced by three different mechanisms: (1) inadequate heat dissipation from the skin, (2) excessive heat production, and (3) alteration in hypothalamic regulation. The first two are not involved in allergic reactions; indeed, if anything, cutaneous allergic reactions would tend to promote heat dissipation.

The third mechanism is responsible for most kinds of fever. Thermosensitive neurons in the preoptic region of the anterior hypothalamus are responsible for the regulation of body temperature. They act essentially as a thermostat, regulating physiologic reactions that control the production (shivering) and dissipation (sweating and vasodilation) of heat. So-called *pyrogens* act indirectly or directly by raising the temperature at which the hypothalamic control reaches equilibrium.

INDIRECT PYROGENS

Microorganisms exert their pyrogenic effect either through the release of endotoxin or simply by being phagocytosed. Endotoxins are lipopolysaccharides that form part of the cell wall of gram-negative bacteria. They are potent pyrogens; as little as 0.0001 μg/kg will produce detectable fever (Atkins and Bodel, 1974). Endotoxin is thought to be responsible for the fever in the Jarisch-Herxheimer reaction that may complicate the treatment of syphilis (Gelfand et al., 1976). There is some biologic variation in the endotoxin effect. For example, brucella endotoxin has a latent period of several hours, while typhoid endotoxin produces fever only 30 to 60 minutes after injection (Abernathy and Spink, 1958).

Gram-positive bacteria do not contain endotoxin, and only the group A streptococcus and a few strains of *Staphylococcus aureus* produce soluble pyrogens. However, the most important reaction responsible for fever is phagocytosis of intact bacteria; disrupted cells are not pyrogenic unless antibody to some constituent of the cell is present. Phagocytosis also is necessary for the pyrogenic effect of cryptococcal cells and various nonbacterial colloidal particles (Snell, 1972). Some classes of virus are pyrogenic when given intravenously to rabbits; the literature on virus-induced fever has been reviewed recently by Atkins and Bodel (1974).

Although several drugs can produce fever pharmacologically, the only ones that act as chemical pyrogens are steroids such as etiocholanolone and bile acids with a 5β-H ring. Etiocholanolone fever is an interesting model, but there is no convincing evidence that this steroid plays a role in clinical febrile diseases.

That hypersensitivity reactions can be associated with fever has been known since the late 19th century, when serum sickness became a clinical problem. It was only after World War II, however, that experiments were begun that established that antigen-antibody complexes were pyrogenic in experimental animals. These will be discussed later.

ENDOGENOUS PYROGEN

When animals given any of the indirect pyrogens develop fever, a substance appears in the circulation that produces fever almost immediately. This was first reported by

731

Atkins and Wood (1955), who referred to it as an endogenous pyrogen (EP). This turned out to be the same as a pyrogen obtained several years earlier from exudate cells by Beeson, the so-called leukocytic pyrogen. Cells that produce EP include neutrophils, monocytes, eosinophils, Kupffer cells, and other tissue phagocytic cells (Dinarello and Wolff, 1978). Although lymphocytes are not sources of EP, sensitized T cells from rabbits or guinea pigs do produce a type of lymphokine that stimulates EP production by phagocytic cells (Chao et al., 1977).

Activation of leukocytes takes from as little as 15 minutes from completion of phagocytosis, if that is the stimulus, to as much as 6 hours after exposure to etiocholanolone. Further time is required before an appreciable amount of EP is released, because EP production requires the synthesis of new messenger RNA and protein (Dinarello and Wolff, 1978). It is likely that the pyrogenicity of antigen-antibody complexes also depends on phagocytosis, which follows the binding of complexes to Fc and complement receptors on phagocytes.

Endogenous pyrogen is a small molecule, compared to the indirect pyrogens, having a molecular weight of 15,000 daltons. In contrast to endotoxin, it is heat labile and is destroyed by exposure to trypsin or pronase. It is pyrogenic in nanogram concentrations when injected.

THE THERMOREGULATORY CENTER AND MODIFYING FACTORS

When injected into the appropriate region of the hypothalamus, EP is 100 times as potent a pyrogen as when given systemically. It has the same local effect on the center as does cooling. This effect is modulated locally by opposite-acting 5-hydroxytryptamine and by norepinephrine. The former promotes fever in subhuman primates, but the role is reversed in lower animals.

The possibility that EP exerts its effect by stimulating prostaglandin synthesis is a matter of considerable current interest. It is known that E prostaglandins (PG) are pyrogenic at the same site as EP. Acetylsalicylic acid and similar drugs that are inhibitors of PG synthesis, prevent EP fever, but not PG fever. Although this is an attractive concept,

it remains controversial (Veale et al., 1977). If PG does turn out to be involved in the genesis of fever, it may do so by increasing the level of cyclic AMP, which is also thought to be pyrogenic (Dinarello and Wolff, 1978).

HUMAN FEVER

Atopic Disease. The earliest reference to fever in allergic disease had to do with hay fever (Bostock, 1819). More than a half-century went by before Blackley (1873) published the results of his classic experiments that established the association of allergy to pollens and other substances. Among other things, Blackley recorded body temperatures and, though commenting that true fever was rare, also noted that it had occurred after inhalation challenge with one species of tree pollen. Since then, observations on temperature elevation in natural or artificially provoked pollenosis have been conspicuous by their absence; and fever has not even been observed following allergen injections used for hyposensitization (immunotherapy). Shouldn't the term "hay fever" be abandoned then? John Freeman, an early associate of Leonard Noon (who first developed immunotherapy), gave an appropriate response to the question several decades later (1950).

> But why should we tolerate the incorrect "fever" when in uncomplicated hayfever there is no rise in temperature? This well-known error in clinical observation has long been embedded in popular language all the world over (e.g., *heufieber, fièvre du foin, fiebre del heno*, etc.); since it involves no aetiological mistakes it will not embarrass any radical treatment. I think we should lose more than we should gain by trying to correct this popular word; we must not go tilting at every verbal windmill, so "hay-fever" let it continue to be for us.

Actually, pollenosis sufferers often *feel* feverish during the season, so the term, coined by the laity, remains popular today, regardless of the numbers on a thermometer.

In textbooks of 20 or more years ago, several authors stated that it was not uncommon to observe fever in young children with severe asthma and no other identifiable cause of fever. Such general or anecdotal statements were never referenced. In recent years, mention of such fever in asthma has been practically nonexistent, probably because of better success in identifying non-allergic causes such as infection and atelectasis.

Food allergy (not necessarily atopic) also was cited occasionally in the older literature as a cause of fever. One of the most interesting is a baffling case reported to the Association of American Physicians by Janeway in 1908. We now know this patient had periodic polyserositis. She was seen by Cooke in 1916, who placed her on a milk-free diet, with a prompt remission that lasted for the 9 subsequent years of follow-up (Cooke, 1933)! Being aware of this, Siegel (1964) reviewed his experience with 50 such patients. He noted that significantly more were atopic than in a control group, but only two were helped by the elimination of milk. Feigin and Shearer (1976) recently reported on 146 patients with fever of unknown origin (FUO) seen at St. Louis Children's Hospital. The cause in two of them was thought to be milk allergy.

In summary, the only information supporting an association between fever and atopic, or IgE-antibody mediated, reactions is anecdotal.

Serum Sickness. The introduction of horse serum antitoxin for treatment of diphtheria was soon followed by adverse reactions; the first was reported in Germany in 1894. By 1905 the clinical pattern was well established and little has been added since von Pirquet and Schick (1905) published their classic report. They observed that fever was one of the most frequent symptoms and was typically remittent in nature. As in animal experiments, the fever was accompanied by leukopenia with relative lymphocytosis. Fever was a major manifestation also in the immediate and accelerated reactions following readministration of serum.

Xenogenic antiserum therapy reached its peak in the 1930's. Kojis (1942) reported on 6,211 cases treated at the Willard Parker hospital in New York. Of those given diphtheria antitoxin, 27 percent developed fever, while 50 percent reacted to scarlet fever serum. The fever pattern was variable. In addition to the remittent pattern, steplike, typhoidal, persistent, and even doubly remittent reactions occurred.

For a while, convalescent human serum was also used in treatment of diphtheria and other conditions. This usually was taken from donors who had become sensitized to horse serum. One patient given such serum

received intramuscular diphtheria antitoxin 11 days later. In 3 hours a marked local Arthus reaction developed, along with a high fever (Kojis, 1942). Deliberately induced passive serum sickness was actually tried as a therapeutic modality at Willard Parker hospital. Of 62 patients, 65 percent reacted when given 2 to 10 ml convalescent serum intravenously after an earlier injection with horse serum. Several became febrile (Karelitz and Stempien, 1942).

Inhalation Fevers. Inhaled allergens produce bronchospasm without fever in patients with IgE antibodies to those allergens. A comparatively small number of patients respond differently. A typical patient will develop cough, fever, and breathlessness 4 to 6 hours after inhaling the offending agent, usually an organic dust or aerosol to which the patient has become sensitized with the development of serum precipitating antibodies. Such agents include material from various birds and rodents (including gerbils), and fungi that grow in hay, sugar cane, wood, cork, and in air-conditioning and humidifying equipment. The last has received special attention recently as an important public health problem in industry (Leading article, 1978) and is a potential problem in the home as well. Phagocytosis of the antigen-IgG antibody complexes is a sufficient explanation for the fever, but a T cell–derived mechanism also could play a role.

Reactions to Human Blood Products. Allogeneic reactions to red cell antigens are so well known that little comment is necessary. Fever is probably caused by the phagocytosis of red-cell antigen-antibody complexes, resulting in the production of EP. Jandl and Tomlinson (1958) were able to produce fever in normal recipients by passive sensitization, using red cells and anti-Rh antibodies. They noted that the response was invariably associated with leukopenia. The febrile reactions were more striking with relatively weak incompatibilities than with ABO reactions, where the complexes formed are much larger and rapidly sequestered. Most nonhemolytic transfusion reactions are due to alloincompatibility of leukocytes, and are associated with circulating leukoagglutinins. Perkins et al. (1966) found that the number of leukocytes necessary to raise the temperature one degree Celsius per hour was about 10^9. Plasma reactions are rare but do occur, particularly in those who receive multiple transfusions and develop allogeneic

TABLE 58–1 NONALLERGIC CAUSES OF DRUG FEVER

Mechanism	Examples
Endogenous release of bacterial pyrogen	Jarisch-Herxheimer reaction
Administration of exogenous pyrogen	Contaminated fluids or drugs
	"Fever therapy": injection of endotoxin or typhoid vaccine
Release of endogenous pyrogen	Sterile inflammation after intramuscular drug injection
Secondary to another type of adverse reaction producing tissue injury	Hemolysis, hepatitis
Increased tissue metabolism	Uncoupling of oxidative phosphorylation by general anesthetics
Peripheral vasoconstriction and reduced heat loss	Norepinephrine effect
Central effect	Amphetamine intoxication
Hormonal	Etiocholanolone fever

(From VanArsdel, P. P., Jr.: Adverse drug reactions. *In* Middleton, E., Jr., Reed, C. E., and Ellis, E. F. (eds.): Allergy. St. Louis, The C. V. Mosby Co., 1978.)

sensitivity to such determinants as the Gm group on immunoglobulins.

Drug Fever. Perhaps the earliest description of allergic fever produced by a drug was reported by Jadassohn (1896). He described a patient with contact dermatitis who subsequently swallowed a small amount of the offending chemical and several hours later developed fever and generalized erythroderma.

Drugs can produce fever by several mechanisms besides allergy. The nonallergic mechanisms are listed in Table 58–1. In children, *epinephrine as well as norepinephrine can cause fever.* Atropine (even eyedrops) and phenothiazines inhibit sweating, and certain psychotropic drugs can produce profound hyperpyrexia (Feigin and Shearer, 1976).

Fever may be part of drug-induced vasculitis, which may have manifestations similar to serum sickness. It may be the first sign of drug-induced hepatitis, or it may be the only physical manifestation. The patient with drug fever usually lacks the other symptoms associated with a febrile illness. This is a noteworthy feature to recognize when fever due to allergy to an antibiotic appears after resolution of the earlier infectious fever. When treatment with the offending drug is stopped, the temperature almost always drops to normal within 48 hours. Table 58–2 lists drugs reported to cause probable allergic fever without other signs of allergy. Most commonly implicated are the penicillins, cephalosporins, aminosalicylic acid, phenobarbital, quinidine, and iodides. Fever is relatively uncommon among all forms of adverse drug reactions in hospitalized patients but may make up as much as 25 percent of the total number of allergic reactions. Three of the 146 children with FUO cited earlier turned out to have drug fever.

The cause of drug fever in man has not been established. Because the clinical features are consistent with allergy and because fever has been produced in sensitized rabbits by a penicilloyl conjugate (see below), there is a general consensus that drug fever is caused by the release of EP during phagocytosis of complexes of antibody with drug-carrier conjugate.

Miscellaneous Conditions. The role of

TABLE 58–2 CAUSES OF ALLERGIC DRUG FEVER

Antimicrobials

Aminosalicylic acid
Cephalosporins
Chloramphenicol
Erythromycin
Isoniazid
Nitrofurantoin
Penicillins
Pyrazinamide
Quinine
Streptomycin-kanamycin
Sulfonamides
Tetracyclines

Other Drugs

Allopurinol
Heparin
Hydralazine
Iodides
Mercurial diuretics
Methyldopa
Penicillamine
Phenobarbital
Procainamide
Propylthiouracil
Quinidine

(From VanArsdel, P. P., Jr.: Adverse drug reactions. *In* Middleton, E., Jr., Reed, C. E., and Ellis, E. F. (eds.): Allergy. St. Louis, The C. V. Mosby Co., 1978.)

hypersensitivity in the tissue injury of human infection has been a matter for debate throughout this century. Fever, of course, would reflect this tissue injury through the activation of phagocytic cells. As noted earlier, the hypersensitive person will respond with fever to a very small dose of Brucella endotoxin. Tuberculin will produce fever in the sensitive person. However, how much carries over into clinical infection is not known. It is likely that cell-mediated sensitization enhances the inflammatory response to the tubercle bacillus, certain fungi, and some parasites — and thus contributes to the febrile response. Whether fever is enhanced by the action of antigen-antibody complexes in such infections as bacterial endocarditis or hepatitis B is just not known.

Despite the wealth of laboratory information on antibodies in some autoimmune diseases, there is hardly any information about the pathogenesis of fever. It is likely that the antigen-antibody complexes in systemic lupus erythematosus (SLE) activate phagocytes to produce EP, but this possibility has not been tested. Infants of mothers with SLE can harbor maternal antinuclear antibodies for many weeks after birth but develop no fever or any other sign of illness. This may be due to the host's nuclear antigen being inaccessible to the antibody in the absence of substantial cellular injury.

Rheumatoid arthritis in adults is associated with very active antigen-antibody complex phagocytosis in the synovia, yet fever is not a prominent feature except in active disease with vasculitis. By contrast, those children with the systemic form of juvenile rheumatoid arthritis frequently present with high intermittent fever patterns but, paradoxically, do not have circulating antinuclear antibodies or rheumatoid factors (Schaller and Wedgwood, 1972).

Even in conditions in which there is stronger evidence for an immune pathogenesis, such as rheumatic fever and the graft-versus-host reaction, one can only speculate that the mechanism for fever is the same as in experimental animals. A major problem in human investigation is that no one has been able to identify circulating EP in naturally occurring febrile diseases. Now that a very sensitive immunoassay for EP has been developed, more progress in the understanding of fever can be anticipated (Dinarello and Wolff, 1978).

ANIMAL MODELS OF HYPERSENSITIVITY FEVER

Much of the progress in understanding human fever has been made possible by studies in experimental animals; some of the key observations have already been cited.

Although fever was observed with serum sickness produced in rabbits many years ago (Hagebush et al., 1932), little attention was paid to it until after World War II. The stimulus for investigation then developed from studies in several laboratories on the mechanism of fever. A standard method for producing fever was to inject an endotoxin, which we now know acts by stimulating the formation of EP by phagocytic cells. Some investigators thought that the response to endotoxin was due to a naturally acquired hypersensitivity. This idea was found not to be correct, but it led to studies in animals that had been specifically sensitized. Farr and his associates (1954) sensitized rabbits with bovine serum albumin (BSA) and reported that 70 percent developed fever after subsequent injection of BSA intravenously. Stetson (1955) produced fever with old tuberculin given intravenously to sensitive rabbits.

In later work Atkins and various associates, studying tuberculin fever in BCG-sensitized rabbits, were able to induce tolerance with repeated injections and found that tolerant animals were still capable of producing EP from other stimuli. The antigen (old tuberculin) induced the production of EP by blood cells in the presence of plasma from sensitive donors. This suggested that circulating antibody as well as antigen was involved in the pyrogenic reaction (Atkins and Heijn, 1965).

Later, Chusid and Atkins (1972) were successful in producing fever with benzylpenicilloyl (BPO)-protein conjugates in sensitized rabbits containing BPO-specific antibodies. Intravenous penicillin-G had no effect. Antigen and antibody also caused leukocytes to release EP in vitro. Three animals died from anaphylaxis, but IgE antibodies were not looked for.

Wolff and his associates studied fever produced with human serum albumin (HSA) in sensitive rabbits. They reported that the degree of pyrogenic response that could be achieved was distinctly restricted by the small difference between the pyrogenic and anaphylactic dose (Mott and Wolff, 1966).

Febrile reactions were accompanied by leukopenia, thrombocytopenia, and complement consumption, but prior complement depletion did not prevent antigen-induced fever (Mickenberg et al., 1971).

The prime role of antibody in mediating the febrile response has been well established by passive sensitization studies. Grey, Briggs, and Farr (1961), using BSA, were the first to report the successful transfer of pyrogenic sensitivity to normal recipients. Since then, successful passive transfer has been reported for HSA (Mickenberg et al., 1971) and the BPO conjugate (Chusid and Atkins, 1972). In a variation, Root and Wolff (1968) collected blood after antigen challenge but before the development of fever and found this to be pyrogenic in normal recipients in the pattern of a preformed antigen-antibody complex.

Apparently, no attempt has been made to characterize the antibodies responsible for fever, but they probably are of the IgG immunoglobulin class. Those of the IgE class are responsible for anaphylactic reactions; whether they have any role in antigen-induced fever is doubtful, but the possibility has not been ruled out.

Fever can also be part of cell-mediated (delayed) hypersensitivity reactions. This was first reported by Uhr and Brandriss (1958), using four different protein antigens in guinea pigs. Several years later Atkins's group observed febrile responses to dinitrophenyl-protein conjugates in rabbits that had cell-mediated sensitivity to these antigens. They found that when sensitive lymphocytes were incubated with antigen they released a substance that caused EP production by phagocytic cells, indicating the possible role of a lymphokine (Atkins and Bodel, 1974). Recently Chao et al. (1977) in Atkins's laboratory, produced delayed hypersensitivity to bovine gamma globulin (BGG) in guinea pigs and obtained similar results, reinforcing the concept that lymphokines are involved in the fever of cell-mediated reactions.

Fever produced by microorganisms or their products may be related to cellular, as well as humoral, sensitivity. Tuberculin sensitivity appears to involve both mechanisms, while staphylococcal and cryptococcal reactions in rabbits appear to be due exclusively to cell-mediated sensitivity (Snell, 1972; Atkins and Bodel, 1974).

References

Abernathy, R. S., and Spink, W. W.: Studies with brucella endotoxin in humans: The significance of susceptibility to endotoxin in the pathogenesis of brucellosis. J. Clin. Invest. 37:219, 1958.

Atkins, E., and Bodel, P.: Fever. In Zweifach, B. W., Grant, L., and McCluskey, R. T. (eds.): The Inflammatory Process III. 2nd ed. New York, Academic Press, 1974. Chapter 11.

Atkins, E., and Heijn, C., Jr.: Studies on tuberculin fever. III. Mechanisms involved in the release of endogenous pyrogen in vitro. J. Exp. Med. 122:207, 1965.

Atkins, E., and Wood, W. B., Jr.: Studies on the pathogenesis of fever. II. Identification of an endogenous pyrogen in the blood stream following the injection of typhoid vaccine. J. Exp. Med. 102:499, 1955.

Blackley, C. H.: Experimental researches on the causes and nature of catarrhus aestivus (hay-fever or hay-asthma), 1873. Reprinted, London, Dawson's, 1959.

Bodel, P. T., and Atkins, E.: Studies in staphylococcal fever. V. Staphylococcal filtrate pyrogen. Yale J. Biol. Med. 38:282, 1965.

Bostock, J.: Case of a periodical affection of the eyes and chest (1819). In Samter, M. (ed.): Excerpts from Classics in Allergy. Columbus, Ohio, Ross Laboratories, 1969. p. 8.

Chao, P., Francis, L., and Atkins, E.: The release of an endogenous pyrogen from guinea pig leukocytes in vitro. A new model for investigating the role of lymphocytes in fevers induced by antigen in hosts with delayed hypersensitivity. J. Exp. Med. 145:1288, 1977.

Chusid, M. J., and Atkins, E.: Studies on the mechanism of penicillin-induced fever. J. Exp. Med. 136:227, 1972.

Cooke, R. A.: Gastrointestinal manifestations of allergy. Bull. N.Y. Acad. Med. 9:15, 1933.

Dinarello, C. A., and Wolff, S. M.: Pathogenesis of fever in man. New Engl. J. Med. 298:607, 1978.

Farr, R. S., Campbell, D. H., Clark, S. L., Jr, and Proffitt, J. E.: The febrile response of sensitized rabbits to the intravenous injection of antigen (abstract). Anat. Record 118:385, 1954.

Feigin, R. D., and Shearer, W. T.: Fever of unknown origin in children. Current Problems in Pediatr., Vol. 6, #10, Aug. 1976.

Freeman, J.: Hay-fever, A Key to the Allergic Disorders. London, Heinemann, 1950.

Gelfand, J. A., Elin, R. J., Berry, F. W., and Frank, M. M.: Endotoxemia associated with the Jarisch-Herxheimer reaction. New Engl. J. Med. 295:211, 1976.

Grey, H. M., Briggs, W., and Farr, R. S.: The passive transfer of sensitivity to antigen-induced fever. J. Clin. Invest. 40:703, 1961.

Hagebush, O. E., Robben, F. J., Fleisher, M. S., and Jones, L.: Serum sickness in rabbits. III. Reactions of body temperature and leukocytic curves. J. Immunol. 22:373, 1932.

Jadassohn, J. (1896): In Samter, M. (ed.): Excerpts from Classics in Allergy. Columbus, Ohio, Ross Laboratories, 1969, p. 27.

Jandl, J. H., and Tomlinson, A. S.: The destruction of red cells by antibodies in man. II. Pyrogenic, leukocytic and dermal responses to immune hemolysis. J. Clin. Invest. 37:1202, 1958.

Karelitz, S., and Stempien, S. S.: Studies on the mechanism of serum sickness. I. Passive serum sickness. J. Immunol. 44:271, 1942.

Kojis, F. G.: Serum sickness and anaphylaxis. Am. J. Dis. Child. 64:93, 313, 1942.

Leading Article: Inhalation fevers. Lancet 1:249, 1978.

Mickenberg, I. D., Snyderman, R., Root, R. K., Mergenhagen, S. E., and Wolff, S. M.: Immune fever in the rabbit: The relationship of complement consumption to immune fever. J. Immunol. 107:1466, 1971.

Mott, P. D., and Wolff, S. M.: The association of fever and antibody response to rabbits immunized with human serum albumin. J. Clin. Invest. *45*:372, 1966.

Perkins, H. A., Payne, R., Ferguson, J., and Wood, M.: Nonhemolytic febrile transfusion reactions. Quantitative effects of blood components with emphasis on isoantigenic incompatibility of leukocytes. *Vox Sang. 11*:578, 1966.

Root, R. K., and Wolff, S. M.: Pathogenetic mechanisms in experimental immune fever. J. Exp. Med. *128*:309, 1968.

Schaller, J., and Wedgwood, R. J.: Juvenile rheumatoid arthritis. A review. *Pediatrics 50*:940, 1972.

Siegel. S.: Familial paroxysmal polyserositis. Analysis of fifty cases. Amer. J. Med. *36*:893, 1964.

Snell, E. S.: Hypersensitivity fever. *In* Dash, C. H., and Jones, H. E. H. (eds.): *Mechanisms in Drug Allergy.* Baltimore, Williams and Wilkins Co., 1972, Chapter 9.

Stetson, C. A., Jr.: Studies on the mechanism of the Schwartzman reaction. J. Exp. Med. *101*:421, 1955.

Uhr, J. W., and Brandriss, M. W.: Delayed hypersensitivity. IV. Systemic reactivity of guinea pigs sensitized to protein antigens. J. Exp. Med. *108*:905, 1958.

Veale, W. L., Cooper, K. E., and Pittman, Q. J.: Role of prostaglandins in fever and temperature regulation. The Prostaglandins (New York) *3*:145, 1977.

Von Pirquet, C. F., Schick, B.: *Serum Sickness.* Baltimore, Williams and Wilkins Co., 1951, 130 pp. (Translation of 1905 edition).

59

Oscar L. Frick, M.D., Ph.D.

Controversial Concepts and Techniques with Emphasis on Food Allergy

DELAYED-ONSET REACTIONS TO FOODS (DELAYED-ONSET FOOD ALLERGY)

Delayed onset food reactions ("allergy"), as used in this chapter, refer to onset of symptoms *2 or more hours* after ingestion of an offending food. The gastrointestinal tract (nausea, vomiting, abdominal pain, diarrhea, and constipation), respiratory tract (rhinorrhea, cough, and wheezing) and skin (erythematous rashes and urticaria) are most commonly involved. Less frequent symptoms include urinary urgency, incontinence, enuresis, headaches, and mental confusion. Often symptoms are low grade or subclinical and may be recognized only after an offending food is eliminated.

Other symptoms ascribed by some to food intolerance include "allergic toxemia" (Kahn, 1927), meaning fatigue, pallor, and difficulty in concentration occurring in patients with severe hay fever; "cerebral allergy" (Rowe, 1950) designating mental symptoms, drowsiness, and interference with concentration, thinking and memory; confusion, depression, irritability, emotional instability, nervous tension and disturbed sleep and/or muscular pain and stiffness, especially of the neck, shoulders, back and legs (Randolph, 1951).

Baker (1898) noted that school children with chronic rhinitis and cough often were fatigued, had short concentration spans, and learning disabilities. Similarly, Shannon in 1922 described several children who were hyperirritable, slept poorly, and were unable to concentrate until apparent offending foods were eliminated from their diets.

Allergic tension fatigue syndrome was a name given by Speer (1954) to a condition that occurred in allergic children, consisting of alternating periods of tension and excessive fatigue (Table 59-1). These children slept restlessly and often had nightmares and nightsweats. Nasal congestion, infraorbital circles secondary to nasal venous congestion, and pallor were almost always present along with abdominal pains, headache, leg muscle aches ("growing pains"), enuresis, and occasionally severe depressions alternating with almost manic hyperactivity and nervous tics. He reported that elimination of particular foods (such as cow milk, chocolate, cola, corn, wheat, and egg) from the diet often resulted in a remarkable improvement in symptoms, which returned when the suspected foods were reintroduced.

Pathogenesis. Double-blind studies of children with suspected immediate type food allergy have resulted in gastrointestinal, skin, and respiratory symptoms within 2 hours of food challenge (May, 1976*a*; Bock et al., 1978*a*). These children showed positive immediate skin tests, and some also showed antigen-specific leukocyte histamine release,

738

which correlated with the challenge tests (Bock et al., 1978b). However, in this study, children whose food challenge resulted in delayed onset intestinal symptoms had negative prick and histamine release tests. A recent double-blind cross-over study of delayed onset food allergy at the University of California Medical Center was inconclusive, but the study was limited by the quantity of food that can be administered in capsule form (Pfuetze et al., 1978).

An immune basis for delayed onset food allergy, if one exists, has yet to be defined. As with other antigens, foods may induce hypersensitivity by various immune mechanisms. For example, symptoms of delayed onset food allergy may be caused by IgE-mediated hypersensitivity, with antigen absorbed more slowly than in the usual immediate response, or new antigenic determinates may be released or formed *de novo* during the digestion of such substances as bovine β-lactoglobulin (Spies, 1970). Studies using the RAST technique in patients with clinical cow milk allergy have shown that some may have positive tests only to trypsin digests of β-lactoglobulin and not to the original protein (Haddad et al., 1979).

Buisseret et al. (1978) demonstrated marked or complete protection against food-induced intestinal symptoms by pretreatment with aspirin or other prostaglandin synthetase inhibitors. In a patient anaphylactically sensitive to shellfish, food challenge induced severe vomiting and diarrhea, and was associated with a sharp rise in both plasma and stool PGE_2 and $PGF_{2\alpha}$. Rectal administration of indomethacin promptly stopped the reactions. Subsequent pretreatment with ibuprofen prevented symptoms following challenge. This suggests that PGE_2 and $PGF_{2\alpha}$ may be mediators of food intolerance in some patients. Small bowel biopsy has been employed to study histopathologic features of food intolerance. Harris et al. (1977) biopsied seven infants whose "colic" improved on changing from cow milk to soy formula and found a significant reduction in the number of IgE-bearing plasma cells when the infants were on soy formula. Shiner et al. (1975) demonstrated mast cell degranulation after cow milk ingestion in children with milk allergy, followed in 11 hours by a predominance of IgM-bearing plasma cells in the lamina propria. These findings suggest an immediate IgE-mediated reaction that is subsequently followed by a late reaction, such as an immune complex and/or complement-mediated (C3a and C5a) anaphylatoxin reaction.

Galant et al. (1973) conducted an immunologic study of a group of patients who had immediate reactions to foods and a study of a second group, who had delayed reactions. Of 14 patients with immediate respiratory or skin symptoms, food-induced leukocyte histamine

TABLE 59–1 ALLERGIC TENSION FATIGUE SYNDROME

Tension
  MOTOR (hyperkinesis)
    Overactivity
    Clumsiness
    Poor manual control
    Inability to relax
  SENSORY (hyperesthesia)
    Irritability
    Insomnia
    Oversensitivity
    Photophobia
    Hypersensitivity to pain and noise

Fatigue
  MOTOR
    Fatigue
    Sluggishness
  SENSORY
    Torpor
    Achiness

Associated Systemic Signs
  Almost always present
    Pallor
    Infraorbital circles
    Nasal stuffiness
  Common
    Infraorbital edema
    Increased salivation
    Increased sweating
    Abdominal pain (2/3)
    Headache (1/2)
    Enuresis
    Musculoskeletal pains

Less Common Mental and Nervous Symptoms
  Mental depression
  Feeling of unreality
  Bizarre, irrational behavior
  Paranoid ideas
  Inability to concentrate
  Nervous tics

After Speer, F.: Allergic tension-fatigue syndrome. Ped. Clin. North Am. *1*:1029, 1959.

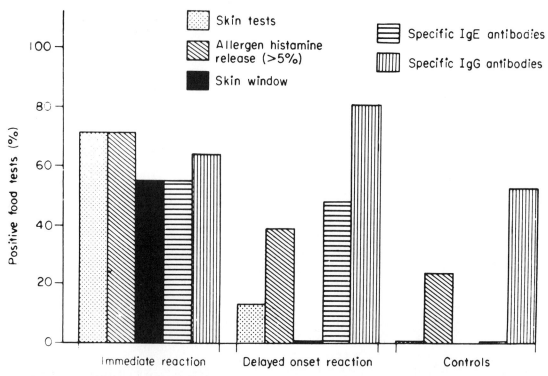

FIGURE 59–1. Incidence of positive immunologic tests in patients with immediate and delayed onset food allergy and in non-atopic controls. (From Galant, S. P., et al.: An immunological approach to the diagnosis of food allergy. Clin. Allergy 3:363, 1973.)

release was positive in 11, direct skin tests were positive in 10, and skin window eosinophilia in 7. However, in 23 patients with delayed onset food allergy, food-induced histamine release was positive in 9, skin tests were positive in 3, and skin window eosinophilia was negative in all. Seven of these 23 patients fit Speer's criteria for tension-fatigue syndrome. Patients with immediate allergy reacted to a variety of foods, whereas patients with delayed onset symptoms reacted primarily to milk and/or chocolate. Figure 59–1 compares the immunologic tests in these two groups of patients with a control group. IgG antibodies to foods could be demonstrated by radioprecipitin techniques in all groups.

Leukocyte inhibition factor (LIF) assay was carried out in patients with delayed onset food allergy who had negative tests for immediate IgE-type allergy (Minor and Frick, 1975). Twenty-one of 30 patients had positive LIF to cow milk protein compared to 2 out of 24 controls (p <0.01) (Fig. 59–2); and 5 of 11 had positive tests to corn, while all control tests were negative. These results suggest that another immune mechanism

may be present in patients with delayed food allergy, involving either a cell-mediated immune mechanism or granulocyte adherent immune complexes (Packaten and Wassermann, 1971).

One can speculate that food antigens may form immune complexes with IgM or IgG antibodies to activate complement and to induce symptoms. Sandberg et al. (1977) reported a fall in C3 in some nephrotic children following ingestion of milk. May (1976b) observed a high level of spontaneous leukocyte histamine release in patients with food allergy and suggested that circulating immune complexes might be the cause of these high values. Although immune mechanisms may well be operative in delayed onset reactions to foods, it also should be recognized that nonimmune mechanisms may account for so-called "allergic" symptomatology, especially headache and fatigue or tension-fatigue syndrome (see also Chapter 15). Tyramine is a vasoactive amine derived from tyrosine and is metabolized by oxidases to inactive p-hydroxyphenyllactic acid. Patients on monoamine oxidase inhibitor drugs, e.g., certain antidepressants and antihypertensives, who eat foods high in tyramine content (chocolate, aged cheeses, wine, beer, yeasts and pickled meats) experience migraine-type headaches (Holloman, 1972). In addition, one may speculate that inborn enzymatic deficiency of monoamine oxidase in patients on high tyramine diets (chocolate and dairy products) might develop headache and fatigue ("tension-fatigue"). Similarly, nitrites in processed meats (e.g., hot dogs, cured bacon, Spam) may induce headaches ("hot dog headaches") (Henderson and Raskin, 1972). Foods rich in monosodium glutamate may induce a "Chinese restaurant syndrome" — burning skin of the neck, facial pressure, chest tightness, and headache — by a nonimmune mechanism (Schaumberg et al., 1968; Kwok, 1968).

CONTROVERSIAL TECHNIQUES IN THE DIAGNOSIS AND MANAGEMENT OF FOOD ALLERGIES

A number of techniques for diagnosis and treatment of food allergy based on empirical observations have become very controversial in medicine. These include: *in vitro* leu-

kocytotoxic food tests; hyposensitization to foods by sublingual antigen administration; subcutaneous injections of foods for hyposensitization, with dose selection based on provocative injections and end-point skin reaction titration; and neutralization of symptoms with injections of weaker antigenic solutions. Double-blind studies on several of these tests have failed to establish objective support for their validity (Golbert, 1975). Nevertheless, such procedures continue to have strong empirical support from a considerable number of physicians. The intensity of feeling concerning these procedures is evident in a 1975 editorial:

Controversial procedures must undergo appropriate evaluation. However, those who hold them to be invalid will hardly be willing to devote time and effort either to validate or to discredit them. On the other hand, proponents are usually satisfied with the status quo and see no need to demonstrate once more what seems obvious to them. The matter can hardly rest there. Who, then, is to see that such trials are undertaken? There can be but one answer. He who makes the claim. (Lowell, 1975)

Leukocytotoxic Test. Vaughan (1934) observed a drop in total leukocyte count

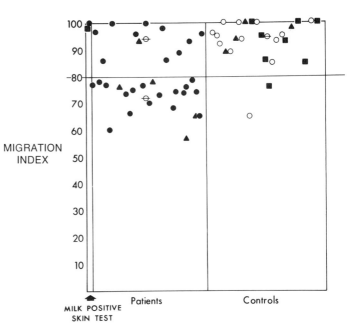

FIGURE 59–2. Incidence of positive and negative LIF tests to whole cow milk or milk products (proteins) in patients with delayed onset food allergy and in non-atopic controls. (From Minor, J. D., and Frick, O. L.: Leukocyte inhibition factor (LIF) production in delayed onset food allergy. J. Allergy Clin. Immunol. 55:88, 1975.)

WHOLE COW'S MILK OR MILK PRODUCTS

after ingestion of allergen in apparently food-sensitive individuals, and he proposed that a "leukopenic index" could be used to determine food hypersensitivity. Cytolysis of leukocytes in the presence of serum from a food-sensitive individual and antigen, observed by Black (1956), was modified by Bryan and Bryan (1960). In leukocytotoxicity testing, buffy coat leukocytes are suspended in one drop of water, and four to eight drops of serum are placed on a slide with dried antigen under a coverslip. After 2 hours the leukocytes are examined for lytic changes. Proponents of this test report that 80 to 85 percent of their patients improve by elimination of foods associated with a positive test.

However, two double-blind controlled studies were inconsistent and did not correlate with clinical symptoms (Lieberman et al., 1975; Benson and Arkins, 1975). This test appears to be difficult to reproduce in a given patient, and it does not correlate well with "immediate" (IgE-mediated) food-induced symptoms.

End-Point Intracutaneous Test Titration. Originated by Phillips (1926) for seasonal pollen therapy for hay fever, this test determines the "optimal dose" of antigen for hyposensitization, using wheal size induced by intradermal injection of various antigen concentrations. An optimal dose produced a wheal 20 to 30 mm in diameter and relieved symptoms. Rinkel (1963) refined the technique and applied it, in addition, to other inhalants and to foods. Nine or more fivefold dilutions of antigen are used, starting with highest dilutions (lowest concentrations), until a 7 mm wheal reaction is obtained (erythema is disregarded); this "end-point" is the starting dose for allergy therapy and purportedly is a safe starting point and "within a close range of effective therapeutic relief" (Rinkel, 1963). Many exceptions or bizarre whealing response patterns have been described, and a number of modifications have been made by Rinkel's students (Rinkel, 1963; Williams, 1971; Willoughby, 1974).

Subcutaneous Provocation Testing. As commonly performed (Willoughby, 1965), 0.1 ml of 1:100 dilution of concentrated extract (dilution No. 1) of suspected allergen (e.g., food) is injected subcutaneously into one site above the elbow, and the patient is observed closely for 20 minutes for signs and symptoms. Any of the following symptoms may be induced: rhinorrhea, sneezing, and wheezing; gastrointestinal reactions; skin eruptions and itching; headache and generalized aches, drowsiness or anxiety. If none develop, the test is considered negative and another food is tested.

Symptoms induced by a positive provocation test are relieved by injecting the optimal neutralizing dose, starting with 0.1 ml of fivefold dilutions, and increasing the concentration serially at 10-minute intervals until the "end-point neutralization" is attained. After provocation and neutralization with one food antigen, the next suspected food may be tested.

Sublingual Provocation Testing. The principle is the same as for subcutaneous provocation testing. In the sublingual method, three drops of "Dilution No. 1" (1:100) in 50 percent glycerin is placed under the tongue, and the patient is observed for symptoms for 10 to 20 minutes. If symptoms occur, neutralization is attempted with various antigen dilutions. Dilution No. 6 (1:312,500) is claimed often to be successful (Williams, 1966).

If an offending food, so identified, cannot be eliminated from the diet completely, "desensitization" is carried out with sublingual drops or subcutaneous injections of antigen, which my be administered just before a meal that includes the offending food (Lee et al., 1969).

Double-blind evaluations, and subcutaneous or sublingual provocation testing to date have failed to validate these procedures (Caplin, 1973; Breneman, 1973; Breneman, 1974).

Orthomolecular Therapy. Orthomolecular therapeutic approaches to many illnesses, including asthma and other allergies, have received wide publicity. Such measures as high doses of vitamins, especially Vitamin C and B complex, and minerals, such as calcium and zinc, have strong advocates. Interest in the role of Vitamin C in asthma was stimulated by the report of Zuskin and others (1973) that ascorbic acid can antagonize histamine- and $PGF_{2\alpha}$-induced tracheal smooth muscle contraction in guinea pigs. They also showed that pretreatment with 500 mg ascorbic acid reduced airway responses to inhaled hemp dust and histamine in healthy human subjects and to inhaled textile dust in patients with byssinosis (Zuskin and Bouhuys, 1975; Zuskin et al., 1976). Possible mechanisms were by ascorbic acid augmentation of synthesis of PGE_2 or of cortisol in stress situations. However, Kreisman and colleagues (1977) in the same laboratory later could not confirm these observations even with 2 gm ascorbic acid daily for 3 days before histamine inhalation challenge. Neither could Cockcroft and others (1977) find protection against bronchospasm with 1 gm ascorbic acid from histamine inhalation challenge in asthmatic patients. Finally, Kordansky and colleagues (1979) failed to find protection with 500 mg ascorbic acid for 7 days against bronchospasm induced by ragweed inhalation in ragweed-sensitive asthmatics. Although these orthomolecular approaches are interesting, much experimental work in animals and allergic patients must be done before they can be accepted as valid medications in the treatment of allergic conditions.

FOOD ADDITIVES, ALLERGY, AND HYPERKINESIS

Food additives, such as dyes and flavorings, have been implicated in allergic reactions since the report of Lockey (1959) who observed three patients with urticaria from tartrazine yellow dye in steroid medications. Michaelsson and Juhlin (1973) found that in 35 patients with chronic urticaria caused by aspirin, 19 also reacted to tartrazine and 22 to sodium benzoate. Patients with aspirin-induced asthma also were shown to develop asthma after ingesting tartrazine and sodium benzoate (Chaffee and Settipane, 1967; Juhlin et al., 1972). In Stenius and Lemola's study (1976), 25 of 140 asthmatics developed bronchoconstriction following tartrazine ingestion, although 64 percent were unaware of this sensitivity. "Tang" and orange drinks with sulfur dioxide preservative and benzoates may also cause asthma, rhinitis, and urticaria in susceptible individuals (Freedman, 1977).

The mechanism of these reactions is unknown, although it probably is not immunologic. Current opinion favors an action through the prostaglandins, SRS-A, or both.

Feingold (1975) related hyperactivity in school children to artificial food colorings and flavors, and claimed substantial improvement when they were fed diets free of these substances. The resulting Feingold Kaiser-Permanente (K-P) diet (Table 59–2) has received widespread publicity and acceptance

although it has yet to be validated scientifically. The publicity accorded these claims and the current vogue for natural, organically grown foods, which reinforced the public clamor for further regulation of chemicals in foods, prompted the food industry to study them through the Nutrition Foundation and the Food and Drug Administration. The initial Nutrition Foundation Committee report (National Advisory Committee, 1975) concluded the following:

1) controlled studies have not shown that hyperkinesis is related to ingestion of food colors; 2) a significant reduction of hyperactive behaviors when children are given the K-P diet has not been demonstrated experimentally; 3) the diet should be used only with competent medical supervision.

The results of controlled studies are now appearing in the literature, with no final conclusion yet reached. An uncontrolled Australian study (Salzman, 1976) reported that mothers scored marked improvement in 10 out of 15 school children on the K-P diet. However, there was no control group in this study, diet monitoring was inadequate, and no standardized rating scores were used, thus not excluding placebo effect in the study.

Connors (1970) developed observation-rating scales for parents and teachers of hyperactive children and carried out a

TABLE 59–2 ITEMS TO BE AVOIDED IN THE FEINGOLD K-P DIET

almonds	frankfurters
apples	oil of wintergreen
apricots	toothpaste and powder
blackberries	mint flavors
cherries	lozenges
currants	mouthwash
grapes and raisins	jam and jelly
nectarines	lunch meats (salami,
oranges	bologna)
peaches	gin and all distilled beverages (except vodka)
plums and prunes	
raspberries	cider and cider vinegar
strawberries	wine and wine vinegar
cucumbers and pickles	Kool-aid and similar
tomatoes	beverages
ice cream	soda pop (all soft drinks)
margarine	tea
cloves	beer
cake mixes	diet drinks and supplements
bakery goods	
jello	all medicines containing aspirin
candies	
gum	perfumes

double-blind cross-over study of the K-P diet on 15 hyperactive schoolboys (Connors et al., 1976). A statistically significant reduction in hyperactivity (reported by teachers but not by parents with children on the K-P diet) occurred only in the group given the control diet first, followed by the K-P diet. This reduction did not appear when the diet sequence was reversed.

Goyette et al. (1978) selected 50 hyperactive children who improved on one month of an additive-free diet. This double-blind phase of the study employed parent and teacher scoring and visual-motor tracking tests. The children were given chocolate cookies that contained food coloring. Dye-free cookies were used as controls. The overall results showed no difference in test performances of children receiving dye-containing or dye-free cookies. However, a few children did show consistent improvement on the dye-free diet; these may represent a small subgroup of children sensitive to food dyes.

Harley et al. (1978) conducted the most extensive double-blind cross-over study to date, in which 36 school-age and 10 preschool hyperactive boys were evaluated by an interdisciplinary team of researchers, consisting of physicians, psychologists, dietitians, and statisticians. They employed neurologic examination, EEG, parent-teacher evaluation questionnaires (Connors, 1970), and a battery of 12 neuropsychiatric tests. Dietary compliance was insured by removing *all* food from each household and supplying *all* the food for the entire family for the 8 week trial.

Whether or not food additives were included in the diet was not known to those scoring the children. No consistent relationship between diet and behavior was observed either by teachers, psychologists, or parents of school-age children. Only in the preschool children, for whom there was no teacher evaluation, was there a suggestion that behavior improved on a dye-free diet.

Harley and coworkers (1978) subsequently selected nine children who appeared to respond to the K-P diet for further challenge study. Only one of the nine showed a consistent reaction to the additives.

A conclusive assessment of the importance of artificial food colorings and flavors is not yet possible. The preponderance of scientific evidence suggests that dyes play only a minor role in causing hyperactivity in children, although there may be individual children for whom elimination of dyes may be helpful. Further investigation should evaluate the effect of larger doses of dyes, approaching actual daily intake (75 to 100 mg), and should avoid chocolate, which may complicate the trial. Investigations should also make more use of appropriate tests for concentration and attention span. More scientific studies are needed to shed light on these crucial issues before government regulators are called upon to effect further controls on the food industry.

References

Baker, S.: Fatigue in school children. Educa. Rev. *15*:341, 1898.

Benson, T. A., and Arkins, J. A.: Clinical correlation and reproducibility of the cytotoxic test for food allergy. J. Allergy Clin. Immunol. *55*:89, 1975.

Black, A. P.: A new diagnostic method in allergic disease. Pediatrics *17*:716, 1956.

Bock, S. A., Lee, W. Y., Remigio, L. K., and May, C. D.: Studies of hypersensitivity reactions to foods in infants and children. J. Allergy Clin. Immunol. *62*:327, 1978*a*.

Bock, S. A., Lee, W. Y., Remigio, L. K., Holst, A., and May, C. D.: Appraisal of skin tests with food extracts for diagnosis of food hypersensitivity. Clin. Allergy *8*:559, 1978*b*.

Breneman, J. C., et al.: Report on the Food Allergy Committee on the Sublingual Method of Provocative Testing in Food Allergy. Ann. Allergy *31*:382, 1973.

Breneman, J. C., et al.: Final Report of the Food Allergy Committee of the American College of Allergists on the Clinical Evaluation of Sublingual Provocative Food Testing Method for Diagnosis of Food Allergy. Ann. Allergy *33*:164, 1974.

Bryan, W. T. K., and Bryan, M. P.: The application of *in vitro* cytotoxic reactions to clinical diagnosis of food allergy. Laryngoscope *70*:810, 1960.

Buisseret, P. D., Heinzelmann, D. I., Youlton, L. J. F., and Lessof, M. H.: Prostaglandin-synthesis inhibitors in prophylaxis of food intolerance. Lancet *1*:906, 1978.

Caplin, I.: Report of the Committee on Provocative Food Testing. American College of Allergists. Ann. Allergy *31*:375, 1973.

Chaffee, F. H., and Settipane, G. A.: Asthma cause by FD and C approved dyes. J. Allergy *40*:65, 1967.

Cockcroft, D. W., Killian, D. N., Adrian-Mellon, J. J., and Hargreave, F. E.: Protective effect of drugs on histamine-induced asthma. Thorax *32*:429, 1977.

Connors, C. K.: Symptom patterns in hyperkinetic, neurotic, and normal children. Child. Dev. *41*:667, 1970.

Connors, C. K., Goyette, C. H., Southwick, D. A., Lees, J. M., and Andrulonis, P. A.: Food additives and hyperkinesis: A controlled double-blind experiment. Pediatrics *58*:154, 1976.

Feingold, B. F.: *Why is Your Child Hyperactive?* New York, Random House, 1975.

Freedman, B. J.: Asthma induced by sulfur dioxide, benzoate, and tartrazine contained in orange drinks. Clin. Allergy *7*:407, 1977.

Galant, S. P., Bullock, J. D., and Frick, O. L.: An immunological approach to the diagnosis of food allergy. Clin. Allergy *3*:363, 1973.

Golbert, T. M.: A review of controversial diagnosis and therapeutic techniques employed in allergy. J. Allergy Clin. Immunol. 56:170, 1975.

Goyette, C. H., Connors, C. K., Petti, T. A., and Curtis, L. E.: Effects of artificial colors on hyperactive children: A double-blind challenge study. Psychopharmacol. Bull. 14:39, 1978.

Harley, J. P., Ray, R. S., Tomasi, L., Eichman, P. L., Mathews, C. G., Chun, R., Cleeland, C. S., and Traisman, E.: Hyperkinesis and food additives: Testing the Feingold hypothesis. Pediatrics 61:818, 1978.

Haddad, Z. H., Kalra, V., Verma, S.: IgE antibodies to peptic and peptic-tryptic digests of betalactoglobulin: Significance in food allergy. Ann. Allergy 42:368, 1979.

Harris, M. J., Petts, V., and Penny, R.: Cow's milk allergy as a cause of infantile colic: Immunofluorescent studies of jejunal mucosa. Aust. Paediatr. J. 13:276, 1977.

Henderson, W. R., and Raskin, N. H.: "Hot dog" headache: Individual susceptibility to nitrite. Lancet 2:1162, 1972.

Holloman, J. D.: Relation of headaches to allergy. In Patterson, R. (ed.): Allergic Diseases, Diagnosis and Management. Philadelphia, J. B. Lippincott Co., 1972, p. 509.

Juhlin, L., Michaelsson, G., and Zetterstrom, O.: Urticaria and asthma induced by food-and drug-additives in patients with aspirin hypersensitivity. J. Allergy Clin. Immunol. 50:92, 1972.

Kahn, I. S.: Pollen toxemia in children, J.A.M.A. 88:241, 1927.

Kordansky, D. W., Rosenthal, R. R., and Norman, P. S.: The effect of Vitamin C on antigen-induced bronchospasm. J. Allergy Clin. Immunol. 63:61, 1979.

Kreisman, H., Mitchell, C., and Bouhuys, A.: Inhibition of histamine-induced airway constriction: Negative results with oxtriphylline and ascorbic acid. Lung 154:223, 1977.

Kwok, R. H. M.: Chinese restaurant syndrome. New Engl. J. Med. 278:796, 1968.

Lee, C. H., Williams, R. I., and Binkley, E. L.: Provocative testing and treatment for foods. Arch. Otolaryngol. 90:87, 1969.

Lieberman, P., Crawford, L., Bjelland, J., Connell, B., and Rice, M.: Controlled study of the cytotoxic food test. J.A.M.A. 231:728, 1975.

Lockey, S. D.: Allergic reactions to FD and C yellow No. 5 tartrazine aniline dye used as a coloring and identifying agent in various steroids. Ann. Allergy 17:719, 1959.

Lowell, F. C.: Editorial. Some untested diagnostic and therapeutic procedures in clinical allergy. J. Allergy Clin. Immunol. 56:168, 1975.

May, C. D.: Objective clinical and laboratory studies of immediate hypersensitivity reactions to foods in asthmatic children. J. Allergy Clin. Immunol. 58:500, 1976a.

May, C. D.: High spontaneous histamine release in vitro from leukocytes of persons hypersensitive to food. J. Allergy Clin. Immunol. 58:432, 1976b.

Michaelsson, G., and Juhlin, L.: Urticaria induced by preservatives and dye additives in food and drugs. Brit. J. Dermatol. 88:525, 1973.

Minor, J. D., and Frick, O. L.: Leukocyte inhibition factor (LIF) production in delayed onset food allergy. J. Allergy Clin. Immunol. 55:88, 1975.

National Advisory Committee on Hyperkinesis and Food Additives. Report of the Nutrition Foundation. New York, Nutrition Foundation, 1975.

Packaten, T., and Wassermann, J.: Inhibition of migration of normal guinea pig blood leukocytes by homologous immune gamma globulin in the presence of specific antigens. Int. Arch. Allergy 41:790, 1971.

Pfuetze, B. L., Jones, R. F., and Frick, O. L.: Double-blind study of delayed onset food allergy. Second International Food Allergy Symposium, American College of Allergists, Mexico City, Mexico, 1978.

Phillips, E. W.: Relief of hayfever by intradermal injections of pollen extract. J.A.M.A. 86:182, 1926.

Phillips, E. W.: Intradermal pollen therapy during the attack. J. Allergy 5:29, 1933.

Randolph, T. M.: Allergic myalgia, J. Mich. M. Soc. 50:487, 1951.

Rinkel, H. J., Randolph, T. G., and Zeller, M.: Food Allergy, Springfield, Ill. Charles C Thomas, 1951, p. 90–112.

Rinkel, H. J.: The management of clinical allergy. II. Etiological factors and skin titration. Arch. Otolaryngol. 77:42, 1963. III. Inhalant allergy therapy. Ibid. 77:205, 1963. IV. Food and mold allergy. Ibid. 77:302, 1963.

Rowe, A. H.: Food allergy: Its manifestations, diagnosis and treatment, J.A.M.A. 89:1623, 1928.

Rowe, A. H.: Allergic toxemia and fatigue. Ann. Allergy 8:72, 1950.

Salzman, L. K.: Allergy testing, psychological assessment and dietary treatment of the hyperactive child syndrome. Med. J. Aust. 2:248, 1976.

Sandberg, D. H., Bernstein, C. W., McIntosh, R. M., Carr, R., and Strauss, J.: Severe steroid-responsive nephrosis associated with hypersensitivity. Lancet 1:388, 1977.

Schaumberg, H. H., Byck, R., Gerstl, R., and Mashman, J. H.: Monosodium L-glutamate: Its pharmacology and role in the Chinese restaurant syndrome. Science 163:826, 1969.

Shannon, W. R.: Neuropathic manifestations in infants and children as a result of anaphylactic reactions to foods contained in their diets. Am J. Dis. Child. 24:89, 1922.

Shiner, M., Ballard, J., and Smith, M. E.: The small intestinal mucosa in cow's milk allergy. Lancet 1:136, 1975.

Speer, F.: Allergic tension-fatigue syndrome. Ped. Clin. North Am. 1:1029, 1954.

Spies, J. R., Stevan, M. A., Stein, W. J., and Coulson, E. J.: The chemistry of allergens. XX. New antigens generated by pepsin hydrolysis of bovine milk proteins J. Allergy 45:208, 1970. XXI Eight new antigens generated by successive pepsin hydrolysis of bovine B-lactoglobulin. J. Allergy Clin. Immunol. 50:82, 1972.

Stenius, B. S. M., and Lemola, M.: Hypersensitivity to acetylsalicyclic acid (ASA) and tartrazine in patients with asthma. Clin. Allergy 6:119, 1976.

Vaughan, W. T.: Further studies on the leukopenic index in food allergy. J. Allergy 6:78, 1934.

Williams, J. I., Cram, D. M., Tausig, F. T., and Webster, E.: Relative effects of drugs and diet on hyperactive behaviors: An experimental study. Pediatrics 61:311, 1978.

Williams, R. I.: Modern concepts in clinical management of allergy in otolaryngology. Laryngoscope 76:1389, 1966.

Williams, R. I.: Skin titration testing and treatment. Otolaryngol. Clin. North Am. 3:507, 1971.

Willoughby, J. W.: Serial dilution titration skin tests in inhalant allergy. A clinical quantitative assessment of biologic skin reactivity to allergenic extracts. Otolaryngol. Clin. North Am. 7:579, 1974.

Willoughby, J. W.: Provocative food test technique. Ann. Allergy 23:543, 1965.

Zuskin, E., Lewis, A. J., and Bouhuys, A.: Inhibition of histamine-induced airway constriction by ascorbic acid. J. Allergy Clin. Immunol. 51:218, 1973.

Zuskin, E., and Bouhuys, A.: Byssinosis: Airway responses in textile dust exposure. J. Occup. Med. 17:357, 1975.

Zuskin, E., Valic, F., and Bouhuys, A.: Byssinosis and airway responses due to exposure to textile dust. Lung 154:17, 1976.

60

R. Michael Sly, M.D.

Allergy and School Problems

The purpose of the school is to provide education under conditions that facilitate effective learning. Any chronic illness can cause a variety of problems. Overprotection can lead to understimulation, dependency, and development of a poor self-image, which can impair motivation, and result in underachievement.

Allergy affects the child at school much in the same way as it does at home, but the demands of school are likely to make disabilities more evident; and classmates and teachers are likely to be less tolerant of symptoms and less able to be of assistance than the family. Furthermore, school is such an important part of any child's life that difficulties in adjustment there may have adverse effects upon behavior elsewhere and the consequences may be lifelong.

The allergic child's achievement and adjustment at school may be affected by absenteeism, fatigue, irritability, exercise-induced asthma, need for special diets or medications, and side effects of medications. Behavioral changes secondary to allergic disorders may be misinterpreted as primary psychologic problems. The extent to which learning may be impaired by conductive hearing loss due to secretory otitis media is unknown; but the condition has been shown to affect learning and speech development. Allergic medical emergencies at school, such as bee sting anaphylaxis, may necessitate prompt treatment.

ABSENTEEISM

The National Health Survey of 1959–61, based upon household interviews, disclosed that among chronic conditions asthma accounted for 22.9 percent of days reported lost from school in children less than 17 years old. Additional time is lost from school because of acute hives, severe exacerbations of allergic rhinitis, and complications of respiratory allergy, such as sinusitis, otitis media, and chronic coughing. Even when the child is not ill, he may miss school during inclement weather because of the parents' fear that it might provoke an asthmatic attack. Visits to physicians for diagnosis and treatment may increase absenteeism significantly.

When severe allergy does necessitate frequent or prolonged absences, it is essential for the child's welfare that the teacher and school officials understand the nature of the problem. This may require a more extensive physician's letter than the usual brief excuse requested by the parents. Every effort must be made to secure cooperation from teachers so that the student can make up missed work and keep up with the rest of the class.

A less obvious effect of excessive school absenteeism relates to the child's psychologic adjustment to his or her peer group. The child who misses considerable school is often excluded from the peer group. This ostracism may contribute further to loss of school time because the child may prefer to remain at home in comfortable surroundings rather than to return to school, only to be excluded socially from peer groups.

A major goal in treating the allergic child should be to prevent or to reduce school absenteeism. The number of days missed from school should be recorded in initial and follow-up history sheets as a way of monitoring absenteeism.

Loss of time from school is minimized by appropriate medical management, which should enable most asthmatic children to tolerate exposure to cold or rainy weather. Two important factors are education of parents and school officials in ways of alleviating the child's anxieties that add to school absenteeism and attempts by physicians to schedule patient visits during nonschool hours. When frequent office visits for allergy injections are necessary, for example, these can usually be scheduled not to conflict with school attendance. The child may need further parental and teacher support to encourage her or him to rejoin the peer group.

FATIGUE

Fatigue may result from loss of sleep, may be a manifestation of the allergic reaction, or may occur as a side effect of medications. Loss of sleep may also be a side effect of medications or it may be due to the illness itself.

Fatigue reduces attention span and impairs concentration. The child may even sleep throughout much of the day, with nearly the same effects as school absenteeism. The physician must be cognizant of potential undesirable effects of medication. Only by inquiring directly may he learn that the antihistamine is causing drowsiness or difficulty in concentrating in school or that the bronchodilator or the dosing schedule that controls the child's asthma so effectively is interfering with sleep.

Most teachers resent sleeping students, but parents may become aware of the problem only when the child receives a poor grade report. To forestall misunderstandings, teachers and parents must communicate. If the parents have been warned by their physician of this possible problem, they can ask the teacher to tell them when the

student appears fatigued. Recognition of the teacher as a person concerned with the child's welfare rather than as an adversary can allay misunderstandings and facilitate the cooperation essential for optimal medical management as well as the child's education. Most teachers are eager to be helpful when they know the facts and when their cooperation is sought. Accommodations such as additional tutoring or special assignments may be possible to supplement classroom instruction when fatigue interferes with schoolroom performance. The parents must be willing to cooperate and the physician should be reinforcing when the teacher recommends additional assistance.

IRRITABILITY

Irritability can result either from loss of sleep or side effects of medications. Headaches, abdominal pain, or unrelenting symptoms of allergic rhinitis, asthma or atopic dermatitis, even if mild, also can cause the child to become irritable. The physician should take seriously the mother's or father's complaints that a medication is causing a personality change. An alternative medication should be prescribed if possible. Both fatigue and irritability have been described as manifestations of the allergic tension-fatigue syndrome (see Chapter 59).

Irritability also has adverse effects upon attention span, concentration, and relationships with classmates and teachers. If the teacher does not understand the nature of the problem, he or she may erroneously ascribe it to rebellion or a lack of discipline and may even react with hostility. The teacher whose cooperation has been solicited, on the other hand, may be the source of information indicating the need for some modification of therapy for optimal management.

EXERCISE-INDUCED ASTHMA

Physical education is found in almost all school curricula. Furthermore, much of the social life and many opportunities for leadership depend upon participation in intramural or interscholastic sports in secondary school. On the one hand, participation is important to the physical and emotional health of the child, but on the other hand, strenuous exercise can provoke asthma (see Chapter 46).

Exercise can provoke bronchospasm in most asthmatic children. The response depends upon such factors as the type of exercise, its duration, the ambient temperature, air pollution levels, presence of airborne allergens, and use of medications. Asthma is more likely to follow running than any other form of exercise and is least likely to follow swimming. The thrust of therapy is to control bronchospasm optimally while avoiding exercise restrictions as much as possible. Exercise-induced asthma can be relieved by bronchodilators or prevented or minimized by administration of theophylline, sympathomimetics, or cromolyn sodium before exercise. On the other hand, the necessity for taking medicine prior to exercise may be so embarrassing that the child refuses to take it, even though it is effective.

It is essential that athletic coaches, physical education instructors, and teachers be familiar with the symptoms of exercise-induced asthma, not only so they may recognize the source of a child's exercise-associated problem, but also so that they can alert the parent to the condition, which frequently is unappreciated at home. Once parents understand the problem, appropriate recommendations can be sought from the child's physician. The physician must not only be aware of the proper medication but also must be aware of the circumstances under which the child must take it and must recommend a medication schedule satisfactory to the patient.

addition, the child should be permitted to take medication inconspicuously, so as not to be "different." Occasionally, children live close enough to school to permit a parent to administer midday doses of medications, but this is best avoided if possible, especially for older children, since it singles out the child. Even when the medication is administered by the child himself, school officials should be informed to avoid misunderstandings.

Use of sustained-release preparations may obviate the need for administration of medications during school.

Even when medications are given only at home, the teacher should be asked to report any side effects that may affect the child's achievement. Sedation is the commonest side effect of antihistamines, but irritability or central nervous system stimulation may also occur. Irritability can also be a side effect of theophylline or sympathomimetics such as ephedrine, pseudoephedrine, or metaproterenol. The commonest side effect of terbutaline is muscle tremor, a general side effect of $beta_2$ adrenergic drugs taken orally. This may be extreme enough to have a serious effect upon penmanship and coordination and may expose the child to ridicule by peers and criticism by teachers.

When side effects are recognized, they can often be controlled by an adjustment in dosage or by substituting an alternate drug. In other cases, it may be necessary to seek the teacher's understanding and cooperation in accepting minimal side effects as an alternative to more severe allergic symptoms, since uncontrolled sneezing or coughing in the classroom can be even more disruptive than side effects of medications.

MEDICATIONS

The responsible child can carry single doses of antihistamine, decongestant, bronchodilator, or cromolyn sodium to school for self-administration when necessary. Such medications can usually be taken most conveniently immediately before or with lunch. Special arrangements can sometimes be made to permit administration of medications by a teacher or school nurse; this may require the direct intervention of the physician, since a letter from the parent is often not sufficient in some school systems. In

DIETS

When food allergy necessitates dietary restrictions, the school lunch usually offers children their most serious challenge. This is often best met by supplying the lunch from home, even though the parents' ingenuity may be severely taxed by efforts to pack an attractive, nutritious lunch without milk, egg, or wheat. Soup can be carried in a thermos, and fruit and vegetables can be wrapped in foil or sent in a wide-mouthed thermos. Responsible children can be taught to avoid allergens as they select their lunches in the school cafeteria, when dietary restrictions are not extensive or when they include only obvious foods. Occasionally one must seek cooperation from the school dietitian.

LEARNING DISABILITY

Learning disability is a somewhat poorly defined syndrome that manifests itself as scholastic underachievement due to various combinations of impaired perception, conceptualization, language, or memory and in loss of control of attention, impulses, or motor function. As many as 3 percent of children have been estimated to suffer from learning disability. Learning disability can be due to hearing loss, medications, fatigue, or somatopsychic factors. Evidence for and against the possible role of food additives is discussed in Chapter 59.

Children with learning disability must be evaluated with a thorough history, careful physical examination, and ophthalmologic and audiologic examinations. Psychometric and psychologic evaluations may also be necessary.

HEARING LOSS

It is estimated that 3 percent of elementary school children have some impairment of auditory acuity. The majority of these have conductive hearing loss, often due to serous or secretory otitis media. Although it is unknown how often conductive hearing loss is due to allergy in the general population, it occurs frequently, in up to 33 percent of children, with allergic rhinitis (Gupta and Sly, 1977; Bierman and Furukawa, 1978).

Recent studies indicate that even a moderate hearing loss (15 to 25 Db) has a profound effect on speech development and learning in preschool children (Chap. 38). Most serious effects occur in preschool children — the children in whom secretory otitis media occurs most frequently. Fortunately, tympanometry affords objective evidence of middle ear disease even in this young age group; and as tympanometry is applied more widely, it should permit more effective treatment of secretory otitis media and more extensive assessment of the effects of untreated disease upon learning.

Advantages of tympanometry over audiometry for routine screening in school children include the need for only very minimal cooperation, the lack of need for a soundproof room, and the very short time necessary for completion of the study.

The child with impairment of auditory acuity or an abnormal tympanogram is in need of medical attention, even if only for removal of impacted cerumen. When associated allergy is found, appropriate treatment is indicated. The disadvantage at which such a child is placed for learning may necessitate special seating in the classroom, special attention from the teacher, a hearing aid, or supplemental speech and lip reading instruction. Persistent, severe impairment of auditory acuity may necessitate enrollment in a special class or a special school.

COSMETIC PROBLEMS

The presence of obvious stigmata of allergic disease may result in ridicule or ostracism. The child with an "allergic facies," a "barrel chest," or the obvious lesions of atopic dermatitis or chronic urticaria is likely to be self-conscious even when accepted by his peers, although the problem is rarely brought to the attention of the physician by the child or parent.

Appropriate therapy may partly reverse many of these abnormalities, but they often continue to concern the child, if not his peers, unless completely controlled. Manifestations include a dislike of school, irritability, fighting with peers, and poor academic achievement.

When possible, it is appropriate to reassure the patient that improvement is expected to follow therapy. In extreme cases special counseling may become necessary.

It may also be necessary to reassure teachers that lesions of severe atopic dermatitis or chronic urticaria are not due to an infectious process.

EMERGENCIES

Children subject to sudden, severe asthmatic attacks must carry appropriate bronchodilators for self-administration, unless arrangements have been made for treatment by the teacher or the school nurse.

Children with allergies that predispose to systemic anaphylaxis following bee stings or ingestion of specific drugs or foods should wear emblems identifying their problem.* School officials should also be warned of the possibility of such reactions, so that the nurse or teacher can be prepared to administer epinephrine by subcutaneous injection in an emergency. In many states, enactment of legislation may be necessary to permit administration of epinephrine by a teacher in such an emergency. The child should then be rushed to the nearest emergency room or his physician's office for further observation or treatment.

SUMMARY

The physician is not likely to recognize the presence of many of these problems without specific inquiry, and parents, coaches, and teachers often fail to recognize allergy or prescribed medications as the cause of behavior erroneously ascribed to a perverse temperament.

Just as the education and cooperation of the parents of the allergic child are essential for optimal management, so are the education and cooperation of teachers and school officials, who are often responsible for the child during most waking hours.

When the special needs and problems of the allergic child are explained fully and when their solution is understood to be essential to advancing the school's goal of facilitating effective learning, it is only the very rare teacher who is unwilling to cooperate. Physicians and parents must seek the cooperation of school officials, however, and must be willing to take the time to educate them. "Tips for Teachers," a pamphlet available from the Asthma and Allergy Foundation of America,* is a useful supplement to the more specific instructions regarding a particular child.

*Available from Medic Alert Foundation, P.O. Box 1009, Turlock, California 95380

*Asthma and Allergy Foundation of America, 19 West 44th Street, New York, N.Y. 10036.

References

Bierman, C. W., and Furukowa, C. T.: *Medical management of serous otitis in children.* Pediatrics *61*:768, 1978.

Committee on School Health: *School Health: A Guide for Health Professionals,* American Academy of Pediatrics, Evanston, Illinois, 1977.

Gupta, D., and Sly, R. M.: *Tympanometry in allergic children.* Ann. Allergy, *36*:105, 1977.

Sly, R. M.: *Pediatric Allergy.* Garden City, N.Y., Medical Examination Publishing Company, 1980.

Robert J. Dockhorn, M.D. # 61

Genitourinary Problems

When physicians and patients think about allergy, there is a natural tendency to focus on the skin and respiratory tract, sometimes overlooking involvement of other systems, including the genitourinary tract. "Allergic" genitourinary problems have been reported by numerous investigators over a time span of greater than 50 years. The implication of allergy in genitourinary problems has been based for the most part on observations of a higher than normal incidence of allergy in patients with genitourinary disease, the presence of eosinophils in urine or in urinary tract tissue, and a response to antiallergic treatment, including allergy injection therapy.

HISTORICAL PERSPECTIVE

In 1917, Longcope and Rackemann reported renal involvement in six patients with urticaria; in four of these patients, hypersensitivity to one or more foreign proteins could be demonstrated. A few years later, Duke (1923) described various urinary tract symptoms in a group of patients, which were attributed to allergy to foods. In 1930, Vaughan and Hawke described a patient with angioedema, with joint, respiratory tract, and nervous system involvement, associated also with cystitis. Eisenstadt (1951) as well pointed out that generalized allergic responses may include urinary tract involvement or that the urinary tract may be the target of an isolated reaction. Rowe (1933)

previously had indicated also that the genitourinary tract may be the focus of a localized allergic reaction, the bladder being the component most commonly affected. Dysuria, frequency, lower quadrant pain (Kindall and Nickels, 1949); hematuria, renal colic, enuresis, interstital cystitis (Hand, 1949; Kittredge and Johnson, 1949; Burkland, 1951; Breneman, 1959); vulvovaginitis (Walter, 1958); recurrent urinary tract infections (Horesh, 1976a and b); Henoch-Schönlein purpura, and nephrosis (see Chapter 67) all have been claimed to be caused by or aggravated by allergy over the years. Most commonly the reactions are attributed to allergy to foods (Rowe, 1933; Kindall and Nickels, 1949; Eisenstadt, 1951; Breneman, 1959; Unger, 1959), but various other allergens, including inhalants and drugs, have been implicated. On the other hand, Siegel et al. (1976) found no relationship between respiratory allergy, enuresis, and urinary tract infections in a group of 234 children.

Kindall and Nickels (1949) reported that a urethral biopsy revealed mucosal eosinophilia in a patient with urinary tract symptoms related to the ingestion of foods. Powell and Powell (1954) investigated 154 female patients with urinary tract problems, 114 of whom had transurethral bladder neck resections. Bladder eosinophilia was shown in five of these patients, all of whom had a positive allergic history. Horowitz et al. (1972) reported an asthmatic patient with eosinophilic cystitis that lead to unilateral loss of renal functions, with contralateral hydronephrosis and chronic renal failure, related in turn to structure of the urethral ostia. Corticosteroids or ACTH produced only temporary amelioration of the problem. The basis of the eosinophilic cystitis was considered to be the same as the allergic basis of the patient's asthma.

ENURESIS

Enuresis, or involuntary emptying of the bladder beyond the age when bladder control normally has been established, may be nocturnal or diurnal. Nocturnal enuresis is more common and is present in about 10 to 15 percent of otherwise normal 5-year-old children. There is a familial tendency, and it is slightly more common in boys.

Organic disorders that cause nocturnal enuresis include nocturnal epilepsy; urinary tract infection; increased urinary volume in diabetes mellitus and diabetes insipidus and in any condition in which the ability to concentrate urine is impaired; obstructive uropathy; and chronic renal failure.

Few disorders affect so many children for so great a time as enuresis, and enuresis (and the parents' and patient's reaction to it) can exert an important influence on the maturing personality of the child. Parental concern for an enuretic child often is little relieved by most available medical advice, which frequently, in fact, is conflicting.

Frequent failure of the usual pediatric management of enuresis has promoted other considerations in management of this disorder. Breneman (1959) found that some patients with enuresis responded when food allergens were isolated and restricted from their diets. The foods commonly involved with enuresis were milk, wheat, eggs, corn, chicken, oranges, and tomatoes.

Crook (1974) also reported an association between enuresis and allergy, allergy to foods in particular. Food allergens implicated (in order of importance) were milk, corn, chocolate, cola drinks, citrus fruits, and food colors. He reported that inhalants, particularly pollens and molds, were occasional causes of enuresis, too, and that these cases dramatically improved with allergy injection therapy. Although there is some correlation between serum IgE levels and allergic disease, IgE levels have not been found to be elevated in enuretic children (Kaplan, 1973).

RECURRENT URINARY TRACT INFECTIONS

In evaluating patients with recurrent urinary tract infections for a possible underlying allergic problem, determination of the presence or absence of other allergic diseases such as atopic dermatitis, hay fever, or asthma may be a helpful clue. Eosinophilia of the blood and urine is a useful sign if present, but the lack of eosinophils does not rule out urinary tract allergy (Horesh, 1976a and b). An elevated total serum IgE and identification of IgE antibody to various allergens provides only circumstantial evidence of a possible allergic etiology and, as with other allergic diseases, does not in itself establish an allergic basis for the condition.

Symptoms of acute allergic involvement of the lower urinary tract are those of inflammation: burning, frequency, dysuria, and possibly hematuria. Fever is not a symptom, and there is no pyuria (Powell et al., 1970). The presence of mucosal edema and eosinophils in histologic sections of the urinary tract may be indicative of an allergic process involving that system. However, numerous mast cells normally are found in subepithelial locations and in smooth muscle of the ureter, bladder, and urethra, as well as deposits of eosinophils (Selye, 1965). Therefore, the finding of eosinophils in urine and urethral discharge must be interpreted with caution, since it may represent a washout phenomenon, regardless of the cause of the inflammation.

HEMATURIA

Immune reactions leading to hematuria are well known. Besides hematuria in Henoch-Schönlein purpura and other immune glomerulonephritis, there also is an isolated form of hematuria that Coca described in 1930 as "allergic hematuria," in which the absence of protein and erythrocyte casts make a glomerular origin unlikely (Ammann and Rossi, 1966). Allergens suspected most commonly in allergic hematuria include foods, drugs, and inhalants. Others feel that "allergy" is not involved in this condition, which they term "essential hematuria."

EOSINOPHILIC CYSTITIS

Eosinophilic infiltration involving the soft tissues of the lower urinary tract are infrequent. Wenzel et al. (1964) reported an unusual case of cystitis characterized by proliferative and ulcerative vesical lesions composed largely of eosinophilic infiltrates. Nine reported cases of chronic eosinophilic cystitis, two occurring in association with asthma, were summarized by Horowitz et al. (1972), who reported an additional case in a patient whose urinary symptoms were associated with an exacerbation of asthma. This patient's disease progressed to renal failure in spite of corticosteroid treatment. Allergy has not been proven to be a cause of eosinophilic cystitis.

ALLERGY OF EXTERNAL GENITALIA

Allergic reactions occasionally involve the external genitalia. Girls with enuresis often have an associated vulvovaginitis and occasional cystitis. Boys may develop dermatitis of the tip of the penis, possibly due to contact sensitivity.

Though some authors have speculated that foods such as milk, corn, chocolate, cola,

citrus, and food colors may cause allergic reactions of the external genitalia, this has not been proven. On occasion, contact with pollen allergens may induce seasonal vulvovaginitis in young girls, which may respond to hyposensitization therapy (Berman, 1964).

GENITOURINARY ALLERGY— A PERSPECTIVE

Management of genitourinary "allergy" is, in principle, similar to management of other allergic disorders. Once a cause and effect relationship between contact with a substance and genitourinary symptoms is established, avoidance of the substance is the mainstay of therapy. Use of pharmacotherapy and allergy injection therapy to alleviate unavoidable inhalant allergens can be considered if appropriate. If the genitourinary tract symptoms are a part of the overall allergic disease, genitourinary tract symptoms usually improve along with other allergic symptoms. Does this then mean that the genitourinary symptoms were primarily allergic? Not at all. If the patient's general health improves and sleep patterns become normal, the problem of enuresis may diminish or cease altogether.

From our current knowledge, it is evident that further detailed studies are needed to define the role of IgE-mediated allergy in genitourinary tract disease.

References

Ammann, P., and Rossi, E.: Allergic hematuria. Arch. Dis. Child. 41:539, 1966.
Berman, B. A.: Seasonal allergic vulvovaginitis caused by pollen. Ann. Allergy 22:594, 1964.
Breneman, J. C.: Allergic cystitis: The cause of nocturnal enuresis. GP. 20:84, 1959.
Burkland, C. E.: Manifestations of hypersensitivity in the genitourinary system. Urol. Cutan. Rev. 55:290, 1951.
Coca, A. F.: Specific sensitiveness as a cause of symptoms in disease: Essential hematuria and localized retinal edema as possible allergic symptoms, Bull. N. Z. Acad. Med. 6:593, 1930.
Crook, W. G.: Genito-urinary allergy. In Speer, F. and Dockhorn, R. J. (eds.); Allergy and Immunology in Childhood. Springfield, Ill.: Charles C Thomas, 1974.
Duke, W. W.: Food allergy as a cause of irritable bladder. J. Urol. 10:173, 1923.

Eisenstadt, J. S.: Allergy and drug sensitivity of the urinary tract. J. Urol. 65:154, 1951.
Hand, J. R.: Interstitial cystitis: Report of 223 cases. J. Urol. 61:291, 1949.
Horesh, A. J.: Allergy and recurrent urinary tract infections in childhood (Part I). Ann. Allergy 36:16, 1976a.
Horesh, A. J.: Allergy and recurrent urinary tract infections in childhood (Part II). Ann. Allergy 36:174, 1976b.
Horowitz, J., Slavin, S., and Pfau, A.: Chronic renal failure due to eosinophilic cystitis. Ann. Allergy 30:502, 1972.
Kaplan, G. W.: Allergic origin of enuresis seen possible, but unlikely. Pediatr. News 7:12, 1973.
Kindall, L., and Nickels, T. T.: Allergy of the pelvic-urinary tract in the female. A preliminary report. J. Urology 61:222, 1949.
Kittredge, W. E., and Johnson, C.: Allergic hematuria due to milk. New Orleans Med. Surg. J. 101:419, 1948–49.

Longcope, W. T., and Rackemann, F. M.: Severe renal insufficiency associated with attacks of urticaria in hypersensitive individuals. J. Urol. *1*:351, 1917.

Powell, N. B., and Powell, B. B.: Vesical allergy in females. Southern Med. J. *47*:841, 1954.

Powell, N. B., Boggs, P. B., and McGovern, J. P.: Allergy of the lower urinary tract. Ann. Allergy *28*:252, 1970.

Rowe, A. H.: The present status of food allergy. Northwest Med. *32*:217, 1933.

Selye, H.: *The Mast Cells*. Washington, D.C., Butterworths, Inc. 1965, p. 111.

Siegel, S., Rawitt, L., Sokoloff, B., and Siegel, B.: Relationship of allergy, enuresis and urinary tract infections in children 4 to 7 years of age. Pediatrics *57*:526, 1976.

Unger, D. L., Kubik, F., and Unger, L.: Urinary tract allergy. J.A.M.A. *70*:1380, 1959.

Vaughan, W. T., and Hawke, E. K.: Angioneurotic edema with some unusual manifestations. J. Allergy *2*:125, 1930.

Walter, C. K.: Allergy as the cause of genitourinary symptoms: Clinical considerations. Ann. Allergy *16*:158, 1958.

Wenzl, J. E., Greene, L. F., and Harris L. E.: Eosinophilic cystitis. J. Pediatr. *64*:746, 1964.

Bettina C. Hilman, M.D. **62**

Surgery in Allergic Patients

Surgical risks in allergic patients include hypersensitivity and other adverse reactions to drugs given in association with surgery and to foods inadvertently given to patients hypersensitive to them. Reactions to drugs and foods are discussed elsewhere. Patients with asthma pose additional problems at surgery. This chapter will address the evaluation of risks and management of asthmatic patients before, during, and immediately after surgery.

The risks of surgery for the asthmatic patient depend on: the severity of the underlying asthma, the type and extent of surgery, the control of asthma when the operation is performed, and the effectiveness of therapy to prevent postoperative pulmonary complications.

Although there are no detailed studies of risks in children with asthma, preoperative risks have been assessed in adults with obstructive airway disease (Diament and Palmer, 1967; Stein et al., 1962). Up to 20 percent of patients who undergo abdominal or thoracic surgery have clinically significant postoperative complications. Segmental atelectasis is the most common complication (Stein and Abdel-Rassoul, 1976). Patients with asthma have an increased risk of postoperative atelectasis because of plugging of airways from increased secretions and/or bronchospasm. Though adequate hydration in the asthmatic patient may minimize inspissated mucous plugs, overhydration can predispose to pulmonary edema. A prolonged period in a supine position adds to the risk in the asthmatic patient, since the diaphragm and the intercostal and accessory muscles of respiration are at mechanical disadvantage in this position. When considering the risks of surgery in an individual patient, the timing of

surgery is important. If surgery is elective, optimal control of asthma should be achieved prior to surgery. The more severe the asthma, the more important its preoperative control becomes.

Evaluation and management of asthmatic patients undergoing surgery will be discussed under the following sections:

1. Preoperative assessment
2. Preoperative management
3. Operative management
4. Postoperative evaluation and management

PREOPERATIVE ASSESSMENT

Preoperative assessment of the asthmatic patient should include a careful review of the history and a complete physical examination.

The history should include details of the severity of asthma and the drugs used in its control, the multiple factors that may play a role in precipitating or aggravating it, and the relative importance of each of these factors. It is important to inquire about the association of asthma with specific extrinsic allergens or with irritants such as cold air and tobacco smoke. The medication history should include the patient's current asthma medication dosage and times of administration, response to other drugs in the past, and history of idiosyncratic or allergic reactions to medications. A thorough history for food hypersensitivity is of particular importance in pre- and postoperative management.

On physical examination, note the presence of wheezing on quiet and on forced expiration. In younger children, wheezing may be elicited by having the child play a game of blowing a sheet of paper to produce a forced expiration. An increased anterior-posterior (AP) diameter of the chest due to hyperinflation is a sign of obstructive lung disease. The use of accessory muscles of respiration, especially retractions of sternocleidomastoid muscles, correlates with abnormal pulmonary function (McFadden et al.,1973). Chest roentgenograms (AP and lateral views) are helpful in evaluating the degree of air-trapping (hyperinflation) and the presence of pulmonary and extrapulmonary complications such as infection, atelectasis, pneumothorax, and pneumomediastinum. All asthmatic patients should have a preoperative chest x-ray examination.

Pulmonary function studies offer an objective means of evaluating airway obstruction. In children, there are marked intrasubject and intersubject variations in pulmonary function, owing to growth, as well as to the degree of cooperation and training in the performance of the studies. The "best test," rather than the average of two or three performances, should be compared to the mean or predicted normal value for the patient's standing height (see Chapter 42). The detection of abnormalities in preoperative pulmonary function enables the anesthesiologist to anticipate problems during surgery and provides a baseline with which to compare postoperative lung function tests. Pulmonary function abnormalities indicating significant small airway disease can be the harbinger of postoperative respiratory problems and increased risk of postoperative complications. The MEFR (maximal expiratory flow rate), probably indicating the adequacy of cough, gave the best prediction of postoperative complications in a study assessing the preoperative pulmonary status of 63 adults (Stein et al., 1962). In younger children, the peak expiratory flow rate with the Wright Peak Flow Meter* may be the only practical, noninvasive pulmonary function test that is feasible for baseline and follow-up evaluation of lung function in the preoperative and postoperative periods. It should be interpreted cautiously, however, because it is so effort-dependent. In older children, a spirogram from which the FVC (forced vital capacity), FEV_1 (one second vital capacity), and $FEF_{25-75\%}$ can be determined provides a useful baseline.

In moderately severe or severe asthmatics it is important to determine arterial blood gases preoperatively, to evaluate the degree of hypoxemia. Arterial blood gases may also be the only practical method to assess pulmonary status preoperatively in the child too young to perform lung function tests.

PREOPERATIVE MANAGEMENT

Preoperative management will vary in individual asthmatic patients depending upon: age (airway size), timing of surgery (elective, semi-elective, emergency), type of surgery (e.g., thoracic, abdominal) and severity and reversibility of asthma.

If a child or adolescent with mild asthma is in remission at the time of surgery and has normal pulmonary function, bronchodilators may not be necessary in the preoperative period. If bronchospasm develops in the postoperative period, aminophylline can be administered with the intravenous fluids and/or aerosolized adrenergic agents such as isoproterenol can be administered with a nebulizer driven by oxygen or compressed air.

The patient with moderate or severe asthma who has pulmonary function abnormalities requires more extensive preoperative management, and optimal bronchodilation should be achieved before surgery. Theophylline can be administered orally or aminophylline intravenously. Theophylline serum concentration should be in the range of 10 to 20 μg/ml before surgery. If emergency surgery is necessary in a patient who has not received bronchodilators, aminophylline should be given intravenously, with a loading dose followed by a maintenance dosage (see Chapters 23 and 45). Patients who require continuous bronchodilator therapy for control of their asthma should receive theophylline intravenously when they are on nothing-by-mouth regimens (preoperative, operative and postoperative periods), to maintain serum theophylline in the optimal therapeutic range.

Patients with severe asthma may require corticosteroids in addition to theophylline. The use of steroids at the time of surgery is mandatory for patients who have needed steroids for control of asthma within the 6 months before surgery, because of possible suppressed adrenal pituitary axis responsiveness. Such patients should receive large doses the day before and the day of surgery and at least for 2 days postoperatively. The steroid dosage is tapered to the preoperative

---

*Armstrong Industries, Inc., Northbrook, Illinois, U.S. Distributors for Airmed Ltd., London.

dose on the third or fourth postoperative day, if no exacerbation of asthma occurs as a result of the surgical stress. The exact corticosteroid regimen varies. A plasma 17-hydroxycorticosteroid level in excess of 100 $\mu g/100$ ml has been recommended in adults, based on studies (Dwyer et al., 1967) that suggested that this concentration of corticosteroids was needed to control acute episodes of asthma in patients with chronic asthma. Double-blind, controlled studies (McFadden et al., 1976; Britton et al., 1976) have not substantiated the need for higher doses of steroids in the treatment of severe asthma in adults.

Controlled studies (Pierson et al., 1974) in children with status asthmaticus revealed significant improvement in recovery from arterial hypoxemia with each of the following regimens:

Hydrocortisone hemisuccinate intravenously, 7 mg/kg bolus, followed by 7 mg/kg/24 hr by continuous infusion.
Dexamethasone intravenously, 0.3 mg/kg bolus, followed by 0.3 mg/kg/24 hr by continuous infusion.
Betamethasone intravenously, 0.3 mg/kg bolus, followed by 0.3 mg/kg/24 hr by continuous infusion.

Both betamethasone and dexamethasone appeared to have the advantage over hydrocortisone of higher unbound pharmacologically active corticosteroid levels.

The type of premedication given the asthmatic can also influence the dose of steroids needed to achieve an optimal serum concentration. Short-acting barbiturates frequently are used as preoperative medications. Since barbiturates are potent microsomal enzyme inducers and can increase metabolic clearance of steroids, steroid dosage should be increased when barbiturates are prescribed. An intravenous line is mandatory in preparation for surgery to assure an easy access route for the administration of theophylline and steroids, if needed during surgery. In severe asthmatics, a baseline electrocardiogram also should be obtained.

An arterial line for monitoring blood gases is desirable in all patients with severe asthma but essential to optimal management of the patient with severe asthma who is symptomatic when lengthly surgery is necessary.

Adequate preparation of the asthmatic patient prior to and following surgery includes the clearing of airway secretions. Segmental bronchial drainage and chest physical therapy are physical maneuvers utilized to encourage removal of secretions. Segmental bronchial drainage is a technique that uses gravity and other physical maneuvers to prevent or relieve bronchial obstruction due to secretions; this technique often has been referred to as *postural drainage*. The term *segmental bronchial drainage* emphasizes the importance of accurate positioning of the patient. The segment to be drained is placed uppermost, with the segmental bronchi in optimal position to allow gravity to assist in the flow of secretions into the main stem bronchi and trachea where they can be expectorated or swallowed. Figure 62–1 shows the correct drainage positions for the right middle lobe (RML). A complete set of instructions for accurate positioning in infants and children has been prepared by the author and can be obtained from the Cystic Fibrosis Foundation.*

Clapping is another physical maneuver used to assist gravity in the movement of secretions and is thought to set up vibrations that are transmitted to the bronchi, stimulating the movement of secretions and dislodging secretions adhering to the bronchial walls. Clapping is done with the cupped hand on the chest wall. The hand is cupped by flexing the fingers together at the metacarpophalangeal joints so that the contour of the cupped hand conforms with the chest wall. The technique of cupping tends to collect a cushion of air between the hand and chest wall, which softens the impact of the clapping (Fig. 62–2). A plastic mask such as the one shown in Figure 62–2 can be useful in clapping on very small children and for individuals who have difficulty in achieving a "cupped" hand position.

Vibration also is a physical manuever that may loosen secretions from the walls of the bronchi and assist gravity in the movement of secretions; this manuever is done with the flattened hand pressed firmly on the chest wall. The therapist tenses the muscles of the upper arm and shoulder and vibrates while the patient exhales.

The use of an inhaled adrenergic drug as a bronchodilator prior to bronchial drainage usually is beneficial. Aerosolized agents should be administered by a nebulizer rather than by intermittent positive pressure

___
*Segmental Bronchial Drainage, available from Cystic Fibrosis Foundation, 6000 Executive Boulevard, Suite 309, Rockville, Maryland 20852.

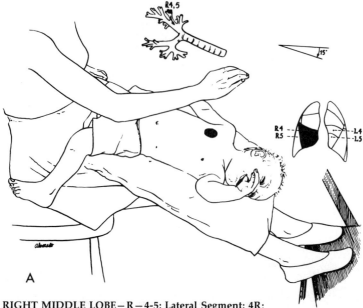

A

RIGHT MIDDLE LOBE—R—4-5: Lateral Segment: 4R;
Medial Segment: 5R

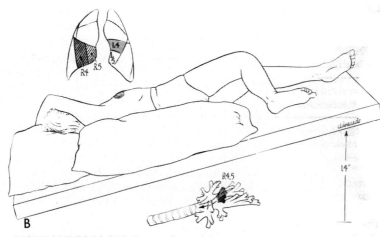

B

RIGHT MIDDLE LOBE, R—4-5: Lateral Segment:
4R; Medial Segment: 5R

FIGURE 62–1. *A,* The infant is placed over the extended legs of the therapist. A pillow may be placed over the extended legs. The infant lies head down on the left side and is rotated 1/4 turn backwards. The therapist claps over the right nipple. The area for clapping of the right middle lobe, R—4-5, is shown in the diagram.

B, The foot of the table or bed is elevated 14 inches (about 15°). The patient lies head down on the left side and rotates 1/4 turn backwards. A pillow may be placed behind the patient (from shoulder to hip). The knees should be flexed. The therapist claps over the right nipple. In females with breast development or tenderness, use cupped hand with heel of hand under armpit and fingers extending forward beneath the breast. The area for clapping of the right middle lobe, R—4-5, is shown in the diagram.

breathing (IPPB) because IPPB increases the risk of pneumothorax and/or pneumomediastinum in the pediatric patient with asthma.

The asthmatic patient is more likely to develop bronchospasm during endotracheal intubation, because of reflex bronchoconstriction due to stimulation of vagal receptors. Since the incidence of vagally mediated arrhythmias during intubation can be reduced by having the patient well anesthetized before attempting intubation, it would seem logical that this practice might be helpful in preventing vagally-mediated bronchospasm. Atropine administration preoperatively also decreases reflux broncho-

constriction, but should be used cautiously since it can increase the danger of airway mucous plugging because of its drying effects. Adequate preoxygenation before intubation also may decrease the risks of arrhythmias due to hypoxemia in a myocardium sensitized by catecholamines.

It is important to choose carefully preoperative medications for the patient with asthma. Avoid barbiturates if possible, as well as histamine-releasing drugs such as codeine, morphine, meperidine, curare and d-tubocurarine. Pancuronium is the muscle relaxant of choice preoperatively and operatively in the asthmatic.

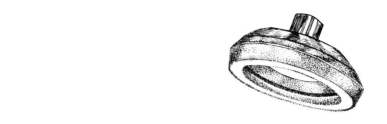

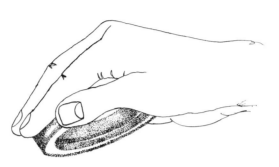

FIGURE 62–2. For small infants or when the therapist has difficulty in cupping, a small plastic mask can be substituted for the cupped hand in clapping on the chest.

The choice of an anesthetic agent is of prime importance. *The anesthetic recommended for asthmatic patients is halothane, because it is less irritating and has bronchodilating properties* (Gold and Helrich, 1970). Ketamine is best avoided, because it may cause endogenous release of catecholamines. Diethyl ether has potent smooth muscle relaxant properties; however, it has the distinct disadvantage of increasing bronchial secretions. The newer steroid intravenous anesthetics such as 3α hydroxy-5α pregnane-11, 20 dione and 21-acetocy-3α hydroxy-5α pregnane-11, 20 dione (Althesin) allow smooth induction (Woo et al., 1976).

OPERATIVE MANAGEMENT

The operative management of bronchospasm includes intravenous theophylline in therapeutic concentrations and the judicious use of steroids. The hazard of aspiration can be minimized by cricoid pressure after the patient is asleep but prior to intubation. The importance of adequate preoxygenation before endotracheal intubation has been noted.

The patient with severe asthma should have electrocardiographic monitoring during surgery and continued into the immediate postoperative period. Arrhythmias are more likely to develop in the severe asthmatic who becomes hypoxemic. Arrhythmias can be precipitated by many other factors, including: bronchospasm, electrolyte imbalance, catecholamine airways sensitization of the myocardium, and stimulation of hyperirritable airways during intubation or endotracheal suctioning. Arterial blood gases also should be monitored in patients with severe asthma, especially in those with evidence of hypoxemia or significant small airway disease on the preoperative assessment. If curare-like drugs are used during surgery, neostigmine can be used at the end of surgery to reverse these drug effects. A sufficient dose of atropine should be given to block its muscarine effects. During surgery, it is necessary to provide adequate ventilation by oxygenation and proper placement of the endotracheal tube.

POSTOPERATIVE EVALUATION AND MANAGEMENT

Therapeutic decisions for the asthmatic patient during the postoperative period include the timing of extubation, the need for bronchodilator and steroid therapy, the use of pulmonary therapy to remove secretions to prevent postoperative pulmonary complications, and the management of those complications if they develop.

The patient should be evaluated before the endotracheal tube is removed. Early extubation is desirable so that normal coughing can occur. When intubated, the glottis cannot close and the patient cannot develop the high intrathoracic pressures needed to cough effectively (Hudson, 1975). Accepted parameters for weaning from assisted to spontaneous ventilation include a dead space-tidal volume (V_D/V_T) ratio of less than 0.6, alveolar-arterial oxygen tension gradient less than 350 mm Hg on 100% oxygen, and vital capacity of at least 10 ml per kg of body weight.

Atelectasis is the most common postoperative pulmonary complication. It may present with cyanosis and tachypnea, with or without fever, and is diagnosed by x-ray examination.

Postoperative changes in both lung mechanics and pulmonary gas exchange vary with the anesthetic, intubation, and type and duration of surgery. They may include a decrease in total lung capacity (TLC), a decrease in functional residual capacity (FRC), a decrease in compliance, an increase in work of breathing and arterial hypoxemia due to intrapulmonary shunting (perfusion of nonventilated alveoli). Generally, these changes become most severe 48 to 72 hours after surgery and return to normal within 7 days. Often they are subclinical and do not cause symptoms, but they can progress to atelectasis and pneumonia. Though the causes of these pulmonary abnormalities are not known, shallow, even, nonsighing tidal breathing appears to be an important factor. It is related to preoperative medication, prolonged or deep anesthesia, postoperative pain, and medications for pain. Numerous postoperative respiratory maneuvers recommended to decrease postoperative pulmonary complications include voluntary coughing; coughing induced by tracheal catheter; blowing into a balloon, glove or tube; blowing into blow bottles; breath holding; carbon dioxide-induced hyperventilation; voluntary sustained maximal inspiratory maneuvers; and intermittent positive pressure breathing (IPPB). Though IPPB frequently is used in postoperative management, it does not appear to be effective in either preventing or treating atelectasis and may increase postoperative risks of pneumothorax, pneumomediastinum, and nosocomial infections.

Voluntary maximal inhalation, (deep-breathing exercises emphasizing sustained inspiration to total lung capacity), on the other hand, have been effective in inflating collapsed alveoli and reducing or preventing postoperative pulmonary complications (Bartlett, 1973). These respiratory maneuvers can be achieved by the use of a device called the *incentive spirometer*,* which aids the patient in performing a sustained maximal inspiration to total lung capacity with the glottis open and provides a reproducible, physiologically appropriate respiratory maneuver.

In the postoperative period, the asthmatic child may need additional bronchodilators, chest physiotherapy, or both. If preventive measures fail, early detection of postoperative pulmonary complications and prompt treatment should minimize morbidity and reduce hospital stay.

*Triflo II Incentive Deep-Breathing Exerciser, available from Chesebrough-Ponds, Inc., Greenwich, Connecticut 06830.

References

Bartlett, R. H., Gazzaniga, A. B., et al.: Respiratory maneuvers to prevent postoperative pulmonary complications. J.A.M.A. 224:1017, 1973.

Britton, M. G., Collins, J. V., Brown, D., et al.: High-dose corticosteroids in severe acute asthma. Br. Med. J. 2(6027):73, 1976.

Diament, M. L., and Palmer, K. N. V.: Spirometry for preoperative assessment of airways resistance. Lancet 1:1251, 1967.

Dwyer, J., Lazarus, L., et al.: A study of cortisol metabolism in patients with chronic asthma. Aust. Ann. Med. 16:297, 1967.

Gold, M. I., and Helrich, M.: Pulmonary mechanics during general anesthesia: V. Status asthmaticus. Anesthesiology 32:422, 1970.

Hudson, L. D.: The asthmatic patient who needs surgery. In The Asthmatic Patient in Trouble. Greenwich, Conn., Upjohn Company, pp. 41–47, 1975.

McFadden, E. R., Jr., Kiser, R., deGroot, W. J., et al.: A controlled study of the effects of single dose of hydrocortisone on the resolution of acute attacks of asthma. Am. J. Med. 60:52, 1976.

McFadden, E. R., Jr., Kiser, R. and deGroot, W. J.: Acute bronchial asthma: Relations between clinical and physiologic manifestations. N. Engl. J. Med., 288:221, 1973.

Pierson, W. E., Bierman, C. W., and Kelley, V. C.: A double-blind trial of corticosteroid therapy in status asthmaticus. Pediatrics 54:282, 1974.

Stein, M., Koota, G. M., and Simon, M.:Pulmonary evaluation of surgical patients. J.A.M.A., 181:765, 1962.

Stein, M., and Abdel-Rassoul, M. I.: Preoperative and postoperative considerations in patients with bronchial asthma. In Weiss, E. B., and Segal, M. S. (eds.): Bronchial Asthma: Mechanisms and Therapeutics. Boston, Little, Brown and Co., 1976, pp. 991–997.

Woo, Sybil W.; Malhotra, I. V., and Hedley-Whyte, J.: Anesthetic considerations. In Weiss, E. B., and Segal, M. S. (eds.): Bronchial Asthma: Mechanisms and Therapeutics. Boston, Little Brown and Co., 1976, pp. 999–1006.

Abraham H. Eisen, M.D. **63**

Eosinophilia

Cases of hypereosinophilia without explanation are rare in children. The more common presentation is a child with a clear history of skin or respiratory allergy, in whom, during the course of routine investigation, eosinophilia is noted. If the eosinophilia is modest (less than 10 per cent), it usually can be attributed to the underlying allergic state, especially if the patient has eczema, or it may be due to transient postinfection eosinophilia. If the eosinophilia is higher and/or is persistent, a complete investigation is indicated.

Table 63–1 describes two methods for counting eosinophils in peripheral blood. Table 63–2 lists a differential diagnosis of the *more common* conditions in which peripheral eosinophilia may be a feature. Most of the diseases listed in the differential diagnosis will be apparent by a careful history and physical examination. When the diagnosis is not apparent after history and physical examination, the following laboratory investigation is indicated:

1. The hemogram and total eosinophil count (TEC) first should be repeated at weekly or 2-week intervals to confirm the level and persistence of eosinophilia.
2. A chest x-ray should be obtained to check for infiltrates and hyperinflation.
3. At least two fresh stool specimens should be examined for ova and parasites, and a search should be made for pinworms. *(Toxocara ova are not found in stool.)*

TABLE 63–1 METHODS FOR COUNTING EOSINOPHILS IN PERIPHERAL BLOOD

Smear Technique

1. Prepare a thin smear (free flowing blood from fingertip).
2. Air dry the smear.
3. Fix smear in methylhydrate for 3 minutes.
4. Stain with Wright's stain for 3 minutes.
5. Place in phosphate buffered solution ph 6.8 for 3 minutes.
6. Under high dry power, count at least 100 white blood cells.
7. Normal up to 5% eosinophils.

Direct Count

1. Use Unopett (test 5877 Becton-Dickenson) for eosinophil determination for manual methods.
2. Draw 25 lambda blood into Unopett (free flowing blood from fingertip).
3. Inject blood into eosinophil stain and mix. After thorough mixing, discharge $1/4$ of blood-stain mixture.
4. Fill both sides (full but not overflowing) of a Fuchs-Rosenthal chamber, using special cover slip for manual counting of eosinophils.
5. Allow cells to settle for 10 minutes.
6. Count all cells under both ruled areas.
7. Calculation:

$$\frac{\text{Number of cells} \times 20 \ (1{:}20 \ \text{dilution})}{3.2 \ (\text{area under square})}$$
$$= \text{eosinophils per cu. mm.}$$

8. Normal = 40–440 eosinophils per cu. mm.

TABLE 63–2 EOSINOPHILIA – DIFFERENTIAL DIAGNOSIS

Atopic disorders—asthma, atopic dermatitis, seasonal allergic rhinitis

Drug hypersensitivity reactions

Parasitic infestation

Pulmonary infiltrates with eosinophilia (PIE syndrome)

Collagen vascular diseases (e.g., polyarteritis)

Dermatologic conditions—pemphigus, dermatitis herpetiformis

Acute infections (postinfectious stage)

Malignancies, e.g., Wilms' tumor, Hodgkin's disease

Hematologic disorders—pernicious anemia, chronic myelocytic anemia, eosinophilic leukemia, post-infectious mononucleosis.

Immunodeficiency

Irradiation

Familial eosinophilia

Miscellaneous—allergic gastroenteropathy, sarcoid, graft versus host disease

Idiopathic

4. Blood should be obtained for:
   a. A sedimentation rate, for nonspecific evidence of an inflammatory process.
   b. IgG, IgM, and IgA levels, for evidence of immune stimulation or aberration.
   c. IgE level, which may be elevated in parasitic infestation, atopic disorders or in bronchopulmonary aspergillosis.
   d. Autoimmune markers: ANF, RF, helpful in certain collagen vascular diseases (see Chapter 65).
   e. Liver function tests (appropriate when the diagnosis of sarcoid or graft versus host disease is being entertained).
5. Allergy skin tests to common allergens are considered if the history is consistent with or suggestive of an allergic state. Skin testing for immediate reactivity to

Aspergillus species also is important in establishing the diagnosis of bronchopulmonary aspergillosis.

6. Other studies such as biopsy of skin, muscle or gastrointestinal tract; IVP; and bone marrow aspiration should be done as indicated by the clinical condition.

A chest x-ray, examination of stools for ova and parasites, and skin test for aspergillosis will help diagnose the major causes of profound eosinophilia.

EOSINOPHIL COUNTS IN THE MANAGEMENT OF ALLERGIC PROBLEMS IN CHILDREN

The TEC often is normal in allergic children, as is diurnal variation in counts. The TEC falls 4 to 8 hours after oral prednisone and may drop after systemic beta adrenergic stimulators (isoproterenol, metaproterenol, terbutaline, salbutamol) are administered. Theophylline, cromolyn sodium, and inhaled steroids in normal doses do not affect the TEC. Children receiving steroids on alternate days show normal diurnal variation on the day *off* steroids (Blumberg and Buckley, 1976).

In adults with nonallergic (intrinsic) asthma, pulmonary function tests vary inversely with TEC, and the TEC reportedly has been useful in anticipating severe attacks and also in assessing therapy (Horn et al., 1975). This may apply as well to selected severely asthmatic children.

TEC may be of value in provocative drug trials. In one study, TEC declined immediately after provocation in drug-sensitive individuals and increased 24 to 48 hours later (Stubb, 1976).

References

Blumberg, M. Z., and Buckley, J. M.: The total eosinophil count in asthmatic children. J. Allergy Clin. Immunol. *57*:493, 1976.

Horn, B. R., Robin, E. D., Theodore, J., and Van Kessel, A.: Total eosinophil count in the management of bronchial asthma. New Engl. J. Med. *292*:1152, 1975.

Stubb, S.: Blood leukocytes with special reference to basophils and eosinophils during provocative tests on fixed eruption and drug exanthems. Acta Derm. Venereol. (Suppl) 56(76):1, 1976.

Helen M. Emery, M.D.
Jane G. Schaller, M.D.

64

Rheumatic Diseases

Allergy and rheumatic diseases are sometimes discussed together because both are thought to be mediated by immune pathways. In allergy, these pathways are becoming increasingly well-defined. However, in rheumatic diseases, pathogenetic mechanisms are still poorly understood. Nevertheless, the role of host response to what may be commonly encountered environmental factors may be critical in initiating and perpetuating these diseases. There is, however, no evidence that rheumatic diseases are allergic in the ordinary sense, nor has any increased incidence of atopic allergy been proved in rheumatic disease patients or their families.

Rheumatic diseases are relatively common and are estimated to affect between 250,000 and 500,000 children in the United States. Over recent years there has been a marked decline in rheumatic fever, once the most common disease in this category, and an increasing interest in diseases formerly considered uncommon, such as juvenile rheumatoid arthritis. This chapter deals with the clinical features and management of juvenile rheumatoid arthritis, ankylosing spondylitis, systemic lupus erythematosus, dermatomyositis, scleroderma, mixed connective tissue disease, rheumatic fever, and vasculitis (Table 64–1). It should be noted that there are a number of other conditions that may mimic rheumatic diseases that should be excluded before a firm diagnosis is made (Table 64–2).

JUVENILE RHEUMATOID ARTHRITIS

An estimated 200,000 children in the United States have juvenile rheumatoid arthritis (JRA). This disorder is defined as the presence of inflammation of at least one joint for

TABLE 64–1 SYSTEMS OFTEN AFFECTED IN VARIOUS RHEUMATIC DISEASES

	Skin	Joints	Heart	Kidney	Skeletal Muscle	Gastro-Intestinal	Eye	Central Nervous System
Juvenile rheumatoid arthritis	+	+	+	−	+	−	+	−
Lupus erythematosus	+	+	+	+	+	+	+	+
Rheumatic fever	+	+	+	−	−	−	−	+
Schönlein-Henoch vasculitis	+	+	−	+	−	+	−	−
Dermatomyositis	+	+	−	−	+	+	−	−
Scleroderma	+	+	+	+	+	+	−	−

TABLE 64–2 CONDITIONS CAUSING OR SIMULATING CHILDHOOD ARTHRITIS

Rheumatic Diseases

Juvenile rheumatoid arthritis; juvenile chronic arthritis
Ankylosing spondylitis
Reiter's syndrome
Arthritis of inflammatory bowel disease
Psoriatic arthritis
Rheumatic fever
Systemic lupus erythematosus
Dermatomyositis
Vasculitis syndromes
Scleroderma
Mixed connective tissue disease

Infectious Diseases

Septic arthritis
Viral-related arthritis
"Reactive" arthritis
Osteomyelitis

Childhood Malignancies

Leukemia
Neuroblastoma
Lymphoma, Hodgkin's disease
Others

Noninflammatory Conditions of Bones and Joints

Limb pains ("growing pains")
Psychogenic musculoskeletal pain or dysfunction
Musculoskeletal trauma
Avascular necrosis
Miscellaneous orthopaedic conditions (slipped capital femoral epiphysis, Osgood-Schlatter's disease, chondromalacia patella syndrome, discitis, etc.)
Genetic and congenital malformations

Miscellaneous Conditions

Sarcoidosis
Hemoglobinopathies

more than three months in which underlying causes have been excluded. (See Table 64–2). Infectious diseases (septic arthritis, osteomyelitis, viral-related arthritis), malignancies, and various noninflammatory conditions of bones and joints must be considered in the differential diagnosis. JRA has been classified into several categories based on the pattern of disease in the first three to six months of disease; these include: (1) systemic onset, (2) polyarticular, and (3) pauciar-

ticular (Schaller and Wedgwood, 1972; Schaller, 1977). Table 64–3 lists the clinical manifestations of the different subgroups.

Systemic Onset JRA

This form of disease is characterized by high fever, evanescent rash, and arthritis and occurs in about 20 percent of children with JRA. Fever is over 39° C, usually highest in the evening, and returns to normal between peaks. While febrile, patients may appear toxic and experience marked myalgia, arthralgia, and malaise. An evanescent rash consists of small pink or red macules up to 0.5 cm in diameter, often with central clearing; it accompanies febrile episodes in the majority of patients and may occur anywhere in the body. It often is pronounced in areas of skin trauma, such as where skin and clothing rub, and sometimes becomes confluent. Individual lesions generally clear within hours.

Arthritis, arthralgia, and myalgia may be transient early in the disease, often coinciding with fever. However, objective arthritis should persist for three consecutive months before a firm diagnosis of JRA is made (Table 64–2).

Polyserositis in the form of pleuritis or pericarditis occurs in about 50 percent of patients. Symptoms and signs include chest pain and dyspnea. Life-threatening cardiac involvement, such as cardiac tamponade or cardiac failure from pericarditis or myocarditis, occur rarely. Interstitial lung changes resembling viral pneumonia are sometimes present, and abdominal pain, probably resulting from peritonitis or mesenteric adenitis, occurs in some patients. Lymphadenopathy, splenomegaly, and hepatomegaly (at times accompanied by abnormal liver function tests) are common findings. Iridocyclitis is rarely, if ever, found in systemic onset JRA.

When classic fever, rheumatoid rash, and arthritis are present, the diagnosis of systemic onset JRA is not difficult to make. However, infectious disease and malignancy must be considered in the differential diagnosis, particularly in patients with atypical presentations.

Laboratory Findings. There are no diagnostic laboratory tests. Anemia is common and sometimes severe. White blood cell counts usually are elevated with a predomi-

TABLE 64–3 SUBGROUPS OF JUVENILE RHEUMATOID ARTHRITIS

Subgroup	Sex	Age at Onset	Joints Affected	Laboratory Tests	Extra-Articular Manifestations	Prognosis
Systemic onset	60% boys	Any age	Any joints	*ANA neg **RF neg	Prominent: High fever, rash, and others	25% severe arthritis
Seronegative	90% girls	Any age	Any joints	ANA 25% RF neg	Few	10–15% severe arthritis
Seropositive	80% girls	Late childhood	Any joints	ANA 75% RF 100%	Rheumatoid nodules, Rheumatoid vasculitis	50% severe arthritis
Pauciarticular Type I	80% girls	Early childhood	Few large joints (Hips and sacroiliac joints spared)	ANA 50%	Chronic iridocyclitis 50%	Severe arthritis uncommon. 10–20% ocular damage from iridocyclitis
Pauciarticular Type II	90% boys	Late childhood	Few large joints (Hip and sacroiliac involvement common)	ANA neg RF neg †HLA-B27 75%	Acute iridocyclitis 5–10%	Some have ankylosing spondylitis at follow-up

*ANA = antinuclear antibody
**RF = rheumatoid factor
†HLA-B27 = histocompatibility antigen-B27

nance of early forms of PMN's. Sedimentation rates generally are elevated, and thrombocytosis sometimes is seen. Tests for rheumatoid factors and antinuclear antibodies are negative.

Treatment. Fever and arthritis usually are well-controlled by salicylates, although two or three weeks of therapy may be necessary before there is a clinical response. In small children (under 25 kg body weight), aspirin in a dose of 100 mg per kg per day usually results in therapeutic levels of 20 to 30 mg per 100 ml. In heavier children, a total daily dose of 40 to 60 grains (2400 to 3600 mg) usually is sufficient. Aspirin is given four times a day, with each meal and at bedtime. Patients and parents should be aware of signs of salicylate toxicity, such as hyperventilation, excessive drowsiness, irritability, or peculiar behavior (tinnitus and hearing loss are common complaints in children). Gastric upset, urticaria, bronchospasm, and bleeding tendency are other possible aspirin side effects that are not related directly to dosage. Corticosteroids may be required for severe pericarditis or myocarditis, severe anemia, or debilitating febrile episodes unresponsive to salicylates. A single morning dose of 1 to 2 mgm per kg of prednisone initially should control these signs; prednisone should be gradually tapered off and discontinued within six months.

The arthritis associated with systemic onset JRA should be managed as that of polyarticular JRA (see next section). Steroids should be avoided in managing joint manifestations alone because of their side effects.

Prognosis. Episodes of fever and rash may last several months if untreated, but usually are self-limited. Recurrences of systemic complaints may occur after periods of quiescent disease. Arthritis may persist in the absence of systemic symptoms and can be severe, resulting in functional limitation in up to 25 percent of patients. Growth retardation also may follow chronic, uncontrolled inflammation, even in the absence of steroid treatment. In some parts of the world amyloidosis is a major complication in this and other subgroups of JRA, but this rarely occurs in the United States.

Polyarticular JRA

Patients who have inflammation of more than five joints in the first six months of disease without the febrile manifestations of systemic onset JRA are included in this category. As seen in Table 64–1, there are two main groups, divided by the presence or absence of serum rheumatoid factors.

SERONEGATIVE POLYARTICULAR JRA

Children present with inflammation of both large and small joints, often symmetrical in distribution. Morning stiffness, joint swelling, and limitation of joint movement are common findings. Pain may not be a prominent complaint, as children often avoid movements that precipitate pain. Some patients have malaise, low-grade fever, mild anemia, mild adenopathy or hepatosplenomegaly, and growth retardation. Rheumatoid rash and polyserositis are not characteristic, nor are patients at increased risk for chronic iridocyclitis.

Laboratory Findings. Mild anemia and elevation of the sedimentation rate are common but nonspecific findings. Rheumatoid factors are not present. About 25 percent of patients have positive tests for antinuclear antibodies.

Joint radiographs show few changes early in disease other than soft tissue swelling and periarticular osteoporosis. In patients with severe disease, loss of articular cartilage and damage to periarticular bone may be visible later in the course of the disease. Premature fusion of epiphyses in the short bones of the hands and feet may occur with resultant metacarpal or metatarsal shortening. Mandibular undergrowth can result from temperomandibular arthritis. Epiphyseal overgrowth around inflamed knees and ankles may result in lengthening of affected limbs.

Treatment. In all types of JRA, salicylates are the drugs of choice. The majority of seronegative patients will respond well to the same therapeutic levels described in the treatment of systemic disease, and other drugs generally need not be considered in the first six months of treatment.

A number of other nonsteroidal anti-inflammatory medications are available for adults with rheumatoid arthritis, including indomethacin, ibuprofen, and tolmetin. However, experience with these drugs in children is limited, and only tolmetin is available currently in the United States for use in children. These drugs appear to be therapeutically equivalent to aspirin, but some patients may respond better to one drug than to another.

Gold salts (sodium thiomalate or thioglucose) and antimalarial agents, such as hydroxychloroquine, are the next drugs of choice in arthritis that is not adequately controlled by salicylates or other nonsteroidal anti-inflammatory agents. Gold salts must be given intramuscularly; side effects include skin rashes, mucosal ulcers, renal toxicity (proteinuria or hematuria), and bone marrow suppression (leukopenia or thrombocytopenia). The chief hazard of antimalarial drugs is retinal toxicity. Parents should be warned that irreversible cardiac and respiratory depression may occur with an acute overdose of antimalarial drugs. All patients receiving these drugs must be evaluated carefully and frequently during therapy. With gold therapy, monitoring includes complete blood count, urinalysis, and physical examination *before* each injection; with an antimalarial, ophthalmologic surveillance should be carried out every three months.

Maintenance of good range of motion and function of joints and good muscle strength are of great importance in the management of JRA. A program of coordinated physical and occupational therapy should be planned. Both range of motion and muscle strengthening exercises are required. Heat, such as from a hot bath, often reduces morning stiffness. Moving inflamed joints, though sometimes painful, will not damage them, and activities such as tricycle riding and swimming are both fun and therapeutic. Splints worn at night will keep joints in functional positions and can also reduce flexion contractures.

Prognosis. As cartilaginous changes and bony destruction occur late and tend to be mild, the outcome is good for about 90 percent of patients with seronegative JRA when joint function is maintained during acute disease.

SEROPOSITIVE POLYARTICULAR JRA

Patients with this type of arthritis usually are older than eight years at onset, and their disease resembles that of adults with severe rheumatoid arthritis. The distribution of joint involvement is similar to that of seronegative JRA, but the severity of the arthritis and the resulting joint destruction frequently are much greater than in seronegative disease. Patients often show subcutaneous rheumatoid nodules over pressure points such as the extensor surfaces of the elbows. They are also at risk for extra-articular manifestations, such as rheumatoid vasculitis, Sjögren's syndrome (parotitis, keratoconjunctivitis sicca) and Felty's syndrome (hypersplenism, leukopenia).

Laboratory Findings. Rheumatoid factor tests are consistently positive, often in high titers. Patients also frequently have positive tests for antinuclear antibodies. Joint radiographs often show erosive and destructive changes about joints, sometimes in the first year of disease.

Treatment. Inflammation often is difficult to control. Salicylates remain the first drug of choice. However, most patients require aggressive treatment with salicylates in combination with gold salts or other agents.

Penicillamine appears to have similar efficacy and side effects to gold salts but can be given orally. Experience in children is limited, and this agent still is considered experimental.

Cytotoxic drugs including azathioprine, cyclophosphamide, and chlorambucil have been used in adults, but side effects, both short-term (bone marrow suppression, increased susceptibility to infection) and long-term (infertility, malignant changes) must seriously limit their use in children.

Prognosis. Children with seropositive polyarticular JRA frequently have joint destruction and deformity. About half will have long-active disease and residual functional limitation in spite of aggressive therapy. Surgical joint replacements may be effective in relieving pain and increasing mobility in patients with severe joint destruction and disability; however, they usually are reserved for children who have achieved full growth.

Pauciarticular Onset JRA

Patients with inflammation of five or fewer joints for at least three months after exclusion of other underlying diseases are classified into the pauciarticular category. Consideration of two subgroups is helpful in evaluating patients with this disease: (1) young onset (mean two years), predominantly girls (Type I); and (2) older onset (over eight years), predominantly boys (Type II).

PAUCIARTICULAR DISEASE TYPE I

Girls are predominantly affected, and the age at onset is early, usually before the fifth birthday. As in other forms of arthritis, patients usually present with joint swelling, limitation of movement, loss of joint function, and morning stiffness. However, this distribution of arthritis is "spotty," but not symmetrical. Large joints, such as knees, ankles, and elbows, are predominantly af-

fected; some small joints are occasionally involved as well. Hip and sacroiliac joint involvement are unusual.

Chronic iridocyclitis is a major risk in this type of disease. It is insidious and asymptomatic at onset and can lead to irreversible scarring of the iris, band keratopathy, cataract formation, and glaucoma. It is particularly important to perform routine slit lamp examinations every three months in all pauciarticular patients, as early detection of this complication is essential to successful therapy.

Laboratory Findings. No test is specific for this type of disease. Sedimentation rates may be elevated. Anemia is not common. Tests for rheumatoid factors are negative. More than half of these patients have positive tests for antinuclear antibodies (ANA), which correlate strongly with risk of chronic iridocyclitis; 80 percent of patients with iridocyclitis have ANA.

As destruction of cartilage occurs late if at all in patients with pauciarticular JRA, joint radiographs rarely show destructive changes. However, prolonged joint inflammation may lead to accelerated bone growth at the epiphysis of long bones.

Treatment. Response to aspirin and physical therapy generally is good, and seldom are other anti-inflammatory regimens necessary.

Chronic iridocyclitis usually is controlled by topical steroids and mydriatics, although sometimes when it is severe, subconjunctival or systemic steroids may by required. Careful ophthalmologic follow-up is essential to monitor disease activity and to adjust medications, as the iridocyclitis may be intermittently active for many years, even when joint disease is no longer active.

Prognosis. In these younger onset children, the outlook for joint range and function is very good. The major long-term morbidity is that of eye disease.

PAUCIARTICULAR DISEASE TYPE II

The second subgroup of patients with pauciaritcular JRA consists mainly of boys over the age of eight years at onset. There may be a family history of ankylosing spondylitis or other spondyloarthropathy or of acute iritis.

Symptoms are similar to the first group of patients, but joint involvement frequently is confined to the lower extremities, including hips and sacroiliac joints. Heel pain and Achilles tendinitis may occur also. Disease in some patients will progress over a period of years to classic ankylosing spondylitis. A number of patients will have attacks of acute self-limited iridocyclitis.

Laboratory Findings. Patients do not have antinuclear antibodies or rheumatoid factors, but they have been found to carry histocompatibility antigen HLA-B27 in a much higher frequency than expected. This may correlate with the development of ankylosing spondylitis and acute iritis.

Radiographs of peripheral joints show few early changes other than soft tissue swelling. In about half of the patients, radiographic evidence of sacroiliitis appears either early or late in the disease. If full-blown ankylosing spondylitis develops, sacroiliitis and other spinal changes consistent with that disease will be found; destruction of hip joints is frequent.

Prognosis. In some children, episodes of arthritis are transient and may represent a "forme fruste" of ankylosing spondylitis. In others, disease may be long-standing with progressive spondyloarthropathy.

Treatment. Salicylates generally control symptoms adequately, but in older children who are unresponsive to salicylates, a trial of one of the other nonsteroidal anti-inflammatory agents may be warranted. Physical therapy programs should include back mobility exercises as well as standard range and strengthening regimens for affected joints.

ANKYLOSING SPONDYLITIS

Ankylosing spondylitis is an inflammatory condition affecting primarily joints and ligamentous structures of the axial skeleton, clinically characterized by limited mobility of the lumbosacral spine, with evidence of sacroiliitis on radiographic examination (Schaller et al., 1969).

Although the etiology is unknown, an interesting association has been demonstrated with the histocompatibility antigen HLA-B27, which has been identified in over 90 percent of patients with ankylosing spondylitis, and also in a large percentage of patients with other spondyloarthropathies (Reiter's syndrome and the spondylitis of psoriasis and inflammatory bowel disease). This antigen is found in about 8 per-

cent of the general Caucasian population. Although the antigen itself probably is not responsible for initiating the disease, it may be closely linked to the genes that in some way determine susceptibility, possibly by influencing the immune response.

Clinical Features. The diagnosis of ankylosing spondylitis is made most frequently in young adult males. However, as previously discussed, children as young as eight years may present with pauciarticular arthritis, which progresses to ankylosing spondylitis over a number of years. Classic ankylosing spondylitis affects about eight times as many men as women; however, it is possible that more women are afffected mildly.

Symptoms characteristically include low back pain, which often is worse at night and in the early morning and which may be relieved by movement. There may be inflammation of peripheral joints, such as knees, ankles, hips, shoulder, and temperomandibular joints. In the spine, the sacroiliac joints usually are involved first, with inflammation then ascending in variable degrees through the lumbar, thoracic, and cervical regions. By contrast, rheumatoid arthritis affects the cervical spine and occasionally the sacroiliac joints but almost always spares the rest of the spine. The inflammation results in fusion (ankylosis) of the apophyseal joints of the spine and also in calcification of various spinal ligaments, resulting in the so-called "bamboo spine." Limitation of flexion and rotation in the spine and decreased chest expansion (from costovertebral joint involvement) are characteristic.

Extra-articular manifestations include acute iridocyclitis and aortitis (usually in adulthood). Pulmonary function may be compromised if chest wall mobility is affected.

Laboratory Findings. As in other rheumatic diseases, there is no laboratory test specific for ankylosing spondylitis. The blood count usually is normal, but the erythrocyte sedimentation rate is elevated. Tests for rheumatoid factors and antinuclear antibodies are negative. Over 90 percent of patients will have HLA-B27, but of all people with this antigen, probably only a low percentage (probably 15 to 20 percent) will develop overt spondylitis (Schaller et al., 1976).

Radiographic changes of the sacroiliac joints are essential for diagnosis. Initially, periarticular erosions may give an appearance of widening of the joints, but later sclerosis leads to fusion. With long-standing ascending inflammation, fusion of the spinal apophyseal joints and calcification of paraspinal ligaments are seen. Periostitis may occur at sites of tendon attachment, commonly on the os calcis ("heel spurs") and the pelvis.

Treatment. Salicylates frequently are sufficient to control symptoms. Indomethacin also is an effective anti-inflammatory agent but has not been approved for use in children in the United States. Other nonsteroidal drugs such as tolmetin are still being evaluated in ankylosing spondylitis. Gold and antimalarials are not thought to be helpful.

Exercises to maintain joint and spinal position and muscle strength are of great importance. In addition, an upright posture while standing and sitting and sleeping flat on a firm mattress should be encouraged to prevent kyphosis.

Prognosis. Most patients have active inflammation for many years but have a good outlook if functional posture is maintained. In some patients, however, destruction and ankylosis of peripheral joints occur, particularly in the hips. In such patients, surgical joint replacements may be required. Although attacks of acute iridocyclitis are common, permanent ocular damage is unusual.

SYSTEMIC LUPUS ERYTHEMATOSUS (SLE)

SLE is a serious and potentially life-threatening disease when it occurs in childhood. It usually presents with inflammatory changes of multiple organ systems. Antinuclear antibodies invariably are present in the blood, and antibodies to many cell types (e.g., platelets, red cells, and lymphocytes) and cell components (e.g, RNA and DNA) and IgG also may be present (Cook et al., 1960). It appears that a major component of cell damage is mediated by deposition of circulating antibody–antigen complexes, particularly DNA–anti-DNA. Mechanisms triggering such aberrant antibody with immune complex formation are not understood. However, abnormal host response and certain environmental agents appear to be important. For example, patients with deficiencies of complement components are at increased risk of developing SLE, and

mothers of children with chronic granulomatous disease also have a high incidence of SLE-like illness, suggesting a role for impaired host response mechanisms. Many drugs (e.g., procaine amide, most anticonvulsants, and hydralazine) can induce SLE in certain individuals (see Chap. 54). A role for viruses in inducing SLE is also suggested by identification of viral-type inclusions by electron microscopy in human SLE tissues. In the animal model of SLE in NZB mice, viruses appear to play a role in pathogenesis. However, many aspects of etiology and pathogenesis of SLE are yet poorly understood.

Clinical Features. Children presenting with SLE usually are ill with fever, malaise, and weight loss. Multiple system involvement is characteristic of the childhood disease. Skin findings include the classic malar rash, a helpful diagnostic sign when present. Other cutaneous findings include nonspecific rashes, vasculitis, and alopecia.

Musculoskeletal involvement is frequent. Arthritis may be chronic, resembling rheumatoid arthritis (except that deformity and joint destruction are unusual), or transient as in rheumatic fever. Some patients have only joint pain (arthralgia), with few objective joint changes. Other musculoskeletal findings include myositis and avascular necrosis (either from SLE itself or from steroid treatment).

Hematologic abnormalities are frequent. Anemia may result from the bone marrow suppression of chronic illness or from antibody-mediated hemolysis of red cells. Thrombocytopenia mediated by anti-platelet antibodies may be severe. Some patients present with apparent idiopathic thrombocytopenic purpura. Leukopenia also is common. Circulating anticoagulants may occur and should be sought before any biopsy or surgical procedures are planned.

Generalized lymphadenopathy and hepatosplenomegaly are common. Patients appear to have increased susceptibility to infections because of both their underlying disease and the drugs used in therapy.

Renal involvement is common in children. The most frequent early findings are microscopic hematuria, pyuria, cylinduria, or proteinuria. Hypertension, the nephrotic syndrome, or renal insufficiency may be apparent clinically, and renal function studies may reveal decreased renal function. Renal histologic changes vary from mild mesangial deposition of immune complexes to diffuse proliferative glomerulonephritis or membranous nephritis. Renal biopsy is invaluable in defining the nature and extent of damage when devising treatment plans. If renal function deteriorates, dialysis or transplant procedures can be successful in controlling uremia and hypertension, but fortunately with good early medical management, this rarely is required.

Polyserositis is frequent in SLE, commonly presenting as pericarditis or pleuritis. Other possible cardiovascular changes include myocarditis and verrucous (Libman-Sacks) endocarditis. Peripheral small vessel vasculitis is common. Some patients also exhibit digital vascular spasm in response to cold (Raynaud's phenomenon). Pulmonary disease may be severe, resulting from vasculitis, inflammatory infiltrates, or fibrosis; superimposed infection always must be excluded before attributing pulmonary changes to SLE alone.

Central nervous system involvement is quite common but may be difficult to diagnose. When seizures, strokes, overt psychosis, or objective motor or sensory losses can be detected, an area of cerebritis or infarction can be suspected. However, evaluation of the role of active SLE in the less specific thought disorders or behavioral changes that occur in patients is more difficult. Central nervous system involvement is not always reflected in procedures such as lumbar puncture, brain scan, or electroencephalograph, though such tests are warranted when there is suggestive brain involvement.

Laboratory Findings. The clinical diagnosis of SLE is confirmed by a positive test for antinuclear antibodies performed by indirect immunofluorescence utilizing frozen tissue sections (e.g., rat or mouse liver) as a source of nuclei (see Chap. 65). The LE preparation is a less sensitive method for detecting one type of ANA. In active disease, there may be evidence for complement consumpton (a decrease in total hemolytic complement activity or in complement components such as C3, C4). Antibodies to double-stranded DNA are relatively specific for SLE and are often elevated in active disease. The combination of lowered hemolytic complement and elevated DNA antibodies is indicative of active immune complex disease, particularly with nephritis. Antibodies to red cells (positive Coombs' test) often can be identified, and leukopenia

or thrombocytopenia may be present. Immunoglobulin levels usually are increased, and rheumatoid factors (IgM antibodies against IgG) are frequent.

Patients with SLE should be evaluated extensively at time of presentation to establish the degree of organ involvement in the blood (by red cell counts and indices, Coombs' test, bleeding and clotting screen, and white cell and platelet counts), lungs (by chest radiograph and pulmonary function tests), the cardiovascular system (by electrocardiograph, chest radiograph, and echocardiogram if available), kidney (by several careful urinalyses, serum creatinine, creatine clearances, quantitative protein excretion, and possibly renal biopsy) and the central nervous system (by EEG, perhaps lumbar puncture, and brain scan). Serum complement studies and DNA antibody assays give useful information about disease activity and severity. These studies also can be used to monitor therapeutic response.

Treatment. For patients with mild disease, such as only arthritis and rash, salicylates, alone or in conjunction with antimalarials, may provide adequate control. However, most children have major system involvement at the time of diagnosis and require corticosteroids, sometimes in large doses (2 mg per kg per day of prednisone in divided dose) initially. Treatment is directed at relieving clinical symptoms and returning complement and anti-DNA antibody levels to normal. Prednisone may then be slowly tapered to a single daily dose sufficient to control clinical and serologic parameters but low enough to preclude cushingoid changes in appearance (usually 5 to 10 mg per day) if possible. In some patients, however, this cannot be achieved. Regimens of higher dose alternate day steroids may be tried to avoid steroid side effects. When side effects are severe or when disease activity continues after an adequate trial of steroids, additional agents are considered. These include antimalarials or the various anticancer drugs. Azathioprine, chlorambucil, and cyclophosphamide all have been used, but controlled studies have yet to confirm their efficacy. In addition, the risks of bone marrow suppression with their use, increased susceptibility to untreatable infections, predisposition to malignancy, and decreased fertility should be considered carefully before initating such therapy, particularly in children.

Prognosis. At one time diagnosis of SLE

in a child implied a fatal outcome. With the advent of antibiotics and corticosteroids, however, the outlook improved considerably. Now, with laboratory parameters available to monitor disease activity and means to treat severe hypertension and renal failure, the prognosis is still better. However, flares of active disease and complications of therapy still occur, and the outlook must be guarded. Deaths still occur from infection (often with opportunistic agents such as viruses, fungi, or Pneumocystis carinii), renal disease, CNS disease, pulmonary lupus, and myocardial infarction.

DERMATOMYOSITIS

Childhood dermatomyositis is characterized by a violet scaly rash, usually over the face (particularly the eyelids and malar area) and the extensor prominences of the hands and limbs, and inflammation of striated muscle. Unlike its adult counterpart, it has no association with underlying malignancy. Before the introduction of steroid treatment, this disease had a high mortality rate, and many surviving patients were severely disabled. However, with early recognition and treatment the outlook is now good for most patients (Sullivan et al., 1972; Schaller, 1973).

Clinical Features. Onset of this disease may be either abrupt or insidious. Muscle weakness, often accompanied by pain, tenderness, or edema is the usual presenting symptom. Proximal muscle groups, such as those of the hip and shoulder girdle and of the trunk and neck, are affected predominantly. Occasionally other more distal muscle groups are involved as well. Weakness is variable, ranging from difficulty in climbing stairs to total inability to move against gravity. Muscles controlling swallowing and respiration also may be affected, and aspiration and respiratory failure are major causes of death in severe disease. Rarely, myocarditis occurs, reflected in abnormal cardiac function and conduction tests.

Vasculitis has been reported in many organs but usually is clinically apparent only in the gut, where bleeding, perforation, and necrosis can result. Subcutaneous calcification may occur in affected muscles or over fingertips or elbows.

Laboratory Findings. The basic pathologic lesion is inflammation of muscle and small blood vessels, and although the mechanism of this inflammation is unclear, it is possible that it is mediated by lymphokines. Nonspecific indicators of inflammation, such as sedimentation rate, may be elevated or normal. The most useful tests both for diagnosis and continuing management are the muscle enzymes. Those commonly available are the transaminases (SGOT or SGPT), aldolase, and creatinine phosphokinase (CPK). None is entirely specific to muscle, however, and the CPK is particularly sensitive to trauma, such as intramuscular injection or even physical activity. Tests for antinuclear antibodies and rheumatoid factors generally are negative.

Electromyogram (EMG) and muscle biopsy also may provide useful information. However, the EMG findings (drop-out of muscle units, low voltage potentials, and positive wave patterns) are common to all myopathic processes, and the muscle biopsy, while showing inflammation, also is nonspecific. With both these tests, care must be taken to choose an involved muscle for study.

Treatment. In few rheumatic diseases do children respond so dramatically to treatment. Steroids usually are used in high doses initially (prednisone 2 to 3 mg per kg. in divided daily doses), then tapered to maintain clinical and serologic ("muscle enzyme") remission for the duration of the natural history of the disease, which is about two years. Both clinical and serologic parameters must be followed carefully to avoid a flare of muscle inflammation. After approximately two years of clinical remission, steroids may be gradually discontinued with warnings to the patient and family of risks of adrenal insufficiency associated with withdrawal of steroid therapy.

Physical therapy also is important in managing acute dermatomyositis. All joints must be ranged passively if necessary, as these patients may develop flexion contractures very early. As inflammation decreases, strengthening exercises will allow return of function as quickly as possible. In the few patients who show progressive muscle inflammation or severe vasculitis in spite of steroid treatment, cytotoxic agents, such as methotrexate, azathioprine, and cyclophosphamide, have been used. However, because of toxicity and potential long-term effects, the use of these drugs is warranted only in the most severely ill patients.

Care must be taken to monitor patients for palatal–respiratory insufficiency, aspiration, and gastrointestinal bleeding or perforation. There is no known effective therapy for calcinosis.

Prognosis. With appropriate early therapy of corticosteroids, airway protection, and physical therapy, most children will return to normal function. In a few patients, disease recurs after apparent remission, or muscle destruction sufficient to result in permanent disability occurs. Extensive calcification of subcutaneous and muscle tissues has been noted as a late occurrence in some patients.

SCLERODERMA

This rare disease is characterized by excessive amounts of collagen, primarily in skin but also in other organs. There are two main types of scleroderma: localized (morphea or linear scleroderma) and generalized (progressive systemic sclerosis). Unlike other rheumatic diseases, overt inflammation is not a major feature (Winkelmann, 1971).

Clinical Features. In localized scleroderma (morphea and linear scleroderma), thickening of the skin occurs in well-circumscribed areas. Affected skin may be edematous initially with progression to hard patches with either hyperpigmentation or hypopigmentation. Contractures may result if these changes occur across joints.

In systemic scleroderma, generally termed "progressive systemic sclerosis" (PSS), pathologic changes are similar to those in localized forms of scleroderma, but the process is not well-circumscribed and also may involve other organ systems, Raynaud's phenomenon is common and may be severe enough to cause digital ulceration. Longstanding changes result in tapering of fingers from loss of bone and soft tissue (sclerodactyly). Arthritis is frequent in both large and small joints. In mild cases, changes may be limited to the fingers, but skin involvement may progress to the face and trunk. In addition to cutaneous changes, other organs may be involved. Dysphagia, reflecting esophageal dysmotility, usually is the first sign of gastrointestinal involvement. However, sclerosis may extend through the small bowel and colon with secondary stasis and malabsorption. Renal vascular disease is common with hypertension and fulminant or chronic renal function.

Pulmonary involvement may be primary (progressive fibrosis) or secondary to aspiration from esophageal dysfunction. Myocardial sclerosis and cor pulmonale also occur. Growth retardation may occur in some children.

Laboratory Findings. Blood counts and sedimentation rates usually are normal. Many patients have positive tests for antinuclear antibodies and rheumatoid factors, often in high titers. Urinalyses may be abnormal, and electrocardiograms and chest films reflect cardiopulmonary involvement. Serum albumin and carotene levels may be lowered if malabsorption is present.

Treatment and Prognosis. Although treatment with many drugs has been tried in both localized and systemic scleroderma, none have been successful in controlling severe disease. For patients who show progressive disease, a trial of corticosteroid, penicillamine, or a cytotoxic agent such as cyclophosphamide may be warranted. Topical steroids may soften affected areas of localized morphea or linear scleroderma. Physical therapy should be directed to maintaining mobility of joints and other soft tissues.

MIXED CONNECTIVE TISSUE DISEASE (MCTD)

For many years, occasional patients have been reported to have features of more than one rheumatic disease, for example, systemic lupus erythematosus, scleroderma, and dermatomyositis. Many of these patients have very high titers of antinuclear antibodies, directed against ribonucleoprotein, a ribonuclease-digestible extractable nuclear antigen (ENA). This antibody appears on routine ANA tests as high titered ANA of a "speckled pattern." MCTD has now been defined as a clinical "overlap" syndrome with laboratory evidence of high titer antibody reactive with ribonucleoprotein (Sharp et al., 1972).

Clinical Features. Polyarticular arthritis resembling rheumatoid arthritis, diffuse swelling of hands, and Raynaud's phenomenon are the presenting complaints in about 90 percent of patients. Dysphagia and gastrointestinal involvement like that of scleroderma also are frequent; myositis with weakness and muscle tenderness is present in three quarters of patients. Skin rashes may resemble those of systemic lupus erythematosus or dermatomyositis. Polyserositis (pleuritis and pericarditis) occurs in about one-fourth of patients. Lymphadenopathy may be so prominent that lymphoma is suspected. Early reports of this syndrome emphasized the low incidence of renal disease compared with systemic lupus or scleroderma, but now that the disease has been studied over longer periods of time, nephritis has been found in approximately 25 percent of patients.

Laboratory Findings. In patients presenting with MCTD, all major organ systems should be evaluated, as in SLE. Diagnosis requires the typical high titer of speckled ANA already described, as well as the more specific test for antibodies to ribonucleoprotein. Anemia, leukopenia, thrombocytopenia, hypergammaglobulinemia, and elevated sedimentation rates are common, and tests of specific organs, such as muscle enzymes, electrocardiograms, and pulmonary function studies, also may be abnormal. In contrast to active SLE, antibodies to double-stranded DNA are unusual, and serum complement levels generally are normal.

Treatment. MCTD has been thought to be usually responsive to corticosteroid therapy, unlike scleroderma. In patients who present primarily with arthritis, adequate control may be achieved at times with salicylates and antimalarials. Systemic symptoms, such as polyserositis, thrombocytopenia, or renal disease, require more vigorous therapy. Physical therapy is important in management of the musculoskeletal system.

Prognosis. Mixed connective tissue disease has been recognized as a separate entity for only a short time. Originally its course appeared to be benign, but now that reports of life-threatening complications such as vasculitis and renal disease are appearing, it is apparent that more years of experience are needed before the true prognosis and character of this "disease" can be adequately defined.

VASCULITIS

With the exception of Henoch-Schönlein purpura (discussed in Chapter 66), vasculitis is a rare condition in childhood. Vasculitis is seen in childhood as part of other rheumatic disease syndromes (particularly SLE, dermatomyositis, and scleroderma): There are a few types of vasculitis that present independently, such as polyarteritis nodosa and its variants, infantile polyarteritis, Kawasaki disease or mucocutaneous lymph node syndrome, and granulomatous angiitis (Wegener's disease and its variants).

Polyarteritis.

In polyarteritis, inflammation of small and medium-sized arteries occurs with secondary inflammation and tissue injury that may involve multiple organ systems (Owano, et al., 1963).

Etiology. In most cases the cause of vascular inflammation is not known. In some individuals an association between hepatitis B antigenemia and polyarteritis has been documented. In serum sickness, vasculitis results from an immune complex disease of foreign antigen and antibody.

Clinical Features. In childhood, two apparently distinct syndromes of arteritis have been described. Infantile polyarteritis usually involves children in the first two years of life. It presents with a high fever accompanied by maculopapular rashes, upper respiratory symptoms and conjunctivitis and may be difficult to differentiate from an acute infection. There may be little evidence for vascular involvement unless coronary arteries are affected, which results in thrombosis or aneurysm formation and sometimes sudden death. Renal abnormalities may be present in about one-third of cases, and other large central vessels may be involved. Frequently the diagnosis is only made postmortem.

Adult type polyarteritis occurs in older children and resembles the adult syndrome of multiple organ system involvement, which presents with fever, malaise, and weight loss. Gastrointestinal symptoms include abdominal pain, vomiting, diarrhea, and (occasionally) ascites. Half the patients have symptoms or signs of renal disease with hypertension, oliguria, or abnormal urine sediment due to involvement of intrarenal arterioles, glomeruli, or both. Seizures, coma, or focal neurologic abnormalities occur frequently, and some children may develop peripheral neuritis. Skin rashes commonly consist of maculopapular erythematous areas that become frankly hemorrhagic and persist for several weeks. Ulceration of the mucous membrane of the mouth and nose, arthritis and arthralgias, and muscle involvement also occur. Pulmonary findings may include asthma, rhinitis, or pulmonary infiltrates, and cardiac involvement also may occur.

Laboratory Findings. Anemia, leukocytosis, and elevated sedimentation rates are common, but there is no serologic test specific for polyarteritis. Histologic confirmation of vasculitis by biopsy of an affected area is the only diagnostic study. Renal biopsy may be useful. Angiography of the hepatic renal or mesenteric vessels may demonstrate vascular changes and be helpful diagnostically.

Differential Diagnosis. The most difficult differentiation is between Henoch-Schönlein purpura and polyarteritis, and many argue that they are part of the same disease spectrum. In Henoch-Schönlein purpura, however, the rash generally is limited in distribution to the lower extremities and buttocks, and lesions appear in crops over several weeks; abdominal pain is more colicky, and renal involvement usually is self-limited and rarely leads to renal failure. The lungs and nervous system usually are not affected.

Treatment. Corticosteroids in high doses may be successful, at times in combination with cytotoxic agents, such as azathioprine and cyclophosphamide. Complications, such as hypertension and renal failure, require appropriate supportive management.

Prognosis. Many cases of polyarteritis in childhood have been fatal, particularly the infantile form. However, if the diagnosis can be confirmed and treatment instituted early, the outlook appears much better at least for individuals with classic "adult type" polyarteritis nodosa (PAN). Long-term remissions have now been reported even after therapy has been discontinued.

MUCOCUTANEOUS LYMPH NODE SYNDROME (MCLNS, KAWASAKI DISEASE)

A new syndrome, first noted in Japan but later reported elsewhere, appears to be a variant of polyarteritis (Kawasaki et al., 1974). A relationship between this disease and infantile polyarteritis has been suggested (Landing and Larson, 1977).

Clinical Features. The peak age incidence is 12 to 18 months, 80 percent of patients being under five years of age. High fever is prominent and is unresponsive to antibiotics. Mucous membrane involvement includes nonpurulent conjunctivitis, redness of the oral mucosa, strawberry tongue, and red, dry, fissured lips. Skin involvement usually is limited to the hands and feet, with early reddening and induration and later desquamation from the fingertips and toes, although sometimes there may be nonspecific generalized exanthem. Often one or more cervical lymph nodes are massively enlarged but are nonpurulent. Transient arthralgia and arthritis are common. Cardiac involvement is found only in a small number of patients, but more serious is the coronary artery involvement (aneurysm and thrombosis), which leads to sudden death in 1 to 2 percent of cases.

Laboratory Findings. Mild anemia, leukocytosis, elevated sedimentation rate, and nonspecific acute phase reactants are found. Proteinuria and pyuria have been reported, as have mild changes in liver function tests. There is elevation of serum IgE levels.

Treatment. Steroids do not appear to be helpful. Salicylates in therapeutic doses offer symptomatic relief and are the preferred treatment for this disease.

Prognosis. In over 95 percent of children, the disease is self-limited with resolution within a few weeks. However, a fatality rate of 1 to 2 percent is due to coronary arteritis with aneurysm formation and thrombosis causing sudden death, usually within the first few weeks of disease. Unfortunately, premortem chest films and EKGs have not been good predictors of this complication. Angiographic studies of the coronary vessels have shown that over half of children with Kawasaki disease have coronary vasculitis.

RHEUMATIC FEVER

Until recent years, young patients with arthritis usually were assumed to have rheumatic fever. As a result, rheumatic fever was overdiagnosed, and other important forms of childhood arthritis were overlooked. Since the 1940s, the incidence of acute rheumatic fever has decreased steadily for reasons that are still unclear. Improvements in standards of living probably are of prime importance, as the decline had begun before the introduction of antibiotics.

Although the relationship between preceding infection with β-hemolytic streptococcus has been well known for many years, the exact mechanisms by which it initiates rheumatic fever still are unknown (Markowitz and Gordis, 1972).

Clinical Features. The accurate diagnosis of rheumatic fever is essential for both immediate medical management and its prognostic implications. The Jones criteria (Table 64-4) have long been valuable aids. The presence of two major criteria or one major and two minor criteria associated with supporting evidence of a recent group A β-hemolytic streptococcal infection strongly suggests the diagnosis. However, other rheumatic diseases, such as systemic lupus erythematosus and juvenile rheumatoid arthritis, also fulfill the criteria and should be considered in the differential diagnosis.

Rheumatic fever is most common in the five to fifteen year age group and is rare under the age of four. It has no predilection for either sex. There may be a history of sore throat before the onset of acute symptoms, but in many cases the association with streptococcal infection can be demonstrated only serologically. Moderate fever may persist for several weeks in untreated patients and may be accompanied by epistaxis or abdominal pain.

Acute migratory polyarthritis usually involves large joints, such as knees, ankles, and wrists, and may last up to several days in each joint. Arthritis can last for several weeks. Arthralgia may be more prominent in some joints than true arthritis, although the time course is the same.

Carditis is the most serious manifestation of rheumatic fever, occurring in almost half of the patients. Persistent tachycardia or new or changing murmurs indicate cardiac involvement. Frequent careful auscultation by experienced examiners is essential during the acute phase. Cardiomegaly (reflecting myocarditis, cardiac failure, or both) and pericarditis may occur. Mitral, aortic, or tricuspid stenosis are late complications and may not be apparent for years after the attack. Both subcutaneous nodules and skin rashes are rare now. Subcutaneous nodules, firm, nontender lumps up to 1 cm diameter commonly found over pressure points such as extensor surfaces of elbows and the scalp, are associated with carditis and longstanding or repeated attacks.

Erythema marginatum, a raised, pink, ser-

TABLE 64-4 MODIFIED JONES CRITERIA*

Major Criteria	Minor Criteria
Carditis	Fever
Polyarthritis	Arthralgia
Chorea	Prolonged PR interval
Subcutaneous nodules	Increased ESR or CRP†
Erythema marginatum	Preceding group A streptococcal infection
	Previous rheumatic fever

*From American Heart Association, Committee on Standards and Criteria for Programs of Care of the Council on Rheumatic Fever: Jones criteria (modified) for guidance in diagnosis of rheumatic fever. Mod. Conc. Cardiovasc. Dis., *24*:291–293, 1955.

†ESR = erythrocyte sedimentation rate; CRP = C-reactive protein.

piginous rash, often elicited by heat, which waxes and wanes over hours, is found in only 10 percent of cases.

Chorea is most common in females and may occur late in the disease, after other signs have subsided. Sometimes it is the only manifestation of rheumatic fever. The involuntary purposeless movements can be distressing to patients but usually resolve spontaneously within a few months. Patients with a history of chorea have an increased incidence of later cardiac sequelae.

The acute attack usually lasts three to four weeks, although a small proportion of patients may have a so-called "chronic" course with persistence of either carditis or arthritis, or rebound after attempted withdrawal of anti-inflammatory drugs.

Laboratory Findings. The most important laboratory finding is the documentation of a recent group A β-hemolytic streptococcal infection by throat culture, by rising antistreptococcal antibody titers, or both. The antistreptolysin O (ASO) titer has been replaced in many laboratories by the streptozyme test, which screens for several other streptococcal antibodies as well. Other specific tests for particular streptococcal antigens also are available.

Abnormal hematologic tests, such as mild anemia, an elevated white count, and elevated sedimentation rate, are nonspecific.

The electrocardiogram frequently shows prolongation of the P–R interval and low voltages with elevation of ST segments suggestive of pericarditis. Chest radiographs may show cardiomegaly due to either myocarditis or pericardial effusion.

Treatment. Therapy should not be initiated until the diagnosis has been established, as the typical syndrome may be suppressed, resulting in later uncertainty about management, particularly concerning antibiotic prophylaxis and likelihood of valvular problems.

If carditis is present, corticosteroids are the treatment of choice in doses of 2 mg per kg per day. Generally they will suppress carditis and arthritis within a few days. Medication is slowly tapered off after about four weeks. Supportive measures, such as diuretics or digoxin, may also be needed depending on the type and extent of cardiac involvement. Aspirin is the drug of choice when carditis is absent and is tapered off after about four weeks.

Chorea does not appear to respond to anti-inflammatory medications, although drugs such as chlorpromazine or haloperidol may reduce its severity.

The role of bed rest is controversial. It is almost impossible to maintain bed rest in a child who does not feel ill unless he or she is heavily sedated. Its role in preventing later heart disease is unknown. In general, in the absence of active carditis, few limitations are necessary, and only patients with cardiac residua need subsequently to restrict activity.

Prevention. The prevention of rheumatic fever depends on the diagnosis and treatment of the preceding streptococcal pharyngitis. In first attacks the prior infection may go unnoticed. Patients who have had documented rheumatic fever should receive long-term penicillin prophylaxis preferably by monthly intramuscular injections of long-acting penicillin. Oral penicillin prophylaxis also can be effective, but compliance may be a major problem. In penicillin allergic patients, erythromycin is a satisfactory alternative.

Additional prophylaxis against bacterial endocarditis before dental or surgical procedures is required if valve damage already exists.

Prognosis. Cardic damage most often results from recurrent attacks with subsequent valvular scarring and destruction — hence, effective prophylaxis is crucial to good cardiac outcome. Some adult patients present in middle age with late rheumatic valve disease (usually affecting mitral and aortic valves) often without a documented history of previous carditis. Therefore, prevention of β-hemolytic streptococcal infection is vital in reducing the long-term effects of rheumatic heart diseases.

References

GENERAL

Proceedings of the First American Rheumatism Association Conference on the Rheumatic Diseases of Childhood, chaired by Schaller, J. G. and Hanson, V.: Arthritis Rheum. (Suppl. 2) *20*: 145–611, 1977. Part I: Juvenile Rheumatoid Arthritis: General Aspects. Part II: Juvenile Rheumatoid Arthritis: Specific Aspects. Part III: Childhood SLE, Dermatomyositis, Scleroderma, and Related Syndromes. Part IV: Rheumatic Fever, Vasculitis Syndromes, AS, Reiter's Syndrome, Psoriatic Arthritis, and the Arthritis of Inflammatory Bowel Disease. Part V: Immunologic, Infectious, and Genetic Aspects of the Rheumatic Diseases of Childhood. Part VII: Juvenile Infectious Arthritis. Part VIII: Pediatric Rheumatology Education; Care of the Juvenile Patient.
Note: This publication presents an in-depth update on all aspects of rheumatic diseases in childhood. The reader interested in specific aspects of the subjects covered by this chapter is advised to consult this reference. Since there are so many excellent papers in this issue, they will not be referenced specifically.

SPECIFIC REFERENCES OTHER THAN THE SYMPOSIUM

Cook, C. D., Wedgwood, R. J., Craig, J. M., et al.: Systemic lupus erythematosus. Description of 37 cases in children and a discussed of endocrine therapy in 32 of the cases. Pediatrics *26*:570, 1960.
Kawasaki, T., Kosaki, F., Okawa, S., et al.: A new infantile acute febrile mucocutaneous lymph node syndrome (MLNS) prevailing in Japan. Pediatrics *54*:271, 1974.

Landing, G. H., and Larson, E. J.: Are infantile periarteritis nodosa with coronary artery involvement and fatal mucocutaneous lymph node syndrome the same? Comparison of 20 patients from North America with patients from Hawaii and Japan. Pediatrics, *59*:651, 1977.
Markowitz, M., and Gordis, L.: Rheumatic Fever–Diagnosis, Management and Prevention, 2nd ed. Philadelphia, W. B. Saunders Co., 1972.
Owano, I. R., and Sueper, R. H.: Polyarteritis nodosa — A syndrome. Am. J. Clin. Pathol. *40*:527, 1963.
Schaller, J. G.: Dermatomyositis. J. Pediatr. *83*:699, 1973.
Schaller, J. G.: The diversity of JRA: A 1976 look at the subgroups of chronic arthritis. Arthritis Rheum. *20*:S52, 1977.
Schaller, J., Bitnun, S., and Wedgwood, R. J.: Ankylosing spondylitis with childhood onset. J. Pediatr. *74*:505, 1969.
Schaller, J. G., Ochs, H. D., Thomas, E. D., et al.: Histocompatibility in childhood-onset arthritis. J. Pediatr. *88*:926, 1976.
Schaller, J., and Wedgwood, R. J.: Is juvenile rheumatoid arthritis a single disease? A review. Pediatrics *50*:940, 1972.
Sharp, G. C., Irvin, W. S., Tan, E. M., et al.: Mixed connective tissue disease: An apparently distinct rheumatic disease syndrome associated with a specific antibody to an extractable nuclear antigen (ENA). Am. J. Med. *52*:148, 1972.
Sullivan, D. B., Cassidy, J. T., Petty, R. E., et al.: Prognosis in childhood dermatomyositis. J. Pediatr. *80*:555, 1972.
Winkelmann, R. K.: Symposium on scleroderma. Mayo Clin. Proc. *46*:77, 1971.

J. Roger Hollister, M.D.

65

Laboratory Tests in the Diagnosis of Collagen-Vascular Disease

Laboratory tests of practical value in the diagnosis and management of collagen-vascular ("rheumatic") diseases should aid, but cannot replace, clinical judgment. Some tests, such as erythrocyte sedimentation rate, are simple and have been in use for decades; others, such as the fluorescent band test, have been developed only recently. This chapter describes diagnostic tests useful in collagen-vascular disease and provides a perspective on the clinical usefulness of each.

CBC AND ESR

The complete blood count and erythrocyte sedimentation rate are among the oldest laboratory procedures in clinical medicine. Abnormal findings in these tests provide important — though rarely specific — information in collagen-vascular diseases.

An elevated white blood cell count, with a predominance of neutrophils and early forms such as bands, occurs in several rheumatic conditions. Elevated white cell counts in systemic juvenile rheumatoid arthritis (JRA) may approach leukemoid levels, and bone marrow examination may be required for differential diagnosis. Systemic lupus erythematosus (SLE), on the other hand, is characterized by neutropenia and lymphocytopen-

ia. In patients treated with alternate-day corticosteroids there is a neutrophilia following steroid administration, which returns to normal levels on the "off" day (Dale et al., 1974). Only clinical assessment can distinguish bacterial or viral infection from active collagen-vascular disease.

Though anemia occurs regularly in rheumatic diseases, hematocrits below 20 percent are rare and should suggest other causes. Anemia usually is due to bone marrow hypoproliferation caused by the systemic inflammatory disease (Zucker et al., 1974). Erythrocytes appear normochromic and normocytic and reticulocyte counts are normal or low. Although iron deficiency may coexist, treatment rarely will normalize the hematocrit or hemoglobin, because inflammation depresses bone marrow function. Coombs' test–positive, hemolytic anemia is due to autoimmune destruction in SLE. Vigorous treatment of the anemia in SLE may be required, but the hypoproliferative anemia associated with the other conditions usually will improve with treatment of the inflammatory state.

Elevated platelet counts are a concomitant of JRA and may aid in the differentiation from leukemic states. The thrombocytosis apppears to be nonspecific and related to active systemic inflammation. SLE may present with thrombocytopenia as its main

777

manifestation. Few patients in the typical age group of childhood idiopathic thrombocytopenic purpura develop multi-organ disease on follow-up.

The ESR is a sensitive indicator of systemic inflammation but is nonspecific. The increased rate of red cell sedimentation is due to protein coating of the cells. Fibrinogen, α_1 globulins, and gamma globulins are increased as acute phase reactants and are the proteins responsible for causing the elevated ESR. On the other hand, infections of differential diagnostic concern also have elevated ESR, whereas self-limited fevers of unknown origin do not (Pizzo et al., 1975). Similarly, in patients with ill-defined arthralgias, myalgias, fatigue or other symptoms, a normal sedimentation rate suggests a benign cause of such symptoms. However, ESR occasionally is normal in obvious clinical rheumatoid arthritis or dermatomyositis. Correlation with disease activity is not as accurate in collagen-vascular disease as in other infectious processes, such as osteomyelitis.

RHEUMATOID FACTORS

Tests for rheumatoid factors have been a source of confusion in the diagnosis of collagen-vascular disease. Although these autoantibodies were demonstrated first in patients with adult rheumatoid arthritis, their presence is not sufficiently disease-specific to establish the diagnosis of rheumatoid arthritis. The rheumatoid factor test detects antibodies directed against IgG immunoglobulin. This autoantibody is seen less frequently in JRA than in adults with rheumatoid arthritis. Its presence appears to correlate with the age of the patient at onset of the disease (Hanson et al., 1969). With a low frequency of 5 percent in 2-year-olds with JRA, the incidence approaches that in the adult (70 percent) if JRA begins when the patient is an adolescent. Patients with systemic JRA rarely, if ever, have demonstrable rheumatoid factors. The specificity of the test is only fair, as patients with other collagen-vascular diseases may be positive. Chronic infections such as tuberculosis and subacute bacterial endocarditis also may have positive tests. Although the titre of rheumatoid factor does not correlate with

disease activity, a positive test does augur a more serious prognosis in patients with JRA. The latex fixation test clinically used to detect rheumatoid factors is most sensitive for IgG autoantibodies. Newer radioimmunoassays that detect other classes of rheumatoid factors may offer increased sensitivity, but the tests are not yet sufficiently specific to be generally helpful.

ANTINUCLEAR ANTIBODIES (ANA)

ANA is detectable in nearly 100 percent of patients with clinically active SLE, and the ANA test has replaced the less sensitive LE cell test (which is positive in 70 to 80 percent of patients with clinically active SLE). A negative test effectively excludes the diagnosis of SLE, but a positive test does not prove that SLE is the cause. Other diseases associated with a positive ANA include pauciarticular JRA in young females, in whom significant titres may be present in 30 percent of the cases. These children do not progress to SLE on follow-up. Drug-induced lupus is unusual in childhood, as causative agents are not used frequently in this age group. However, anticonvulsants (the hydantoins, trimethodione, and ethosuximide) have produced ANA's and clinical symptomatology (Beernink and Miller, 1973). Antinuclear antibodies are detected most accurately by a fluorescent antibody technique with frozen tissue sections. In addition, a description of the pattern of fluorescence in the nucleus may provide additional information as to the disease responsible for the autoantibody. High titred ANA's increase the specificity of the test for SLE. Mixed connective tissue disease (MCTD) invariably is associated with high titred ANA's, and the specific test for the antibody to ribonuclear protein (RNP) found in MCTD need not be performed if the ANA is negative (Singsen et al., 1977). In the future, the detection of antinuclear antibodies to nuclear constituents such as nuclear acidic protein, and nuclear histones may help establish and diagnose specifically associated collagen-vascular disease (Notman et al., 1975). The ANA frequently is positive in the neonatal period of children born of mothers with SLE, owing to placental transfer of maternal IgG antibody, but overt disease is extremely rare in such infants.

ANTI-DNA ANTIBODIES

The detection of the autoantibody to desoxyribonucleic acid (aDNA) has been a major advance in laboratory tests in SLE. Antibodies to double-stranded or native DNA are highly specific for SLE and serve to distinguish patients with a positive ANA test from one another. On the other hand, antibodies to denatured or single-stranded DNA are not specific and may be seen in viral infections and other collagen-vascular diseases in the absence of antinuclear antibodies. Antibodies to DNA have been recovered from diseased kidneys in SLE, suggesting a pathogenetic role for this autoantibody. Antibodies to DNA (aDNA) are detectable in only 60 to 70 percent of patients with SLE, and, similar to complement, aDNA is associated with renal, CNS, and skin involvement.

In addition to the specificity of aDNA, the level of these antibodies correlates well with disease activity in SLE (Schur and Sandson, 1968). Figure 65–1 demonstrates that when SLE is active, levels of aDNA are elevated but subsequently diminish as the disease responds to therapy or becomes quiescent. Rises in antibody levels to DNA may precede a recrudescence of the disease. Clinical judgment must be used before altering therapy in response to laboratory test fluctuations. In patients who are clinically well but maintain persistently abnormal autoantibodies and complement levels, further investigation, including renal biopsy, may be necessary. If no renal or CNS disease is apparent, therapy should be reduced in spite of abnormal tests.

COMPLEMENT

Lowered levels of complement in serum or pathologic fluid offer strong support that immune complexes are operative in the patient's symptomatology. Except in patients with hereditary deficiencies of individual complement components, lowered complement levels indicate activation and consumption of the proteins in the complement cascade. In body fluids other than serum, the complement level should be corrected for the protein content of the fluid relative to serum.

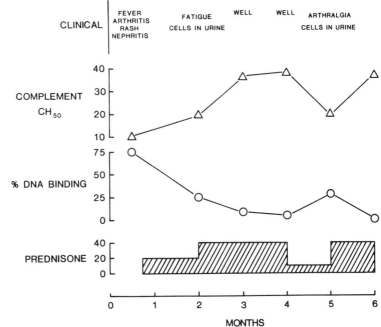

FIGURE 65–1. Immunologic parameters in systemic lupus erythematosus.

Several complement assays currently are available. C3 levels can be performed accurately on serum frozen at $-20°C$. C4 and total hemolytic complement activity (CH50), however, involve highly heat-labile components, and the serum should be stored at $-70°C$ (i.e., in dry ice) until the assay is performed. As the correlation between C3 and CH_{50} is good, it is practical to use the former as a reflection of total complement activity. Although complement levels are a static measurement of a dynamic process involving anabolism and catabolism, lowered levels almost always reflect excessive utilization of complement. Other materials may directly activate complement, but in the clinical setting, immune complexes are the activating agents in such diseases as SLE, the prodromal syndrome of Australia antigen hepatitis, or poststreptococcol glomerulonephritis. In addition to the diagnostic value in certain immune complex diseases, complement levels provide useful laboratory confirmation of disease activity. In Figure 65–1, active untreated lupus nephritis is associated with reduced levels of complement as well as with elevated levels of aDNA. With treatment and waning of disease activity, complement utilization is reduced, and the serum values return to normal.

Lowered levels of complement can also be demonstrated in pleural or pericardial fluid in patients with immune complex disease. Despite considerable effort, no reliable complement or autoantibody assay on cerebrospinal fluid has been found for patients with CNS lupus. The best correlates currently useful in this disease process are generalized disease activity and a lowered serum complement. Other tests, such as flow brain scans and EEG findings, may or may not show abnormalities.

Recently, techniques to determine split products of C3 have been developed that may provide additional information about complement activation. Activation of the complement cascade by either the classic or alternative pathways results in cleavage of C3 into fragments with different electrophoretic mobilities. However, aged serum or trypsin-like activity can produce similar changes, and experience currently is too limited to assess the future clinical usefulness of this assay.

FLUORESCENT BAND TEST

A new fluorescent technique performed on small skin biopsies is a useful addition to the diagnostic tests for SLE. Punch biopsies are snap-frozen and sectioned and then are mounted on slides for fluorescent staining. As with the ANA, a fluorescent anti–human immunoglobulin or complement reagent is applied; the sections are washed and examined with ultraviolet microscopy. The localization of human gamma globulin and complement components along the dermal-epidermal junction is highly specific for SLE. Occasional "false-positives" occur with other collagen-vascular diseases, but in normal individuals and patients with other disease entities, the test virtually always is negative (Wertheimer and Barland, 1976). It is of interest that in SLE the band test is positive on clinically uninvolved skin as well as on areas with rash, whereas discoid lupus demonstrates deposits only where the rash exists. Although a correlation with active nephritis has been found in some patients, the band test cannot replace a renal biopsy for accurate assessment. In addition, anti-DNA antibodies and complement levels in serum more accurately reflect overall disease activity.

MUSCLE ENZYMES

The diagnosis and management of patients with dermatomyositis and polymyositis is aided by measurement of muscle enzymes in serum. Although elevations of creatin phosphokinase (CPK) have been described most frequently, aldolase and SGOT may be the only abnormal values. It is most important to detect an elevated muscle enzyme level because this laboratory test accurately reflects disease activity with muscle damage and release of enzyme into serum (Sullivan et al., 1972). As demonstrated in Figure 65–2, improvement of muscle enzyme levels with treatment occurs prior to a return of strength in patients with dermatomyositis. Similarly, with flares of disease or withdrawal of steroid therapy, muscle enzymes become elevated prior to muscle weakness. In longstanding disease or in the presence of severe

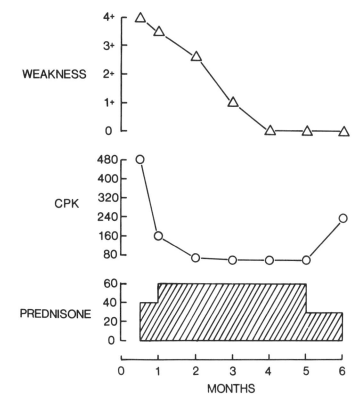

FIGURE 65–2. Muscle enzymes in dermatomyositis.

muscle atrophy, muscle enzyme levels are a less reliable guide to disease activity. In addition, the clinician should be aware that strenuous muscle exertion may elevate serum muscle enzymes.

OTHER TESTS

Streptozyme and/or ASO. Both tests detect serum antibodies against components of β-hemolytic streptococcus. The significance in either case is the association with a preceding streptococcol infection. Neither test is disease-specific. The tests are only indicative of streptococcol infection. A rising titre in either test indicates recent infection as opposed to residual serum antibodies from antigen stimulation remote in time from the present illness. Although streptococcol infection appears pathogenetic in acute rheumatic fever, its can also occasionally serve as a stimulant for chronic inflammatory diseases such as JRA, SLE, or Henoch-Schönlein purpura. The diagnosis of acute rheumatic fever depends on the clinical assessment of carditis, arthritis, chorea, and other clinical findings rather than on a positive streptozyme or ASO result.

Cryoprecipitates. Certain protein combinations or aggregates are considerably less soluble at 4° C. In particular, immune complexes of antigen, antibodies, and complement components will precipitate upon cold exposure for 48 to 72 hours. It is important to maintain the blood and to separate the serum at 37° C before exposure to the cold. Cryoprecipitates are a rough index of immune complex disease, and may be found in SLE, Australia antigen hepatitis, infectious mononucleosis, and SBE. A test for cryoprecipitates is of value as a screening test, but disease specificity depends on sophisticated analysis of individual antigens or antibodies.

Mitogen Stimulation. Stimulation of peripheral blood lymphocytes with phytomitogens, such as PHA, concanavalin A, or pokeweed, provides investigators with *in vitro* information about lymphocyte reactivity. These tests are of research interest but have so far not reached clinical diagnostic significance.

Detection of Immune Complexes. Several tests are becoming available as indica-

TABLE 65–1 EFFECTIVENESS OF LABORATORY TESTS IN
COLLAGEN-VASCULAR DISEASE

	JRA*	SLE*	DM*	Scleroderma	ARF*	MCTD*
Rheumatoid factors	+	±	−	−	−	±
Complement	nl or ↑	↓↓	nl	nl	nl	nl
aDNA	−	+++	−	−	−	−
ANA	±	+++	−	±	−	+++
Muscle enzymes	±	±	+++	−	−	±
Streptozyme ASO	±	−	−	−	+++	−

+frequently positive
±occasionally positive
+++strongly positive or disease specific
*JRA = juvenile rheumatoid arthritis
SLE = systemic lupus erythematosus
DM = dermatomyositis
ARF = acute rheumatic fever
MCTD = mixed connective tissue disease

tors of soluble immune complexes in serum. The Raji cell assay and CIq binding test are positive in SLE and other immune complex diseases. Until isolation of putative antigens is possible, these tests will lack disease specificity, however. On the other hand, the quantitation of immune complexes offers promise of significant correlation with disease activity or response to therapy.

In summary, laboratory tests in collagen-vascular disease have helped the diagnosis and management of SLE and dermatomyositis, but they have not replaced clinical judgment. Scleroderma, JRA, and overlap syndromes still lack sensitive, disease-specific tests. Table 65–1 summarizes the usefulness of various laboratory tests in relation to collagen-vascular disease.

References

Beernick, D. H., and Miller, J. J., III: Anticonvulsant-induced antinuclear antibodies and lupus-like disease in children. J Pediatr. 82:113, 1973.
Dale, D. C., Fauci, A. S., and Wolff, S. M.: Alternate-day prednisone. N. Engl. J. Med. 291:1154, 1974.
Hanson, V., Drexler, E., and Kornreich, H.: The relationship of rheumatoid factor to age of onset in juvenile rheumatoid arthritis. Arthritis Rheum. 12:82, 1969.
Notman, D. D., Kurata, N., and Tan, E. M.: Profiles of antinuclear antibodies in systemic rheumatic diseases. Ann. Int. Med. 83:464, 1975.
Pizzo, P. A., Lovejoy, F. H., and Smith, D. H.: Prolonged fever in children: Review of 100 cases. Pediatrics 55:468, 1975.
Schur, P. H., and Sandson, J.: Immunologic factors and clinical activity in systemic lupus erythematosus. N. Engl. J. Med. 278:533, 1968.
Singsen, B. H., Bernstein, B. H., Kornreich, H. K., King, K. K., Hanson, V., and Tan, E. M.: Mixed connective tissue disease in childhood. Pediatrics 90:893, 1977.
Sullivan, D. B., Cassidy, J. T., Petty, R. E., and Burt, A.: Prognosis in childhood dermatomyositis. Pediatrics 80:555, 1972.
Wertheimer, D., and Barland, P.: Clinical significance of immune deposits in the skin SLE. Arthritis Rheum. 19:1249, 1976.
Zucker, S., Friedman, S., and Lysik, R. M.: Bone marrow erythropoiesis in the anemia of infection, inflammation, and malignancy. J. Clin. Invest. 53:1132, 1974.

Charles S. August, M.D.
Jeffrey Greene, M.D.

66

Diseases of Erythrocytes, Leukocytes, and Platelets

AUTOIMMUNE HEMOLYTIC ANEMIA

Immune hemolysis is defined as the destruction of red cells by mechanisms that involve antibody, complement, or both. *Autoimmune hemolysis* occurs when an individual forms antibodies against his own red cells. *Isoimmune hemolysis* occurs when antibodies formed in one person destroy cells from another, as in transfusion reactions or erythroblastosis fetalis.

The diagnosis of immune hemolysis depends upon demonstration of accelerated destruction of red cells and on demonstration of immunoglobulins, complement components, or both on the red cell membrane.

Pathogenesis. Patients with autoimmune hemolytic anemia (AHA) display a wide variety of immunohematologic abnormalities. Antibodies found on red cells and in sera of patients with AHA are heterogeneous with respect to immunoglobulin class, serologic properties, biologic activities, and associated clinical disease.

Warm and Cold Autoantibodies. Traditionally, autoantibodies to red blood cells have been divided into two groups according to the temperature at which maximum binding takes place. "Warm antibodies" bind maximally at 37° C; "cold antibodies" bind maximally at 4° C, and hardly at all at temperatures above 30° C.

"Complete" and "Incomplete" Agglutinins. Antibodies also are characterized as "complete" or "incomplete" with regard to their ability to agglutinate red blood cells. Agglutination, or clumping of red cells (Fig. 66–1), occurs when two or more red cells are bound together by antibody. A "complete" agglutinin causes clumping of red cells directly (e.g., anti-A or anti-B isohemagglutinins). Cross-linking of red cells by antibody directly is facilitated under conditions of high antigen concentration on the red cell surface and when IgM (molecular weight 900,000 daltons) is the antibody involved.

"Incomplete" agglutinins bind to red cells, but agglutination occurs only in the presence of an additional, amplifying antibody. The most common method of detecting red cells coated with incomplete antibodies employs an anti–human globulin antibody (Coombs reagent) produced in rabbits. Red cells coated with incomplete antibodies are incubated with a Coombs reagent: the rabbit antibody binds to the antibody globulin on red blood cells, resulting in agglutination that may be seen grossly or detected by microscopic examination. This constitutes the "direct" Coombs test; a positive direct Coombs test is the *sine qua non* of immune hemolysis.

The "indirect" Coombs test detects antibody to red cells that exist in serum. The test is performed by incubating normal red blood cells with a patient's serum, washing, and then exposing the cells to the Coombs reagent. If the red cells agglutinate, the in-

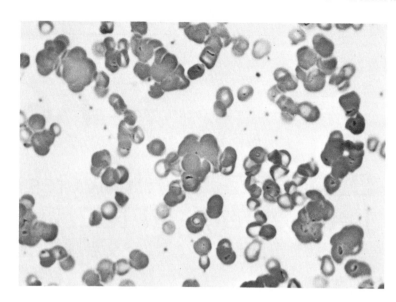

FIGURE 66–1. Agglutination of red blood cells by antibody as might be seen in the peripheral blood smear of a patient with autoimmune hemolytic anemia. (×430).

direct Coombs test is positive, which constitutes evidence, therefore, that the patient's serum contains antibody to red cells (Coombs et al., 1945).

Complete agglutinins usually are IgM and incomplete agglutinins usually are IgG antibodies. It must be noted, however, that there are exceptions to this general rule, and the distinction between complete and incomplete agglutinins cannot be made solely on the basis of antibody class.

Hemolysins. Antibodies capable of inducing red cell lysis are termed "hemolysins." Hemolysins activate the complete sequence of complement components (classic pathway), resulting in prompt destruction of red cells *in vitro* or *in vivo*.

Thus, three types of serologic reactions are possible: complete agglutination, incomplete agglutination, and hemolysis. Antibodies giving all three types of reactions *in vitro* may mediate rapid red cell destruction *in vivo*. Hemolysins, however, cause intravascular hemolysis, whereas agglutinins mediate destruction of red cells by promoting their phagocytosis, primarily by phagocytic cells of the liver, spleen, bone marrow, and lymph nodes. Antibodies that behave primarily as agglutinins may activate some but, by definition, never all of the components of complement. AHA in children most often is associated with warm, incomplete autoagglutinins (Hathaway and August, 1980).

Antibody Characteristics. The classes of immunoglobulins that have been found to be associated with autoimmune hemolysis have been studied by several investigators. Although results differ somewhat, it appears that approximately one third of patients have IgG antibody alone on red cells, one third have complement component alone (usually C4 or C3), and the remainder have mixtures of antibodies and complement components. IgA has been found only rarely on red cells. IgG antibodies mediate erythroblastosis fetalis since only members of this class of immunoglobulin cross the placenta.

In many instances when attempts are made to determine the specific red cell antigen(s) to which antibodies involved in AHA are directed, specificity cannot be defined. Such antibodies are considered to be "panagglutinins." However, when specificity can be demonstrated, the antibodies usually are directed against antigens of the Rh system, in particular c and e (Habibi et al., 1974). Cold agglutinins almost always show anti-I specificity. If available, studies to define red cell antigen specificity should be undertaken, for they aid in the selection of blood donors if transfusions become necessary.

Effects of Antibody and Complement on Red Cells. The biologic consequences of immune reactions occurring on surfaces of red blood cells also have been the subject of considerable investigation. Such reactions may be divided into three types: those involving antibody alone, those involving antibody plus components of serum complement, and those involving complement alone.

In general, when antibodies bind to red

cells, the overall electrical charge present on the red cell membrane decreases, thus diminishing electrostatic forces that tend to repel cells from each other. Agglutination occurs when the distance between cells that is imposed by electrostatic charges can be bridged by antibodies. Studies with the scanning electron microscope have shown that during agglutination the surfaces of red cells roughen and then develop finger-like protrusions that link the cells together. When "cold agglutinins" are involved, these events occur at low temperatures — the process reversing itself when the mixture of antibodies and red cells is warmed to 37° C. Incomplete antibody produces similar changes, albeit more slowly, but cross-linking of cells does not occur.

Whereas it is easy to understand how hemolysis can occur when one in dealing with agglutinating and hemolytic antibodies, it is more difficult to understand the pathophysiology of incomplete antibody–induced red cell destruction. Some insight into this problem was provided in 1938 by Dameshek and Schwartz, who observed spherocytosis and increased osmotic fragility of the red cells of patients with AHA. More recently, it has been shown that macrophages possess membrane receptors for IgG. It now is thought that when red cells coated with incomplete IgG antibody pass through the reticuloendothelial system, they bind to macrophages via IgG receptors. At points of contact with macrophages, injury to red cell membranes occurs, resulting in the formation of spherocytes. These cells are relatively inelastic and are promptly trapped in the sinusoids of the reticuloendothelial system (RES), where they ultimately are destroyed.

The crucial role of the spleen and the RES has been inferred from the fact that patients without spleens may not have spherocytes or increased osmotic fragility. Moreover, incubating normal red cells with antibody *in vitro* induces neither spherocyte formation nor changes in osmotic fragility.

The sequential reactions of some or all of the nine components of serum complement are responsible for many of the serologic and clinical phenomena associated with AHA. As described earlier, some patients have lytic antibodies (hemolysins) that activate all the components of complement. However, the majority of immune reactions occurring on the surface of the red cells involving complement do not proceed through a complete lytic sequence and acute intravascular hemolysis is a rare clinical event. Macrophages also possess receptors for C3b, a portion of the third component of complement. Complement-coated red cells passing through the RES probably suffer the same fate as red cells coated with IgG.

Complement may be detected on the surface of the red cell by a variation of the direct Coombs test by using a Coombs reagent that contains antibody directed against one or another component of complement, rather than to human immune globulin. This is called the "non-gamma" Coombs test.

Etiology. At present, there is no single explanation for the cause of AHA. Current theories center around four major mechanisms, namely: modification of red cell antigens, development of cross-reacting antibodies, formation of "forbidden clones" of antibody-forming cells, and the failure of immunoregulatory mechanisms (presumably mediated by T lymphocytes) that control the function of B lymphocytes capable of forming autoantibodies.

Antigen Modification. This can occur if an exogenous antigen such as a virus or drug adsorbs to the red cell membrane and behaves as a hapten. The combination of the hapten and the red cell membrane may create a new antigen against which the patient can form antibody (Zuelzer et al., 1974; Dacie and Worlledge, 1969).

Cross-Reacting Antigens. Certain natural substances or microorganisms contain antigens that are similar to those found on red cells. If an individual formed antibodies to such antigens, the antibodies so formed might also react against the patient's own red cells. This may be a partial explanation for the elevated titers of cold agglutinins with anti-I specificity that follow mycoplasma infection.

Forbidden Clones. This theory holds that AHA results from the sudden appearance, by somatic mutation, of clones of cells capable of forming antibodies against the individual's own red cells (Mackay and Burnet, 1963). Normally, such clones are eliminated by the host's T lymphocytes. However, if such clones are themselves malignant (as in lymphoproliferative diseases) and escape immune surveillance, AHA would result.

Failure of Immunoregulation. Another possible mechanism for the development of AHA relates to failure of immunoregulation by suppressor T lymphocytes. Animal models for AHA exist in which suppressor T lymphocytes disappear as the afflicted animals grow older, with a corresponding increase in the incidence of AHA (Krakauer, 1978).

Diagnosis and Clinical Manifestations. AHA is rare but occurs in children of all ages. The clinical features that characterize the onset of disease are determined largely by the rate of hemolysis. Rapid hemolysis occurs intravascularly and is associated with shaking chills, fever, and frequently pain in the back and abdomen. Pallor and weakness may progress to the point of prostration or even shock. In addition, the patient may pass urine varying in color from pink to red to dark brown. If the syndrome is caused by a cold-reacting antibody (paroxysmal cold hemoglobulinuria or cold agglutinin disease), the development of the syndrome can be related to a recent exposure to cold. Physical examination usually does not disclose the presence of enlarged liver, spleen or lymph nodes; and jaundice is not prominent (Pirofsky, 1976).

More commonly, hemolysis occurs more slowly and erythrocytes are destroyed extravascularly in the RES. Patients so afflicted will become symptomatic gradually, and their pallor and weakness will be determined by the depth of their anemia. Jaundice and low-grade fever are common. In addition to the above, physical examination usually reveals the presence of an enlarged spleen. The liver may be moderately enlarged, but lymph nodes generally are not (Smith, 1966). This is the most common presentation of warm antibody–mediated AHA.

The laboratory findings in AHA reflect the red cell destruction and the attempt by the body to compensate for the destruction. The hemoglobulin may vary from the lower limits of normal to profoundly low values. The reticulocyte count usually is elevated in proportion to the severity of hemolysis.

Examination of the peripheral blood smear is the most important simple test that can be performed. This usually discloses the presence of fragmented RBC's microspherocytes, large bluish reticulocytes, and occasionally nucleated red cells (Fig. 66–2). In

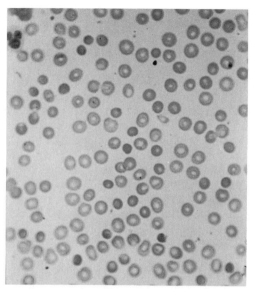

FIGURE 66–2. Peripheral blood smear from a patient with autoimmune hemolytic anemia. Note microspherocytes and macrocytes. (×430). (From Hathaway, W. E. and August, C. S.: Hematologic Disease. *In* Stiehm, E. R., and Fulginiti, V. A. (eds.): Immunologic Diseases in Infants and Children. Philadelphia, W. B. Saunders Co., 1973, p. 484.)

newborn infants, pronounced macrocytosis and the presence of normoblasts at many stages of maturation are characteristic (Fig. 66–3). In acute intravascular hemolysis, leukocytosis with a shift to young forms may be present. Examination of the bone marrow usually reveals erythroid hyperplasia and phagocytosis of red cells by monocytes and macrophages; the other elements are normal. Occasionally, megaloblastic changes will be found that may reflect a relative deficiency of folic acid due to the increased demand.

The direct Coombs test usually will be positive. The indirect Coombs test may be positive, in which case the antibody titer should be estimated. On occasion, the Coombs test will be negative in the presence of typical clinical findings of AHA. One reason for this is that the patient may have too little antibody bound to the red cells to be detected by commercial Coombs reagents. In addition, if the antibody in question is IgA or IgM, the Coombs test will usually be negative because commercial reagents usually react only with IgG and complement.

The absence of haptoglobin in the serum is one of the most reliable signs of hemolysis. Haptoglobin forms soluble complexes with hemoglobin. Such complexes are rapidly

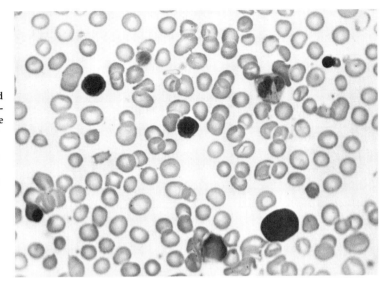

FIGURE 66–3. Peripheral blood smear from an infant with erythroblastosis fetalis. Note the variation in size and shape of the red blood cells. All the mononuclear cells except the one at 6 o'clock (which is lymphoid) are red cell precursors at various stages of maturation. (×430).

taken up and degraded by the RES. Because the liver makes haptoglobin slowly, relatively little hemolysis will consume most or all of the serum haptoglobin. Haptoglobin determinations are less useful in infants. Synthesis begins in the first week of life, but it is only after one year of age that normal adult values are achieved (Javid, 1967).

AHA may be the presenting sign or a complication of another disease. The clinical conditions that may be associated with autoimmune destruction of red cells are numerous (Table 66–1) and include viral and bacterial infections; broader autoimmune diseases, e.g., lupus erythematosus; tumors, particularly lymphoreticular; and immune deficiency syndromes. Since the presence or absence of the associated conditions is an important determinant of prognosis, it is important to consider the differential diagnosis carefully and search assiduously for these other conditions.

Treatment. Treatment is directed toward stopping hemolysis and supporting the patients. Most AHA in children is of the "warm" antibody type and occurs without complicating underlying disease. However, the evaluation and treatment of children with AHA may be complex. We recommend referring children who have associated disease or who have been symptomatic more than 3 months to appropriate specialists. Initially, transfusions may be necessary. These should only be used in life-threatening situations.

Blood banks usually report difficulty in typing and cross-matching with blood from patients with AHA; and, at times, transfusions must be performed with blood that is only partially compatible.

Therapeutically, the drugs of choice are adrenocortical steroids. Patients are given prednisone orally at a dose of 1 to 2 mg per kg body weight per day. Equivalent intravenous doses of hydrocortisone, prednisolone, or dexamethasone may be used. Since some patients recover rapidly from a single episode of AHA, steroids should be used only for short courses and tapered rapidly. One should monitor the hemoglobin or hematocrit, reticulocyte count, and Coombs test. If the patient relapses, the steroids should be reinstituted and administered every other day if possible. Should steroids fail to diminish the rate of hemolysis, the patient should be referred to an appropriate consultant.

Some experienced clinicians use antimetabolites (6-mercaptopurine or azathioprine) if steroids fail to control hemolysis. Others recommend splenectomy (Bowdler, 1976). Before splenectomy, however, it is desirable to obtain evidence that the spleen is playing a predominant role in the red cell destruction; this is likely to be so if the autoantibody involved is IgG (as in most cases of childhood AHA). Additionally, the spleen and liver may be scanned after the intravenous administration of ^{51}Cr labeled red cells. It must be remembered, however,

TABLE 66–1 UNDERLYING DISEASES ASSOCIATED WITH AUTOIMMUNE HEMOLYTIC ANEMIA*

Infections
  Viral
    Hepatitis
    Herpes simplex
    Infectious mononucleosis
    Viral pneumonia
    Cytomegalovirus
  Bacterial
    Typhoid
    Streptococcus
    E. coli
    Staphylococcus aureus
    Tuberculosis

Other Autoimmune Diseases
  Systemic lupus erythematosus
  Rheumatoid arthritis
  Periarteritis nodosa
  Ulcerative colitis
  Dermatomyositis
  Idiopathic thrombocytopenia purpura
    (Evans syndrome)

Tumors
  Leukemia
  Lymphoma
  Hodgkin's disease
  Reticulum cell sarcoma
  Miscellaneous carcinomata
  Ovarian teratoma
  Dermoid cyst
  Kaposi's syndrome

Immune-Deficiency State
  Wiskott-Aldrich syndrome
  Congenital, X-linked agammaglobulinemia
  Partial DiGeorge syndrome
  Common variable immunodeficiency syndromes

*From Hathaway and August (1980)

that splenectomy places patients at risk of overwhelming sepsis. We therefore recommend the administration of polyvalent pneumococcal vaccine before splenectomy, and the prophylactic daily use of antibiotics (e.g., penicillin or trimethoprim-sulfa) afterwards.

Prognosis. In trying to predict the outcome of AHA, the most important step is to define the illness as thoroughly as possible (Zuelzer, 1970; Habibi et al., 1974; Buchanan et al., 1976; Dausset and Colombani, 1959). AHA in conjunction with neutropenia, low reticulocyte count, collagen vascular disease, or altered immune mechanism will have the prognosis of the underlying disease. Acute AHA tends to be an isolated illness, and in contrast to chronic AHA, its onset frequently is associated with a viral infection. Acute AHA usually resolves in 3 months. Chronic AHA, unassociated with an underlying disease may last for many months, but the ultimate outcome is favorable. Table 66–2 presents a comparison of the clinical features of acute and chronic AHA.

DRUG-INDUCED HEMOLYTIC ANEMIA

Drug-induced AHA is rare (Worlledge, 1969). Probably the most common mechanism whereby this occurs is the adsorption of antigen-antibody complexes onto the red cell membrane with the subsequent activation of complement and opsonization or lysis of red cells. In this situation, the red cell is an innocent bystander.

Another mechanism involves the incor-

TABLE 66–2 AUTOIMMUNE HEMOLYTIC ANEMIA IN CHILDREN: COMPARATIVE FEATURES

	"Acute"	"Chronic"
Onset	Acute	Insidious, gradual, or acute
Association with viral infection	Usual	Rarely
Response to steroids	Good	Variable
Recovery	Three months or less	Variable, may last years
Coombs test	Complement (non-gamma)	Either gamma or mixed
Deaths*	3 of 58 patients (5%)	20 of 73 patients (27%)

*From Zuelzer et al., 1970; Habibi et al., 1974; Buchanan et al., 1976.

TABLE 66–3 DRUGS ASSOCIATED WITH HEMOLYTIC ANEMIA

Alpha-methyl dopa
Cephalothin
Chlorpromazine
Mefenamic acid
PAS
Penicillin
Phenacetin
Quinidine
Quinine
Rifampicin
Sulfonamides
Sulfonylurea drugs

poration of the drug into the red cell membrane, where it functions as a hapten. Antibodies are then formed against the new antigen, and ultimately the red cell is destroyed. This appears to explain the hemolytic anemia seen with administration of large doses of penicillin.

Unfortunately, these two mechanisms do not account for hemolytic reactions seen with all drugs, and many are still largely unexplained. Table 66–3 presents a list of those drugs used in children which have been shown to cause AHA.

ISOIMMUNE HEMOLYSIS

Erythroblastosis Fetalis

Erythroblastosis fetalis, or hemolytic disease of the newborn, represents isoimmune hemolytic anemia caused by placental transfer of maternal IgG antibodies directed against the red blood cells of the fetus. Antibodies other than IgG may be found in the serum of the mother, but these do not cross the placenta. In most cases, the antibodies are directed against the antigens of the Rh group (CDE/cde), and secondarily against the antigens of ABO system. Rarely, hemolytic disease may be caused by antibodies to other red cell antigens (Mollison, 1972).

Pathogenesis. Approximately 15 percent of white persons and 7 percent of black persons do not have the D antigen and are designated Rh negative. During pregnancy, if as little as 1 cc of D-positive blood passes from an infant into its D-negative mother, the mother will develop anti-D antibodies. This sensitization can occur during a normal pregnancy, during abortion, or at delivery. If the second baby also possesses the D antigen, IgG from the mother will cross the placenta and cause hemolysis in the infant. When the ABO system is involved, the mother may have IgG antibodies at the time of her first pregnancy if she is type O, A, or B. In practice, most instances of hemolysis occur when the mother is type O and the baby is type A_1.

Diagnosis. Clinically, the range of hemolysis may be mild, with only slight elevations of serum bilirubin, to severe hemolysis with compensatory hyperplasia of hematopoietic tissue both inside and outside the bone marrow. Thus, the liver and spleen may be markedly enlarged. "Hydrops fetalis" is the term used when the severe anemia has resulted in heart failure, massive edema, and death of the baby. Generally, Rh incompatibility is associated with more severe and ABO incompatibility with milder disease. The diagnosis is made by demonstrating blood group incompatibilities between mother and baby and a positive direct or indirect Coombs' test. In Rh incompatibility, the peripheral blood smear shows marked variation in the size and shape of the red cells and red cell precursors at different stages of maturation (Fig. 66–3). In ABO incompatibility, the changes are milder and the peripheral smear may show only spherocytes.

Prevention. Human anti-D antibody (Rhogam), given to an Rh negative mother at times when fetal red cells leak into the maternal circulation can prevent primary sensitization. Specifically, Rhogam should be administered to Rh negative women within 72 hours of an abortion, or live birth if the baby is known to be D positive. With the administration of Rhogam, the risk of initial sensitization of Rh negative mothers has been reduced from between 10 and 20 percent, to less than 1 percent. With the continued use of this agent, it is to be hoped that the risk of erythroblastosis fetalis will be reduced even further.

IMMUNE NEUTROPENIAS

Neutropenia may be defined as an absolute polymorphonuclear leukocyte (PMN) count of less than 2500/mm³ in older children and adults. Infants display leukocytosis at birth, and PMN counts less than 6000/mm³ may represent significant neutropenia for the first day or two of life. During the first 2 weeks of life, the PMN count drops gradually; and by 7 days of life, the lower range of normal is 1500/mm³. Neutrophil counts usually stabilize between 2 and 17 weeks of age (Lalezari and Radel, 1974). Oski and Naiman (1966) have emphasized the wide variation seen in PMN counts of newborn babies. Thus, multiple determinations of the absolute PMN count are required to establish a diagnosis of neutropenia in the neonatal period.

Immune neutropenias may be divided into two groups: autoimmune and isoimmune. Autoimmune neutropenias are rare. The antigens involved usually are neutrophil-specific, antigens NA1, NA2, and NB1. Most cases occur in adults and may be associated with lupus erythematosus or with the administration of a variety of drugs (Weitzman et al., 1978). The serum of such patients opsonizes normal PMN's and facilitates their ingestion by phagocytes. IgM, IgG antibodies, and complement are involved in a manner identical to that found in AHA. Rarely, a newborn infant will become neutropenic due to the transplacental passage of maternal IgG antibody.

Isoimmune neonatal neutropenia usually is associated with infection of the skin, respiratory, and urinary tracts. Antibiotics often are necessary, and transfusions of compatible (maternal) PMN's are given if the infections are severe.

IMMUNE THROMBOCYTOPENIA

Definition. Thrombocytopenia is defined in most laboratories as a platelet count less than 150,000 platelets/mm.³ Immune thrombocytopenia (referred to in most discussions as idiopathic thrombocytopenia purpura, or ITP) occurs when platelets are coated with antibody and, as a consequence, undergo accelerated removal from the circulation.

Etiology. Antiplatelet antibodies associated with immune thrombocytopenia can be divided into two groups, isoimmune and autoimmune. Isoimmune anti-platelet antibodies are found in patients who have received antibody passively or who have become sensitized following exposure to incompatible platelets. An example of the former is "neonatal purpura" which occurs with maternal immunization to paternal platelet antigens possessed by the fetus. Maternal IgG antibodies cross the placenta and cause fetal thrombocytopenia. An example of the latter mechanism occurs in patients who have received multiple red blood cell or platelet transfusions. Isoimmunization may become manifest when the platelet counts in such patients fail to rise after transfusions of random-donor platelets. In these cases, sensitization usually is found to be directed toward HLA antigens, which are represented on platelets as well as on leukocytes.

Autoimmune antiplatelet antibodies may be found in children as well as in adults with ITP. (Dixon and Rosse, 1975). Drug-specific antiplatelet antibodies may be found in patients whose thrombocytopenia follows exposure to a drug. In this situation the drug functions as a hapten.

Antiplatelet antibodies that have been defined usually are IgG and may be found free in the serum and bound to patient's platelets. They appear to be produced in the spleen and to promote platelet phagocytosis by splenic macrophages. Thus, thrombocytopenia is due to the sequestration of antibody-coated and damaged platelets in the spleen and occasionally in the liver. In this condition, the bone marrow can increase platelet production as much as eightfold.

Diagnosis. Children with ITP usually experience the acute onset of easy bruising, petechiae, epistaxis, and occasionally melena, and hematuria. Life-threatening intracranial bleeding occurs in less than 1 percent of patients (McClure, 1975). ITP follows an acute viral illness in 50 percent of cases. A careful history must be taken to rule out drug ingestion (e.g., quinine, Dilantin, quinidine, chloroquine, digitoxin); toxic agents (e.g., pyrethrins, petroleum hydrocarbons); heparin; a familial or congenital thrombocytopenia (e.g., Wiskott-Aldrich syndrome); and a variety of disorders, including chronic infections, infectious mononucleosis, collagen-vascular or other autoimmune diseases.

Physical examination is usually unremarkable except for evidence of bleeding. The presence of enlarged lymph nodes, spleen, or liver should alert the physician to consider diagnostic possibilities other than ITP.

Laboratory tests will reveal a decreased platelet count, no anemia (except in cases of severe bleeding), and a normal or slightly elevated white count. Platelets are often large in size. Except for prolongation of the bleeding time, routine coagulation tests (thrombin time, prothrombin time, partial thromboplastin time) are normal. The bone marrow shows normal red blood cell and PMN precursors and increased numbers of megakaryocytes. A Coombs test (direct and indirect) should be performed, and other autoimmune diseases (e.g., lupus erythematosus) should be ruled out.

Treatment. Since childhood ITP usually is self-limited and rarely recurs, a conservative approach to treatment is warranted. If bleeding is not severe, no specific therapy is necessary. It is advised that the patient avoid trauma, contact sports, and the ingestion of aspirin or any other drug known to decrease platelet function. In spite of the findings of several retrospective studies that indicate that corticosteroids may not influence the morbidity of the disease (McLure, 1975; Cohn, 1976), most consultant hematologists advise corticosteroids for repeated episodes of skin bleeding, epistaxis, internal bleeding, intracranial hemorrhage, or platelet counts <5000/mm^3. Corticosteroids are given for their possible antibleeding effect, their effect on splenic function, or their effect on the production of antiplatelet antibody itself. If the decision is made to use corticosteroids, prednisone (1 to 2 mg per kg of body weight per day) is given for 2 weeks. Although the platelet count often rises rapidly, it has not been possible to show that this therapy prevents intracranial bleeding. Drug dosage is then tapered rapidly (4 to 7 days) and discontinued. If the platelet count falls and symptoms recur, it is advisable to refer the patient to a consultant. The usual therapeutic maneuver at this point is to find the lowest effective dose of prednisone and use an alternate day schedule of administration. Long-term steroid therapy (daily or, if possible, alternate day) may be necessary in the small number of older children or adolescents who have chronic or adult-type ITP.

Splenectomy is performed in two situations. In cases of intracranial hemorrhage, emergency splenectomy is performed and the patient is treated with corticosteroids and platelet transfusions. In chronic ITP (thrombocytopenia for longer than 6 to 12 months), elective splenectomy sometimes has a beneficial effect on the course of the disease. Indications for splenectomy depend in part on the severity of the clinical bleeding associated with the patient's thrombocytopenia and in part on the existence of dangerous or bothersome side effects of prolonged corticosteroid therapy. It should be remembered, however, that the risk of overwhelming infection is increased in splenectomized individuals, particularly in the very young.

Platelet transfusions (1 unit per 5 to 6 kg of body weight) may be used to provide hemostasis for a few hours while steroid therapy is being instituted in patients with life-threatening hemorrhage, and occasionally during surgery. Immunosuppressive therapy (e.g., azathioprine) rarely is used in children, although a few favorable results have been recorded.

Neonatal purpura due to isoimmunization rarely causes significant bleeding. However, in babies who are symptomatic, a double volume exchange transfusion to remove antibodies followed by a transfusion of *maternal* platelets is recommended (Adner et al., 1969).

MISCELLANEOUS

Aplastic Anemia

Idiopathic acquired aplastic anemia is a disease of unknown cause that is characterized by severe anemia, leukopenia, thrombocytopenia, and failure of normal hematopoiesis in the bone marrow. The best treatment at present is prompt bone marrow transplantation from a histocompatible (HLA-A, B, and D identical) sibling (Camitta, 1975). A number of patients have been described whose own bone marrows have recovered following profound immunosuppression and rejection of engrafted marrow. This phenomenon has prompted physicians in some centers to treat patients lacking histocompatible marrow donors with immunosuppression alone — usually in the form of antithymocyte globulin — and some favorable results have been reported (Speck et al., 1977). The inference that may be drawn from these clinical experiences is that some cases of aplastic anemia may have an autoimmune basis, and indeed, experimental evidence supporting this idea exists. However, the number of patients with "autoimmune" aplastic anemia remains to be determined.

TRANSFUSION REACTIONS

Adverse reactions to blood tranfusions include hemolytic reactions, febrile reactions, and allergic reactions.

Hemolytic Reactions. Hemolytic reactions can be immediate or delayed. Immediate hemolysis is most commonly due to an incompatibility in the ABO system, though the Rh and Kell systems also have been involved. In these reactions the offending antigen is on the donor's red cells and the antibody is in the recipient's serum. Symptoms may include fever, low back pain, hypotension, nausea, vomiting, and the sensation of constriction of the chest. Occasionally, symptoms may be limited to as little as urticaria and a low-grade fever. Abnormal bleeding also may occur as a result of a consumptive coagulopathy. Considering the diversity of symptoms, any unusual reaction in a patient receiving a transfusion must be considered a hemolytic reaction unless proven otherwise.

Confirmation of a hemolytic reaction rests upon the demonstration of hemolysis along with the presence of antibodies directed against donor cells. In practice, urine is tested for the presence of hemoglobin and serum is visually examined for the presence of free hemoglobin, which is pink, or methemalbumin, which is brown. In addition, the patient's blood is immediately sent to the blood bank for a direct Coombs test, antibody screen (indirect Coombs test), and for retyping against the donor blood. The donor blood also is returned to the blood bank to be re-cross-matched and for an antibody screen. Both patient and donor blood is cultured, and a peripheral smear is examined for the presence of spherocytes. If a coagulation problem is suspected a prothrombin time, a partial thromboplastic time, a fibrinogen level, and a platelet count are obtained.

The treatment of a transfusion reaction begins with the early recognition of the reaction. The transfusion should be terminated immediately, and steps instituted to prevent shock, bleeding, and to maintain renal circulation. Osmotic diuresis should be initiated with mannitol; but in the face of a falling renal output, it must be presumed that acute tubular necrosis has occurred and mannitol should be stopped. Thereafter, treatment is directed toward treating acute renal failure, with attention paid to the hemoglobin level.

Delayed hemolytic reactions can occur 4 to 14 days after a transfusion. The patient may already have been sensitized to donor blood antigen, but the level of antibodies in such cases presumably is too low to cause an immediate reaction. Within days, however, the formation of increased amounts of antibodies occurs and induces hemolysis. The diagnosis can be made on the basis of a positive Coombs' test and identification of the blood group specificity of the antibody involved.

Febrile Reactions. Febrile reactions occur as the result of bacterial contamination, sensitivity to leukocyte or platelet antigens, and hemolytic reactions; in many cases, however, there is no identifiable cause. Reactions from bacterial contamination are minimal, owing to the use of disposable transfusion equipment. Reactions to platelet and leukocyte antigens occur mainly in patients who have had repeated transfusions or pregnancies.

Allergic Reactions. Allergic reactions consist of urticaria, generalized pruritus, bronchospasm, and generalized anaphylaxis. The latter reaction is most commonly seen in profoundly IgA deficient patients who have received blood containing IgA. The recipient develops an anti-IgA antibody that activates complement, and allergic symptoms ensue. Occasionally an individual may develop antibodies against donor IgG or IgA if they are of a different allotype; however, this is a much less common occurrence.

References

Adner, M. M., Fisch, G. R., Starobin, S. B., and Aster, R. H.: Use of "compatible" platelet transfusions in treatment of congenital isoimmune thrombocytopenic purpura. New Engl. J. Med. *280*:244, 1969.

Bowdler, A. J.: The role of the spleen and splenectomy in autoimmune hemolytic disease. Sem. Hematol. *13*:335, 1976.

Buchanan, G. R., Boxer, L. A., and Nathan, D. G.: The acute and transient nature of idiopathic immune hemolytic anemia in childhood. J. Pediatr. *88*:780, 1976.

Camitta, B. M., Thomas, E. D., Nathan, D. G., Santos, G., Gordon-Smith, E. C., Gale, R. P., Rappeport, J. M., and Storb, R.: Severe aplastic anemia: A prospective study of the effect of early marrow transplantation on acute mortality. Blood *48*:63, 1976.

Cohn, J.: Thrombocytopenia in childhood: An evaluation of 433 patients. Scand. J. Haemat. *16*:226, 1976.

Coombs, R. R. A., Mourant, A. E., and Race, R. R.: A new test for the detection of weak and "incomplete" Rh agglutinins. Br. J. Exp. Pathol. *26*:255, 1945.

Dacie, J. W., and Worlledge, S. M.: Autoimmune hemolytic anemias. Prog. Hematol. *6*:82, 1969.

Dameshek, W., and Schwartz, S. O.: Hemolysis as cause of clinical and experimental hemolytic anemias with particular reference to nature of spherocytosis and increased fragility. Amer. J. Med. Sci. *196*:769, 1938.

Dausset, J., and Colombani, J.: The serology and the prognosis of 128 cases of autoimmune hemolytic anemia. Blood *14*:1280, 1959.

Dixon, R. H., and Rosse, W. F.: Platelet antibody in autoimmune thrombocytopenia. Br. J. Haematol. *31*:129, 1975.

Habibi, B., Homberg, J. C., Schaison, G., and Salmon, C.: Autoimmune hemolytic anemia in children. A review of 80 cases. Am. J. Med. *56*:61, 1974.

Hathaway, W. E., and August, C. S.: Hematologic Disorders. *In* Stiehm, E. R., and Fulginiti, V. A.: *Immunologic Disorders in Infants and Children.* 2nd ed. Philadelphia, W. B. Saunders Co., 1980.

Javid, J.: Human serum haptoglobins. A brief review. Sem. Hematol. *4*:35, 1967.

Krakauer, R. S.: Disorders of the suppressor cell system in autoimmunity (p. 233). *In* Waldmann, T. A. (moderator): Disorders of suppressor immunoregulatory cells in the pathogenesis of immunodeficiency and autoimmunity. Ann. Int. Med. *88*:226, 1978.

Lalezari, P., and Radel, E.: Neutrophil-specific antigens: Immunology and clinical significance. Sem. Hematol. *11*:281, 1974.

Mackay, I. R., and Burnet, F. M.: *Autoimmune Diseases.* Springfield, Ill.: Charles C Thomas, Publisher, 1963.

McClure, P. D.: Idiopathic thrombocytopenic purpura in children: Diagnosis and management. Pediatrics. *55*:68, 1975.

Mollison, P. L.: *Blood Transfusion in Clinical Medicine,* 5th ed. Oxford, Blackwell Scientific Publications, Inc., 1972.

Oski, F. A., and Naiman, J. L.: Hematologic Problems in the Newborn. Philadelphia. W. B. Saunders Co., 1966. p. 14.

Pirofsky, B.: Clinical aspects of autoimmune hemolytic anemia. Sem. Hematol. *13*:251, 1976.

Smith, C. H.: *Blood Diseases of Infancy and Childhood,* 2nd ed. St. Louis: C. V. Mosby Co., 1966.

Speck, B., Gluckman, E., Hoak, H. L., and van Rood, J. J.: Treatment of aplastic anaemia by antilymphocyte globulin with and without allogeneic bone marrow infusions. Lancet *II*:1145, 1977.

Weitzman, S. A., Stossel, T. P., and Desmond, M.: Drug induced immunological neutropenia. Lancet *I*:1068, 1978.

Worlledge, S. M.: Immune drug-induced haemolytic anemias. Sem. Hematol. *6*:181, 1969.

Zuelzer, W. W., Mastroangelo, R., Stulberg, C. S., Poulik, M. D., Page, R. I., and Thompson, R. I.: Autoimmune hemolytic anemia: Natural history and viral immunologic interactions in childhood. Am. J. Med. *49*:80, 1970.

67

Dana P. Rabideau, M.D.
Rawle M. McIntosh, M.D.

Renal Diseases

Immune mechanisms play a role in a variety of diseases of the kidney and may be responsible for injury to the glomerulus, tubules, interstitium, and vessels. Immune insult results in a variety of clinical syndromes and histologic alterations. It is important to recognize that identical etiopathogenetic mechanisms may be expressed in different clinical and pathologic manifestations. Experimental animal models exist for several forms of immune pathology in the kidney; clinical and laboratory studies in human renal disease have established several as the clinical correlates of these experimental analogs.

In this chapter, an approach to diagnosis and management of children with renal disease is outlined. Although a complete discussion of immune-mediated renal disease is beyond the scope of this chapter, the more commonly encountered renal diseases of infancy, childhood, and adolescence will be considered.

STRUCTURE AND FUNCTION OF THE KIDNEY

Glomerulus. Each human kidney contains about 1.3 million glomeruli (Allen, 1963). The glomerulus consists of a complex capillary tuft surrounded by a capsule (Fig. 67–1); the capillary tuft is a capillary network lined by endothelial cells. These cells contain fenestrae, or pores, with a mean diameter of about 700 Å (Jorgensen, 1966). The fenestrae serve as a coarse filter, keeping cells away from the underlying basement membrane during the processes of glomerular filtration of plasma. The underlying basement membrane, which is thinner in infants and children than in adults and approaches adult width by about the age of 3 years, has three electron-microscopically distinct layers (Jorgensen and Bentzon, 1968; Vernier, 1964). The central lamina densa (1200 Å) is surrounded by less dense areas on both sides—the lamina rara interna (800 Å) and the lamina rara externa (1000 Å). The lamina densa surrounds the capillary loop except at the mesangium, and the lamina rara interna merges with the mesangial matrix. The basement membrane is composed of a collagen-like protein rich in hydroxylysine and hexose and noncollagenous glycoprotein rich in glycine, galactose, mannose, fucose, and sialic acid (Kefalides, 1973). The basement membrane also functions as a coarse filter during the formation of the glomerular filtrate. Visceral epithelial cells (podocytes) cover the basement membrane. Trabeculae extend out from the main cell bodies, forming foot processes that interdigitate leaving gaps of 200 to 400 Å. A thin membrane bridges the gap between adjacent foot processes (slit diaphragm). Each foot process is covered with a thin coat of glycoprotein rich in sialic acid (glycocalyx). This negatively charged surface appears to be important in maintaining separation of the foot processes, and alterations in charge may play a role in the development of proteinuria. The slit diaphragm appears to be the fine filter during glomerular filtration. Capillary loops derive

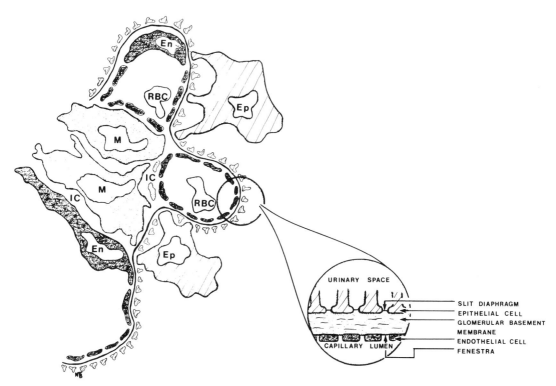

FIGURE 67–1. Schematic representation of a glomerulus (inset: details glomerular basement membrane). En = endothelial cell; Ep = epithelial cell; M = mesangium.

their structural support from the mesangial cells, which also may serve a phagocytic function. The glomerular capillary tuft is enclosed in Bowman's capsule, a layer of squamous epithelial cells, and basement membrane. The structure of the renal glomerulus is schematically represented in Figure 67–1.

Tubules The first portion of the tubular system is the proximal convoluted tubule, which consists of the pars convoluta and the pars recta. Both contain a brush border (microvilli) covering the apical or luminal surface of the tubular cells. The basement membrane is continuous with that of Bowman's capsule and the thin descending limb of the loop of Henle. The composition of the tubular basement membrane is similar to that of the glomerular basement membrane, although it is not as well characterized. The thin limb of the loop of Henle descends into the medulla, makes a sharp hairpin turn, and ascends back toward the glomerulus as the thin and thick ascending limbs of the loop of Henle. Cells in the loop of Henle lack the prominent, well developed microvillous cov-

ering seen in proximal tubules. When the ascending limb of the loop of Henle (ALH) meets the glomerulus, the tubule becomes the distal convoluted tubule (DCT). The DCT becomes the collecting duct when joined by another DCT. The collecting duct then traverses the medulla and empties on the surface of the papilla.

The tubules serve to regulate acid-base and fluid and electrolyte balance, in addition to reclaiming albumin, proteins, and carbohydrates filtered at the glomerulus. The structure of the tubules is schematically represented in Figure 67–2.

Interstitium. In both the cortex and medulla of the normal kidney, the tubules are compact, separated only by delicate interstitium and by vascular structures. The interstitial space of the medulla, however, usually is much greater than that seen in the cortex. Two types of interstitial cells are discernible in the cortex. The majority of cells resemble fibroblasts and contain a well developed Golgi apparatus. Fewer cells resemble monocytes, with an abundance of lysosomes and phagocytic vacuoles. The remaining intersti-

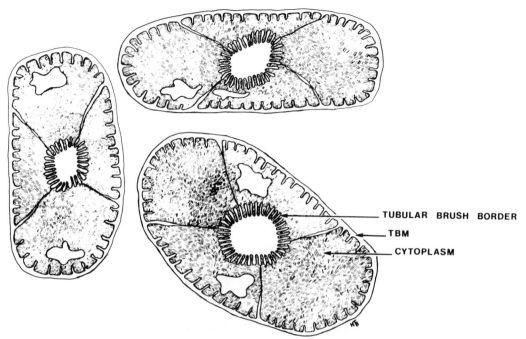

TUBULAR BRUSH BORDER

TBM

CYTOPLASM

FIGURE 67–2. Schematic representation of tubules. TBM = Tubular basement membrane.

tial space is occupied by a flocculent material with low electron density, containing cellular debris, lipid droplets, basement membrane–like material, and collagen. The function of the interstitium appears to be the production of prostaglandins, and phagocytosis (McGiff et al., 1974; McIntosh et al., 1977).

CLINICAL ASSESSMENT OF RENAL FUNCTION

The assessment of immune-mediated renal injury begins with a *thorough history and physical examination*. The basic history and physical examination of the child with suspected renal impairment are detailed later and will not be discussed here; only particular points will be emphasized as specific disease entities are discussed.

Only after a *careful urinalysis*, performed by the physician himself, should other, more expensive and invasive procedures be considered. Important information that may be obtained from the urinalysis includes: (1) the ability to concentrate or dilute the urine (osmolality and specific gravity), (2) the ability to acidify the urine (pH), (3) the presence of hematuria, proteinuria, glycosuria, or ke-

tonuria, and (4) the presence of cellular elements (WBC's, RBC's, casts, epithelial cells). Proteinuria, when detected by dipstick, should be followed by quantitation on a timed urine specimen. Proteinuria greater than 200 mg per 24 hours, which does not significantly clear with recumbency, warrants detailed investigation and consideration of the disorders listed in Table 67–1.

In general, the two most clinically useful tests for evaluating the glomerular filtration rate as an index of renal function are the *creatinine clearance* obtained on a timed urine specimen and the *serum creatinine*. In the same patient, once creatinine clearance has been determined, the serum creatinine may be a reasonable reflection of changes in the glomerular filtration rate.

The technique of *percutaneous renal biopsy*, when performed by an experienced and accomplished physician, may yield valuable information that will allow the establishment of a specific diagnosis and direct the course of treatment. Reported complications of the procedure include gross hematuria (10 to 40 percent, usually painless and subsiding with bed rest), and hematomas (0.2 percent). Rarely (0.06 percent), nephrectomy may be required; and death (0.07 percent) can occur.

TABLE 67–1 PROTEINURIA: DIAGNOSTIC CONSIDERATIONS

Glomerular
Minimal change disease
Acute glomerulonephritis: idiopathic, post-strep, post-infectious
Rapidly progressive glomerulonephritis: idiopathic, post-strep, anti-GBM
Chronic glomerulonephritis: proliferative, membranous, membrano-proliferative, systemic lupus erythematosus, anaphylactoid purpura, idiopathic mixed cryoglobulinemia, polyarteritis, neoplasia
Miscellaneous glomerular diseases: focal sclerosis, Berger's disease
Metabolic diseases: diabetes, amyloidosis, accelerated hypertension
"Mechanical": congestive heart failure, pericarditis, renal vein thrombosis
Toxins: heavy metals, allergens (bee sting, poison ivy, poison oak), drugs (trimethadione, penicillamine, paramethadione)

Tubular
Congenital tubulopathies: RTA, Fanconi's syndrome, Alport's syndrome, oculocerebral renal dystrophy, familial asymptomatic tubular proteinuria, nephrogenic, diabetes insipidus
Systemic diseases with tubular defects: Wilson's disease, galactosemia, oxalosis with nephrocalcinosis, cystinuria with lithiasis, laxative hyperkaluria, heritable connective tissue disorders
Inflammatory: interstitial nephritis, pyelonephritis
Toxins: cadmium, Balkan nephropathy
Renal transplant

In centers with vast experience, the complications are considerably lower than reported mean figures.

DISEASES OF THE RENAL GLOMERULUS

Mechanisms of Immune-Mediated Glomerular Injury

This subject has been reviewed in detail in a number of recent publications (McIntosh et al, 1977; Cochrane and Koffler, 1973; Wilson and Dixon, 1976).

Anti-GBM disease. Historically, the earliest model of immune renal disease was produced by the passive administration to rats of antiserum from rabbits immunized by repeated injections of rat kidney (Masugi, 1934). Other experimental models subsequently employed active immunization with homologous or heterologous glomerular basement membrane (GBM), chemically or immunochemically similar membranes (lung, placenta, choroid plexus) or a urinary glycoprotein thought to originate from the GBM (Steblay, 1959; Lerner and Dixon, 1968). In these models, immunoglobulin (anti-GBM antibody) and complement can be demonstrated lining the GBM of the host's kidney in a linear pattern by immunofluorescent staining (Fig. 67–3). Electron microscopy exhibits electron-dense material in the lamina densa area of the GBM. Light microscopy reveals a diffuse, active proliferative glomerulonephritis. These findings are identical to those of human anti-GBM disease, found in Goodpasture's syndrome (nephritis and pulmonary hemorrhage) and in some cases of rapidly progressive nephritis.

In man, as in the experimental analogs, circulating antibody to GBM can be detected in the serum, and cell mediated immunity to GBM components is demonstrable (Rocklin et al., 1970). Injury to the GBM is mediated

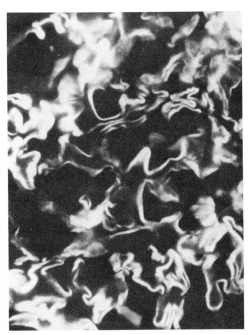

FIGURE 67–3. Photomicrograph of immunofluorescent staining of a glomerulus from a patient with anti-GBM nephritis, showing smooth linear deposits of IgG.

by activation of the complement system, which in turn leads to chemotaxis of polymorphonuclear cells and subsequent release of proteolytic enzymes. However, this sequence of events is not seen in all animal models of anti-GBM disease. Moreover, in approximately 24 percent of human cases of anti-GBM disease, no complement component is demonstrable on the GBM by immunofluorescent staining. The mechanism of tissue injury in such cases is not defined. There is some evidence that the coagulation system and the kinin system (circulating vasoactive polypeptides) are involved in certain models (Vassalli and McClusky, 1971).

Anti-GBM nephritis rarely is documented in the pediatric age group, and among all ages it accounts for only about 5 percent of cases of immune-mediated glomerulonephritis (Wilson and Dixon, 1973). Hydrocarbons, penicillamine, thermal injury, influenza A_2 virus, and dermatologic and pulmonary diseases have been reported to be associated with anti-GBM antibodies and with anti-GBM disease (McIntosh et al, 1977).

Immune Complex Disease. A far greater number of immune-mediated renal diseases either are proven or suspected to be secondary to injury by immune complexes. By definition, this is renal disease produced by the deposition of soluble circulating complexes of antibody and antigen in the glomerulus, where structural and functional derangements are produced by one or several mediators of inflammation. Several experimentally induced and naturally occurring animal prototypes exist, and immune complex mechanisms appear to be responsible for several human diseases.

The administration of a large, single dose of foreign protein, e.g., bovine serum albumin (BSA), to the rabbit results in a reproducible series of events (Cochrane and Koffler, 1973): The onset of a rapid decline in serum concentration of the foreign antigen on day 8 to 10 corresponds to the production of rabbit antibody and the appearance of immune complexes in the serum. These complexes deposit in blood vessels, joints, and glomeruli, resulting in clinical arteritis, arthritis, and glomerulonephritis. At 12 to 14 days, free antibody becomes detectable in the serum, indicating that all the antigen has been complexed. The antibody titer progressively increases with time if the animal survives the acute insult; clinical and pathologic evidence of arteritis and glomerulonephritis resolves as the antibody level rises.

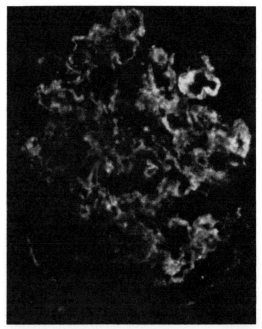

FIGURE 67–4. Photomicrograph of a glomerulus from a patient with glomerulonephritis, showing granular deposits of IgG along the glomerular basement membrane — granular pattern considered characteristic of immune complex glomerulonephritis.

At the peak of the acute reaction, light microscopy of the kidney reveals diffuse endothelial swelling. Immunofluorescent studies demonstrate host immunoglobulin and complement, as well as BSA antigen, in a granular ("lumpy-bumpy") pattern along the GBM (Fig. 67–4). Electron microscopy may reveal electron-dense deposits in the GBM. Histology of the vessels demonstrates a severe necrotizing vasculitis, with polymorphonuclear infiltration, endothelial proliferation, and fibrinoid necrosis. Vascular immunofluorescent findings of immunoglobulin, complement, and antigen are transient, owing to rapid phagocytosis of the complexes by infiltrating polymorphonuclear leukocytes.

Chronic serum sickness may be produced in the rabbit by repetitive, daily administration of BSA in a dose sufficient to prevent the animal from achieving a state of antibody excess and complete antigen elimination (Cochrane and Koffler, 1973). Consequently, there is persistent formation and tissue deposition of immune complexes. The rabbits develop a progressive, chronic glomerulonephritis, which may be either membranous or proliferative, depending on host factors discussed later. In contrast to the "single-shot" model of acute disease, in the chronic proliferative variety, deposits of antigen, immunoglobulin, and complement are demonstrable in a granular pattern along the subepithelial aspects of the GBM. Subepithelial deposits are seen by electron microscopy.

These models have enabled investigators to define a number of critical factors in the development of immune complex disease. It is readily apparent, when one comprehends the number of immune reactions that occur through natural exposure to foreign antigens throughout the lifetime of man or the experimental animal, that a small minority of antibody-antigen reactions result in pathogenetic complexes of clinical significance. Physical factors that are critical to pathogenetic capacity include immune complex size, solubility, and quantity. In turn, size of immune complexes is determined by antigen size, numbers and arrangement of antigenic determinants, antibody size and binding sites, and antibody-antigen affinity.

In general, complexes of less than one million daltons remain soluble in the circulation and have the capacity to deposit along the GBM and produce disease. If such complexes have a sedimentation rate smaller than 19S, however, they are nonpathogenetic and do not localize in the glomerulus. At the other extreme, complexes much larger than one million daltons are readily cleared from the circulation by phagocytosis by the reticuloendothelial system, and therefore do not produce deposits in the glomerular basement membrane. It should be mentioned, however, that the glomerular mesangium, in addition to its structural and supportive functions, may harbor monocytes with phagocytic capabilities, possibly accounting for the presence of certain intermediate size complexes in this area of the glomerulus. Complexes formed under conditions of moderate antigen excess, such as in the experimental models of chronic serum sickness, tend to be soluble, pathogenetic agents. In several naturally occurring states in animals and man, a

poor antibody response to an inciting antigen may result in such complexes.

Other host factors are equally important determinants in the development of immune complex disease. Hemodynamic factors such as increased total renal blood flow and renal arterial pressure are influential in the glomerular deposition of complexes (Cochrane and Koffler, 1973). Conversely, an increase in pressure in Bowman's space, as in hydronephrosis, acts to inhibit the deposition of complexes on the GBM.

Active factors of the host also may be involved. Vasoactive substances, including histamine, serotonin, and epinephrine, enhance the deposition of inert markers such as colloidal carbon in the vascular basement membrane of experimental animals (Wilson and Dixon, 1976). Immune complexes, when passively administered, are capable of producing the same effect, presumably through activation or release of the vasoactive substances in vivo. The importance of vasoactive materials in the pathogenesis of immune complex disease is further supported by the fact that pretreatment of animals with antihistamines prevents the deposition of immune complexes in vascular walls, including deposition in glomeruli and development of chronic glomerulonephritis (Masugi, 1934). Also, preliminary studies in humans receiving heterologous antitoxin have demonstrated a beneficial effect of antihistamines in reducing the incidence of clinically overt serum sickness. Platelets are repositories of vasoactive amines in rabbits, while mast cells serve a similar function in man.

The propagation of disease following the deposition of immune complexes also involves a number of active host factors. Removal of neutrophils or complement in vivo inhibits the development of the lesions of the systemic vasculitis of acute serum sickness, although the glomerulonephritis proceeds unaltered (Wilson and Dixon, 1976). The glomerulonephritis of chronic serum sickness, on the other hand, appears to be more dependent on neutrophil infiltration, and, by implication, on the activation of complement.

Antigens implicated in immune complex disease may be classified as exogenous, endogenous, or autologous. Exogenous antigens can induce acute or chronic nephritis, whereas endogenous and autologous antigens usually are associated with chronic disease.

Exogenous Antigens. These antigens usually are associated with an acute self-limited process. The main exogenous antigens identified have been microorganisms. Exposure to the antigen usually is brief, and antigen is eliminated by host defense mechanisms or by therapeutic measures. Immune complexes are formed and deposited in the glomerulus during the period of immune elimination, a situation reminiscent of acute "one shot" serum sickness in the experimental animal. Mild hematuria and abnormalities of the urinary sediment may be observed. These alterations, previously attributed to "the febrile episode" or "toxic factors," are probably the result of an immune complex glomerulitis.

On the other hand, chronic infection due to chronic bacteremia or to viremia as a result of inability to eliminate the microorganism either because of ineffective therapy or impaired host defense (as with chronic osteomyelitis, chronically infected ventriculoatrial shunt, syphilis, and chronic hepatitis antigenemia) results in a chronic rather than acute nephritic syndrome. In this instance there is a constant source of antigen, and patients with the critical level of immune response constantly form immunopathogenic complexes.

In man, a variety of drugs or foreign proteins, (e.g., horse antitoxin, anti-lymphocyte serum) may provoke immune complex nephritis, either by their own immunogenicity or through haptenic binding to host protein. In addition, several bacterial and protozoal infections have been associated with immunohistologic evidence of immune complex glomerulonephritis. Moreover, in addition to immunohistologic demonstration of immunoglobulin and complement in a granular immunofluorescent pattern along the GBM and/or mesangial area, supportive evidence of immune complex disease has been provided by demonstration of the suspected antigen in the glomerulus in a pattern similar to the experimental analog. More definitive evidence requires elution of immunoglobulin from the kidney specimen by exposure to acid buffers or chaotropic ions, and demonstration of the specificity of the eluted an-

tibody for the suspected antigen by one or more standard antibody-antigen reactions.

Additional proof lies in detection of antibody-antigen complexes in the circulation. A variety of tests for such complexes exist. These include: examination of the serum for cryoglobulins, which frequently represent circulating immune complexes precipitable at 4°C; precipitation of complexes by rheumatoid factor; several modifications of complement fixation techniques; and the use of cells with surface complement receptors to bind antibody-antigen-complement immune complexes *in vitro* (McIntosh et al., 1977). Although any individual test may suffer from a lack of sensitivity or specificity, they have been successfully employed to demonstrate the etiopathogenesis of a number of immune complex mediated diseases in man. These include: the glomerulonephritides associated with *Staphylococcus albus* ventriculoatrial shunt infections; *Enterococcus, Staph. albus,* and *Corynebacterium* subacute bacterial endocarditis; secondary syphilis; acute hepatitis B infection; malaria; and other bacterial or parasitic diseases (McIntosh et al., 1977). On the other hand, the pathogenesis of several suspected immune complex–mediated renal diseases remains controversial. Included in this category are the common post-streptococcal acute glomerulonephritis and acute nephritis associated with pneumococcal infection. Detection of glomerular-bound bacterial antigen in both diseases has been variable, and evidence exists for alternate forms of immune injury (McIntosh et al., 1977). Several other infections may have an associated glomerulonephritis with immunohistologic findings suggestive of immune complex disease; however, antigen identification and other proof of etiopathogenesis is lacking.

Autologous Antigens. Autologous antigens also may become immunogenic under special circumstances. This may involve exposure of a hitherto sequestered antigen to the immune system by tissue damage, or alteration in the physical or chemical structure of a tissue protein by microbial or toxic interaction to render it immunogenic.

The earliest model of immune complex nephritis induced by autologous antigens was produced by Heymann (Heymann et al., 1959), who repetitively immunized rats with homologous renal tissue in Freund's adjuvant. This resulted in the typical findings of an immune complex glomerulonephritis; the antigen responsible was identified as a lipoprotein from the brush border of the proximal renal tubular epithelial (RTE) cell (Wilson and Dixon, 1973). As is characteristic of autologous immune complex disease in general, once the process is initiated, the glomerular disease progresses by virtue of continued release or exposure of antigen from host tissue secondary to damage by antibody. Toxic damage to tubules, such as has been demonstrated with mercuric chloride in rats, or ischemic damage, as suggested in nephropathy associated with sickle cell disease in man, may result in release of RTE antigen and consequent immune complex glomerulonephritis (McIntosh et al., 1977). In addition, an autologous immune complex pathogenesis has been suggested in a number of cases of "idiopathic" membranous nephropathy (McIntosh et al., 1977). The inciting agent to RTE release, however, has not been identified in these cases.

Another interesting autologous antigen–induced disease for which a human correlate also recently has been demonstrated is the induction of glomerulonephritis in rabbits with chemically altered rabbit thyroglobulin. The rabbits develop an immune-mediated thyroiditis, and complexes of thyroglobulin and anti-thyroglobulin antibody deposit in the kidney. Human examples of this situation have recently been described in patients with thyroiditis. Immune complex nephritis also has been produced with intestinal antigens (McIntosh et al., 1977).

Endogenous Antigens. For theoretical considerations, we classify as endogenous antigens those which are chronically and intimately associated with host tissue, either by virtue of intracellular location, as with some viruses, or by actual derivation from normal host tissue, as with neoplastic disorders. The foundation for this theoretical classification is in the multitude of life-long, often vertically transmitted, chronic viral illnesses occurring spontaneously in animals, and associated with chronic glomerulonephritis. These viruses include several murine oncornaviruses, lymphocytic choriomeningitis, lactate dehydrogenase and polyoma virus in mice, the virus of Aleutian mink disease, hog cholera virus, and equine infectious anemia virus (Wilson and Dixon, 1976). In the

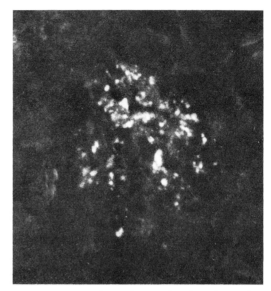

FIGURE 67–5. Photomicrograph of a glomerulus, showing mesangial deposits of IgA.

case of the oncornaviruses (murine leukemia virus), chronic infection also is associated with neoplastic lymphoproliferative disorders. Antigens involved in immune complex formation in this instance may be viral, tumor, or "viral-transformed" host cell antigen (Wilson and Dixon, 1976).

Mesangial Deposit Disease. Until relatively recently, it was generally accepted that a diffuse pattern of tissue response (glomerular capillary wall thickening and proliferation of endothelial cells, epithelial cells, and occasionally mesangial cells) was characteristic of all immune complex–induced glomerulonephritis. However, another pattern—characterized by the primary deposition of immunoglobulins in the mesangium, a proliferation of mesangial cells and matrix, or both—has been recognized (Fig. 67–5).

The mesangium has several roles. It serves as a structural support for the glomerulus, and it may have a phagocytic function. Although many questions remain unanswered concerning mesangial deposit disease, several facts are clear (Shibata et al., 1976; Germuth and Rodriguez, 1973; Stilmant et al., 1975). It is the *site* of deposition of immune complexes rather than the size of the complexes per se that determines the type of tissue response. Although complexes larger than one million daltons tend to be cleared from the circulation by phagocytosis and to localize in the mesangial area rather than in the GBM, there is evidence that many immune complexes deposit initially in the mesangium and that GBM deposition occurs as the phagocytic capacity of the mesangium is "fatigued." Variables influencing size of the immune complexes are the molecular weight of the antibody, the ratio of antibody and antigen, the avidity of the antibody, the size of the antigen, and the interaction of complexes with components of the complement system and rheumatoid factor. Hemodynamic factors may be important in mesangial immune complex localization. How the material deposits in the mesangium is unclear. Circulating antibody may react with a mesangial-fixed antigen by virtue of the mesangial phagocytic function or, alternatively, the complexes may form within the circulation.

The route these immunoglobulins take into the mesangium remains to be clarified. Complexes may be swept from subepithelial sites into the mesangium, they may pass directly from the circulation into the mesangium; or they may be removed from the subepithelial to the subendothelial sites as part of the GBM turnover. Using immune electron microscopy investigators have studied the uptake and disposal of aggregated human albumin injected intravenously into mice. Aggregated human albumin gained access to the mesangium via spaces between endothelial cells and, within 4 hours, occupied a complex series of channels within the mesangial matrix.

Experimental models of mesangial deposits include the intravenous administration of colloidal carbon, thorotrast, ferritin, and heat aggregated human IgG, IgA, or albumin. If antibody to human IgG is administered following the localization of human IgG in the mesangium, extensive mesangial and endothelial cell swelling develops, with infiltration by polymorphonuclear leukocytes and deposition of complement and fibrinogen. In mice repeatedly immunized with ferritin, a glomerulonephritis with mesangial proliferation and mesangial deposits of IgG, C3, and ferritin develops. Mesangial proliferation and sclerosis has been induced in rabbits by injecting ferritin into hyperimmunized animals. Chronic progressive mesangial glomerulonephritis has been induced in rats

given a water-soluble renal glycoprotein. In contrast to the above examples of experimental immune deposit mesangial disease, most spontaneous or experimentally induced mesangial immune depostis are not associated with significant glomerular disease.

Sensitization of mice with orally administered ferritin has been demonstrated. The animals show an IgA serum antibody to ferritin which is produced predominantly in intestinal mucosal lymphoid tissue.

Human forms of mesangial deposit disease include: (1) conditions in which the immune deposits are restricted in large part to the mesangium and (2) autologous forms, in which there are deposits in other areas of the glomerulus. Examples of the first group of conditions include IgG-IgA nephropathy (focal segmental proliferative glomerulonephritis with deposition of IgG, IgA, and sometimes complement in the mesangial region of all glomeruli) and anaphylactoid purpura. Systemic lupus erythematosus and membranoproliferative glomerulonephritis are examples of the latter. In SLE, immune complexes of a wide spectrum of sizes are produced and deposited throughout the glomerulus and mesangium. Membranoproliferative glomerulonephritis with mesangial cell hyperplasia and matrix increase also has a curious interposition of mesangial cell processes between the GBM and the capillary endothelial cell.

The mesangium has been a relatively "ignored" portion of the glomerulus until recently. With animal models that closely simulate human mesangial deposit diseases and with renewed interest in the mesangium and its role in disease, major advances in the understanding of these forms of glomerulonephritis should be forthcoming (Shibata et al., 1976; Germuth and Rodriguez, 1973; Stilmant et al., 1975).

Glomerular Fixed Antigens. Antibody may combine with antigen in the circulation, as occurs in circulating immune complex disease; or the antibody may combine with antigen "fixed," to tissue leading to the in situ formation of immune complexes (McIntosh et al., 1977; Golbus and Wilson, 1977; Shibata et al., 1976). These "glomerular-fixed" antigens may be glomerular basement membrane glycoproteins, substances that share immunologic similarities to other autologous or exogenous antigens, or foreign substances that become fixed to the glomerulus.

Experimental evidence in animals supports the role of glomerular fixed antigens in anti-GBM nephritis as well as in the production of mesangial deposit disease by renal glycoproteins, and mesangial proliferative disease evolving to membranous nephropathy by a renal glycoprotein. In humans, diseases involving glomerular fixed antigens may include poststreptococcal glomerulonephritis, certain cases of mesangial deposit disease, membranous nephropathy, diseases with subepithelial deposits, and the membranous nephritis of SLE. It has been suggested that in SLE there first is localization of nuclear antigens in the glomerular capillary walls, followed by the deposition of antibody on the trapped antigens. Furthermore, specific biochemical binding of nuclear proteins to GBM substances has been demonstrated *in vitro*. This area is in its early stages of development and promises exciting insights into the pathogenesis of immune-mediated glomerulonephritis.

Cell mediated immunity, the role of IgE, and mediators of inflammation are discussed under specific disease entities.

Clinical Entities

Acute Poststreptococcal Glomerulonephritis. The acute nephritic syndrome is characterized by hematuria, oliguria, and hypertension of sudden onset accompanied by decreased glomerular filtration rate. Although it may follow a variety of microbial infections and can be associated with a number of defined clinical entities, acute poststreptococcal glomerulonephritis is the most common cause of the acute nephritic syndrome in childhood.

Acute poststreptococcal glomerulonephritis is most common between the ages of 3 and 7 years. It is rare under age 2 years, and the incidence decreases with each decade. It usually is preceded by an acute streptococcal infection with certain (nephritogenic) types of streptococci (Types 1, 2, 4, 12, 18, 25, 49, 55, 57, 60). In the United States, 80 percent follow respiratory infections (pharyngitis, tonsillitis, and otitis media) and 5 to 10 percent follow skin infections. There is a 7 to 14 (mean = 10) day latent period between the onset of infection and clinical signs of nephritis. During an acute infection, hematuria and/or proteinuria is present in a third of patients. This usually disappears, only to recur later. If microscopic hematuria is present during an acute streptococcal infection, glomerulonephritis is more likely to develop.

The patient usually presents with a history of an upper respiratory infection or impetigo 2 weeks previously. Loss of appetite and occasional abdominal pain have been reported. There usually is moderate edema, especially of the orbits and dorsa of the hands and feet. Hypertension commonly is mild or moderate but sometimes may be rapid in onset and, on occasion, may cause sudden seizures or cardiac failure. Gross hematuria or "smoky urine" usually is present; but in subclinical cases, hematuria may be minimal or absent. Occasionally, oliguria or even anuria and acute renal failure may be present.

Evidence of a recent streptococcal infection sometimes is obtained by recovery of the organism. (It should be remembered that some forms of nephritogenic streptococci do not show β hemolysis.) The serologic diagnosis of a recent streptococcal infection is best determined by a battery of tests: Anti-streptolysin O (ASO) and anti-nicotine adenine dinucleotidase (ANADase) are helpful diagnostically but usually are not markedly elevated with streptococcal skin infections. Anti-desoxyribonuclease B (ADNase) is higher in acute glomerulonephritis than in acute rheumatic fever. Anti-hyaluronidase (AH) and anti-streptokinase (ASK) also are useful. A practical and inexpensive laboratory test is the Streptozyme test, which utilizes five enzymes (ASO, AH, ASK, ADNase, ANADase).

Urinalysis usually reveals hematuria with red cell, hyaline and granular casts. Proteinuria is common but not usually severe, and glomerulonephritis-associated nephrotic syndrome is rare in children. The hematocrit may be decreased and serum sodium levels low due to volume overload. The BUN and creatinine may be slightly elevated, and some patients have frank azotemia.

Serum levels of IgG are moderately to markedly elevated. Total hemolytic complement is extremely low; C1 and C4 are only moderately depressed. Multicomponent cryoglobulins and C1q-binding immune complexes are detected in the sera early in the disease. Antiglobulins and rheumatoid factor titers are moderately to markedly increased.

The complement profile is unique—not strictly representative of strictly classic or alternative pathway activation. C1q usually is normal, C4 is reduced early but returns to normal before C3. C2 and C4 levels are reduced less than in SLE. C3 and C5 are markedly decreased.

Only under unusual circumstances is renal biopsy necessary. Histologically, proliferation of glomerular cells and infiltration of inflammatory cells in the glomerulus are observed. Immunohistologic studies show immunoglobulin components in a granular pattern along the GBM, and, in some cases, properdin and fibrin in the glomerulus. Tubular, granular, or linear deposits of immunoglobulins also have been localized. The differential diagnosis includes all causes of the acute nephritic syndrome. Acute exacerbation of poststreptococcal glomerulonephritis usually is differentiated by the latent period (usually shorter than one week), the clinical history, and also the presence of marked funduscopic changes, left ventricular hypertrophy, or marked anemia. Other considerations must include SLE, IgG-IgA nephropathy, diffuse angiitis, and the vasculitis syndromes.

Although the epidemiologic relationship between streptococcus and nephritis has long been recognized, the sequence of events in the pathogenesis is unclear (Zabriskie et al., 1973; Rodriguez-Iturbe et al., 1980). Streptococcal antigens have been identified only occasionally within the glomerulus. When demonstrable, streptococcal material usually is present in the mesangium; no streptococcal material has been identified in the characteristic subepithelial humps, despite the presence of IgG and C3. In addition, there is considerable disagreement as to the exact nature of this streptococcal material. Some investigators suggest that the material is M protein, while others claim it is a water-soluble, non-M protein (endostreptosin). Although the majority of evidence favors an immune complex pathogenesis (cryoglobulinemia, circulating immune complexes, and the granular glomerular deposition of IgG and C3), a glomerular fixed-antigen pathogenesis or an "anti-GBM" pathogenesis due to streptococcal-GBM cross reactivity remain as possibilities. Evidence that the pathogenesis may involve an autologous immune complex mechanism includes the finding in poststreptococcal glomerulonephritis of cryoproteins with IgG lacking sialic acid, the demonstration that streptococcal material alters IgG (particularly with reference to sialic acid) and that this IgG is autoimmunogenic and can induce cryoglobulinemia and nephritis in experimental animals. In addition, we have demonstrated antiglobulins in the serum and glomerulus of patients with acute poststreptococcal glomerulonephritis and have shown that the eluate of a diseased kidney contains antiglobulin activity.

Mortality is approximately 1 percent and continues to decrease, owing to improved treatment of complications (CNS complications, cardiovascular disease, and acute renal failure). There is no convincing evidence that clinical features of the acute phase determine ultimate outcome. Within one year most patients destined to heal do not have significant proteinuria.

There are numerous problems in assessing long-term prognosis. The pathogenesis is still unknown. There are pitfalls in diagnosis; definition of criteria is variable (clinical, morphologic, and immunohistologic); and there apparently are many subclinical cases. In epidemics, the rate of complete healing of acute poststreptococcal glomerulonephritis is high in both adults and children. However, in sporadic cases the long-term prognosis is controversial. Most observers report a favorable outcome in children, whereas in adults the prognosis is more guarded.

The factors that lead to progression are poorly understood. A continuing immune complex mechanism seems unlikely; a secondary autologous immune complex pathogenesis related to a neoantigen or a primary autologous immune complex mechanism is most plausible. Cell mediated immunity also has been implicated in some cases, but not in others; and information on the possible participation of cellular immune mechanisms is conflicting.

It must be kept in mind that the acute nephritic syndrome may be associated with numerous etiologic factors other than the streptococcus and may be the mode of presentation of clinical entities with less favorable prognoses. Percutaneous renal biopsy has revealed that there are different types of renal lesions in patients with the acute nephritic syndrome, even in those of presumed poststreptococcal etiology. In order of frequency these include: (1) diffuse endocapillary proliferative glomerulonephritis; (2) endo- and extracapillary glomerulonephritis (cresenteric), and (3) mesangiocapillary glomerulonephritis.

The prognosis is least favorable in the mesangiocapillary glomerulonephritis and most favorable in the endocapillary proliferative type. The number of glomeruli affected by extracapillary proliferation is directly related to the long-term prognosis in the endo- and extracapillary form.

After careful clinical and laboratory assessment and observation of the patient's clinical course, a renal biopsy may be of value for prognostic implications. This should be performed by an experienced physician and in a center where optimal examination and interpretation of tissue are possible.

Treatment is based mainly on treatment of renal failure, hypertension, and cardiovascular and CNS complications. There is no evidence for therapeutic value of steroids, antimetabolites, or prophylactic penicillin

Anaphylactoid Purpura. Anaphylactoid purpura (AP Henoch-Schönlein purpura) includes skin, gastrointestinal, articular, and renal manifestations. The dermatologic lesions are the most characteristic, consisting of an initial urticarial lesion evolving into palpable purpuric macules chiefly involving the lower extremities and buttocks. Abdominal manifestations include vomiting, melena, hematemesis, and pain. Nonmigratory transient arthralgias, occasionally with effusions, particularly of the ankle and knee joints, may be present. The disease is more common in males, and the peak incidence is in the winter months. Hepatitis B infection may be associated with a clinical picture indistinguishable from anaphylactoid purpura.

The incidence of nephropathy (22 to 70 percent) is difficult to estimate and varies with the population studied and the criteria used (Meadow et al., 1972; Levy et al., 1976). Nephropathy is a particularly important element in this syndrome, since the prognosis of the disease is based on the severity of the

renal lesion. (The severity of dermal, GI, and arthritic manifestations bears no relationship to severity of the renal disease). A higher incidence of renal involvement has been observed in children developing the disease after age 5 years. Evidence of renal disease is most commonly present from a few days to 4 weeks after the onset of initial symptoms. However, renal involvement may first appear more than 2 years after the onset of disease; and, occasionally, symptoms referable to the kidney may precede other signs. Renal manifestations include gross or microscopic hematuria, proteinuria, and, occasionally, acute renal failure. Approximately 50 percent of patients have the nephrotic syndrome, which may be a presenting manifestation or may develop later. Hypertension has been reported as an initial finding in approximately 13 percent of children.

Renal biopsy is an important diagnostic tool in patients with renal involvement. The indications for renal biopsy in anaphylactoid purpura include the presence of the nephrotic syndrome, renal insufficiency, persistent proteinuria, or a clinical picture not readily explained by anaphylactoid purpura but that may represent vasculitis or SLE.

Despite the early association of the disease with food allergens, bee stings, and bacterial infections, no consistent relationship between antecedent events and the disease has been established. There is a strong history of allergy in approximately 25 percent of patients and several cases have been described with recurrent bouts of acute nephrotic syndrome apparently related to food allergy. Although a history of upper respiratory infection in the preceding 1 to 3 weeks has been noted in 75 percent of patients and antistreptolysin 0 titers are moderately elevated, there is no convincing evidence linking this syndrome with Group A streptococcal infection. Other reported predisposing causes include drugs, vaccination, primary tuberculous infection, and insect bites. Acute toxoplasmosis has been associated with findings similar to those of anaphylactoid purpura. There is a tendency for frequent relapses, occasionally following exposure to cold and after respiratory illnesses. Successive attacks may be accompanied by further renal complications, and episodes of acute nephrotic syndrome may occur in the absence of other manifestations of the disease.

There are no characteristic laboratory abnormalities in anaphylactoid purpura. Serum complement levels usually are normal, but depressed C3 has been reported on rare occasions. Recent studies have shown that, although C3 levels remain normal throughout the course of the disease, C1q, C4, C5, and C3 PA levels are decreased mainly after the initial phase. The complement profile suggests activation of the alternative pathway (Levy et al., 1976). Reported levels of serum immunoglobulins have been variable, IgA being most commonly elevated. However, elevated IgA levels do not appear to correlate with the prognosis. Cryoglobulinemia (predominantly IgA immunoglobulin) may be observed, and other serum immune complex laboratory studies may be positive in active disease. In our preliminary observations, there is a high incidence of circulating antibodies to bovine proteins (bovine gamma globulin and casein) and simultaneous presence of these antigens. Urinary fibrin degradation products frequently have been observed, the higher levels being present in association with more severe glomerular lesions and persistence indicating disease progression.

The etiology and pathogenesis of anaphylactoid purpura remain obscure. Immunohistologic studies reveal predominantly mesangial deposits of IgA and, to a lesser extent, fibrinogen, complement (alternative pathway pattern), IgG, and IgM. These and serologic findings suggest an immune complex pathogenesis. The predominance of IgA in the glomerulus may represent an IgA response to oral, respiratory, or even skin sensitization.

In general this syndrome is a benign self-limited disorder, although there may be episodic bouts of rash, arthralgias, gastrointestinal symptoms, and hematuria for several months or even years after the initial onset.

The long-term prognosis of the disease is almost exclusively related to the renal disease. Death from renal failure occurs either in the first few months or after many years. Initial renal failure and decreased GFR are not necessarily poor prognostic signs. The histologic type of lesion, the degree of proteinuria, and the presence and persistence of the nephrotic syndrome are the best prognostic guides. The severity of the nephropathy can best be evaluated at the end of the third month of anaphylactoid purpura. At this time, patients having proteinuria of more than 1 gm per day have a poor outcome (Levy et al., 1976). An unfavorable course is more common in those patients presenting with signs of severe nephropathy at onset or in those who have an exacerbation of their nephropathy during recurrences of their disease.

The predominant renal lesion observed is a focal and segmental proliferative glomerulonephritis. Habib has emphasized the importance of renal biopsy in the prognosis of anaphylactoid purpura (Levy et al., 1976). The morphologic types observed include the following:

1. Minimal lesion
2. Focal and segmental endocapillary glomerulonephritis
3. Diffuse endocapillary proliferation
4. Endocapillary and extracapillary proliferation
5. Membranoproliferative glomerulonephritis.

The endocapillary and extracapillary form of glomerulonephritis with > 30 percent crescents and membranoproliferative glomerulonephritis is associated with a poor prognosis.

Treatment generally is held to be ineffective in altering the course of the renal disease. The frequency of spontaneous remissions, the generally favorable course, and the lack of a tendency of the focal lesion to progress do not demand an aggressive management program. However, patients with the more ominous extracapillary proliferative lesion have been treated with steroids, immunosuppressive agents, and anticoagulants. These usually have been used in an uncontrolled fashion and results are difficult to assess. The International Study of Kidney Disease in Children is conducting a controlled study on the efficacy of these drugs. At the present time most observers agree that immunosuppressive therapy may be indicated in life-threatening nephritis.

Recurrent Hematuria (IgA-IgG Nephropathy, Berger's Disease). Interest in the mesangium was fostered by Berger's description of an IgA-IgG nephropathy associated with recurrent hematuria (Levy et al., 1973). Clinically, patients often present with recurrent episodes of gross hematuria, sometimes associated with flank pain, and often occurring during or shortly after an upper respiratory tract infection or exercise. Moderate proteinuria may be present during the attack and may

TABLE 67–2 HEMATURIA: DIAGNOSTIC CONSIDERATIONS

Glomerular
Membranoproliferative
Proliferative
Focal segmental
IgA-IgG: Berger's recurrent hematuria
Alport's syndrome
Familial benign recurrent hematuria
Allergic hematuria

Nonglomerular
Malformations of the urinary tract
Trauma
Tumor of the urogenital sinus
Renal tuberculosis
UTI: cystitis, trigonitis, urethritis
Schistosomiasis
Lithiasis (metabolic work-up)
Wilms' tumor
Vascular: angioma, telangiectasis
Hemophilia, thrombocytopenia, disorders of platelet function
Sickle cell anemia, leukemia
Renal vein thrombosis
Toxins: cytoxan, sulfa, methicillin, ASA, turpentine
Iatrogenic: catheter, renal biopsy
Psychologic: emotional stress, masturbation, instrumentation

persist between attacks along with microscopic hematuria. Histologic examination of kidney tissue reveals a focal and segmental proliferative glomerulonephritis. Immunofluorescent studies show diffuse abnormalities, with deposition of IgA, IgG, and sometimes complement in the mesangial region of all glomeruli. The finding of immunoglobulin localized to the mesangium without as yet demonstrable antigen has led to speculation about the etiopathogenesis of this condition. The postulated etiopathogenic mechanisms have been alluded to previously in considerations of mesangial deposit disease.

This disease appears to have a good prognosis, particularly in children. It is likely that many cases of "benign" hematuria described in the past prior to the advent of routine immunohistology were in fact IgA-IgG nephropathy. General diagnostic considerations related to hematuria are listed in Table 67–2.

Nephrotic Syndrome. The "nephrotic syndrome" is a term used to describe a spectrum of clinical disorders of diverse etiologies characterized by heavy proteinuria (chiefly albumin and usually greater than 3.5 grams per 24 hours) and hypoalbuminemia (usually less than 3.0 grams per dl). Other features of the syndrome may include lipiduria, elevated serum lipids (cholesterol, triglycerides, or both), and edema.

Several classification schemes of the nephrotic syndrome have been used. One is primary or secondary (the renal manifestation of a systemic disorder). Another relies on the distinction between steroid response and steroid resistance. A third, and perhaps the most popular at the current time, is based on glomerular pathology as detected by light, electron, and immunofluorescent microscopy in renal biopsy specimens.

Physical examination always should include accurate blood pressure determination and evaluation of signs and symptoms of growth retardation, ocular and auditory abnormalities, and other associated developmental deformities.

The laboratory evaluation of the patient with the nephrotic syndrome should be guided by the differential diagnosis in Table 67–1, narrowed significantly by the history and physical examination. After the basic urinalysis, quantitation, and characterization of the proteinuria and the determination of the glomerular filtration rate, more specific "diagnostic" tests may be warranted. These special immunologic tests are detailed later.

The physician should be particularly cognizant of the decreased intravascular volume status of the patient. This may be associated with significant orthostatic hypotension and a decreased glomerular filtration rate. A hypercoagulable state frequently is present, increasing the risk of renal vein thrombosis, peripheral venous thrombosis and pulmonary embolization. The large loss of IgG in the urine also increases the patient's susceptibility to pneumococcal sepsis, peritonitis, or both.

Idiopathic Nephrotic Syndrome of Childhood (Minimal Change, Nil Disease). Minimal change disease most commonly, but not exclusively, presents in children under the age of 5 years with nephrotic syndrome, and without hematuria, hypertension, or azotemia. Study of the renal histopathology by light microscopy reveals either a normal glomerulus or mild mesangial cell proliferation. There generally is no evidence of immunoglobulin or complement deposition by immunofluorescence, and there is the nonspecific finding of epithelial cell foot-process fusion by electron microscopy. The vast majority of these patients respond to prednisone therapy, although many have frequent relapses requiring repeated courses of therapy. A small number will not respond initially to prednisone. Immunosuppressive therapy (cyclophosphamide or chlorambucil) usually is successful in the treatment of these patients, as well as in inducing prolonged remission in patients who have been frequent relapsers (Grupe et al., 1976).

Renal biopsy is not necessary in the majority of children with idiopathic nephrotic syndrome (INS) before steroid therapy is started. Because 50 to 75 percent of children with INS have minimal change disease, a therapeutic trial of steroid therapy will spare many children the potential hazards of biopsy. Indications for renal biopsy prior to steroid treatment are systemic hypertension, gross hematuria, age greater than 8 to 10 years, persistently low serum C3, elevated antistreptolysin O titer, or azotemia. Biopsy may be performed after steroid treatment if there is steroid resistance or frequent relapse with unacceptable steroid toxicity.

Although minimal change nephrosis was one of the earliest described renal syndromes of childhood, its pathogenesis remains an enigma (McIntosh et al., 1977). Renal tissue of most patients show no evidence of either anti-GBM, immune complex, or complement mediated disease. There are, however, some clinical and laboratory findings in select groups of patients that suggest the participation of the immune system (McIntosh et al., 1977; Shalhoub, 1974; Sandberg et al., 1977). Antigenic stimulation may be important, as suggested by exacerbations or recurrences of nephrotic syndrome repeatedly associated with upper respiratory tract or other viral infections. In addition, there have been a number of patients reported over the past two decades in whom proteinuria has been associated with exposure to food or inhalant allergens, bee sting, or contact dermatitis. Suggestive evidence for the role of hypersensitivity in this disease has been the detection of glomerular-bound IgE in some of these patients, and of elevated serum IgE levels in others. However, the failure to verify these findings in subsequent studies suggests that these abnormalities may apply to only a particular subgroup of nephrotic patients. Elevated IgM levels and decreased IgG and IgA levels have been observed. Whether this represents a preexistent immunologic abnormality or is evidence of active immune-mediated disease is unknown. The primary defect may be a deficiency in T cell function that mediates conversion of B cell synthesis of IgM to IgG, since the immunoglobulin pattern is similar to that in X-linked immunodeficiency with increased IgM. The response of most of these patients to steroids and immunosuppressants, as well as remissions following infection with measles (T cell function depressor), suggests a role for T cell dysfunction. In summary, it is probable that multiple etiologies exist for what now is considered to be a single disease entity.

Focal Glomerulosclerosis. Focal glomerular sclerosis is responsible for approximately 10 to 20 percent of cases of childhood idiopathic nephrotic syndrome (Habib, 1973). This disease may closely mimic the minimal change lesion at onset. However, the subsequent course typically is marked by poor response to therapy and progressive renal insufficiency. These patients, often slightly older than most patients with minimal change disease, frequently have early hematuria, hypertension, or azotemia.

Histopathology distinguishes these patients from those with lesions of minimal change disease. Sclerosed, hyalinized lesions are seen within glomeruli throughout the kidney. Early in the disease, the lesions may be limited to the juxtamedullary glomeruli. Some glomeruli appear normal. In addition, the morphology may be divided into two distinct forms. In focal segmental glomerular sclerosis, only a portion of the affected glomerulus is involved. In the second form, focal glomerular obsolescence (or focal global fibrosis), all of the involved glomerulus is scarred and hyalinized. The first variety appears to have a poorer clinical course. Immunoglobulin M, IgG, and complement may be seen in an irregular, granular, or nodular distribution in the sclerosed segments.

The etiology of focal glomerular sclerosis is as obscure as that of minimal change disease. It has been suggested that the two disorders are on opposite ends of a spectrum of a single disease. The fact that this lesion begins in the juxtamedullary cortex and only deep cortical biopsies will show its early presence may explain the apparent "progression" from the minimal change lesions to focal sclerotic lesions.

The frequently reported clinical or histopathologic recurrence of disease in transplanted kidneys in these patients suggests a role for systemic, possibly immune, factors. However, electron microscopy generally shows no evidence of immune complex deposition.

Membranous Nephropathy. Idiopathic membranous nephropathy refers to a distinctive clinicopathologic entity usually associated with the nephrotic syndrome, appearing in the absence of systemic disease or known precipitating factors. It is unusual in children and adolescents, usually being initially diagnosed in patients over the age of 40. The onset typically is insidious, with hypertension and azotemia occurring as late manifestations. The glomerular basement membrane is thickened without an accompanying inflammatory response. Subepithelial, intramembranous, or subendothelial electron-dense deposits may be seen. Immunoglobulin G and complement are deposited in a granular pattern throughout the capillaries but are not present in the mesangium. The serum complement level almost always is normal.

The etiology of idiopathic membranous nephropathy, as the name suggests, remains unknown. The granular deposition of IgG and C3 strongly suggests an immune complex disease, but the nature of the antigen is unclear. A small percentage of these patients have detectable circulating immune complexes. The disease pursues an indolent but slowly progressive course punctuated by spontaneous clinical remissions. These remissions are more likely in children early in the course of the disease.

It is this variable nature of the disease that makes evaluation of therapy difficult. Short-term, high-dose prednisone therapy in adults with idiopathic membranous nephropathy and the nephrotic syndrome has been reported to slow the progression to renal failure, although no significant change in proteinuria in the treated group was seen when compared to controls. No consistent benefit of cytotoxic agents has been shown.

Hypocomplementemic Membranoproliferative Glomerulonephritis (MPGN). As with Berger's disease, the description and

examination of this relatively recently reported clinical entity (MPGN) has stimulated research into new areas of renal immunopathology.

As discussed earlier, complement is an important mediator of inflammation and tissue injury in most immune complex disease. Complexes of antigen and IgG or IgM activate complement via the classic pathway. A variety of substances, including bacterial endotoxin, yeast, zymosan, and inulin, as well as aggregated IgA, activate the alternative complement pathway (see Chapter 5). Recent evidence suggests that the human glomerulus may possess complement receptors that facilitate the binding of complement-containing immune complexes, as well as of C3 activated through the alternative complement pathway.

A great deal of attention has been focused on a human glomerulonephropathy commonly seen in adolescence which demonstrates evidence for renal injury secondary to complement activation by the alternative pathway (West, 1976; Habib et al., 1975). The histologic picture of diffuse proliferation associated with apparent GBM thickening on light microscopy has led to the designation of hypocomplementemic membranoproliferative glomerulonephritis. As this actually is a general term which may apply as well to certain cases of systemic lupus erythematosus or acute poststreptococcal glomerulonephritis, further designations have been applied. Electron microscopy has helped in the differentiation of two varieties of this condition. In the first, there is evidence of interposition of mesangial cell processes between the GBM and capillary endothelial cell, leading to the descriptive term of mesangiocapillary glomerulonephritis (Type I MPGN). Electron-dense material, closely resembling immune complex deposits in other diseases, is seen in the mesangium and subendothelial space. Immunofluorescence usually demonstrates immunoglobulins and early complement components as well as C3 and components consistent with alternative pathway activation. The serum complement component profile suggests lowering of classic as well as alternative pathway components. In summary, there is the suggestion that immune complex formation may actually be involved in Type I MPGN.

In Type II MPGN, immune complexes do

not appear to be involved. Electron microscopy demonstrates the presence of large deposits of electron-dense material within the GBM as well as in Bowman's capsule and in the tubular basement membrane. This is the so-called *Dense Deposit Disease*. These deposits do not have the appearance of immune complexes. Immunofluorescence usually demonstrates abundant C3 with little or no immunoglobulins or early complement components. The serum complement profile is more distinctly one of activation of the alternative complement pathway. Some investigators have demonstrated a serum factor capable of triggering complement activation in the circulation of these patients (C3 nephritic factor). There is evidence for reduced C3 synthesis as well. The origin of the dense deposits and the mechanism of glomerular injury are matters of current speculation and research.

Clinical differences also exist between these two diseases. The dense deposit variety is most common in children. Total hemolytic complement levels are more consistently and persistently low in Type II; levels in Type I vary with time. Both varieties may present acutely with edema, macroscopic hematuria, hypertension and azotemia; or the onset may be documented by only microscopic abnormalities on urinalysis. Both diseases pursue a relentless, progressive course; but patients with intramembranous dense deposits appear to have a more rapid progression to renal failure. One study reported 40 percent of patients dead or on chronic hemodialysis at an average follow-up time of slightly over four and a half years. Furthermore, there are increasingly frequent reports of the recurrence of glomerulonephritis in transplanted kidneys in these patients. Histologic evidence of recurrence seems to correspond to persistence or recurrence of hypocomplementemia and is particularly common in dense deposit disease.

In general, investigations into the pathogenesis of this disease have focused on the peculiar complement abnormalities. It still is not known whether an etiologic link exists between the hypocomplementemia and glomerular damage; the possibility remains that the two events are pathogenetically unrelated.

Many therapeutic regimens have been tried in patients with membranoproliferative glomerulonephritis. Neither steroids nor cytotoxic agents have been shown to be of therapeutic value.

IMMUNE-MEDIATED TUBULOINTERSTITIAL NEPHRITIS

Until recently attention has been focused on anti-glomerular basement membrane disease and immune complex mediated glomerulonephritis. Little consideration was given to the possibility that there may be immunologically mediated damage directly involving renal tubules or interstitial tissue. Experimental animal models and observations in man provide compelling evidence that tubular and interstitial disease can result from immunologic injury (autoimmune or immune complex) (Andres and McCluskey, 1975; McCluskey and Colvin, 1978). Moreover, it appears that the renal interstitium is an area where cell mediated immune reactions can occur, accounting for some forms of interstitial nephritis.

The tubules and interstitium contain several antigenic components, including the following: tubular basement membrane (TBM), renal tubular epithelial antigen (RTE), tubular cytoplasm, cellular components of tubules, collecting duct, and the loop of Henle. The tubular basement membrane antigens appear to be of two distinct varieties: In one, anti-glomerular basement membrane antibodies cross-react with TBM antigen. Saturation of the GBM may lead to TBM deposits. The other TBM antigen is distinct and does not react with anti-GBM antibodies. Renal tubular epithelial antigen is found in the brush border of the proximal tubule as well as in several other epithelial tissues.

Human anti-TBM disease has been seen in a number of clinical situations as part of anti-GBM disease (linear deposits of IgG and C3 on the TBM and circulating anti-TBM antibodies), in renal allograft patients (in both the allograft and host kidney), in association with drugs (methicillin), and as a manifestation of immune complex disease (poststreptococcal glomerulonephritis).

Tubular and interstitial immune complex disease has been observed in association with SLE glomerulonephritis. In 50 to 60 percent of patients with SLE nephritis, granular or interstitial tubular deposits of IgG and

C3 are observed in the proximal tubule, tubular basement membranes, and interstitium. Nuclear antigen components (cytidine and thymidine) have been demonstrated in the tubules in association with the immunoglobulin and complement, suggesting that these deposits are immune complexes similar to those observed in the glomerulus in this disease. Other diseases and syndromes in which tubular and interstitial immune complex disease have been observed include renal allografts, Sjögren's syndrome, idiopathic interstitial nephritis, glomerulonephritis with cryoglobulinemia, membranoproliferative glomerulonephritis, and rapidly progressive glomerulonephritis.

A role for cell mediated immunity in tubulointerstitial nephritis is suggested by the presence of interstitial mononuclear cells. Other supporting evidence for immunopathogenetic mechanisms is the eosinophilic interstitial infiltrate, elevated serum IgE, peripheral eosinophilia, deposition of IgG, IgE, and fibrinogen in the renal interstitium, skin rash, and arthritis seen in some patients. The etiologic agents suspected were penicillin and its analogues, barbiturates, furosemide, and thiazides. The finding of elevated serum IgE, plasma cells containing IgE together with eosinophils, IgG and IgE in the renal interstitium, and eosinophilia in some patients suggest that allergen IgE type antibody complexes are involved.

Although immunoglobulin and complement are deposited in these disorders and infiltration by leukocytes has been observed, the functional significance of the histologic injury has not been clearly defined.

EVALUATION OF THE PATIENT WITH RENAL DISEASE

Various considerations referable to the history, physical examination, and laboratory tests available in evaluating patients with renal disease are listed in Table 67–3.

The primary care physician has been required to evaluate and treat an increasing number of children with proteinuria and hematuria since the advent of simple dipstick methods for detecting urinary abnormalities. A logical and stepwise approach to these patients helps to assure a thorough evalua-

tion, proper treatment, and referral of those patients requiring more specialized diagnostic procedures. Three main categories of urinary abnormalities are easily recognized: (1) hematuria with minimal or no proteinuria, (2) proteinuria with no hematuria, and (3) hematuria and proteinuria.

Hematuria. The most commonly encountered abnormality is isolated hematuria — less than 10 to 20 mg of protein per deciliter of urine, in the absence of gross hematuria.

It becomes imperative to confirm by history and physical examination that the hematuria is not part of a systemic illness. The physician should confirm the absence of rashes (Henoch-Schönlein purpura), dysuria (urinary tract infections), recent upper respiratory illnesses (Berger's disease), coagulation abnormalities, or a family history of deafness or renal disease (Alport's syndrome). Laboratory tests should include a blood urea nitrogen (BUN) and/or creatinine test as an index of renal function, a TB skin test, a urine culture, streptozyme, serum C3 and/or total hemolytic complement activity test, and an intravenous pyelogram. The family members should be checked for microhematuria and proteinuria. If no proteinuria is detected on *multiple* urine samples and the other laboratory tests are normal, the hematuria may be the result of a condition referred to as benign hematuria. Nevertheless, the physician should continue to examine the urine for blood and protein and to assess renal function periodically. If the laboratory tests are abnormal, the physician may want to discuss them and detail a further diagnostic plan in consultation with a nephrologist (see Table 67–2).

Proteinuria. The second main category of urinary abnormality is isolated proteinuria. The most common conditions leading to this finding in children are orthostatic proteinuria and idiopathic nephrotic syndrome. Again, it is important to be certain that the patient is asymptomatic. A simple test for orthostatic proteinuria may be supervised by the child's parents at home. The patient is instructed to void immediately before retiring. A specimen of urine is then collected in the morning while the subject is still in bed, and a second specimen is collected after the child has been up and about. Each container is clearly labeled for the physician, and the

TABLE 67–3 EVALUATION OF THE PATIENT WITH RENAL DISEASE

History of possible etiologic factors
  Atopic allergy
  Medications
  Drug allergies
  Drug abuse: heroin, amphetamines
  Infections: pharyngitis, impetigo, urinary tract
    infection, hepatitis
  Photosensitivity
  Raynaud's phenomenon
  Vaccinations
  Immunizations

Other historical factors
  Age at onset
  Symptoms of multisystem involvement: CNS,
    peripheral nerves
  Family history of renal disease

Physical examination
  Systemic hypertension and funduscopic evi-
    dence of hypertension or vasculitis
  Skin involvement: urticaria, petechiae, palpa-
    ble purpura, rash, impetigo
  Abdominal masses
  Edema
  Signs of multisystem involvement: CNS, pul-
    monary, joints, peripheral nerves

Laboratory examination
  General: CBC, throat culture
  Related systems: bilirubin, alkaline phos-
    phatase, SGOT, SGPT, LDH, CPK
  Renal: urinalysis, creatinine clearance, quanti-
    tative protein excretion, serum electrolytes,
    BUN, creatinine, total protein, albumin

Laboratory examination (Continued)
  Immunologic (available in most laboratories):
    Serum protein electrophoresis
    Immunoelectrophoresis
    Quantitative immunoglobulins: IgG, IgM,
      IgA
    Complement: CH50, C4, C3
    Antibodies:
      ANA (pattern and titer)
      DNA binding (anti-DNA) titer
      ASO, AH, ASK, ADNase B, ANADase
      Streptozyme
      HB_sAg and antibody to HB_sAg
      Rheumatoid factor
      Cryoglobulins
  Renal biopsy: examination of tissue by light,
    electron microscopy and immunofluores-
    cence
  Skin biopsy: examination by light and immuno-
    fluorescence microscopy (looking for the
    "lupus band" or IgA deposits)
  Immunologic (available by consultation with
    specialized laboratories):
    Anti-GBM antibodies: immunofluorescence,
      hemagglutination, radioimmunoassay
    Tests for circulating immune complexes:
      fluid and solid phase C1q binding assays,
      Raji cell radioimmunoassay, cryoglobulins
      (antigen and antibody content)
    Serum C3 nephritic factor activity
    Renal elution studies and specialized renal
      immunohistology

test is performed at least three times. The absence of protein in the recumbent specimen and the presence of protein in the second specimen suggests orthostatic proteinuria. If the proteinuria is not orthostatic, further evaluation is necessary. Tests to assess renal function, serum protein and cholesterol, and C3 and/or total hemolytic complement should be performed. If the child is under 6 years of age and renal function, complement level, and blood pressure all are normal, the urinalysis is negative for red blood cells or cellular casts, but serum cholesterol is elevated, a presumptive diagnosis of minimal change nephrotic syndrome is entertained. A therapeutic trial of prednisone may be instituted. Prednisone in a dose of 60 mg/meter^2 per day in divided doses for 4 weeks followed by 40 mg/meter^2 every second day usually is used. Most chil-

dren with the minimal change nephrotic syndrome will respond with a marked decrease in urinary protein (less than 4 mg/meter^2 per hour of urine protein). If edema is a problem, salt restriction and bed rest usually are helpful. Fluids may be given ad lib. Initial steroid nonresponders, frequent relapsers, and those patients with hypertension, impaired renal function, hypocomplementemia, or cellular urinary casts should be discussed with a nephrologist.

Combined Hematuria and Proteinuria. The third category of patients includes those with both hematuria and proteinuria. These patients usually have glomerulonephritis, and a renal biopsy often is indicated in the course of the diagnostic evaluation. Consultation with a nephrologist therefore is frequently required (see Table 67–1).

References

Allen, A. C.: *The Kidney: Medical and Surgical Diseases.* New York, Grune and Stratton, 1963.

Andres, G. A., and McCluskey, R. T.: Tubular and interstitial renal disease due to immunologic mechanisms. Kidney Int. *7*:271, 1975.

Cochrane, C. G., and Koffler, D.: Immune complex disease in experimental animals and man. Adv. Immunol. *16*:185, 1973.

Germuth, F. G., Jr., and Rodriguez, E.: *Immunopathology of the Renal Glomerulus: Immune Complex Deposit and Anti-basement Membrane Disease.* Boston: Little, Brown, and Company, 1973, p. 57.

Golbus, S., and Wilson, C .B.: Glomerulonephritis produced by the in situ formation of immune complexes on the glomerular basement membrane. Kidney Int. *12*:513 (Abstract), 1977.

Grupe, W. E., Makker, S. P., and Inglefinger, J. R.: Chlorambucil treatment of frequently relapsing nephrotic syndrome. New Engl. J. Med. *295*:746, 1976.

Habib, R.: Focal glomerular sclerosis. Kidney Int. *4*:355, 1973.

Habib, R., Gubler, M. C., Loirat, C., Maiz, H. B., and Levy, M.: Dense deposit disease: A variant of membranoproliferative glomerulonephritis. Kidney Int. *7*:204, 1975.

Heymann, W., Hackel, D. B., Harwood, J., Wilson, S. G. F., and Hunter, J. L. P.: Production of the nephrotic syndrome in rats by Freund's adjuvant and rat kidney suspection. Proc. Soc. Exp. Biol. Med. *100*:660, 1959.

Jorgensen, F.: The ultrastructure of the normal human glomerulus. Copenhagen, Ejnar Munksgaard, 1966.

Jorgensen, F., and Bentzon, M. W.: The ultrastructure of the normal human glomerulus — Thickness of the glomerular basement membrane. Lab. Invest. *18*:42, 1968.

Kefalides, N. A.: Structure and biosynthesis of basement membranes. Int. Rev. Connect. Tissue Res. *6*:63, 1973.

Lerner, R. A., and Dixon, F. J.: The induction of acute glomerulonephritis in rabbits with soluble antigen isolated from homologous and autologous urine. J. Immunol. *100*:1277, 1968.

Levy, M., Beaufils, H., Gibler, M. C., and Habib, R.: Idiopathic recurrent microscopic hematuria and mesangial IgA-IgG deposits in children (Berger's disease). Clin. Nephrol. *1*:63, 1973.

Levy, M., Broyer, M., Arsan, A., Levy-Bentolila, D., and Habib, R.: Anaphylactoid purpura nephritis in children: natural history and immunopathology. Adv. Nephrol. *6*:183, 1976.

Masugi, M.: Über die experimentelle Glomerulonephritis durch das spezifische Antinierenserum. Ein Beitrag zur Pathogenese der diffusion Glomerulonephritis. Beitr. Pathol. *92*:429, 1934.

McCluskey, R. T., and Colvin, R. B.: Immunological aspects of renal tubular and interstitial diseases. Ann. Rev. Med. *29*:191, 1978.

McGiff, J. C., Crowshaw, K., and Itskovitz, H. D.: Prostaglandins and renal function. Fed. Proc. *33*:39, 1974.

McIntosh, R. M., Allen, J. E., Rabideau, D., Garcia, R., Rubio, L., and Rodriguez-Iturbe, B.: The role of interactions between streptococcal products and immunoglobulins in the pathogenesis of glomerular and vascular injury. *In* Zabriskie, J., et al. (eds.): *The Streptococcus and the Immune Response.* Academic Press. In press, 1980.

McIntosh, R. M., Carr, R. I., and Kohler, P. F.: Etiology, epidemiology, and pathogenesis of renal disease. Pathobiology Annual. *7*:143, 1977.

Meadow, S. R., Glasgow, E. F., White, R. H. R., Moncrieff, M. W., Cameron, J. S., and Ogg, C. S.: Schönlein-Henoch nephritis. Quarterly J. of Med. New Series. *XLI*(163):241, July 1972.

Rocklin, R. E., Lewis, E. J., and David, J. R.: Glomerulonephritis: Cellular hypersensitivity to basement membrane antigens. New Engl. J. Med. *283*:497, 1970.

Rodriguez-Iturbe, B., Garcia, R., Rubio, L., Carr, R. I., Allen, J. E., Rabideau, D., and McIntosh, R. M.: Etiologic, pathogenic, clinical, and immunopathologic considerations in acute post-streptococcal glomerulonephritis. *In* Zabriskie, J., et al. (eds.): *The Streptococcus and the Immune Response.* Academic Press. In press, 1980.

Sandberg, D. M., McIntosh, R. M., Bernstein, C. W., Carr, R. I., and Strauss, J.: Severe steroid responsive nephrosis associated with food hypersensitivity. I. Demonstration of the role of food allergens in exacerbation of disease activity. Lancet *1*:388, 1977.

Shalhoub, R. J.: Pathogenesis of lipoid nephrosis. A disorder of T-cell function. Lancet *2*:556, 1974.

Shibata, S., Sakaguchi, H., and Nagasawa, T.: Induction of chronic progressive glomerulonephritis with immunofluorescent "mesangial pattern" in rats. Nephron *16*:241, 1976.

Steblay, R. W.: Glomerulonephritis induced in sheep by injection of heterologous glomerular basement membrane and Freund's complete adjuvant. J. Exp. Med. *109*:1, 1959.

Stilmant, M. M., Couser, W. G., Cotran, R. S.: Experimental glomerulonephritis in the mouse associated with mesangial depositon of autologous ferritin immune complexes. Lab. Invest. *32*:746, 1975.

Vassalli, P., and McCluskey, R. T.: The pathogenic role of the coagulation process in glomerular diseases of immunologic origin. Adv. Nephrol. *1*:47, 1971.

Vernier, R. L.; Electron microscopic studies of the normal basement membrane. *In* Siperstein, M. D., A. R., Colwell, Sr., and K. Heter: *Small Blood Vessel Involvement in Diabetes Mellitus.* Publication 57. American Institute of Biological Sciences. Arlington, Virginia, 1964.

West, C. D.: Pathogenesis and approaches to therapy of membranoproliferative glomerulonephritis Kidney Int. *9*:1, 1976.

Wilson, C. B., and Dixon, F. J.: Antiglomerular basement membrane induced glomerulonephritis. Kidney Int. *3*:74, 1973.

Wilson, C. B., and Dixon, F. J.: The renal response to immunological injury. *In* Brenner, B. M., and Rector, F. C. (eds.): The Kidney, Vol. II. Philadelphia: W. B. Saunders Co., 1976.

Zabriskie, J. B., Utermohlen, V., Read, S. E., and Fischetti, V. A.: Streptococcus related glomerulonephritis. Kidney Int. *3*:100, 1973.

INDEX

Numbers in italics refer to illustrations; numbers followed by (t) refer to tables.